P9-CFK-393

Principles and Practice of Nuclear Medicine

PAUL J. EARLY, DABSNM, ABMP

Director, NMA Medical Physics Consultation,
Mallinckrodt Medical, Inc.,
Cleveland, Ohio

D. BRUCE SODEE, M.D., F.A.C.P.

Associate Professor of Radiology,
Case Western Reserve University;
Section Chief, Nuclear Medicine and Ultrasound,
MetroHealth Medical Center, Department of Radiology,
Cleveland, Ohio

SECOND EDITION

with 549 illustrations

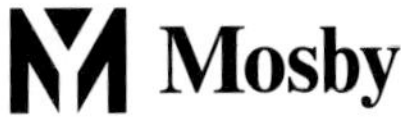

An Affiliate of Elsevier

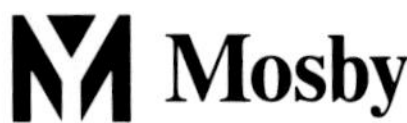

An Affiliate of Elsevier

Managing Editor: Jeanne Rowland
Associate Developmental Editor: Lisa Potts
Project Manager: Linda Clarke
Project Supervisor: Allan S. Kleinberg
Design: Sheilah Barrett

On the cover:

The top image depicts a three-dimensional surface rendering of a SPECT brain image. A malignant tumor has been removed from the right frontal lobe.

The bottom is a wire-frame, computer-generated representation of the same image.

SECOND EDITION

Printed in the United States of America

Mosby
11830 Westline Industrial Drive
St. Louis, Missouri 63146

Library of Congress Cataloging-in-Publication Data

Principles and practice of nuclear medicine / [edited by] Paul J.
Early, D. Bruce Sodee.—2nd ed.
p. cm.
Includes bibliographical references and index.
ISBN 0-8016-2577-7
1. Nuclear medicine. 2. Medical—laboratory technology.
I. Early, Paul J. II. Sodee, D. Bruce
[DNLM: 1. Nuclear Medicine. 2. Diagnostic Imaging—methods.
3. Radiotherapy. WN 440 P956 1994]
R895.P75 1994
616.07'575—dc20
DNLM/DLC 94–4425

04 05 06 07 08 / 13 12 11 10 9

CONTRIBUTORS

Abass Alavi, M.D.
Professor of Radiology, Chief, Division of Nuclear Medicine, Hospital of the University of Pennsylvania, Philadelphia, Pennsylvania

Naomi P. Alazraki, M.D.
Professor of Radiology and Co-Director, Division of Nuclear Medicine, Emory University School of Medicine and VA Medical Center, Atlanta, Georgia

John H. Baughman, B.A., ARRT(NM), CNMT
Product Manager, Nuclear Medicine Division, Medical Consultants Imaging Co., Cleveland, Ohio

Marshall Brucer, M.D.†
Tucson, Arizona

B. David Collier, M.D.
Director of Nuclear Medicine, Medical College of Wisconsin, Milwaukee, Wisconsin

Carlo Giuntini, M.D.
Professor of Respiratory Pathophysiology, Chief, Pulmonary Unit, CNR Institute of Clinical Physiology and II Medical Clinic, Univerisity of Pisa, Pisa, Italy

Mark A. Green, Ph.D.
Associate Professor of Medicinal Chemistry, Division of Nuclear Pharmacy, Department of Medicinal Chemistry, School of Pharmacy, Purdue University, West Lafayette, Indiana

Milton D. Gross, M.D.
Professor of Internal Medicine, Department of Internal Medicine, Division of Nuclear Medicine, University of Michigan Medical Center, Director/Chief, Nuclear Medicine Service, Department of Veterans Affairs, Ann Arbor, Michigan

Albert V. Heal, Ph.D.
Associate Professor of Radiology, Department of Radiology and Nuclear Medicine, University of South Florida School of Medicine/Tampa VA Hospital, Tampa, Florida

Kimberly G. Hoffman, CNMT
Program Director, Nuclear Medicine Technology, Harry S. Truman Memorial Veterans Hospital, University of Missouri-Columbia School of Health Related Professions, Columbia, Missouri

Richard A. Holmes, M.D.
Professor of Medicine, Radiology, Nuclear Engineering, Chief, Nuclear Medicine, University of Missouri-Columbia School of Medicine and Harry S. Truman Memorial Veterans Hospital, Columbia, Missouri

Ban An Khaw, Ph.D.
George D. Behrakis Professor of Pharmaceutical Sciences, Director, Center for Drug Targeting and Analysis, Bouve College of Pharmacy and Health Sciences, Northeastern University, and Associate Professor, Department of Radiology, Harvard Medical School and Massachusetts General Hospital, Boston, Massachusetts

James H. Larose, M.D., FACNP
Clinical Associate Professor of Radiology (Nuclear Medicine), University of Alabama, Birmingham, Alabama

Myron L. Lecklitner, M.D., FACNP
Professor and Director, Diagnostic Imaging Division, Department of Radiology, University of South Alabama, Mobile, Alabama

H. L. Malinoff, M.D.
Fellow, Division of Nuclear Medicine, University of Michigan Medical Center, Ann Arbor, Michigan

David P. Mihalic, B.A., CNMT, ARRT
Computer Consultant, Cleveland, Ohio

William H. Miller, B.S., DABSNM
Formerly Senior Consultant, Nuclear Medicine Associates, Mallinckrodt Medical Inc., Cleveland, Ohio

†Deceased.

Jagat Narula, M.D.

Associate Director, Center for Drug Targeting and Analysis, Bouve College of Pharmacy and Health Sciences, Northeastern University, and Research Fellow, Department of Radiology, Harvard Medical School and Massachusetts General Hospital, Boston, Massachusetts

Richard A. Nickel, M.S.

Regional Manager, Diagnostic Imaging Services, Mallinckrodt Medical Inc., St. Louis, Missouri

Richard B. Noto, M.D.

Director, Division of Nuclear Medicine, Rhode Island Hospital, Clinical Assistant Professor, Brown University School of Medicine, Providence, Rhode Island

James K. O'Donnell, M.D.

Associate Professor of Radiology, Division of Nuclear Medicine, Department of Radiology, Case Western Reserve University, University Hospitals, Cleveland, Ohio

Michael D. Okerlund, M.D.†

Nuclear Medicine Section, Department of Radiology, The Medical Center at the University of California, San Francisco, California

Antonio Palla, M.D.

Assistant Professor of Respiratory Pathophysiology, CNR Institute of Clinical Physiology and II Medical Clinic, University of Pisa, Pisa, Italy

Steven C. Port, M.D.

Professor of Medicine, University of Wisconsin Medical School; Director, Nuclear Cardiology, Sinai Samaritan Medical Center, Milwaukee, Wisconsin

David F. Preston, M.D.

Professor of Diagnostic Radiology (Nuclear Medicine), Department of Diagnostic Radiology, Division of Nuclear Medicine, University of Kansas Medical Center, Kansas City, Kansas

David C. Price, M.D.

Professor of Radiology and Medicine, Chief, Nuclear Medicine, Radiology Service, Nuclear Medicine Section, The Medical Center at the University of California, San Francisco, California

†Deceased.

John Reilley, CNMT

Division of Nuclear Medicine, Department of Radiology, Hospital of the University of Pennsylvania, Philadelphia, Pennsylvania

Ralph G. Robinson, M.D.

Professor of Diagnostic Radiology, Head, Division of Nuclear Medicine, The University of Kansas Medical Center, Kansas City, Kansas

Ronald J. Scala, M.S.

Certified Radiological Physicist, Iron City Medical Physics Inc., Pittsburgh, Pennsylvania

Brahm Shapiro, M.B., Ch.B., Ph.D.

Professor of Internal Medicine, Division of Nuclear Medicine, Department of Internal Medicine, University of Michigan Medical Center and Department of Nuclear Medicine, Ann Arbor VA Medical Center, Ann Arbor, Michigan

James C. Sisson, M.D.

Professor of Internal Medicine, Division of Nuclear Medicine, The University of Michigan Medical Center, Ann Arbor, Michigan

Richard P. Spencer, M.D., Ph.D.

Professor and Chairman, Department of Nuclear Medicine, The University of Connecticut Health Center, Farmington, Connecticut

H. William Strauss, M.D.

Vice President, Diagnostic Drug Discovery, Pharmaceutical Research Institute, Bristol-Myers Squibb, Princeton, New Jersey

Andrew Taylor, Jr., M.D.

Professor of Radiology, Co-Director, Division of Nuclear Medicine, Department of Radiology Emory University School of Medicine, Atlanta, Georgia

Sabah S. Tumeh, M.D.

Clinical Professor of Radiology, Georgetown University, Department of Radiology, DePaul Medical Center, Norfolk, Virginia

Michael G. Velchik, M.D.

Department of Radiology, Division of Nuclear Medicine, Fairfax Hospital, Falls Church, Virginia

Richard L. Wahl, M.D.

Professor of Internal Medicine and Radiology, Director, General Nuclear Imaging, The University of Michigan Medical Center, Ann Arbor, Michigan

Michael J. Welch, Ph.D.

Professor of Radiology, Director, Division of Radiation Services, Mallinckrodt Institute of Radiology, Washington University Medical Center, St. Louis, Missouri

Tsunehiro Yasuda, M.D.

Assistant Professor, Department of Radiology, Harvard Medical School and Massachusetts General Hospital, Boston, Massachusetts

Jack Ziffer, M.D., Ph.D.

Department of Radiology, Baptist Hospital, Miami, Florida

TECHNICAL ASSISTANCE

Michael Ballistrea, B.S., CNMT, RT(N)(ARRT), NMT(ASCP)

Manager, Nuclear Medicine Department, Meridia Hillcrest Hospital, Mayfield Heights, Ohio

John H. Baughman, B.A., ARRT(NM), CNMT

Product Manager, Nuclear Medicine Division, Medical Consultants Imaging Co., Cleveland, Ohio

ILLUSTRATOR

Susan Nicolet Greene

FOREWORD

In the remaining few weeks as president of the American College of Nuclear Physicians I welcome this opportunity to give my view of the need for up-to-date textbooks in Nuclear Medicine. *Principles and Practice of Nuclear Medicine* is a timely addition to the contemporary reference resources in educational textbooks available in Nuclear Medicine.

Changes in healthcare delivery with increased managed care, declining reimbursements, and looming healthcare reforms by the federal government have many of us asking about the future of Nuclear Medicine. These changes are occurring at a time, I believe, when Nuclear Medicine contributes more to the health care of patients than ever before. It is very important for technologists and physician practitioners to be knowledgeable about the refinements that have occurred in many established procedures such as myocardial perfusion imaging, infection evaluation in AIDS patients, dementia evaluations with brain SPECT, and gallbladder function evaluations with gallbladder scintigraphy. Significant recent advances using monoclonal antibody imaging for colorectal and ovarian carcinoma and strontium-89 for the relief of painful bone metastases have created the need for up-to-date textbook information. Those of us practicing Nuclear Medicine and those studying to practice Nuclear Medicine will continue to see the Nuclear Medicine benefits to patients being referred either by primary care physicians or specialists. Regardless of healthcare reform, Nuclear Medicine procedures, when practiced by individuals with the most up-to-date information, contribute significantly to the health and welfare of patients.

I challenge trainees and practitioners of Nuclear Medicine to continue to update their skills and correlate Nuclear Medicine studies with the clinical and diagnostic information available on patients. Who is in a better position to judge the significance of Nuclear Medicine results than a Nuclear Medicine specialist? Be as specific as possible in answering the clinical question when reporting diagnostic study results.

Paul Early and Bruce Sodee have gathered a superb faculty as contibutors to this textbook. New chapters in this textbook dealing with refinements in many of the existing procedures and discussions of recently offered procedures, updates on new regulations affecting Nuclear Medicine, and information about marketing Nuclear Medicine procedures help to make this a valuable addition to any Nuclear Medicine library.

Conrad E. Nagle, M.D.
President, American College of Nuclear Physicians
Chief, Nuclear Medicine Services
William Beaumont Hospital
Troy, Michigan

January 5, 1994

PREFACE

Nuclear medicine is a constantly changing specialty whose database has grown exponentially with the input of nuclear medicine specialists, technologists, nuclear radiologists, cardiologists, psychiatrists, neurologists, surgeons, internists, engineers, computer specialists, radiopharmacists, and physicists.

Computer power, single photon emission tomography, new diagnostic and therapeutic radiopharmaceuticals, monoclonal antibodies, and advanced engineering concepts have almost completely changed many aspects of procedures in nuclear medicine.

This updated and expanded edition of *Principles and Practice of Nuclear Medicine* offers new chapters in these growing areas: planar imaging, SPECT, PET, parathyroid imaging, the adrenal gland, and monoclonal antibodies—to name just a few. To help the practitioner stay current in this changing field, this second edition presents dozens of new laboratory applications in the most innovative areas. Sprinkled throughout the text, laboratory applications offer practical, step-by-step instructions on successfully performing numerous procedures.

Principles and Practice of Nuclear Medicine is divided into two sections, giving the reader complete and timely discussions on both the principles and the clinical applications that make nuclear medicine what it is today. The first section presents the basic physics, chemistry, instrumentation, and nuclear medicine regulations (NRC) utilized in nuclear medicine. The second section presents the anatomy, physiology, pathophysiology, nuclear medical procedures, and basic interpretation guidelines of nuclear procedures.

Education of those in the field is an ongoing, constantly changing process as we attempt to keep abreast of the current procedures and practices in nuclear medicine. With respect we thank the nuclear medicine educators, technology students and practitioners with whom we have had contact over the years and whose practices have formed the basis of nuclear medicine. We also wish to thank the past and present contributors for their presentations, the technologists for procedural formation and case material preparation, the illustrator, and the secretaries for their invaluable contribution to the manuscript.

We would also like to pay tribute to two dear friends and colleagues who have passed away, Michael D. Okerlund, M.D., and Marshall Brucer, M.D. We acknowledge the important contributions they both made to nuclear medicine. Michael and Marshall will be remembered and missed by all.

Paul J. Early
D. Bruce Sodee

CONTENTS

Part One

PRINCIPLES OF NUCLEAR MEDICINE

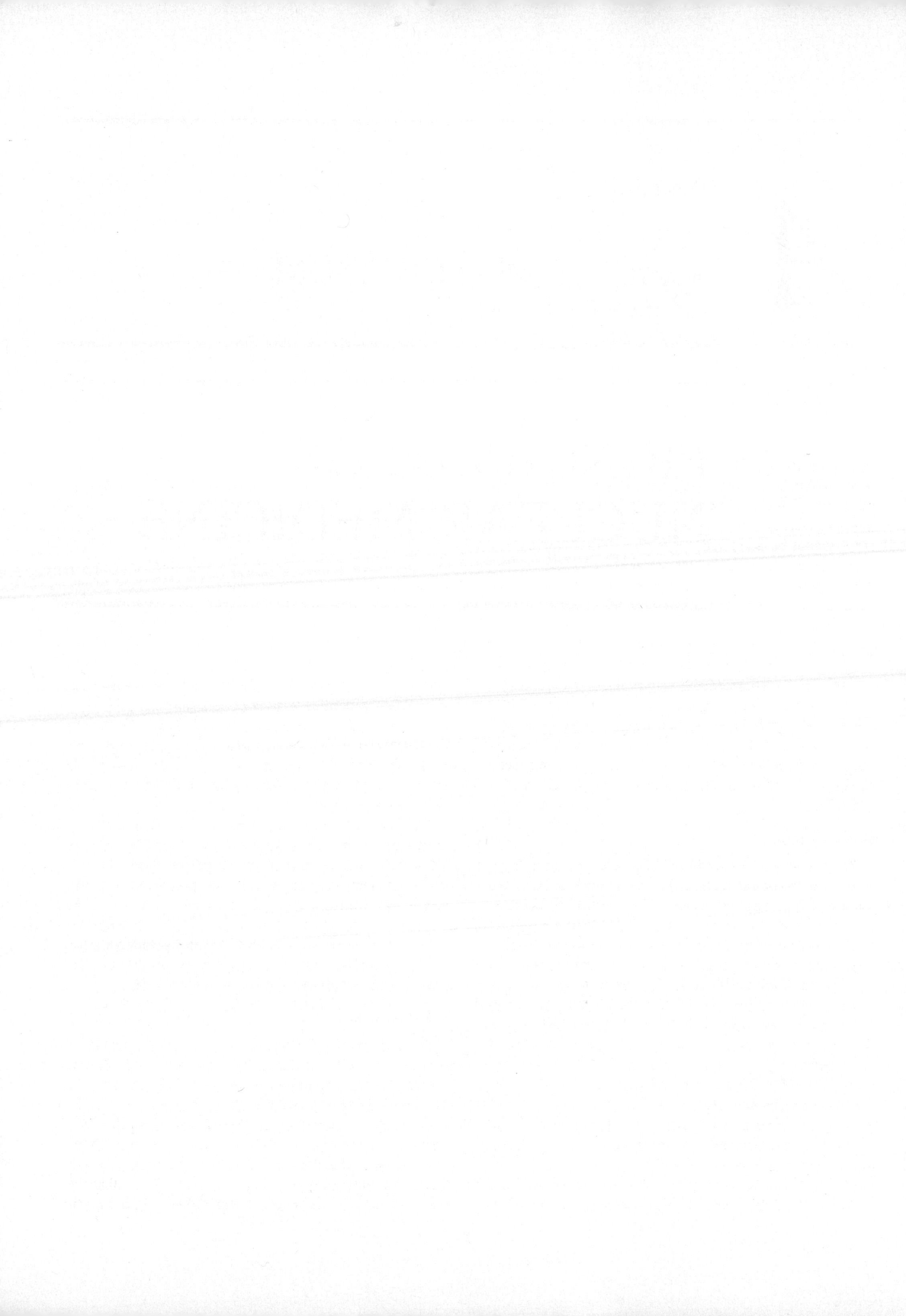

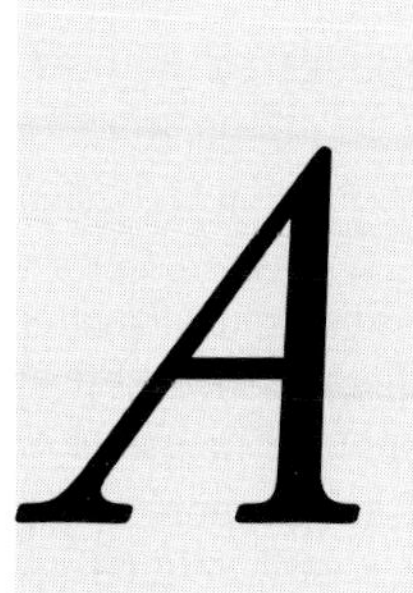

Chapter 1

NATOMY OF THE ATOM

PAUL J. EARLY

In any treatise on the basic sciences a detailed discussion of the structure of matter, molecules, and the constituent atoms must first be presented. In any treatise on the basic *nuclear* sciences a discussion of the constituent parts of the atom should be presented, since these parts play such an important role in the understanding of the nuclear sciences. All the parts of the atom that are important to the nuclear sciences, particularly to nuclear medicine, are presented in this chapter.

Table 1-1. Mass and charge of particles of the atom

Particle	Charge	Mass
Electron	Negative	1*
Proton	Positive	1,836
Neutron	Neutral	1,840
Neutrino	Neutral	~0

*Reference mass.

■ NATURE OF MATTER

The atom is composed of a central positively charged core known as a *nucleus*. Traveling in a path around the nucleus are one or more smaller, negatively charged particles of mass called *electrons*. Bohr compared this arrangement to a miniature solar system—the nucleus representing the sun, and the electrons representing the planets circling the sun.

■ The electron

Definition and description. The electron is a high-velocity extranuclear particle that has a more or less fixed elliptic path around the nucleus. The electron possesses a known mass that remains constant for electrons of all atoms. The number of electrons that are circling the nucleus is a variable, which in an electrically neutral atom is dictated by the constituents of the nucleus. Two criteria may be used to differentiate the electron particle from other particles in the atom: *mass* and *electrical charge* (Table 1-1). With the electron as a reference point, the electron has a relative mass of 1 and a negative charge. This negative charge apparently cannot be separated from the electron. Possessing a negative charge, the electron exhibits forces of attraction or repulsion to other charged particles. These forces were first noticed by Coulomb, and the principle is now an accepted principle of physics. Coulomb's law states in part that *like charges repel; unlike charges attract*.

Mystery of the electron. Because of Coulomb's law and the fact that negative electrons circle the positive nucleus, the question of what effect all this has in the atom may well be asked. A repulsion effect between electrons is exhibited as a distribution in space as they circle the nucleus. The mystery arises in the lack of attraction of the electrons to the nucleus. What prevents the electron from being attracted to the nucleus?

The attraction is prevented through the action of two phenomena working simultaneously. (1) Since the electron is a particle circling the nucleus at high velocities, the electron counteracts the attraction by the nucleus to a certain degree by centrifugal force, the force of inertia that tends to make rotating bodies move away from the center of rotation. (2) A much larger amount of energy from the atom known as *binding energy* is expended for no other reason than to retain the electron in its preordained orbit.

■ The nucleus

On learning of the existence of the nucleus, scientists became intrigued with the fact that the nucleus contained almost all of the weight attributed to the atom. The nucleus therefore became a primary target of research. The effort to discover the composition and function of the nucleus still continues. Many aspects of the nucleus are known; others are unknown, but theories have been formulated about them. One fact that is considered indisputable is that the nucleus itself is made up of small particles. The two particles most important to students of nuclear medicine are the *proton* and the *neutron*. These particles are normal constituents of the nucleus and are commonly referred to as *nucleons*. This positively charged core of every atom contains almost the entire mass of the atom but only a small part of its volume. It has been calculated that the nucleus is only 1/100,000 the size of the entire atom, but it is so dense that a child's marble of the same density would weigh approximately 36,400,000 tons. The nucleus is very stable and is impervious to chemical or physical changes; however, radiation can cause changes within it.

The proton. The proton (p) possesses a known mass, which remains constant. It has a positive charge associated with it that cannot be separated from it. The charge is equal in magnitude to the negative charge of the electron. It is because of the presence of these protons within the nucleus that the nucleus possesses a positive charge. In fact, in the hydrogen atom, the proton *is* the positive nucleus. In all other atoms the proton is one of the constituents. The mass of the proton is much greater than that of the electron. The proton has a mass 1836 times that of the electron (Table 1-1). The number of protons within the nucleus determines the type of atom; for example, all carbon atoms have 6 protons, and all atoms containing 6 protons are carbon atoms.

The neutron. The neutron (n) also possesses a known mass that remains constant. This mass is just slightly greater than the mass of a proton (1840). This particle, as the name implies, has no electric charge. Because of the neutral charge it cannot attract or repel charged particles. In fact, it is this very property that makes the neutron important. With a lack of charge, the neutron cannot be affected by the charged particles in the atom and can penetrate right into the heart of the atom. Under proper conditions the neutron can actually be incorporated into the nucleus or disrupt it. The former is referred to as neutron activation; the latter is referred to as fission. Both phenomena will be discussed later.

Mystery of the nucleus. The nucleus can be considered to be an aggregate of positive charges because of its proton constituents. According to Coulomb's law, the protons should repel one another, and the repulsive effects of the positive charges should cause the nucleus to fragment. However, this does not seem to be the case. An explanation is that the protons—and therefore the nucleus—are contained through binding energy. The nucleus expends a large amount of energy to keep the nucleons bound to one another.

The neutrino/anti-neutrino. The neutrino or antineutrino cannot be considered a normal constituent of the nucleus but is the result of interactions within the nucleus. These particles play a more or less important role in nuclear medicine, since they are emitted during several methods of atomic decay. Currently, only a description of the particles are warranted. The neutrino (υ) or antineutrino ($\bar{\upsilon}$) is, as the name would indicate, a particle possessing a neutral charge. Its mass approaches zero mass.

The mass and charge of all these particles are summarized in Table 1-1.

■ Energy shells

The atom has been defined as the smallest unit of matter that exhibits the chemical properties of an element. It is composed of a nucleus containing protons and neutrons of varying numbers and is surrounded by one or more negatively charged electrons circling in rather well-defined orbits, or *energy shells*. The number of electrons in each energy shell varies according to the chemical element. Each shell can contain only a certain number of electrons. That number is defined by the *$2n^2$ formula,* in which n is the number of the energy shell. The energy shells are numbered beginning with that shell closest to the nucleus and proceeding outward numerically. According to the $2n^2$ formula, the first energy shell can contain no more than 2 electrons. The second energy shell can contain no more than 8 electrons, the third energy shell can contain no more than 18 electrons, the fourth energy shell can contain no more than 32 electrons, and so on. Rather than being designated by numbers, the shells are labeled alphabetically beginning with K and proceeding outward. Therefore the K shell can have no more than 2, the L shell no more than 8, and the M shell no more than 18 electrons. A more lengthy discussion of energy levels, orbital as well as nuclear, will be found at the end of Chapter 2.

■ NUCLEAR SHORTHAND

In every phase of business and professional life, there is a need to express oneself in concise, definitive terminology. Nuclear physics is no different. For this reason, a shorthand system has been devised to specify every atom and every form of that atom. This identification process is carried out with the aid of the *chemical symbol,* the *atomic number,* and the *mass number* in accordance with the following format:

$$^{A}_{Z}X$$

X = Chemical symbol
A = Mass number
Z = Atomic number

The *mass number* (A) has the superscript position immediately preceding the chemical symbol and indicates the number of protons and neutrons in the nucleus. (In the past, this number held the superscript position immediately following the chemical symbol.) The *atomic number* (Z) has the subscript position immediately preceding the chemical symbol and indicates the number of protons in the nucleus just as it does on the periodic chart of the atoms. Since the proton number of any element is synonymous with the element itself, this shorthand method has been shortened even further by indicating only the element and the mass number. These two terms are sufficient to identify the atom. The *neutron number* (N) can be found by subtracting the atomic number from the mass number:

$$N = A - Z$$

■ THREE SIMPLEST ATOMS

In a detailed study of the three simplest atoms—hydrogen, helium, and lithium—some basic principles can be learned of the nature of the more complex atoms that occur in nature (Fig. 1-1). These principles will be delineated after the discussion of each of these atoms.

■ Hydrogen

The simplest of all atoms is the hydrogen atom (H). This element is a colorless, odorless gas that occurs throughout all living material. It represents 10% of the body weight of the biochemical standard man. Hydrogen, the simplest atom in the periodic chart of the atoms, possesses the atomic number 1, indicating 1 proton and therefore 1 electron. The number of neutrons in the nucleus of any atom can be learned by rounding off the atomic weight and subtracting the atomic number. The rounding off of the atomic weight of hydrogen, 1.0079, would result in the number 1. Since the atomic number is 1, there are no neutrons in the most abundant form of the hydrogen atom. The symbol for this form is ${}^{1}_{1}H$.

■ Helium

Helium (He), occupying the next position on the periodic chart, is also a colorless and odorless gas. It has an atomic number of 2 and an atomic weight of 4.0026. The helium nucleus consists of 2 protons and 2 neutrons, accounting for the symbol ${}^{4}_{2}He$.

For the helium atom to be electrically neutral, 2 orbiting electrons are required because there are 2 protons in the nucleus. This same pattern is followed throughout all the atoms.

■ Lithium

Lithium (Li) is a metal considered not essential for biologic materials. Lithium occupies the next position in the order of complexity, having an atomic number of 3 and an atomic weight, when rounded off, of 7. This would indicate that the lithium atom has 3 protons, 4 neutrons, and, in an electrically neutral atom, 3 orbiting electrons, as shown in the symbol ${}^{7}_{3}Li$.

■ Principles

In studying these three simplest atoms, four important principles are demonstrated:

1. To maintain electrical neutrality, the number of orbiting electrons must equal the number of protons within the nucleus. Hydrogen has 1 proton and therefore 1 electron. Helium has 2 protons and therefore 2 electrons. Lithium has 3 protons and therefore 3 electrons.
2. The mass of the electron lends little to the total mass of the atom under study. In the hydrogen atom the nucleus consists of 1 proton. Since the proton is 1836 times greater in mass than the electron, the nucleus is of the same order of magnitude. In the helium atom the nucleus is 7350 times greater in weight than the electron. The mass of any atom is closely equal to

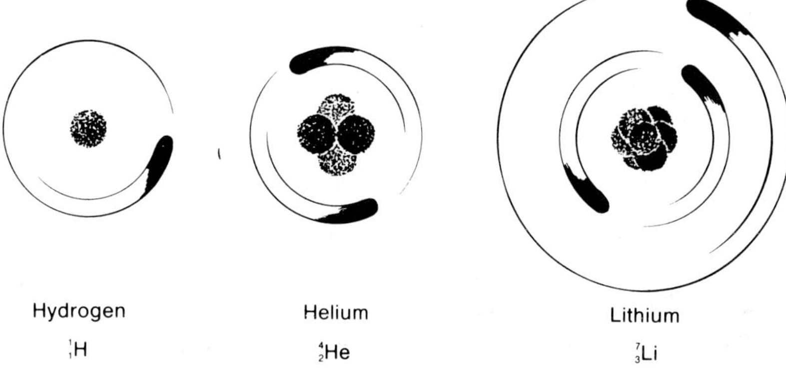

Fig. 1-1. Nuclear components and electron configurations of the three simplest atoms—hydrogen, helium, and lithium. These atoms have not been drawn proportionally. If the constituents of the hydrogen atom, for example, were depicted correctly, it would be impossible to display the atom on the page. It has been calculated that if the nucleus of the hydrogen atom were the size of a baseball, the electron would be circling in an orbit wide enough to encompass New York City. It should also be remembered that atoms are three-dimensional. The electrons do not circle the nucleus in a flat field relationship as depicted here, but they can circle the nucleus from an infinite number of angles. Further, they orbit the nucleus in pathways that are more or less elliptical.

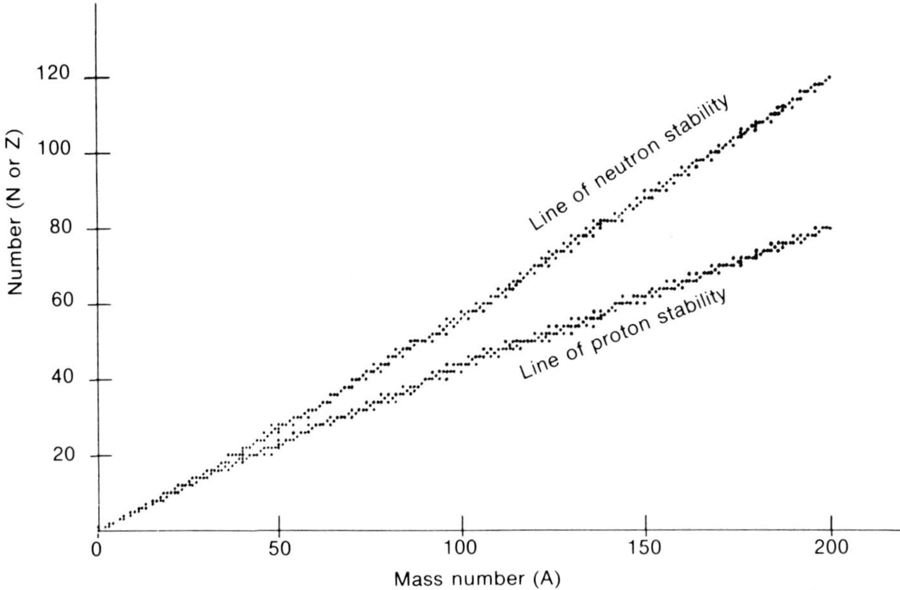

Fig. 1-2. Number of neutrons to the number of protons for all known stable forms of an element and plotted against their mass number. Graph displays neutron and proton lines of stability. Graph also illustrates the fact that as atoms become more complex, more neutrons are required to maintain stability.

the sum of the masses of the protons and the neutrons comprising its nucleus. The mass of the orbital electrons can in general be disregarded.

3. The electron configuration of each atom has a certain order. In hydrogen the electron is added to the K shell. In helium the second electron is added to the K shell, thereby completing that shell's full complement of electrons according to the $2n^2$ formula. In the lithium atom the third electron must be added to the L shell, because the K shell has received its full complement of electrons. A somewhat similar orderly progression continues throughout the entire chart of the atoms, although many irregularities exist, especially beyond potassium (K).
4. The number of neutrons within the nucleus varies with respect to the number of protons that exist within the nucleus. In the case of hydrogen there are no neutrons. Helium contains an equal number of protons and neutrons. Lithium has a larger number of neutrons than protons. In fact, proceeding from lithium in complexity, the number of neutrons must increase at a faster rate than the number of protons to maintain nuclear stability, that is, to maintain a nonradioactive status (Fig. 1-2). This relationship begins to express itself as early as the third atom in the order of complexity. It continues until an atom such as polonium 210, which contains 84 protons and 126 neutrons, is reached. Even with this obvious abundance of neutrons, the nucleus cannot maintain stability, and the atom is subject to radioactive decay.

BIBLIOGRAPHY

Bernier, D.R., Langan, J.K., and Wells, L.D.: Nuclear medicine technology and techniques, ed. 2, St. Louis, 1989, Mosby–Year Book.

Blahd, W.H.: Nuclear medicine, New York, 1965, McGraw-Hill Book Co.

Bogardus, C.R., Jr.: Clinical applications of physics of radiology and nuclear medicine, St. Louis, 1969, Warren H. Green, Inc.

Boyd, C.M., and Dalrymple, G.V.: Basic science principles of nuclear medicine, St. Louis, 1974, Mosby–Year Book.

Chandra, R.: Introductory physics of nuclear medicine, ed. 4, Philadelphia, 1992, Lea & Febiger.

Chase, G.D., and Rabinowitz, J.L.: Principles of radioisotope methodology, ed. 3, Minneapolis, 1967, Burgess Publishing Co.

Goodwin, P.N., and Rao, D.V.: An introduction to the physics of nuclear medicine, Springfield, Ill., 1977, Charles C Thomas, Publisher.

Gottschalk, A., and Potchen, E.J.: Diagnostic nuclear medicine, Baltimore, 1976, The Williams & Wilkins Co.

Hendee, W.R.: Medical radiation physics, ed. 2, Chicago, 1979, Year Book Medical Publishers, Inc.

Johns, H.E., and Cunningham, J.R.: The physics of radiology, ed. 4, revised edition, Springfield, Ill., 1983, Charles C Thomas, Publisher.

King, E.R., and Mitchell, T.G.: A manual for nuclear medicine, Springfield, Ill., 1961, Charles C Thomas, Publisher.

Pizzarello, D.J., and Witcofski, R.L.: Medical radiation biology, ed. 2, Philadelphia, 1982, Lea & Febiger.

Prasad, K.N.: Human radiation biology, New York, 1974, Harper & Row, Publishers.

Quimby, E.H., and Feitelberg, S.: Radioactive isotopes in medicine and biology, ed. 2, Philadelphia, 1963, Lea & Febiger.

Rocha, A.F.G., and Harbert, J.C.: Textbook of nuclear medicine: basic science, Philadelphia, 1978, Lea & Febiger.

Rollo, F.D.: Nuclear medicine physics, instrumentation, and agents, St. Louis, 1977, Mosby–Year Book.

Shilling, C.W.: Atomic energy encyclopedia in the life of sciences, Philadelphia, 1964, W.B. Saunders Co.

Sorenson, J.A., and Phelps, M.E.: Physics in nuclear medicine, ed. 2, New York, 1987, Grune & Stratton, Inc.

Schleien, B.: The health physics and radiological health handbook, rev. ed., Silver Springs, Md., 1992, Scinta, Inc.

Wagner, H.N.: Principles of nuclear medicine, Philadelphia, 1968, W.B. Saunders Co.

Wang, C.H., and Willis, D.L.: Radiotracer methodology in biological science, Englewood Cliffs, N.J., 1965, Prentice-Hall, Inc.

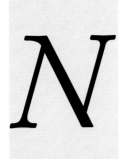

Chapter 2

UCLIDES AND RADIONUCLIDES

PAUL J. EARLY

In recent years the terms *isotope* and *radioisotope* have fallen into disfavor. These two terms had been used for many years to describe all forms of all elements. Since this is not entirely correct usage of the two terms, they have been replaced by the terms *nuclide* and *radionuclide,* respectively. The term *nuclide* was proposed as a more precise term than isotope because the meaning of nuclide is any nucleus plus its orbital electrons. The term *isotope* refers to two or more forms of the same element. It would be incorrect to say ^{127}I is the only stable isotope of iodine, because there is only one stable form, not two or more. It would be more meaningful to describe ^{127}I as the only stable nuclide of iodine. Furthermore, it would be improper to refer to ^{99m}Tc and ^{131}I as radioactive isotopes (radioisotopes). They are actually radioactive nuclides (radionuclides) because they are two different elements. A correct usage of the term *radioisotopes* would be that ^{123}I and ^{125}I are radioisotopes because they are two forms of the same element.

■ ISOTOPES

■ Definition

An isotope may be defined as one of two or more forms of the same element having the same atomic number *(Z),* differing mass numbers *(A),* and the same chemical properties. These different forms of an element may be stable or unstable (radioactive). However, since they are forms of the same element, they possess identical chemical properties. These chemical properties remain the same even though, if unstable, their radioactive properties differ. Another way of defining isotopes is that they are forms of the same element, but each form has a different weight because of the varying number of neutrons in the nucleus (Fig. 2-1).

There are over 270 known nuclidic forms of stable elements; 40 of these exist in nature and are termed *naturally occurring* nuclides. In addition to these, more than 900 radionuclides have been produced artificially.

■ Three isotopes of hydrogen

The periodic chart lists atomic numbers (chemical numbers) as whole numbers and atomic weights as decimal fractions. It would seem that if the nucleus consists of protons and neutrons and each nucleon represented one unit of atomic weight (the electrons not adding significantly to the weight of the atom), then all atoms should have an atomic weight that would be a multiple of one. However, this is not the case. For example, hydrogen has an atomic weight of 1.008. This must have caused great concern to early investigators, because the earliest known form of hydrogen had only 1 proton and should have had an atomic weight of 1.000. This not being the case, early investigators found it necessary to hypothesize the existence of some other form of the element that reacted identically to hydrogen but was heavier. This would cause the resultant weight to be something greater than 1.000, the degree being dependent on the weight and abundance of this heavier form. The existence of isotopes was postulated as one of the possible factors in this obvious discrepancy. Hydrogen was found to occur in nature in two different forms, ordinary hydrogen and deuterium, thus proving the hypothesis.

Hydrogen. Ordinary hydrogen, $^{1}_{1}H$ (sometimes called *protium*), is the most abundant form of the element hydrogen. Its nucleus has only 1 proton ($Z = 1$) and no neutrons ($A = 1$) (Fig. 2-2). It is naturally occurring and stable.

Deuterium. Another isotope of hydrogen is deuterium. Deuterium, $^{2}_{1}H$, consists of 1 proton ($Z = 1$) and 1 neutron ($A = 2$) and is the least abundant form. It occurs in a ratio of 8 parts to every 1000 parts of ordinary hydrogen. Deuterium is naturally occurring and stable. It has also been called *heavy hydrogen.* Since ordinary hydrogen has 1 proton and deuterium has 1 proton plus 1 neutron, deuterium is twice the weight of the most abundant form.

It is interesting to note that deuterium occurs at a ratio of 8 : 1000 parts of all hydrogen atoms in nature. This ratio of abundance would justify the atomic weight differential

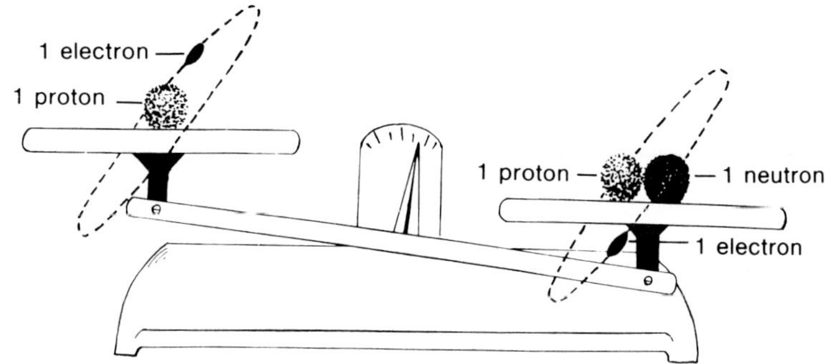

Fig. 2-1. Difference between two nuclides can be expressed as a weight differential caused by an increased number of neutrons in their nuclear configurations.

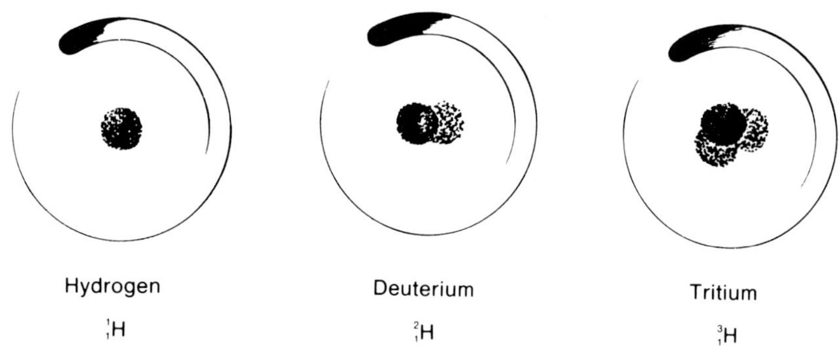

Fig. 2-2. Three nuclides of hydrogen: ordinary hydrogen, deuterium, and tritium. Number of protons and electrons remains the same for all three forms, but the neutron number increases.

of the hydrogen atom as 1.008. The atomic (chemical) weight of an element is derived from all the *stable* forms of the element, considering the atomic weight of each form of the element and its percent abundance in nature. For example, if both forms occurred in nature at a rate of 50:50, and since ^{2}H is twice the weight of ^{1}H, the atomic weight would be 1.500.

Tritium. There is a third isotope of hydrogen, but it does not occur naturally. It is the artificially produced tritium, $^{3}_{1}H$. This isotope contains 1 proton ($Z = 1$) and 2 neutrons ($A = 3$) and is therefore three times the mass of the most abundant form. It is sometimes referred to as *extra-heavy hydrogen*. Since hydrogen is an intimate part of body chemistry, the use of tritium plays an important role in medical and agricultural research. It is also used as one of the nuclides measured in the Nuclear Regulatory Commission's stratospheric sampling program. It is formed by neutron bombardment of nitrogen 14 after the detonation of an atomic device, yielding carbon 12 and tritium.

All three forms of hydrogen have only 1 proton in their nuclei and only 1 electron in their orbits (Fig. 2-2). Since the electrons determine the chemical characteristics and their number is the same on all three forms, these isotopes, whether stable or unstable, react identically in a chemical situation. The difference in mass is caused solely by the number of neutrons within the nucleus.

■ Neutron to proton ratio

From studying these isotopes of hydrogen, the principle of neutron to proton ratio and nuclear stability can be observed. In the cases of ordinary hydrogen and deuterium, the presence or absence of 1 neutron does not alter the stability of the nucleus. In both cases the nucleus is nonradioactive. However, the incorporation of 1 more neutron into the nucleus, as in the case of tritium, exceeds the bounds of nuclear stability. Why the nucleus becomes unstable at that point is not clearly understood, but tritium becomes an unstable or radioactive nuclide of hydrogen because there are too many neutrons.

This principle is also true with all other nuclides. Each element has its own unique ratio(s) or combination(s) of neutrons and protons. Any deviation from this, either too few neutrons and too many protons or too many neutrons and too few protons, results in nuclear instability.

The method by which a nuclide decays (changes into another nuclide) is one that will result in the nucleus becoming stable or closer to stability. If the decay process contains only one step, then the resultant new nuclide is stable. If the decay process contains many steps, then the nuclide formed after the first step will be unstable and more than one step is necessary before a stable form of an element is reached.

■ OTHER "ISOS"

■ Isobar

By definition, isobars are 2 atoms that have the same mass number but different atomic numbers and therefore different chemical properties. To state it another way, the nucleus of each of these atoms contains the same sum of protons and neutrons, but the division between protons and neutrons is different. An example of isobars would be lithium 7($^{7}_{3}$Li) and beryllium 7($^{7}_{4}$Be). Both nuclides have a total of 7 nucleons. Lithium has 3 protons and 4 neutrons, and beryllium has 4 protons and 3 neutrons. Isobars in nuclear medicine are of no particular importance per se.

■ Isotone

Isotones are nuclides having the same number of neutrons. In no other way are 2 isotones similar. They differ in atomic number, mass number, and chemical properties. They are mentioned primarily because the trilinear chart of the nuclides has been formulated on the basis of isotopes, isobars, and isotones. An example of isotones would be $^{131}_{53}$I and $^{132}_{54}$Xe. In each case $N = 78$.

Table 2-1 summarizes the differences between isotopes, isobars, and isotones.

■ Isomer

An isomer is one of two or more nuclides that has the same mass number and atomic number as the others but exists for measurable times in the excited state. When a nucleus is in an excited state and decays by gamma emission, the transition from the higher to the lower energy usually takes less than 10^{-13} seconds. Nuclei that take longer than 10^{-12} seconds are called *isomers*. Two examples of isomers are technetium 99m (^{99m}Tc) and strontium 87m (^{87m}Sr).

■ ATOMIC ENERGY LEVELS

Both x-rays and gamma rays represent energy releases as a result of changes in energy levels either within the nucleus or in the extranuclear structure. X-rays are releases of energy as a result of changes within the orbital pattern of the electron. Gamma rays are releases of energy as a result of changes occurring within the nucleus itself. To understand these energy releases an explanation of both the orbital energy levels and the nuclear energy levels is warranted.

■ Orbital energy levels

Although it has been said that an electron is more or less assigned to a definite orbit, the analogy of an atom to a miniature solar system is to some degree an oversimplification. Unlike the planets circling the sun, the electron can actually exist anywhere, although it is most often found in its regularly assigned orbit. In contrast to the usual illustrations of the atom, it has been suggested that the electron does not follow a circular path around the nucleus but makes more nearly an elliptical path—an imprecisely defined "region of space." In fact, some scientists subscribe to the theory that the K shell electron(s) has such an elliptical pattern that the orbit of the K shell electron actually passes through the nucleus. Furthermore, since the like charges repel one another, the electrons repel each other in their respective orbits so that these electrons are actually arranged in space symmetry. There are two types of energies involved in the course of an electron, and each plays a definite role in the action and subsequent reaction of electron disturbance. These energies are the binding energy and the energy state of the electron itself.

Binding energy. The binding energy of the electron is the energy required to remove the particle from its orbit. If the binding energy of a K shell electron of a particular atom were 70,000 electron volts (70 keV), as in Fig. 2-3, that electron would need to be supplied with an energy equal to or greater than 70 keV to remove it from its energy shell. This energy could be supplied to that electron by a high-energy particle or photon radiation, at which time the energy of the interacting particle or ray would be decreased in energy by an amount equal to the binding energy. The same principle is true for an L shell electron except that less energy is required to remove it, since the binding energy becomes less as the electron is positioned farther away from the nucleus. In a typical atom, in which the K shell electron would have a binding energy of 70 keV, the binding energy of the L shell electron may be reduced to as lit-

Table 2-1. Summary of the differences between isotopes, isobars, and isotones

	Atomic number (Z)	Mass number (A)	Neutron number (N)	Chemical properties
Isotopes	Same	Different	Different	Same
Isobars	Different	Same	Different	Different
Isotones	Different	Different	Same	Different

tle as 11 keV, the M shell electron to 2.5 keV, and the N shell electron ≈0, the latter being the case with all outer shell electrons. In each of these cases, energy equal to or greater than that of the binding energy of the electron must be supplied to remove that electron from its orbit.

Energy state of the electron. The energy state of an orbital electron can perhaps best be described by a crude analogy that compares it to a racetrack (Fig. 2-4). For each car to stay abreast with the others it must possess a different speed (energy). According to the illustration, the car on the outside track (the M track) must travel at 75 mph to keep abreast with the car on the inner track (the K track) traveling at 65 mph. Therefore the 75 mph car has a greater energy state than does the car on the inner track. Should the car on the inside track drop from the race, either the car in the middle track or the car on the outside track would have the ability to take its place. To do so, each car must decrease its speed, that is, decrease its energy state to maintain its position in the race.

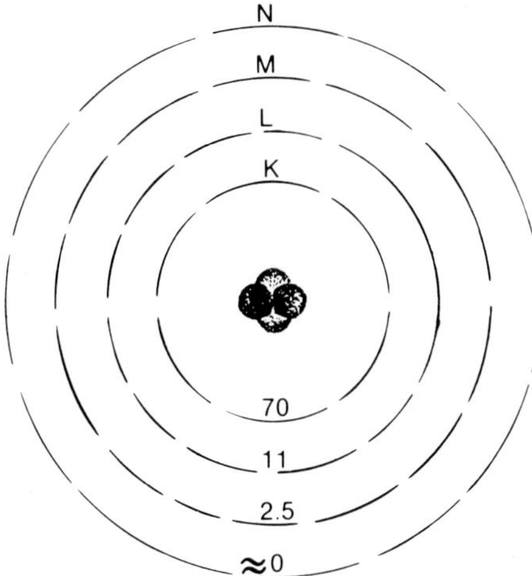

Fig. 2-3. Representative electron-binding energies of a hypothetical atom. Binding energy is larger for those electrons circling closer to the nucleus. To remove an electron from its orbit, removing force must possess energy equal to or greater than binding energy.

Such is also the case of the orbiting electrons. Should the K shell electron be removed from its orbit for some reason, the L or the M shell electron would take its place. To do so, there would necessarily have to be a decrease in the energy state of that orbiting electron. At the same time there would be an increase in the binding energy, since the electron is assuming the role of the K shell electron that possesses more binding energy. Should a K shell electron be removed, the probability that that space would be filled by the L electron and the L space filled by the M electron would be greater than that of the M falling down into the K shell electron. In any case, just as nature abhors a vacuum, an electron shell abhors a vacancy. By depicting the energy states of the electrons as analogous to a racetrack, the intention is to simplify the phenomena of *optical radiation* and *characteristic radiation*.

Optical radiation. The ability of atoms under certain conditions to emit radiations that fall into the visible spectrum allowed scientists a means of identifying the atom by identifying the color of the light. This type of radiation is termed *optical radiation*. It results from the fact that when an atom is given a certain amount of energy (termed *excited state*), the electron will move to a certain correspond-

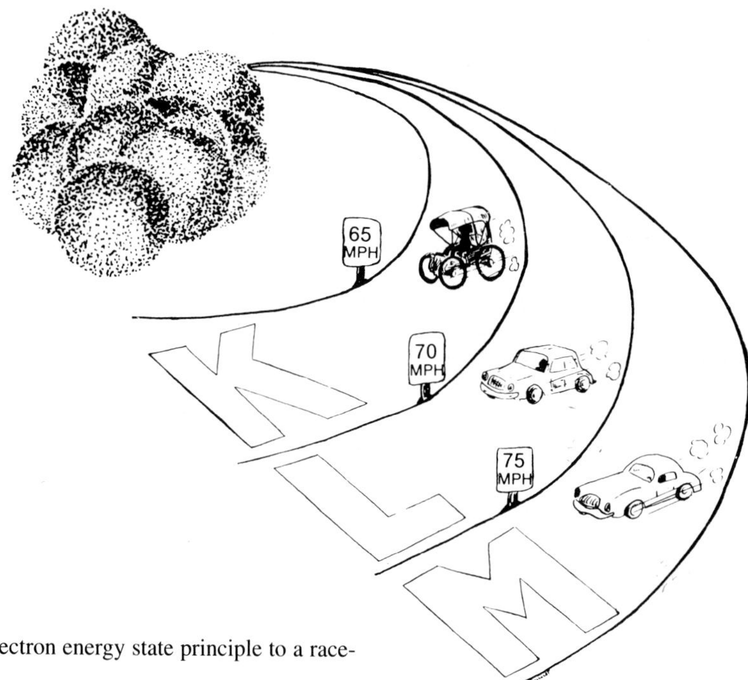

Fig. 2-4. Comparison of electron energy state principle to a racetrack.

ing path (subshell) farther from the nucleus. This energy would not be enough to move the electron into another orbit. (In the case of the racing car, the car would not move into the 80 mph racetrack but would move into a suborbit that might correspond to the outer portion of the 75 mph track, thereby necessitating the car to go 77 mph to keep aligned.) To go to this subshell, the electron would have to assume additional energy, just as would the racing car. As soon as the source of energy is removed, the electron drops back to the original orbit and emits a photon of an energy corresponding to the energy loss by the electron. The photon would be of a frequency and wavelength equal to some form of the visible light spectrum, thereby serving as a means of color identification.

This same principle applies to *excitation* of an atom by a passing particle (α or β) or electromagnetic radiation (γ- or x-radiation). An orbital electron is raised in energy state with the subsequent release of that energy when the electron drops into its normally occupied energy shell.

Characteristic radiation. The same principle holds true for electrons falling into an energy shell closer to the nucleus. In the event that a K shell electron would be removed, the vacancy would be filled by either the L shell electron or the M shell electron. Since the L shell electron would have to decrease in energy state by assuming the role of a K shell electron, the energy differential must be released in the form of x-radiation. This is known as characteristic radiation, or *fluorescent radiation.* It is important to note that these emissions are not known as gamma radiation. The only difference between gamma radiation and x-radiation is their source, or origin. X-rays originate from the orbital structure of the atom, and gamma rays always originate from the nucleus. At no time could these characteristic radiations be referred to as gamma rays. The term *characteristic radiation* has been applied because the energy of the resultant x-ray is characteristic of the energy loss by an electron falling from an orbit distant from the nucleus to an orbit closer to the nucleus. All electrons falling into the K shell, regardless of their origin, would emit x-rays, called *characteristic K-radiation;* all electrons falling into the L shell would emit characteristic L-radiation and so on.

The actual situation is considerably more complex than that described previously. Electrons are capable of rotating about and moving back and forth with respect to their position with the nucleus. The energy pathways in which these electrons travel and still stay within their primary energy shells are called *subshells.* The total subshells for each primary energy shell are known, as well as is the number of electrons to be found on each subshell (Fig. 2-5 and Table 2-2). Changes between subshells (within the same primary energy shell) occur constantly, so that physicists avoid trying to predict the exact location of any electron at any time. They attempt to predict only the probability that an electron is at a given energy level. For each change, a discrete amount of energy is released. Changes between primary energy shells can also occur; however, it requires an electron vacancy in a lower level or a degree of excitation sufficient to overcome the binding energy of that electron. Whenever changes in electron position of this magnitude occur, the resultant release of energy falls usually in the x-ray portion of the electromagnetic spectrum (Chapter 3).

The laws of physics forbid the movement of some electrons of one energy shell to another shell. A discussion of these rules are not within the scope of this textbook, however. Suffice it to say that the changes that are permitted result in energy emissions bearing names such as "Kαl x-ray." A Kαl x-ray is the energy released as a result of the L_{III} electron dropping into the K shell, called a *K-L_{III} transition.* A listing of all such transitions worthy of note follows:

X-ray	Transition
Kα1	K-L_{III}
Kα2	K-L_{II}
Kβ1	K-M_{III}
Kβ2	K-N_{II}
Kβ3	K-M_{II}
Lα1	L_{III}-M_V
Lα2	L_{III}-M_{IV}
Lβ1	L_{II}-M_{IV}

■ Nuclear energy levels

The concept of energy states regarding the orbital structure is also applicable to the nucleus, except that releases of energy resulting from changes within the nucleus are of much greater magnitude than those of the electrons. There are two possible results of an elevation in energy state (excited state) by the nucleus. There may be particle emission as the result of conditions involving binding energy or photon (gamma) emission caused by conditions involving the energy state of the nucleus.

Binding energy. Just as there is a binding energy involved with the orbiting electrons, so also is there a binding energy involved with the nucleus. The binding energy in the nucleus is the energy required to remove a single proton, neutron, or alpha particle from the nucleus. The existence of binding energy can be demonstrated by comparing the mass relationship of an intact helium 4 nucleus (2 protons, 2 neutrons) to the weight of 2 protons and 2 neutrons weighed separately (Fig. 2-6). The intact helium 4 atom actually weighs less than the sum of its constituent parts because some of the actual mass of the helium 4 nucleus has been converted to energy (binding energy). The nuclear binding energy is the equivalent energy difference between the sum of the masses of the protons and neutrons as they would exist separately and the equivalent energy of the mass of the nucleus itself. This difference is also called *mass defect* (Chapter 3).

It is believed that the protons and neutrons are in a constant state of motion. When energy is supplied to an atom, the degree of motion increases. This condition can be

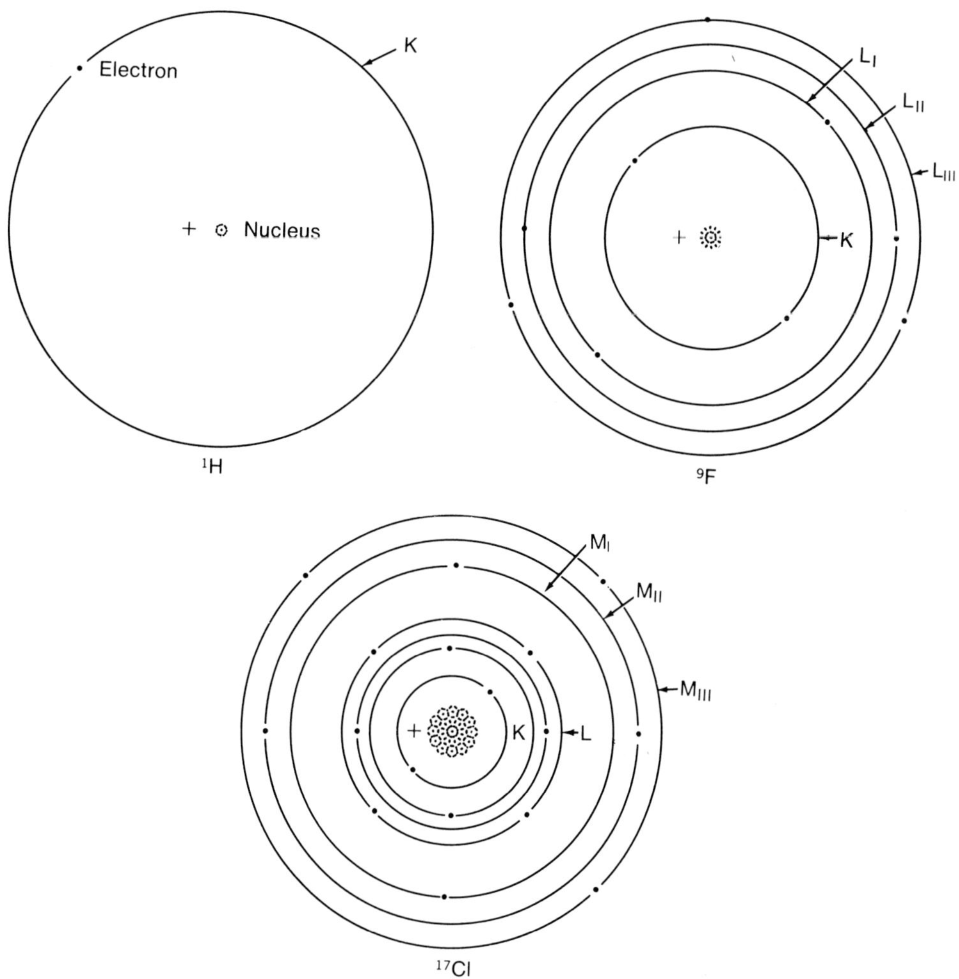

Fig. 2-5. Subshell arrangements of three different-size atoms.

Table 2-2. The occupation capacities of the electron shells of the atom

n	Primary shell letter designation	Subshell designation I	II	III	IV	V	VI	VII	Total capacity
1	K	2	—	—	—	—	—	—	2
2	L	2	2	4	—	—	—	—	8
3	M	2	2	4	4	6	—	—	18
4	N	2	2	4	4	6	6	8	32
5	O	2	2	4	4	6	6	8	32

caused by the absorption of a photon, collisions with other particles or systems, or the natural radioactivity of the nucleus.

Since the nucleons are in motion, there are many chances for collisions between nuclear particles. When energy is added to the nucleus, the number of collisions increases. When a collision occurs, some or all of the energy of the colliding particle is transferred to the particle into which it collides. By this transfer of energy, the particle receives and retains an inordinate amount of energy until such time as it would lose that energy by a subsequent collision. If the energy that the particle receives exceeds the binding energy of that particle in the nucleus, the particle will be subject to ejection from the nucleus if no subsequent collision occurs. This would then constitute *particle emission*.

This phenomenon could be compared to a pool table. A

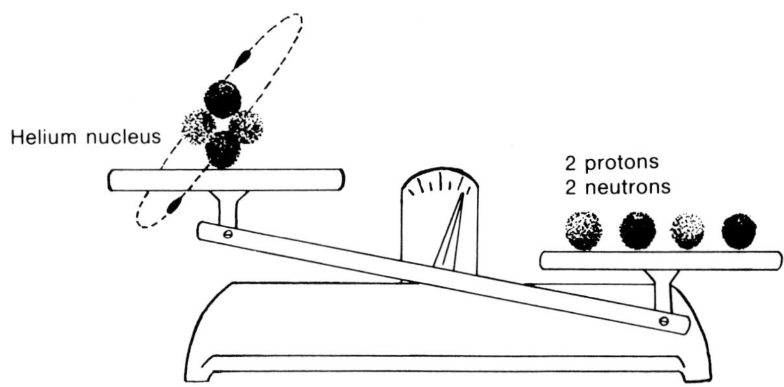

Fig. 2-6. Proof of nuclear binding energy. Intact helium 4 nucleus weighs less than individual components weighed separately. This suggests that some nuclear mass has been converted to binding energy.

dormant cue ball can be supplied with energy when striking it with a cue stick. As the cue ball is propelled over some distance of the pool table, it collides with other balls. Through this collision the cue ball transfers some or possibly all of its energy to other balls on the table. Should the energy transferred to another ball on the table be sufficient, the ball could possibly exceed the limits of the rebound cushions and be ejected from the pool table. In particle emission, energies transferred to the nucleons that exceed their binding energy result in the loss of a particle from the nucleus, just as energy transferred to the pool balls, sufficient to overcome the containing effect of the table cushions, results in the loss of a pool ball from the table. This analogy typifies exactly one mode of decay. The analogy must be altered somewhat for other modes of decay that result in the production of particles other than protons and neutrons. These "foreign" particles, then, receive high energies with their subsequent emission from the nucleus.

Energy state of the nucleons. The concept of energy state of the electron is also applicable to that of the nucleus. When energy is added to the nucleus, but not enough to cause particle emission, the nucleus may merely be raised to another energy state. The most frequent cause for this is particle emission. The particle does not require all the energy given to the nucleus to bring about its ejection. Therefore energy remains in the nucleus, raising it to an excited state. Actually, both the protons and the neutrons have their own set of discrete energy levels to which either nucleon can be raised if sufficient energy is supplied to the nucleus. A nucleus is in its *ground state* when all of its lower energy levels are filled. This can be compared to stepladders with several missing rungs (Fig. 2-7). Only the intact rungs in the ladder would be representative of energy levels to which the nucleons could be raised. If each rung of the ladder represented 100 keV, the nucleons could be raised only to an energy level of 200, 400, 500, or 800 keV. In Fig. 2-7, *A*, the nucleus is in its ground state because all the nucleons occupy the lowest rungs (or energy level). In Fig. 2-7, *B*, an excited state of the nucleus is represented in which a nucleon has been raised to an excited level of 500 keV. When this occurs, the nucleus instantaneously returns to ground state and releases energy corresponding to the energy differential. This energy release is known as gamma radiation. The return to ground state could occur as a one-step, one-gamma affair (monoenergetic), as in Fig. 2-7, *B*, or as a series of jumps with more than one gamma being released, as in Fig. 2-7, *C*. It is possible that in exciting the nucleus the nucleus would not receive sufficient energy to raise the excitation state of the neutron to 500 keV but may only raise it to 400 keV. The reverse could also be true; the nucleus may have received a greater amount of energy, thereby raising the nucleus to 800 keV. It is impossible to predict which particular atom in a given sample of atoms would receive more energy or less energy so that these variations in neutron and proton excitation levels would be known. It is possible, however, to predict the percentages of nuclei receiving these varying energies. It is also possible to predict the percentages of gamma emissions having specific energies. The gamma energy that occurs the most times is referred to as the *primary energy peak,* that is, ^{131}I = 364 keV. This does not mean that ^{131}I has gamma emissions of only one energy. It means simply that the gamma emission of 364 keV occurs the greatest number of times for any given number of ^{131}I atoms undergoing the "de-excitation" process.

The concept of atomic energy levels is extremely complex. The analogies of racetracks, pool tables, and ladders can undoubtedly be considered oversimplifications. There are no perfect analogies, and the ones used here are certainly no exceptions. They are included to assist the student of nuclear medicine to understand these highly complicated principles. Any one of these analogies could be subject to criticism should it be extended beyond its intended purpose.

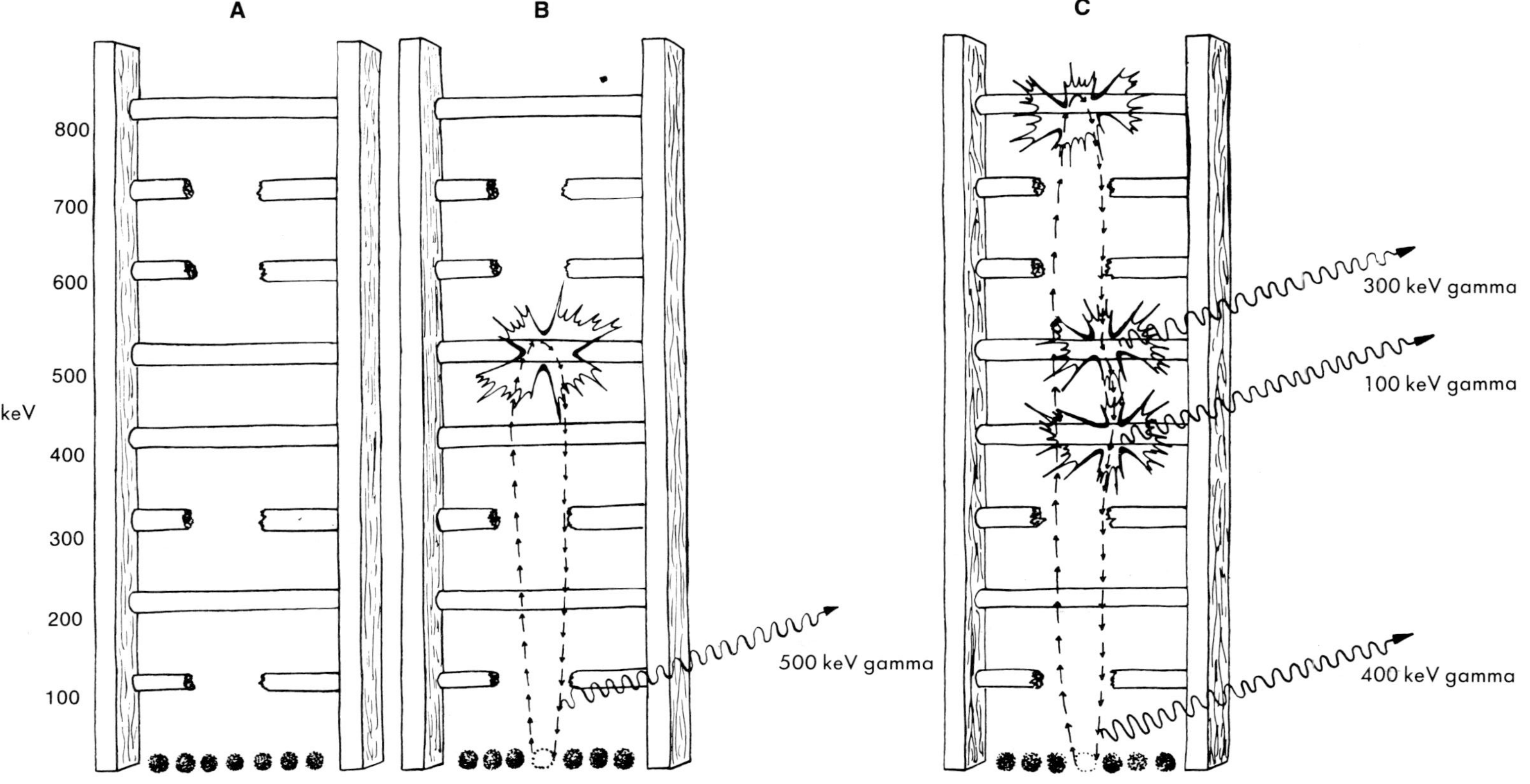

Fig. 2-7. Comparison of nuclear energy state principle to a ladder. **A,** Nucleus at ground state. **B,** Emission of a monoenergetic gamma. **C,** More complex decay scheme.

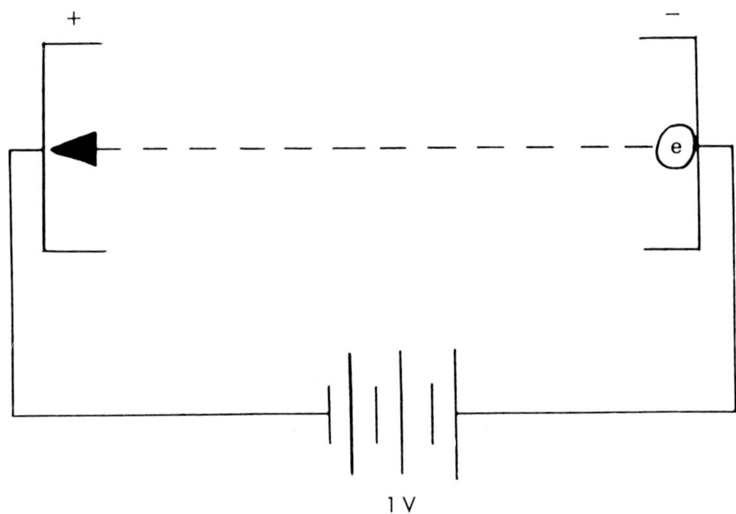

Fig. 2-8. One electron volt (eV).

■ ELECTRON VOLT

In all references to the fundamentals of physics and electricity, terms that have become commonplace include *volt, ampere,* and *erg*. In nuclear medicine the unit of definition seems to center on the term *electron volt* (eV). As the name implies, an electron volt has a relationship to an electron and to the volt. In physics the fundamental unit of work is the *joule*. A more useful energy unit for nuclear medicine purposes is the electron volt with its multiples, thousand electron volts (keV) and million electron volts (MeV). The electron volt is defined as the amount of kinetic energy acquired when an electron falls through a potential difference of 1 volt (Fig. 2-8). In some instances keV is similar to kV (used on x-ray equipment). If 1 electron falls through a potential difference of 1 V, it is equivalent to 1 eV; therefore, if 1 electron falls through a potential difference of 1000 V, it is equivalent to 1000 eV (1 keV). In this instance both kV and keV relate to 1000 V potential difference. In other instances keV is completely different from kV; if 1000 electrons fall through a potential difference of 1 V, it is also equivalent to 1000 eV (1 keV). In this example the potential difference is 1 V and quite unlike kV.

The amount of work performed by 1 eV, expressed in joules, is found to be the product of the charge of the electron (in coulombs) and the potential difference through which it falls. The charge of 1 electron is known to be 1.60×10^{-19} coulombs. Therefore:

$$1 \text{ eV} = 1.00 \times 1.60 \times 10^{-19} \text{ coulombs} = 1.60 \times 10^{-19} \text{ joules}$$

Thus 1 eV has the capacity to do the work of 1.60×10^{-19} joules. Through the use of this formula the electron volt has been converted to the joule, a fundamental unit of work. This conversion figure will be used in the following chapters.

BIBLIOGRAPHY

Bernier, D.R., Langan, J.K., and Wells, L.D.: Nuclear medicine technology and techniques, ed. 2, St. Louis, 1989, Mosby–Year Book.

Blahd, W.H.: Nuclear medicine, New York, 1965, McGraw-Hill Book Co.

Bogardus, C.R., Jr: Clinical applications of physics of radiology and nuclear medicine, St. Louis, 1969, Warren H. Green, Inc.

Boyd, C.M., and Dalrymple, G.V.: Basic science principles of nuclear medicine, St. Louis, 1974, Mosby–Year Book.

Chandra, R: Introductory physics of nuclear medicine, ed. 4, Philadelphia, 1992, Lea & Febiger.

Chase, G.D., and Rabinowitz, J.L.: Principles of radioisotope methodology, ed. 3, Minneapolis, 1967, Burgess Publishing Co.

Goodwin, P.N., and Rao, D.V.: An introduction to the physics of nuclear medicine, Springfield, Ill., 1977, Charles C Thomas, Publisher.

Gottschalk, A., and Potchen, E.J.: Diagnostic nuclear medicine, Baltimore, 1976, The Williams & Wilkins Co.

Hendee, W.R.: Medical radiation physics, ed. 2, Chicago, 1979, Year Book Medical Publishers, Inc.

Johns, H.E., and Cunningham, J.R.: The physics of radiology, ed. 4, revised edition, Springfield, Ill., 1983, Charles C Thomas, Publisher.

King, E.R., and Mitchell, T.G.: A manual for nuclear medicine, Springfield, Ill., 1961, Charles C Thomas, Publisher.

Prasad, K.N.: Human radiation biology, New York, 1974, Harper & Row, Publishers.

Quimby, E.H., and Feitelberg, S.: Radioactive isotopes in medicine and biology, ed. 2, Philadelphia, 1963, Lea & Febiger.

Rocha, A.F.G., and Harbert, J.C.: Textbook of nuclear medicine: basic science, Philadelphia, 1978, Lea & Febiger.

Rollo, F.D.: Nuclear medicine physics, instrumentation, and agents, St. Louis, 1977, Mosby–Year Book.

Shilling, C.W.: Atomic energy encyclopedia in the life sciences, Philadelphia, 1964, W.B. Saunders Co.

Sorenson, J.A., and Phelps, M.E.: Physics in nuclear medicine, ed. 2, New York, 1987, Grune & Stratton, Inc.

Schleien, B.: The health physics and radiological health handbook, rev. ed., Silver Springs, Md., 1992, Sienta, Inc.

Wagner, H.N.: Principles of nuclear medicine, Philadelphia, 1968, W.B. Saunders Co.

Wang, C.H., and Willis, D.L.: Radiotracer methodology in biological science, Englewood Cliffs, N.J., 1965, Prentice-Hall, Inc.

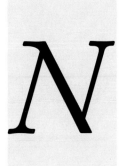

Chapter 3

ATURE OF RADIATION

PAUL J. EARLY

Every human being is exposed daily to a variety of radiations whether he recognizes it or not. The popular concept of radiation is somehow synonymous only with radiations emanating from an x-ray tube, from radioactive materials, or from fallout. In addition to these, however, there are several other types of radiations, all of which manifest themselves in different ways. Some of these radiations can be felt, such as the radiant energy whereby heat is transferred. Other radiations are audible, or at least the devices that receive these radiations, such as the radio, translate them to audible sound. Other radiations can be seen, such as light, which, when focused through a prism, can be further subdivided into all the colors of the spectrum.

There are other radiations that can neither be heard, seen, felt, nor otherwise perceived by the human senses. Examples of these are x-rays and gamma rays. All of these radiations are among the members of the electromagnetic spectrum and are spoken of in terms of waves of energy. Note that none of these radiations are affected by electrical or magnetic properties of matter; hence the name *electromagnetic*.

■ ENERGY WAVES AND THEIR CHARACTERISTICS

A wave in the electromagnetic spectrum is not unlike a wave resulting from a disturbance within a body of water. Throwing a rock into a large body of water would result in the familiar ripples, beginning at the point where the rock touched the water and progressing outward in a circular fashion. Close inspection of these waves would reveal that each wave is an entity in itself, each having a definite length. Those waves occurring near the point of impact occur more frequently than those at a distance from the point of impact, and they travel away from the point of impact. The *wavelength* is defined as the distance from a point on one wave to the same point on the subsequent wave. It could be said that the wavelength of those waves at the point of impact is shorter than those at a distance. The *frequency* is defined as the number of wave formations per unit time. It could be said that the frequency of waves would be greater near the point of impact than the frequency of those distant from the point of impact. The *velocity* is defined as the speed at which these waves travel.

All electromagnetic waves possess these same three characteristics of wavelength, frequency, and velocity. The velocity *(c)* of an electromagnetic wave is a constant. All waves travel at the same velocity regardless of their position on the electromagnetic spectrum. The speed of light waves is 186,000 miles per second (3.0×10^{10} cm/sec), and all members of the electromagnetic spectrum travel at this velocity. Wavelength (λ) and frequency (n) are variables and are *inversely proportional* to one another. This is readily apparent in Fig. 3-1. If the wavelength is decreased, the frequency with which that wave would occur per unit time would necessarily increase (Fig. 3-1, *B*).

The following formula shows a very important relationship between wavelength, frequency, and velocity for electromagnetic waves:

$$c = n \times \lambda$$

c = Velocity in cm/sec
n = Frequency in waves (vibrations)/sec
λ = Wavelength in cm

Since $c = 3 \times 10^{10}$ cm/sec, that value can be substituted immediately. If the frequency is known, the wavelength can be calculated, or, conversely, if the wavelength is known, the frequency can be calculated. Since the wavelength of radiations of interest to nuclear medicine personnel is extremely small, the angstrom unit (Å) has been devised as an expression of length, rather than the centimeter. The angstrom unit has a value of 10^{-8} cm.

■ ELECTROMAGNETIC SPECTRUM

The electromagnetic spectrum is usually displayed on the basis of wavelength in angstrom units. It could also be displayed in terms of frequency or energy. Figure 3-2 illus-

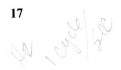

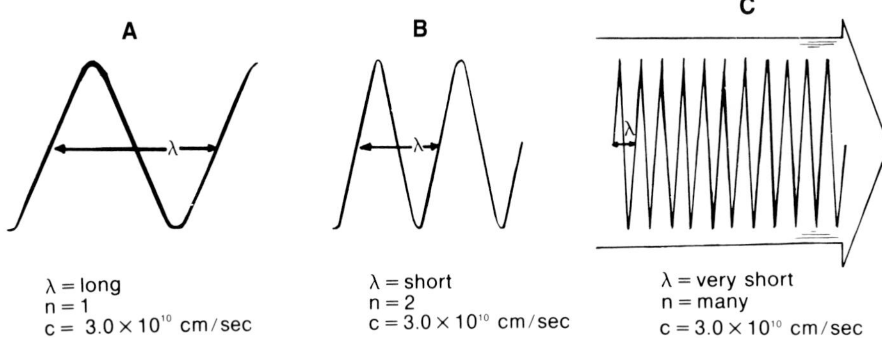

Fig. 3-1. Characteristics of electromagnetic waves. **A,** Wavelength, frequency, and velocity of a wave. **B,** As the wavelength decreases, the frequency increases and velocity remains unchanged. **C,** Quantum nature of radiation; the wave behaves like a bundle of energy, having direction and traveling at the speed of light.

trates an attempt to incorporate all three variables with a display of the electromagnetic spectrum.

The spectrum may best be discussed by imagining ourselves in a room containing a variety of electrical and electronic instrumentation, seated before an instrument that has a capacity of dialing in wavelengths ranging from 10^{17} to 10^{-5} Å. By setting the dial of the instrument at 10^{17} Å, the operator would feel heat, because heat waves occur at this wavelength. If the dial were turned slightly to decrease the wavelength, the radio would begin to play. A further turn of the dial would allow reception from the television set. When the dial is turned even further to allow reception of even shorter wavelengths, the radar monitoring scope would begin to indicate reception of information. With another turn of the dial an intense and deeply penetrating heat in the form of infrared radiation from the heat lamp would be experienced. As the dial is turned further, the room would become illuminated by a deep red light. Subsequent turns of the dial would change the color of the light from red to orange, orange to yellow, yellow to green, green to blue, blue to indigo, and indigo to violet. Eventually the sunlamp will glow, allowing exposure to ultraviolet radiation. Up to this point, changes in wavelengths have demonstrated phenomena that, with appropriate aids, could be felt, seen, or heard. Further changes in wavelength, indicating reception of even shorter waves, cannot be perceived by the human senses. The first of these that would be encountered would be x-rays, next would be gamma rays, and finally, at the shortest wavelength setting possible, cosmic radiation. In this hypothetical situation a variety of waves of energy would be experienced, all of which differ from one another in wavelength, frequency, and energy.

It is important to note that although emissions from radioactive materials are spoken of in terms of alpha particles, beta particles, and gamma rays, alpha and beta particles do not appear on the electromagnetic spectrum. Only gamma rays exist as electromagnetic waves. Alpha particles and beta particles are particulate matter and therefore possess mass. They are not waves of energy and for this reason are not seen on the spectrum, even though these particles sometimes behave as waves of energy and waves of energy sometimes behave as particles.

■ Relationship of wavelength to frequency

Since the electromagnetic spectrum is based on wavelength, it is apparent that the wavelengths of the various entities must be known. Red light, which has the longest wavelength of the visible light spectrum, has a value of 0.00007 cm or 7000 Å. Green light is known to have a wavelength of 5000 Å, and blue light has a wavelength of 4000 Å. If the wavelength of the radiation is greater than 7000 Å or shorter than 4000 Å, the radiations are no longer visible to the human eye and fall into the infrared and ultraviolet ranges, respectively. The frequency of radiation from blue light (4000 Å) can be calculated by **(3-1)**

$$n \times \lambda = c$$

$$n = \frac{c}{\lambda} = \frac{3.0 \times 10^{10}}{0.00004} = 7.5 \times 10^{14} \text{ waves/sec}$$

Proceeding further up the electromagnetic spectrum, the wavelength begins to become very short and the corresponding frequency begins to become very great. At this point the quantum nature of radiation must be considered.

Quantum nature of radiation. Sometimes electromagnetic waves produce results that cannot be explained by the action of waves of energy. A question arises as to whether these waves can actually be regarded as mass. This is especially true with such waves as x rays, gamma rays, and cosmic rays, which have very short wavelengths. These waves can assume properties, not of waves, but of particles, as is seen in Fig. 3-1, *C*. They can be likened to bullets possessing great energy and traveling in a given direction. This bundle of energy is called a *quantum* or a *pho-*

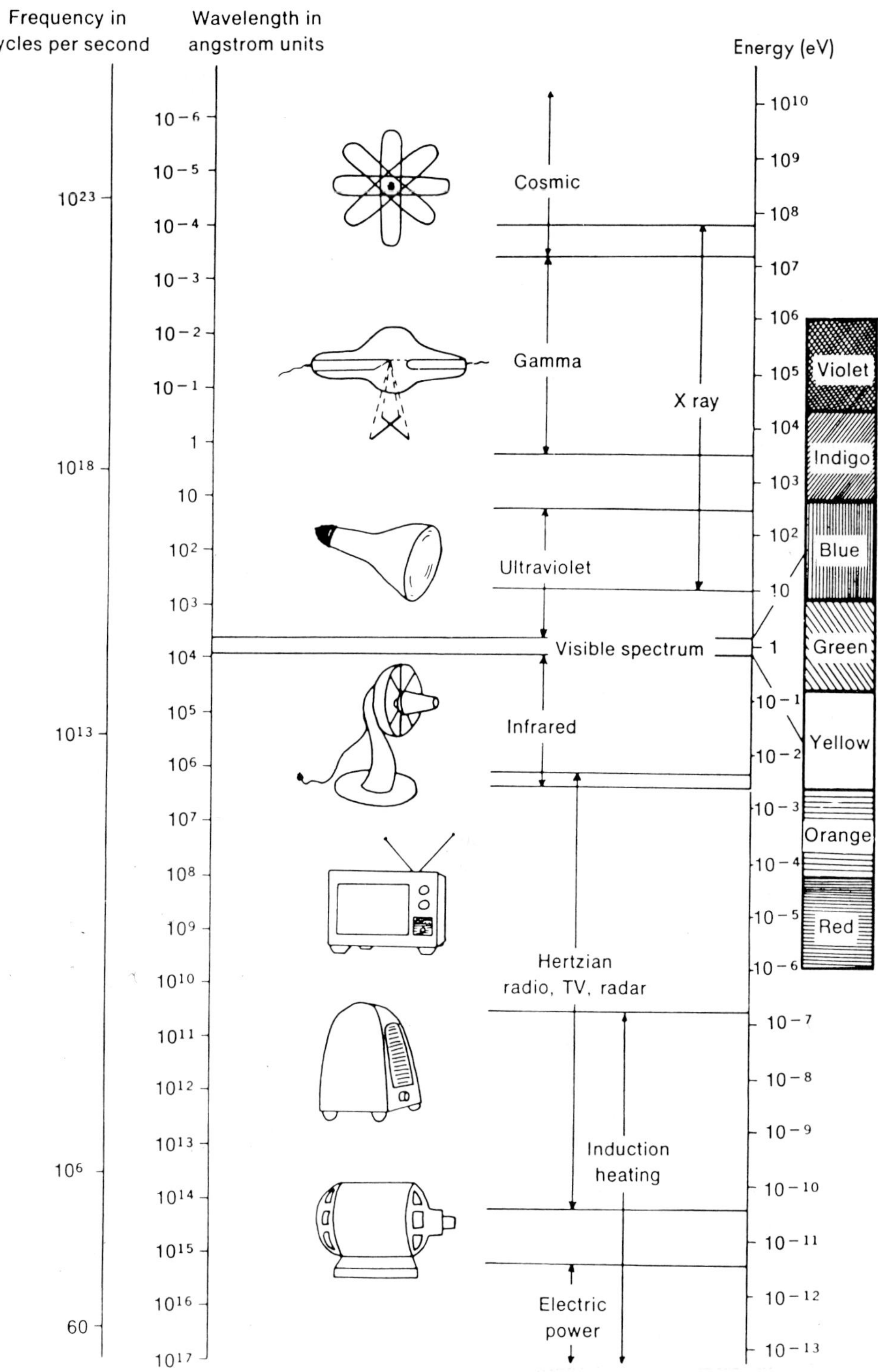

Fig. 3-2. Electromagnetic spectrum.

ton, and the amount of energy carried by the photon depends on the frequency of the radiation. The frequency, in turn, is an inverse function of wavelength. The *energy of the photon is directly proportional to frequency* as indicated by **(3-2)**

$$E = h \times n$$

E = Energy in joules
h = Planck's constant in joule sec = 6.61×10^{-34} joule sec
n = Frequency in seconds

Since the energy of the photon is directly proportional to frequency and frequency is inversely proportional to wavelength, then *energy is inversely proportional to wavelength* also. As the wavelength decreases, the energy of the photon increases, and vice versa.

■ Relationship of wavelength to energy

It has already been demonstrated in formula 2-1 that 1 eV is equal to 1.6×10^{-19} joules. With this value and formulas 3-1 and 3-2 it is possible to calculate the energy of any photon of radiation, given the wavelength. To express a photon with a wavelength of 1.0 Å in terms of energy, three steps are required:

1. Convert wavelength to frequency (formula 3-1):*

$$c = n \times \lambda$$

$$n = \frac{c}{\lambda} = \frac{3 \times 10^{10}}{10^{-8}} = 3 \times 10^{18} \text{ waves/sec (equivalent to 1 Å)}$$

2. Convert frequency to energy in joules (formula 3-2):*

$$E = h \times n$$
$$E = 6.61 \times 10^{-34} \times 3 \times 10^{18}$$
$$E = 19.83 \times 10^{-16} \text{ joules (equivalent to 1 Å)}$$

3. Convert joules to electron volts by comparing it to the value of 1 eV, that value being 1.6×10^{-19} joules:

$$1 \text{ Å} = \frac{19.83 \times 10^{-16}}{1.6 \times 10^{-19}} = 12.4 \times 10^{3} \text{ eV (or 12.4 keV)}$$

With these formulas, given the wavelength of any type of radiation, it is possible to convert wavelength to energy in electron volts or, conversely, energy in electron volts to wavelength. Since energies of the various radionuclides are known, it is possible to place them in their proper positions on the electromagnetic spectrum.

If a photon with a wavelength of 1.0 Å has an energy of 12.4 keV as just determined, then a photon with a wavelength of 0.01 Å has an energy of 1240 keV, or 1.24 MeV. This relationship holds true for any wavelength. Since this is the case, another relationship can be formulated whereby wavelength can immediately be converted to energy in electron volts without going through the three steps just discussed: **(3-3)**

$$E = \frac{12{,}400}{\lambda}$$

E = Energy in electron volts
λ = Wavelength in angstrom units

*Since formula 3-1 is $n = \frac{c}{\lambda}$ and formula 3-2 is $E = hn$, formula 3-1 can be substituted into formula 3-2 to read $E = \frac{hc}{\lambda}$.

■ MASS-ENERGY EQUIVALENCE

For centuries it was believed by all that mass was mass and energy was energy; no thought was given to the possibility that the two were interconvertible. It was not until the current century that the possibility was advanced and proved. Einstein's contribution to nuclear science was an extremely important one and helped explain some of the phenomena of nuclear disintegration. He explained that mass is really a form of energy and that mass and energy could be converted from one to the other with formula 3-4: **(3-4)**

$$E = mc^2$$

E = Energy in joules
m = Mass weight in kg
c = Velocity of light in m/sec

By this equation it is possible to calculate the amount of energy released if 1 gm of matter were completely destroyed and converted to energy:

$$E = 10^{-3} \times (3 \times 10^{8})^2$$
$$= 10^{-3} \times 9 \times 10^{16}$$
$$= 9 \times 10^{13} \text{ joules}$$

The conversion of joules to the more useful electron volt would yield an immense number, not of particular importance at this time.

More important, just as one can convert 1 kg of mass to energy, so also can one calculate the energy released should an atom become annihilated or, even more appropriately, should a subatomic particle (a proton, neutron, or electron) be converted to energy. This is accomplished by the use of the *atomic mass unit* (amu). The atomic mass unit is defined as one twelfth of the arbitrary mass assigned to carbon 12 ($^{12}_{6}C$). It is known that 1 amu is equal to 1.49×10^{-10} joules. According to formula 2-1, 1 eV is equal to 1.6×10^{-19} joules, and 1 MeV is equal to 1.6×10^{-13} joules; therefore it follows: **(3-5)**

$$1 \text{ amu} = \frac{1.49 \times 10^{-10}}{1.6 \times 10^{-13}} = 0.9312 \times 10^{3} \text{ MeV, or 931.2 MeV*}$$

*A proportion:

$$\frac{1 \text{ MeV}}{1.6 \times 10^{-13} \text{ joules}} = \frac{x}{1.49 \times 10^{-10} \text{ joules}}$$
$$1.6 \times 10^{-13}\, x = 1.49 \times 10^{-10}$$
$$x = 931.2 \text{ MeV}$$

This figure (931.2) becomes of value as a conversion factor to convert mass to an equivalent amount of energy whenever a loss of mass has been observed after any nuclear reaction or interaction. Examples of its use in a nuclear reaction will be shown in Chapter 4. An example other than a nuclear reaction is that of a helium atom. It has previously been discussed that the intact helium atom actually weighs less than the sum of its constituent parts weighed separately because some of the mass has been converted to binding energy. The actual energy realized by such a loss of mass can be calculated by the use of this relationship between atomic mass units and energy. Helium 4 is composed of 2 protons, 2 neutrons, and 2 electrons. It has an amu value of 4.003874. The sum of its component particles, however, is as follows:

$$\begin{aligned} \text{amu of protons} &= 1.007277 \times 2 = 2.014554 \\ \text{amu of neutrons} &= 1.008665 \times 2 = 2.017330 \\ \text{amu of electrons} &= 0.000549 \times 2 = \underline{0.001098} \\ \text{sum of components} &= 4.032982 \end{aligned}$$

Based on these values, the component particles of helium 4 weighed separately are heavier than the intact helium 4 atom by 0.030379 amu (4.032982 − 4.002603 = 0.030379 amu). Since 1 amu has been determined to be equal to 931.2 meV (formula 3-5), the binding energy within the atom of helium 4 is equal to 28.2898 MeV in accordance with the following calculation:

$$E = 0.030379 \times 931.2 \text{ MeV} = 28.2898 \text{ MeV}$$

What has actually occurred is that the atom, to keep itself intact, must convert 0.03 units of atomic mass into 28.3 MeV of energy. The atom uses a small fraction of this energy as binding energy to keep the electrons in their energy shells. The major part of this energy is used by the nucleus to keep its nucleons (primarily the protons carrying the positive charges) from repelling one another to the point of disrupting it.

The fact that the nucleus possesses the ability to convert units of mass to pure energy tends to place the entire phenomenon in the realm of sheer fantasy. The possibility of having a piece of matter in one instance converted to invisible energy in another instance is a fact that sometimes seems difficult to understand. However, this same type of phenomenon occurs almost every time a reaction or interaction occurs in a nucleus.

A better example of the conversion of mass to energy is that of the reaction between a positron and an electron. It is known that when these 2 units of mass collide, they completely annihilate one another, and all of their mass is converted to energy according to the following calculations:

$$\begin{aligned} \text{amu of electron} &= 0.000549 \\ \text{amu of positron} &= \underline{0.000549} \\ & 0.001098 \\ 0.001098 \times 931.2 &= 1.02 \text{ MeV} \end{aligned}$$

The resultant energy of the annihilation reaction between a positron and an electron is 1.02 MeV. Actually the energy is not represented as 1 photon of 1.02 MeV but as 2 photons of 0.51 MeV emitted in exactly opposite directions from one another (see Fig. 4-8).

■ GENERAL CLASSIFICATIONS OF RADIOACTIVITY

In general, there are two classifications of radioactivity and of radioisotopes: natural and artificial. Naturally occurring radionuclides are those nuclides that emit radiation spontaneously. No additional energy is necessary to place them in an unstable state. Artificial radioactivity is that radioactivity resulting from man-made unstable nuclides. Such nuclides are made unstable by bombarding stable nuclides with high-energy particles. Both types of radioactivity play an important role in nuclear medicine.

■ Natural radioactivity

It has been suggested that particles within the atom are in a constant state of motion. This motion within the nucleus results in collisions between nucleons whereby energy is transferred to other nucleons. This transfer of energy sometimes results in a nucleon achieving energy greater than the binding energy, in which case the particle is allowed to escape the nucleus. This particle escape is termed a *disintegration*. The process of *decay* and the act of particle escape allow the nucleus to reduce the number of protons or neutrons or both to a point at which the binding energy can contain the remainder of the nucleons. In this way, stability is eventually achieved.

All nuclides with an atomic number greater than 82 are radioactive because they possess an unstable number of protons or neutrons. Many of these are naturally occurring. There are also instances of naturally occurring radionuclides of lesser atomic number, such as potassium 40 and carbon 14.

These naturally occurring radionuclides are found in all parts of the world; therefore all the peoples of the world are subjected to their radiation effects. The amount of radiation caused by these nuclides would vary from place to place based on local geographic conditions. Some genetic mutations are attributable in part to such exposures to naturally occurring radioactivity. These radiations could also have contributed to some of the phases of the evolutionary process. The source of these radiations is both extraterrestrial and terrestrial. Cosmic rays arising from outside the earth's atmosphere constitute the radiations of extraterrestrial origins. Those of terrestrial origin are found in the earth's crust, and radioactive materials in gaseous form are found in the air.

Generally, in the process of decay only a few steps are necessary before a stable ratio of neutrons to protons is reached. Occasionally, however, the process of achieving stability will require as many as 18 different steps. Such a sequence of events is called a *radioactive series*. There are currently four such series in existence: the thorium series, decaying to stable lead 208; the actinium series, decaying to stable lead 207; the uranium series, decaying to lead 206; and the neptunium series, decaying to bismuth 209. It has been suggested by some scientists that there may have been more radioactive series that existed at some point in time, but they have all since attained stability.

■ Artificial radioactivity

Artificial radioactivity is the same as natural radioactivity, except that the radionuclides are man-made. It is possible to subject stable nuclides to high-energy particles to produce instability. This instability can be effected by subjecting a stable nuclide to such devices as a cyclotron or a nuclear reactor (pile), wherein the stable nuclides are bombarded with neutrons, protons, deuterons, or alpha particles. In such bombardment, some of these bombarding particles will be absorbed by the nucleus of the target material. In each case an alteration has occurred in the proton to neutron relationship. By such changes in the nucleus the number of particles within the nucleus is altered to a point at which the binding energy can no longer contain them. Accordingly, a particle is ejected from a nucleus and a new nuclide, which may be either radioactive or stable, is formed. If it is a stable nuclide, the reaction ends. The manner in which these artificial radionuclides are produced will be discussed in Chapter 5.

BIBLIOGRAPHY

Bernier, D.R., Langan, J.K., and Wells, L.D.: Nuclear medicine technology and techniques, ed. 2, St. Louis, 1989, Mosby–Year Book.

Casarett, A.P.: Radiation biology, Englewood Cliffs, N.J., 1968, Prentice-Hall, Inc.

Chandra, R.: Introductory physics of nuclear medicine, ed. 4, Philadelphia, 1992, Lea & Febiger.

Johns, H.E., and Cunningham, J.R.: The physics of radiology, ed. 4, revised edition, Springfield, Ill., 1983, Charles C Thomas, Publisher.

Rollo, F.D.: Nuclear medicine physics, instrumentation, and agents, St. Louis, 1977, Mosby–Year Book.

Shilling, C.W.: Atomic energy encyclopedia in the life sciences, Philadelphia, 1964, W.B. Saunders Co.

Wagner, H.N.: Principles of nuclear medicine, Philadelphia, 1968, W.B. Saunders Co.

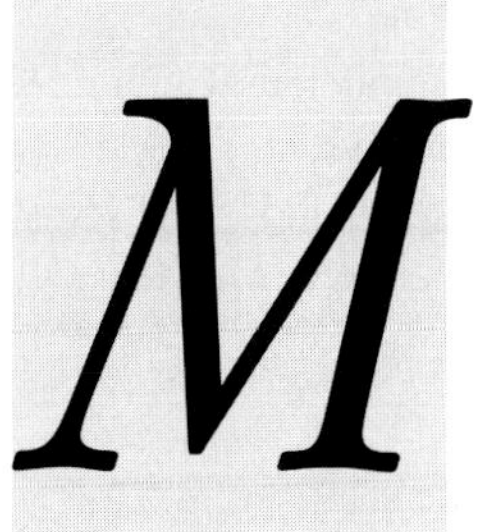

Chapter 4

METHODS OF RADIOACTIVE DECAY

PAUL J. EARLY

■ IDENTIFICATION OF EMISSIONS

There are basically three emissions from radionuclides—alpha particles, beta particles, and gamma rays. A means of identifying these radiations had to be devised. This problem became the doctoral thesis of Mme Marie Curie around the turn of the century. To carry out the experiment of identification, Mme Curie devised a simple technique. She took a large block of lead with a hole in its center into which she placed a source of radium. In this manner, since the radiations emanate at an infinite number of angles from the source, those that did not radiate upward through the hole would be absorbed by the surrounding lead. A piece of photographic film was placed above the lead block. In this way, radiations emanating from the radium source and going through the hole in the lead block would be detected by an area of darkening on the film. In an effort to learn if these radiations had electrical charges, Mme Curie included a magnetic field in a direction perpendicular to the direction of the emissions (Fig. 4-1). She reasoned that, if charged, the positively charged emissions would be deflected to the right according to the rule of physics for positive charges in a magnetic field, and the negatively charged emissions would be deviated to the left. Those with no charge would remain unaffected by the magnetic field. Furthermore, in the presence of the magnetic field, if all three types of emissions were present, three areas of darkening would be seen on the photographic plate. Since Mme Curie did detect three areas of darkening, she arbitrarily labeled the emissions after the first three letters of the Greek alphabet. Those that were deflected to the right and had a positive charge were called *alpha* emissions, those that were deflected to the left and negatively charged were called *beta* emissions, and those that remained undeflected with no charge were called *gamma* emissions.

■ CHARACTERISTICS OF EMISSIONS

Many experiments have been performed to learn more about radioactivity. In addition to the conclusions of Mme Curie's experiment, many other characteristics are now known.

It is an accepted fact that a radioactive nuclide will emit one, two, or all three of these basic radiations. There are comparatively few radionuclides that possess the ability to decay by both alpha and beta emission with the subsequent release of a gamma ray. Most radionuclides decay by either alpha emission or beta emission. In either case, gamma emission could be a subsequent reaction. Those radionuclides that decay by alpha emission only or beta emission only are termed *pure alpha emitters* and *pure beta emitters,* respectively.

It is also known that the process of decay creates other nuclides that may be either radioactive or stable. (Note the word *nuclides,* not isotopes.) ^{131}I, for instance, does not eventually decay to ^{125}I (an isotope); it decays by beta-gamma emission to ^{131}Xe (another nuclide). This is called *transmutation,* the conversion of one element into another.

Another indisputable fact is that the process of decay is a series of random events. It is impossible to predict exactly which atom is going to undergo disintegration at any given time. However, it is possible to predict, on the average, how many atoms will disintegrate during any interval of time. Because of this predictability, the rate of disintegration can be used as a method of quantitative analysis. These disintegrations can be detected, those detected can be counted, and the results can be expressed as counts per unit time.

It has also been demonstrated that temperature, pressure, and chemical combination have absolutely no effect on the rate of decay. Radioactive materials can be placed in a

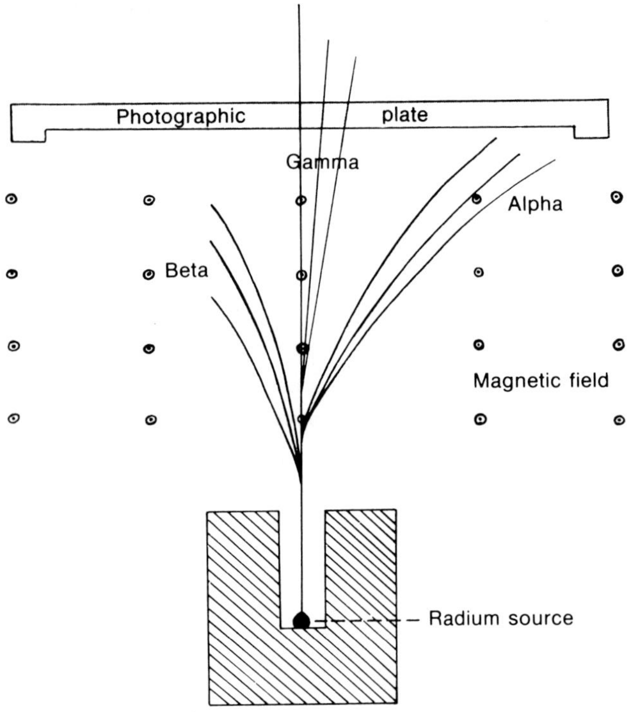

Fig. 4-1. Electric properties of radioactive emissions. Mme Curie's experiment to prove that alpha emissions are positively charged, beta emissions are negatively charged, and gamma emissions are neutrally charged.

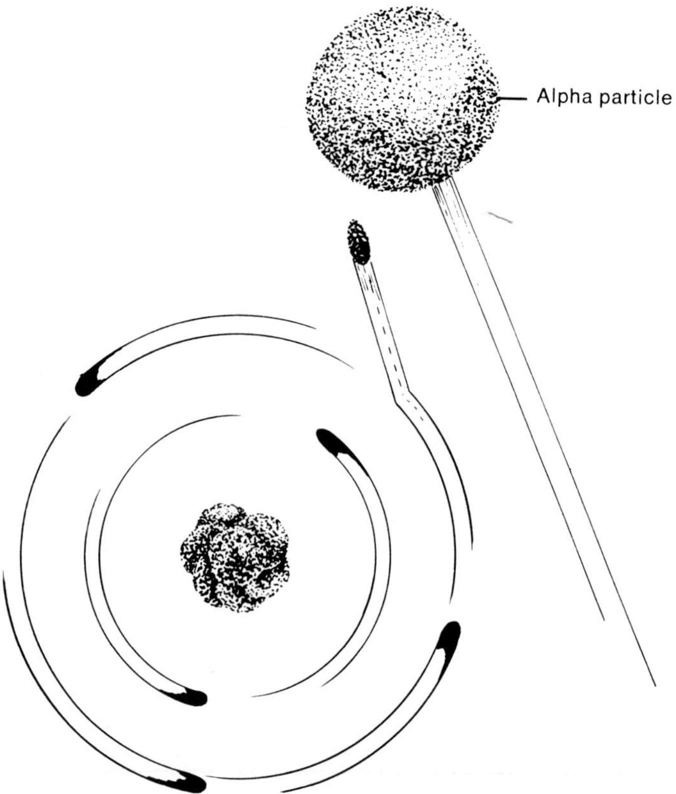

Fig. 4-2. Ionization of matter by a passing alpha particle. Note that the artist's concept is misleading, because alpha particles are approximately 7400 times larger than the mass of the electron.

freezer without any demonstrable change in the half-life. The same is true should a source of radioactivity be subjected to heat and pressure, as in an autoclave for sterilization purposes.

The fact that chemical combination does not alter the radioactive characteristics is the rationale responsible for labeling or "tagging" chemicals, by replacing stable atoms of a compound with radioactive atoms. ^{11}C-labeled glucose is an example. In labeling this compound the stable form of carbon is replaced by the unstable form. In this way, neither the glucose nor the ^{11}C is altered in any way, and the body reacts to either form similarly.

■ METHODS OF DECAY

The original radionuclide in any method of decay is called a *parent;* the nuclide to which it decays is called a *daughter,* which may be stable or unstable. If a daughter nuclide is stable, the decay process is terminated. If the daughter is unstable, a new decay process begins that may differ entirely from its predecessor.

■ Alpha decay

Definition and origin. The alpha particle (α, $^4_2\alpha$, or ^4_2He) is a helium nucleus consisting of 2 protons and 2 neutrons. It is a highly energetic particle, having discrete energy levels. The alpha particle is the same as the helium atom with the exception that there are no orbital electrons. Because there are no negative charges to neutralize the positively charged nucleus, the alpha particle possesses an electric charge of +2 on emission. Since the particle is without electrons, it will not be satisfied until it acquires 2 electrons, making it an electrically neutral helium atom.

Alpha particles originate in the nuclei of heavier atoms. For the most part, these atoms occupy the upper one third of the chart of the nuclides. It is obvious that if alpha emissions occurred as a result of nuclear changes in the lighter nuclides, the nuclide would be discarding a major portion of its nucleus. Alpha decay is a fast and efficient means of bringing the neutron to proton ratio closer to a stable ratio. Since an alpha particle removes 2 protons and 2 neutrons from the parent nuclide, the new nuclide contains 2 fewer protons and 2 fewer neutrons. In effect, the atomic number (Z) would be decreased by 2, the neutron number (N) would be decreased by 2, and the mass number (A) would be decreased by 4.

Ionization and penetration. Since an alpha particle has an electrical charge of +2, its immediate purpose is to acquire 2 electrons to become electrically neutral. As the alpha particle passes through matter, it attracts electrons from nearby atoms (Fig. 4-2). Because of the strong electrical attraction of the alpha particle (+2), its huge mass (7400 times the size of the electron), and the almost nonexistent binding energy of outer shell electrons, the alpha particle can actually overcome the binding forces of the electron's parent atom, causing the electron to be released in space. As a result the electron is free to ionize other atoms in the surrounding media (provided it has enough energy to do so), to combine with positive ions in the vicinity, or to become one of the free electrons that occur in all matter. This process of removal of an electron from an atom is called *ionization*. The result of this ionization process is the creation of an *ion pair* consisting of a negative ion (the electron) and a positive ion (the atom from which the electron was removed). *Primary ionization* is that produced by the originally charged particle; *secondary ionization* is that subsequently produced by the ions that resulted from the primary event (electrons, primarily).

This process of attracting the electron by the alpha particle causes a slowing down and loss of kinetic energy of the particle itself because the alpha particle uses some of its energy to remove the electron. This process of ionization will continue many, many times with subsequent atoms in the path of the alpha particle. The particle will create more ion pairs until it loses all its kinetic energy and comes to *rest mass*. The particle picks up the 2 electrons necessary for electrical neutrality and comes to rest as a helium atom, a chemically inert gas. At this point it ceases to be of radiobiologic significance.

An alpha particle loses an average of 34 eV per ionization event in air. If energy loss by the alpha particle were the only consideration, this would mean that an alpha particle with 3,400,000 eV of energy (3.4 MeV) would undergo 100,000 ionization events (100,000 ion pairs) before expending all of its energy and coming to rest mass. It would require less than 2 cm of air to expend all the energy of such an alpha particle. As matter increases in density, less distance is required to expend the energy of the alpha particle; therefore penetration decreases.

Range. The *range* of an alpha particle, that is, the distance the charged particle travels from its point of origin to the place where it no longer acts as a destructive radiation particle, is about 4 cm in air. This value changes considerably in tissue, in which the range is reduced to a few thousandths of a centimeter. For this reason, an alpha particle is unable to penetrate the epidermis of the skin. It is not to be assumed, however, that an alpha particle is without injurious radiation effects because it cannot penetrate the skin. The most common methods of alpha contamination are inhalation or ingestion of alpha-laden materials. This is not of particular importance in the usual nuclear medicine laboratory, because alpha emitters are not used in routine nuclear medicine procedures.

Specific ionization. Ionization is often spoken in terms of *specific ionization,* that is, the number of ion pairs formed per unit of path traveled by a moving charged particle through matter. The reason for the term is because two different particles (for example, alpha and beta) of the same energy ionize about the same total number of atoms. However, the ionization events occur much closer together for alpha particles, and therefore their distance traveled (range, penetration) is less. Specific ionization increases with mass and charge and decreases with velocity. The alpha particle has the highest specific ionization, and therefore the highest radiobiologic significance (see discussion of indirect action, Chapter 9), because of its great mass, its two positive charges, and its slow speed. This larger, slow-moving particle simply spends more time in the vicinity of the atom and therefore has a greater chance to ionize it. The specific ionization in air for a 1 MeV alpha particle is about 60,000 ion pairs per centimeter of path traveled. Compare this to the specific ionization of a 1 MeV beta particle (see discussion of beta decay, p. 26).

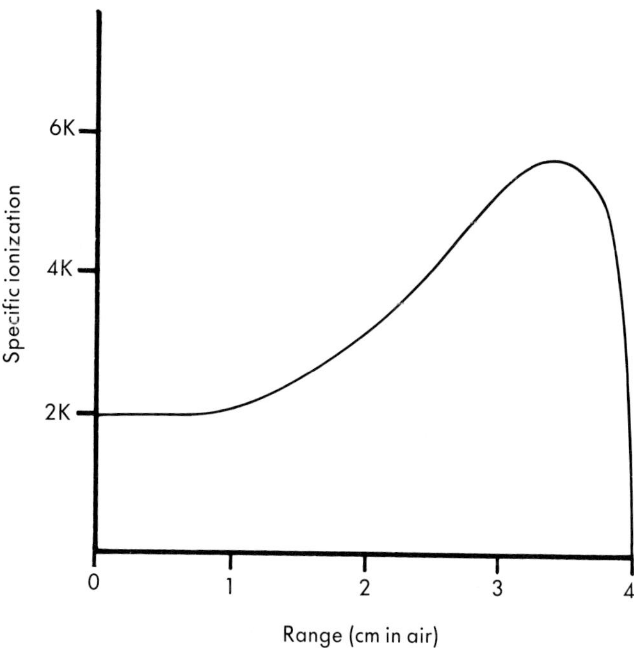

Fig. 4-3. Number of ion pairs formed per centimeter of air along track of alpha particle. *Bragg ionization peak* is demonstrated.

Since ionization causes a reduction in the energy of the ionizing particle, and since mass does not change, the reduction in energy is necessarily a reduction in velocity. As velocity decreases, the probability of ionization increases, and the result is a marked increase in ionization density near the end of its track. This peak in ionization density at the end of the particle track is called the *Bragg ionization peak* (Fig. 4-3).

Excitation. An alpha particle is also capable of *excitation* of an atom as it approaches or passes through it. To excite an atom is to increase the energy state of an orbital electron by the transfer of some of the energy of the alpha particle to the electron. By increasing the energy state the electron assumes a new suborbit distant to the nucleus. The electron cannot stay in this excited state, so it immediately releases the excess energy and returns to its original orbit.

Example. Since an alpha particle consists of 2 protons and 2 neutrons, there would necessarily be 2 fewer protons and 2 fewer neutrons in the parent atom. A typical alpha emitter is $^{226}_{88}Ra$. Following is the reaction of alpha emission:

$$^{226}_{88}Ra \rightarrow {}^{222}_{86}Rn + {}^{4}_{2}He$$
$$\text{(radium)} \rightarrow \text{(radon)} + \text{(alpha)}$$

Accordingly, the new nuclide, radon 222, has a mass number reduced by 4 and an atomic number reduced by 2.

■ Beta decay

A beta particle (β) is a high-velocity electron ejected from a disintegrating nucleus. The particle may be either a negatively charged electron, termed a *negatron* (β^-), or a positively charged electron, termed a *positron* (β^+). Both types of beta particles have the same mass, regardless of their charge. Although the precise definition of "beta emission" refers to both β^- and β^+ particles, the common usage of the term refers only to the β^- particle, as distinguished from positron emission, which refers to the β^+ particle.

Definition and origin. The beta particle (β^-) is a high-velocity, negatively charged electron emitted from a nucleus of an atom undergoing disintegration. The beta particle is identical to the orbital electron in mass and electrical charge. Both possess a charge of −1 and a mass 1/1836 that of a proton and equivalent to 0.000549 amu.

Since a β^- particle is defined as being ejected from the nucleus, the question arises of how an electron can be emitted from the nucleus when there is no electron in the nucleus. What actually happens is that a neutron is converted into a proton, an electron (β^-), and an antineutrino* as follows:

$$\text{Neutron} \rightarrow \begin{cases} \text{Proton} \\ + \\ \text{Electron } (\beta^-) \\ + \\ \text{Antineutrino } (\bar{\upsilon}) \\ + \\ \text{Energy} \end{cases}$$

The immediate result of the neutron breakdown is that the electron (β^-) and the antineutrino are ejected from the nucleus, whereas the proton remains. The parent atom is increased in atomic number by 1, with no change in mass number. (Mass number is protons plus neutrons, and one has been converted to the other, so there is no change in the total number.)

Examples. An example of a beta emitter is ^{32}P. It decays to ^{32}S with the emission of a beta particle and an antineutrino according to the following:

$$^{32}_{15}P \rightarrow {}^{32}_{16}S + \beta^- + \bar{\upsilon}$$

In this reaction no gamma particles are released; therefore ^{32}P is a *pure* beta emitter. Others are carbon 14 ($^{14}_{6}C$), cesium 137 ($^{137}_{55}Cs$), and tritium ($^{3}_{1}H$).

An example of a beta-gamma emitter is ^{131}I. ^{131}I decays by beta emission to ^{131}Xe according to the following:

$$^{131}_{53}I \rightarrow {}^{131}_{54}Xe + \beta^- + \bar{\upsilon} + \gamma$$

Other beta-gamma emitters are xenon 133 ($^{133}_{54}Xe$), iron 59 ($^{59}_{26}Fe$), molybdenum 99 ($^{99}_{42}Mo$), and sodium 24 ($^{24}_{11}Na$).

Debit mass and credit energy. It is important to realize that whenever the disintegration of a nucleus occurs, regardless of the method of decay, there is a release of energy. The source of this excess energy is the nucleus itself because of a disparity in the mass of the new nuclide. This unaccounted mass is expressed in atomic mass units (amu) in the calculations of the ^{32}P reaction that follow (amu values taken from Appendix C:

amu $^{32}_{15}P$	31.973910
less amu 15 electrons = 0.000549 × 15 =	0.008235
amu of $^{32}_{15}P$ nucleus	31.965675(A)
amu $^{32}_{16}S$	31.972074
less amu 16 electrons = 0.000549 × 16 =	0.008784
amu of $^{32}_{16}S$ nucleus	31.963290(B)
amu of $^{32}_{15}P$ nucleus	31.965675(A)
less amu of $^{32}_{16}S$ nucleus	31.963290(B)
mass difference	0.002385
less β^- mass	0.000549
less antineutrino mass	0.000000
unaccounted mass	0.001836

It was not until Einstein that this question of what happened to the rest of the mass could be answered. He said that mass or energy could not be destroyed but that each could be converted into the other. In these reactions some mass is always lost, but an equivalent amount of energy is always gained. It has already been shown (formula 3-5) that 931.2 is the conversion factor to convert mass (amu) to energy expressed as MeV. Therefore the energy released from decay of ^{32}P to ^{32}S is as follows:

$$\text{Energy released in MeV} = 0.00183 \times 931.2 = 1.70 \text{ MeV}.$$

The energy resulting from this neutron breakdown is expended in three different ways: (1) Some of the energy goes to the electron so that it may be ejected from the nucleus. (2) Some of the energy goes to the antineutrino so that it may be ejected from the nucleus. (3) In any radionuclide other than a pure beta emitter, some of the energy is retained by the nucleus. The latter elevates a nucleon to a new energy level. The consequence of this elevated energy level or excited state is that, with the exception of isomeric transition (p. 32), the excess energy is instantaneously released in the form of gamma radiation. The energy levels

*Antineutrino has opposite spin of the neutrino.

to which the excited nucleus is elevated are discrete energy levels and are well known. Therefore the energy released in the form of gamma radiation is also well known. This is not the case with the β^- particle and the neutrino. The amount of energy that is expended on the beta particle or the antineutrino is unpredictable from one atom to another, but the energy distribution is known based on percentages.

Energy distribution of a pure beta emitter. Unlike alpha particles, beta particles do not have discrete energy levels. The energy of beta particles from the same radionuclide varies from approximately zero to its maximum energy, the latter being a variable between radionuclides but not between different atoms of the same radionuclide.

As shown in the examples, some radionuclides are pure beta emitters, while others have an accompanying gamma emission. In the pure beta emitter all the energy resulting from a neutron breakdown is expended on the beta particle and antineutrino to eject them from the nucleus. There is no elevated energy state of the nucleus and therefore no subsequent gamma emission. Figure 4-4 shows the distribution of energy to the ^{32}P beta particle as a function of energy plotted on the abscissa (horizontal axis) versus frequency of occurrence on the ordinate (vertical axis). As indicated, the maximum energy (E_{max}) of any beta particle from this radionuclide is that of 1.7 MeV. The number of atoms in a given sample producing a beta particle of 1.7 MeV is extremely low. Conversely, the number of atoms in the given sample producing a beta particle of 0.6 MeV is much higher. E_{max} indicates that the maximum energy resulting from the neutron breakdown is 1.7 MeV. Since all the energy in a pure beta emitter is expended on either the beta particle or the antineutrino, whatever portion of the energy that the beta particle does not receive, the antineutrino receives. Therefore an atom that supplies the beta particle with all the energy resulting from the neutron breakdown would have an antineutrino that has just enough energy to be ejected from the nucleus. However, one of its sister atoms in the same sample that gives only 0.6 MeV of energy to the beta particle would have an antineutrino possessing the energy difference of 1.1 MeV. According to Fig. 4-4, the situation in which a beta particle receives 0.6 MeV and the antineutrino receives 1.1 MeV of energy occurs much more frequently than that in which the beta particle receives the total energy and the antineutrino very little or vice versa. This whole concept of energy distribution can be crudely summed up as whatever energy the beta particle does not use, the antineutrino receives. If this were actually the case, the beta particle must be considered as most charitable. Most of the beta particles receive only about one third of the available energy, leaving the other two thirds for the antineutrino. This energy value is generally considered to be its average energy represented by the symbol $\overline{E}_\beta$. Since it is approximately equivalent to one third of all the available energy, $\overline{E}_\beta \approx \frac{1}{3}E_{max}$. In any nuclide that is not a pure beta emitter the nucleus would contribute some of its energy to the nucleus itself. Energy distribution between the beta particle and the antineutrino would remain similar.

Purpose. When a nucleus undergoes beta disintegration, the daughter nuclide possesses a nucleus with an atomic number increased by 1 and the mass number remains

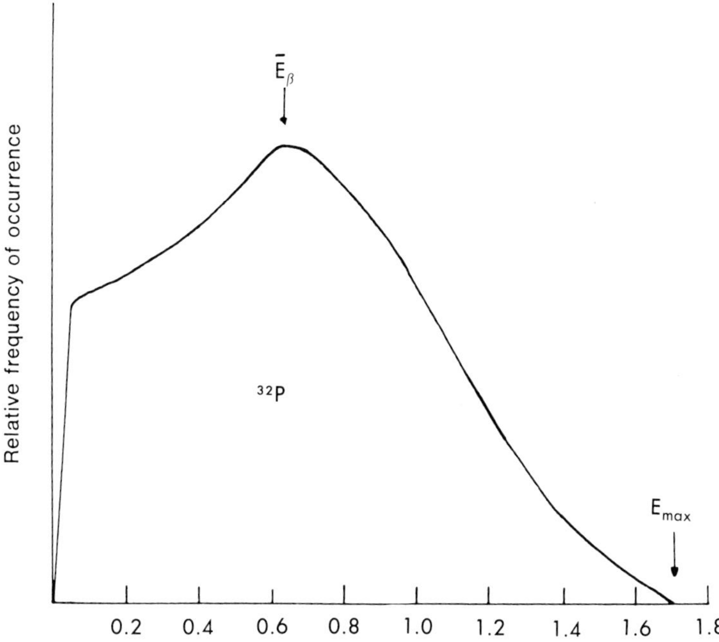

Fig. 4-4. Distribution of resultant energy to ^{32}P beta particles following conversion of neutron to proton with expulsion of electron and antineutrino from the nucleus.

the same. A neutron has been changed into a proton; therefore the proton number is increased by 1. However, the mass number has not been changed because what has been lost in neutrons has been gained in protons. This type of decay would occur in any nuclide having too many neutrons or too few protons or both. Beta decay is the only method available to such an unstable nucleus. The neutron number is decreased, and the proton number is increased in an attempt to achieve stability. It may be, however, that the new nuclide may also be unstable for the same reason, and it may subsequently disintegrate by the same method. This process will continue until a stable proportion of neutrons and protons exists. (Disintegration of a nucleus means only that it changes in composition, not that it no longer exists.)

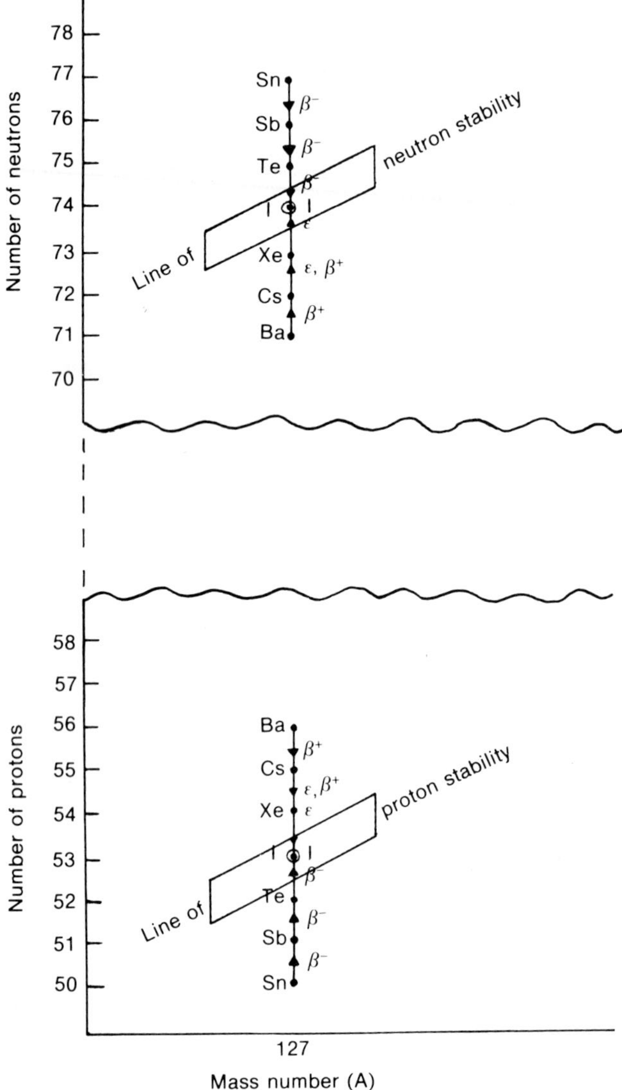

Fig. 4-5. Magnification of Fig. 1-2 at level of A = 127, demonstrating that unstable atoms decay to stability by whatever method is required to achieve a stable ratio of neutrons to protons.

This situation exemplifies the conditions that exist in every atom of tin 127 ($^{127}_{50}$Sn) (Fig. 4-5). ^{127}Sn contains 77 neutrons and 50 protons. For some reason not completely understood, this neutron to proton ratio is unstable because there are too many neutrons and too few protons. Its only course of action is beta decay. In decaying by beta emission, ^{127}Sn becomes antimony 127 ($^{127}_{51}$Sb); this nucleus with 76 neutrons and 51 protons is still unstable. Consequently, it decays by beta emission to tellurium 127 ($^{127}_{52}$Te), and this nucleus with 75 neutrons and 52 protons is unstable also. Finally it decays by beta emission to iodine 127 ($^{127}_{53}$I), which has a stable ratio of 74 neutrons to 53 protons, and the decay series ends. ^{127}I happens to be the only stable isotope of iodine and is the form of the element that is found in iodized salt, fish, and so on.

Since the unstable parent atom decays by beta emission to a daughter atom that has the same mass number but a different atomic number and therefore different chemical properties, it can be said that beta decay gives rise to an isobar. The process is termed *isobaric transition.*

Ionization and penetration. Beta particles also possess the ability to excite or ionize atoms or both. The method of ionization, however, is somewhat different from the ionization of alpha particles. An alpha particle attracts an orbital electron and thus creates an ion pair. The beta particle repels the orbital electron from its energy shell to create an ion pair (Fig. 4-6). Each ion pair produced by the β^- particle represents a loss of energy by the beta particle. These processes of excitation and ionization continue until

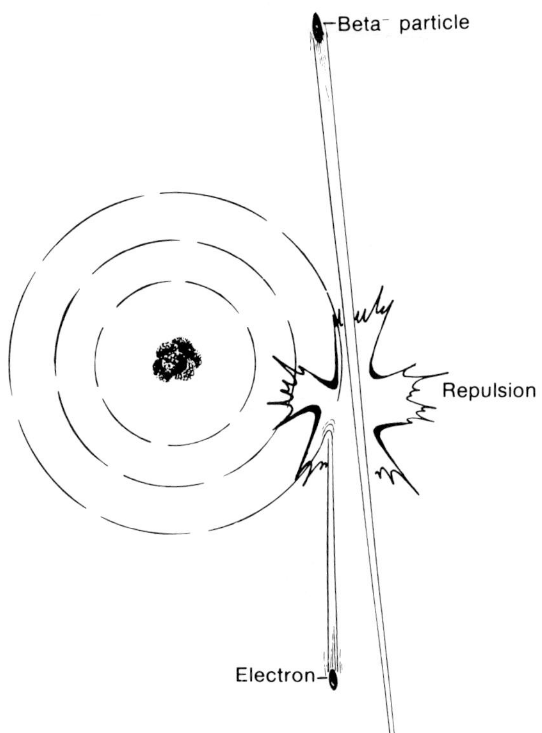

Fig. 4-6. Ionization of matter by a passing beta particle.

the beta particle loses all its kinetic energy. At this point the beta particle is said to have attained rest mass. It can now combine with some positively charged ion to make it a neutral atom once again. This process is termed *deionization*. It can also become a free electron, in which capacity it does not combine with anything. The specific ionization of a 1 MeV beta particle in air is about 45 ion pairs per centimeter of path traveled. Compared to an alpha particle, the specific ionization of a beta particle is greatly reduced. This is largely because the charge of an alpha particle is twice as much as and its mass 7400 times that of a beta particle. Furthermore, an alpha particle has a lower velocity than a beta particle and is in the area of any one atom for a longer period of time, which increases its probability of attracting an orbital electron to it.

As with alpha particles, beta particles lose an average energy of 34 eV per ionization event. Similarly, considering only the loss of particle energy, a 3.4 MeV beta particle would undergo 100,000 ionization events before losing its radiobiologic significance. It differs from the alpha particle, however, in its penetration. As the specific ionization values indicate, a beta particle incurs fewer ionization events per unit of path traveled, so it travels farther than an alpha particle of equal energy. The penetrating power of beta particles is approximately 1000 times as great as that of alpha particles. However, the penetration power of beta particles is only a small fraction of that of gamma rays. Alpha particles are completely absorbed by a thin sheet of paper, whereas an inch of wood or 1/25 inch of aluminum is required to stop a beta particle. In tissue a 1 MeV beta particle has a range of 0.42 cm. However, this particle is not harmless from a radiobiologic standpoint. It is well to remember that phosphorus 32, a pure beta emitter, is used as a therapeutic agent for such clinical states as leukemia, polycythemia, and ascites. In each case the epidermis is bypassed either by intravenous or intracavitary administration.

Bremsstrahlung. *Bremsstrahlung* is the German word for braking radiation. Bremsstrahlung is the production of electromagnetic radiation by the deceleration (actually, negative acceleration) that a fast, charged particle undergoes when it is deflected by another charged particle. The charged particles in the case of Bremsstrahlung are the beta particle and the nucleus of an atom near which the beta particle passes. When a beta particle passes near an atomic nucleus, its path of travel will be changed somewhat in the direction of the nucleus because of the attraction of unlike charges. This change in direction is spoken of as acceleration, but it is a negative acceleration. The beta particle slows down and loses kinetic energy. In these instances the energy lost is released in the form of x-rays (Fig. 4-7). These x-rays are equal in energy to that energy lost by the beta particle. This is one of the phenomena that occur in x-ray tubes and their subsequent x-ray production. In the case of x-ray machines, however, electrons are used rather than beta particles.

Bremsstrahlung is also the reason that high Z material, such as lead, is not always the answer to radiation protection. With beta emitters, the amount of Bremsstrahlung increases with the density of the material through which it passes. Therefore, because Bremsstrahlung is x-ray it is not as easily shielded as is the beta particle. It is considered a better practice during the administration of these pure beta emitters to use some low Z material, such as plastic or lucite, as an adequate barrier for the beta particle and to re-

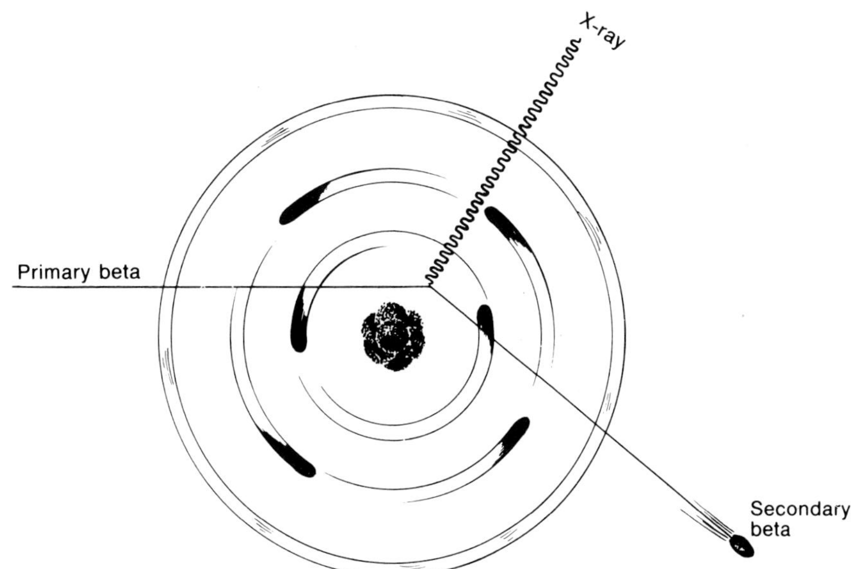

Fig. 4-7. Bremsstrahlung. Beta particle passes near the nucleus of an atom and is attracted to it. This results in a loss of energy and change in direction. That loss of energy is expressed as *x-ray*, or *Bremsstrahlung*.

duce the amount of Bremsstrahlung produced in the shielding material. In fact, the plastic syringe used in the administration of the material is usually adequate shielding.

■ Positron decay

Definition and origin. The positron (β^+) is a high-velocity, positively charged electron emitted from the nucleus of an atom undergoing disintegration. The positron differs from the electron and the beta particle only in that it has an opposite electrical charge. It has the mass of an electron but the electrical charge of a proton. The nuclear origin of the positron is the proton. A proton, under the influence of all the nucleons in its nucleus, is converted into a neutron, an electron with a positive charge (positron), and a neutrino, as follows:

$$\text{Proton} \rightarrow \begin{cases} \text{Neutron} \\ + \\ \text{Electron } (\beta^+) \\ + \\ \text{Neutrino} \\ + \\ \text{Energy} \end{cases}$$

The immediate result of the proton breakdown is that the positive electron (β^+) and the neutrino are ejected from the nucleus while a neutron remains. The parent atom is reduced in atomic number by 1, with no change in mass number. (Similar to beta decay, one of the units comprising the mass number is converted to the other so that there is no change. In positron decay, however, it is the opposite of beta decay; a proton becomes a neutron.)

Examples. An example of a positron emitter is nitrogen 12. It decays to carbon 12 with the emission of a β^+ particle and a neutrino according to the following:

$${}^{12}_{7}\text{N} \rightarrow {}^{12}_{6}\text{C} + \beta^+ + \upsilon$$

In this reaction no gamma particles are released; therefore ^{12}N is a pure positron emitter; ^{18}F is another.

Five examples of other positron emitters more useful to nuclear medicine are as follows:

1. ${}^{11}_{6}\text{C} \rightarrow {}^{11}_{5}\text{B} + \beta^+ + \upsilon$
2. ${}^{13}_{7}\text{N} \rightarrow {}^{13}_{6}\text{C} + \beta^+ + \upsilon$
3. ${}^{15}_{8}\text{O} \rightarrow {}^{15}_{7}\text{N} + \beta^+ + \upsilon$
4. ${}^{18}_{9}\text{F} \rightarrow {}^{18}_{8}\text{O} + \beta^+ + \upsilon$
5. ${}^{82}_{37}\text{Rb} \rightarrow {}^{82}_{38}\text{Kr} + \beta^+ + \upsilon$

Debits and credits. Just as with beta decay, the disintegration of a nucleus with the subsequent emission of a positron yields energy as a result of loss through conversion of mass. The mass-energy equivalence can be calculated because amu values are known. A calculation of the ^{12}N reaction follows:

amu ${}^{12}_{7}$N	12.018641
less amu 7 electrons = 0.000549 × 7 =	0.003843
amu of ${}^{12}_{7}$N nucleus	12.014798 (A)

amu ${}^{12}_{6}$C	12.000000
less amu 6 electrons = 0.000549 × 6 =	0.003294
amu of ${}^{12}_{6}$C nucleus	11.996706 (B)

amu of ${}^{12}_{7}$N nucleus	12.014798 (A)
less amu of ${}^{12}_{6}$C nucleus	11.996706 (B)
mass difference	0.018092
less β^+ mass	0.000549
less neutrino mass	0.000000
unaccounted mass	0.017543

Having determined the mass difference, the mass-energy equivalence can be determined as follows:

$$\text{Energy released (MeV)} = 0.017543 + 931.2 = 16.33 \text{ MeV}$$

Purpose. By undergoing positron decay the proton number is decreased by 1, and the neutron number is increased by 1. This would result in a daughter product having 1 less atomic number and the same mass number, another example of isobaric transition. This type of decay is exactly opposite to beta decay. This type might occur in an unstable nucleus in which there are too many protons and/or too few neutrons to bring the number of neutrons and protons to a stable ratio. In many instances positron emission is in competition with electron capture (p. 31), because both methods of decay have identical results.

It may be, however, that positron emission will only bring the neutron to proton ratio closer to stability. This is the case with barium 127 (${}^{127}_{56}$Ba) (Fig. 4-5). ^{127}Ba contains 71 neutrons and 56 protons. This ratio of neutrons to protons is not stable, so it decays by β^+ emission to cesium 127 (${}^{127}_{55}$Cs). ^{127}Cs is still unstable, so it decays by β^+ emission or electron capture (primarily the latter) to xenon 127 (${}^{127}_{54}$Xe). ^{127}Xe still contains an unstable ratio of neutrons and protons, and it decays entirely by electron capture to iodine 127 (${}^{127}_{53}$I). The series has finally reached stability at this point because iodine 127 has 74 neutrons and 53 protons, and these are the numbers necessary for stability.

It is of particular importance to learn what happens to the positron once it is ejected from the nucleus. Three reactions are of importance: ionization, Bremsstrahlung, and the annihilation reaction.

Ionization. The degree of ionization and Bremsstrahlung is similar to that which occurs with the beta particle for as long as the positron survives. The methods, however, are different because of an opposite electrical charge. Ionization occurs when the positron attracts the negatively charged orbital electron from its orbit; the beta particle repels it from its orbital path.

Bremsstrahlung. Bremsstrahlung differs also, since the nucleus has a preponderance of positive charges and the positron is also positive. The negative acceleration seen in the Bremsstrahlung phenomenon would be that of a repulsion away from the nucleus rather than an attraction toward it. This negative acceleration is, as in the beta particle, a loss of energy to that positron, and this energy is released in the form of an x-ray. The x-ray is equal in energy to the energy lost by the positron particle.

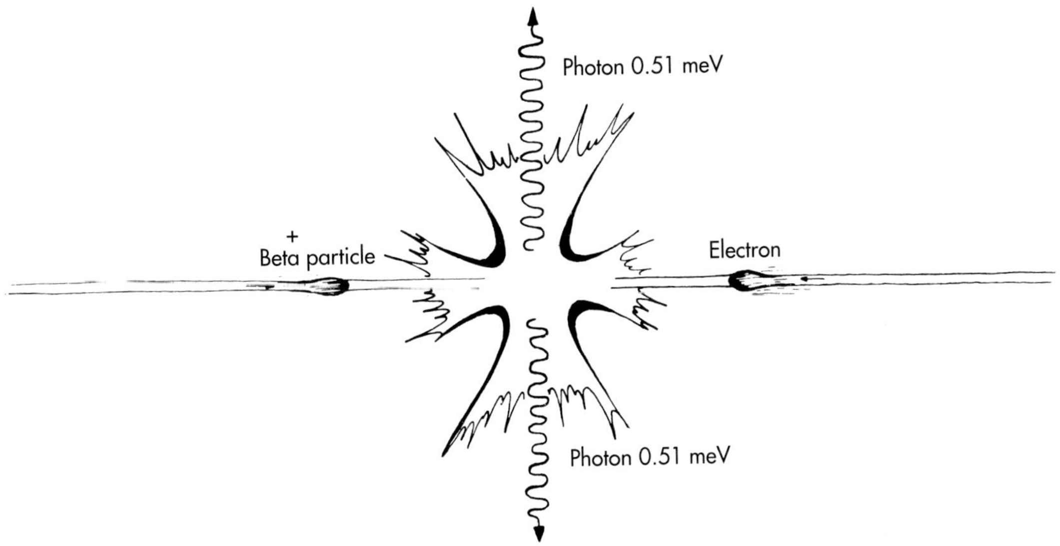

Fig. 4-8. Annihilation reaction. A positron at rest mass (0 keV) is attracted to an electron at rest mass (0 keV), whereon both particles are annihilated and converted to energy (2 gamma photons each with an energy of 0.511 MeV).

Annihilation reaction. The most important reaction of the positron after ejection is the annihilation reaction. It is for this reason that the positron is short lived; the average life is approximately 10^{-9} seconds. The annihilation reaction is the result of a collision between the positively charged positron that has lost all its kinetic energy and an always-present, negatively charged electron that is also at "0" kinetic energy. The masses of both particles are completely annihilated. Accordingly, energy must be released equivalent to the masses of 1 electron and 1 positron. That mass energy equivalence is 1.022 MeV of energy:

$$\begin{aligned} \text{amu of electron} &= 0.000549 \\ \text{amu of positron} &= \underline{0.000549} \\ & 0.001098 \\ 0.001098 \times 931.2 \text{ meV} &= 1.022 \text{ MeV} \end{aligned}$$

The energy that results is not 1 photon with an energy of 1.022 MeV but 2 photons of 0.511 MeV radiating in exactly opposite directions of one another. The available energy is equally divided between the 2 photons. This reaction is seen in Fig. 4-8.

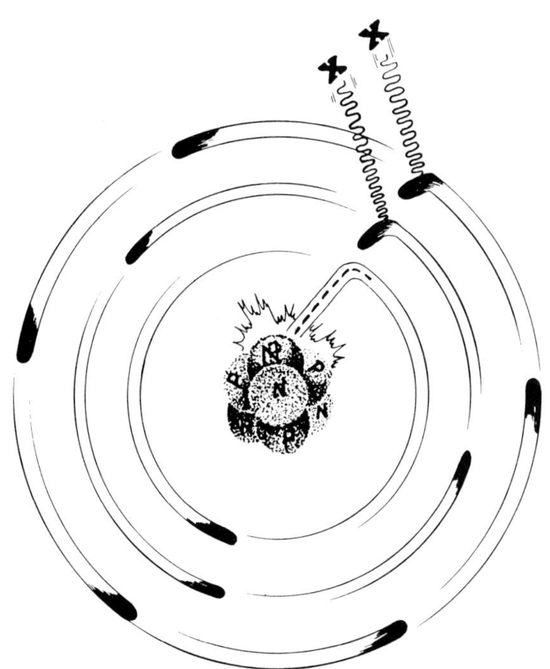

Fig. 4-9. Electron capture. The nucleus attracts an orbital electron, which combines with a proton to form a neutron. Secondary process of filling the orbital vacancy results in emission of characteristic x-radiation.

■ Electron capture

Another mode of radioactive decay used by unstable nuclei having too few neutrons and too many protons is that of electron capture (ϵ). As stated previously, it is generally believed that energy shells are not perfectly circular around the nucleus but are more elliptic in shape. It is even thought that possibly the K shell electron passes through the nucleus during one of its orbits and is captured by the nucleus. Whatever the case, it is known that one of the orbiting K shell electrons is captured by the nucleus. When this electron is captured, the nucleus transforms a proton into a neutron and a neutrino is ejected (Fig. 4-9). It is usually the K shell electron that is captured by the nucleus (K capture). This method of decay is known to exist with electrons from the L energy shells as well. In these cases the phenomenon is known as L capture. Capture of unbound (free) electrons by nuclei has not been observed to date. Whatever electron is captured, a vacancy will exist in that shell that must be filled. Electrons fall down into the vacancy, and characteristic x-radiation results, as described in Chapter 2.

By the decay process of electron capture, the parent nucleus produces a daughter nucleus with a neutron number increased by 1 and a proton number decreased by 1. In so doing, the daughter product becomes an isobar of the parent. This is the third method of isobaric transition. Chromium 51 ($^{24}_{51}Cr$) is an example of electron capture; its decay scheme is shown at the end of this chapter (p. 46). Other pertinent radionuclides that decay by electron capture are iodine 123 ($^{123}_{53}I$), iodine 125 ($^{125}_{53}I$), cobalt 57 ($^{57}_{27}Co$), and thallium 201 ($^{201}_{81}Te$).

Electron capture is similar to positron decay in that the end results are similar, but the methods used to achieve these ends differ. The difference is that positron decay usually occurs among lighter nuclides, while electron capture usually occurs among those that are heavier. As is evident, positron emission and electron capture are competing modes of decay. The difference can be explained on the basis of "available energy." Positron decay requires that the available energy be greater than 1.022 MeV. Further, in heavier atoms, the orbital structure of the electrons tends to be more compact, placing the electrons closer to the nucleus and therefore easier to capture.

■ Isomeric transition

An isomer, in nuclear terms, is one of the 2 nuclides having the same mass number and the same atomic number that can exist for measurable times in the excited state. This differs from the chemical meaning of the term. It has been stated before that in most cases this state of excitation must be instantaneously relieved by the emission of a gamma ray. In some radionuclides, however, this does not occur instantaneously. Isomeric transition is the radioactive transition from one nuclear isomer to another of low energy. It is part of the decay process of certain radionuclides. An example of this would be molybdenum 99 ($^{99}_{42}Mo$). ^{99}Mo decays by beta-gamma emission to technetium 99 ($^{99}_{43}Tc$). In the process of decay a point is reached at which the nucleus is able to retain its excited level (142 keV) for a half-life period of 6 hours. Since the molybdenum nucleus has ejected the beta particle and the neutrino, it has already lost 1 neutron and gained 1 proton. It is no longer ^{99}Mo, but ^{99}Tc. Furthermore, it can only be ^{99}Tc when the nucleus is at ground state, which it is not. It acts as though it were another radionuclide, a semistable ^{99}Tc atom. For this reason, the atom that can exist in this increased energy state of the nucleus is referred to as being in a *metastable* state. This state is signified by *m* after the mass number (^{99m}Tc). Not until the nucleus loses that energy is it known as a true ^{99}Tc atom. Isomeric transition is regarded by some as a form of decay because of the emission of the gamma ray. However, it only represents a change in energy state, not a change in nuclear composition. Other pertinent radionuclides that decay by isomeric transition include indium 113m (^{113m}In) and barium 137m (^{137m}Ba).

■ Gamma emission

Radioactive decay by alpha emission, beta emission, positron emission, or electron capture usually leaves some of the energy resulting from these changes in the nucleus. As a result, the nucleus is raised to an excited level. None of these excited nuclei (with the exception of isomeric transition) can remain in this high-energy state. They must instantaneously release this energy so that the nucleus can return to ground state or its lowest possible energy state. This energy is released in the form of gamma radiation, and the gamma ray has an energy equal to the change in energy state of the nucleons. These photons are members of the electromagnetic spectrum and have a wavelength corresponding to very short x-rays. As stated previously, a gamma ray differs from an x-ray only in its origin—gamma rays originate in the nucleus; x-rays originate in the orbital electron structure. Although of different origin, gamma rays and x-rays can have precisely the same characteristics. Their powers of excitation, ionization, and penetration can be exactly the same. For this reason they are used interchangeably in medical diagnosis and treatment.

Gamma rays carry no electrical charge; therefore they are not subject to forces of attraction or repulsion as are alpha, beta, and positron particles. Unlike these particles, gamma rays are the only emissions from an unstable nucleus that are members of the electromagnetic spectrum. Since they are not particles, the postemission product differs from the preemission form of the element only in a decreased energy state. There is no change in atomic number, neutron number, or mass number. Furthermore, some nuclear reaction or interaction must have preceded the gamma emission for the nucleus to be in an excited state. Reactions include neutron bombardment and charged particle bombardment. Interactions include alpha decay, beta decay, and positron decay.

Ionization and penetration. Gamma rays are also capable of producing ionization. It is referred to as *indirect* ionization, however. Gamma photons are capable of striking orbital electrons, thereby ejecting them from their orbits at high velocities. These rapidly moving secondary electrons ionize the atoms in the surrounding media. The same is true of x-rays.

The degree of penetration by a gamma ray is much greater than that of the other nuclear emissions. Penetration is such that, theoretically, enough shielding could never be provided to entirely stop all gamma rays. Even with a mile of lead there would be some gamma rays not totally absorbed but passing its full length. The degree of absorption or degree of attenuation can be predicted.

Interactions with matter. There are seven ways that gamma and x-ray photons can interact with matter: Compton effect, photoelectric effect, pair production, internal conversion, production of Auger electrons, triple production, and coherent scattering. Only the first five are important to nuclear medicine. All methods result in the loss of energy by the photon, and its eventual absorption.

Compton effect. The Compton effect (Fig. 4-10) (also called incoherent scattering) occurs when an incident gamma ray (primarily of medium energy) interacts with a free or loosely bound (outer shell) electron. In this interaction with matter a portion of the energy of the incident gamma ray is transferred to the electron. The energy expended depends on the angle at which the incident gamma ray hits the electron. If the electron is hit head-on, then a major portion of the energy is given to the electron. If the hit is one of a glancing nature, little of the energy is transferred to the electron. As a result, the electron (Compton electron) is ejected from the orbital structure, and a gamma ray of reduced energy *(secondary, Compton,* or *scatter)* emerges from the atom with a change in direction. The incident gamma ray has been reduced in energy by two factors. First, it has had to use some of its energy to overcome the binding energy of the electron that was removed. Second, it has transferred some of its energy to that electron. Therefore the energy of the secondary gamma ray is equal to the energy of the incident gamma ray, less the binding energy of the electron released, less the energy given to that electron. The energy of the scattered photon (E_{sc}) can be calculated by the following relationship:

$$E_{sc} = \frac{E_i}{1 + \left(\frac{E_i}{0.511}\right)(1 - \text{Cos } \theta)}$$

E_{sc} = Energy of the scattered photon
E_i = Energy of the incident photon
θ = Scattering angle (Fig. 4-10)

Inasmuch as this secondary gamma emission is changed in direction and is of reduced energy, it becomes of extreme importance to nuclear medicine. (Without knowledge of instrumentation—spectrometry—and Compton scatter, results from scanning techniques and function studies could be misinterpreted. This will be discussed in greater detail in Chapter 10.)

Photoelectric effect. The photoelectric effect (Fig. 4-11) occurs when an incident gamma ray (primarily of low energy) interacts with an inner-orbital electron. When this reaction occurs, the entire energy of the gamma ray is transferred to the electron, and the gamma is totally absorbed. The electron, called a *photoelectron,* is released from its energy shell and the atom. Since the electron had a binding energy to contain it within its orbit, energy had to be used by the incident gamma ray to overcome that binding energy. Therefore the electron would have the energy of the gamma ray less the amount of energy required to overcome the binding energy. Since a vacancy exists within that inner orbit, other orbital electrons will fall into that vacancy with a subsequent emission of characteristic x-rays.

In the process of absorption of gamma rays, the gamma ray usually goes through a series of Compton collisions, progressively reducing it in energy until it can finally be totally absorbed by the photoelectric process.

Pair production. Pair production is the third way in which gamma rays interact with matter. This phenomenon occurs when high-energy gamma rays interact in the vicin-

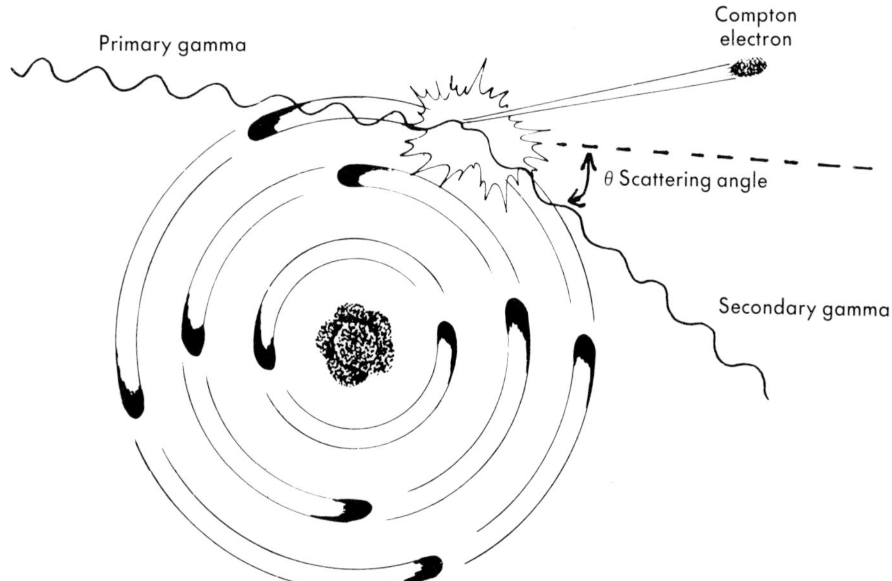

Fig. 4-10. Compton effect. Gamma photon of medium energy strikes outer orbital electron and releases it from its orbit. This results in production of a secondary gamma of reduced energy.

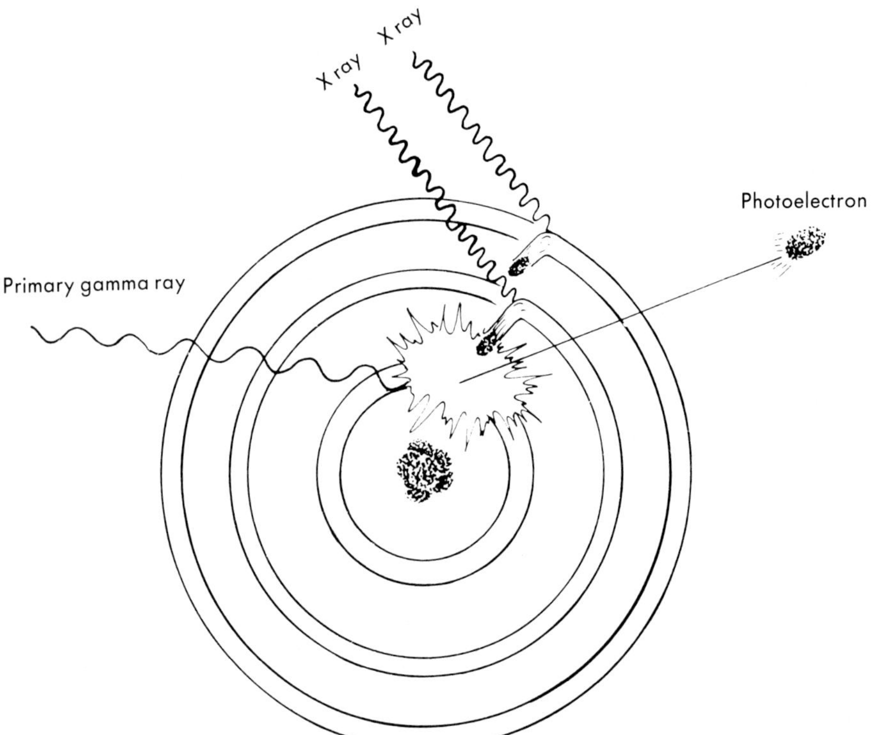

Fig. 4-11. Photoelectric effect. Low-energy gamma photon strikes inner orbital electron and releases it from its orbit, which effects total absorption of the gamma photon. Characteristic x-radiation results from the filling phenomenon.

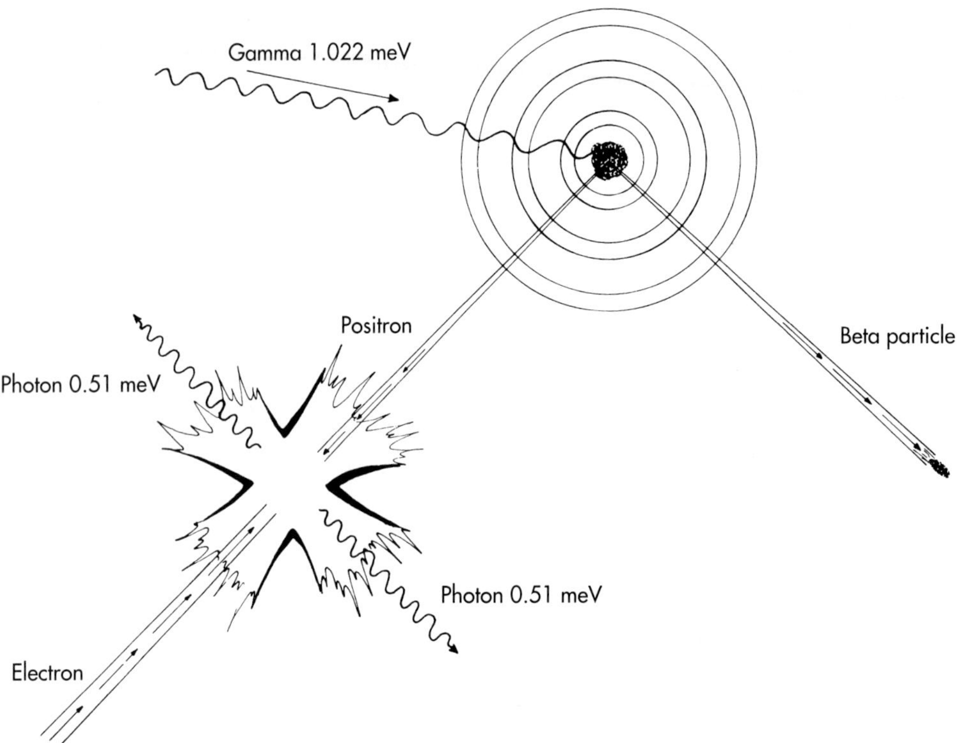

Fig. 4-12. Pair production. High-energy gamma ray interacts near the nucleus, producing two particles, a beta particle (negatron) and a positron. Positron annihilates almost immediately.

ity of the nucleus. In pair production the energy of the gamma ray is completely absorbed in the vicinity of the strong electrical field of the nucleus with a subsequent production of a negatron and a positron (Fig. 4-12). For this to occur the incident gamma ray must have a minimum energy of 1.022 MeV. If these conditions are met, the positron and the negatron are ejected from the atom. The beta particle acts as other beta particles in that it passes through matter, creating ion pairs along its path, until such time as it is incorporated into an atom or becomes a free electron. The positron, however, almost instantaneously collides with an electron. This results in the subsequent annihilation of both particles and the emission of 2 gamma rays of 0.511 MeV. Since the conversion of the mass of 2 beta particles is equal to 1.022 MeV and since the amount of energy is equally divided between the 2 annihilation photons regardless of the energy of the incident gamma ray (provided it is greater than 1.022 MeV), the energy of the annihilation gamma rays would always be equal to the 0.511 MeV. If the incident gamma ray is greater in energy than 1.022 MeV, the excess energy is given to the β^+ and β^- as kinetic energy that must be lost before the β^+ can undergo annihilation. Regardless of the energy of the incident gamma ray (provided it is 1.022 MeV or greater), the energy of the annihilation photon is always 0.511 MeV. This gamma interaction represents an energy-to-mass-to-energy relationship. The reaction was begun with energy (gamma) and was converted to mass ($\beta^- + \beta^+$), which in turn was converted to energy (2 photons of 0.511 MeV).

Internal conversion. After almost all nuclear interactions the nucleus is left in an excited state. This elevated energy state is usually decreased to ground state immediately by the emission of a gamma ray equal to the change in energy level. In some cases, however, when this gamma ray emerges from the nucleus, the gamma ray can be naively regarded as transferring all its energy to one of its own orbital electrons, usually the K shell electron. The electron is then ejected from the atom and possesses an energy equal to that of the gamma ray less the binding energy (Fig. 4-13). The gamma ray has internally converted its own atom, hence the name internal conversion. The electron that is ejected from the atom is called the *internal conversion electron* (ICE). Since these electrons have energy and are capable of ionizing other atoms, it must be a consideration in the calculations of radiation dose from internal emitting radionuclides. This reaction occurs most with high Z materials.

Production of Auger electrons. Another process resulting from changes in energy state and changes in electron configuration in the orbital shells is the release of Auger electrons. It can occur when a vacancy is created in an inner shell. Fluorescent (characteristic) radiation is then emitted as an electron assumes the lower energy state necessary to fill that vacancy. If this energy release (in the form of an x-ray) possesses the capability of interacting with and removing electrons from neighboring atoms (that is, photoelectric and Compton interactions), then it also possesses the capability of removing its own electron from orbit. This electron, given energy from the fluorescent radiation and removed from its orbit, is an *Auger electron* (Fig. 4-14). As with internal conversion electrons, these electrons have energy and are capable of ionizing other atoms; therefore

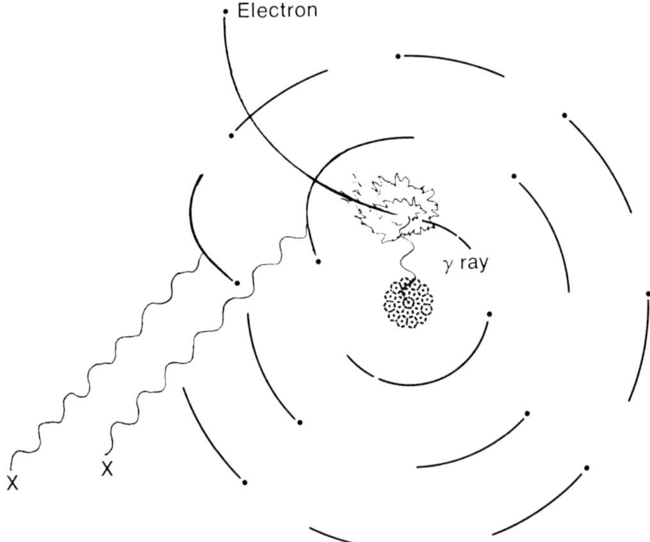

Fig. 4-13. Internal conversion. Gamma ray being released from nucleus strikes and ejects K shell electron. Characteristic x-ray emissions are a result of the loss of energy by other orbital electrons falling into the vacancy created by the ejected electron.

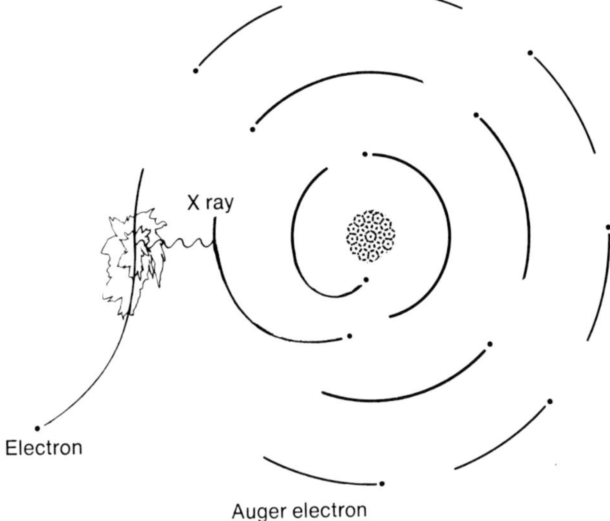

Fig. 4-14. Auger electron. Characteristic x-ray emitted from one of the orbital electrons as it assumes a lower energy state strikes another orbital electron and removes it from orbit.

they must be a consideration when calculating internal radiation dosimetry. This interaction occurs with low Z materials.

Auger electrons are known as to their frequency and average energy for all of the radionuclides. Further, they can be identified not only as to the energy shell from which they are ejected, but by the change of electron position that caused the characteristic radiation as well. For instance, an Auger electron can be identified as a KLL Auger e, which means that it is an Auger electron emitted from the L shell as a result of the transition of another L shell electron to a vacancy in the K shell. Other appellations are as follows: KLX Auger e = an Auger electron emitted from the X shell, when X stands for any shell higher than the L shell, as a result of the transition of an L shell electron to a vacancy in the K shell; KXY Auger e = an Auger electron emitted from the Y shell as a result of the transition of an X shell electron to a vacancy in the K shell, when X and Y each stand for any shell higher than the L shell; LMM Auger e = an Auger electron emitted from the M shell as a result of the transition of another M shell electron to a vacancy in the L shell; MXY Auger e = an Auger electron emitted from the Y shell as a result of the transition of an X shell electron to a vacancy in the M shell, when X and Y each stand for any shell higher than the M shell.

Triple production. This is another photon interaction with matter; though not important to nuclear medicine, it is included in the interest of completeness. Triple production is similar to pair production except that it requires a photon of very high energy (greater than 2.04 MeV) to interact in the field of an orbital electron causing the following three changes: (1) creation of a negatron, (2) creation of a positron, and (3) the removal of the electron from orbit. Since radionuclides with such high energies are not routinely used in nuclear medicine, this interaction phenomenon has little importance to this text.

Coherent scattering (Thomson scattering). This also is an interaction with matter not necessarily important to nuclear medicine but included here in the interest of completeness. Coherent scattering occurs when the photon of very weak energy is absorbed by an orbital electron. In the process of absorption, the electron begins to vibrate, thereby releasing electromagnetic waves of the same energy as the incident photon. Except that it differs in direction, the resultant photon is no different from the incident photon with respect to wavelength, frequency or energy. This is the only interaction with matter in which the photon is "scattered" without losing any energy. This phenomenon is not important to nuclear medicine because it occurs only with photons of very low energy.

The neutron. Since the neutron has no charge and is a comparatively large particle, it is unaffected by other particles containing electrical charges. The neutron can penetrate through the orbital structure directly into the nucleus where it is either absorbed, as in the case of neutron capture and transmutation (Chapter 5), or possibly disrupts the nucleus, as in the case of fission. Another special consideration of neutrons is that they are produced in enormous quantities in the fission process, either controlled as in the case of a nuclear reactor, or uncontrolled as in the detonation of a nuclear bomb. Neutrons can have energies from as low as 0.025 eV (thermal neutrons) to higher than 1 million eV (fast neutrons).

The ionizing effects of neutrons are greater than those of gamma or x-rays. They also have one special feature regarding their ability to ionize hydrogen that is a major constituent of all biologic materials. Ordinary hydrogen has a nucleus composed of only 1 proton, which is less in mass than the neutron. On subjecting biologic materials to neutron bombardment, the neutron possesses the unique quality of ionizing its hydrogen atoms by removing the nucleus, rather than the usual orbital electron.

■ PRINCIPLES OF RADIOACTIVE DECAY

When radiopharmaceuticals are introduced into a biologic system, two processes are usually taking place to reduce the amount of radioactivity in the body. One that is always present is the reduction of radioactivity because of the physical decay of the radionuclide. There is no way to stop, slow, or speed up this process. The other, which may or may not be present, is the biologic elimination of the material. Most materials introduced into the body will at some time be eliminated. Some materials, however (such as ^{99m}Tc–labeled sulfur colloid), are removed from circulation by the reticuloendothelial system and are never excreted by any elimination system. The units of measurement by which these radioactivity reduction times are defined are physical half-life, biologic half-life, and effective half-life. Physical half-life is specifically defined by the use of the term *curie*.

■ The curie

When a radioactive nucleus changes to another nucleus, the change is called decay, or disintegration. The rate of decay is spoken of in terms of number of disintegrations per unit of time, usually in seconds or minutes. The curie (Ci) is defined as a unit of radioactivity in which the number of disintegrations per second is 3.7×10^{10}. By multiplying this unit by 60 the definition can be expressed as disintegrations per minute (dpm), 2.2×10^{12} dpm. Multiples and submultiples of the curie unit can be expressed similarly in disintegrations per second and disintegrations per minute according to Table 4-1.

At the meeting of the International Commission on Radiation Units and Measurements (ICRU) in July 1974, it was recommended that within a period of not less than about 10 years the curie be replaced with the new Si unit,* the reciprocal second (sec^{-1}). This new unit is to be used

*An abbreviation for Système International d'Unités, an international system of units designed to end the confusion of various units of length and weight used by various countries.

Table 4-1. Multiples and submultiples of the curie

Units	Disintegrations per second (dps)	Disintegrations per minute (dpm)	Becquerels
Megacurie	3.7×10^{16}	2.2×10^{18}	37 PBq
Kilocurie	3.7×10^{13}	2.2×10^{15}	37 TBq
Curie (Ci)	3.7×10^{10}	2.2×10^{12}	37 GBq
Millicurie (mCi)	3.7×10^{7}	2.2×10^{9}	37 MBq
Microcurie (μCi)	3.7×10^{4}	2.2×10^{6}	37 kBq
Nanocurie (nCi)	3.7×10 or 37	2.2×10^{3} or 2,200	37 Bq
Picocurie (pCi)	3.7×10^{-2}	2.2	37 mBq

to express the unit of activity as a function of the rate of spontaneous nuclear transformations of radionuclides, as one per second (dps, as we are used to thinking of it). Further, it was suggested that this new unit of activity be given the name *becquerel,* bearing the symbol *Bq*. The becquerel, therefore, would be equal to 1 dps or approximately 2.703 $\times 10^{-11}$ Ci. A 15 mCi dose of ^{99m}Tc would then be referred to as 555 megabecquerels (555 MBq). (Refer to Appendix H for other conversions.)

The conversion to the use of the SI units has been slow in the United States. For this reason, SI units will appear as a parenthetical expression, when appropriate, throughout the remainder of this text; for example, 20 mCi (740 MBq).

■ Physical half-life

The physical half-life ($T_{1/2}$ or T_p) is often called the *radioactive half-life*. It is defined as the length of time required for one half of the original number of atoms in a given radioactive sample to disintegrate. This reduction of the number of atoms through disintegration of their nuclei is known as radioactive decay and is inherent in all radioactive materials. The rate of decay of a given isotope remains constant. It cannot be influenced by temperature, pressure, or chemical combination. Furthermore, every atom in a radioactive sample has the same probability of disintegrating.

Because of decay, all radioactivity decreases with time, since fewer atoms are left as some atoms decay. Since the fraction of nuclei disintegrating per unit time is always the same and since progressively fewer atoms are left, the fraction of remaining atoms represents fewer and fewer atoms with the passage of time. This fraction of the remaining number of atoms that decay per unit of time is called the *decay constant* (λ). The larger the fraction, the faster the process of decay. Stated another way, the larger the decay constant, the shorter the half-life. Therefore $T_{1/2}$ is inversely proportional to λ. If one were to plot on linear paper the number of atoms present in a given radioactive sample versus time, the curve shown in Fig. 4-15, *A,* would be obtained. It is apparent that the same length of time is required for 100 atoms to decay to 50 atoms as for 50 atoms to decay to 25 atoms. The length of time during which the number of atoms diminish to one half is referred to as the half-life. Half-lives range in value from thousandths of a second to millions of years. Notice that the curve approaches the abscissa asymptotically, which would imply that some atoms live forever in their excited state. This is not true. If an atom is excited, it must relieve that excitation with the emission of a gamma ray at some point in time. This decay curve is only applicable to large numbers of atoms. If the same curve were plotted on semilogarithmic paper with the number of atoms on the logarithmic scale and time on the linear scale, a straight line would be obtained (Fig. 4-15, *B*). The rate of decay can therefore be said to have an exponential function.

Figure 4-16 also exemplifies the concept of decay constant. It shows that one half of the atoms decay per unit time (in this case the unit of time is one half-life). In the first unit of time 100 atoms decay to 50 atoms; in the second unit of time the 50 atoms remaining decay to 25 atoms. In each unit time the fraction of the number of atoms remaining in the sample is constant at one half (decay constant).

Average life expectancy (mean life). The active life of any particular radioactive atom can have any value between zero and infinity. However, the *mean life* of a large number of atoms is a definite quantity. It is related to the decay constant, being equal numerically to its reciprocal ($1/\lambda$). It can be described as the period of time that it would take for all the atoms of a radionuclide to decay provided they decayed at the initial rate of decay until all the atoms were gone. Although one half of all nuclei decay in one half-life, the average life becomes longer because in the subsequent half-lives, nuclei live longer. The average life expectancy is always equal to 1.443 times the physical half-life (Fig. 4-16). In Fig. 4-16, the number of nuclei originally in the sample (N_0) is plotted against time in half-lives. Accordingly, after one half-life has elapsed, only one half of the original radioactive nuclei are still present in the sample. After two half-lives, only one fourth of the original radioactive nuclei are present in the sample. If one were to extend the slope of the curve received at the initial rate of decay until it intercepted the abscissa, the extension would

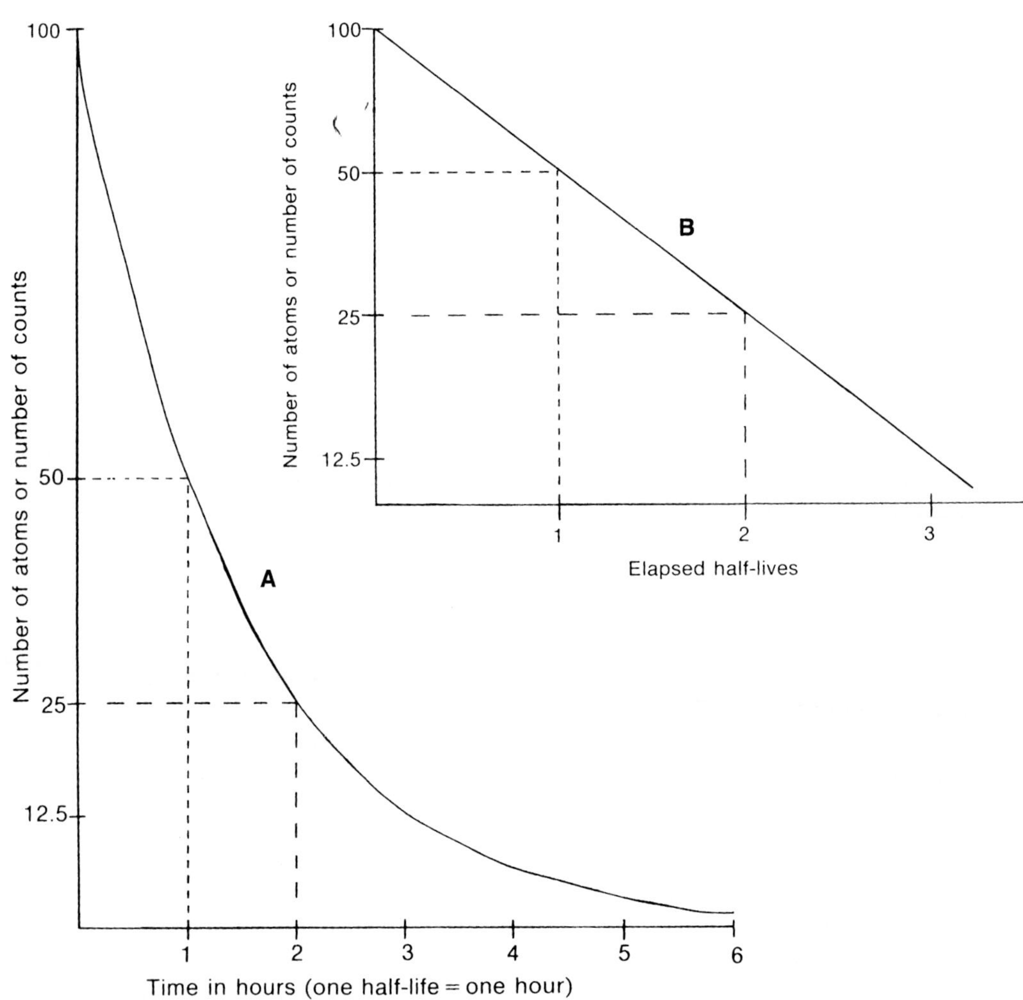

Fig. 4-15. Physical decay of radionuclide, plotting elapsed time versus number of atoms remaining or number of counts received. **A,** This relationship on linear graph paper. **B,** Semilogarithmic paper. This can be used as a universal decay table to be applied to any radionuclide, provided units of time are appropriately placed.

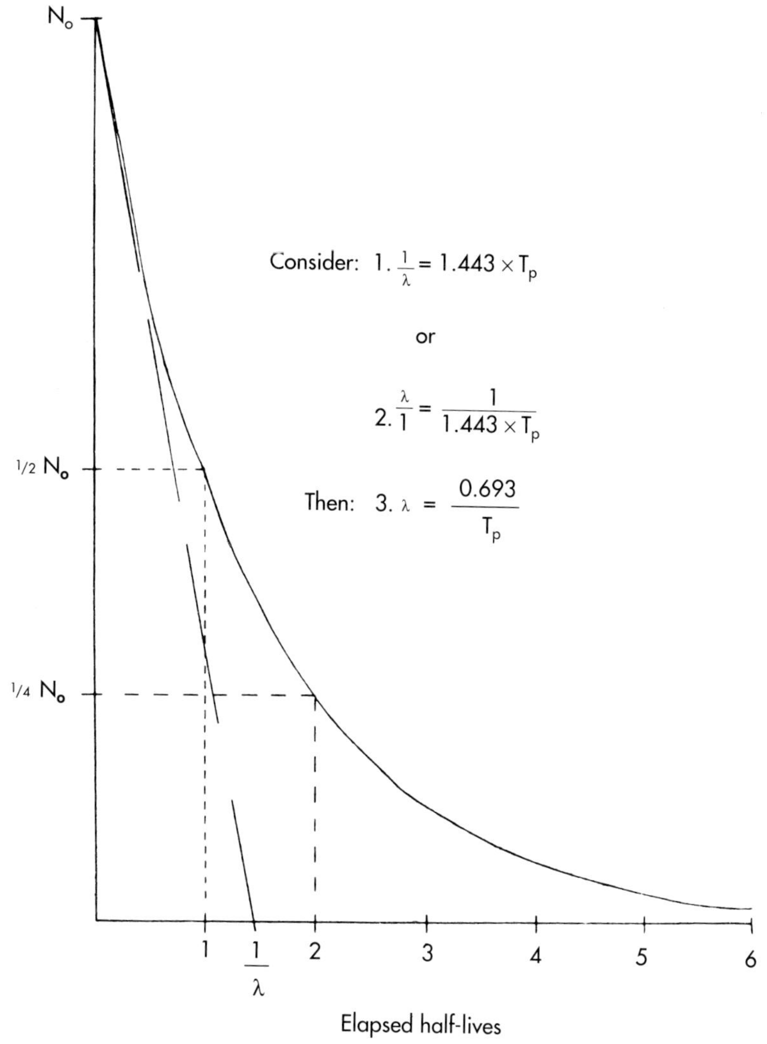

Fig. 4-16. Radioactive decay demonstrating average life expectancy of each atom in the sample.

intercept at 1.443 half-lives. This is the life expectancy of each radioactive atom and is the reciprocal of the decay constant ($1/\lambda$).

Decay formula. The curve for radioactive decay can be expressed by the following equation:

$$N_t = N_o e^{-\lambda t}$$

N_t = Number of atoms at some point in time
N_o = Number of atoms originally present
e = Base of the natural logarithm, 2.718
λ = Decay constant
t = Time elapsed

Minus sign indicates that the number of atoms are decreasing.

λ can be proved mathematically to be equal to $\frac{0.693}{T_p}$ (Fig. 4-14).

Substituting:

$$N_t = N_o e^{-\frac{0.693t}{T_p}}$$

This formula can be expressed similarly in terms of activity as follows:

$$A_t = A_o e^{-\frac{0.693t}{T_p}}$$

A_t = Activity after a period of elapsed time
A_o = Activity in the original sample

The use of the last formula is seen in the following problem:

A sample of ^{131}I was known to have an activity of 10 mCi (370 MBq) on January 14 at 12 noon CST. What would the activity be on January 15 at 3 PM EST? (Note: Calculations of elapsed time must also include variations in time zones. The elapsed time in this case is exactly 50 hours.)

A_o = 10 mCi
t = 50 hr
T_p = 8.1 days or 194 hr—both time units (t and T_p) must be the same

Solve for A_t by

$$\begin{aligned} A_t &= A_o e^{-\frac{0.693t}{T_p}} \\ &= 10 \text{ mCi} \times e^{-0.693 \times \frac{50 \text{ hr}}{194 \text{ hr}}} \\ &= 10 \times e^{-\frac{34.65}{194}} \\ &= 10 \times e^{-0.18*} \\ &= 10 \times 0.84 \\ &= 8.4 \text{ mCi } (310.8 \text{ MBq}) \end{aligned}$$

*The value for e^{-x} can be found in Appendix E.

Accordingly, the activity of the sample on January 16 at 3 PM EST is 8.4 mCi (310.8 MBq).

Decay tables. The factor found on any decay table for iodine 131 with an elapsed time of 2 days plus 2 hours (50 hours) is 0.84, or it may be listed at 84% remaining, the result of $e^{-0.693t}/T_p$. In either case, the original activity is multiplied by 0.84 to find the present activity. All decay tables for the various radionuclides are nothing more than the complication of these values for various periods of elapsed time. Appendix B shows a universal decay table.

Since decay tables are more convenient to use, most nuclear medicine personnel prefer them to the use of the decay formula. Two practical problems involving their use should be mentioned: (1) How is the decay table used when an aliquot of the radioactive solution is needed before the calibration date and (2) How is the decay table used when the decay factors do not cover a sufficient period of time?

The first problem could present itself when an order of radioactive material is received from a supplier before its calibration date. If the new source is to be used, it becomes necessary to first calculate the amount of activity on hand (this will be larger than that indicated on the label); then the volume that will represent the desired dose must be calculated. (Some tables include these factors.) The following problems will demonstrate the correct use of decay tables.

Problem. A 10 mCi (370 MBq) source of ^{131}I in a volume of 10 ml, calibrated for June 10 at 12 noon EST, was received on June 9. What would be the activity on June 9 at 12 noon EST?

Solution (using decay table). Decay factor for ^{131}I after one day of elapsed time = 0.918. This factor may be used, but instead of multiplying the activity by the decay factor, divide the decay factor:

$$\frac{10 \text{ mCi}}{0.918} = 10.9 \text{ mCi } (403.3 \text{ MBq})$$

Similarly, using concentration:

$$\frac{1 \text{ mCi/ml}}{0.918} = 1.09 \text{ mCi/ml } (40.3 \text{ MBq/mL})$$

Expressing it another way:

To determine activity on hand *before* calibration date:

$$A_t = A_o \div \text{DF}$$

A_t = Activity on hand
A_o = Activity indicated on the vial
DF = Decay factor

Table 4-2. Decay factors for ^{99m}Tc

	Minutes			
Hours	**0**	**15**	**30**	**45**
0	1.000	0.972	0.944	0.917
1	0.891	0.866	0.841	0.817
2	0.794	0.771	0.749	0.727
3	0.707	0.687	0.667	0.648
4	0.630	0.612	0.595	0.578
5	0.561	0.545	0.530	0.515
6	0.500	0.486	0.472	0.459
7	0.445	0.433	0.420	0.408
8	0.397	0.385	0.375	0.364
9	0.354	0.343	0.334	0.324
10	0.315	0.306	0.297	0.289
11	0.281	0.273	0.264	0.257
12	0.250			

Problem. The second problem involving decay tables presents itself when the decay factors given do not cover a sufficient period of time.

A 10 mCi (370 MBq) source of ^{99m}Tc has an elapsed time of 15 hours from time of calibration, and the decay table has values only to 12 hours (see Table 4-2). What is the activity on hand?

Solution. The easiest approach in this case is to correct for two half-lives knowing that ^{99m}Tc has a 6-hour half-life. Then using the decay factor representative of the time differential from 2 half-lives (12 hrs) to the remaining period of elapsed time (15 hours), that is, 3 hours (15 hours–12 hours), multiply by one fourth of the original activity:

1. Activity at time zero (A_o) = 10 mCi (370 MBq)
2. Activity at 12 hours or 2 half-lives = 2.5 mCi (92.5 MBq)
3. Elapsed time = 15 hr
4. Elapsed time = 2 × T_p (in this case) + 3 hours remaining time
5. Decay factor for remaining time = 0.707
6. Using the activity at 2 half-lives: 2.5 mCi × 0.707 = 1.77 mCi (65.5 MBq) activity on hand

Accordingly, the original vial of 10 mCi (370 MBq) ^{99m}Tc would contain 1.77 mCi (65.5 MBq) 15 hours later.

Expressing it another way:

$A_t = A_{2 \times T_p} \times$ DF (for remaining time)
A_t = Activity on hand
$A_{2 \times T_p}$ = Activity after two half-lives*
DF = Decay factor for total elapsed time (two half-lives*)

This would also apply to concentrations, if this was the desired method of record keeping.

*This could also be the value after 2 or more half-lives, depending on the circumstances.

■ Biologic half-life

Biologic half-life (T_b) is the time required for the body to eliminate one half of the dose of any substance by the regular processes of elimination. This time is the same for both stable and radioactive isotopes of any given element. The principal methods of elimination are by way of urine, feces, exhalation, and perspiration. Biologic half-life is an important consideration when attempting to predict radiation damage to the human body from internal emitters. Any radionuclide that is retained by the body for only a short period of time will have a relatively small radiobiologic effect, regardless of whether it has a long physical half-life or a short physical half-life.

■ Effective half-life

Because both the physical and biologic half-lives must be taken into consideration when predicting the amount of radiation that is absorbed per unit mass of tissue, a third term is used to express the combined effect of the two. This is called the *effective half-life*. This term is defined as the time required for the body to eliminate one half of the dose of any *radioactive* substance. This is the result of the combined action of radioactive decay and loss of the material by biologic elimination. The effective half-life (T_e) is usually experimentally determined.

A relatively simple example of experimentally determining effective half-life is that of iodine 131 in the thyroid gland. Iodine 131, labeled sodium iodide, is administered to the patient, and an uptake is determined at 24 hours after administration by a standard thyroid uptake counter. Uptakes are continued every subsequent 24-hour period. By plotting the count on day 1 and comparing subsequent daily counts, one may find the activity in the thyroid reaches 50% at 6 days, even though the physical half-life of iodine 131 is approximately 8 days. Obviously, biologic elimination has acted on the iodine 131 in the thyroid gland so that the 50% rate is reached before the physical half-life. The effective half-life in this case is something less than the physical half-life. The biologic half-life always decreases the effective half-life to a value less than that of the physical half-life. The only time that this would not be the case is in the event of no biologic elimination, as with technetium 99m–labeled sulfur colloid in the liver. In this case the effective half-life is equal to the physical half-life. In no case is the effective half-life larger than the physical half-life. If the biologic half-life is known, the effective half-life can be mathematically calculated by the following expression:

$$T_e = \frac{T_p \times T_b}{T_p + T_b}$$

The usual case, however, is that both the effective half-life (experimentally determined) and the physical half-life are known. Using these two values the biologic half-life can be determined by the following formula:

$$T_b = \frac{T_p \times T_e}{T_p - T_e}$$

■ DECAY SCHEMES

A decay scheme provides a ready reference for a variety of data. Quick identification of such information as mode of decay, energy states of the nuclei and their subsequent gamma emissions, and the nuclide to which the radionuclide decays is possible. These decay schemes have a wide variation in complexity. Those that decay directly to the daughter product without emitting electromagnetic radiation are the simplest forms. These would include the pure alpha emitters and pure beta emitters. Those decay schemes with resultant electromagnetic radiation vary greatly in complexity. Some, such as ^{60}Co, have a simple decay scheme. Others, such as ^{131}I and ^{99}Mo, have extremely complex decay schemes.

Decay schemes are patterned by placing the parent nucleus at the top of the decay scheme. Diagonal lines extending from the right or the left of the parent indicate the mode of decay. Those diagonal lines that angle to the right represent the mode of decay whereby the daughter nuclide is of higher atomic number than the parent. Those diagonal lines that angle to the left represent the modes of decay whereby the daughter nuclide is of lower atomic number than the parent. Alpha decay, positron decay, and electron capture all result in the daughter nuclide being of lower atomic number than is the parent. Beta decay is the only method resulting in a daughter nuclide of higher atomic number than that of the parent.

A pure beta emitter is an example of the simplest form of decay. ^{32}P is representative of such a scheme. The "Input Data" box* (p. 42, top) indicates that the parent radionuclide, phosphorus 32, has a 14.3-day half-life and decays by β^- directly to sulfur 32, which is stable. One hundred percent (mean number/disintegration = 1.0000) of all ^{32}P nuclei decay by this method; the maximum energy is 1.7100 MeV. All the energy is distributed to the beta particle and the neutrino. The nucleus does not receive any energy from this reaction; therefore neither is the nucleus raised to an excited level nor is there a subsequent gamma emission. Note that in this mode of decay the diagonal line is angled to the right, indicating an increase in atomic number by the daughter. The atomic number of phosphorus 32 is 15 decaying to sulfur 32 with an atomic number of 16. Simple decay schemes can also be represented by pure alpha emitters, by pure positron emitters, or in nuclides that undergo 100% electron capture. In these cases all diagonal lines would be angled to the left because in all cases the daughter has a lower atomic number than does the parent.

In general, the scintillation crystals used in routine diagnostic nuclear medicine procedures detect only gamma emissions. For the nuclide to be of importance to diagnostic nuclear medicine, gamma emission must be a part of its decay scheme. There are exceptions to this, such as beta emitters used with liquid scintillation detectors and positron

*"Output Data" box will be explained in Chapter 7.

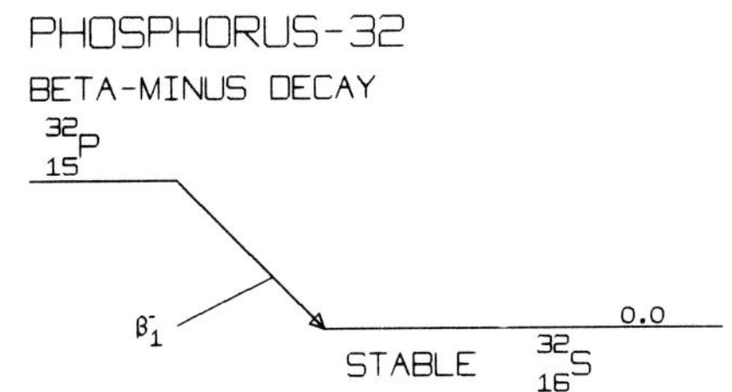

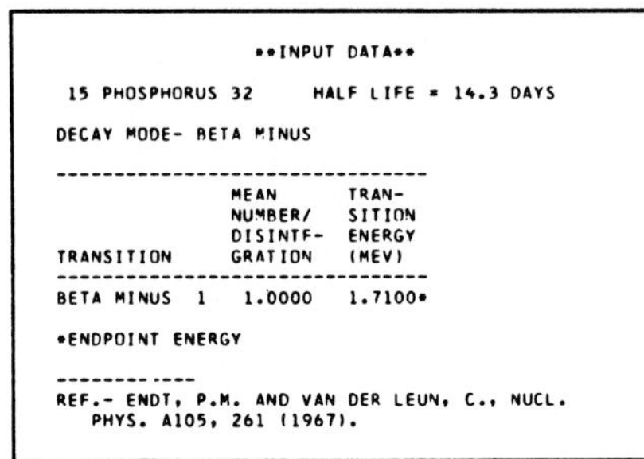

INPUT DATA

15 PHOSPHORUS 32 HALF LIFE = 14.3 DAYS

DECAY MODE- BETA MINUS

TRANSITION	MEAN NUMBER/ DISINTE- GRATION	TRAN- SITION ENERGY (MEV)
BETA MINUS 1	1.0000	1.7100*

*ENDPOINT ENERGY

REF.- ENDT, P.M. AND VAN DER LEUN, C., NUCL. PHYS. A105, 261 (1967).

OUTPUT DATA

15 PHOSPHORUS 32 HALF LIFE = 14.3 DAYS

DECAY MODE- BETA MINUS

RADIATION	MEAN NUMBER/ DISINTE- GRATION n_i	MEAN ENERGY/ PAR- TICLE $\bar{E}_i$ (MeV)	EQUI- LIBRIUM DOSE CONSTANT Δ_i (g-rad/ µCi-h)
BETA MINUS 1	1.0000	0.6948	1.4799

Courtesy Dillman L.T., and Von der Lage F.C.: MIRD Pamphlet No. 10, New York, 1975, Society of Nuclear Medicine.

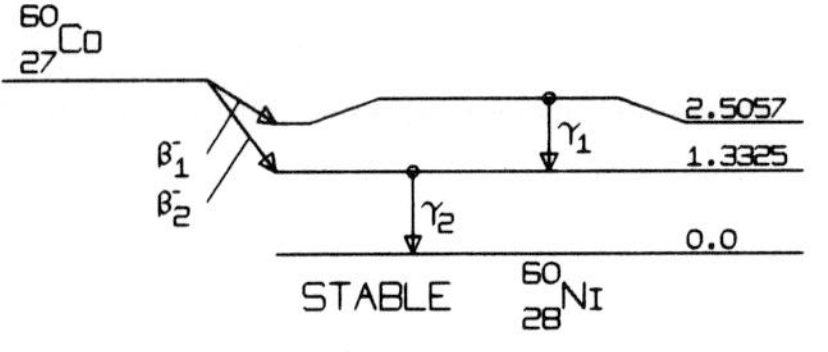

COBALT-60

BETA-MINUS DECAY

INPUT DATA

27 COBALT 60 HALF LIFE = 5.26 YEARS

DECAY MODE- BETA MINUS

TRANSITION	MEAN NUMBER/ DISINTE- GRATION	TRAN- SITION ENERGY (MEV)
BETA MINUS 1	0.9980	0.3130*
BETA MINUS 2	0.0012	1.4860*
GAMMA 1	0.9980	1.1732
GAMMA 2	1.0000	1.3324

*ENDPOINT ENERGY

REF.- LEDERER, C.M. ET AL, TABLE OF ISOTOPES, 6TH. ED.

OUTPUT DATA

27 COBALT 60 HALF LIFE = 5.26 YEARS

DECAY MODE- BETA MINUS

RADIATION	MEAN NUMBER/ DISINTE- GRATION n_i	MEAN ENERGY/ PAR- TICLE $\bar{E}_i$ (MeV)	EQUI- LIBRIUM DOSE CONSTANT Δ_i (g-rad/ µCi-h)
BETA MINUS 1	0.9980	0.0941	0.2000
BETA MINUS 2	0.0012	0.6243	0.0015
GAMMA 1	0.9978	1.1732	2.4935
K INT CON ELECT	0.0001	1.1648	0.0004
GAMMA 2	0.9998	1.3324	2.8378
K INT CON ELECT	0.0001	1.3241	0.0003

Courtesy Dillman LT and Von der Lage FC: MIRD Pamphlet No. 10, New York, 1975, Society of Nuclear Medicine.

emitters. For gamma rays to be emitted, the radionuclide must decay in such a way that only part of the energy involved in the transition from parent to daughter is distributed in the ejection particles. When this occurs, the nucleus is raised to an excited energy state, and in returning to ground state this energy is emitted in the form of gamma rays. These increases in energy state are represented by horizontal lines drawn between the parent and daughter nuclide and are representative of the various energy levels to which the nucleus can be raised. These horizontal lines would be analogous to the rungs on the stepladder used previously to describe the nuclear energy levels. A relatively simple example of such a decay scheme involving gamma emission would be that of ^{60}Co. ^{60}Co is an unstable nucleus with a half-life of 5.26 years, and it decays by beta decay to the stable ^{60}Ni. In this transition, however, only a portion of the energy resulting from the change within the nucleus is distributed to the beta particle and the neutrino. The remainder of the energy is retained by the nucleus, which is raised to an excited state. The energy state to which the nucleus is raised varies depending on whether the nucleus of the particular ^{60}Co atom decays by $\beta^-{}_1$ or $\beta^-{}_2$. As the "Input Data" box above indicates, 99.8% of all ^{60}Co atoms decay by $\beta^-{}_1$, which itself has an emission energy (transition energy) of 0.313 MeV. The rest of the atoms of ^{60}Co (1.2%) decay by $\beta^-{}_2$, which has an emission energy of 1.486 MeV. The energy state to which the nucleus of ^{60}Co is raised after the emission of $\beta^-{}_1$ is 2.5057 MeV. Rather than decaying from this elevated energy state with one release of energy to achieve ground state, it releases 2 gamma quanta to achieve ground state. In jumping from 2.5057 MeV to 1.3325 MeV energy state, there is a release of a gamma photon (γ_1) of 1.1732 MeV in energy, the energy difference between the two energy states. Note that this occurs in 99.8% of all atoms, which is to be expected because only 99.8% of all ^{60}Co atoms decay by $\beta^-{}_1$ and therefore reach this level of excitation. This release of energy is followed immediately by another release of energy of 1.3324 MeV (γ_2) representative of the change in energy state from the 1.3324 MeV level to the ground state. Note that this transition energy occurs 100% of the time. The reason is that all atoms of ^{60}Co, whether they decay by $\beta^-{}_1$ or $\beta^-{}_2$, have their nuclei excited to an energy state of 1.3324 MeV at some time during their decay. The total energy involved in the transition of ^{60}Co to ^{60}Ni is 2.818 MeV regardless of whether it decays by $\beta^-{}_1$ or $\beta^-{}_2$.

Decay schemes are simplified methods to describe the mode of decay and subsequent energy release in the form of gamma radiation produced by changes in an unstable nucleus. The directions of the arrows that represent the modes of decay, although not intended, assume a similarity to the Mme Curie experiment discussed at the beginning of this chapter. The negatively charged particle, representing the beta decay, is angled in one direction; the positively charged particles, representing alpha decay and positron decay (also electron capture), are angled in the opposite direction; the gamma ray with no charge is drawn perpendicular to the parent nucleus.

■ Alpha decay

Alpha decay can be represented by the decay of ^{224}Ra (at right). Ninety-four and eight-tenths percent of the atoms of ^{224}Ra (Z = 88) decay by an alpha particle of 5.7837 MeV to ^{220}Rn (Z = 86). Since an alpha particle is a helium nucleus, the parent atom loses 2 protons and 2 neutrons (an atomic number of 2 and a mass number of 4) to become ^{220}Rn. Five and two-tenths percent of all atoms of ^{224}Ra decay by an alpha particle that leaves the nucleus in an excited state with a new energy level of 0.2410 MeV. The atom instantaneously emits a gamma ray of 0.2410 MeV to become ^{220}Rn. The daughter product has a decreased atomic number, so the angle of the schematic is to the left. ^{220}Rn itself is an unstable nucleus and an inert gas. Being unstable, it continues to decay and does so by alpha emission. This is a portion of the series that eventually decays to stable ^{214}Pb. This chain of decay can be easily followed by referring to Brucer's trilinear chart of the nuclides, a portion of which appears on p. 61. ^{224}Ra has a simple alpha decay scheme. There are others much more complex in nature.

■ Beta (beta-minus) decay

The decay scheme of a pure beta emitter, ^{32}P, has already been discussed on page 41. This is a simple decay scheme in which no electromagnetic radiation is emitted. As energies to the beta particles vary and as energy states of the nucleus vary, the decay scheme becomes increasingly complex.

Gold 198. A more complex decay scheme involving 3 beta particles of different energies and 3 gamma photons of different energies is that of ^{198}Au. ^{198}Au (Z = 79) decays by beta decay to stable ^{198}Hg (Z = 80). The percentage of all ^{198}Au atoms that decay with a beta particle having a maximum energy of 0.9612 MeV (β_2) is 98.6%. This leaves the nucleus in an excited energy state of 0.4117 MeV. This state of excitation is instantaneously relieved by the emission of a gamma ray of 0.4117 MeV (γ_1). This path of decay represents an energy differential between parent and daughter nuclei of 1.37 MeV; the beta particle has a maximum energy of 0.9612 MeV, and the gamma has an

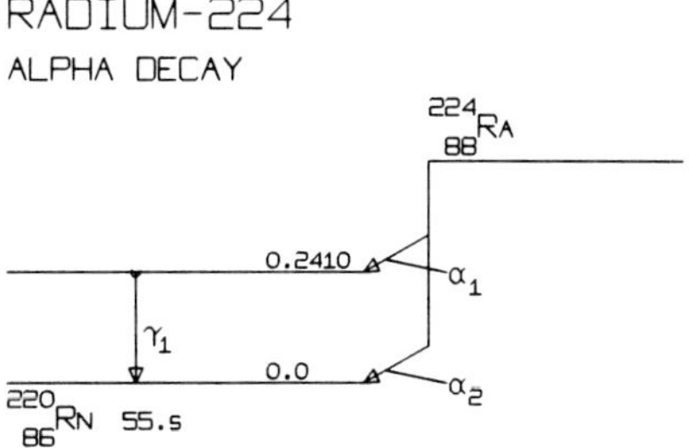

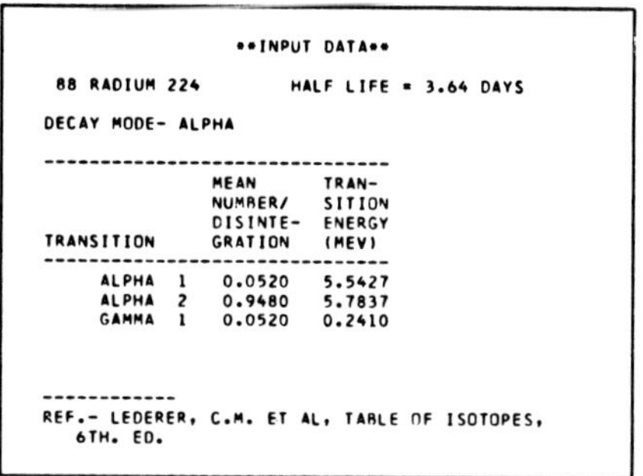

INPUT DATA

88 RADIUM 224 HALF LIFE = 3.64 DAYS

DECAY MODE- ALPHA

TRANSITION	MEAN NUMBER/ DISINTE- GRATION	TRAN- SITION ENERGY (MEV)
ALPHA 1	0.0520	5.5427
ALPHA 2	0.9480	5.7837
GAMMA 1	0.0520	0.2410

REF.- LEDERER, C.M. ET AL, TABLE OF ISOTOPES, 6TH. ED.

OUTPUT DATA

88 RADIUM 224 HALF LIFE = 3.64 DAYS

DECAY MODE- ALPHA

RADIATION	MEAN NUMBER/ DISINTE- GRATION n_i	MEAN ENERGY/ PAR- TICLE E_i (MeV)	EQUI- LIBRIUM DOSE CONSTANT Δ_i (g-rad/ μCi-h)
ALPHA 1	0.0520	5.4472	0.6033
RECOIL ATOM	0.0520	0.0990	0.0109
ALPHA 2	0.9480	5.6840	11.4773
RECOIL ATOM	0.9480	0.1033	0.2086
GAMMA 1	0.0400	0.2410	0.0205
K INT CON ELECT	0.0044	0.1425	0.0013
L INT CON ELECT	0.0056	0.2242	0.0026
M INT CON ELECT	0.0018	0.2374	0.0009
K ALPHA-1 X-RAY	0.0020	0.0837	0.0003
K ALPHA-2 X-RAY	0.0011	0.0810	0.0002
K BETA-1 X-RAY	0.0007	0.0948	0.0001
LMM AUGER ELECT	0.0052	0.0097	0.0001
MXY AUGER ELECT	0.0170	0.0035	0.0001

DAUGHTER NUCLIDE, RADON 220 IS RADIOACTIVE AND MAY CONTRIBUTE TO THE DOSE.

Courtesy Dillman LT and Von der Lage FC: MIRD Pamphlet No. 10, New York, 1975, Society of Nuclear Medicine.

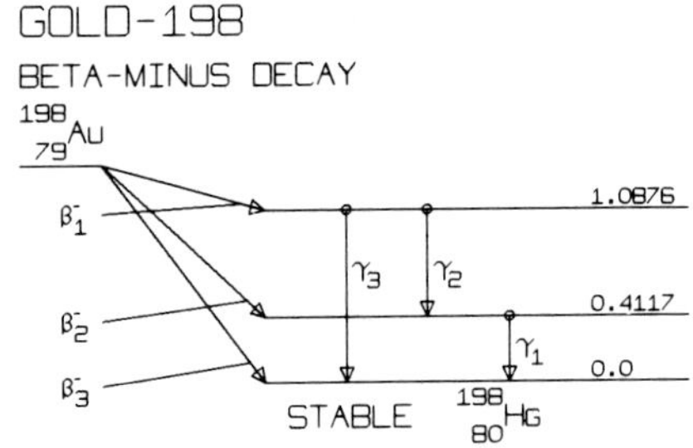

INPUT DATA

79 GOLD 198 HALF LIFE = 2.69 DAYS

DECAY MODE- BETA MINUS

TRANSITION	MEAN NUMBER/ DISINTE- GRATION	TRAN- SITION ENERGY (MEV)
BETA MINUS 1	0.0130	0.2900*
BETA MINUS 2	0.9860	0.9612*
BETA MINUS 3	0.0002	1.3710*
GAMMA 1	0.9970	0.4117
GAMMA 2	0.0110	0.6758
GAMMA 3	0.0023	1.0876

*ENDPOINT ENERGY (MEV).

REF.- NUCLEAR DATA B6, 328 (1971).

OUTPUT DATA

79 GOLD 198 HALF LIFE = 2.69 DAYS

DECAY MODE- BETA MINUS

RADIATION	MEAN NUMBER/ DISINTE- GRATION n_i	MEAN ENERGY/ PAR- TICLE $\bar{E}_i$ (MeV)	EQUI- LIBRIUM DOSE CONSTANT Δ_i (g-rad/ μCi-h)
BETA MINUS 1	0.0130	0.0811	0.0022
BETA MINUS 2	0.9860	0.3163	0.6643
BETA MINUS 3	0.0002	0.4648	0.0002
GAMMA 1	0.9555	0.4117	0.8380
K INT CON ELECT	0.0287	0.3286	0.0201
L INT CON ELECT	0.0095	0.3979	0.0081
M INT CON ELECT	0.0031	0.4089	0.0027
GAMMA 2	0.0107	0.6758	0.0154
K INT CON ELECT	0.0002	0.5927	0.0003
GAMMA 3	0.0022	1.0876	0.0053
K ALPHA-1 X-RAY	0.0139	0.0708	0.0021
K ALPHA-2 X-RAY	0.0076	0.0688	0.0011
K BETA-1 X-RAY	0.0048	0.0802	0.0008
K BETA-2 X-RAY	0.0013	0.0831	0.0002
L ALPHA X-RAYS	0.0060	0.0099	0.0001
L BETA X-RAYS	0.0056	0.0118	0.0001
LMM AUGER ELECT	0.0206	0.0081	0.0003
MXY AUGER ELECT	0.0622	0.0028	0.0003

Courtesy Dillman LT and Von der Lage FC: MIRD Pamphlet No. 10, New York, 1975, Society of Nuclear Medicine.

energy of 0.4117 MeV.

The percentage of all ^{198}Au atoms that emit a beta particle with a maximum energy of 0.29 MeV (β_1) is 1.3%. The energy state of the nucleus is raised to 1.0876 MeV. There are two ways to relieve this excited state. The nuclei may reach ground state immediately by the emission of a gamma ray of 1.0876 MeV (γ_3), or they may do it in a two-step fashion by the emission of a gamma ray of 0.6758 MeV (γ_2) plus a gamma ray of 0.4117 MeV (γ_1). Both paths represent an energy differential between parent and daughter of 1.37 MeV just as the β_2-γ_1 route does.

There is also a possibility that 0.02% of all ^{198}Au atoms would distribute all their energy to the beta particle and the antineutrino, in which case the atom decays directly by beta decay (β_3) to stable ^{198}Hg with no emission of electromagnetic radiation. The maximum energy of such a beta particle would be 1.37 MeV, the energy differential between parent and daughter.

The largest number of beta particles (98.6%) decay in such a manner as to elevate the nucleus to an energy state of 0.412 MeV. This being the case, the energy used in detecting ^{198}Au with radiation detection devices is 0.412 MeV. In addition to the 98.6%, contributions are received from $\beta^-{}_1$ since one of its paths in relieving its excited state is by the 0.412 MeV route, which further increases the percentage of atoms decaying by that energy emission to 99.7%. In looking at a gamma spectrum of ^{198}Au, if the detection device was sensitive enough, three gamma peaks would be displayed: a very large peak at 0.412 MeV and two much smaller peaks at 0.676 MeV and 1.088 MeV. The peak of choice in any study using ^{198}Au would be the peak of 0.412 MeV.

Iodine 131. An even more complex beta-gamma spectrum is that of ^{131}I. ^{131}I decays by beta decay to stable ^{131}Xe by way of metastable state of ^{131}Xe at 0.1639 MeV energy state. The nuclei of ^{131}I can decay by six different methods represented by six different beta particles all varying in energy. The differential between parent and daughter is 0.970 MeV, regardless of which beta-gamma pathway is calculated. Since 89.8% of all nuclei of ^{131}I decay by the β_5^--γ_9 pathway and γ_9 has an energy of 0.364 MeV, the energy used to detect ^{131}I is 0.364 MeV. With ^{131}I there are no contributors from other beta pathways to increase the percentage of 0.364 MeV gammas, as was the case of ^{198}Au. In fact, the opposite is true. The β_5^- pathway results in two different gammas (γ_4 and γ_9), each having different energies. In effect, this would actually reduce the percentage of nuclei giving the 0.364 MeV gamma. This is realized by the study of gamma percentages of the 89.8% of ^{131}I atoms that decay by the β_5^- route; only 83.8% continue the decay process by the γ_9 route (0.364 MeV); the remaining 6% decay by the γ_4 route.

■ Electron capture

Iodine 125. A simple decay scheme representing the electron capture phenomenon is that of ^{125}I ($Z = 53$). ^{125}I decays by electron capture to an excited state of ^{125}Te. One-hundred percent of all atoms of ^{125}I achieve this excited state in the process of their transition, which is relieved by the emission of a gamma photon of 35 keV (0.0354 MeV), an energy that represents the change in energy state from excited to ground. The daughter, ^{125}Te, has an atomic number that is less than the parent, so the diagonal line is angled to the left.

An interesting phenomenon regarding this particular radionuclide is shown in the examination of the "Output Data." As previously noted, electron capture necessarily involves the production of x-rays because of the "filling" phe-

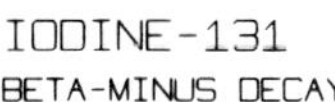

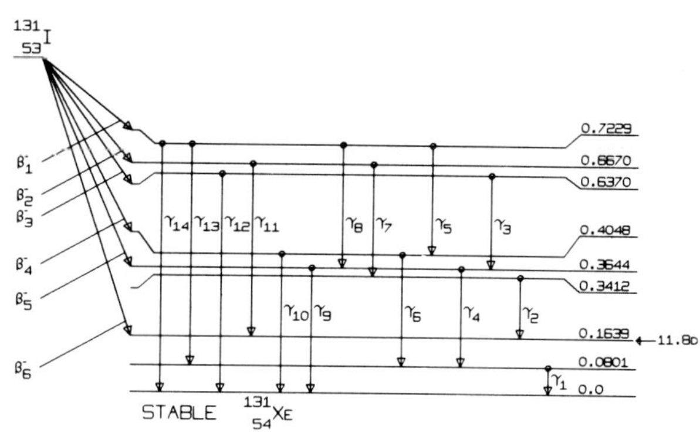

INPUT DATA

53 IODINE 131 HALF LIFE = 8.06 DAYS

DECAY MODE- BETA MINUS

TRANSITION	MEAN NUMBER/ DISINTE- GRATION	TRAN- SITION ENERGY (MEV)
BETA MINUS 1	0.0200	0.2470*
BETA MINUS 2	0.0067	0.3030*
BETA MINUS 3	0.0664	0.3330*
BETA MINUS 4	0.0000	0.5650*
BETA MINUS 5	0.8980	0.6060*
BETA MINUS 6	0.0080	0.8060*
GAMMA 1	0.0660	0.0801
GAMMA 2	0.0035	0.1772
GAMMA 3	0.0006	0.2723
GAMMA 4	0.0607	0.2843
GAMMA 5	0.0011	0.3180
GAMMA 6	0.0003	0.3250
GAMMA 7	0.0037	0.3257
GAMMA 8	0.0001	0.3585
GAMMA 9	0.8380	0.3644
GAMMA 10	0.0006	0.4048
GAMMA 11	0.0029	0.5029
GAMMA 12	0.0657	0.6367
GAMMA 13	0.0014	0.6430
GAMMA 14	0.0174	0.7228

*ENDPOINT ENERGY (MEV).

REF.- GRAEFFE, G. AND WALTERS, W.R., PHYS. REV. 153, 1321 (1967).
LEDERER, C.M. ET AL, TABLE OF ISOTOPES, 6TH. ED.

OUTPUT DATA

53 IODINE 131 HALF LIFE = 8.06 DAYS

DECAY MODE- BETA MINUS

RADIATION	MEAN NUMBER/ DISINTE- GRATION n_i	MEAN ENERGY/ PAR- TICLE $\bar{E}_i$ (MeV)	EQUI- LIBRIUM DOSE CONSTANT Δ_i (g-rad/ µCi-h)
BETA MINUS 1	0.0200	0.0691	0.0029
BETA MINUS 2	0.0067	0.0867	0.0012
BETA MINUS 3	0.0664	0.0964	0.0136
BETA MINUS 5	0.8980	0.1916	0.3666
BETA MINUS 6	0.0080	0.2859	0.0048
GAMMA 1	0.0258	0.0801	0.0044
K INT CON ELECT	0.0343	0.0456	0.0033
L INT CON ELECT	0.0043	0.0751	0.0007
M INT CON ELECT	0.0014	0.0792	0.0002
GAMMA 2	0.0029	0.1772	0.0011
K INT CON ELECT	0.0004	0.1426	0.0001
GAMMA 3	0.0006	0.2723	0.0003
GAMMA 4	0.0578	0.2843	0.0350
K INT CON ELECT	0.0023	0.2497	0.0012
L INT CON ELECT	0.0004	0.2792	0.0002
GAMMA 5	0.0010	0.3180	0.0007
GAMMA 6	0.0003	0.3250	0.0002
GAMMA 7	0.0036	0.3257	0.0025
GAMMA 8	0.0001	0.3585	0.0001
GAMMA 9	0.8201	0.3644	0.6366
K INT CON ELECT	0.0147	0.3299	0.0103
L INT CON ELECT	0.0023	0.3594	0.0017
M INT CON ELECT	0.0007	0.3635	0.0006
GAMMA 10	0.0006	0.4048	0.0005
GAMMA 11	0.0029	0.5029	0.0031
GAMMA 12	0.0653	0.6367	0.0886
K INT CON ELECT	0.0002	0.6021	0.0003
GAMMA 13	0.0014	0.6430	0.0020
GAMMA 14	0.0173	0.7228	0.0267
K ALPHA-1 X-RAY	0.0249	0.0297	0.0015
K ALPHA-2 X-RAY	0.0128	0.0294	0.0008
K BETA-1 X-RAY	0.0068	0.0336	0.0004
K BETA-2 X-RAY	0.0014	0.0345	0.0001
KLL AUGER ELECT	0.0041	0.0244	0.0002
KLX AUGER ELECT	0.0018	0.0285	0.0001
LMM AUGER ELECT	0.0477	0.0031	0.0003
MXY AUGER ELECT	0.1147	0.0009	0.0002

DAUGHTER NUCLIDE, XENON 131M IS RADIOACTIVE AND MAY CONTRIBUTE TO THE DOSE.
BRANCHING TO 0.1639 MEV, 11.8 DAY HALF LIFE, ISOMERIC LEVEL IN XENON-131 IS 0.0144 PER DISINTEGRATION OF IODINE-131.

Courtesy Dillman LT and Von der Lage FC: MIRD Pamphlet No. 10, New York, 1975, Society of Nuclear Medicine.

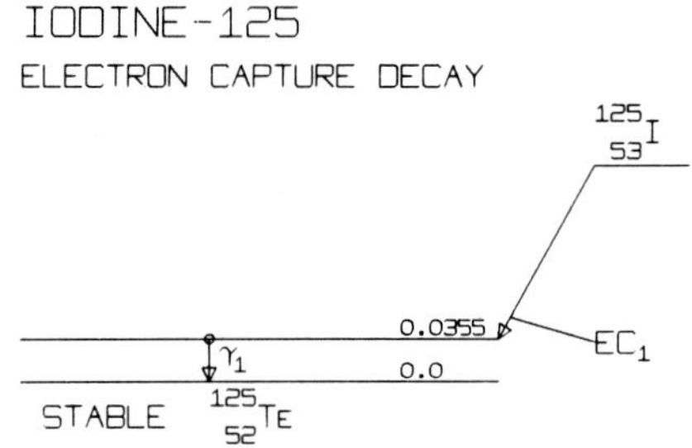

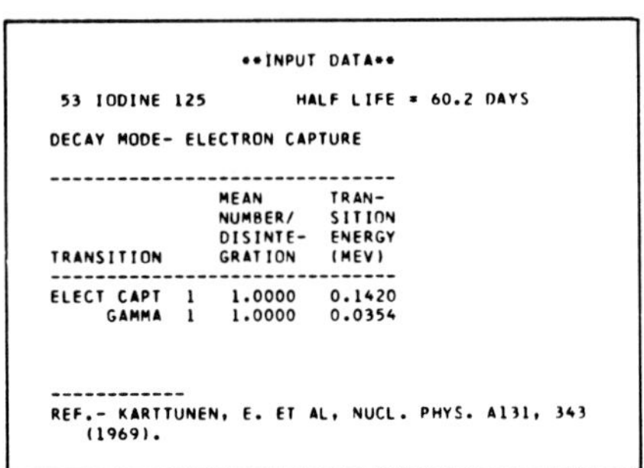

INPUT DATA

53 IODINE 125 HALF LIFE = 60.2 DAYS

DECAY MODE- ELECTRON CAPTURE

TRANSITION	MEAN NUMBER/ DISINTE-GRATION	TRAN-SITION ENERGY (MEV)
ELECT CAPT 1	1.0000	0.1420
GAMMA 1	1.0000	0.0354

REF.- KARTTUNEN, E. ET AL, NUCL. PHYS. A131, 343 (1969).

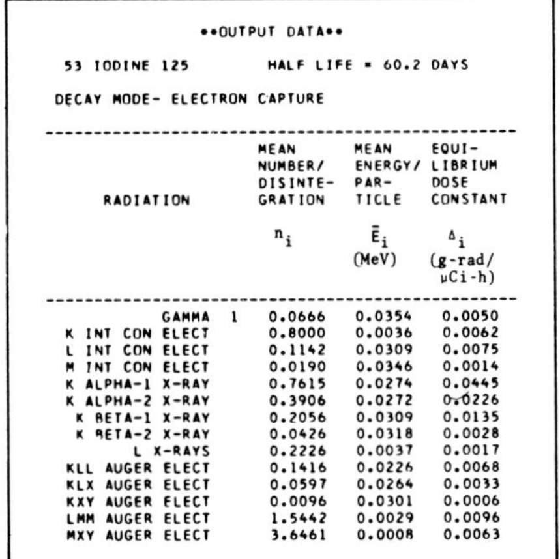

OUTPUT DATA

53 IODINE 125 HALF LIFE = 60.2 DAYS

DECAY MODE- ELECTRON CAPTURE

RADIATION	MEAN NUMBER/ DISINTE-GRATION n_i	MEAN ENERGY/ PAR-TICLE $\bar{E}_i$ (MeV)	EQUI-LIBRIUM DOSE CONSTANT Δ_i (g-rad/ μCi-h)
GAMMA 1	0.0666	0.0354	0.0050
K INT CON ELECT	0.8000	0.0036	0.0062
L INT CON ELECT	0.1142	0.0309	0.0075
M INT CON ELECT	0.0190	0.0346	0.0014
K ALPHA-1 X-RAY	0.7615	0.0274	0.0445
K ALPHA-2 X-RAY	0.3906	0.0272	0.0226
K BETA-1 X-RAY	0.2056	0.0309	0.0135
K BETA-2 X-RAY	0.0426	0.0318	0.0028
L X-RAYS	0.2226	0.0037	0.0017
KLL AUGER ELECT	0.1416	0.0226	0.0068
KLX AUGER ELECT	0.0597	0.0264	0.0033
KXY AUGER ELECT	0.0096	0.0301	0.0006
LMM AUGER ELECT	1.5442	0.0029	0.0096
MXY AUGER ELECT	3.6461	0.0008	0.0063

Courtesy Dillman LT and Von der Lage FC: MIRD Pamphlet No. 10, New York, 1975, Society of Nuclear Medicine.

CHROMIUM-51
ELECTRON CAPTURE DECAY
51 24 CR
0.3200
EC1
γ1
0.0
EC2
STABLE
51 23 V

INPUT DATA

24 CHROMIUM 51 HALF LIFE = 27.7 DAYS

DECAY MODE- ELECTRON CAPTURE

TRANSITION	MEAN NUMBER/ DISINTE-GRATION	TRAN-SITION ENERGY (MEV)
ELECT CAPT 1	0.1020	0.4310
ELECT CAPT 2	0.8980	0.7550
GAMMA 1	0.1020	0.3200

REF.- RIBORDY, CL. AND HUBER, O., HELVETICA PHYSICA ACTA 43, 345 (1970).

OUTPUT DATA

24 CHROMIUM 51 HALF LIFE = 27.7 DAYS

DECAY MODE- ELECTRON CAPTURE

RADIATION	MEAN NUMBER/ DISINTE-GRATION n_i	MEAN ENERGY/ PAR-TICLE $\bar{E}_i$ (MeV)	EQUI-LIBRIUM DOSE CONSTANT Δ_i (g-rad/ μCi-h)
GAMMA 1	0.1018	0.3200	0.0694
K ALPHA-1 X-RAY	0.1289	0.0049	0.0013
K ALPHA-2 X-RAY	0.0659	0.0049	0.0006
K BETA-1 X-RAY	0.0224	0.0054	0.0002
KLL AUGER ELECT	0.5614	0.0044	0.0052
KLX AUGER ELECT	0.1240	0.0048	0.0012
LMM AUGER ELECT	1.5323	0.0004	0.0014
MXY AUGER ELECT	3.2177	0.0000	0.0002

Courtesy Dillman LT and Von der Lage FC: MIRD Pamphlet No. 10, New York, 1975, Society of Nuclear Medicine.

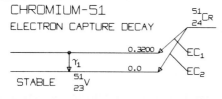

nomenon; it can also result in the production of x-rays as a result of *internal conversion*. While this is a phenomenon common to many radionuclides, it is of particular interest with ^{125}I, since the energies of all of these x-rays (see mean energies $\overline{E}_1$ of K alpha and K beta x-rays in "Output Data") are close to the transition energy of the gamma photon (see Gamma-1 in "Input Data") and therefore indistinguishable with the use of routine nuclear medicine laboratory counting equipment. Further, since many of these events occur, for all practical purposes, at the same time, a second energy peak can be found around 55 to 60 keV, representing a coincident counting of these simultaneous events. Since these simultaneous counting events occur as a constant percentage of the number of disintegrating atoms, it is considered proper to include these counts in the windows used for in vitro counting. This relationship could be destroyed, of course, if the amount of radioactivity in the sample were greater than the counting capacity of the instrument. See Chapter 12 for a discussion of this matter.

Chromium 51. Another radionuclide used in nuclear medicine procedures that involves electron capture is ^{51}Cr. ^{51}Cr decays to ^{51}V by two methods of electron capture. Eighty-nine and eight-tenths percent of all atoms of ^{51}Cr decay by electron capture to the ground state of ^{51}V, whereas 10.2% leave the nuclei in an excited energy state. The 10.2% that decay by way of the excited nucleus do so by raising its nuclear energy state to 0.320 MeV. That energy state is instantaneously relieved by the release of a gamma photon equivalent to the change in energy state (0.320 MeV). ^{51}V is a stable form of the element vanadium.

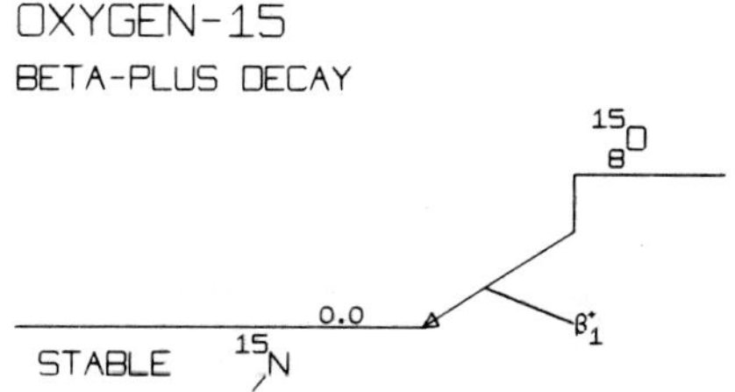

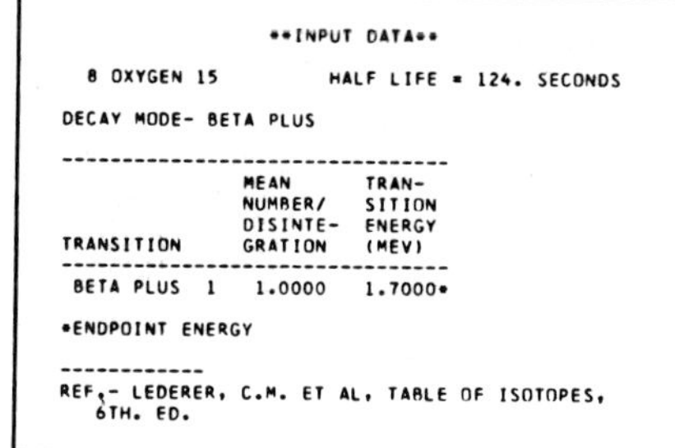

INPUT DATA

8 OXYGEN 15 HALF LIFE = 124. SECONDS

DECAY MODE- BETA PLUS

TRANSITION	MEAN NUMBER/ DISINTE- GRATION	TRAN- SITION ENERGY (MEV)
BETA PLUS 1	1.0000	1.7000*

*ENDPOINT ENERGY

REF.- LEDERER, C.M. ET AL, TABLE OF ISOTOPES, 6TH. ED.

OUTPUT DATA

8 OXYGEN 15 HALF LIFE = 124. SECONDS

DECAY MODE- BETA PLUS

RADIATION	MEAN NUMBER/ DISINTE- GRATION n_i	MEAN ENERGY/ PAR- TICLE $\bar{E}_i$ (MeV)	EQUI- LIBRIUM DOSE CONSTANT Δ_i (g-rad/ μCi-h)
BETA PLUS 1	1.0000	0.7206	1.5349
ANNIH. RADIATION	2.0000	0.5110	2.1768

Courtesy Dillman LT and Von der Lage FC: MIRD Pamphlet No. 10, New York, 1975, Society of Nuclear Medicine.

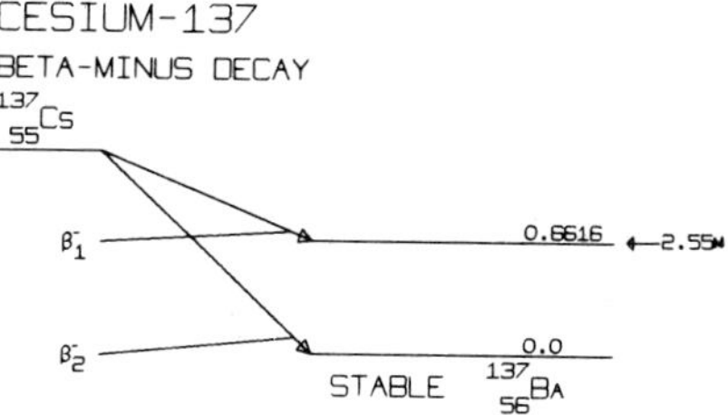

INPUT DATA

55 CESIUM 137 HALF LIFE = 30.0 YEARS

DECAY MODE- BETA MINUS

TRANSITION	MEAN NUMBER/ DISINTE- GRATION	TRAN- SITION ENERGY (MEV)
BETA MINUS 1	0.9460	0.5140*
BETA MINUS 2	0.0540	1.1760*

*ENDPOINT ENERGY (KEV).

REF.- HANSEN, H.H. ET AL, Z. PHYSIK 218,425 (1969).
KARTASHOV, V.M. ET AL, SOV. J. NUCL. PHYS. 6, 656 (1968).

OUTPUT DATA

55 CESIUM 137 HALF LIFE = 30.0 YEARS

DECAY MODE- BETA MINUS

RADIATION	MEAN NUMBER/ DISINTE- GRATION n_i	MEAN ENERGY/ PAR- TICLE $\bar{E}_i$ (MeV)	EQUI- LIBRIUM DOSE CONSTANT Δ_i (g-rad/ μCi-h)
BETA MINUS 1	0.9460	0.1747	0.3520
BETA MINUS 2	0.0540	0.4269	0.0491

DAUGHTER NUCLIDE, BARIUM 137M IS RADIOACTIVE AND MAY CONTRIBUTE TO THE DOSE.
BRANCHING TO 0.6616 MEV, 2.55 MINUTE HALF LIFE, ISOMERIC LEVEL IN BARIUM-137 IS 0.946 PER DISINTEGRATION OF CESIUM-137.

Courtesy Dillman LT and Von der Lage FC: MIRD Pamphlet No. 10, New York, 1975, Society of Nuclear Medicine.

As with the decay of ^{125}I to ^{125}Te, ^{51}Cr produces a daughter nuclide that is reduced in atomic number; therefore the diagonal of the decay scheme is angled to the left. It is interesting to note that this gamma peak of 320 keV represents only 10.2% of all the available atoms of chromium in any sample. The other 89.8% go undetected by standard detection methods. This also explains the unusual readings on dose calibrator constancy checks when ^{51}Cr is measured using a constancy source.

■ Positron (beta-plus) decay

Oxygen 15. ^{15}O is an example of a positron emitter. ^{15}O (Z = 8) decays to ^{15}N (Z = 7), which is stable. One-hundred percent of all atoms of ^{15}O decay directly to their

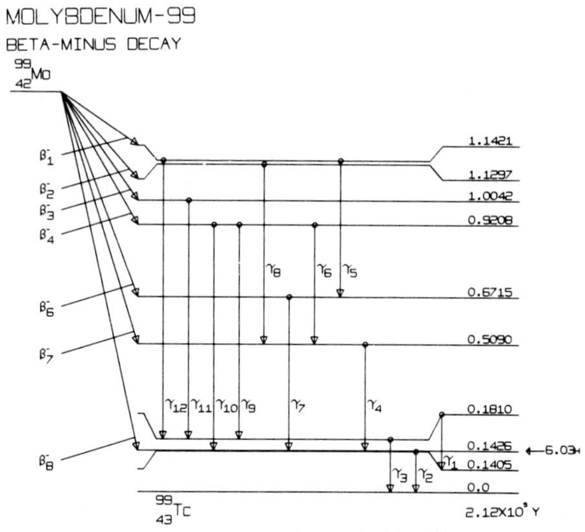

INPUT DATA

42 MOLYBDENUM 99 HALF LIFE = 66.7 HOURS

DECAY MODE- BETA MINUS

TRANSITION	MEAN NUMBER/ DISINTE- GRATION	TRAN- SITION ENERGY (MEV)
BETA MINUS 1	0.0012	0.2340*
BETA MINUS 2	0.0001	0.2470*
BETA MINUS 3	0.0014	0.3730*
BETA MINUS 4	0.1850	0.4560*
BETA MINUS 5	0.0001	0.6150*
BETA MINUS 6	0.0004	0.7050*
BETA MINUS 7	0.0143	0.8680*
BETA MINUS 8	0.7970	1.2340*
GAMMA 1	0.0630	0.0405
GAMMA 2	0.0633	0.1405
GAMMA 3	0.0760	0.1810
GAMMA 4	0.0145	0.3664
GAMMA 5	0.0001	0.3807
GAMMA 6	0.0002	0.4115

INPUT DATA

42 MOLYBDENUM 99 (CONTINUED)

TRANSITION	MEAN NUMBER/ DISINTE- GRATION	TRAN- SITION ENERGY (MEV)
GAMMA 7	0.0005	0.5289
GAMMA 8	0.0002	0.6207
GAMMA 9	0.1370	0.7397
GAMMA 10	0.0480	0.7782
GAMMA 11	0.0014	0.8231
GAMMA 12	0.0011	0.9610

*ENDPOINT ENERGY (MEV).

REF.- VAN EIJK, C.W. ET AL, NUCL. PHYS. A121, 440 (1968).

OUTPUT DATA

42 MOLYBDENUM 99 HALF LIFE = 66.7 HOURS

DECAY MODE- BETA MINUS

RADIATION	MEAN NUMBER/ DISINTE- GRATION n_i	MEAN ENERGY/ PAR- TICLE $\bar{E}_i$ (MeV)	EQUI- LIBRIUM DOSE CONSTANT Δ_i (g-rad/ μCi-h)
BETA MINUS 1	0.0012	0.0658	0.0001
BETA MINUS 3	0.0014	0.1112	0.0003
BETA MINUS 4	0.1850	0.1401	0.0552
BETA MINUS 6	0.0004	0.2541	0.0002
BETA MINUS 7	0.0143	0.2981	0.0090
BETA MINUS 8	0.7970	0.4519	0.7673
GAMMA 1	0.0130	0.0405	0.0011
K INT CON ELECT	0.0428	0.0195	0.0017
L INT CON ELECT	0.0053	0.0377	0.0004
M INT CON ELECT	0.0017	0.0401	0.0001
GAMMA 2	0.0564	0.1405	0.0168
K INT CON ELECT	0.0058	0.1194	0.0014
L INT CON ELECT	0.0007	0.1377	0.0002
GAMMA 3	0.0657	0.1810	0.0253
K INT CON ELECT	0.0085	0.1600	0.0029
L INT CON ELECT	0.0012	0.1782	0.0004
M INT CON ELECT	0.0004	0.1806	0.0001
GAMMA 4	0.0143	0.3664	0.0112
GAMMA 5	0.0001	0.3807	0.0000
GAMMA 6	0.0002	0.4115	0.0002
GAMMA 7	0.0005	0.5289	0.0005
GAMMA 8	0.0002	0.6207	0.0003
GAMMA 9	0.1367	0.7397	0.2154
K INT CON ELECT	0.0002	0.7186	0.0003
GAMMA 10	0.0479	0.7782	0.0794
K INT CON ELECT	0.0000	0.7571	0.0001
GAMMA 11	0.0014	0.8231	0.0024
GAMMA 12	0.0011	0.9610	0.0022
K ALPHA-1 X-RAY	0.0253	0.0183	0.0009
K ALPHA-2 X-RAY	0.0127	0.0182	0.0004
K BETA-1 X-RAY	0.0060	0.0206	0.0002
KLL AUGER ELECT	0.0087	0.0154	0.0002
KLX AUGER ELECT	0.0032	0.0178	0.0001
LMM AUGER ELECT	0.0615	0.0019	0.0002
MXY AUGER ELECT	0.1403	0.0004	0.0001

DAUGHTER NUCLIDE, TECHNETIUM 99M IS RADIOACTIVE AND MAY CONTRIBUTE TO THE DOSE.
BRANCHING TO 0.1426 MEV, 6.03 HOUR HALF LIFE, ISOMERIC LEVEL IN TECHNETIUM-99 IS 0.860 PER DISINTEGRATION OF MOLYBDENUM-99.

Courtesy Dillman LT and Von der Lage FC: MIRD Pamphlet No. 10, New York, 1975, Society of Nuclear Medicine.

ground state, with no energy remaining to excite the nucleus and, consequently, no gamma photon emission. The energy differential between the daughter and parent is 1.7000 MeV, which is seen in the "Input Data" box as the transition energy of the positron particle. This energy is shared with the neutrino as they are both ejected from the nucleus, much the same as in beta decay. The daughter product has a decrease in atomic number so that the diagonals are angled to the left. Since this radionuclide is a pure positron emitter, the only way that it is useful to photon-sensitive (gamma or x-rays) counting equipment, such as that found in routine nuclear medicine departments, is through the eventual annihilation of the positron and the subsequent release of two gamma photons.

■ Isomeric transition

Cesium 137. A simple example of a decay scheme representing isomeric transition is ^{137}Cs. ^{137}Cs ($Z = 55$) decays by 2 beta particles of 0.514 MeV and 1.1760 MeV. The beta particle having a maximum energy of 0.514 MeV (β_1^-) represents 94.6% of all ^{137}Cs atoms; the 1.1760 MeV beta particle (β_2^-) represents only 5.4% of all the atoms of ^{137}Cs. β_2^- decays directly to ground state ^{137}Ba ($Z = 56$), which is stable. β_1^- decays to an excited state of the nucleus. Unlike other forms of decay in which there is an excited state of the nucleus, this excitation state can be held for a half-life of 2.55 minutes. This isomeric state is known to be ^{137m}Ba ($Z = 56$). The isomer decays to ground state, ^{137}Ba, releasing a gamma photon of 0.662 MeV. The transition from parent to daughter represents an energy differential of 1.176 MeV. The daughter product has an increased atomic number, so the diagonals are angled to the right.

Molybdenum 99. A more complex decay scheme representing isomeric transition and pertinent to nuclear medicine is ^{99}Mo. All atoms of ^{99}Mo ($Z = 42$) have a 66.7-hour half-life and decay by 1 of 8 beta particles to ^{99}Tc ($Z = 43$) through the isomeric state of ^{99m}Tc. This isomeric state has a half-life of 6.03 hours and is the form of the radionuclide that is of interest in nuclear medicine procedures. ^{99}Mo decays primarily (79.7%) by a beta particle (β_8^-) having an energy of 1.234 MeV to the metastable form of technetium with an increased nuclear energy state of 0.1405 MeV. It relieves that energy state by the emission of a gamma photon (γ_2) of 0.1405 MeV. The transition from ^{99}Mo to ^{99}Tc represents an energy change of 1.376 MeV, regardless of which pathway the nucleus decays. ^{99}Tc is itself unstable, having a half-life of 2.12×10^5 years, and decays by beta decay, with no electromagnetic radiation, to ^{99}Ru, a stable form of that element.

BIBLIOGRAPHY

Bernier, D.R., Langan, J.K., and Wells, L.D.: Nuclear medicine technology and techniques, ed. 2, St. Louis, 1989, Mosby–Year Book.

Blahd, W.H.: Nuclear medicine, New York, 1965, McGraw-Hill Book Co.

Bogardus, C.R., Jr.: Clinical applications of physics of radiology and nuclear medicine, St. Louis, 1969, Warren H. Green, Inc.

Casarett, A.P.: Radiation biology, Englewood Cliffs, N.J., 1968, Prentice-Hall, Inc.

Chandra, R.: Introductory physics of nuclear medicine, ed. 4, Philadelphia, 1992, Lea & Febiger.

Dillman, L.T., and von der Lage, F.C.: Radionuclide decay schemes and nuclear parameters for use in radiation-dose estimation, MIRD Pamphlet No. 10, New York, 1975, Society of Nuclear Medicine.

Goodwin, P.N., and Rao, D.V.: An introduction to the physics of nuclear medicine, Springfield, Ill., 1977, Charles C Thomas, Publisher.

Gottschalk, A., and Potchen, E.J.: Diagnostic nuclear medicine, Baltimore, 1976, The Williams & Wilkins Co.

Hendee, W.R.: Medical radiation physics, ed. 2, Chicago, 1979, Year Book Medical Publishers, Inc.

Johns, H.E. and Cunningham, J.R.: The physics of radiology, ed. 4, revised edition, Springfield, Ill., 1983, Charles C Thomas, Publisher.

King, E.R., and Mitchell, T.G.: A manual for nuclear medicine, Springfield, Ill., 1961, Charles C Thomas, Publisher.

Quimby, E.H., and Feitelberg, S.: Radioactive isotopes in medicine and biology, ed. 2, Philadelphia, 1963, Lea & Febiger.

Rocha, A.F.G., and Harbert, J.C.: Textbook of nuclear medicine: basic science, Philadelphia, 1978, Lea & Febiger.

Rollo, F.D.: Nuclear medicine physics, instrumentation, and agents, St. Louis, 1977, Mosby–Year Book.

Shilling, C.W.: Atomic energy encyclopedia in the life sciences, Philadelphia, 1964, W.B. Saunders Co.

Shapiro, J.: Radiation protection: A guide for scientists and physicians, ed. 2, Cambridge, Mass., 1981, Harvard University Press.

Sorenson, J.A., and Phelps, M.E.: Physics in nuclear medicine, ed. 2, New York, 1987, Grune & Stratton, Inc.

Wagner, H.N.: Principles of nuclear medicine, Philadelphia, 1968, W.B. Saunders Co.

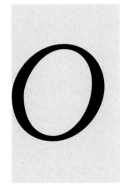

Chapter 5

RIGIN OF NUCLIDES

PAUL J. EARLY
MARSHALL BRUCER

Following is a discussion (by PJE) of six methods whereby nuclides are produced, not all of which are currently used to obtain the nuclides needed in a nuclear medicine department.

■ FISSION

Fission, stated simply, is the production of small nuclei from a large nucleus. It may be strictly defined as an exergonic (energy-liberating) process of splitting certain heavy nuclei into two more or less equal fragments. These fragments are known as fission products. Fission may occur spontaneously or may be induced by the capture of bombarding particles, primarily neutrons. In addition to fission fragments, neutrons and energy in the form of gamma rays are usually by-products. The fission products from such reactions are generally from atomic numbers 42 (molybdenum) to 56 (barium) but may range from atomic numbers 30 through 64. Approximately 200 different radioactive nuclides are formed as fission products in the detonation of a nuclear device (atomic bomb). Uranium and plutonium are generally used in a nuclear reactor to produce some of the radioactive materials used in nuclear medicine. There are 40 or more different ways in which the nuclei of uranium and plutonium can split when fission occurs so that 80 or more different fission products can be produced.

Fission is a process that can either be controlled (the energy released does not reach explosive quantities) or uncontrolled as in an atomic device. The latter results in a nuclear explosion. The controlling of a fission reaction is based primarily on the slowing down of the highly energetic neutrons released from the reaction. Following is a typical example of a fission reaction:

^{235}U absorbs a neutron to become ^{236}U, liberating 2 neutrons plus energy in the form of gamma photons. ^{236}U splits into approximately two equal parts to begin two fission chains. One of these chains begins with ^{99}Mo and continues to stable $^{99}_{44}Ru$; the other begins with ^{131}Sn and continues to the stable ^{131}Xe. Involved in these two fission chains are several radionuclides, other forms of which are used in nuclear medicine procedures (radioisotopes of molybdenum, tin, iodine, and xenon). Obviously, this could be one method of producing radionuclides for use in nuclear medicine. This is currently the method of producing ^{99}Mo for fission generators, the parent of the "fission moly" generators.

According to this reaction, each fission process liberates 6 neutrons. Assuming that each neutron generates another identical fission process, 36 neutrons would be released in the second generation. If each of these neutrons generated an identical fission process, the third generation would release 216 neutrons; the fourth, 1296 neutrons; and so on. Should this fission process go uncontrolled, the amount of energy and continued production of neutrons would reach the point of explosion. Such is the case of the atomic bomb. It has been calculated that in fewer than 90 generations the neutron yield would be sufficient to cause the fission of every nucleus in 110 pounds of uranium. This would result in the liberation of the same amount of energy as in the explosion of 1 million tons of TNT. If uncontrolled, this ninetieth generation will be attained in less than one-millionth of a second.

■ Nuclear reactors

What takes place in a nuclear reactor is an example of the control of fission resulting in a self-sustaining reaction.

$$
\begin{array}{lll}
 & & \nearrow {}^{99}_{42}\mathrm{Mo} \xrightarrow{\beta^-} {}^{99}_{43}\mathrm{Tc} \xrightarrow{\beta^-} {}^{99}_{44}\mathrm{Ru}\ \text{(stable)} \\
{}^{235}_{92}\mathrm{U} + {}^{1}_{0}\mathrm{n} \longrightarrow {}^{236}_{92}\mathrm{U} & & \qquad + 6\,{}^{1}_{0}\mathrm{n} + \text{energy} \\
 & & \searrow {}^{131}_{50}\mathrm{Sn} \xrightarrow{\beta^-} {}^{131}_{51}\mathrm{Sb} \xrightarrow{\beta^-} {}^{131}_{52}\mathrm{Te} \xrightarrow{\beta^-} {}^{131}_{53}\mathrm{I} \xrightarrow{\beta^-} {}^{131}_{54}\mathrm{Xe}\ \text{(stable)}
\end{array}
$$

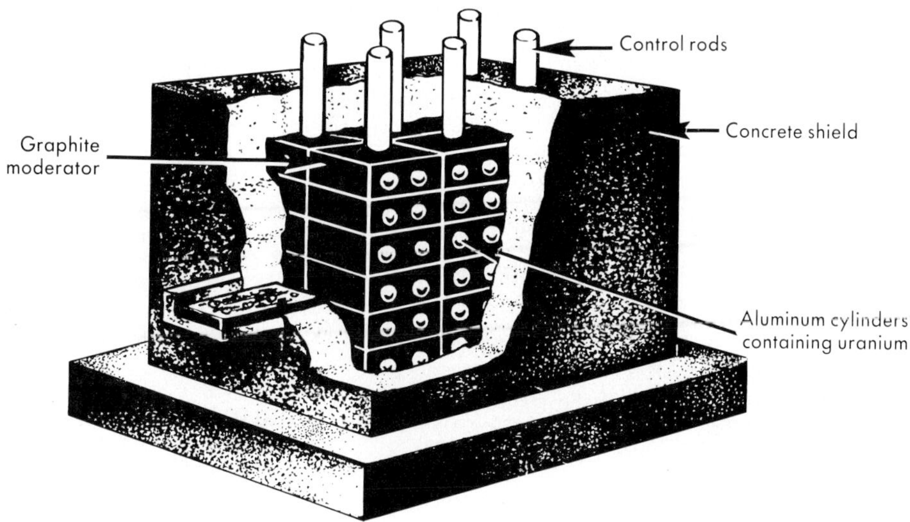

Fig. 5-1. Nuclear reactor.

A nuclear reactor (Fig. 5-1) consists of a central core surrounded by water and/or a graphite reflector. The core consists of (1) the fuel element (for example, uranium 235) as the fissionable material, arranged as plates or cylinders; (2) moderators, composed of low *Z* material, to reduce the energy of the neutrons; and (3) control rods, composed of materials, such as boron and cadmium, which have a high efficiency for absorbing neutrons, thereby preventing a nuclear melt-down. These rods are positioned in the core as needed to control the sustained reaction.

The moderators are necessary because the neutrons that are released from the fission process are of the high-energy type. As such, they become inefficient in sustaining the fission process, which requires low-energy (thermal) neutrons. The job of the moderator is to slow down the neutrons so that they can be effective in the fission process. Further, it is important that the moderator material does not have a high absorption capability for neutrons. Graphite, heavy water, and beryllium are examples of good moderator materials.

With any nuclear reaction, heat is generated. The heat within the nuclear reactor is dissipated by cooling the core with water. The graphite reflector is used to reduce the escape of neutrons by causing the neutrons to be scattered randomly many times. In this way most of them are returned to the core.

When reactors are used to produce radionuclides (by transmutation or neutron activation), stable forms of the required elements are also positioned inside the core of the reactor and allowed to be irradiated.

The first self-sustaining nuclear reaction was carried out on December 2, 1942, under the bleachers of the football stadium at the University of Chicago. When the football stadium was torn down some time later, the reactor was moved to Argonne National Laboratory.

■ NEUTRON ACTIVATION (NEUTRON CAPTURE)

One of the most common production methods of radioactive materials used in nuclear medicine departments is neutron activation (neutron capture). Neutron activation involves the capture of a neutron into a stable nucleus with the subsequent emission of a gamma ray. This process is usually referred to as an (n, γ) process. Production of ^{32}P from ^{31}P by neutron activation is written as follows:

$$^{31}P + {}^{1}_{0}n \rightarrow {}^{32}P + \gamma$$

Following is a shorthand method for indicating this neutron activation phenomenon:

$$^{31}P\ (n, \gamma)\ {}^{32}P$$

The product is always an isotope of the target element, but since it has incorporated a neutron into its nucleus, the product has a mass number increased by 1. The process usually involves neutrons of relatively low energy called *slow neutrons,* or *thermal neutrons.* The bombardment of stable forms of an element by neutrons is generally carried out in nuclear reactors.

Neutron activation, in addition to being a means of obtaining radionuclides, has also become a dynamic tool in research and is developing into an exciting new field in medicine. Many areas of use have not even been touched yet. Some, however, are well known. Neutron activation is used not only in medicine but also in the field of crime detection. Neutron activation analysis has been used to determine the presence of heavy metal poisons in tissues. This has been extremely valuable in medical-legal problems. It can also be used to quantitate very small quantities of elements in serum and other biologic samples. A human hair can be subjected to neutron activation for purposes of identification, chemical analysis, and so on. A paper chromatograph of a serum sample can be subjected to neutron activation analysis in an effort to determine the constituents of the serum. These are just a few current applications of neutron activation.

Since the product of such a reaction is an isotope of the target element, there is no possible way to separate these on a chemical basis. Furthermore, it is impossible to create a situation in the reactor whereby all atoms of ^{31}P incorporate a neutron to become ^{32}P. The material that is removed from the reactor after bombardment is necessarily a mixture of the two isotopes. For this reason, the ^{32}P administered to a patient will also have a certain amount of stable ^{31}P. The latter is referred to as a *carrier*.* To inform the user of the quantity of ^{31}P in the ^{32}P dose, the terms *specific weight* and *specific activity* are often used.

■ Specific weight

It is often the problem of the researcher to determine the specific weight of the material introduced into the human body. Knowing the specific weight becomes valuable from the standpoint of toxicity, in that the researcher does not want to approach the toxic dose of any material to successfully perform the study. Also, the "load" introduced into the human body must not upset the normal physiologic balance of the material. For example, if in any thyroid diagnostic procedure the amount of iodine exceeds the normal daily intake, the normal physiology of the thyroid is altered.

■ Problem

An ^{131}I dosage of 50 μCi (1.85 MBq) is used as an uptake and scanning dose. How much ^{131}I is introduced into the iodine pool? (^{131}I is used as the example because it is carrier-free.)

■ Solution

The determination of specific weight involves two mathematical procedures: (1) determination of the number of atoms in the sample and (2) determination of the specific weight. These are calculated as follows:

1. Determine the number of atoms by the formula:

$$\lambda N = A$$

A = Activity in disintegrations per minute (1 μCi or 37 kBq = 2.22×10^6 dpm; so 50 μCi or 1.85 MBq = 1.11×10^8 dpm)

$\lambda = \frac{0.693}{T_p}$ (since A is in minute units, so must T_p)

N = Number of atoms

*The amount of carrier present in radiopharmaceuticals is usually too small to be measured by ordinary chemical or physical means. Since materials in such small amounts are known to sometimes behave chemically in an unpredictable manner, carriers in the form of nonradioactive isotopes are sometimes added during processing to permit ease of handling. This is referred to as *carrier-added*. However, amounts of these carriers must be kept to a minimum to prevent undesirable physiologic reactions.

Solving for N:

$$\frac{0.693}{8.1 \text{ days} \times 24 \text{ hr/day} \times 60 \text{ min/hr}} \times N = 1.11 \times 10^8 \text{ dpm}$$

$$\frac{0.693}{11{,}664} N = 1.11 \times 10^8$$

$$5.94 \times 10^{-5} N = 1.11 \times 10^8$$
$$N = 1.87 \times 10^{12}$$

2. Determine specific weight of the sample by the formula:

$$W = \frac{A \times N}{K}$$

W = Weight of sample (grams)
A = Atomic weight of radionuclide
N = Number of atoms
K = Avogadro's number = 6×10^{23}

Solving for W:

$$W = \frac{131 \times 1.87 \times 10^{12}}{6 \times 10^{23}}$$

$$= \frac{244.97 \times 10^{12}}{6 \times 10^{23}}$$

$$= 40.83 \times 10^{-11} \text{ grams or } 4 \times 10^{-7} \text{ mg or } 4 \times 10^{-4} \text{ μg}$$

It has been determined that a 50 μCi (1.85 MBq) dosage introduces 0.0004 μg of ^{131}I into the iodine pool. Since the daily adult intake of iodine is considerably more than this,* the iodine pool remains physiologically unaltered. Furthermore, approximately 20 mCi (740 MBq) could be administered without altering the iodine pool.

■ Specific activity

Another parameter of interest in nuclear medicine and one that relates activity to weight is specific activity. Specific activity is strictly defined as the ratio of activity to the specific weight of the radionuclide. It is usually expressed as millicuries per milligram or curies per gram. Using the information just determined on specific weight and the strict definition of specific activity, the preparation in the problem just given would have a specific activity of:

$$\frac{50 \text{ μCi}}{40 \times 10^{-8} \text{ mg}} = \frac{50 \times 10^{-3} \text{ mCi}}{40 \times 10^{-8} \text{ mg}}$$
$$= 1.25 \times 10^5 \text{ mCi/mg (or 4.6 TBq/mg)}$$

The strict definition of specific activity is rarely used with commercial preparations of radionuclides, however. The specific weight used in their formula is sometimes the weight of the stable nuclide or, more commonly, the weight

*In 1969 the average diet in the United States contained approximately 150 μg/day. By 1974 the average was estimated to have increased to 450 μg/day for males and 382 μg/day for females. Data suggest that these levels may eventually reach 1050 μg/day. (Data from Talbot, J.M., Fisher, D.K., and Carr, C.J.: A review of the effects of dietary iodine on certain thyroid disorders. Fed. Am. Soc. Exp. Biol. 7:11-13, 1976.)

of the chemical compound to which the radionuclide is labeled. This information regarding specific activity is found on all radiopharmaceutical labels.

Even though neutron activation is the most common method of obtaining radionuclides, the inability to separate the stable form of the element (carrier) from the unstable increases the problems of chemical toxicity levels. To obtain a desired level of radioactive material in a patient, it may be necessary to introduce an undesirable level of the element or an undesirable level of the labeled compound. (A compound is said to be labeled when it consists in part of radioactive atoms, such as ^{131}I-labeled iodohippurate sodium [Hippuran].)

Specific activity is not to be mistaken for concentration. This information is also found on all radiopharmaceutical labels. Concentration is defined as the ratio of activity to volume. It is usually expressed in units of millicuries per milliliter or microcuries per milliliter. A vial containing 10 mCi (370 MBq) activity in a volume of 10 ml will be expressed as having a concentration of 1.0 mCi/ml (37 MBq/ml). As with specific activity, this value is only true at the date and time of calibration.

■ TRANSMUTATION

Transmutation can be described as a process in which one element is converted into another. More specifically, it is the transformation of a nuclide of one element into a nuclide of a different element by nuclear reaction. Transmutation is often referred to as the answer to the alchemist's dream. Hundreds of years ago a group of "scientists" tried in vain to change common metals into gold. Their object was to bring about transmutation. Now, after years of investigation and accumulated knowledge of the nature of radioactive materials, the process of conversion from one element to another element by decay is well known. However, in the case of radionuclide production, transmutation applies specifically to converting one stable element into another unstable element. An example of such a reaction is the conversion of stable ^{32}S into radioactive ^{32}P. This is accomplished by bombarding ^{32}S with neutrons in such a manner as to eject a proton from its nucleus. In this manner, an element having one more neutron and one less proton is produced—^{32}P. This process is described as an *(n, p)* reaction according to the following:

$$^{32}_{16}S + ^{1}_{0}n \rightarrow ^{32}_{15}P + ^{1}_{1}p$$

The shorthand method is written as follows:

$$^{32}_{16}S(n, p)^{32}_{15}P$$

Like neutron activation, transmutation also involves neutron bombardment (as well as bombardment with protons, deuterons, and alpha particles). In the case of transmutation, however, rather than being bombarded with a slow neutron, the target element is bombarded with a fast neutron. The incorporation of a *fast neutron* into the nucleus is immediately followed by the emission of a proton. The advantage of the transmutation process is that the target and the product are no longer isotopes but are nuclides. Being two different elements, they are subject to separation by standard chemical techniques. ^{32}P can easily be separated from the ^{32}S. In this way a pure product of ^{32}P, referred to as *carrier-free,* is obtained. In a shipment of ^{32}P from a radiopharmaceutical supplier the specific activity on the label will indicate *C.F.* for carrier-free. Ideally, this would be the method of producing all radiopharmaceuticals, but methods by which to produce all radiopharmaceuticals in this manner are not known.

■ PARTICLE ACCELERATORS

Under the usual conditions that prevail in the atom, charged particles are unable to enter and/or interact with nuclei of other atoms because they have insufficient energy to penetrate the orbital electrons or the nucleus. A negatively charged particle, as it nears an atom, is repelled by the negatively charged orbital electrons. Likewise, a positively charged particle would be repelled by a positively charged nucleus. However, if sufficient energy is supplied to these charged particles, they can overcome these repulsion effects and penetrate the nucleus, causing an interaction. Devices that provide the energy necessary to perform this action are called *particle accelerators.* There are two basic types: the type that moves the particle in a straight path, called the *linear accelerator,* and the type that moves the particle in a circular path, such as a *cyclotron, betatron,* and *synchrotron.* Such devices can accelerate particles to the point at which they possess energy from 1 million to 1 billion eV.

■ Linear accelerator

The linear accelerator is a high-energy particle accelerator consisting of cylinders of increasing lengths arranged in a straight line. These linear accelerators can be 2 miles or more in length. The particle acceleration is provided by means of a pulsing electrostatic or magnetic field.

One explanation of the function of linear accelerators is as follows. If a positively charged particle such as an alpha particle, proton, or deuteron (nucleus of deuterium atoms) were used at the beginning of the linear accelerator and the first cylinder was charged negatively, the particle would be attracted by electrostatic attraction through the first cylinder, thereby gaining energy. As the particle nears the second cylinder, which is increased slightly in length, the charge of the cylinder through which it has just passed is reversed to a positive charge and the cylinder toward which it is approaching is charged negatively. The particle is attracted by the unlike charge in the second cylinder and repelled by the like charge in the cylinder through which it has just passed. This process of reversal of charges between cylinders continues throughout the entire length of the linear accelerator; each time it occurs the particle is acceler-

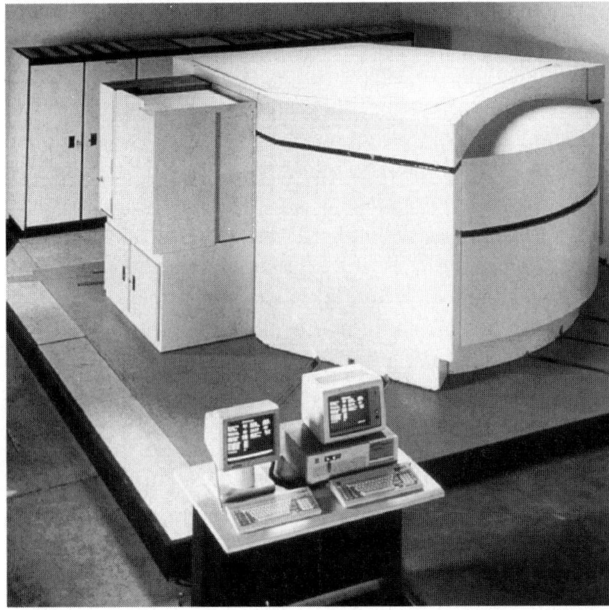

Fig. 5-2. "Baby" cyclotron (RDS cyclotron) in completely shielded state. Cyclotron can be serviced by rolling sections of the shield outward on the tracks seen on the floor. (Courtesy of Siemens Medical Systems, Inc.)

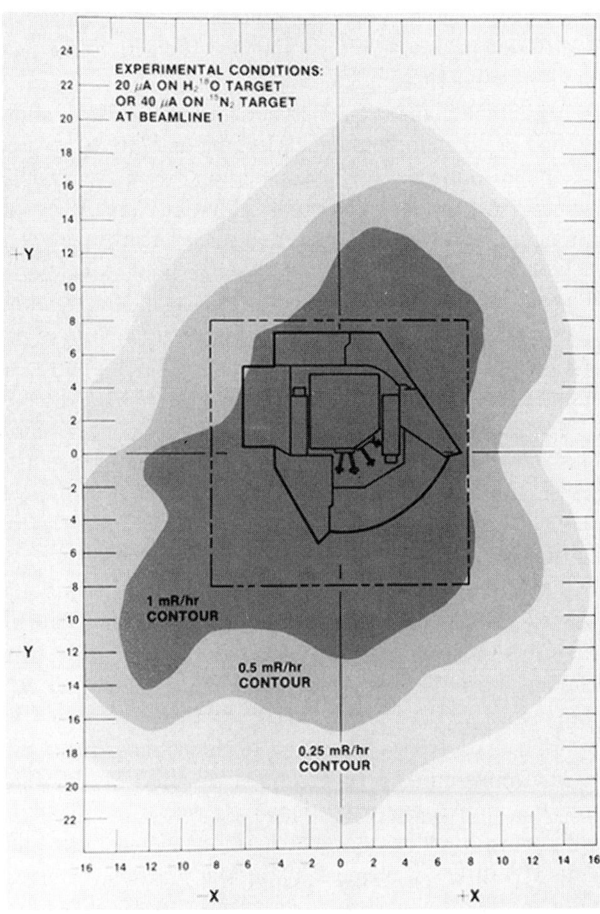

Fig. 5-3. Radiation isocontours around "baby" cyclotron during operation. (Courtesy of Siemens Medical Systems, Inc.)

ated further. In this way the particle can achieve tremendous energy levels. By achieving such high energies, the particles can overcome the repulsive effects of the nucleus and actually interact with it. In this way, stable nuclei are made unstable and accelerators become a source of radionuclides.

Another explanation of the internal workings of the linear accelerator is that electrons are fed into one end of the tube down which an electromagnetic wave of radiofrequency is traveling. The electrons are carried forward on this wave not unlike a surfboard being carried by an ocean wave. Linear accelerators of this type are used for radiotherapy. In this way very high energy electrons (4 to 8 MeV) may be produced through a distance of 1 to 2 m. It is important that charged particles are used. Higher energies are possible with greater distance. Neutrons, gamma rays, and neutrinos are unacceptable as a bombarding material in this type of unit.

■ Cyclotrons

The principle of reversed electromagnetic charges is also used in the cyclotron. The cyclotron was first described in 1931 by Lawrence and Livingston as a type of particle accelerator. In the past, cyclotrons were extremely large devices requiring thousands of square feet of floor space and tons of shielding. Current versions of cyclotrons for medical purposes, called "baby" cyclotrons, are self-contained and can be housed in a room 500 square feet (20 by 25 ft) (Fig. 5-2). The neutron and gamma attenuation properties of its polyethylene-loaded concrete (80 cm) and lead (20 cm) self-contained shield will maintain 2 mr/hr or less outside the shield during routine operation of the cyclotron (Fig. 5-3).

In the cyclotron the particles are repeatedly accelerated through intermediate voltages to achieve high energies. The cyclotron consists of two hollow semicircular pieces of metal with a gap between them. Each semicircular piece of metal is called a *dee* because of its shape, although recent versions use two quarter-circle wedges affixed opposite each other (Fig. 5-4). The dees are mounted between the poles of the large electromagnet which cause the electrons to move in a circle. The particles used as the bombarding material are introduced into the cyclotron at the center of the system. These particles are usually positively charged particles, such as protons. Their source is a small amount of hydrogen placed in the center of the cyclotron. The hydrogen is then bombarded with electrons from a tungsten filament. This action removes the single electron in the orbit of the hydrogen atom and leaves the positive ion in the source. Another technique is to place the hydrogen in a strong electrical field, thereby stripping off the single electron and leaving the proton, since the nucleus of the hy-

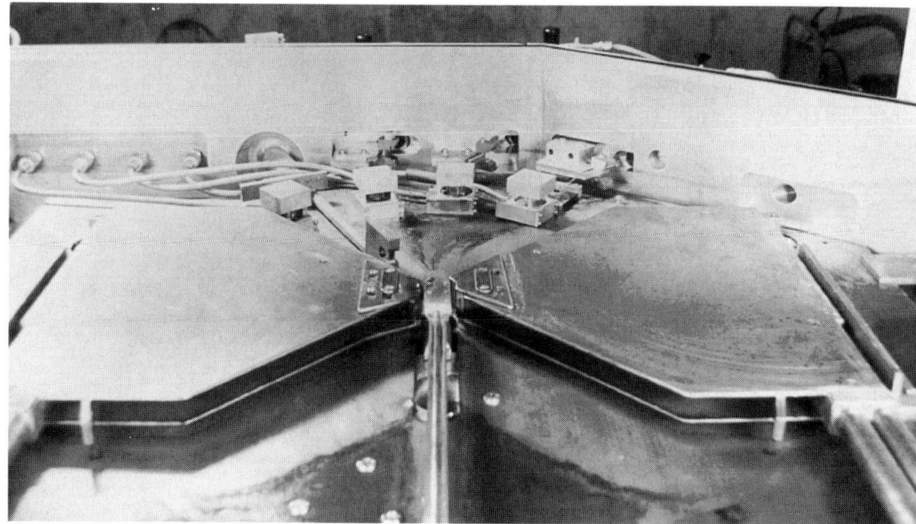

Fig. 5-4. Cutaway of a cyclotron displaying the two dees through which the charged particles are accelerated. (Courtesy of Siemens Medical Systems, Inc.)

drogen atom is a proton. Recent advances in cyclotron technology use the theory of accelerating negative ions (H^-) (Fig. 5-5) and then stripping off the two electrons of this hydrogen atom through the use of stripping foils before it bombards the target. The advantage to this technique is that the components of the cyclotron do not become radioactive as they do in accelerating positive hydrogen ions (H^+).

The process of acceleration is one in which the particles are attracted into the first dee that has an opposite electrical charge. The particle moves through the dee in a circular pattern (because of the influence of the magnetic fields) until it reaches the gap. At this point the electrical fields are reversed. The dee through which the particle just passed changes in charge so as to have a repulsive effect, and the dee into which it will now move will have an attractive effect. In this way the particle is accelerated and because of its increasing velocity makes a larger and larger circle. This process continues throughout the extent of the cyclotron until the particle reaches the target material. The particle now possesses extremely high energies and interacts with the target material to produce an altered nucleus, which is unstable. The source of the particles is arranged in the center of the circle formed by the two dees, and the particles proceed outward in a spiral fashion until they reach the target material.

The cyclotron is generally a more versatile device compared with a reactor or a linear accelerator. It has an advantage over the linear accelerator because space does not present the problem for a cyclotron that it does for a linear accelerator. It has more advantages over a nuclear reactor because of the wider variety of nuclear particles it can employ. Another major advantage is that it is capable of producing certain useful radionuclides, primarily short-lived, that are not produced in significant quantities in nuclear reactors. A further advantage over reactors is that radioisotopes may be produced with much higher specific activity; they are often carrier-free. The disadvantage is that many of the radionuclides are very short-lived, and therefore require a cyclotron on the premises, or nearby if they are to be used for medical purposes. This is especially true with PET radionuclides, such as ^{11}C, ^{13}N, ^{15}O and ^{18}F. Their half-lives are 20.4 min, 9.96 min, 2.04 min, and 110 min, respectively. With the possible exception of ^{18}F, an immediate supply must be on hand for their utility. For these reasons, the process of cyclotron production has taken on new

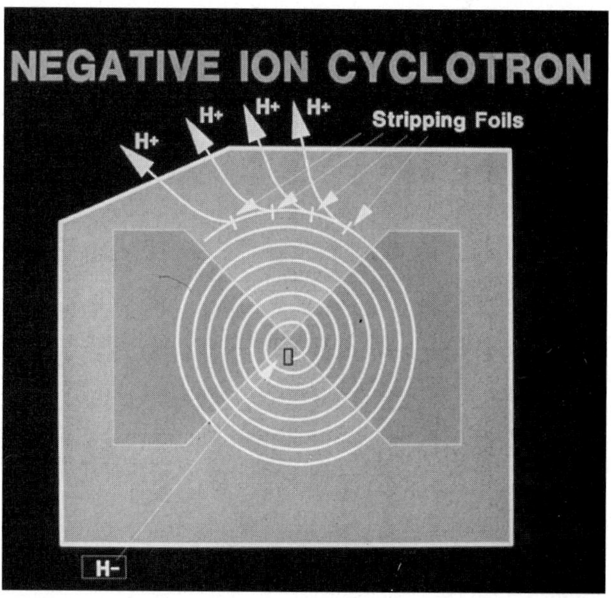

Fig. 5-5. Pathway of a charged particle through a cyclotron (Courtesy of Siemens Medical Systems, Inc.)

Table 5-1. ^{123}I production techniques

Reaction	Radionuclide impurities	At TOC*	At TOC +6 hrs	At TOE**
^{124}Xe *(p, 2n)* ^{123}I	^{123}I	99.9	99.85	99.5
	^{124}I	0.0	0.0	0.0
	^{125}I	0.007	0.0095	0.035
**TOE = 30 hrs	^{126}I	0.0	0.0	0.0
	^{201}Tl	<0.1	0.135	0.455
^{127}I *(p, 5n)* ^{123}I	^{123}I	98.4	97.70	92.45
	^{124}I	0.0	0.0	0.0
	^{125}I	1.6	2.17	7.14
**TOE = 30 hrs	^{126}I	0.0	0.0	0.0
	^{201}Tl	<0.1	0.135	0.43
^{124}Te *(p, 2n)* ^{123}I	^{123}I	94.0	92.85	85.0
	^{124}I	<5.0	6.5	13.5
	^{125}I	0.0	0.0	0.0
**TOE = 24 hrs	^{126}I	0.0	0.0	0.0
	^{24}Na	<0.5	0.67	1.5

*Time of calibration
**Time of expiration

significance as a result of the recent rapid acceptance of PET (Positron Emission Tomography) (see Chapter 15).

Further, production methods using cyclotron are becoming refined. Iodine 123 can be made from a number of targets (^{124}Xe, ^{127}I and ^{124}Te). The importance of each is not that the ^{123}I product is any different, but that the radionuclidic purity of the product varies greatly with the production method. This is of extreme importance since radionuclide impurities affect the patient radiation dose and image quality (Table 5-1). In the case of ^{123}I from the ^{124}Te *(p, 2n)* reaction, the radionuclidic impurity is the high-energy, gamma-emitting ^{124}I, which interferes greatly with nuclear medicine images. The level of impurity increases to 13.5% at 30 hours. Contrast that to the material produced by the ^{124}Xe *(p, 2n)* reaction. This material has the low-energy contaminants of ^{121}Te and ^{125}I, which present no imaging problems. The same is true with the ^{123}I product produced by the ^{127}I *(p, 5n)* reaction.

■ GENERATORS

Another method of radionuclide production is the generator (Fig. 5-6). The generator has become a convenient method of obtaining short-lived radionuclides at places distant to large-scale production sites. Short-lived radionuclides have gained wide acceptance in the field of nuclear medicine because, by their use, larger doses of radiopharmaceuticals can be injected with resultant decreased radiation dose to the patient and organs of interest. In addition, they provide increased statistics that are necessary for more meaningful imaging results, and a continuous availability of a short-lived radionuclide in the nuclear medicine laboratory. Examples of these short-lived radionuclides are $^{99}Mo/^{99m}Tc$ generators and $^{82}Sr/^{82}Rb$ generators.

■ Physical characteristics

All generators are modifications of a basic physical arrangement. The generator consists of a small glass column containing an ion exchange material. The parent nuclide is firmly affixed (adsorbed) onto this material. The column of ion exchange material is held by a porous glass frit at the bottom of the column and a plastic ring at the top. An outer plastic housing is usually provided to guard against breakage during shipment and handling. Both ends of the system should be sealed to preserve sterility and pyrogen-free conditions within the column.

■ Principle of operation

$^{99}Mo/^{99m}Tc$ generator. The basis of operation for this radionuclide generator is that a relatively long-lived parent nuclide continually produces through radioactive decay a shorter-lived daughter nuclide. Separation of the daughter nuclide can be performed easily and repeatedly, usually on the basis of chemical separation techniques. This separation process, or "milking," is referred to as *elution*.

The daughter nuclide is eluted from the parent nuclide (which remains on the ion exchange medium) and collected at the bottom of the column. Other elution processes are known, such as distillation, solvent extraction (MEK, methyl ethyl ketone), and precipitation; however, the simplicity of ion exchange media lends itself well to the routine nuclear medicine laboratory. The daughter is eluted by introducing the recommended reagent through the top of the column and collecting the product solution from the bottom of the column. The product is then assayed for concentration of daughter nuclide.

This process of elution can be repeated as many times as is thought necessary; however, the percent yield will

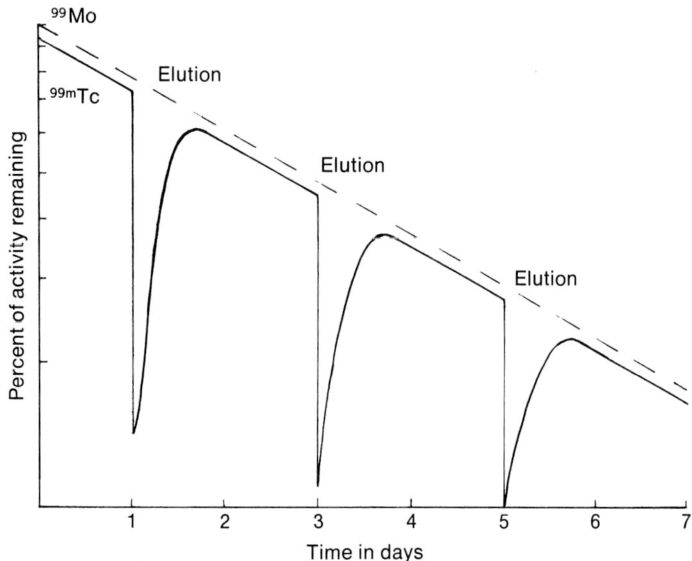

Fig. 5-6. Elution of generator. Plot of ^{99}Mo/^{99m}Tc generator with ^{99}Mo decay shown as dotted line and ^{99m}Tc decay shown as solid line. Generator is eluted on days 1, 3, and 5, changing in no way the course of the decay of ^{99}Mo. Following each elution, it requires approximately four physical half-lives to return to equilibrium. Regeneration is an exponential function with approximately 50% regeneration during the first half-life, 25% more during the second half-life, and so on. Daughter activity (^{99m}Tc) never reaches 100% parent activity (^{99}Mo), because 7.6% of all ^{99}Mo atoms decay to ^{99m}Tc, bypassing the metastable state.

vary. After the daughter has been eluted, the daughter activity remaining on the column is low but begins to increase (regenerate) until it eventually approximates the activity of the parent again (Fig. 5-6). At this point, if undisturbed, the activity of the daughter nuclide appears to assume the half-life of the parent. The next elution repeats the cycle. (The parent continues to decay also but at a much slower rate than the daughter.) If the column has completely regenerated, the usual yield is approximately 70% of the parent activity. In the case of the ^{99}Mo/^{99m}Tc generator, regeneration requires approximately 24 hours. Any elutions that are performed before that time will result in lower yields per elution; however, a large net yield can be realized if several premature elutions are performed over any period of time. For example, one elution per day (at 8 AM) will yield ^{99m}Tc between 70% and 90% of the activity of the ^{99}Mo, whereas two elutions per day (at 8 AM and 2 PM) will yield ^{99m}Tc at approximately 105% to 120% of the activity of ^{99}Mo. This is caused by the exponential buildup of the daughter product after elution. This increased net yield carries with it a sacrifice of concentration.

The principle of generators becomes almost impossible to believe because the question always arises as to how the generator can regenerate when 1 atom of ^{99}Mo with a 67-hour half-life decays to ^{99m}Tc with a 6-hour half-life. The question is best answered not on a one-atom-to-one-atom basis but with many atoms. An analogy may help clarify the situation.

Radioactive decay (Chapter 4) can be compared to a reservoir of water with an outlet at its base (Fig. 5-7). The molecules of water flowing through the outlet represent atoms undergoing the decay process, whereas the molecules in the tank represent radioactive atoms that have not yet decayed. The rate of flow of water molecules in both tanks is controlled only by the height of the column of water (flow rate is proportional to height of column), since the size of their outlets is the same. As the height of the column decreases by one half, the flow rate decreases proportionally. This is also true in a sample of radioactivity; as the number of atoms in the original sample is reduced to one half (half-life), the rate of decay is reduced proportionally.

It becomes clear from this analogy that for 2 radionuclides having two different half-lives but the same number of disintegrations per unit time, the radionuclide having the longer half-life must have a larger number of atoms in the sample.* This situation is represented by the two reservoirs of water, tank A and tank B in Fig. 5-7. Since the flow rate (or disintegration rate) is exactly the same in both reservoirs, tank B will reach half height (half-life) in a shorter

*It is as simplistic as this: the difference in the number of atoms is related to the difference in half-life. ^{99}Mo has a half-life that is 10 times longer than ^{99m}Tc; therefore ^{99}Mo has 10 times the number of atoms for the same amount of radioactivity. The first formula (p. 52) bears out this relationship. This is also one of the reasons why longer-lived radionuclides deliver a larger radiation dose than do shorter-lived radionuclides.

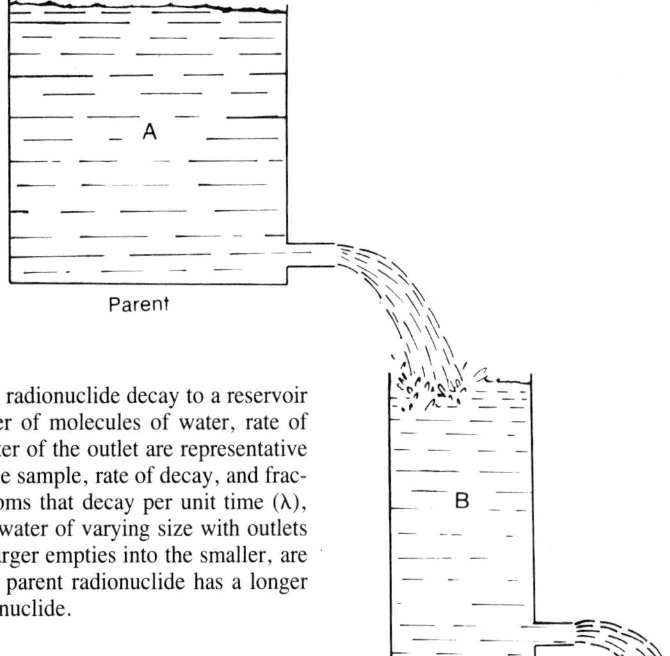

Fig. 5-7. Illustration comparing radionuclide decay to a reservoir of water with an outlet. Number of molecules of water, rate of flow from the outlet, and diameter of the outlet are representative of number of atoms in radioactive sample, rate of decay, and fraction of remaining number of atoms that decay per unit time (λ), respectively. Two reservoirs of water of varying size with outlets of the same size, in which the larger empties into the smaller, are analogous to a generator whose parent radionuclide has a longer half-life than the daughter radionuclide.

period of time because it has less water (fewer atoms).

Figure 5-7 also demonstrates the probability of decay. It is impossible to predict which water molecules flowing from tank A to tank B will, in turn, flow from tank B. Some water molecules will flow immediately to the outlet and out of tank B, whereas others will flow inside tank B before being expelled. The overriding principle is that it is possible to predict which water molecules will flow out of tank B per unit time. The same is true with a radioactive series of unstable parent and daughter atoms. The radioactive daughter atom may decay immediately on being transmuted or may exist in its unstable state for a longer period of time. Although it is impossible to predict which atom will decay immediately, it is possible to predict how many atoms will decay from a given radioactive sample per unit time.

The analogy of reservoirs can also be extended to the operation of a generator. Since generators currently in use are those of relatively long-lived parents and relatively short-lived daughter products, the reservoirs of Fig. 5-7 accurately depict the situation. At the time of the initial elution, both reservoirs are full to capacity and the flow rates (decay rates, activity, disintegrations per unit time) are the same. The first elution decreases tank B to $\approx$ 30% capacity, and tank A remains undisturbed. Because the height of the column of water has been reduced, the flow rate has also been reduced, analogous to decreased activity of the daughter product. As tank A continues to flow at the same rate into tank B, tank B will begin to fill up; at the same time, the outflow continues at an increasingly greater rate because the column of water increases in height. The same is true in the generator. The parent nuclide continues to decay at the same rate, but because tank B has fewer atoms after elution, the rate of decay is decreased. After elution, and because the parent nuclide continues to decay to the daughter at the same rate, the number of daughter atoms becomes increasingly greater and therefore the number of disintegrations per unit time (activity) becomes increasingly greater also. Eventually a point is reached at which tank B is filled to the same height as tank A and the flow rates of both reservoirs are again equal. The same point of complete regeneration is reached in the generator when the activity of the daughter nuclide is the same as the parent nuclide. Furthermore, because the decay of the parent nuclide to the daughter nuclide is at the same rate as the daughter nuclide is to its successor, the half-life of the daughter appears to be the same as the parent. This is not true, of course, because the removal of the daughter from the parent allows the daughter to display its own characteristic half-life. The point at which the ratio of the two activities remains constant and both appear to decay with the half-life of the parent is called *equilibrium*.

Two terms are used to describe two different types of equilibrium: *transient* equilibrium and *secular* equilibrium. Transient equilibrium is a condition that exists when the parent radionuclide has a physical half-life that is not much longer than that of the daughter nuclide. A good example of this type of equilibrium is the ^{99}Mo/^{99m}Tc generator system. Secular equilibrium, on the other hand, is a condition that exists when the parent radionuclide has a physical half-life that is considerably longer than that of the daughter nuclide. An example of this type of equilibrium is the 82Sr/^{82}Rb generator system.

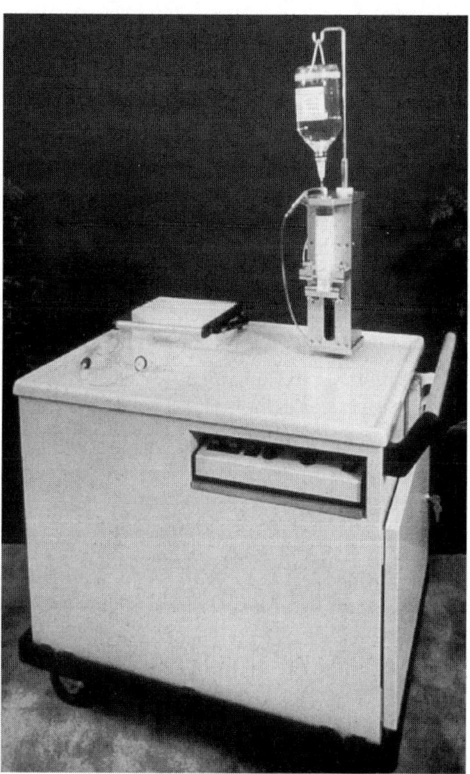

Fig. 5-8. Rubidium 82 Infusion System, housing a $^{82}Sr/^{82}Rb$ generator. The system is automated to provide desired radioactivity, volumes, and infusion rates for myocardial blood flows. (Courtesy of Siemens Medical Systems, Inc.)

$^{82}Sr/^{82}Rb$ infusion system. With the recent advances in Positron Emission Tomography (PET) and the recent interest within the nuclear medicine community, it became necessary to make available a good positron emitter for the physicians not situated close to a cyclotron. Such was rubidium 82. ^{82}Rb is a radioactive daughter of strontium 82; these have physical half-lives of 75 seconds and 25 days, respectively. ^{82}Rb has been shown to be useful for myocardial blood-flow studies. Since ^{82}Rb is a daughter of the long-lived ^{82}Sr, the combination was acceptable as a generator system.

The $^{82}Sr/^{82}Rb$ generator is inserted into an automated infusion system (Fig. 5-8). The total dose of ^{82}Rb activity to be administered, the total volume, and the infusion rates are preselected by push buttons on the control panel. Intravenous delivery is started by pushing the "inject button," which turns off automatically once the preselected dose of radioactivity has been delivered. A total permissable dose is 120 mCi (4440 MBq). Such a system will be usable for clinical studies for a period of 4 to 6 weeks.

As stated above, $^{82}Sr/^{82}Rb$ is an example of a generator in secular equilibrium. As such, the parent activity decreases very little with time in comparison with the daughter radionuclide.

■ TRILINEAR CHART OF THE NUCLIDES

Marshall Brucer, M.D.

At the beginning of the twentieth century the main problem in chemistry was the periodic table. The table was filling rapidly, but some puzzling inconsistencies occurred among the naturally radioactive elements. Some thorium substances with very different physical properties could not be separated chemically. Uranium was geochemically related to lead, but there seemed to be more than one atomic weight for lead, all with the same chemical properties.

Kasimer Fajans, a German physical chemist, developed a "displacement law" to explain the pattern of radioactive decay. In 1912 he found a way to explain the puzzling inconsistencies, but the explanation demanded more than one "element" in one place on the periodic table. Frederick Soddy, a physical chemist in Glasgow, generalized this solution to the entire periodic table. During the nineteenth century "atomic weight" was not a true "mass" but was a relative "proportional number" of each element balanced against the others in ordinal progression up the periodic table. Atomic weight, thus, could be an average of all the atomic numbers making up a chemical element. Soddy called these the "isotopes" of the element. A few years later (1917) he pointed out that if some substances had equal atomic number (chemical properties) but different atomic weight (a physical property), then there must also be substances with equal weight but different atomic number. Eventually, the latter were called *isobars*.

The number of electrons in an atom had already (in 1913) been related to the number of positive charges (protons) in the nucleus of the atom. This was the atomic number *(Z)*. It was postulated in 1920 that the remainder of the nucleus was made up of uncharged particles much like the proton but neutral in charge (neutrons). Chadwick, in England, discovered these in 1932. The atomic number was the number of protons (iodine has 53, hence $_{53}I$). The atomic weight was the number of protons plus neutrons (one of the iodines was 53 plus 78, hence $^{131}_{53}I$). If there are isotopes with equal proton number and isobars with equal mass, then there should also be substances with an equal number of neutrons. Replace the "p" (for proton) in isotope with an "n" (for neutron) and the word becomes *isotone*.

In 1921 Otto Hahn, a German chemist, while trying to straighten out some difficulties in the uranium chain of decay, found two substances that had entirely different half-lives but were the same isotope, isobar, and isotone. By 1935, in the search for new radioisotopes, physicists were finding more of these unusual species. In 1936 Lisa Meitner, the long-time physicist-associate of Hahn, called these *nuclear isomers*.

■ Discovery of the artificial radioisotopes

Atom smashing to study atomic structures was popular around 1933. In Paris, Frederick Joliot and his wife, Irene

Curie (the daughter of Marie Curie), noticed that the aluminum target they were bombarding with polonium alpha particles remained radioactive after the bombardment stopped. After careful investigation, on Feb. 10, 1934, Joliot and Curie published a note on the production of a new artificial isotope of phosphorus ($^{30}_{15}P$). Thirty-six years after she and her husband had discovered the first naturally radioactive element (polonium), Curie's mother, Marie Curie, had the pleasure of hearing her daughter and son-in-law announce the discovery of the first artificial radioactive substance made with alpha particles from her own first discovery in 1898.

On reading the announcement of the discovery of artificial radioactive isotopes, Enrico Fermi, at the University of Rome, thought that the newly discovered neutron would be a better bombardment projectile than alpha particles. Within 2 months of the production of the first ^{30}P, he had bombarded many elements and found 33 radioisotopes (and 13 others that were probably also radioactive). Physicists immediately began the search for others.

■ Terminology

During World War II, Fermi's nuclear reactor and the newer cyclotrons were used to create still different nuclear reactions to produce even more radioactive nuclides. By 1947 there were about 800 known species; it was becoming too complex to talk about an *isotope-isobar-isotone-isomer*. In 1947 Turner, an American physicist, proposed the word *nuclide* to signify any specific arrangement of protons and neutrons. The term was quickly adopted, and this branch of science became nuclear, not isotope, physics; chemistry became nuclear, not isotope, chemistry. However, before World War II the nuclear sciences had revolved around the chemical similarity of reactions of isotopes. The first chemical and then biologic use of a nuclide had been because of its chemical isotopy. The name *isotopes* took hold with physicians and political administrators who did not know the historical background; newspapers picked up the catchword. By the time medical personnel began to use radionuclides, the improper term *radioisotopes* was embedded in the language.

Yet the medical and tracer personnel were not using isotopes. Once they had obtained, for example, an isotope of iodine, they measured its decay to xenon; they were using isobar relationships. The nuclear reactor personnel were using isotone relationships. With the founding of the first medical society of physicians using these nuclear reaction products, the improper use of the term "radioisotopes" was corrected and physicians adopted the name *nuclear medicine*.

■ Development of the trilinear chart of the nuclides

In 1946 William H Sullivan, one of the chief chemists at Oak Ridge, Tennessee, put all the known radioactive and stable nuclides onto a trilinear chart of many hexagons. Each hexagon represented one nuclide. One axis of the hexagonal array signified isotopes, the second axis signified isobars, and the third axis signified isotones. Production, chemistry, physics, or medical use did not matter to Sullivan. He had plotted the first trilinear chart that showed all the nuclides in their true structural relationship.

Every physicist who looked at Sullivan's trilinear chart of 1946 knew that there were more nuclides to be discovered. There were 800 nuclides known in 1947; by 1968 about 1800 had been found; by December 1978 there were almost 2452, and a few more seemed necessary to make the chart symmetric. If each hexagon is to be a complete designation of a nuclide, a tremendous amount of data is involved—much too much for a simple chart. Also, the fine details are changing with each increase in accuracy. Summary *Tables of Isotopes* are out of date before they are published, and a special journal, *Nuclear Data,* is published periodically to keep researchers up to date.* Physicists and chemists need the complete tabular data. Clinical physicians need only a small fragment; this much can be put in chart form. Figure 5-9 shows 15 of the nearly 2500 nuclides.

The central box in each hexagon gives the proper name of the nuclide. All of the iodines (I) have the same number of protons ($_{53}I$). One nuclide of iodine has 76 neutrons and 53 protons, which equals 129 nucleons ($^{129}_{53}I$); one has 79 neutrons ($^{132}_{53}I$). Iodines 115 to 141 have been demonstrated, and there may be a few more. Six of the 27 known iodine nuclides have isomers of appreciable half-life; hence, there are more than 33 different kinds of iodine. Only one kind is stable ($^{127}_{53}I$). Each hexagon on the trilinear chart shows not only a nuclide (and maybe an isomer) but also its isobaric, isotopic, and isotonic relationship to its neighbors in the periodic table.

■ Choice of data

By the time Sullivan's chart had gone through a few editions, the data had become so complex that Sullivan had to leave something out. He wanted to make a medical chart; but with the rapid changes in medical demands, he did not know which data were important (and neither did anyone else). However, some items were obviously important to physicians.

Half-life. Half-life is so important in medical use that it was put immediately above the name plate. For example, iodine 141 has a half-life of 0.43 seconds; iodine 129 has a half-life of 15.7 million years. The amount of any nuclide that can be given to a patient is probably the first consideration of a clinician. However, is "amount" the physical dose of radiation or the chemical dose of a nuclide? "Dose" of a radionuclide is usually measured in millicuries (a mCi is the number of atoms that will result in 37 million disintegrations per second). Because the disintegrations of

**Nuclear Data,* Section B, New York, 1967 to date, Academic Press, Inc.

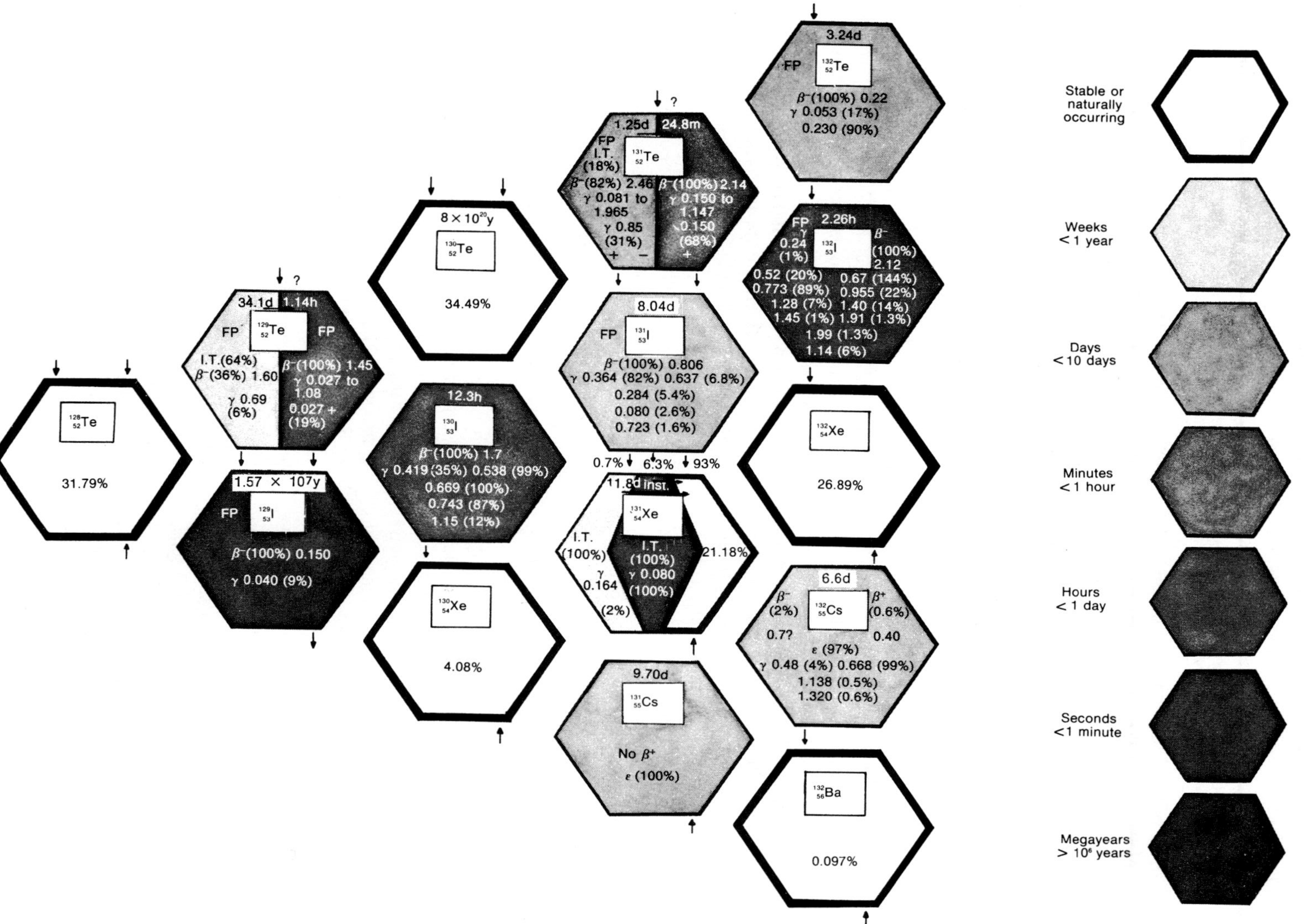

Fig. 5-9. Portion of trilinear chart of nuclides demonstrating arrangement and information content of chart. (Courtesy Mallinckrodt Inc., St. Louis, Mo.)

^{129}I occur over such a long time span, it would take about 62 gm of chemical to produce 1 mCi of radiation; a proper large chemical dose is in the milligram range. But only femtograms of ^{141}I are needed for a millicurie. (A femtogram is 1/1000 of a picogram, which is 1/1000 of a nanogram, which is 1/1000 of a microgram, which is 1/1000 of a milligram, which is 1/1000 of a gram.) A true "tracer" chemical dose of the short-lived iodines (hours to weeks) can be given with extremely large physical doses of radiation. Both concepts of "amount" are implied in half-life.

A 24-hour thyroid uptake could be measured with short-lived ^{132}I. But, even if a full millicurie were given, at 24 hours there would only be one half of ½ of ½ of ½. . . (10 half-lives) left, and approximately three fourths of this would have been excreted. To administer the original millicurie, a day's shipping time from the pharmaceutical house would have to be allowed. A curie would be ordered to give a millicurie to measure a fraction of a microcurie—this is feasible and has been done, but it is not practical.

Radiation characteristics. Just as important as half-life is whether the energy of radiation emission is highly penetrating or below the limits of the detecting instruments. The trilinear chart gives the energy of ^{132}I as 773 keV plus many other energies. This is supervoltage radiation that demands tremendous shielding. On a complete table of isotopes, many nuclides are described that have a clinically convenient half-life but emit energies in the multimillion volt range. No matter what their biologic specificity, the tremendous shielding necessary in their use might be impractical in a busy clinical laboratory and might be completely unacceptable to clinical instruments.

A high-energy gamma ray has little chance of being stopped by a piece of tissue. If it is stopped, however, it has great effect. A low-energy gamma ray will not cause as much effect, but it is more likely to be stopped. The same is true in a radiation-measuring instrument. Gamma rays much under 0.1 MeV or much over 0.5 meV cause problems in the clinical laboratory. This is why most medical nuclides are selected from the medium range, for example, ^{131}I = 0.364 MeV and ^{99m}Tc = 0.140 MeV. With the development of the thin crystal, fast gamma camera, the low energy nuclides (0.1 to 0.2 MeV) have a great advantage in detection sensitivity.

Pattern of decay. The concept of milking a short-lived daughter nuclide from a long-lived parent was already in medical use before World War I. ^{226}Ra with a half-life of 1600 years decays to 3.8-day ^{222}Rn. For many medical uses the shorter-lived (and less expensive) radon is more valuable than the longer-lived radium. Early in the 1920s G. Failla, a New York medical radiation physicist, devised a method to milk (elute) the radom from a large radium source and gave it the expressive name "radon cow."

^{132}Te has a 3.24-day half-life; its daughter nuclide, 2.26-hour ^{132}I, can be milked from a well-shielded tellurium source in the laboratory. This first artificial nuclide cow (the euphemism is "generator") was devised in the early 1950s. It was valuable in the development of the concept of dual nuclide studies. Shielding, contamination, cost, transportation, procurement, and many problems connected with half-life can be solved by the use of a cow system. In 1964 the ^{99}Mo/^{99m}Tc generator revolutionized radiopharmaceuticals, and over 200 cow systems are now theoretically available for development.

^{131}I, the most common radionuclide of early nuclear medicine had a surprisingly complex decay scheme. Only 93% decays to stable ^{131}Xe. Once its beta emission has occurred, the ^{131}I atom becomes ^{131}Xe in a metastable state. Eight hesitations can occur during the emission of gamma rays before the xenon achieves stability. Seven of these hesitations have nanosecond and picosecond durations and hence are of no medical concern, but 0.42% of the decays are through an 11.9-day isomer of ^{131}Xe; this half-life is longer than that of the original 8-day ^{131}I. Although 0.42% is too small to be of any concern in routine clinical work, during a long-term iodine retention study, within a few weeks there may be more ^{131m}Xe than there is ^{131}I in a closed system. To some extent absorption in fat makes the body a closed system for xenon.

The gamma emission of ^{131}I at 364 keV can now easily be distinguished from the gamma emission of ^{131m}Xe at 164 keV. The older ^{131}I literature, before spectroscopy, lists the ^{131}I half-life at 8.08, 8.07, or 8.05 days (now 8.04). Some of the confusion was caused by measurement in an open system (^{131}I only) or in a closed system (^{131}I + ^{131m}Xe).

The 6.6-day ^{132}Cs nuclide shown in Fig. 5-9 decays with the emission of either a negatron (β^-) or a positron (β^+). The negatron decay yields ^{132}Ba; the positron decay yields ^{132}Xe. A double decay pattern is more common at the upper end of the periodic table where decay can be partially alpha and partially beta emission. It is not very serious in routine medical pharmacology, but it can be very serious in precise chemical work.

When multiple daughters are present in a decay system, the succeeding daughters can confuse counting problems in routine work. The same confusion can be caused by multiple nuclides produced by almost every production technique. Even a negligible chemical impurity can be a significant radiation impurity. The first iodine radionuclide used in thyroid therapy (1939) was ^{130}I. It was the preferred isotope because of its relative radiochemical purity. ^{131}I was then made from the cyclotron bombardment of tellurium, and at least 10 different isotopes of iodine were produced. It is now impossible to determine which of the isotopes were being measured in some of the early studies of iodine metabolism.

When fission product ^{131}I first became available in 1946, it was the first of the iodine nuclides to have a relative radiochemical purity. But then, when higher specific activity was thought to be desirable, ^{131}I could be made even more cheaply in a nuclear reactor by neutron bombardment of ^{130}Te. The pharmaceutical manufacturer bought 1.25-day ^{131}Te, which decays to 8-day ^{131}I during shipment. A simple final chemical extraction of iodine yielded a very pure and very high specific activity ^{131}I.

■ Medical trilinear chart

For ordinary clinical laboratory work, half-life, decay pattern, and proportion and energy of beta and gamma emission are all that can be included on a simplified chart of the nuclides. Some of the details that are essential to physicists and chemists are also essential in pharmaceutical research. Neutron cross sections might be of great importance in diagnostic procedures involving neutron activation analysis. The average beta emission energy is essential in initial radiation dosage estimates. Alternative production methods invariably present the toxicologic problems of contaminating activities. However, there is no room for such data on a simplified chart. The trilinear chart does show the pattern of decay and the great diversity of radionuclides that are theoretically available in the practice of nuclear medicine.

LABORATORY APPLICATION

1

CHART OF THE NUCLIDES

Purpose

This exercise will familiarize you with the chart of the nuclides so that it may become an effective tool in your radionuclide laboratory.

Theory

The trilinear chart of the nuclides is an orderly grouping of all known nuclides and represents a concentration of data that have been compiled over many years. It has been designed so that the nuclides are presented visually, illustrating the relationship between isotopes, isotones, and isobars. In addition, data particular to each individual nuclide are included in the hexagon set aside for it.

Individual nuclides and their isotopes are placed in diagonal rows extending from lower left to upper right as atomic weight increases. Each different elemental row is similarly angled but is displaced from upper left to lower right as proton number increases. With this arrangement all nuclides found in a vertical row are isobars, and all nuclides found in a diagonal row from upper left to lower right are isotones.

Nuclide identification by proton number, symbol, and atomic weight ($^{A}_{Z}X$) is within each hexagon. If the nuclide is stable, only its percent abundance in a sample of the element from nature is added. If the nuclide is radioactive, the half-life, mode of decay, and energy and abundance of emitted particles and photons are included. Outside the hexagons are arrows. These arrows point to the route a nuclide takes as it decays toward stability. Some nuclides may have several arrows pointing from them. This multiplicity reflects the fact that some nuclides decay by two or more modes, sometimes resulting in different products. Isomeric transitional states (IT) are represented by hexagons with two or more divisions. The IT form of the nuclide always appears on the left of the hexagon. The letters *FP* to the left of the square block within the hexagon signify "fission product."

The hexagons are color coded, reflecting approximate half-lives. The natural decay series of thorium, actinium, uranium, and neptunium is also identified with lines that connect the daughter nuclides produced while en route to stability.

All the mass numbers *(A)* are listed at the top of the chart in ascending sequence from left to right. A nuclide bearing that *A* number can be found in the vertical column of isobars below. Elemental symbols are listed at the bottom of the chart in ascending atomic numbers *(Z)* from left to right. A nuclide bearing that Z number may be found in the diagonal column of isotopes above. Other symbol information may be found by referring to the explanatory note key.

Procedure

Materials

Trilinear chart of the nuclides.

Continued.

Technique

By inspecting the trilinear chart of the nuclides, answer the following questions (the first four questions have already been answered for you):

1. What is the half-life of ${}^{198}_{79}Au$? (2.696 days)
2. What is the mode of decay? (β^-, γ)
3. Identify the particles and/or the photons emitted plus their energies and percent abundance. (β^-: 1.371 meV, 100%; 3γ : 0.412 − 1.087 meV (0.412 ≅ 100%)
4. What is the daughter product? (${}^{198}_{80}Hg$)
5. How many stable nuclides of oxygen exist?
6. How many stable nuclides contain 8 protons?
7. In a fission reaction a zinc (Zn) fragment is produced. Which one of the 13 nuclides of Zn is this?
8. Are there any stable forms of uranium (U)?
9. What is the heaviest known nuclide of uranium?
10. Which uranium nuclide is the most abundant?
11. What is the stable isotope of iodine (as found in table salt)?
12. Technetium 99m (left half of block) decays to what? Is this stable?
13. What is the principal gamma energy of the following nuclides? (The first two are answered for you.)
    (a) ${}^{137}Cs$ (no γ, daughter ${}^{137m}Ba$ emits 0.662 meV γ); *(b)* ${}^{131}I$ (0.364 meV); *(c)* ${}^{99m}Tc$; *(d)* ${}^{125}I$; *(e)* ${}^{133}Xe$; *(f)* ${}^{67}Ga$; *(g)* ${}^{99}Mo$; *(h)* ${}^{32}P$; *(i)* ${}^{201}Tl$; *(j)* ${}^{3}H$; *(k)* ${}^{57}Co$; *(l)* ${}^{60}Co$
14. When ${}^{51}Cr$ decays, what is the daughter product?
15. When ${}^{32}P$ decays, what is the daughter product?
16. What are the half-lives of the following nuclides? (The first one is answered for you.)
    (a) ${}^{137}Cs$ (30 years); *(b)* ${}^{131}I$; *(c)* ${}^{99m}Tc$; *(d)* ${}^{125}I$; *(e)* ${}^{133}Xe$; *(f)* ${}^{67}Ga$; *(g)* ${}^{99}Mo$; *(h)* ${}^{32}P$; *(i)* ${}^{201}Tl$; *(j)* ${}^{3}H$; *(k)* ${}^{57}Co$; *(l)* ${}^{60}Co$

BIBLIOGRAPHY

Brucer, M.: Vignettes in nuclear medicine, St. Louis, 1967-1979, Mallinckrodt, Inc.

Chandra, R.: Introductory physics of nuclear medicine, ed. 4, Philadelphia, 1992, Lea & Febiger.

Gottschalk, A., and Potchen, E.J.: Diagnostic nuclear medicine, Baltimore, 1976, The Williams & Wilkins Co.

Johns, H.E. and Cunningham, J.R.: The physics of radiology, ed. 4, revised edition, Springfield, Ill., 1983, Charles C Thomas, Publisher.

Quimby, E.H., and Feitelberg, S.: Radioactive isotopes in medicine and biology, ed. 2, Philadelphia, 1963, Lea & Febiger.

Rollo, F.D.: Nuclear medicine physics, instrumentation, and agents, St. Louis, 1977, Mosby–Year Book.

Shilling, C.W.: Atomic energy encyclopedia in the life sciences, Philadelphia, 1964, W.B. Saunders Co.

Wagner, H.N.: Principles of nuclear medicine, Philadelphia, 1968, W.B. Saunders Co.

Chapter 6

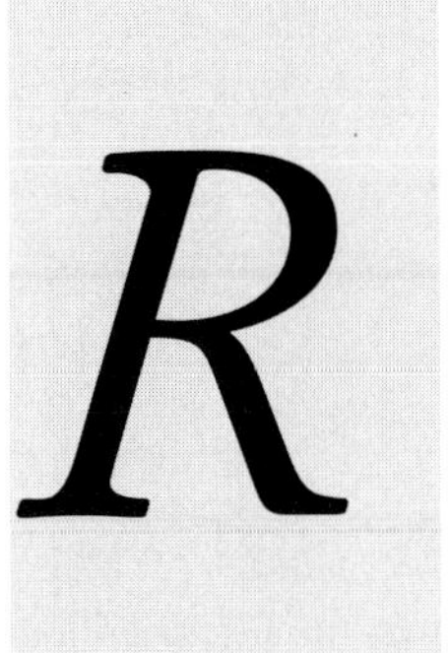

RADIATION MEASUREMENT AND PROTECTION

PAUL J. EARLY

The many aspects of radiation measurement and consequent protection should become a primary consideration any time radioactive materials are used. The actual effects of radiation are not completely known, but it can generally be stated that all radioactivity can be injurious; therefore steps must be taken to prevent unnecessary exposure. A number of factors include type and energy of radiation, penetration power, ionization ability, radioactive half-life, biologic half-life, and effective half-life. In addition, personnel who use radioactive materials must be introduced to the various units of radiation measurement and recognize the necessity for certain limitations to radiation exposure.

■ MEASUREMENT OF RADIATION

■ Radiation units

Basically, two dimensions are used to define the various terms of radiation measurement: the ionization of matter by radiation and the energy absorbed by matter from radiation. From these two basic concepts three kinds of radiation measurements have been derived: (1) the roentgen (R)*, (2) the radiation absorbed dose (rad)*, and (3) the roentgen equivalent, man (rem).* A fourth unit describes the number of atoms that disintegrate per unit time, the curie* and its submultiples. All of these are used or have been used in the past as units of radiation measurement. The curie is described on p. 36.

Coulombs/kg. The *roentgen (R)* was originally defined as the amount of x-radiation that produces 1 electrostatic unit (esu) of charge as a result of interactions in 1 cc of dry air at standard temperature and pressure. It is now defined in equivalent units as 2.58×10^{-4} coulombs/kg of air. At the meeting of the International Commission on Radiation Units and Measurements (ICRU) in July 1974, it was recommended that within a period not less than about 10 years this unit of exposure be replaced with a new unit—the coulomb per kilogram (C/kg or C kg^{-1}) recommended by the International System of Units (SI Units). This new unit of exposure would then be equal to 3876 R in the old terminology. No name other than C/kg was recommended for this new unit at that July 1974 meeting.

Regardless of its name, there are two important items to be emphasized regarding the definition of this exposure unit. First, the exposure unit is a measure of the total exposure and does not involve the time over which exposure is administered. Second, it is a unit only of x rays or gamma rays and only in air.*

Gray. The *radiation absorbed dose (RAD)* was developed to provide a measurement for radiation other than photons and in a medium other than air. It is a measure of the amount of energy imparted to matter by ionizing radiation per unit mass of irradiated material at the place of interest. One rad is equal to 100 ergs of absorbed energy per gram of absorbing material. There are two areas that warrant emphasis in this definition. First, a rad includes any ionizing radiation, as distinguished from the roentgen, which applies only to x rays or gamma rays. Second, the rad is only a measure of the energy absorbed by the material of interest and is not directly related to quantity or intensity of the radiation field. The rad also came under scrutiny at the ICRU meeting in July 1974. It was suggested that a new unit of the International System of Units be assigned to this unit of dose, that it be called the *joule per kilogram* when used for ionizing radiation, and that it be given the name *gray,* with the symbol *Gy*. This new unit of dose would then be equal to 100 rad, using the old terminology.

Relative biologic effectiveness. *RBE* is a term used to indicate that different types of radiation have different effects in biologic materials or systems. More specifically, it is the ratio of an absorbed dose of x rays or gamma rays to the absorbed dose of any radiation required to produce an

*See Appendix G for SI equivalents and relationships.

*The restriction to x rays has been dropped. The roentgen is now considered to include all photons with energies below 3 MeV.

identical biologic effect. This definition can be written as a formula:

$$\text{RBE} = \frac{\text{Dose in rad to produce some effect with x rays or gamma rays}}{\text{Dose in rad to produce same effect with radiation under investigation}}$$

For example, it is known that an absorbed dose of 0.05 rad of alpha radiation produces the same biologic effect as an absorbed dose of 1 rad of x-radiation or gamma radiation. The RBE for an alpha particle would be determined by the following:

$$\text{RBE} = \frac{1.0 \text{ rad}}{0.05 \text{ rad}} = 20$$

Accordingly, the RBE value for an alpha particle is 20. Although all ionizing radiations are capable of producing similar biologic effects, the effect varies from one type of radiation to another based on the absorbed dose (Table 6-1). This RBE of physically different ionizing radiations depends solely on the number of ionization events, commonly referred to as linear energy transfer (LET). Since the LET is a function of the charge and velocity of the ionizing particle, it requires less alpha radiation to produce the same biologic effect as x-radiation or gamma radiation.

Seivert. The *roentgen equivalent, man (REM),* was the unit of human biologic dose as a result of exposure to one or many types of ionizing radiation.* It is equal to the absorbed dose in rad times the RBE of the particular type of radiation being absorbed. The new SI unit for the rem is the Seivert (Sv); 100 rems is the equivalent of 1 Sv. Another way of expressing it is as follows:

$$\text{Radiobiologic dose in rem*} = \text{Dose in rad} \times \text{RBE}$$

If the radiation being measured is x-radiation, gamma radiation, or beta radiation greater than 30 keV, the rem value would be equal to the rad value, since the RBE value of all three types of emissions is 1.

There is a distinct difference between the three major forms of radiation measurement. The roentgen is considered the unit of exposure dose, the rad is a unit of absorbed radiation dose, and the rem is a unit of biologic dose. All three units are used in various situations in nuclear medicine. The roentgen, or more commonly its submultiple the milliroentgen, is used as a value for most survey meter readings. The rad is used as a unit to describe the amount of exposure received by the organ of interest on injection of a radiopharmaceutical; the rem is the unit used to express exposure values of some personnel monitoring devices (film badges, for example).

Considerable confusion has arisen regarding the use of the RBE and therefore the rem. It is obvious from the preceding discussion that different ionizing radiations cause different biologic effects. What is not so obvious (without highly controlled animal experiments) is that even though Table 6-1 attempts to do it, there is no single RBE value that can be used for all tissue by any one category of radiation. RBE values for the same type of radiation vary from tissue to tissue. A very high RBE has been found for cataracts in mice, whereas a very low RBE has been found for testicular atrophy, all with the same type of radiation.

The concept of RBE or rem dose is a unit now limited to use in radiation biology. This was at the suggestion of the ICRU in their Report No. 11 in 1968. Jacob Shapiro in his text *Radiation Protection* suggests in a footnote that "the term RBE was originally used as a multiplication factor of 'rads' to give 'rem' but this practice is no longer employed." The term that is similar to the RBE and currently used is the *quality factor (Q).*

Quality factor. *Q* is another name for expressing the LET dependent response by a biologic system and was initially intended to be used specifically for radiation protection. If the biologic response per rad of two different types of radiation are the same, *Q* is the same. A distinction may be made between the two terms; the measurement made for determining the relative effectiveness of two different types of radiations is the RBE; the factor expressing this relative effectiveness is the *Q*. *Q* values are usually determined by animal experiments.

Another problem in attempting to determine biologic effectiveness is distribution of the dose. Internally administered radionuclides are not uniformly distributed within the body. Therefore the dose delivered to that body would have a greater or lesser effect, depending on the distribution of the material for the same amount of dose. Therefore the dose distribution factor (DF) is also a consideration. Another way of expressing all these factors is as follows:

$$\text{Radiation protection dose in rem*} = \text{Dose in rad} \times Q \times \text{DF}$$

Specific ionization (SI). *SI* is the average number of ion pairs (primary or secondary) that are produced per unit of path traveled by the incident radiations. As mentioned in the section of this text on alpha decay, a 1.0 MeV alpha particle causes the formation of approximately 60,000 ion pairs per centimeter (air), expending an average of 34 eV

Table 6-1. RBE and *Q* values for various types of radiation

Radiation	RBE	*Q*
Alpha	20	20
Beta	1	1.0
Gamma	1	1.0
X-	1	1.0

*Referred to as *RBE dose (rems).*

*Referred to as *dose-equivalent* or *DE (rems).*

of energy per ion pair. (Energy is also lost as a result of the excitation of nearby atoms. It is estimated that 2.2 atoms are excited by the ionization of a neighboring atom in air.) With this information the LET can be computed.

Linear energy transfer (LET). *LET* differs from SI in that it is the average loss in energy per unit of path traveled by the incident radiations. The two dimensions are closely related. One deals with the number of events, the other with the deposition of energy in each segment of tissue. LET is simply the product of the SI and the average energy expended on the production of each ion pair. Expressed as a formula:

$$\text{LET} = \text{SI} \times \text{Energy expended per ion pair produced}$$

Therefore

$$\begin{aligned}\text{LET of a 1.0 MeV alpha} &= 60{,}000 \text{ ion pairs/cm (air)} \\ &\quad \times 34 \text{ eV energy expended/pair} \\ &= 2.04 \text{ MeV/cm (air)}\end{aligned}$$

The distance that any incident radiation can travel (range) can be determined knowing the energy of the incident radiation and LET of the material through which it is passing, according to the following mathematic relationship:

$$\text{Range} = \frac{E}{\text{LET}}$$

Therefore

$$\begin{aligned}\text{range of a 1.0 MeV } \alpha \text{ in air} &= \frac{1.0 \text{ MeV}}{2.04 \text{ MeV/cm (air)}} \\ &= 0.49 \text{ cm of air}\end{aligned}$$

As LET increases or energy decreases, the range decreases.

■ Relationships of units

When LET and SI units were discussed, they were expressed as the *average*. These two units are not constant throughout the medium through which the incident radiation is passing. An alpha particle passing through tissue has ionization events spaced farther apart at its entrance into the tissue than at the end of its pathway (Fig. 6-1, *A*). As the alpha particle progresses into the tissue, the speed with which the particle is traveling becomes slower and slower because of the loss of energy through its ionization activities. As the particle nears the end of its pathway, SI increases tremendously as a result of the very slow speed of the particle and its probable influence on almost each atom that it passes. The same relationship exists for LET and RBE (Fig. 6-1, *B* and *C*). This is called the *Bragg curve*.

■ Conversions between radiation units

Conversions can be made among all of these units but usually only through rather complicated mathematic manipulations; roentgens can be calculated in rad, rad can be calculated in rems, and so on. The Nuclear Regulatory Commission regulations state that roentgens, rad, and rems and their SI counterparts are almost identical, and for all practical purposes x-radiations, gamma radiations, and beta radiations are treated as having identical values. Precise conversion methods are not within the scope of this book. However, there is one conversion that may find practicality in the nuclear medicine laboratory. This is the conversion of units of activity (millicuries) to exposure rate (milliroentgens per hour: mR/hr). This correlation can be used to calibrate survey meters.

If there is a known source of activity, the exposure rate can be calculated from any gamma point source by the following formula:

$$\text{mR/hr} = \frac{n \times I_\gamma}{s^2}$$

n = Number of millicuries
I_γ = mR/hr at 1 m/mCi
s = Distance in meters

Since this formula is for any gamma point source, a point source of cobalt 60 can be used as a calibration source. The formula and the I_γ values can be found in the *Health Physics and Radiological Health Handbook*.* These values are constant for each gamma source. In the case of cobalt 60, $I_\gamma = 1.32$. Other I_γ values are ^{226}Ra = 0.825, ^{137}Cs = 0.33, ^{131}I = 0.21, ^{99m}Tc = 0.072, and ^{125}I = 0.067.

The formula just given can be used to find a survey meter reading for a 5 mCi (185 MBq) point source of cobalt 60 at a distance of 1 m:

$$\begin{aligned}\text{mrem/hr} &= \frac{5 \times 1.32}{1^2} \\ \text{mrem/hr} &= 6.60\end{aligned}$$

This formula may prove beneficial to persons working in the nuclear medicine department because continuous calibration of survey meters is necessary. In some cases a calibration check source is provided with the survey meter. For others one must be provided. The values of the calibration check source should be known and checked at each use. Should the value vary, the survey meter should be recalibrated with a National Institute of Standards and Technology (NIST) traceable standard. Too often this source is used solely to check for functional batteries.

■ TOTAL EFFECTIVE DOSE EQUIVALENT (TEDE)

Since radiation is generally thought to be harmful to human beings, the ideal would be no radiation exposure at all. However, the use of radiation and radioactive materials in many instances has proved to be beneficial to humans. Since humans are therefore going to use these radiation-emitting materials, some methods must be devised to allow their use within safe limits. This establishment of a compromise is the issue addressed by the International

*Published by Scinta, Inc., 2421 Homestead Dr., Silver Springs, MD 20902, 1992.

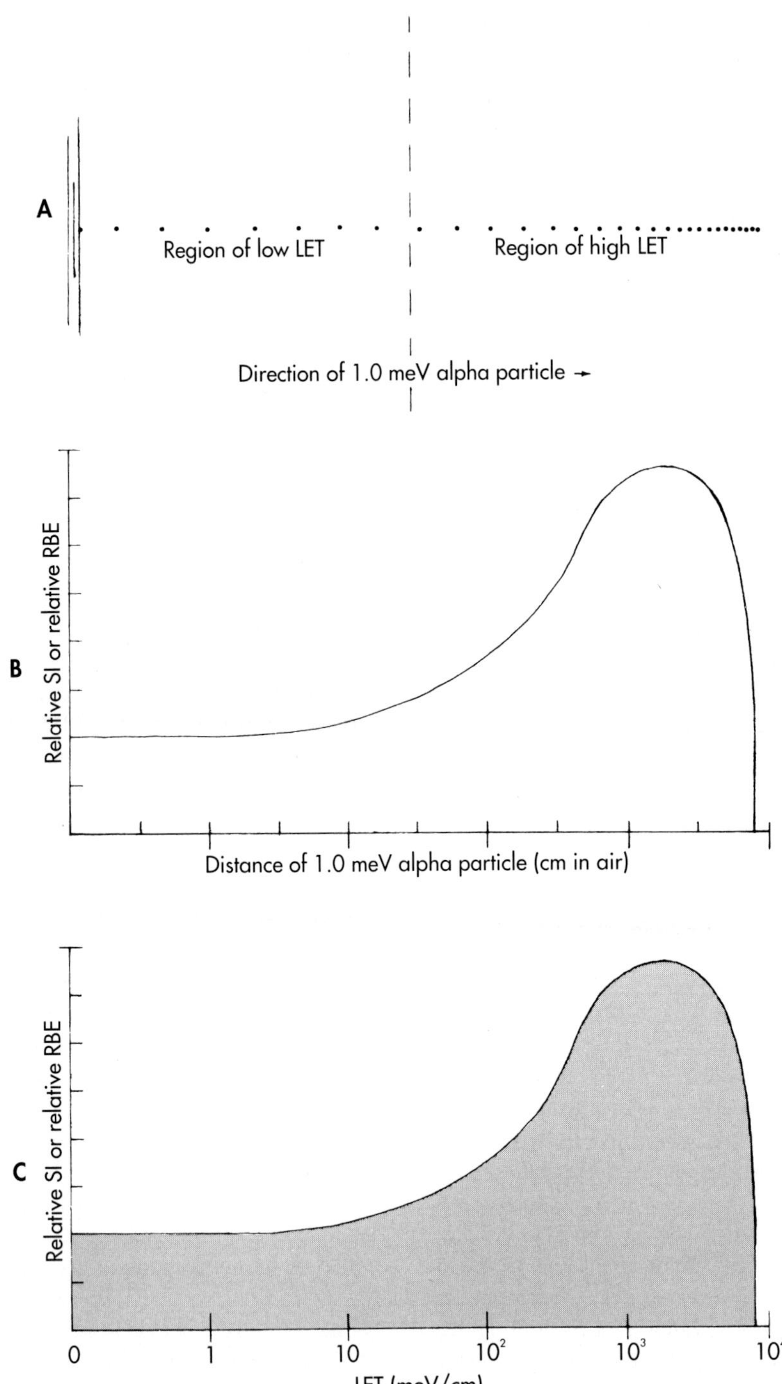

Fig. 6-1. A, Relationship of interaction of an alpha particle as it passes through matter (air). **B,** Relationship of the specific ionization (SI) (or relative biologic effectiveness [RBE]) of a 1.0 MeV alpha particle to distance. The reason the SI decreases near the termination of the alpha pathway is that the alpha particles have been slowed to the point that they capture electrons, reducing their charge and thus their ionization capabilities. **C,** Relationship of RBE to linear energy transfer (LET) for a 1.0 MeV alpha particle in air. The reason the RBE decreases near the termination of the alpha pathway is that at this point more energy than is necessary has been deposited in the tissue to fulfill some desired response—usually cell death.

Council on Radiation Protection (ICRP) and the National Council on Radiation Protection and Measurements (NCRP). The ICRP speaks for the global community, while the NCRP speaks for the United States. Because of their differences in spheres of influence, there are slight differences in their recommendations. The U.S. Nuclear Regulatory Commission (NRC) uses these recommendations to generate their regulations as they apply to the use of by-product radioactive materials. All three bodies work in concert to establish the dose of ionizing radiation that, in light of current knowledge, is not expected to cause appreciable bodily injury to a person at any time during his lifetime.

Concern for radiation protection falls into two general categories: (1) those effects that get more severe with increasing dose and for which a threshold is believed to exist—called *nonstochastic,* and (2) those effects where the probability of the effect (rather than the severity) gets worse with increasing dose and which have no threshold—called *stochastic*. Examples of nonstochastic effects include cataracts, blood changes, and sperm production. These are effects that arguably are produced only beyond a certain threshold, and the severity of the effect is increased with increasing exposure to ionizing radiation. Examples of stochastic effect are cancer and genetic effects. These are effects that can be produced at low absorbed doses of ionizing radiation.

The purpose of radiation protection practices then is twofold: (1) to prevent, as much as possible, the development of nonstochastic diseases by setting dose equivalent limits well below the threshold limit such that these limits will not be reached even for the total period of one's working life; and (2) to limit the risks of stochastic diseases to a frequency no greater than risks in nonradiation occupations. To keep risks at a minimum, the NRC highly recommends the subscription to the ALARA program.

The acceptance of any dose involves the acceptance of a risk as well because a possibility exists that the radiation dose will manifest itself during the lifetime of the exposed person or in subsequent generations. However, the probability is so low that the risk is acceptable to the average individual. The new term relating risk to dose and the term that reflects the changes in philosophy regarding radiation is the *total effective dose equivalent* (TEDE). This term replaces the *maximum permissible dose* (MPD $= 5\ (N - 18)$ rem) established prior by the NCRP and used by the NRC until their rewrite of 10CFR20, effective 1/1/94. The definition of this new term (TEDE) is the sum of the *deep-dose equivalent* (DDE)—for *external whole body* exposures at a tissue depth of 1 cm—and the *committed effective dose equivalent* (CEDE)—from *internal exposures*.

$$\text{TEDE} = \text{DDE} + \text{CEDE}$$

The DDE is the same as the whole body deep dose with which occupational workers are familiar (see below). The CEDE is an internal dose to each irradiated organ and/or tissue from an intake of radioactive material by an individual during the 50-year period following the intake (called the *committed dose equivalent* or CDE), corrected for the stochastic risk to the whole body via the *weighting factor* (w_T). The CEDE is calculated as the sum of the CDEs multiplied by their respective weighting factors. Since the internal dose has rare applicability to a routine nuclear medicine worker, (with the possible exception of volatilized $Na^{131}I$ or $Na^{125}I$), the TEDE is essentially the DDE. These new terms reflect the new philosophy of the various councils on radiation protection by converting our thinking from organ doses and/or whole body doses to equivalent stochastic risks to the whole body.

Dose-equivalent (DE or H_T) is defined as the product of the absorbed dose (D) and the quality factor (Q) and any other modifying factor (N):

$$\text{DE} = \text{D} \times \text{Q} \times \text{N}$$

where D is the dose (energy absorbed per unit mass of irradiated material), Q is a factor to express the difference in biologic effectiveness of different types of radiation (Table 6-1), and N represents any other modifying factors. The units of dose-equivalents are the rem and sievert. Because external exposures to nuclear medicine personnel are due to beta and gamma radiation, where $Q = 1$ for both, and with no other modifying factors, DE reduces to D, or dose, which can be expressed (under whole body exposure conditions) as deep dose equivalent at 1 cm (DDE), shallow dose equivalent at 0.007 cm (SDE), or eye dose equivalent at 0.3 cm (LDE) and reported as such on the film badge report.

Another term, the *effective dose-equivalent* (EDE) or H_E, is an extension of the DDE. EDE is the sum of the deep dose-equivalents (DDE) for the various irradiated tissues and/or organs multiplied by their weighting factors. This manipulation expresses the mortality risk from cancer and the risk of severe hereditary effects in the first two generations due to the irradiation of different organs and/or tissues. EDE (H_E) is expressed as

$$\text{EDE} = \text{DDE} \times w_T$$

where w_T is a weighting factor (Table 6-2) representing the proportionate risk (stochastic) of tissue, T, under conditions of uniform whole-body irradiation* and DDE is the mean dose-equivalent received by tissue, T. Multiplying the dose to the organ by w_T results in the dose that would produce the same stochastic risk to the whole body. Because external exposures to nuclear medicine personnel are uniform to the whole body, the net result of multiplying all of the organs by their weighting factors results in a value of 1. Therefore, for external exposures:

$$\text{EDE} = \text{DDE}$$

*In conditions other than uniform whole-body exposures, EDE $=$ DE $\times\ w_T$.

That would not be the case for internal exposures, however, due to the fact that all of the organs and/or tissues would not recieve the same amount of radiation. In the case of inhaling volatilized $Na^{131/125}I$, the DE (or for longer effective-lived radionuclides, the CDE) would be modified primarily by the thyroid w_T value of 0.03 (from Table 6-2) in order to determine the CEDE. In so doing, the CEDE would be changed to reflect the proportionate amount of stochastic risk contributed by that thyroid to the whole body. Appendix C and its associated scenario is an attempt to simplify these difficult concepts.

Hands, forearms, feet, ankles, and lenses of the eyes are excluded from the H_E calculations. These are limited to the annual nonstochastic dose equivalent limits (Table 6-3) or 15 rems (150 mSv) to the lens and 50 rem (500 mSv) to extremities. Assuming a weighting factor of 0.01 applied to the skin (ICRU*), the annual dose-equivalent limit for skin is 50 rem (500 mSv).

A distinction is made between stochastic and nonstochastic effects with respect to annual dose equivalent limits; however, compliance with the stochastic effective dose-equivalent limits will necessarily allow for compliance with the nonstochastic dose-equivalent limits (e.g., stochastic effect limit for gonads is 5 rem [50 mSv], whereas their nonstochastic effect limit is 50 rem [500 mSv]). This simplistic approach becomes more complex when considering internal doses or ALI (annual limit on intake) and DAC (derived air concentrations).

The NCRP and the NRC recommend the discontinuance of the age proration formula of $5(N - 18)$ rem but continues the use of the annual 5 rem (50 mSv) limit. The cumulative exposure should not exceed $N \times 1$ rem ($N \times 10$ mSv), where N is age in years.

The fetus is always of concern in these dose-limiting discussions. The ICRP, NCRP, and NRC (in the new Part 20, specifically 20.1208) has retained its total dose limit at 0.5 rem (5 mSv) *once the pregnancy is declared.* If the pregnancy is never declared, the RSO is absolved of all responsibilities to the fetus. Once the pregnancy is declared (in writing, to include her estimated date of conception) and if fetal exposures have exceeded 0.5 rem (5 mSv), or are within 0.05 rem (0.5 mSv) of this dose, exposures to the fetus will not exceed 50 mrem (0.5 mSv) during the remainder of the pregnancy. Methods for the calculation of radiation dose to the embryo/fetus can be found in NRC Regulatory Guide 8.36. Should these limits threaten the job se-

*International Commission on Radiation Units and Measurements.

Table 6-2. Recommended weighting factors*

Tissue *(T)*	W_T
Gonads	0.25
Breast	0.15
Red bone marrow	0.12
Lung	0.12
Thyroid	0.03
Bone surfaces	0.03
Remainder	0.30
Whole body **Total:**	**1.00**

*Table expanded in NCRP60 to include more tissues and changes some values; however, the NRC uses this version.

Table 6-3. NRC dose-limiting recommendations (1994)

A. Occupational exposures (annual)		
1. Whichever is more limiting:		
a. TEDE (stochastic), or	5 rem	(50 mSv)
b. Sum of DDE and CDE to any organ/tissue except lens of the eye (non-stochastic)	50 rem	(500 mSv)
2. Eye dose equivalent (LDE)	15 rem	(150 mSv)
3. Shallow dose equivalent (SDE) to skin/extremity	50 rem	(500 mSv)
4. Minors (occupational)	10% of above	10% of above
B. Public exposures		
1. TEDE (annual)	0.1 rem	(1 mSv)
2. Dose in unrestricted area (in any one hour)	2 mrem/hr	(0.02 mSv/hr)
C. Embryo-fetus exposures		
1. Total dose (if pregnancy declared)	0.5 rem	(5 mSv)
2. Dose limit for remainder of pregnancy if dose $>$ 0.5 rem or within 0.05 rem (0.5 mSv) of that dose at time of declaration	0.5 rem	(0.5 mSv)
D. Planned special occupational exposure		
1. In any year	As in A	As in A
2. In individual's lifetime	5 × A	5 × A

curity of the occupational worker, she may "undeclare" her pregnancy (in writing) and all fetal restrictions are lifted. It is recommended that special attention be given to the occupational worker of child-bearing age so that exposures are distributed uniformly with time so that the fetus does not receive more than its limit before pregnancy is known. All such records will be preserved for the lifetime of the individual. Regardless of thc method used to calculate occupational personnel radiation exposure, any excesses are considered overexposures and must be reported to the Commission as specified in Title 10CFR20.403.

■ ALARA

The Nuclear Regulatory Commission has continued to attempt to reduce radiation exposure to occupational personnel. As more methods and devices are made available to reduce exposure, the commission has encouraged their use through regulation by making their use a condition of licensure, or by suggestion via regulatory guides.

Such was the reasoning behind the development and publication of NUREG-0267, as a draft in December 1977, by the Office of Standards of the Nuclear Regulatory Commission. The document was entitled, *Principles and Practices for Keeping Occupational Radiation Exposures at Medical Institutions As Low As Reasonably Achievable*. The document has assumed the name *ALARA* as an acronym from the last five words of the title. The document reviews methods for maintaining ALARA exposures in detail. A model program was developed from this document that was to be enacted by each medical institution, effective August 15, 1980. It became a condition of the Nuclear Regulatory Commission license. On 4/1/87, it took on further importance by being incorporated into Title 10 of the Code of Federal Regulations (10 CFR35.20). As of January 1, 1994, ALARA has been incorporated into 10CFR20. By so doing, it becomes an NRC regulation, and binding.

Although the ALARA program deals with a commitment by management as well as the radiation safety committee (RSC) and the radiation safety officer (RSO), the overriding purpose was to develop an increased awareness for occupational exposures. This was accomplished by suggesting two investigational levels for occupational external radiation exposure (Table 6-4) that when exceeded initiate a review or an investigation by the RSO and/or the RSC. The investigational levels that are eventually adopted are set as a function of the RSO in accordance with 10CFR 35.21(b)(4).

If the quarterly exposure for an individual is less than investigational level I, no further action is required. If the personnel exposure is equal to or greater than investigational level I but less than level II, the RSO will review and report the results to the RSC at the next meeting. The RSC compares these results to the exposures of other individuals performing the same tasks as an index of ALARA program quality. If exposures are equal to or greater than investigational level II, the RSO will investigate and take action. The action is reviewed by the RSC and the institution's management. All such records are made available to Nuclear Regulatory Commission inspectors.

■ SPECIFIC FACTORS INVOLVED IN RADIATION PROTECTION

■ Type of radiation

In nuclear medicine three types of emissions are of primary concern: alpha particles, beta particles, and gamma rays. In addition, there are x rays resulting from several phenomena of interaction with matter. Some of these have great impact on patient dosimetry (e.g., characteristic x rays (from ^{201}Hg) in ^{201}Tl decay) while others are very weak and of no consequence, in terms of radiation protection. One fact to be considered is that of external emission versus internal emission—whether the radiation comes from outside the body and penetrates the epidermis into the body or whether the emitters are already inside the body after being introduced by way of ingestion, inhalation, or intravenous injection. Gamma rays and x rays are able to penetrate the epidermis of the skin and therefore present the same hazard whether they are external or internal emitters. Such is not the case with alpha and beta emitters. Alpha and beta particles cannot ordinarily penetrate the outer layers of the skin. As external emitters they do not usually constitute a serious problem with radiation protection. If they are used as internal emitters, however, the problem of alpha and beta radiation damage becomes severe.

Table 6-4. Suggested investigational levels for occupational external radiation exposures according to ALARA

Body part	mrem (mSv)/quarter year	
	Level I	Level II
Whole body; head and trunk; active blood-forming organs; lens of eyes; or gonads	125 (1.25)	375 (3.75)
Hands and forearms; feet and ankles	1875 (18.75)	5625 (56.25)
Skin of whole body*	750 (7.50)	2250 (22.50)

*Not normally applicable to nuclear medicine operations except those using significant quantities of beta-emitting nuclides.

■ Penetration power

As just stated, alpha and beta particles are not generally regarded as radiation hazards if they are external emitters. A 1.0 MeV alpha particle has a range in tissue of 0.0006 cm and in air of 0.49 cm, whereas a 5 MeV alpha particle has a range of 0.0037 cm in tissue. An alpha particle would require an energy of 7.5 MeV to penetrate human skin. Under ordinary circumstances a piece of paper stops an alpha particle.

The penetration power of beta particles is about 100 times that of alpha particles. An inch of wood or 1/25 inch of aluminum is required to stop a beta particle. The range in tissue for a 1 MeV beta particle is 0.42 cm and for a 5 MeV beta particle 2.2 cm. Although an external beta emitter is generally considered not to be of consequence as far as radiation protection is concerned, a beta particle can penetrate from a few millimeters to 1 cm beneath the skin. There is a rapid deceleration of the particle as a result of its interaction with tissue.

Gamma rays have extremely high penetration power and can create radiation hazards as either external or internal emitters. The gamma ray cannot be stopped by paper or small amounts of aluminum or lead. In general, protection is in terms of inches of lead and feet of concrete. In contrast to total absorption of an alpha or beta particle, only 3% of the gamma ray energy is absorbed in 1 cm of tissue. The rest is either absorbed in a much larger volume of tissue or travels through and completely out of the body.

■ Ionization

Ionization in tissue, either directly or indirectly, is thought to be the most important biologic interaction of radiation. Almost all the damage to tissue is as a result of this phenomenon. The ability to ionize varies tremendously among alpha, beta, and gamma emissions. A term that is used to describe this phenomenon is *specific ionization,* discussed previously in this chapter.

There is an important correlation between the ionization ability and the penetration power of the various emissions. The alpha particles are weak in their penetration power, but their ionization ability reaches tremendous proportions. If alpha particles bypass the epidermis, they present a tremendous problem in radiation biology. This is also true of beta emitters. Although beta emitters do not have as great an ionization ability, they have increased penetration power. However, their penetration power is not such that they can penetrate far beyond the skin. Based on their ionization ability, beta emitters can cause tremendous biologic damage, provided the protective layer of the skin is bypassed. It is for this reason that phosphorus 32, a pure beta emitter, is used therapeutically in cases of leukemia and polycythemia. The rationale for its use is based solely on its ability for localized destruction of tissue function. Since most radiopharmaceuticals are beta-gamma emitters, the beta component represents the largest contribution of radiation dose as an internal emitter. In some cases 90% to 95% of the dose is from the beta component. Although alpha and beta particles cannot penetrate the skin, there must still be protection against them. Because of their ability to ionize tissue once they have bypassed the skin, they present more of a radiation hazard than do gamma photons, although the damage is localized.

■ PRACTICAL METHODS OF RADIATION PROTECTION

For personnel involved in the use of radioactive materials, methods of radiation protection should be foremost in their thoughts at all times. The total picture of the actual effects of radiation is not known and may not be known for many centuries to come. However, assuming that all ionizing radiations are potentially harmful, humans can cope with the problem by constantly being alert to methods of protection. Practical limitations established by national and international committees to assist the occupational radiation worker have already been discussed. The rationale for these limits is that even peaceful uses of the atom require some exposure to emissions. It is impossible and impractical to shield workers from them completely. There is also a constant bombardment by cosmic radiation from outside the earth's atmosphere. These cosmic rays are highly energetic; practically speaking, no amount of protection can shield us completely from these rays. Humans have learned to live with these omnipresent cosmic radiations. Complete shielding is also impractical because many beneficial uses of atomic energy would be removed from modern medical technology, such as x-ray and nuclear medicine therapy and diagnosis. For precisely this reason, nuclear medicine personnel must be constantly aware of the practical methods of radiation protection. These methods are distance, shielding, and time. With the judicious use of all three of these methods, the amount of radiation to which the radiation worker is subjected can be kept at a minimum and well within the limitations established by the NCRP.

■ Distance

Distance constitutes one of the best methods of radiation protection and is one of the routine methods used. It is not only an effective means of radiation protection, but in many instances it is the least expensive. As an individual moves away from the source of radiation, it is natural to expect to receive less radiation. The novice might think that as the distance is doubled from the source at a given position, the radiation to the person would be reduced by one half; however, the radiation is reduced to one fourth. This is known as the inverse square law, which states that the amount of radiation at a given distance from a point source is inversely proportional to the square of the distance. By doubling the distance, the dose is one fourth the original;

by halving the distance, the dose is four times the original.

The name of the law defines the nature of the law itself. By increasing the distance by a factor of 2, the dose is decreased by the inverse square of 2 (namely, ¼), according to the following:

Distance factor	Inverse	Inverse square
2	½	$(½)^2$ = ¼

Accordingly, by reducing the distance by a factor of ½, the dose is increased by the inverse square of ½ (namely, 4):

Distance factor	Inverse	Inverse square
½	²⁄₁	$(2/1)^2 = 4/1 = 4$

This relationship is seen in Fig. 6-2.

The inverse square law can also be expressed as a formula. By using this formula and knowing the intensity at a given distance, a person can mathematically determine the intensity at another known distance or the distance at which that person could receive a required intensity. The formula follows:

$$\frac{I}{i} = \frac{d^2}{D^2} \text{ or } ID^2 = id^2$$

I = Intensity at a distance *(D)* from a point source
i = Intensity at a different distance *(d)*

The following examples demonstrate the inverse square law:

1. 300 mrem/hr is measured at 8 cm. What is the dose rate at 2 cm?

$$\frac{x}{300} = \frac{8^2}{2^2}$$

$$x = \frac{8^2}{2^2} \times 300 = \frac{64}{4} \times 300 = 4800 \text{ mrem/hr}$$

2. 600 mrem/hr is measured at 10 cm. What is the distance at which 150 mrem/hr is received?

$$\frac{600}{150} = \frac{x^2}{10^2}$$

$$x^2 = \frac{600}{150} \times 10^2$$

$$x = \sqrt{\frac{600 \times 100}{150}} = \sqrt{400} = 20 \text{ cm}$$

Both examples could have been calculated without the use of the formula. In example 2 the dose rate desired is one fourth of that measured at 10 cm from the point source. According to the inverse square law, this would require twice the distance or 20 cm.

The principle of the inverse square law is easily demonstrated by any survey meter and a point source. If the point source is placed at a distance of 0.5 m from the detector and the reading is recorded by moving the source to a distance of 1 m, the intensity is reduced to one fourth. The inverse square law applies most accurately with the use of gamma emitting point sources; that is, with sources in which the radioactivity is contained in a very small volume. It does not apply to extended sources or to multiple sources.

The inverse square principle explains the suggested use of long-handled tongs and remote-control handling devices with application to large quantities of radiation. It also plays

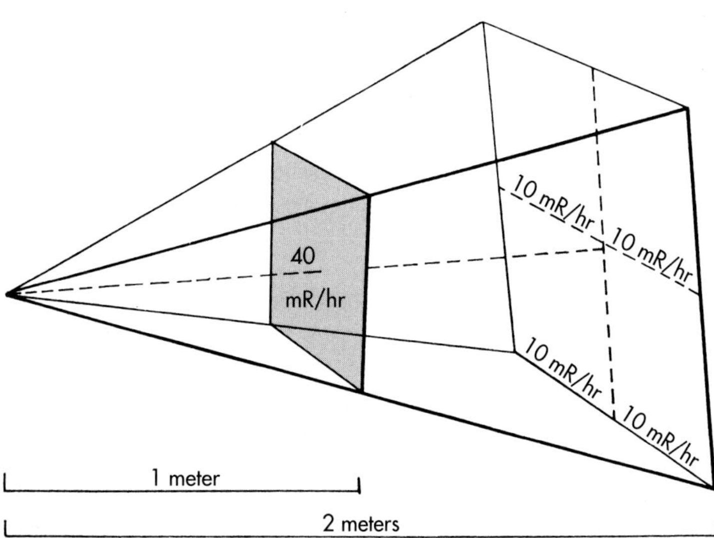

Fig. 6-2. Inverse square law. As radiations are emitted from a point source, an arbitrary area is selected at 1 m, representative of a radiation intensity of 40 mR/hr. At 2 m (twice the distance from the point source) that same radiation field of 40 mR/hr has expanded to an area four times the size of the original area. Consequently, the original area (gray) now receives only one fourth of the entire radiation.

a role in the calculation of visiting time to a recently treated patient. It may be that a patient's family could stay only 10 minutes at the bedside, but by not allowing the visitors within 6 feet, their stay could be prolonged based on inverse square relationships.

■ Exposure

Formula. A formula that might find use in the medical management of a therapy patient is one that can predict the exposure rate at some distance from the treated patient. Since exposure rate is proportional to the emission rate of photons and their energy, and it decreases inversely with the square of the distance, a formula for gamma photons between 70 keV and 4 MeV is as follows:

$$\text{Exposure rate (mR/hr)} = \frac{6\ CEf}{d^2}$$

C = Activity of source in mCi
E = Photon energy in MeV
f = Fraction of atoms yielding E energy photons
d = Distance from source in feet (centimeters can be used by changing 6 to read 5000)

Example. A patient was treated with 100 mg Eq* cesium 137 brachytherapy sources. What is the exposure rate in mrem/hr at a distance of 100 feet? (mg Eq ^{137}Cs must be multiplied by 2.7 to determine mCi.)

$$\text{mrem/hr} = \frac{6 \times 100 \times 2.7 \times 0.662 \times 0.946}{10^2}$$
$$= 10 \text{ mrem/hr (0.1 mSv/hr)}$$

*Eq is equivalent dose to ^{226}Ra therapy.

If the radionuclide used for therapy had several significant photons, each would have to be calculated in this manner and added as in the following example.

Example. Patient was treated with 100 mCi (3.7 GBq) of iodine 131. What is the exposure rate from this patient at 10 feet? (^{131}I has two significant gamma photons, 364 keV [83.8%] and 637 keV [6.6%].)

mrem/hr from 0.364 MeV photons
$$= \frac{6 \times 100 \times 0.364 \times 0.836}{10^2}$$
$$= 1.83 \text{ mrem/hr}$$
mrem/hr from 0.637 MeV photons
$$= \frac{6 \times 100 \times 0.637 \times 0.066}{10^2}$$
$$= 0.25 \text{ mrem/hr}$$
Total exposure rate = 1.83 + 0.25 = 2.08 mrem/hr (or 0.02 mSv/hr)

Another formula to express the same relationship within acceptable agreement is as follows:

$$\text{Exposure rate (rem/hr)} = \frac{\Gamma A}{d^2}$$

Γ* = The specific gamma ray constant expressed in R/mCi/hour at 1 cm and found for each radionuclide in appropriate handbooks
A = Activity in mCi
d = Distance in cm

■ Shielding

Shielding is also a practical method of radiation protection. The use of shielding materials such as lead sheets and

*^{137}Cs = 3.3, ^{60}Co = 13.2, ^{131}I = 2.2, ^{226}Ra = 8.25.

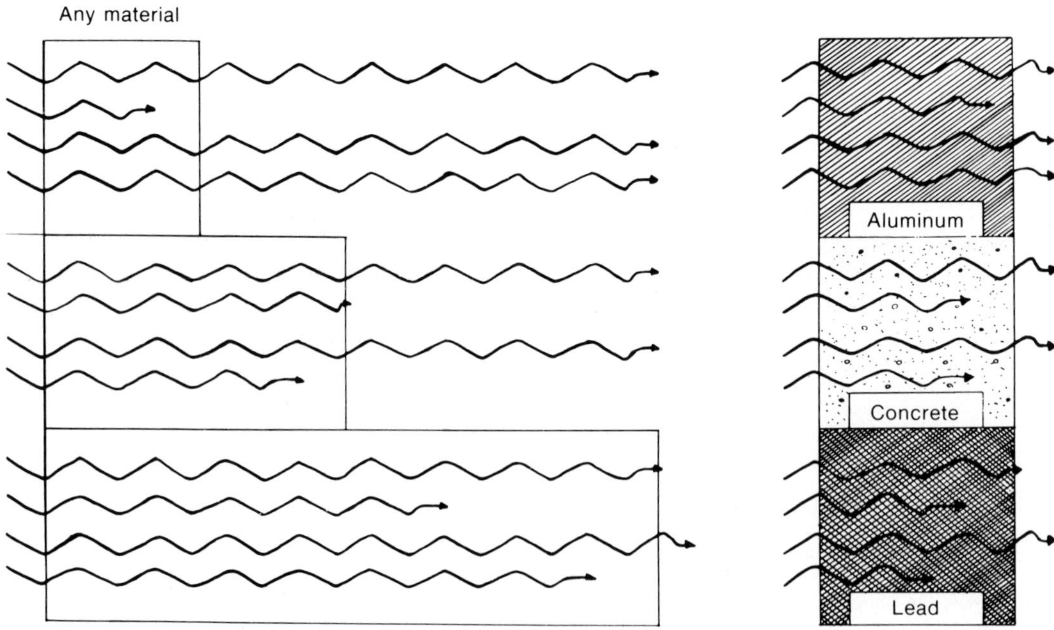

Fig. 6-3. Absorption characteristics of shielding materials. As density and/or thickness of the shielding material increases, the absorption of radioactive emissions by the material also increases.

lead bricks is nothing new to even the most inexperienced radiation worker. This shield is simply a body of material used to prevent or reduce the passage of radiation. In the case of alpha and beta radiation, little shielding is required to absorb the emissions completely. An alpha particle is stopped by a sheet of paper, a beta particle is stopped by an inch of wood, but feet of concrete or inches of lead are necessary to absorb gamma radiation. The general practice is to use enough shielding for complete absorption of alpha and beta particles. However, this is not true with gamma radiation or x-radiation. With these two types of emissions, shielding is used to reduce the amount of radiation.

The shielding aspect of beta particles deserves special consideration. It is known that ¼ inch of plastic stops a beta particle; therefore a syringe provides adequate shielding in itself. For example, if a syringe containing ^{32}P is placed near a scintillation detector, a large number of counts will be received. The detector is actually registering the electromagnetic radiation resulting from Bremsstrahlung.

For radiation to be completely absorbed or reduced in intensity, energy must be lost by the radiations themselves. The energy of charged particles is lost primarily by a series of ionization events or excitation of atoms within the shielding medium. Energy from electromagnetic radiation is lost by three methods: photoelectric effect, Compton effect, or pair production, depending on the energy of the radiation itself. For those gamma rays below 1.02 MeV in energy, the process of absorbing is usually a series of Compton collisions whereby the energy gradually diminishes. Eventually the radiations are sufficiently decreased in energy that total absorption occurs through the photoelectric effect. For those gamma rays above 1.02 MeV of energy, pair production occurs with the eventual formation of two gamma rays of 0.511 MeV. They are eventually absorbed by the Compton and photoelectric interactions.

As far as the shielding material itself is concerned, density and thickness go hand-in-hand in reducing radiation intensity (Fig. 6-3). If a material 1 cm thick with a density of 10 gm/cm^3 (grams per cubic centimeter is a standard unit of density) were placed between a source and a detector, it would have the same stopping power as a material 10 cm thick having a density of 1 gm/cm^3 placed similarly. For this reason, units of *density thickness* have become accepted in grams per square centimeter according to the following:

$$\frac{\text{gm}}{\text{cm}^3} \times \text{cm} = \frac{\text{gm}}{\text{cm}^3} \times \frac{1}{\text{cm}^{-1}} = \text{gm/cm}^2$$

Shielding, however, is considerably more complicated than just these simple concepts in density thickness. It is easy, although hazardous, to suggest a direct relationship of density to atomic number (Z). In general, it is true that the higher the atomic number, the higher the material's density and vice versa. However, there are plenty of exceptions to the rule. Gold and lead are good examples. Gold has a Z of 79 with a density of 19.3 gm/cm^3; lead has a higher Z of 82 and a lower density of 11.0 gm/cm^3. Densities also change when materials assume different physical states, and yet their atomic numbers remain the same. A good example of this is water. It has an effective atomic number of 7.4 but assumes different densities depending on its physical state—whether ice, liquid, or vapor (Fig. 6-4).

Attenuation coefficients. Any discussion of shielding must present some units for measuring the quantity of radiation that is absorbed (attenuated) by some absorber. Two such units are the *linear attenuation coefficient* and the *mass attenuation coefficient*. They differ in that the latter unit considers the density of the attenuating medium.

Linear attenuation coefficient. The linear attenuation coefficient (symbol, μ) is defined as the fraction of the number of photons removed from the radiation field per centimeter of absorber. It is expressed as a constant percentage of photons absorbed, much like the decay constant, λ, in the physical half-life formula. A condition with a μ value of 20% per centimeter (written 0.20 cm^{-1}) would indicate that the remaining number of photons in a photon beam would be reduced in intensity by 20% for each centimeter of the absorbing medium (Fig. 6-5). A μ value is specific for the energy of the photons and the type of absorber. If either change, so also does the linear attenuation coefficient. Table 6-5 lists a variety of linear attenuation coefficients for several photon energies in different media.

Mass attenuation coefficient. The mass attenuation coefficient (symbol, μ/ρ) is another useful unit. It is obtained by dividing the linear attenuation coefficient by the density (ρ) of the absorbing medium. The unit is expressed in terms of cm^2/gm. By the same token, the μ value could be determined by multiplying the mass attenuation coefficient (cm^2/gm) by the density (gm/cm^3).

The relationship between μ and μ/ρ is seen in Fig. 6-4. Since water has a density of unity, μ and μ/ρ are the same. Because density changes with the various physical states of water, the linear attenuation coefficient also changes. The reason is that attenuation by the absorber changes, and this unit reflects only the attenuation by the absorbing medium per centimeter. That is in contrast to the mass attenuation coefficient, which remains the same regardless of the change in the physical state of the medium. The reason is that this unit reflects the density of the entire absorbing medium, not just the thickness. It can also be concluded from this figure that 1 gm of water, ice, or water vapor absorbs the same amount of photons per gram. This relationship is not important in medicine because sizes of human organs do not allow this type of consideration. Further, since the mass attenuation coefficient remains the same for all physical forms of water regardless of density or volume, the mass attenuation coefficient is not important to medicine either. Therefore the shielding formula uses the linear attenuation coefficient.

Attenuation in the photoelectric range. Another interesting phenomenon occurs in the attenuation of various en-

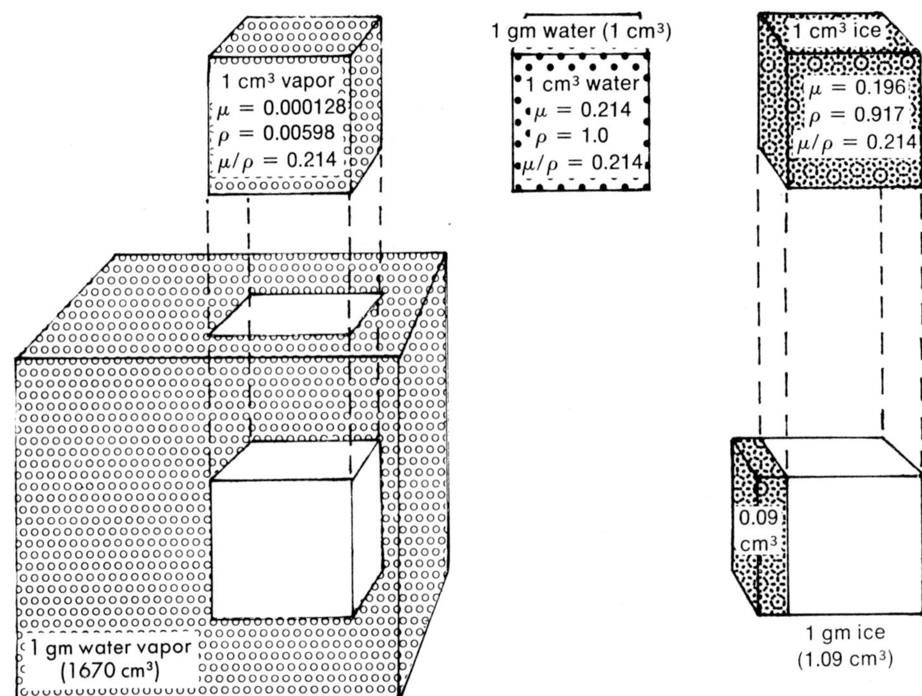

Fig. 6-4. Relationship of mass attenuation coefficients and linear attenuation coefficients for 1 gm of water as it changes its physical state to ice or to water vapor. Values are for a 50 keV monochromatic photon beam. Ice and water vapors are less dense than water so that μ changes proportionally to reflect that density change.

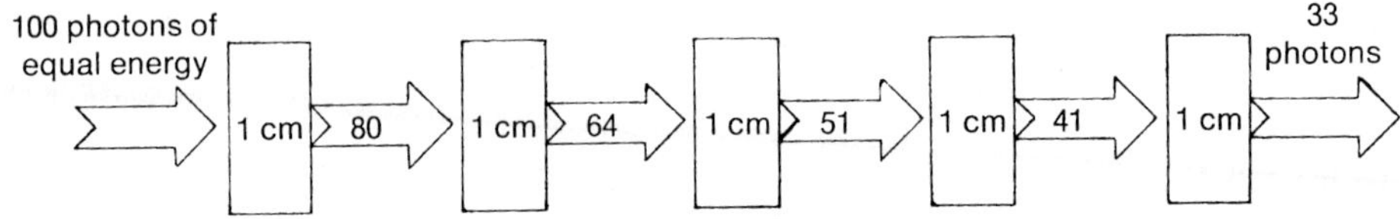

Fig. 6-5. Attenuation of a photon beam through 5 cm of an absorbing medium for which $\mu = 0.20\ cm^{-1}$. Each centimeter of the absorber reduces the remaining number of photons by 20%. Energy is monochromatic. Attenuation of polychromatic beams is much less predictable.

Table 6-5. Linear attenuation coefficients for a variety of media and photon energies

Attenuator with ρ in gm/cm³	Pb 11.34	Al 2.7	H_2O 1.0	NaI 3.67
μ at 20 keV	984.4	9.278	0.711	62.39
μ at 27.4 keV	447.2	3.985	0.434	23.86
μ at 140 keV	27.1	0.386	0.153	2.496
μ at 364 keV	3.164	0.262	0.111	0.459
μ at 511 keV	1.724	0.224	0.096	0.327

Adapted from Gottschalk, A., and Potchen, E.J.: Diagnostic nuclear medicine, Baltimore, 1976, The Williams & Wilkins Co.

ergy photon beams. It is easily understood that as the energy of the photon increases, the probability of attenuation decreases. In other words, the mass attenuation coefficient is changing with the energy, and as the absorbing medium becomes less and less effective, the μ/ρ decreases and the percent transmission increases. Supposedly, a curve generated by plotting mass attenuation coefficient versus photon energy would result in a nice, smooth exponential curve. However, this is not the case. A proper curve used to show this relationship is seen in Fig. 6-6. The curve is not continuous but is broken at specific energy levels. One such break in the curve occurs at 88 keV. The reason for this response is that photons photoelectrically interact with and therefore are absorbed by electrons bearing binding energies closest to their energy. As the energy of the photon increases beyond that binding energy, the probability of the

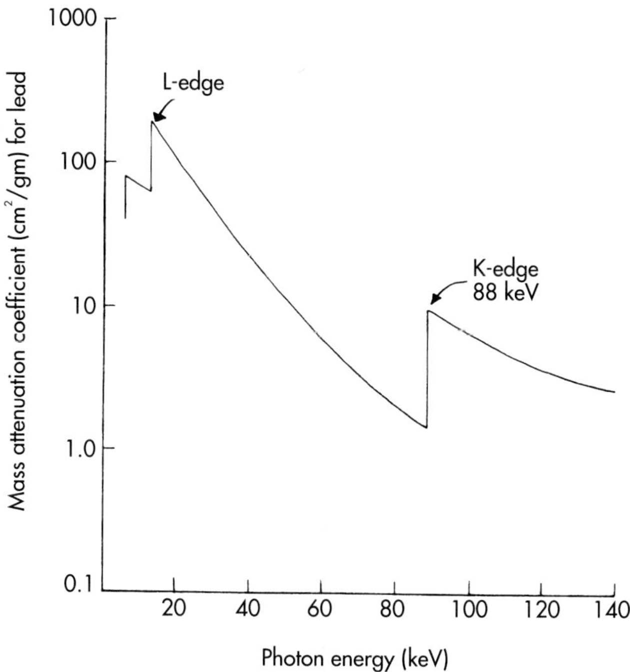

Fig. 6-6. Photoelectric mass attenuation coefficient for lead as related to energy.

photoelectric effect taking place is reduced; therefore percent transmission increases. This fall in attenuation continues until the photon energy reaches the binding energy of the next lowest energy shell, at which point a sharp rise occurs in the mass attenuation coefficient and percent transmission once again is drastically reduced. This point of abrupt change is called the *K-edge* or *L-edge,* depending on the photon energy. The curiosity of this phenomenon is that with two radionuclides of different energy, the amount of lead needed to adequately shield the lower energy radionuclide may be greater. For example, since the K-edge for lead occurs at 88 keV, it would require more lead shielding to satisfactorily attenuate an 81 keV radionuclide (^{133}X) than a 140 keV radionuclide (^{99m}Tc).

Attenuation in the Compton range. Another factor that affects attenuation is the number of electrons per gram. As a general rule, the lower the atomic number, the higher the number of electrons per gram. Just as with the mass attenuation coefficient, even though the term is in units per weight, the unit has little meaning as far as attenuation in the body goes. The number of electrons per gram of water is the same whether it is in the liquid, solid, or gaseous state. To circumvent this problem, the unit should be multiplied by density units to yield electrons per cubic centimeter as follows:

$$\frac{\text{electrons}}{\text{gram}} \times \frac{\text{grams}}{\text{cm}^3} = \frac{\text{electrons}}{\text{cm}^3}$$

In this form the unit has meaning. The number of electrons per cubic centimeter is especially important to attenuation at energy levels at which the Compton reaction predominates. If the photon is not able to be absorbed by way of the photoelectric effect as a result of its high energy, reliance must be placed on the probability that the Compton interaction will occur and recur, eventually reducing the photon energy to a point at which the photoelectric effect will be possible. That probability is directly related to the number of electrons per cubic centimeter. The suggestion by the use of this term is that a less dense material may have the same shielding capabilities as a more dense material because of its increased number of electrons per gram. Or the reverse could be true; a material having fewer numbers of electrons per gram than another material can have significantly different attenuation capabilities associated with differences in the density of the materials, as is evidenced by Table 6-6. This table shows silver (Ag) as being less dense, but as a result of its number of electrons per gram, it is a more effective radiation shield. Needless to say, the cost of silver far outweighs this advantage. The reverse is also true; uranium, which has fewer electrons per gram than lead, is a more effective shield because of the density differences. Depleted uranium is used at the ports of teletherapy units as "trimmers" designed to reduce ineffective radiation to the therapy patient.

Table 6-6. Relationship of density units and electron per gram (e/gm) units to attenuation

Element	Z	e/gm*	Density	e/cm³
Ag	47	2.62×10^{23}	10.5	2.751×10^{24}
Pb	82	2.38×10^{23}	11.35	2.701×10^{24}
U	92	2.33×10^{23}	18.68	4.352×10^{24}

$$\text{*e/gm} = \frac{\text{Avogadro's no. } (6.02 \times 10^{23}) \times Z}{A}$$

Shielding formula. All the factors influencing the effectiveness of the attenuating material can be expressed mathematically as follows:

$$I = I_o e^{-\mu x}$$

I = Radiation intensity after shielding
I_o = Radiation intensity before shielding
e = Base of the natural logarithm, 2.718
μ = Linear attenuation coefficient in cm^{-1}
x = Thickness of shield in cm

Minus sign indicates that the intensity is decreasing

To use the formula it must be assumed that the radiation intensity before shielding is 100 mrem/hr and that the density of the shield (absorber) is such that the fractional decrease (μ) is half the intensity per centimeter (50% per centimeter, or 0.50 cm^{-1}); the intensity after 1 cm shielding would not be 50 mrem/hr as might be expected but greater than that value because of many complicating factors, such

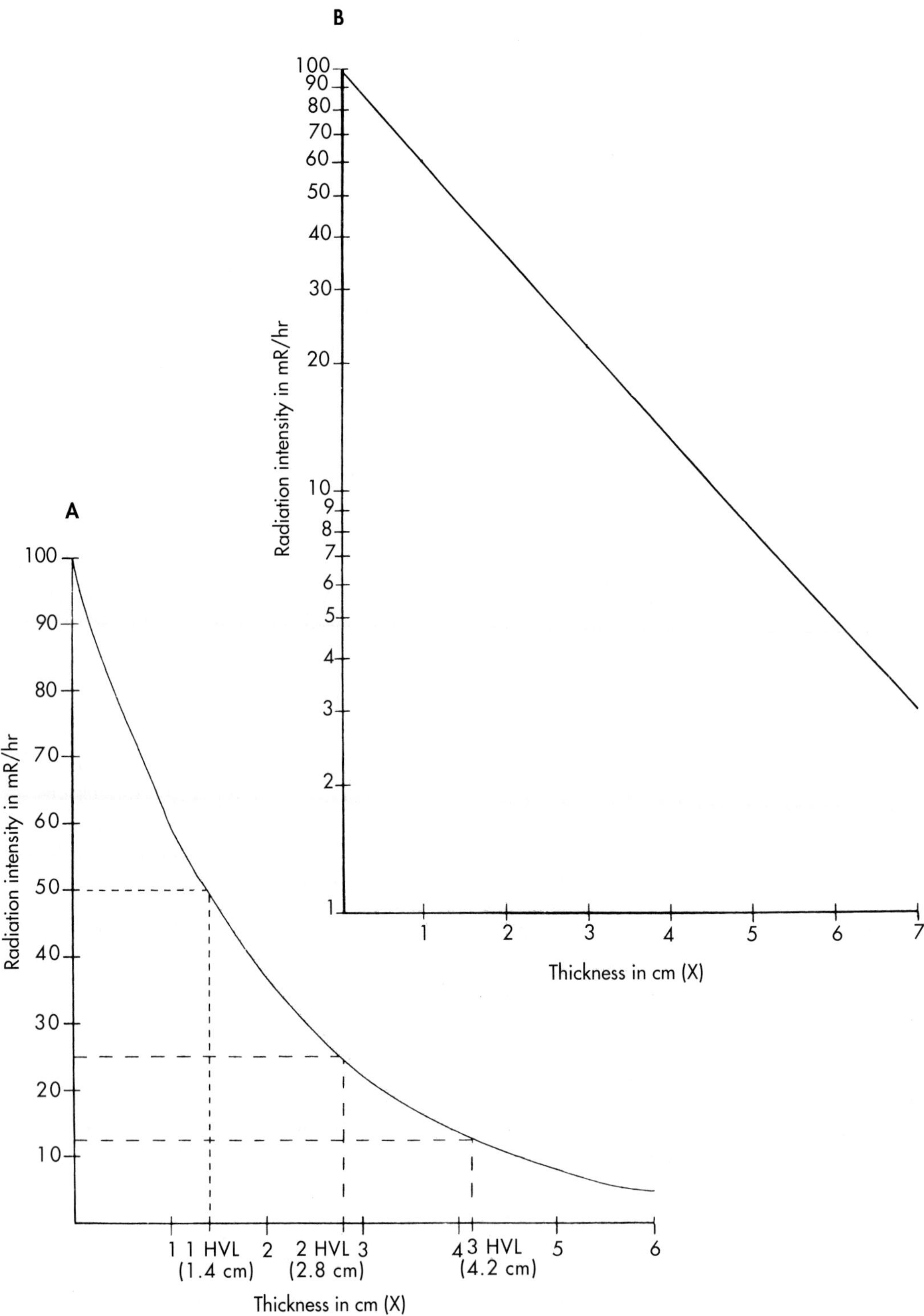

Fig. 6-7. Relationship of thickness of shielding to radiation intensity. **A,** Exponential function of the relationship. **B,** Curve as a straight line plotted on semilogarithmic paper. The half-value layer (HVL) can be ascertained from either part of the graph.

Table 6-7. Half-value layers for a variety of media and photon energies

Attenuator with p in gm/cm^3	Pb 11.34	Al 2.7	H_2O 1.0	NaI 3.67
HVL (cm) at 20 keV	0.0007	0.0747	0.975	0.011
HVL (cm) at 27.4 keV	0.0015	0.174	1.597	0.029
HVL (cm) at 140 keV	0.0256	1.796	4.530	0.278
HVL (cm) at 364 keV	0.2190	2.646	6.245	1.510
HVL (cm) at 511 keV	0.4021	3.094	7.220	2.120

Adapted from Gottschalk, A., and Potchen, E.J.: Diagnostic nuclear medicine, Baltimore, 1976, The Williams & Wilkins Co.

as back-scatter and dose buildup, for which all are accounted in the formula. A micron factor of 0.50 cm^{-1} would result in a decrease in the intensity to only 61 mrem/hr according to the following:

$$I = I_0 e^{-\mu x}$$
$$I = 100 \times e^{-0.50 \times 1}$$
$$I = 100 \times e^{-0.50}$$
$$I = 100 \times 0.61 = 61 \text{ mrem/hr (0.61 mSv/hr) @ 1 cm}$$

Calculations for 2, 3, 4, 5, and 6 cm of the same absorbing media using this formula yield a resultant intensity of 37 mrem/hr, 22 mrem/hr, 13.5 mrem/hr, 8 mrem/hr, and 5 mrem/hr, respectively. By plotting these intensity values versus thickness on linear graph paper, an exponential curve is received (Fig. 6-7, *A*). Plotting the same parameters on semilogarithmic graph paper produces a straight line (Fig. 6-7, *B*).

The formula is not of major practical importance in the field of nuclear medicine. It has value in that it makes possible the prediction of the attenuation of a gamma photon.

Half-value layer. It has already been stated that x-radiation or gamma radiation can be reduced to acceptable limits but theoretically cannot be reduced to zero. As is evidenced by Fig. 6-7, it can be attenuated in a predictable manner. This useful information is referred to as the half-value layer (HVL). By definition HVL is the thickness of any particular material necessary to reduce the intensity of a radiation field to half its original value.

Fig. 6-7 shows that by interposing 1 HVL (1.4 cm) of shielding material between the source and a detector, the radiation field is reduced to half its original intensity (from 100 mrem/hr to 50 mrem/hr). Similarly, by interposing 2 HVLs (2.8 cm), the field is reduced by half again (from 50 mrem/hr to 25 mrem/hr). Because the exponential curve approaches the abscissa asymptotically, it can be theorized that no amount of shielding could completely stop all the photons. Continuous interpositioning of HVLs results in a continuous halving process that becomes infinite.

Half-value layers for most radionuclides in various media are known and can be found in any radiologic handbook. Table 6-7 lists a variety of HVLs for various photon energies in a variety of media. These values provide a quick calculation of the shielding necessary to reduce the radiation intensity to acceptable limits. An example follows.

Table 6-8. Relationship of radiation intensity to barrier thickness

Attenuation (HVL)	Intensity (mrem/hr @ 1 m)	Lead thickness (cm)*
0	24	0
1	12	1.25
2	6	2.5
3	3	3.75
4	1.5	5.0

*Convert to inches: 4.8 cm ÷ 2.54 cm/inch = 1.97 inches. Therefore 2 inches of lead would be adequate to reduce radiation intensity to 2 mR/hr @ 1 m.

Problem. A cobalt 60 calibration source producing a radiation field of 24 mrem/hr at 1 m requires protection. If lead is used as the standard shielding material, how much lead is required to reduce the radiation intensity to acceptable limits? (Pb HVL for ^{60}Co = 1.25 cm.)

Solution. Two inches of lead would be adequate to reduce the intensity to 2 mrem/hr measured at 1 m, the acceptable limit. Table 6-8 demonstrates this relationship.

The respect for half-value layers as a radiation protection device should become tremendously enhanced when it is realized that 1 HVL reduces intensity to one half, regardless of the original intensity. Accordingly, 1.25 cm of lead reduces a cobalt 60 source with an intensity of 1000 rem/hr to 500 rem/hr, just as the same 1.25 cm of lead reduces cobalt 60 from 1 mrem/hr to 0.5 mrem/hr.

By carefully examining the shielding formula and discussion, a number of general statements may be made.

1. Four factors influence the efficacy of shielding: density, electrons per gram, thickness, and energy.
2. As density, electrons per gram, and/or thickness of the attenuating medium increase, the after-shielding intensity decreases.
3. As the energy of the photon or particle increases, the after-shielding intensity increases.
4. Any material regardless of the magnitude of these four factors absorbs some of the radiation and consequently decreases the after-shielding intensity.

5. The type of radiation is also an important consideration. Alpha radiation intensity can be reduced to zero (completely absorbed) by a sheet of paper. Beta radiation intensity can be reduced to zero (completely absorbed) by ¼ inch of plastic or 1 inch of wood. X-radiation and gamma radiation intensity can never be completely reduced, although they can be attenuated in a predictable manner.
6. The shielding material must be of sufficient density and/or thickness to reduce the exposure to acceptable limits. A standard acceptable limit is 2 mrem/hr at 1 m because of the following:

$$2 \text{ mrem/hr} \times 50 \text{ hr/week} \times 50 \text{ week/year}, = 5000 \text{ mrem/year, or } 5 \text{ rem/year}$$

This value is the TEDE for occupational radiation personnel per year. For any length of time, 1 m is a reasonable working distance from any source of radiation.

■ Time

The principle of time is also a practical method of radiation protection. The longer an individual is exposed to a field of radiation the greater is the total exposure. Common sense dictates that time should be used as a control of radiation exposure. In diagnostic applications of nuclear medicine time does not become as important as in therapy.

Three groups of nonoccupational personnel deserve special time considerations: nursing personnel, visitors, and adjacent patients.

For time considerations to become meaningful, reference must be made to the Nuclear Regulatory Commission's regulations on the subject (10CFR20.1301). These regulations stipulate the following:

"Each licensee shall conduct operations so that the TEDE to members of the public . . . does not exceed 0.1 rem (1 mSv) in a year . . . and the dose in any unrestricted area* from external sources does not exceed 0.002 rem (0.02 mSv) in any one hour."

Since these regulations are considerably more restrictive (from 100 mrems/7 days to 100 mrems/year) than old Part 20, time is an important aspect in containing exposure and meeting these new requirements. It should be noted that any member of the public entering a restricted area† (e.g., radiopharmaceutical therapy patient's room) assumes the "risks" of the restricted area and the limits of the occupational personnel. It is inconceivable that they would exceed 5000 mrems TEDE as a visitor or nurse, but time of exposure calculations may be necessary (rare) to determine the need for personnel monitors if 10% of the exposure limits are exceeded (20.1502). It is possible, however, that the adjacent patient may be exposed continuously to radiation from a therapy patient. Time calculations would be necessary to insure that the adjacent patient would be held to 100 mrems per year at a rate not to exceed 2 mrems in any one hour. It may require that the adjacent patient be moved.

It might also be important to indicate that in some therapeutic applications of radiopharmaceuticals this dose rate decreases with time because of large eliminations by way of normal biologic processes. If such is the action of the therapeutic agent, readings taken at various times of the day could extend visitation privileges.

*An "unrestricted area" means an area, access to which is neither limited nor controlled by the licensee.

†A "restricted area" means an area, access to which is limited by the licensee.

BIBLIOGRAPHY

Bernier, D.R., Langan, J.K., and Wells, L.D.: Nuclear medicine technology and techniques, ed. 2, St. Louis, 1989, Mosby–Year Book.

Bogardus, C.R., Jr.: Clinical applications of physics of radiology and nuclear medicine, St. Louis, 1969, Warren H. Green, Inc.

Brodsky, A.: Principles and practices for keeping occupational radiation exposures at medical institutions as low as reasonably achievable. Washington, D.C., 1982, U.S. Nuclear Regulatory Commission.

Chandra, R.: Introductory physics of nuclear medicine, ed. 4, Philadelphia, 1992, Lea & Febiger.

Chase, G.D., and Rabinowitz, J.L.: Principles of radioisotope methodology, ed. 3, Minneapolis, 1967, Burgess Publishing Co.

Goodwin, P.N., and Rao, D.V.: An introduction to the physics of nuclear medicine, Springfield, Ill., 1977, Charles C Thomas, Publisher.

Gottschalk, A., and Potchen, E.J.: Diagnostic nuclear medicine, Baltimore, 1976, The Williams & Wilkins Co.

Hendee, W.R.: Medical radiation physics, ed. 2, Chicago 1979, Mosby–Year Book.

Johns, H.E., and Cunningham, J.R.: The physics of radiology, ed. 4, revised edition, Springfield, Ill., 1983, Charles C Thomas, Publisher.

National Council on Radiation Protection and Measurements: NCRP Report No. 91. Recommendations on limits for exposure to ionizing radiation, Bethesda, Md., 1987.

Quimby, E.H., and Feitelberg, S.: Radioactive isotopes in medicine and biology, ed. 2, Philadelphia, 1963, Lea & Febiger.

Rocha, A.F.G., and Harbert, J.E.: Textbook of nuclear medicine: basic science, Philadelphia, 1978, Lea and Febiger.

Rollo, F.D.: Nuclear medicine physics, instrumentation, and agents, St. Louis, 1977, Mosby–Year Book.

Shapiro, J.: Radiation protection: a guide for scientists and physicians, ed. 2, Cambridge, Mass., 1981, Harvard University Press.

Shilling, C.W.: Atomic energy encyclopedia in the life sciences, Philadelphia, 1964, W.B. Saunders Co.

Shleien, B.: Health physics and radiological health handbook, Silver Springs, Md., 1992, Scinta, Inc.

Sorenson, J.A., and Phelps, M.E.: Physics in nuclear medicine, ed. 2, New York, 1987, Grune & Stratton, Inc.

Wagner, H.N.: Principles of nuclear medicine, Philadelphia, 1968, W.B. Saunders Co.

Chapter 7

DOSIMETRY

PAUL J. EARLY

Perhaps the major consideration in all studies in which radionuclides are administered to human beings is the amount of activity administered to a patient and its consequent radiation dose to vital organs. For the diagnostic uses of such drugs this becomes the limiting factor. All these problems of statistics, time involved in any given study, and so on could be resolved immediately merely by increasing the amount of radioactivity administered. Nuclear medicine procedures are not like x-ray procedures in which millions of photons per second are available for a given study. Because of this factor, many radiographic techniques require only fractions of seconds to complete. The magnitude of photons from a nuclear medicine procedure is on the order of hundreds of thousands of photons; therefore minutes or hours are required to obtain enough counts to make a statistical evaluation of a study. In such studies the radioactive materials become lodged, pooled, or incorporated into selective organs and remain there for periods as short as seconds to as long as months or even years. While the radioactive material is in the organ or is being excreted by the body, it is irradiating the exposed tissues even after the study has been completed. However, x rays originate external to the body and produce effects only during the time that the body or organ or both is exposed to the x-ray unit.

Since this is the case, the radiopharmaceutical user must give thoughtful consideration to the question of radiation dosage caused by the agent during the time that the body and its critical organs are being exposed. It enables the physician to assess benefit versus risk for either a particular radionuclide or a particular application. This is considered important by all three government bodies having at least some form of jurisdiction in the use of radiopharmaceuticals (Nuclear Regulatory Commission, National Institutes of Health, and the Food and Drug Administration). The FDA has authority over all pharmaceutical preparations, whereas the Nuclear Regulatory Commission has authority over only by-products from a nuclear reactor, and the National Institutes of Health has control of blood derivatives.

For years the knowledge of dosimetry was much too fragmentary to establish exact values of dosage to the body and critical organs as a result of the administration of a known amount of radionuclide. The prevailing compromise was to attempt to predict in the approximate order of magnitude the absorbed radiation dose (in rad units) to the whole body, critical organ (organ in which the radionuclide is primarily collected), and the organs of elimination. Many assumptions were incorporated into such a calculation. In many cases when exact values were unknown, it was customary to use pessimistic assumptions. In this way the result represented an acceptable figure but on the upper limit of the true value. If this value were adequate, the true value would represent an even smaller radiation dose.

■ MARINELLI FORMULA

In the past the classic expressions of radiation dosimetry according to Marinelli were as follows:

$$D_\beta = 73.8 \times C \times \bar{E}_\beta \times T_e$$
$$D_\gamma = 0.0346 \times C \times \Gamma \times \bar{g} \times T_e$$

D_β = Dose in rad from beta radiation
D_γ = Dose in rad from gamma radiation
C = Initial concentration of radionuclide in μCi/gm
$\bar{E}_\beta$ = Mean energy of β radiations in MeV ($\cong \frac{1}{3} E_{max}$)
Γ = Gamma dose constant in R/mCi/hr at 1 cm distance
$\bar{g}$ = Geometric factor to account for variations in shape, size, and volume of organ
T_e = Effective half-life in days

The two constants, 73.8 and 0.0346, are conversion factors so that the product appears in rad. $\bar{E}_\beta$ and Γ are parameters that can be found in any handbook of radiation health and in many advanced texts. All other factors are variables. C is a variable because the number of microcuries and the gram weight would both vary among individuals. The adequate calculation of this parameter is compounded when radiopharmaceuticals are used for dynamic function studies, such as ^{99m}Tc DTPA and ^{99m}Tc glucoheptonate studies. T_e varies from person to person. The $\bar{g}$ values are available for a variety of standard geometric configurations, but no human organ exactly resembles a sphere or a cylinder, so this contributes to the value as something removed from the true value. Other complicating factors include unequal distribution of the radioactive material in the organ, energy of the emission (some gammas are so weak that they are betalike as far as dosimetry is concerned), and irradiation from adjacent organs (pancreas and liver) or companion organs (cross irradiation from one lung to the other or one kidney to the other).

In these equations Marinelli and co-workers approached the problem of internal radiation dosimetry from the standpoints of penetrating (D_γ) and nonpenetrating (D_β) radiations but did so by grouping all their constants together and all their variables together and solving for each separately. This necessitated many assumptions, usually erroneously high. The total radiation dose was found by adding the penetrating (p) and the nonpenetrating (np) radiations together.

■ MIRD FORMULA

The current approach to the problems of internal radiation dosimetry as proposed by the Medical Internal Radiation Dose (MIRD) Committee is still to consider both penetrating and nonpenetrating radiations. The MIRD technique, however, groups all physical data for both penetrating and nonpenetrating radiations together. Furthermore, it groups all biologic data and some of the physical data related to time and radionuclide distribution together. Actually, the average absorbed dose from an administered radionuclide can be determined by the grouping of a variety of factors into three categories:

1. The biologic parameters that describe the uptake, distribution, retention, and release of the radiopharmaceutical agent in the body
2. The energy released by the radionuclide and whether it is penetrating or nonpenetrating
3. The fraction of the emitted energy that is absorbed by the target

The average absorbed radiation dose resulting from the administration of internally emitting radionuclides is simply the product of these three groups of information.

■ Biologic parameters

To compute the absorbed dose to an individual from an administered radionuclide, it must be known where the radionuclide goes, how long it takes to get there, how long it stays there, and the masses of the organs involved. Furthermore, there should always be an interest in the total amount of radiation to the target organs for the entire amount of time that the radionuclide is present. Therefore it would be important to determine the cumulative activity ($\tilde{A}$) in this organ from its entrance until its complete elimination from the system. This cumulative activity can be integrated and expressed as follows:

$$\tilde{A} = 1.443 \times A \times T_e{}^{*}$$

$\tilde{A}$ = Cumulative activity in μCi hour
A = Maximum activity in μCi
T_e = Effective half-life in hours

■ Energy released per disintegration

The next consideration is whether the radiations from the internally deposited radionuclide are penetrating or nonpenetrating. Nonpenetrating (np) radiations include alpha particles, beta particles, positrons, conversion electrons, Auger electrons, and x-rays or gamma rays with energies less than 11.3 keV. The penetrating (p) radiations consist of x-rays or gamma rays having energies greater than 11.3 keV and annihilation photons.

To use this information in the MIRD formula it is necessary to know the number of times that the gamma ray or x-ray occurs, termed *fractional abundance* (n_i), as well as its average or mean energies (E_i) in MeV, and add them all together.

The values for n_i and E_i for all the emissions from a variety of radionuclides may be found in MIRD Pamphlets Nos. 4 and 6.† Furthermore, to simplify the mechanics of calculating absorbed doses, the MIRD Committee has defined an equilibrium absorbed dose constant (Δ) as follows:

$$\Delta_i = 2.13 \; n_i \, E_i$$

Δ is in units of $\dfrac{\text{gram} \cdot \text{rad}}{\mu\text{Ci} \cdot \text{hour}}$

n_i = Fraction of quanta emitted per disintegration
E_i = Energy of the emitted quanta (meV)
2.13‡ = Conversion factor so that product appears as gram · rad/μCi · hr · meV

A table of these data as related to ^{99m}technetium can be found in Fig. 7-1. Appendix D contains these data for many radionuclides used in nuclear medicine.

*There are two assumptions in this cumulative activity formula that may or may not be correct. Assumption 1 is that the maximum activity *(A)* is reached in a negligible amount of time. Assumption 2 is that the elimination of the radionuclide is a single exponential curve, but this is often not the case. If Assumption 1 is incorrect, it can usually be corrected by assuming that the uptake of the material to reach maximum activity is approximately exponential in nature. In this case the *A* formula would be altered to read:

$$\tilde{A} = 1.443 \times A \, T_e(1 - T_{uptake}/T_e)$$

If Assumption 2 is incorrect and if more than one exponential curve is apparent, the *A* formula would consist of more than one term. In this way each term would represent another exponential and would be added as follows:

$$\tilde{A} = 1.443 \, (A^1 T_e^1 + A^2 T_e^2)$$

†Available from the Society of Nuclear Medicine, 475 Park Avenue, S., New York, N.Y. 10017.

$$‡2.13 \frac{\text{gram} \cdot \text{rad}}{\mu\text{Ci} \cdot \text{hr} \cdot \text{meV}} = 1.602 \times 10^{-6} \frac{\text{erg}}{\text{MeV}} \times 10^{-2} \frac{\text{rad}}{\text{erg/g}} \times 3.7 \times 10^4 \frac{\text{dis/sec}}{\mu\text{Ci}} \times 3600 \frac{\text{sec}}{\text{hr}}$$

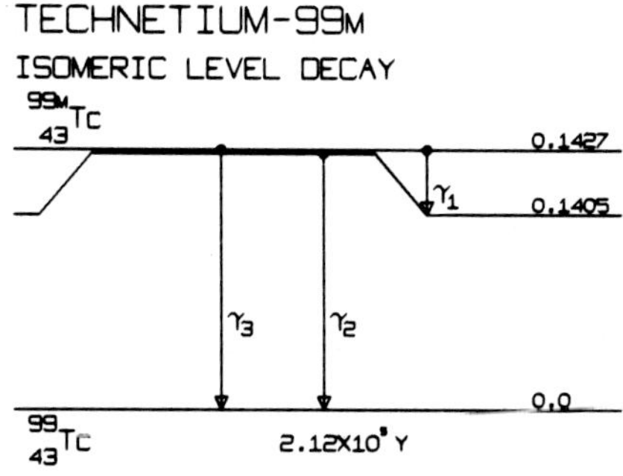

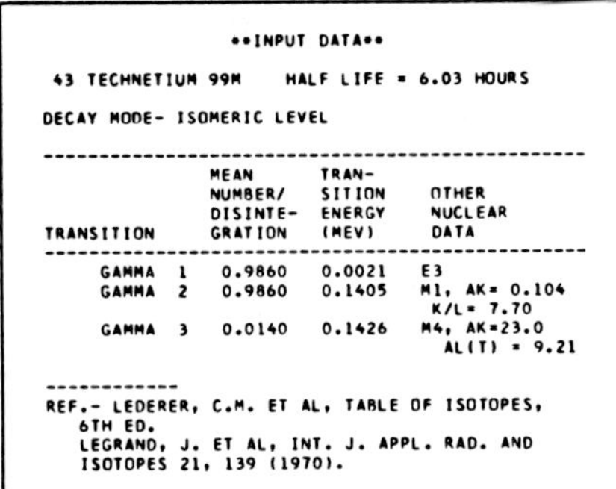

INPUT DATA

43 TECHNETIUM 99M   HALF LIFE = 6.03 HOURS

DECAY MODE- ISOMERIC LEVEL

TRANSITION	MEAN NUMBER/ DISINTE- GRATION	TRAN- SITION ENERGY (MEV)	OTHER NUCLEAR DATA
GAMMA 1	0.9860	0.0021	E3
GAMMA 2	0.9860	0.1405	M1, AK= 0.104 K/L= 7.70
GAMMA 3	0.0140	0.1426	M4, AK=23.0 AL(T) = 9.21

REF.- LEDERER, C.M. ET AL, TABLE OF ISOTOPES, 6TH ED.
LEGRAND, J. ET AL, INT. J. APPL. RAD. AND ISOTOPES 21, 139 (1970).

Fig. 7-1. Radionuclide decay schemes and nuclear parameters for use in radiation dose estimates using ^{99m}Tc. (Courtesy Dillman, L.T., and Von der Lage, F.C.: MIRD Pamphlet No. 10, New York, 1975, Society of Nuclear Medicine.)

OUTPUT DATA

43 TECHNETIUM 99M   HALF LIFE = 6.03 HOURS

DECAY MODE- ISOMERIC LEVEL

RADIATION	MEAN NUMBER/ DISINTE- GRATION n_i	MEAN ENERGY/ PAR- TICLE $\bar{E}_i$ (MeV)	EQUI- LIBRIUM DOSE CONSTANT Δ_i (g-rad/ µCi-h)
GAMMA 1	0.0000	0.0021	0.0000
M INT CON ELECT	0.9860	0.0016	0.0035
GAMMA 2	0.8787	0.1405	0.2630
K INT CON ELECT	0.0913	0.1194	0.0232
L INT CON ELECT	0.0118	0.1377	0.0034
M INT CON ELECT	0.0039	0.1400	0.0011
GAMMA 3	0.0003	0.1426	0.0001
K INT CON ELECT	0.0088	0.1215	0.0022
L INT CON ELECT	0.0035	0.1398	0.0010
M INT CON ELECT	0.0011	0.1422	0.0003
K ALPHA-1 X-RAY	0.0441	0.0183	0.0017
K ALPHA-2 X-RAY	0.0221	0.0182	0.0008
K BETA-1 X-RAY	0.0105	0.0206	0.0004
KLL AUGER ELECT	0.0152	0.0154	0.0005
KLX AUGER ELECT	0.0055	0.0178	0.0002
LMM AUGER ELECT	0.1093	0.0019	0.0004
MXY AUGER ELECT	1.2359	0.0004	0.0011

■ Absorbed fraction of energy (Φ)

The third consideration, the *absorbed fraction* (Φ), is defined as the ratio of energy absorbed by the target to the energy emitted by the source. Since nonpenetrating radiation loses essentially all its energy within 1 cm of its origin, the absorbed fraction *(n)* for these emissions is always 1.0 (or 100%). For penetrating radiation only partial absorption occurs in the tissue containing the radionuclide and in surrounding tissues and organs. The percentages have been determined using a "standard man" phantom.

The phantom has a simple geometric shape that approximates the body shape and dimensions as far as the major forms are concerned (Fig. 7-2). The phantom consists of three principal sections: (1) an elliptical cylinder representing the arms, torso, and hips; (2) a truncated elliptical cone representing both the legs and the feet; and (3) an elliptical cylinder representing the head and neck.

The absorbed fractions were generated by computer techniques relating many photon histories as they pass through an absorbing media. The computer was used to repetitively trace the path of a single photon through an absorbing medium with absorption coefficient data to calculate the energy lost per interaction and the scattering angle. Many such single photon histories were traced to generate a single absorbed fraction value.

The absorbed fraction is a function of photon energy and the size and shape of the tissue containing the radionuclide. Charts are available in MIRD Pamphlets Nos. 3 and 8, which contain absorbed fractions for a variety of organs (see Table 7-10).

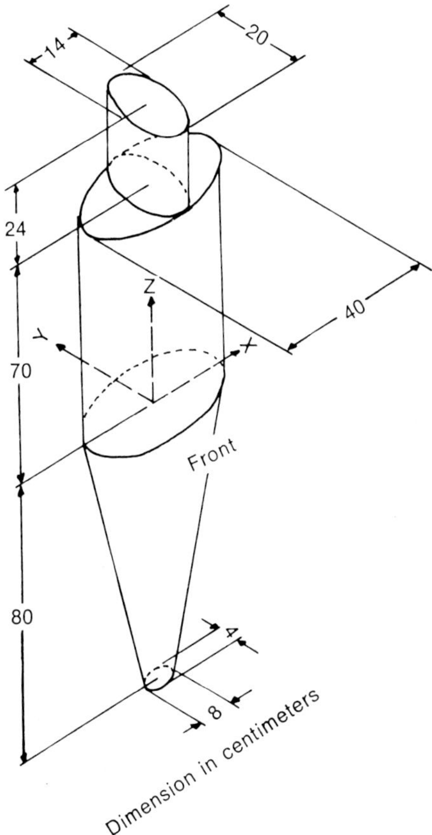

Fig. 7-2. Phantom illustrating approximate body shape and dimensions used by the MIRD Committee to determine absorbed fraction (Φ).

Table 7-1. Effective absorbed energy data for ^{99m}Tc (gray area only) listing all the penetrating and nonpenetrating contributions*

Radiation	η_i	$\bar{E}_i$	$\Delta_i = 2.13\ \eta_i \bar{E}_i$	× Φ_i	= $\Delta_i \Phi_i$
Gamma-1	0.0000	0.0021	0.0000	—	—
M-ice, γ-1†	0.9860	0.0016	0.0035	1.0	0.0035
Gamma-2	0.8787	0.1405	0.2630	0.162‡	0.0426
K-ice, γ-2	0.0913	0.1194	0.0232	1.0	0.0232
L-ice, γ-2	0.0118	0.1377	0.0034	1.0	0.0034
M-ice, γ-2	0.0039	0.1400	0.0011	1.0	0.0011
Gamma-3	0.0003	0.1426	0.0001	0.162‡	—
K-ice, γ-3	0.0088	0.1215	0.0022	1.0	0.0022
L-ice, γ-3	0.0035	0.1398	0.0010	1.0	0.0010
M-ice, γ-3	0.0010	0.1422	0.0003	1.0	0.0003
Kα1 x rays[1]	0.0441	0.0183	0.0017	0.830‡	0.0014
Kα2 x rays[2]	0.0221	0.0182	0.0008	0.830‡	0.0006
Kβ1 x rays[3]	0.0105	0.0206	0.0004	0.784	0.0003
KLL Auger e[4]	0.0152	0.0154	0.0005	1.0	0.0005
KLX Auger e[5]	0.0055	0.0178	0.0002	1.0	0.0002
LMM Auger e[6]	0.1093	0.0019	0.0004	1.0	0.0004
MXY Auger e[7]	1.2359	0.0004	0.0011	1.0	0.0011
					Σ 0.0818
					Σ_{np} 0.0369
					Σ_p 0.0449

*The rest of the data (absorbed fraction, Φ) are compiled for ^{99m}Tc in the liver as a contributor to the radiation dose to the liver.
†Internal conversion electron from M shell as a result of γ-1 interaction.
‡Interpolated values from absorbed fraction tables (Table 7-10).
Key: 1, Kα1 x ray ≡ K-L_{III} transition; 2, Kα2 x ray ≡ K-L_{II} transition; 3, Kβ1 x ray ≡ K-M_{III} transition; 4, KLL Auger e ≡ an Auger electron emitted from the L shell as a result of the transition of another L shell electron to a vacancy in the K shell; 5, KLX Auger e ≡ an Auger electron emitted from the X shell, where X stands for any shell higher than the L shell, as a result of the transition of an L shell electron to a vacancy in the K shell; 6, LMM Auger e ≡ an Auger electron emitted from the M shell as a result of the transition of another M shell electron to a vacancy in the L shell; 7, MXY Auger e ≡ an Auger electron emitted from the Y shell as a result of the transition of an X shell electron to a vacancy in the M shell, where X and Y each stand for any shell higher than the M shell.

■ Calculations

In summary, the absorbed dose to a particular tissue is the product of the three factors just discussed:

Absorbed dose = Cumulative concentration $\left(\frac{\text{Activity}}{\text{Mass*}}\right)$
× Summation of all energies emitted per disintegration
× Their absorbed fractions

Expressed in mathematic form:

$$\bar{D}\ (r_k \leftarrow r_h) = \frac{\tilde{A}_h}{m_k} \Sigma \Delta_i \Phi_i\ (r_k \leftarrow r_h)$$

r_k = Target organ
r_h = Source organ
A_h = Cumulative activity in source organ
m_k = Mass of target organ

Substituting for $\tilde{A}$:

$$D_\infty = \frac{A \times 1.44 \times T_e}{M} \Sigma \Delta_i \Phi_i \text{ rad}$$

*Mass in grams. Masses for all organs (as agreed on by the MIRD Committee) are found in Table 7-11.

Problem 1. A liver scan is to be performed using 2.0 mCi (74 MBq) of ^{99m}Tc sulfur colloid. Approximately 85% of the dose is taken up by the liver, 10% by the spleen, and 5% by the bone. Compute the dose to the liver with both the Marinelli and the MIRD formula. Assume immediate uptake of the colloid by the liver with no biologic elimination; that is, the effective half-life is equal to the physical half-life.

Marinelli. The computation based on the Marinelli formula is as follows:

$$D_\gamma = 0.0346 \times C \times \Gamma \times \bar{g} \times T_e$$

$$= 0.0346 \times \left(\frac{2000 \times 0.85}{1800}\right) \times 0.56 \times 50 \times 0.25^*$$

= 0.23 rad (0.0023 Gy) to each gram of the entire liver

MIRD. The computation based on the MIRD formula requires the calculation on the contribution from three sources: the liver, the spleen, and the bone. These calculations follow on the next several pages.

*NOTE: In the classic Marinelli formula T_e is in units of days, whereas in the MIRD formula T_e is in hours.

Table 7-2. Compressed version of the effective absorbed energy data for ^{99m}Tc (gray area only) in the liver as a contributor to the radiation dose to the liver, listing all the penetrating contributions but combining all the nonpenetrating contributions (compare to Table 7-1)

Radiation	η_i	$\bar{E}_i$	$\Delta_i = 2.13\ \eta_i\bar{E}_i$	× Φ_i	= $\Delta_i\Phi_i$
$\Sigma\eta\rho$			0.0369	1.0	0.0369
Gamma-1	0.0000	0.0021	0.0000	—	—
Gamma-2	0.8787	0.1405	0.2630	0.162	0.0426
Gamma-3	0.0003	0.1426	0.0001	0.162	—
Kα1 x rays	0.0441	0.0183	0.0017	0.830	0.0014
Kα2 x rays	0.0221	0.0182	0.0008	0.830	0.0006
Kβ1 x rays	0.0105	0.0206	0.0004	0.784	0.0003
					$\Sigma\Delta_i\Phi_i$ = 0.0818*

*Once determined, this value, the *effective absorbed energy,* never changes; therefore save these calculations for all future liver calculations using ^{99m}Tc in which values of absorbed energy by the liver from contributions from the liver are required.

Table 7-3. Effective absorbed energy data for ^{99m}Tc in the spleen as a contributor to the radiation dose to the liver

Radiation	η_i	$\bar{E}_i$	$\Delta_i = 2.13\ \eta\bar{E}_i$	× Φ_i	= $\Delta_i\Phi_i$
ηρ—no contribution				0.00	—
Gamma-1	0.0000	0.0021	0.000	0.00	—
Gamma-2	0.8787	0.1405	0.2630	0.00708*	0.0018
Gamma-3	0.003	0.1426	0.0001	0.00708	—
Kα1 x rays	0.0441	0.0183	0.0017	0.000	—
Kα2 x rays	0.0221	0.0182	0.0008	0.000	—
Kβ1 x rays	0.0105	0.0206	0.0004	0.000	—
					$\Sigma\Delta_i\Phi_i$ = 0.0018†

*Interpolated from information on pp. 38-39 of MIRD Pamphlet No. 5.
†*Save for all future determinations.*

Contribution from liver (Table 7-1). The equation is:

$$D_{\infty liver \leftarrow liver} = \frac{2000(0.85) \times 1.443 \times 6^*}{1800} \Sigma_i\Delta_i\Phi_i \text{ rad}$$

To determine $\Sigma\ \Delta_i\ \Phi_i$ for the dose *to* the liver from ^{99m}Tc sulfur colloid *in* the liver, prepare a table as seen in Table 7-1. The table lists all the penetrating and nonpenetrating contributions from ^{99m}Tc (in gray) multiplied by the absorbed fraction (Φ) for each entry. A Φ value of 1.0 means 100% absorbed, a value that applies to all nonpenetrating radiations. Penetrating radiations vary, their value being taken from tables such as Table 7-10 to receive the $\Delta_i\Phi_i$ of each contribution, all of which are summed at the base of the last column. It is this figure that is used in the MIRD calculation. A compressed version of this table is seen in Table 7-2.

Since all nonpenetrating particles and nonpenetrating photons (those less than 11.3 keV) have an assumed absorbed fraction of 1.0, Table 7-1 can be greatly reduced by simply adding all the Δ_i values for these nonpenetrating emissions together. In this way they can be listed as nonpenetrating and the others computed as seen in Table 7-2. (The information in the gray areas is all the same for ^{99m}Tc. This information is always the same for ^{99m}Tc, regardless of the chemical/physical form of its use.) Data for other radionuclides used in nuclear medicine can be found in Appendix D.

With the summation data of Tables 7-1 and 7-2, the dose to the liver as a result of the liver contribution (which accounts for 85% of the dose) is determined by the following formula:

$$D_{\infty liver \leftarrow liver} = \frac{2000\ (0.85) \times 1.443 \times 6}{1800} \Sigma\Delta_i\Phi_i$$
$$= \frac{14{,}719}{1800} \times 0.0818$$
$$= 0.6689 \text{ rad } (0.6689 \text{ cGy})$$

Contribution from spleen (Table 7-3). The contribution from the spleen (assuming the spleen received 10% of dose) is as follows:

$$D_{\infty liver \leftarrow spleen} = \frac{2000\ (0.10) \times 1.443 \times 6}{1800} \Sigma\Delta_i\Phi_i$$
$$= 0.962 \times 0.0018 = 0.0017 \text{ rad } (0.0017 \text{ cGy})$$

Table 7-4. Effective absorbed energy data for ^{99m}Tc in bone as a contributor to the radiation dose to the liver

Radiation	η_i	$\bar{E}_i$	$\Delta_i = 2.13\ \eta\bar{E}_i$ (×)	Φ_i (=)	$\Delta_i\Phi_i$
ηρ—no contribution				0.00	
Gamma-1	0.0000	0.0021	0.0000	0.00	—
Gamma-2	0.8787	0.1405	0.2630	0.00478*	0.0013
Gamma-3	0.003	0.1426	0.0001	0.00478	—
Kα1 x rays	0.0441	0.0183	0.0017	0.00060	—
Kα2 x rays	0.0221	0.0182	0.0008	0.00060	—
Kβ1 x rays	0.0105	0.0206	0.0004	0.00083	—
				$\Sigma\Delta_i\Phi_i$ =	0.0013†

*Interpolated from information on pp. 36-37 of MIRD Pamphlet No. 5.
†*Save for all future determinations.*

Table 7-5. Effective absorbed energy data for ^{99m}Tc in the liver as a contributor to the radiation dose to the uterus

Radiation	η_i	$\bar{E}_i$	$\Delta_i = 2.13\ \eta_i\bar{E}_i$ (×)	Φ_i (=)	$\Delta_i\Phi_i$
ηρ—no contribution					
Gamma-1	0.0000	0.0021	0.0000	0.00	—
Gamma-2	0.8787	0.1405	0.2630	0.000123	0.00003
Gamma-3	0.003	0.1426	0.0001	0.0000	—
Kα1 x rays	0.0441	0.0183	0.0017	—	—
Kα2 x rays	0.0221	0.0182	0.0008	—	—
Kβ1 x rays	0.0105	0.0206	0.0004	—	—
				$\Sigma\Delta_i\Phi_i$ =	0.00003

Contribution from bone (Table 7-4). The contribution from bone (assuming bone received 5% of dose) is as follows:

$$D_{\infty \text{liver} \leftarrow \text{bone}} = \frac{1000\ (0.05) \times 1.443 \times 6}{1800} \Sigma\Delta_i\Phi_i$$
$$= 0.2405 \times 0.0013$$
$$= 0.0003 \text{ rad } (0.0003 \text{ cGy})$$

Total dose to the liver. To determine the total dose to the liver from all implicated organs, the totals of these calculations must be added together as follows:

Contribution from liver = 0.6689 rad
Contribution from spleen = 0.0017 rad
Contribution from bone = 0.0003 rad
Total radiation dose to the liver = 0.6709 rad or 671 mrad (0.6709 cGy)

Problem 2. This MIRD method of dosimetry can easily be extended to other organs as well. Suppose the patient who received this dose of ^{99m}Tc-labeled sulfur colloid revealed at a later date that she was pregnant at the time of the dose administration. The expectant mother now is concerned about the normal maturation of the fetus. The MIRD formula can be used easily to allay her fears as seen in Table 7-5. The dose to the uterus from the liver is as follows:

$$D_{\infty \text{uterus} \leftarrow \text{liver}} = \frac{2000\ (0.85) \times 1.443 \times 6}{80} \Sigma\Delta_i\Phi_i$$
$$= \frac{14{,}719}{80} \times 0.00003 = 0.006 \text{ rad or } 6.0 \text{ mrad}$$
$$= 0.006 \text{ cGy}$$

By this computation the concern of the young mother in this problem can be diminished. A dose of 6.0 mrad (0.006 cGy) should be of minimum concern to the normal maturation of the fetus.

■ S TABLES—ABSORBED DOSE PER UNIT CUMULATED ACTIVITY

As indicated in the footnotes of each of the preceding tabulations, once determined, the effective absorbed energy values should be saved for future determinations. The MIRD Committee has arranged a formula so that tables of factors can be generated for all of the organs (or even parts of organs and contents of some organs) with a variety of radionuclides used in nuclear medicine routinely. Once these factors are generated, that value remains the same regardless of the patient. The only variable in the MIRD formula is the biologic data necessary for the estimation of the cumulative activity, expressed as $\tilde{A}/M$.

The MIRD Committee has even taken it one step farther. It has incorporated the mass of the organ into this single factor, provided the median values for organ weights of a standard 70 kg man can be used and it can be assumed that the activity is uniformly distributed in that organ. That factor is called the S factor and is expressed as the absorbed dose per unit cumulated activity in rad/μCi-hour. These tabulations are referred to as the *S Tables*.* The use of these tables has greatly simplified the problems of internal radiation dosimetry by sparing the clinician the agony of generating all of the tables that preceded this section.

The MIRD formula using these tables (for example, Table 7-6) is expressed as follows:

$\bar{D} = \tilde{A}S$
$\bar{D}$ = Mean dose delivered to target organ
$\tilde{A}$ = Cumulative activity in μCi-hour
$\bar{S}$ = Absorbed dose per unit cumulated activity in rad/μCi-hour

The formula is also written as follows:

$\bar{D}(r_k \leftarrow r_h) = \tilde{A}_h\, S(r_k \leftarrow r_h)$
r_k = Target organ
r_h = Source organ
$(r_k \leftarrow r_h)$ = Dose to target organ as a result of contributions from source organ

The foregoing determination of the total dose to the liver involved the summation of contributions from a number of organs; therefore the total average dose to the target organ is determined by:

$$\bar{D}(r_k) = \sum_h \tilde{A}_h\, S(r_k \leftarrow r_h)$$

■ DOSE CALCULATIONS USING S TABLES (Table 7-6)

Problem 1. Estimate the dose to the *total body*, the *kidneys*, and the *testes* as a result of the presence of 1.0 mCi of ^{99m}Tc in the kidney. Assume that $T_e = T_p$ and there is instantaneous uptake.

Dose to kidney ($\bar{D}_{KID \leftarrow KID}$): (1000 μCi)(1.443)(6.0)
(1.9×10^{-4}) = 1.64 rad (1.64 cGy)

Dose to total body ($\bar{D}_{TB \leftarrow KID}$): (1000 μCi)(1.443)(6.0)
(2.2×10^{-6}) = 0.019 rad (0.019 cGy)

Dose to testes ($\bar{D}_{TES \leftarrow KID}$): (1000 μCi)(1.443)(6.0)
(8.8×10^{-8}) = 0.0007 rad (0.0007 cGy)

Problem 2. Compare the dosimetry of ^{131}I and ^{123}I as used for thyroid evaluation studies. Assume the dose to be 100 μCi with a 20% uptake, the uptake period being negligible. Assume biologic excretion as a single exponential with a biologic half-life (T_b) of 90 days. The solution follows:

*Available as MIRD Pamphlet No. 11 from Society of Nuclear Medicine, 475 Park Ave. S., New York, N.Y. 10017.

1. Convert T_b to T_e (90 days = 2160 hr):

$$^{131}\text{I}: T_e = \frac{8.05 \times 90}{8.05 + 90} = 7.4\text{d} = 178 \text{ hr}$$

$$^{123}\text{I}: T_e = \frac{13 \times 2160}{13 + 2160} = 13 \text{ hr}$$

2. Complete the MIRD formula, given that the only significant dose contribution to the thyroid gland comes from the thyroid tissue itself and the S factors for ^{131}I and ^{123}I as taken from MIRD Pamphlet No. 11 are:

^{131}I = 2.2E-02
^{123}I = 4.0E-03

$^{131}\text{I}: \bar{D}_{thy \leftarrow thy} = 100(0.20) \times 1.443 \times 178 \times 2.2 \times 10^{-2}$
= 113 rad/100 μCi ^{131}I (113 cGy/3.7 MBq ^{131}I)
$^{123}\text{I}: \bar{D}_{thy \leftarrow thy} = 100(0.20) \times 1.443 \times 13 \times 4.0 \times 10^{-3}$
= 1.50 rad/100 μCi ^{123}I (1.50 cGy/3.7 MBq ^{123}I)

To compare the dosimetry for these two radionuclides used to perform identical functions is to justify the use of ^{123}I. The tremendous reduction in radiation dose to the thyroid gland far outweighs the increased cost of ^{123}I.

Compare further the dose to the thyroid gland using ^{99m}Tc for thyroid evaluation studies. Assume the dose to be 1 mCi (37 MBq) with a 4% uptake, the uptake period being negligible. Assume the biologic excretion to be a single exponential with an effective half-life equal to the physical half-life of ^{99m}Tc. Dosimetry is calculated as follows:

$^{99m}\text{Tc}: \bar{D}_{thy \leftarrow thy} = 1000\ (0.04) \times 1.443 \times 6 \times 2.3 \times 10^{-3}$
= 0.8 rad/1 mCi ^{99m}Tc (0.8 cGy/37 MBq ^{99m}Tc)

Although the dosimetry would indicate that ^{99m}Tc would be the agent of choice for thyroid evaluation, many feel that the radiopharmacologic differences would refute this statement.

■ DOSE ESTIMATES FOR THE FETUS

Just as the thyroid can be computed for radiation dose/100 μCi to the thyroid, so also can all other organs be computed similarly. One of the more important areas and certainly the area that produces the most anxiety and concern is the dose to the fetus. This is especially true when the dose is administered unknowingly to a woman shortly after conception.

This was the subject of a scientific paper presented at the Sixteenth Annual Meeting of the Southeastern Chapter of the Society of Nuclear Medicine in Atlanta, Ga., in October 1975 and published in the *Journal of Nuclear Medicine*, volume 17, in 1976. Until this time, the dose to the fetus was considered to be equivalent to the dose to the uterus. In this work S factors were generated with the fetus being the target organ from applicable source organs for a variety of radionuclides (Table 7-7).

The dose per administered activity was calculated for several of the radiopharmaceuticals commonly used in nuclear medicine (Table 7-8). Using tables like this and knowing the amount of activity administered, one can easily estimate the dose to the fetus.

Table 7-6. S absorbed dose per unit cumulated activity (rad/μCi-hour), ^{99m}Tc, half-life 6.03 hours*

Target organs	Source organs									
			Intestinal tract							
	Adrenals	Bladder contents	Stomach contents	SI contents	ULI contents	LLI contents	Kidneys	Liver	Lungs	Other tissue (muscle)
Adrenals	3.1E-03†	1.5E-07	2.7E-06	1.0E-06	9.1E-07	3.6E-07	1.1E-05	4.5E-06	2.7E-06	1.4E-06
Bladder wall	1.3E-07	1.6E-04	2.7E-07	2.6E-06	2.2E-06	6.9E-06	2.8E-07	1.6E-07	3.6E-08	1.8E-06
Bone (total)	2.0E-06	9.2E-07	9.0E-07	1.3E-06	1.1E-06	1.6E-06	1.4E-06	1.1E-06	1.5E-06	9.8E-07
GI (stom wall)	2.9E-06	2.7E-07	1.3E-04	3.7E-06	3.8E-06	1.8E-06	3.6E-06	1.9E-06	1.8E-06	1.3E-06
GI (SI)	8.3E-07	3.0E-06	2.7E-06	7.8E-05	1.7E-05	9.4E-06	2.9E-06	1.6E-06	1.9E-07	1.5E-06
GI (ULI wall‡)	9.3E-07	2.2E-06	3.5E-06	2.4E-05	1.3E-04	4.2E-06	2.9E-06	2.5E-06	2.2E-07	1.6E-06
GI (LLI wall)	2.2E-07	7.4E-06	1.2E-06	7.3E-06	3.2E-06	1.9E-04	7.2E-07	2.3E-07	7.1E-08	1.7E-06
Kidneys	1.1E-05	2.6E-07	3.5E-06	3.2E-06	2.8E-06	8.6E-07	1.9E-04	3.9E-06	8.4E-07	1.3E-06
Liver	4.9E-06	1.7E-07	2.0E-06	1.8E-06	2.6E-06	2.5E-07	3.9E-06	4.6E-05	2.5E-06	1.1E-06
Lungs	2.4E-06	2.4E-08	1.7E-06	2.2E-07	2.6E-07	7.9E-08	8.5E-07	2.5E-06	5.2E-05	1.3E-06
Marrow (red)	3.6E-06	2.2E-06	1.6E-06	4.3E-06	3.7E-06	5.1E-06	3.8E-06	1.6E-06	1.9E-06	2.0E-06
Oth tiss (musc)	1.4E-06	1.8E-06	1.4E-06	1.5E-06	1.5E-06	1.7E-06	1.3E-06	1.1E-06	1.3E-06	2.7E-06
Ovaries	6.1E-07	7.3E-06	5.0E-07	1.1E-05	1.2E-05	1.8E-05	1.1E-06	4.5E-07	9.4E-08	2.0E-06
Pancreas	9.0E-06	2.3E-07	1.8E-05	2.1E-06	2.3E-06	7.4E-07	6.6E-06	4.2E-06	2.6E-06	1.8E-06
Skin	5.1E-07	5.5E-07	4.4E-07	4.1E-07	4.1E-07	4.8E-07	5.3E-07	4.9E-07	5.3E-07	7.2E-07
Spleen	6.3E-06	6.6E-07	1.0E-05	1.5E-06	1.4E-06	8.0E-07	8.6E-06	9.2E-07	2.3E-06	1.4E-06
Testes	3.2E-08	4.7E-06	5.1E-08	3.1E-07	2.7E-07	1.8E-06	8.8E-08	6.2E-08	7.9E-09	1.1E-06
Thyroid	1.3E-07	2.1E-09	8.7E-08	1.5E-08	1.6E-08	5.4E-09	4.8E-08	1.5E-07	9.2E-07	1.3E-06
Uterus (nongrvd)	1.1E-06	1.6E-05	7.7E-07	9.6E-06	5.4E-06	7.1E-06	9.4E-07	3.9E-07	8.2E-08	2.3E-06
Total body	2.2E-06	1.9E-06	1.9E-06	2.4E-06	2.2E-06	2.3E-06	2.2E-06	2.2E-06	2.0E-06	1.9E-06

From Snyder, W.S., and others: "S" absorbed dose per unit cumulated activity for selected radionuclides and organs, MIRD Pamphlet No. 11, New York, 1975, Society of Nuclear Medicine.

*Decay data revised—March 1972.

†The digits following the symbol E indicate the power of 10 by which the number is to be multiplied. For example, 3.1E-03 is equivalent to 3.1×10^{-3} or 0.0031.

‡Abbreviations spelled out in Table 7-11.

Table 7-7. S(fetus ← R_h), absorbed dose per unit cumulated activity (rad/μCi-hour) for several radionuclides and various sources organs R_h with the fetus as the target organ

Source organs	Radionuclides					
	^{99m}Tc	^{111}In	^{113m}In	^{123}I	^{131}I	^{133}Xe
Adrenals	4.0E-07*	1.4E-06	8.6E-07	4.9E-07	1.3E-06	7.0E-08
Bladder contents	1.9E-05	5.7E-05	3.2E-05	2.7E-05	4.9E-05	9.8E-06
Bone (total)	7.6E-07	2.3E-06	1.3E-06	9.0E-07	2.0E-06	2.1E-07
GI tract (stom cont)	9.7E-07	3.0E-06	1.8E-06	1.1E-06	2.8E-06	2.1E-07
GI tract (SI† and cont)	1.1E-05	3.1E-05	1.8E-05	1.4E-05	2.7E-05	4.8E-06
GI tract (ULI cont)	6.1E-06	1.8E-05	9.9E-06	7.4E-06	1.5E-05	2.1E-06
GI tract (LLI cont)	7.6E-06	2.2E-05	1.2E-05	9.2E-06	1.9E-05	2.7E-06
Kidneys	1.2E-06	3.6E-06	2.1E-06	1.4E-06	3.3E-06	2.5E-07
Liver	6.5E-07	2.1E-06	1.3E-06	7.7E-07	2.0E-06	1.3E-07
Lungs	8.4E-08	3.2E-07	2.4E-07	1.1E-07	3.6E-07	1.2E-08
Marrow (red)	2.3E-06	6.6E-06	3.7E-06	2.7E-06	5.8E-06	7.0E-07
Other tissues (muscle)	2.6E-06	8.0E-06	4.6E-06	3.8E-06	6.9E-06	1.3E-06
Ovaries	2.0E-05	5.8E-05	3.3E-05	2.7E-05	5.0E-05	9.9E-06
Pancreas	6.8E-07	2.2E-06	1.3E-06	8.0E-07	2.1E-06	1.3E-07
Salivary glands	4.5E-09	2.4E-08	2.5E-08	7.3E-09	3.9E-08	4.2E-10
Skin	7.0E-07	2.1E-06	1.2E-07	8.3E-07	1.9E-06	1.9E-07
Spleen	5.4E-07	1.8E-06	1.1E-06	6.5E-07	1.7E-06	1.0E-07
Thyroid	4.5E-09	2.4E-08	2.5E-08	7.3E-09	3.9E-08	4.2E-10
Total body	2.8E-06	8.2E-06	8.4E-06	4.1E-06	1.2E-05	5.3E-06

From Smith, E.M., and Warner, G.G.: J. Nucl. Med. 17:836-839, 1976.
*The digits following the symbol E indicate the power of 10 by which the initial number is to be multiplied; for example, 4.0E-07 = 4.0×10^{-7}.
†Abbreviations spelled out in Table 7-11.

Table 7-8. Dose estimates for the fetus

Radiopharmaceutical	Rad per millicurie administered
^{99m}Tc-sulfur colloid (normal)*	0.007
^{99m}Tc-sodium pertechnetate*	
Resting population	0.037
Nonresting population	0.039
^{123}I-sodium iodide (15%)*	0.032
^{131}I-sodium iodide (15%)*	0.10
^{99m}Tc-human serum albumin†	0.018
^{99m}Tc-lung aggregate†	0.035
^{99m}Tc-polyphosphate†	0.036
^{99m}Tc-stannous glucoheptonate†	0.040

From Smith, E.M., and Warner, G.G.: J. Nucl. Med. 17:836-839, 1976.
*Assumed thyroid uptake.
†From Kereiakes, J.G., and Rosenstein, M.: Handbook of radiation doses in nuclear medicine and diagnostic x-ray, 1980, CRC Press, Inc.

Problem 1. Using Table 7-8, estimate the dose to the fetus from an injection of 2.0 mCi ^{99m}Tc-labeled sulfur colloid.

$$\begin{aligned}\text{Fetus dose} &= 2 \text{ mCi} \times 0.007 \text{ rad/mCi}\\ &= 0.014 \text{ rad } (0.014 \text{ cGy})\end{aligned}$$

Extension of tables such as Table 7-8 have been developed. If the radiopharmaceutical does not appear in this table, refer to Appendix F.

Problem 2. Using Table 7-7, estimate the dose to the fetus from an injection of 2 mCi ^{99m}Tc-labeled macroaggregates (MAA). Assume a 100% tagging efficiency and 100% lung uptake with a 6-hour biologic half-life (Tb) in the lungs (= 3 hr T_e) and an infinite half-life in the liver (= 6 hr T_e) once it arrives there from the lungs. Assume the entire dose is sequestered by the liver (a pessimistic assumption, since decay of the radionuclide is occurring while in the lung). The solution is as follows:

$$\begin{aligned}D_{(fetus \leftarrow lung)} &= (2000)\ (1.443)\ (3)\ (8.4 \times 10^{-8}) = 0.0007 \text{ rad}\\ D_{fetus \leftarrow liver)} &= (2000)\ (1.443)\ (6)\ (6.5 \times 10^{-7}) = \underline{0.0113} \text{ rad}\\ \text{Total dose to fetus} &= 0.012 \text{ rad}\\ &\quad (0.12 \text{ mGy})\end{aligned}$$

■ DOSE ESTIMATES FOR NUCLEAR CARDIOLOGY STUDIES

With the rise in nuclear cardiology studies, dosimetry became the concern of nuclear cardiology specialists. Concerns were based on the fact that ^{201}Tl is known to result in significant kidney exposures and to localize in testes and that ^{99m}Tc-labeled methylene diphosphonate (MDP) localizes in the bone marrow. Table 7-9 lists radiation dose estimates to different organs using several radionuclide forms that are used for nuclear cardiology and compares some of them to radiation exposures from catheterization

Table 7-9. Radiation dose estimates to different organs

Tissue	^{201}Tl chloride (rad/mCi)	^{99m}Tc-MDP (rad/20 mCi)	^{99m}Tc-HSA (rad/20 mCi)	Catheterization and angiocardiography (rad examination)
Skeleton	—	0.70	—	—
Bone marrow	0.31	0.56	0.076	1.4
Kidney	1.14	0.62	0.063	—
Liver	0.64	0.16	—	—
Total body	0.22	0.13	0.073	—
Bladder wall	—	—	0.166	—
2-hr void	—	2.60	—	—
4.8-hr void	—	6.20	—	—
Ovaries	—	0.24	—	—
2-hr void	0.59	0.34	—	—
Testes	—	—	0.079	0.025
2-hr void	—	0.16	—	—
4.8-hr void	0.54	0.22	—	—
Heart	0.18	—	—	—
Skin	—	—	—	4.7

From Syed, I.B., and others: Health Phys. 42(2):159-163, 1982.

and angiocardiography procedures. Appendix F contains a greatly expanded version of this table including other radiopharmaceuticals and listing the three most highly exposed organs for each radiopharmaceutical. Perhaps most importantly, this table contains fetal dose estimates.

Problem 1. Using Table 7-9, estimate the dose to the bone marrow using ^{201}Tl chloride and ^{99m}Tc-MDP. Compare this to the radiation dose of catheterization and angiocardiography. The solution is as follows:

$$^{201}\text{Tl chloride: } \overline{D} = 2 \text{ mCi} \times 0.31 \text{ rad/mCi} = 0.62 \text{ rad } (0.62 \text{ cGy})$$

$$^{99m}\text{Tc-MDP: } \overline{D} = 20 \text{ mCi} \times 0.56 \text{ rad/mCi} = 1.12 \text{ rad } (1.12 \text{ cGy})$$

$$\text{Catheterization and angiocardiography: } \overline{D} = 1.4 \ (1.4 \text{ cGy}) \text{ rad per examination}$$

The radiation exposures from MDP and radiographic procedures are similar. Estimates on the risk of leukemia* are on the order of 15 to 25 cases per million persons per rad after a 10-year latent period. However, since these estimates are based on observations following the absorbed dose of 100 rad, it is safe to assume that the risk of leukemia is substantially less with diagnostic doses of 1 to 1.5 rad.

Problem 2. Using Table 7-9, estimate the dose to the testes using ^{201}Tl chloride and ^{99m}Tc-MDP (assuming a 4.8-hour voiding time). Compare to the radiation dose of catheterization and angiocardiography. The solution is as follows:

$$^{201}\text{Tl chloride: } \overline{D} = 2 \text{ mCi} \times 0.54 \text{ rad/mCi} = 1.08 \text{ rad } (1.08 \text{ cGy})$$

$$^{99m}\text{Tc-MDP: } \overline{D} = 20 \text{ mCi} \times 0.22 \text{ rad/mCi} = 4.4 \text{ rad } (4.4 \text{ cGy})$$

$$\text{Catheterization and angiocardiography: } \overline{D} = 0.025 \ (0.025 \text{ cGy}) \text{ rad per examination}$$

As calculated, significant exposures to the testes occur with the use of radionuclide procedures versus catheterization and angiocardiography. Concerns with the use of radionuclide studies are those of genetic mutation. This would be a concern only if the exposed patient would subsequently have children; however, ^{201}Tl procedures are routinely performed on male patients well past what is generally considered to be the reproductive age. Therefore these exposures contribute little to the genetically significant dose.

■ LIMITATIONS OF THE MIRD CALCULATION

The MIRD formula has reduced the number of assumptions necessary to perform the dosimetry calculations over that required by the classic expression of dosimetry. The MIRD formula still has some limitations, however. In the tables in MIRD Pamphlet No. 5, a second set of figures appears next to each absorbed fraction. This number is the coefficient of variation. This is a statistical limitation. A coefficient of variation of 50% or greater represents considerable uncertainty in the estimate of the absorbed fraction (Table 7-10). Other limitations are that the kidney model is not divided into cortex and medulla, and the bladder and stomach are a fixed size (Table 7-11). Furthermore,

*From UNSCEAR 77, United Nations Scientific Committee on the Effects of Atomic Radiation: Sources and effects of ionizing radiation, New York, 1977, United Nations.

Table 7-10. Absorbed fractions (Φ) for different photon energies (E_i) from a uniform source in the liver—photon energy, E_i (MeV)

Target organ	0.010	0.015	0.020	0.030	0.050	0.100	0.200	0.500
Adrenals			0.183E-03	0.440E-03	0.392E-03	0.270E-03	0.237E-03	0.198E-03
Bladder					0.169E-03	0.275E-03	0.389E-03	0.358E-03
Gastrointestinal tract (stomach)			0.171E-03	0.151E-02	0.360E-02	0.300E-02	0.271E-02	0.280E-02
Gastrointestinal tract (SI†)	0.171E-03*	0.495E-03	0.117E-02	0.493E-02	0.108E-01	0.109E-01	0.100E-01	0.971E-02
Gastrointestinal tract (ULI)		0.575E-03	0.927E-03	0.318E-02	0.448E-02	0.401E-02	0.387E-02	0.364E-02
Gastrointestinal tract (LLI)					0.613E-04	0.149E-03	0.211E-03	0.391E-03
Heart		0.112E-03	0.132E-02	0.531E-02	0.762E-02	0.674E-02	0.570E-02	0.573E-02
Kidneys		0.105E-03	0.106E-02	0.437E-02	0.566E-02	0.437E-02	0.390E-02	0.386E-02
Liver	0.967	0.898	0.784	0.543	0.278	0.165	0.158	0.157
Lungs	0.139E-03	0.299E-02	0.859E-02	0.165E-01	0.147E-01	0.101E-01	0.923E-02	0.838E-02
Marrow	0.288E-03	0.182E-02	0.819E-02	0.228E-01	0.325E-01	0.206E-01	0.133E-01	0.107E-01
Pancreas			0.186E-03	0.107E-02	0.130E-02	0.105E-02	0.102E-02	0.822E-03
Skeleton (rib)	0.721E-03	0.447E-02	0.183E-01	0.402E-01	0.366E-01	0.181E-01	0.111E-01	0.867E-02
Skeleton (pelvis)				0.523E-03	0.265E-02	0.308E-02	0.216E-02	0.182E-02
Skeleton (spine)			0.393E-03	0.566E-02	0.217E-01	0.167E-01	0.108E-01	0.857E-02
Skeleton (skull)						0.629E-04	0.140E-03	0.187E-03
Skeleton (total)	0.721E-03	0.458E-02	0.209E-01	0.587E-01	0.803E-01	0.498E-01	0.324E-01	0.260E-01
Skin			0.136E-02	0.468E-02	0.558E-02	0.499E-02	0.507E-02	0.561E-02
Spleen				0.617E-04	0.533E-03	0.606E-03	0.645E-03	0.619E-03
Thyroid								
Uterus					0.564E-04	0.115E-03	0.136E-03	0.130E-03
Trunk	0.996	0.997	0.984	0.905	0.660	0.453	0.413	0.404
Legs					0.159E-03	0.480E-03	0.716E-03	0.141E-02
Head				0.110E-04	0.381E-03	0.493E-03	0.867E-03	0.106E-02
Total body	0.996	0.997	0.984	0.905	0.661	0.454	0.415	0.407

*Read as 0.000171. (E-03, move decimal point 3 places to the left. E-02, move decimal point 2 places to the left and so on.)

†Abbreviations spelled out in Table 7-11.

Table 7-11. Mass of organs used in the MIRD study

Body organs	Abbreviation	Mass (gm)	
		Reference man report	Phantom
Adrenals	AD	14	15.5
Bladder			
Wall	BLADW	45	45.13
Contents	BLADC	200	200
Gastrointestinal tract			
Stomach			
Wall	STW	150	150
Contents	STC	250	246.9
Small intestine and contents	SI	640 wall 400 contents	1,044 wall plus contents
Upper large intestine			
Wall	ULIW	210	209.2
Contents	ULIC	220	200
Lower large intestine			
Wall	LLIW	160	160.1
Contents	LLIC	135	136.8
Kidneys (both)	KI	310	284.2
Liver	LI	1,800	1,809
Lungs (both, including blood)	LU	1,000	999.2
Other tissue	OT	48,000	48,480 (2,800 gm suggested for muscle; 12,500 gm for separable adipose tissue)
Ovaries (both)	OV	11	8.268
Pancreas	PA	100	60.27
Salivary glands	SALG	85	Not represented
Skeleton	SKEL	10,000	10,470
Cortical bone	CORTB	4,000	4,000
Trabecular bone	TRAB	1,000	1,000
Red marrow	RM	1,500	1,500
Yellow marrow	YM	1,500	1,500
Cartilage	CART	1,100	1,100
Other constituents	—	900	1,370
Spleen	SP	180	173.6
Testes	TE	35	37.08
Thyroid	THY	20	19.63
Uterus	UT	80	65.4
Total body	TB	70,000	69,880

From Snyder, W.S., and others: "S" absorbed dose per unit cumulated activity for selected radionuclides and organs, MIRD Pamphlet No. 11, New York, 1975, Society of Nuclear Medicine.

the MIRD formula presupposes that the source is uniformly distributed within a standard-size organ, which is subject to much patient variation. In the case of the dose estimates for the fetus, radioactivity was assumed not to cross the placenta; therefore nonpenetrating activity was not included in the calculations. Authors are quick to point out in all discussions of dosimetry that the user should be aware of all the assumptions and limitations used in the generation of the data. However, as techniques develop and more information on the actual distribution of these radionuclides becomes available, calculations will become increasingly more accurate. Only in this way can the intelligent approach to radiation dosimetry and a reduced radiation dose to the patient be better served.

BIBLIOGRAPHY

Chandra, R.: Introductory physics of nuclear medicine, ed. 4, Philadelphia, 1992, Lea & Febiger.

Dillman, L.T., and von der Lage, F.C.: Radionuclide decay schemes and nuclear parameters for use in radiation-dose estimation, MIRD Pamphlet No. 10, New York, 1975, Society of Nuclear Medicine.

Goodwin, P.N., and Rao, D.V.: An introduction to the physics of nuclear medicine, Springfield, Ill., 1977, Charles C Thomas, Publisher.

Gough, J.H., Davis R., and Stacey, A.J.: Radiation doses delivered to the skin, bone marrow and gonads of patients during cardiac catheterization and angiocardiography, Br. J. Radiol. 41:508-518, 1968.

Hendee, W.R.: Medical radiation physics, Chicago, 1979, Mosby–Year Book.

International Council on Radiation Protection (ICRP), Pamphlet No. 52, Long Island, N.Y., Pergamon Press.

Kereiakes, J.G., and Rosenstein, M.: Handbook of radiation doses in nuclear medicine and diagnostic x-ray, 1980, CRC Press, Inc.

Rao, D.V. and Govelitz, G.F.: Gonadal dose from ^{201}Tl procedures, Med. Phys. **7**(4):430, 1980.

Rocha, A.F.G., and Harbert, J.E.: Textbook of nuclear medicine: basic science, Philadelphia, 1978, Lea & Febiger.

Rollo, F.D.: Nuclear medicine physics, instrumentation, and agents, St. Louis, 1977, Mosby–Year Book.

Smith, E.M., and Warner, G.G.: Estimates of radiation dose to the embryo from nuclear medicine procedures, J. Nucl. Med. 17:836-839, 1976.

Snyder, W.S., and others: Estimates of absorbed fractions for monoenergetic photon sources uniformly distributed in various organs of a heterogeneous phantom, MIRD Pamphlet No. 5, J. Nucl. Med. 10:5-52, 1969.

Snyder, W.S., and others: "S" absorbed dose per unit cumulated activity for selected radionuclides and organs, MIRD Pamphlet No. 11, New York, 1975, Society of Nuclear Medicine.

Sorenson, J.E., and Phelps, M.E.: Physics in nuclear medicine ed. 2, New York, 1987, Grune and Stratton, Inc.

Syed, I.B., and others: Radiation exposure in nuclear cardiovascular studies, Health Phys. 42(2):159-163, 1982.

UNSCEAR 77, United Nations Scientific Committee on the Effects of Atomic Radiation: Sources and effects of ionizing radiation, New York, 1977, United Nations.

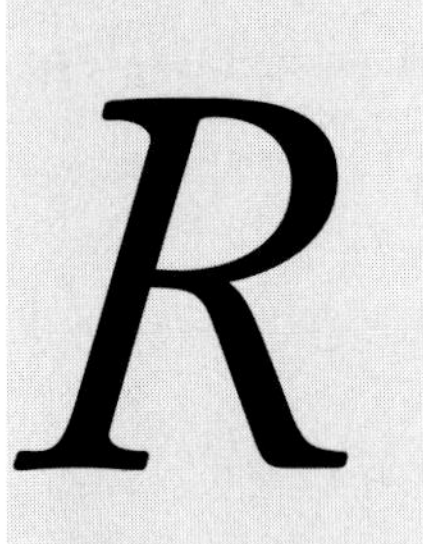

Chapter 8

ADIOPHARMACEUTICALS

RICHARD A. NICKEL

■ DEFINITION

Radiopharmaceuticals are radioactive pharmaceutical agents or drugs used for diagnostic or therapeutic procedures.

One or more of the atoms in the molecular structure of the radiopharmaceutical are unstable. This instability results in emission of alpha, beta, or gamma particles originating within the molecule.

The purpose of using pharmaceutical agents that are radioactive is (1) to follow their absorption, distribution, metabolism, and excretion through the use of appropriate detection devices, or (2) to use the agent to target an organ or tissue for destruction.

An optimal diagnostic radiopharmaceutical agent would be one in which the following apply:

- Readily available
- Easy to prepare
- Short half-life
- Pure gamma emitter
- Localization in only the tissue or organ desired
- No significant radiation exposure to critical organs

■ REGULATORY AGENCIES

For a product to be classified as a radiopharmaceutical agent safe for human use, the preparer must satisfy two branches of the federal government having overlapping jurisdiction: the Nuclear Regulatory Commission (NRC) and the Food and Drug Administration (FDA).

The sponsor or manufacturer of the radiopharmaceutical must first submit the drug to the "IND" process. This process is used to assess a drug's safety and effectiveness before making it generally available for use.

■ IND

The IND is formally known as a "Notice of Claimed Investigational Exemption for a New Drug" and is comprised of FDA forms FD 1571, FD 1572, and FD 1573.

Included in the IND should be the following:

1. Composition of the drug, its source, and all manufacturing data.
2. Any data from preclinical investigations, such as:
   - Pharmacologic profile
   - Animal toxicity data
   - Route of administration
   - Short-term animal studies

   Item no. 2 helps to define the drug's safety, not necessarily its effectiveness.
3. The investigational protocol.
4. Training and experience of the investigators.
5. Copies of the informational material which the sponsor of the IND supplies to each investigator.
6. The sponsor must agree to notify the FDA and all investigators of any adverse effects during animal and human tests.
7. The sponsor must obtain informed consent from the person on whom the drug is to be tested. Copies of the patient consent form must be included.
8. The sponsor must submit annual progress reports to the FDA.

There are three phases in the drug-approval process.

Phase I. In this portion of the investigation, pharmacologic studies are performed to determine:

- Toxicity
- Absorption
- Metabolism
- Excretion
- Other pharmacologic effects
- Preferred route of administration
- Safe dose range

A small number of patients are involved at this stage, and the test is conducted under carefully controlled conditions. The patients undergoing phase I trials should be normal, healthy individuals.

Phase II. A limited number of patients undergo tests for treatment of a specific disease or prevention. Additional animal studies may be necessary to document safety.

Phase III. Clinical trials are performed using larger numbers of patients if the results of Phases I and II demonstrate the drug's safety and effectiveness.

Phase III clinical trials are to further assess the drug's safety and effectiveness, and also to determine the safe dose range.

■ NDA

On successful completion of Phase III clinical trials, the sponsor of the drug may decide to submit a New Drug Application (NDA). The NDA is the final approval procedure that the FDA requires before releasing the drug for general use.

■ PRODUCTION OF RADIOPHARMACEUTICALS

In general, radionuclides may be produced in one of two ways: (1) as a by-product of nuclear fission (by-product material), or (2) through the use of a particle accelerator (e.g., cyclotron). The resultant radionuclides may then be made into radiopharmaceutical agents suitable for administration to humans.

The fission of uranium ^{235}U in a nuclear reactor results in many radionuclides. The desired radionuclide is separated from the by-product material and then used. The neutron flux in the reactor may be used to convert one element into another. By inserting a substance into the core of the reactor, neutron bombardment may produce the desired radionuclide. Examples of radionuclides produced in a reactor include the following: ^{99}Mo, ^{131}I, ^{137}Cs, ^{133}Xe, ^{32}P, ^{51}Cr, and ^{125}I.

In a particle accelerator, charged subatomic particles are accelerated toward a target material. The target material is an isotopically pure element. The radionuclide produced undergoes steps to make it suitable for human use.

In the production of gallium ^{67}Ga citrate, for example, the target material, zinc ^{67}Zn, is bombarded with protons in a cyclotron. The product of the bombardment is gallium ^{67}Ga chloride. Gallium is complexed with citrate ion by adding sodium citrate to the gallium chloride solution. The solution is made isotonic with sodium chloride. The result is a sterile, pyrogen-free solution of gallium ^{67}Ga citrate for intravenous administration. No carrier is added. The cyclotron reaction used for producing ^{67}Ga is sometimes written as ^{67}Zn *(p, n)* ^{67}Ga. Radionuclides produced in a particle accelerator include ^{123}I, ^{57}Co, ^{67}Ga, ^{201}Tl, ^{111}In, ^{127}Xe, and ^{81}Rb.

■ Radionuclide generators

Another source of radiopharmaceuticals is the radionuclide generator system (see Table 8-1). A radionuclide generator system consists of a long-lived parent decaying to a short-lived daughter radionuclide. The daughter is separated from the parent as a result of differences in chemistry. In the $^{99}Mo/^{99m}Tc$ generator system, the daughter, technetium ^{99m}Tc sodium pertechnetate, is separated from ^{99}Mo by eluting with normal saline. The ^{99}Mo parent remains on the generator column, and the technetium ^{99m}Tc sodium pertechnetate is dissolved into the normal saline.

Table 8-1. Radionuclide generator systems

Parent	Daughter	Granddaughter
^{99}Mo	^{99m}Tc	^{99}Tc
^{81}Rb	^{81m}Kr	^{81}Kr
^{195m}Hg	^{195m}Au	^{195}Au
^{113}Sn	^{113m}In	^{113}In

The generator system is sterile and pyrogen-free and produces a sterile, pyrogen-free solution of technetium ^{99m}Tc sodium pertechnetate ready for use.

In the $^{81}Rb/^{81m}Kr$ generator system, either a gas (room air, oxygen) or liquid may be used to elute the ^{81m}Kr daughter.

The decay scheme for a generator radionuclide is as follows:

$$\text{Parent} \rightarrow \text{Daughter} \rightarrow \text{Granddaughter}$$

The granddaughter nuclide is usually very long-lived or stable. Table 8-1 lists several radionuclide generator systems.

■ DOSE FORMS AND ROUTES OF ADMINISTRATION

Radiopharmaceutical agents may be in the form of a solid, liquid, or gas. Depending upon their indicated use and dose form, radiopharmaceutical agents may be swallowed, inhaled, injected, or instilled.

Oral preparations of radiopharmaceutical agents may be capsules or solutions containing a fixed amount of radioactivity at a fixed date and time.

Radiopharmaceutical agents for inhalation may be in the form of a radioactive gas. Xenon ^{133}Xe, xenon ^{127}Xe, and krypton ^{81m}Kr are three examples. They may be in the form of an aerosol for inhalation. Nebulizing a liquid solution of technetium ^{99m}Tc pentetate results in a radioaerosol for inhalation.

Radiopharmaceutical agents for injection must be sterile and pyrogen-free. Generally, they are either true solutions or suspensions. Suspensions may be in the form of colloidal dispersions like technetium ^{99m}Tc sulfur colloid and technetium ^{99m}Tc albumin colloid. They may be suspensions like technetium ^{99m}Tc albumin aggregated.

Technetium ^{99m}Tc sodium pertechnetate solution may be instilled into the bladder through a urethral catheter. It may also be instilled into the eye using a micropipette. Both procedures require the agent to be sterile.

■ ^{99m}Tc BIODISTRIBUTION

Once a radiopharmaceutical agent is administered to a patient, the biodistribution process occurs. This process consists of the substance's absorption, distribution, metabolism, and excretion. When the normal biodistribution pattern of a substance is known, any irregular patterns may suggest the presence of disease.

■ ^{99m}Tc RADIOPHARMACEUTICALS

^{99m}Tc-labeled agents are prepared by adding technetium ^{99m}Tc sodium pertechnetate to a reaction vial. In the reaction vial are the components necessary to bind ^{99m}Tc to the agent. There are no preservatives present so sterile technique must be used throughout the procedure. Most ^{99m}Tc-labeled agents have an expiration time of 6 hours after preparation.

Some products are in the form of a lyophilized powder. When the powder is reconstituted with sodium pertechnetate, the vial should be visually checked for complete dissolution of the powder and for particulate matter.

When eluted from a generator, technetium exists as the sodium pertechnetate salt: $NaTcO_4$. Technetium as pertechnetate is a chemically stable compound and must be reduced to a lower oxidation state to react with and label other substances in the preparation of ^{99m}Tc-radiopharmaceuticals. Technetium may exist as the Tc^{-1} oxidation state through the Tc^{+7} state. As pertechnetate, it exists as Tc^{+7}.

■ STANNOUS REDUCTION

The use of stannous ion (Sn^{+2}) is the predominant method of reducing technetium. The stannous chloride salt ($SnCl_2$) is frequently used.

Most technetium radiopharmaceuticals are chelating agents. They hold metal ions in their chemical "claws." Technetium must be in a reduced oxidation state to react with the chelate.

On complexing with a chelating agent or ligand, the resulting radiopharmaceutical agent is susceptible to oxidation if oxygen is inadvertently introduced into the reaction vial. In addition, stannous ion may be oxidized to stannic ion (Sn^{+4}), which is ineffective as a reducing agent. There is always more than a stoichiometric amount of stannous ion in a ^{99m}Tc-labeled radiopharmaceutical kit. This means that there is enough stannous ion to reduce the technetium in the vial, with more left over. This is to counteract the effect of oxygen which results from introduction of needles into the vial. Multiple-dose vials are particularly vulnerable. During manufacture of a technetium kit, the atmosphere in the reaction vial is replaced with dry nitrogen gas. This prevents oxygen and moisture from degrading the contents before it is mixed with sodium pertechnetate.

When preparing stannous-reduced kits, there are three possible radiochemical forms in which technetium may exist. Thin-layer chromatography is used to quantify the amount of each. The three forms are:

- ^{99m}Tc labeled radiopharmaceutical
- ^{99m}Tc as $NaTcO_4$
- Reduced/hydrolyzed forms of ^{99m}Tc

The $NaTcO_4$ and reduced/hydrolyzed forms are called radiochemical impurities. $NaTcO_4$ results from incomplete reduction of technetium or oxidation of the ^{99m}Tc-labeled radiopharmaceutical agent. The reduced/hydrolyzed form of technetium results from reduced technetium combining with water or incompletely dissolved tin salts. This form of technetium exists as a colloid. If this radiochemical impurity is present in a skeletal-imaging kit, for example, hepatic localization occurs.

■ QUALITY CONTROL OF RADIOPHARMACEUTICALS

The primary responsibility for the quality of radiopharmaceutical agents rests with the manufacturer. Because the final preparation of many radiopharmaceuticals is now performed in the nuclear medicine department or radiopharmacy, it is the responsibility of these latter individuals to ensure that a quality product is dispensed.

Quality control involves many areas. Radionuclidic purity and radiochemical purity are two very important areas. Equipment used to assay doses must be calibrated, and records must be kept.

Since many radiopharmaceuticals are for injection, sterility and apyrogenicity must be maintained. Aseptic technique in the preparation and administration of these agents must be strictly followed.

Quality control may involve certain tests. Non-^{99m}Tc radiopharmaceutical agents are available from the manufacturer in a form that is ready for administration. Assay of the final dose is normally the only test to be done. ^{99m}Tc-labeled radiopharmaceuticals are prepared on-site and require tests to ensure quality.

■ Radionuclidic purity

Each time that a ^{99}Mo generator is eluted, a radionuclidic purity check must be performed to determine molybdenum breakthrough. This test is required by the Nuclear Regulatory Commission. The limits of ^{99}Mo contamination in the ^{99m}Tc generator eluate are 0.15 μCi of ^{99}Mo per 1 mCi of ^{99m}Tc. If the ^{99}Mo contamination exceeds this limit, the technetium ^{99m}Tc sodium pertechnetate cannot be used.

■ ALUMINUM CONTAMINATION TEST

Aluminum contamination is not a frequent problem with commercially available $^{99}Mo/^{99m}Tc$ generators of today. This test should be done, however, because aluminum ions can interfere with the quality of technetium ^{99m}Tc sulfur

LABORATORY APPLICATION

^{99}Mo/^{99m}Tc BREAKTHROUGH TEST

Purpose

The ^{99}Mo breakthrough test is mandated by the NRC to be performed at each elution of the ^{99}Mo/^{99m}Tc generator. There is a simple procedure to assay for molybdenum breakthrough using a dose calibrator.

Procedure

Materials

1. Dose calibrator
2. ^{99}Mo assay canister
3. Elution shield

Technique

1. Elute the generator according to the manufacturer's package insert.
2. Adjust the dose calibrator to assay ^{99}Mo.
3. With the ^{99}Mo assay canister in place, zero the system, or record the displayed background reading if applicable.
4. Transfer the ^{99m}Tc eluate from the elution shield to the ^{99}Mo assay canister and assay.
5. Subtract background activity (step 3) from the displayed reading, and record net ^{99}Mo activity in the log book.
6. Remove the ^{99}Mo assay canister, and readjust the dose calibrator for ^{99m}Tc.
7. Re-zero the system, or record background activity.
8. Using forceps, insert the ^{99m}Tc eluate into the dose calibrator chamber. Subtract background (step 7) from the displayed activity and record the net ^{99m}Tc activity.
9. Calculate the microcuries of ^{99}Mo per millicurie of ^{99m}Tc ratio:

$$\frac{\mu\text{Ci of } ^{99}\text{Mo}}{\text{mCi of } ^{99m}\text{Tc}} = \text{ratio}$$

10. Record the ratio.

colloid and ^{99m}Tc-skeletal agents. The USP has set a limit of 10 μg of aluminum ion (Al^{+3}) per milliliter of eluate. If the Al^{+3} concentration is high, a problem with the generator column may exist.

The aluminum ion test consists of a commercially available test strip and a standard aluminum solution. The test strip is impregnated with a chemical (aurin tricarboxylic acid), which turns pink in the presence of aluminum ion. The intensity of the color increases with aluminum concentration. A bottle containing a concentration of 10 μg/ml of Al^{+3} is included with the test strip. The test strip is spotted with the standard and the generator eluate and the colors compared. If the intensity of the generator eluate is greater than the standard, the eluate must not be used.

■ RADIOCHEMICAL PURITY

Radiochemical purity may be described as the amount of radionuclide in the desired chemical form.

Non-^{99m}Tc radiopharmaceutical agents are available from the manufacturer possessing high radiochemical purity.

^{99m}Tc-labeled agents prepared from "kits" may not be of sufficient radiochemical purity and must be tested. The test used to quantify radiochemical purity is thin-layer chromatography (Table 8-2).

■ ^{99m}Tc-RADIOPHARMACEUTICALS

■ Biodistribution of pertechnetate

Technetium ^{99m}Tc sodium pertechnetate ($NaTcO_4$), procured either prepackaged or from a ^{99}Mo/^{99m}Tc generator system, is chemically a salt. When this salt is placed in water, a solution is formed in which two ions are produced as follows:

$$\text{Na}^{99m}\text{TcO}_4 \rightarrow \text{Na}^+ \text{ and } ^{99m}\text{TcO}_4^-$$

The sodium cations present are required only for electrical neutrality purposes. Any positive ion can serve the same role. When introduced into the body, the positive ion does

LABORATORY APPLICATION

3

CHROMATOGRAPHY

Principle

Thin-layer chromatography is a method of separating different substances through the use of a solvent (mobile phase) passing over a stationary phase. The substances to be separated are spotted on the stationary phase or chromatographic strip. The strip is placed into a solvent tank and allowed to develop. As the solvent moves up the strip through capillary action, the substances travel with different velocities. The velocity of a substance depends upon its solubility in the developing solvent, attraction to the chromatographic strip, and other factors such as pH and molecular weight.

The point at which the radiopharmaceutical is spotted on the strip is called the origin. After the strip is spotted and developed in the solvent, the point at which the solvent stopped is called the solvent front. The R_f value is a ratio used to describe the distance that materials travel on the chromatography strip.

$$R_f = \frac{\text{distance from origin to center of spot}}{\text{distance from origin to solvent front}}$$

Purpose

Thin-layer chromatography is used to quantify the different radiochemical states of technetium that result from the preparation of a ^{99m}Tc radiopharmaceutical. The different radiochemical states that are possible include:

1. ^{99m}Tc-labeled radiopharmaceutical
2. ^{99m}Tc sodium pertechnetate (TcO_4^-)
3. Reduced/hydrolyzed forms of ^{99m}Tc

Procedure

Materials

1. Developing chamber (small glass vial is sufficient)
2. Solvents (methyl ethyl ketone, acetone, saline)
3. Chromatographic strips (paper or silica-gel–coated strips)
4. Well counter or radiochromatogram analyzer

Technique

1. Determine the type of solvent and support to be used.
2. Spot strip with a microdrop of radiopharmaceutical agent at 1 cm from the end. Mark the edge of the strip with a pencil at this point (origin).
3. Place the spotted strip into the developing chamber. The level of the solvent should be below the spot. Cover the chamber.
4. When the solvent migrates a sufficient distance, remove the strip and mark the solvent front with a pencil.
5. After the strip has dried, cut it into two parts: (1) origin (bottom half or one-third of strip) and (2) solvent front (upper half or two-thirds).
6. Place each strip in a counting vial and count in a well counter. The "percent tag" or label can be determined:

$$\%\ \text{Binding} = \frac{\text{Counts on strip A} \times 100}{\text{Counts on strip A} + \text{strip B}}$$

A = Portion of strip containing radiopharmaceutical
B = Portion of strip containing impurity

Radiochemical purity or percent binding should be at least 90% for most ^{99m}Tc-radiopharmaceuticals.

Key points

1. Chromatography should be performed before administration to patients.
2. The spot of radiopharmaceutical agent on the strip should not be allowed to dry before the strip is developed. Oxidation may occur, giving erroneous results.
3. The amount of radioactivity on the strip may be too great for assay in a well counter. Altering the geometry of counting or placing lead absorbers between the detector and chromatography strip may be necessary.

Table 8-2. Systems for analyzing radiochemical purity of ^{99m}Tc radiopharmaceuticals

Radiopharmaceutical	Support	Solvent	Compound	R_f Value
Sodium pertechnetate	Silica Gel TLC	Acetone	Tc (IV)	0
			TcO_4^-	1.0
Sulfur Colloid	Silica Gel TLC	Acetone	Tc Sulf. Coll.	0
			TcO_4^-	1.0
Albumin Colloid	Silica Gel TLC	MEK	Tc Alb. Coll.	0
			TcO_4^-	1.0
Albumin (aggregated)	Silica Gel TLC	Acetone	Tc MAA	0
			TcO_4^-	1.0
Penetrate	Silica Gel TLC	Acetone	Tc DTPA	0
			TcO_4^-	1.0
		Saline	Tc DTPA	1.0
			Tc RH	0
Gluceptate	Silica Gel TLC	Acetone	Tc Gluco	0
			TcO_4^-	1.0
		Saline	Tc Gluco	1.0
			Tc RH	0
Medronate, oxidronate, pyrophosphate	Silica Gel TLC	Acetone	Tc MDP	0
			TcO_4^-	1.0
		Saline	Tc MDP	1.0
			Tc RH	0
Lidofenin, disofenin	Silicic Acid TLC	20% NaCl	Tc Lidofenin	0
			TcO_4^-	1.0
	Silica Gel TLC	Water	Tc Lidofenin	1.0
			Tc RH	0

not follow the biologic pathway of the negative ion.

The pertechnetate anion (TcO_4^-) may be administered either orally or intravenously. If given orally in solution form, the ion will quickly pass from the digestive tract to the bloodstream by the process of simple diffusion. The diffusionary movement to the bloodstream requires only that the gut content concentration be higher than that of the bloodstream.

Movement from the gut contents to the blood requires passage through several layers separating the various fluid compartments of the body.

The passage of pertechnetate ion from gut contents to blood is by simple diffusion. Its absorption begins in the stomach and is completed early in its passage through the small intestine. Gut contents at the time of oral administration govern the rate of absorption to the blood. A normal fasting patient achieves maximum blood levels within 30 minutes following oral administration.

Because of uncertain absorption rates and the resulting variation in blood levels among patients the intravenous administration of pertechnetate is the method of choice. In this way, 100% of the dose is immediately present in the blood. There is no absorption phase. This choice of route also allows for the observation of the initial vascular distribution of the agent seconds after administration and forms the basis for the now-common flow studies.

If blood samples were collected from a patient every minute for several hours after dosing and the samples counted in a well counter, there would be a fall in activity per sample not explained by decay. The overall loss of pertechnetate from the vascular compartment can be explained as the product of many physiologic factors acting independently but simultaneously, resulting in what is known as a disappearance curve. Each physiologic factor contributes to this vascular loss for a different reason and in a different way.

Immediately after injection, pertechnetate ions are partly bound to serum proteins. This binding is reversible but initially accounts for as much as 70% to 80% of the injected dose. Capillary membrane cells lining the vascular compartment are held together by a cellular "glue" that is somewhat porous.

These pores readily allow by simple diffusion the passage of molecules with molecular weights less than 50,000 to 70,000. Molecules larger than these can pass, but it must be by active transport, a much slower process. Pertechnetate-binding serum proteins in general are of a high molecular weight. Because their weights exceed 70,000, they and the pertechnetate they carry are confined to circulate in the vascular compartment.

The unbound pertechnetate ions are small (165 molecular weight). They are not confined to the vascular compartment but rapidly escape through the capillary membranes to the interstitial fluids.

At the same time the free ions are leaving the vascular compartment, it follows that the concentration of these ions in this compartment is falling. As the free ion concentration falls, the protein-bound ion percentage in the vascular fluid is increasing. This is not to say the total percentage bound to protein is increasing but rather that the percentage of the total bound radioions present in the vascular compartment is increasing. This requires a shift in the equilibrium of this situation, favoring release of protein-bound pertechnetate. As these newly freed ions become available, they too can escape the vascular compartment into the interstitial fluid. Thus, there is a mechanism that allows for complete escape from the vascular compartment of the pertechnetate ions injected. The rate of this escape is ultimately governed by the concentration of the radioion in the interstitial spaces.

Since the interstitial fluid volume is three to four times larger than the vascular volume, as much as 75% of the free ions leave the vascular compartment by simple diffusion. Equilibrium or equal concentration of free ions in the vascular compartment and the interstitial fluids is achieved in as little as 2 to 3 minutes. This is the first factor in explaining the initial rapid loss of pertechnetate from the vascular compartment.

Pertechnetate ions arriving in the interstitial fluids can be removed from this fluid compartment in significant quantities by only a few organ systems: the stomach, salivary glands, thyroid, bowel (both small and large), mucous membrane tissue, choroid plexus, sweat glands (to some extent), and last but very important, kidney. All other organ systems exclude pertechnetate from their intracellular fluids, including the brain. The organs just listed provide the second major reason for the loss of pertechnetate from the vascular compartment.

Stomach. The affinity of the stomach for pertechnetate is caused by the ion's similarity to chloride. Both ions are negative one anions. The parietal acid-producing cells of the stomach produce carbon dioxide by normal metabolic pathways. This CO_2 is converted to carbonic acid by enzymatic activity.

Carbonic acid is passed to ducts carrying these secretions to the stomach contents. Here the carbonic acid dissociates into hydrogen ions and bicarbonate, the former taking the place of the pertechnetate in the interstitial fluids of the stomach. The hydrogen along with pertechnetate is secreted into the stomach contents as pertechnic acid in the same fashion as is hydrochloric acid. Thus intravenously administered pertechnetate accumulates quickly in the stomach wall and contents. Within 30 minutes after administration the stomach, because of its size, yields the highest external counting rate. Pertechnetate so secreted into the stomach contents is readily reabsorbed, thus producing an internal cycle.

Salivary glands. Salivary gland accumulation again is produced by the similarity of pertechnetate ions to other anions of similar charge. Saliva is produced in large amounts and contains considerable salts, including negative anions. Pertechnetate escaping the vascular compartments to the salivary gland interstitial fluid is taken up by these cells and secreted into the salivary ducts as a constituent of saliva. Although initially secreted saliva is isotonic to blood, it paradoxically is rendered hypotonic by fluid-secreting cells lining the ducts carrying the saliva from the glands to the mouth. This would lead to the conclusion that overall concentration of pertechnetate in the glands is lower than that of the blood perfusing it. It might further be concluded that the salivary glands should appear as an area of poor uptake on imaging rather than an area of increased uptake. This latter conclusion is false, however. If the salivary glands are seen as a four-compartment system (vascular, interstitial, cellular, and secretion-collecting) and are compared to other tissues not exhibiting a secretory function such as muscle, the reason the salivary glands reveal themselves as "hot" in an imaging procedure can be explained. Muscle tissue and its interstitial fluid surrounding the salivary glands can only achieve a concentration as high as the vascular supply servicing it. Conversely, salivary gland cells permit the entry of pertechnetate anions and in so doing have a concentration as high as the blood and interstitial fluid supply in their vicinity. This anion is then secreted into ducts leaving the salivary gland cells. The fluid in the duct also has a concentration of the anion as high as cells from which it arose. Therefore, in a gram of salivary tissue there are four fluid compartments all containing pertechnetate, whereas in a gram of muscle tissue only two compartments contain the anion. Thus the salivary glands are easily visualized in a sea of muscle.

Classically, the time of imaging is chosen when the target-to-nontarget ratio is the highest. The accumulation of pertechnetate in the salivary glands appears to reach its maximum in less than 10 minutes after dosing. It is at this point that the highest target-to-nontarget ratio is achieved. To wait for vascular clearance is futile, because there is an outflux from the glands of the radionuclide that follows the decrease in vascular pertechnetate. Thus although the ratio remains the same, the count rate differential closes with time. In addition, there is a gradual loss of overall count rate caused by decay, which ultimately results in a lengthened time required to perform the imaging procedure. This is a disadvantage in most cases.

Some clinicians prescribe atropine as an adjunct to salivary gland imaging. Atropine interferes with the discharge of saliva from the gland by blocking the nervous stimulation. Thus saliva formed within the gland is retained. According to some, this should increase the target-to-nontarget ratio. However, the enrichment of salivary gland tissue with pertechnetate depends on the block of two avenues of escape. The release to the oral cavity of the saliva is successfully blocked by atropine, but "obstructed" pertechnetate returns to the vascular compartment by diffusion as the concentration in the blood falls. Atropine is not recommended by all. There may be another and more significant merit to the use of atropine in that the oral cavity contamination buildup of pertechnetate that may obscure the image is avoided.

Secreted saliva that finds its way to the oral cavity is swallowed, passing to the stomach, providing the patient does not permit its loss. The pertechnetate is in effect recycled at this point. It is possible that the unconscious patient will drool on the pillowcase or other bedding. This wetness contains activity that can cause artifacts in subsequent imaging procedures.

Thyroid. An organ that has been successfully studied in so many ways with the iodine radionuclides can also be looked at in a much more limited fashion with the pertechnetate ion. The avidity of the thyroid for iodide ions is well known. Iodide is trapped, oxidized, converted to the positive ionic species, and coupled to the organic molecule thyronine to produce thyroid hormone. Note that only the first step in this sequence can be duplicated with pertechnetate.

Pertechnetate ions are rapidly trapped on arrival at the surface of the acinar cells of the thyroid. This trapping is against a concentration gradient and therefore is a form of active transport. The end result is that the gland has a higher concentration of pertechnetate than the blood supply servicing the organ.

The mechanism of the trap for iodide is not clear, much less the mechanism for the entrapment of pertechnetate. A reasonable hypothesis has been proposed that in two ways supports an explanation for the similarity of the trap between the two ions. First, the iodide ion has a negative one charge; so does the pertechnetate ion. This is apparently partly responsible for the failure of the thyroid to distinguish between the two ions. In addition, other negative one anions are also trapped (for example, perchlorate, ClO_4^-, and iodate, IO_3^-). However, the whole story does not stop here, because there are some negative one ions that are not so avidly accumulated, such as fluoride (F^-) or chloride (Cl^-). A review of an $^{18}F^-$ bone scan, popular before the discovery of today's ^{99m}Tc compounds, failed to reveal the high degree of thyroid uptake normally seen in an iodide or pertechnetate scan.

In an attempt to clarify the picture, the second part of the hypothesis takes into consideration the molecular weight of the ions exhibiting a negative one charge. In examining the list of these ions it is found that among the halogens only iodide (I^-) and astatine (At^-) are significantly trapped. In addition, certain combinations of atoms with overall negative one charges are also trapped, including perchlorate (ClO_4^-, and iodate (IO_3^-), and pertechnetate (TcO_4^-). Those halogens that are trapped and the combination ions just listed have two properties in common. All are negative one anions, and each has an ionic weight of about 100 or more. It is interesting to note that halogen ions (F^-, Cl^-, Br^-) and combination ions (NO_3^-, HCO_3^-) with weights less than 100 are not significantly trapped.

It appears therefore that at least two conditions must be met before the thyroid takes up a substance: negative one charge and ionic weight of more than 100. Many other molecules also fill these qualifications; therefore other properties, such as molecular configuration and ionic volume, probably should be considered.

After trapping, the second step in the iodide conversion to the hormonal state requires its oxidation to I^o. This involves the removal of an electron; that is, $I^- \rightarrow I^o + 1$ electron. At this point, iodide and pertechnetate (along with other oxygen-carrying trap competitors) enter dissimilar pathways. Iodide can be oxidized. Pertechnetate, perchlorate, and others cannot. Thus pertechnetate is accumulated by the thyroid but cannot be further processed. It is instead released from the gland as the pertechnetate (TcO_4^-) ion.

After an intravenous injection of pertechnetate the vascular levels fall rapidly, during which time the thyroid accumulates a portion of the radionuclide. The high efficiency of the trap mechanism yields a thyroid concentration that rises normally to a level approximately 10 times that of the surrounding vasculature. Since the gland is not able to organify the pertechnetate, the trapped ion escapes and diffuses back to the blood. The 10-to-1 ratio is maintained for some time as blood levels fall, with thyroid activity falling proportionately.

Normally accumulation of pertechnetate in the gland is positive throughout the first 10 to 15 minutes after dosing, even though blood levels are falling rapidly. The blood levels are falling because organs such as the thyroid are taking them up. These levels plateau for the next 30 to 45 minutes, during which time blood levels continue to fall; that is, the percentage of the administered dose in the gland remains relatively stable. After 1 hour or so the maximum thyroid-to-blood ratio has been achieved, and a further drop in blood activity results in a proportionate drop in thyroid activity. Total clearance of pertechnetate follows total clearance of the ion from the vascular compartment.

The optimum time for imaging is some time after 20 to 30 minutes following dose administration. To wait longer would serve no purpose because the best target-to-nontarget ratio has already been reached by this time. Further delay would only result in loss of count rate as a result of decay and biologic clearance.

Bowel (small and large). Twenty-four hours after dose administration, the organ system exhibiting the highest concentration of pertechnetate is the large bowel. To follow the distribution of pertechnetate, an understanding of the secretory and absorption function of the bowel in this regard is necessary.

Pertechnetate is found in the stomach contents after either its oral or intravenous injection. (Review the role of the stomach in the secretion of pertechnetate from the vascular volume to the stomach contents.)

Pertechnetate in the stomach and the upper reaches of the small bowel is absorbed by diffusion only so long as blood levels of pertechnetate are lower. When blood levels reach a concentration equal to that of the bowel contents, the absorption of pertechnetate ceases. Because vascular-bound pertechnetate is removed by other organs handling anions, it would appear that absorption would continue indefinitely, cycling back through the stomach as acid and from swallowed saliva. However, the gut content becomes more and more dilute as it passes from the proximal to the distal small bowel because the secretion of fluids exceeds the absorbed volume. Thus pertechnetate becomes less likely to be absorbed by the diffusion process the longer it remains in the gut content, because it is being diluted by the secreted hypotonic fluids.

The ever-more-dilute phenomenon ceases with passage to the large bowel. At this point the liquid chyme begins a process of drying out until by the time the material reaches the descending colon it has attained the semisolid consistency of feces. During this process most of the water and salts to be conserved by the body are being reabsorbed. At this time some pertechnetate is included in those salts that are reabsorbed. As the chyme becomes a solid, however, the remaining pertechnetate is trapped and eventually retained for passage in the stools. This pertechnetate remaining in the fecal mass is partly responsible for the large-bowel activity observed on abdominal images acquired many hours after dose administration.

A second explanation for the activity remaining in the bowel, not as part of its contents but rather as part of the gut wall, rests in the active absorption and secretion processes. The active transport of salts in the gut is well recognized. Water carrying many mineral ions is secreted and absorbed by this process. Pertechnetate is probably handled in this fashion. Since active transport requires the attachment of the absorbed substance to an intracellular carrier that transports the substance from the cell membrane facing one compartment through the cell cytoplasm to the membrane facing the appropriate compartments for release, it allows for a higher cellular concentration than is present in the surrounding fluids. The intestinal mucosa, one of the cellular compartments permitting the entry of pertechnetate, thus retains a portion of the activity when the blood levels have fallen. For this reason, cleaning of the bowel before abdominal imaging is not a completely satisfactory method of removing all bowel activity.

Since so much of the administered pertechnetate is involved with the gastrointestinal tract, it is not surprising to note the high degree of excretion by the fecal route. Estimations have shown that about 30% to 40% of an administered dose of pertechnetate is passed in the stools in the first 48 to 72 hours after dosing. Trace amounts totaling an additional 5% to 10% are added in the succeeding 2 weeks; however, physical decay of ^{99m}Tc does not allow detection after the initial 72 hours.

Choroid plexus. The choroid plexus is composed of a layer of cells found on the interior surfaces of the ventricles of the brain. The function of these cells is to produce the cerebrospinal fluid (CSF) by extracting the required materials from the vascular compartment and secreting it into the CSF spaces. This fluid then bathes the brain tissue and serves, among other purposes, as a protective layer between the brain substance and the skull.

The CSF is continually produced by the choroid but is not absorbed by the same tissue. Instead it flows throughout the many channels of the brain and finally reaches the arachnoidal granulations over the cerebrum where the fluid empties into the venous sinuses.

The composition of the CSF is similar to that of plasma. It contains, among other substances, electrolytes and certain protein materials but no formed elements. The mechanics of the production of CSF by the choroid layer is thought to be primarily one of exuding fluid from the vascular arteriole capillary of the choroid to the CSF space. This should mean that the plasma and CSF composition is the same with regard to electrolytes. However, it has been found that this is not the case. Pertechnetate is caught in the choroid cells but is not transferred to the CSF. This apparent filtering of pertechnetate ions by the choroid cells may be responsible for the increased activity seen in this area during imaging. Clearance of pertechnetate from the choroid requires a drop in blood concentration of the ion whereby it washes out by a diffusionary process. The accumulation of the radioion above that of the surrounding tissue is reached soon after dose administration, and the ratio remains in favor of choroid throughout the succeeding hours as vascular levels fall.

Although the uptake of pertechnetate by the choroid plexus of the brain is an extremely small fraction of the administered dose, the presence of this minute amount has caused great concern among clinicians interpreting brain images. The problem is compounded by the fact that the uptake is variable between patients. In some patients the choroid plexus visualizes, whereas in equal numbers the area does not visualize.

So bothersome is this accumulation of pertechnetate that a great deal of effort has been spent in the development of blocking agents that would prevent this uptake. To date, two agents have found their way into common use as an adjunct to pertechnetate brain imaging.

Lugol's solution, a combination of elemental iodine and potassium iodide, has been used with limited success. Orally administered, Lugol's solution prevents accumulation of pertechnetate in the choroid plexus, apparently by a flooding mechanism whereby stable iodide ions simply dilute the pool of negative one ions available for uptake by this tissue. Unfortunately, clinical use resulted in successful blockage of perhaps only half of those whose choroid would have visualized without the solution. To compound the problems in use of Lugol's solution, the agent has a bad taste, it must be administered before the injection of pertechnetate, and it cannot be given to patients sensitive to iodine or who are unable to take medications orally.

The use of Lugol's solution has given way to the use of potassium perchlorate. This agent administered orally in doses of 200 to 1000 mg has been shown to be more effective but still does not result in a 100% block of all choroid plexus uptakes. On the negative side, perchlorate must be administered orally before pertechnetate administration. It is barely soluble in water (about 7 mg/ml at 20° C), and it is contraindicated in patients with gastric or duodenal disorders.

The solution to the choroid uptake problem lies with the introduction of chelated and other forms of technetium. In these chemical forms the agent no longer accumulates in the choroid plexus, because its negative one charge is altered.

Brain. Brain tissue, with the exception of the choroid plexus, has no effect on the biodistribution of pertechnetate. Brain tissue substance for the most part rejects the entry of the pertechnetate ion into its intracellular compartment.

The unique structural arrangement of brain tissue provides a compact assembly of cells with little if any interstitial space. This clustered arrangement, together with capillaries that have far less permeability than capillaries elsewhere in the body, produces a barrier between the vascular compartment and the brain intracellular compartment commonly called the "blood-brain barrier."

Because the blood-brain barrier rejects the entry of pertechnetate into the brain substance, in the normal patient an image of the brain reveals only the vascular structures. A disruption of the barrier from nearly any cause allows for infiltration by diffusion of the pertechnetate ion from the high concentration of the vascular compartment to the abnormal areas not protected by the blood-brain barrier. Thus immediately after injection and mixing, all vascular compartment fluids should have the same concentrations. Any area exhibiting a high vascular content, such as the heart, placenta, nasal sinuses, or venous sinuses of the brain, is revealed as an area of increased activity over the surrounding tissue. Hypervascular lesions of the brain are often visualized seconds to minutes after injection.

Other lesions not well perfused or in which perfusion is absent accumulate pertechnetate by a slower process, requiring hours in some cases. When blood levels fall, the activity in the lesion remains for some time, producing a favorable target-to-nontarget ratio.

Clearance of pertechnetate from the brain directly follows a vascular clearance. Clearance from abnormal areas follows vascular clearance but at a reduced rate.

Sweat glands. The sweat glands are an organ system that can influence the distribution of pertechnetate.

Water is lost from the body through the skin by two methods: insensible and sensible perspiration. The former involves mere evaporation. Conversely, sensible perspiration requires secretion of fluid by the sweat glands through ducts to the surface of the skin. Perspiration contains essentially the same electrolytes as are found in the extracellular fluid. Since salts are part of the sweat, pertechnetate is included in the materials that are secreted to the surface of the skin.

If active perspiration is not under way, the amount of pertechnetate lost in this fashion is negligible. However, if a patient is actively sweating a normal composition fluid, he can lose a fraction of an administered dose in this manner. The total amount lost in the perspiration depends to a great degree on the electrolyte composition of the extracellular fluid and the amount of sweat being secreted. Therefore skin deposition as a transferable liquid or as a removable dry salt varies greatly among patients.

When sodium iodide ^{131}I, a similarly distributed radionuclide, is administered in therapeutic amounts, linen contamination by perspiration is a factor that must be addressed. This contamination resulted in procedures for monitoring bed linens and possible storage for decay of these articles before laundering. Although pertechnetate given in equal activities to ^{131}I is just as likely to contaminate bed linen, equal concern is not warranted, probably because of its shorter half-life. The fact remains that ^{99m}Tc can be lost in the perspiration. Technicians handling patients and their bed linen do accumulate activity on their fingers. This activity can easily be transferred to glassware, test tubes, and more importantly, camera collimators and controls. Technologists should urge patients receiving pertechnetate not to touch imaging instruments. Wearing gloves and frequent hand washing are advisable for technicians.

Kidney. The kidney plays the most important role in removal of vascular-bound pertechnetate. There is no cycling back to the vasculature once it is removed by the kidneys (unlike the stomach, thyroid, and salivary glands).

Blood arriving at the kidney passes through the renal artery to the afferent arteriole. The afferent arteriole enters the glomerulus, which is composed of about 50 parallel capillaries encased in a structure known as Bowman's capsule. During this passage through the glomerulus, the blood is reduced in volume by about 10%. This reduction is at the expense of the liquid fraction of the blood and not the formed elements. Included in this fraction, which is now known as the glomerular filtrate, is a wide variety of dissolved salts, glucose, amino acids, fats, and a limited amount of some small proteins. Dissolved substances that are vascular bound and larger than 50,000 to 70,000 molecular weight cannot be filtered; they exit the glomerulus by means of an outbound vessel known as the efferent arteriole. All undissolved substances are much too large to be filtered and therefore remain vascular. In addition, a large number of soluble protein molecules and substances that are complexed to protein molecules and whose aggregate molecular weight exceeds 70,000 are also confined to the vascular compartment. The biodistribution of pertechnetate is greatly influenced by these dimensions.

After arrival in the bloodstream, pertechnetate is bound to plasma proteins in significant quantity. These bound ions enter the glomerulus and exit by the efferent arterioles to the peritubular vessels that finally coalesce to form the renal vein.

The free pertechnetate ions that enter the glomerulus are filtered and pass into the tubules that eventually condense to form the ureter. Once in the ureter, these ions are for all practical purposes lost to the body, although they are temporarily stored in the bladder before being discharged in the urine. The blood leaving by the renal vein has a pertechnetate bound-to-free ratio greater than that on entry through the renal artery. This cannot remain because when there is an excess bound pertechnetate in the blood, a portion disassociates to become free. There is then a reestablishment of the same bound-to-free ratio that existed at the time the blood entered the renal artery. The only difference is that the total pertechnetate entering the kidney is reduced by 10% on its exit because of that lost to the glomerular filtrate.

Fifty percent of an administered dose of sodium pertechnetate is removed from the body by the urinary tract in the first 24 hours. The temporary storage of this ion in the bladder cannot be overlooked when this organ becomes part of a pelvic or lower abdominal view. A thyroid uptake with pertechnetate always requires a blood background to be subtracted from the neck count. The thigh is often chosen, and care must be exercised not to include the bladder in the field of view.

■ TECHNETIUM ^{99m}Tc SULFUR COLLOID

Sodium thiosulfate, when boiled in the presence of acid, forms colloidal sulfur. The reaction is as follows:

$$8Na_2S_2O_3 + H^+ \rightarrow 8Na_2SO_3 + S_8 + H^+$$

When technetium ^{99m}Tc sodium pertechnetate is included in the reaction, the technetium combines with sulfur as follows:

$$2TcO_4^+ + 7S + 16H^+ \rightarrow Tc_2S_7 + 8H_2O$$

Since the pertechnetate used in the reaction is carrier-free, the amount of technetium sulfide produced is insufficient to produce even one particle. The latter reaction therefore is assumed, but support is given from studies using rhenium, an element similar to technetium, in which Re_2S_7 was formed.

Since the technetium sulfide is produced in the presence of precipitating elemental sulfur, it is thought that the technetium heptasulfide is coprecipitated with elemental sulfur. Properly synthesized, the reaction allows incorporation of more than 95% of the technetium in the particulate structure and less than 5% remaining as free pertechnetate.

Technetium ^{99m}Tc sulfur colloid is commercially available as the prepackaged agent, or it may be synthesized on site using kits containing all the ingredients except the pertechnetate. The procedure involves mixing pertechnetate, thiosulfate, and an acid in a reaction vial. The reaction vial is then heated in a boiling water bath for about 10 minutes. After cooling, a buffer is added to bring the pH of the preparation to a physiologic level.

An important material present in all sulfur colloid preparations is gelatin. The purpose of this ingredient is to stabilize the colloidal particles formed. The gelatin coats the colloidal particles, and since the particles now absorb water on the surface, the individual particles are kept separate by layers of water. The more gelatin used, the smaller the mean particle size. This can have some influence on the biodistribution of the colloid.

Technetium ^{99m}Tc sulfur colloid preparations contain particles for which diameters range in size from 0.001 to 1 micron. The amount of gelatin used, the heating time, and the presence of contaminants such as aluminum cations (from the generator column) affect the particle size distribution.

On injection, technetium ^{99m}Tc sulfur colloid is confined to the vascular space. The colloidal particles, although much smaller than some blood formed elements, are much larger than any molecule able to escape the vascular compartment. The colloid particles as foreign bodies are removed from the blood by the reticuloendothelial system (RES). The RES is composed primarily of the Kupffer cells lining the liver sinusoids (75% to 80%) and found to a lesser extent in the spleen, with the remainder mostly in the bone marrow. The exact mechanism whereby the liver removes colloid particles from the blood is not clear.

Clearance of technetium ^{99m}Tc sulfur colloid is rapid with a half-time on the order of 2 to 3 minutes. Maximum organ concentrations are achieved in about 10 minutes, at which time circulating colloid is reduced to zero.

The entire RES does not remove foreign particles from the blood with equal efficiency. The spleen tends to favor the accumulation of the larger particles and the marrow smaller particles.

If the mean particle size is reduced, spleen uptake is reduced and marrow uptake is increased. If the mean size is increased, spleen uptake will be increased. If the particles are well above the 1 μm size, trapping occurs in the pulmonary capillary bed. If liver disease is present, the radiocolloid appears in the pulmonary system.

Care must be taken in the preparation of this agent so that it is done in the same manner each day. If not, artifacts in the images may result because of such factors as changes in heating time that result in different particle size distributions.

Technetium ^{99m}Tc sulfur colloid distribution is dependent on blood flow to the RES and the functional ability of these organs to remove foreign particles. A disease state that destroys or alters blood flow or function alters the distribution of the radiocolloid. If the disease is in its early stages, shunting of the activity away from the diseased organ will result in an increased uptake in the remaining organs of the RES. This causes an increase in activity in the normal portion of the RES at the expense of the diseased portion. If the disease process has progressed, the blood clearance time may be extended greatly.

Technetium ^{99m}Tc sulfur colloid trapped by the RES remains indefinitely; it is not biodegradable.

There will still be activity in the urine and stools, however, because of about 5% of the agent being present as soluble technetium heptasulfide.

■ TECHNETIUM ^{99m}Tc ALBUMIN AGGREGATED (^{99m}Tc-MAA)

Human serum albumin extracted from blood sera is a soluble protein. However, this material can be rendered insoluble if merely heated in its water solution with either a little acid or base added. If the conditions of healing are proper and the solution is stirred at the appropriate rate, the protein is precipitated into aggregates with dimensions on the order of 10 to 100 μm. Commercial preparations are rigidly controlled and have a narrower size range. ^{99m}Tc-MAA kits use stannous ion for reduction of technetium.

Human albumin microspheres are similarly synthesized, substituting an oil bath for the aqueous bath in which the protein is denatured. This product is no longer commercially available.

All easily accessible veins lead to the right side of the heart. In going from the site of injection to the heart, the vessel diameter enlarges. From the right side of the heart the blood is pumped through the pulmonary circulation. When the blood reaches the pulmonary artery, the vessel diameter reduces at each branch until at the alveoli level the vessels are approximately 10 to 20 microns.

Aggregates of albumin tagged with ^{99m}Tc are swept along by blood flow to the heart and then to the lungs, where the reduced vessel diameter causes the aggregates to become trapped. Because only a fraction of the vessels become blocked, there is no adverse effect on the patient.

Distribution of ^{99m}Tc-MAA is strictly a function of blood flow. Well-perfused areas show large deposits of activity, whereas poorly perfused areas show less. If a major supply vessel is occluded, all downstream vessels and the areas of the lung they serve will be devoid of trapped particles. This initial distribution and subsequent imaging procedure allows the interpretation of perfusion defects of the lung.

Clearance of the ^{99m}Tc-MAA particles occurs following entrapment. Three processes cause the clearance to occur. First, enzymes in the blood begin immediately to dissolve the particles. Second, respiratory motion continually causes the lung tissue to expand and contract. This motion also elongates and compresses the particles. Third, normal blood pressure is being applied in a rhythmic fashion. Eventually, these processes push the particles out of the capillary bed to the pulmonary vein and into the systemic circulation. The particles clear from the lung with a biological half-life of approximately 6 hours.

Following clearance from the pulmonary system, the particles are cleared from the blood by the RES.

In patients with right-to-left cardiac shunt, the particles do not entirely pass through the pulmonary system upon injection. If aggregates of albumin are in the general circulation, they become trapped in the capillary networks serving other organs. A blockage of capillaries serving the brain could be occluded, for example. In these cases, extreme caution should be taken to administer, to the most practical extent, the least number of particles.

■ TECHNETIUM ^{99m}Tc ALBUMIN COLLOID

Human serum albumin is extracted from blood sera and rendered insoluble in the manufacture of this radiopharmaceutical agent. Human serum albumin particles in the colloid size range are produced and labeled with ^{99m}Tc. The albumin particles in technetium ^{99m}Tc albumin colloid are smaller than those in ^{99m}Tc-MAA and do not become trapped in the lungs under normal conditions.

The technetium ^{99m}Tc albumin colloid uses stannous ion for reduction of technetium. On injection, the albumin colloid is cleared from the plasma by the reticuloendothelial system. Liver and spleen uptake is complete within 15 minutes. The albumin colloid is excreted in the urine.

The indications for this agent are similar to those for sulfur colloid: liver and spleen imaging.

During injection of albumin colloid, back-flushing of the syringe with blood is not recommended, because clot formation may result.

■ TECHNETIUM ^{99m}Tc PENTETATE (^{99m}Tc-DTPA)

DTPA is a molecule that is a chelating agent. Chelating molecules accomplish the binding of metals generally by donating unused electrons to the metal atom from either nitrogen or oxygen without actually giving them up. In this way certain metallic cations in solution attach themselves to the organic molecule and on introduction to the human body are swept along the biopathway of the chelate rather than the free cation.

Many substances in the body perform this same type of task. However, in most cases, the body's chelating substances are large proteins, and in general they and their bound substances are confined to the vascular pool.

The value of DTPA rests with the fact that it is a small molecule (less than 500 mol wt), is soluble, and is stable at physiologic pH. Metallic cations when attached to DTPA do not alter the biodistribution of the parent molecule.

When stannous (Sn^{+2}) ion is mixed with pertechnetate, reduced technetium is formed that joins DTPA. Less than 10% of the technetium added to the reaction is left as free pertechnetate ion. When ^{99m}Tc-DTPA is introduced to the vascular compartment, a rapid equilibrium within the extracellular compartment is established. DTPA, being small, can freely diffuse across the capillary membrane.

The initial disappearance curve for ^{99m}Tc-DTPA is similar to that of pertechnetate. Within 5 minutes after injection and surely by 10 minutes, when mixing is assured, the concentration of the agent is uniformly distributed throughout the extracellular compartment. At this point further bloodstream clearance is produced exclusively by the action of the glomerulus. Since the extracellular compartment is three to four times larger than the vascular compartment, the time required to clear the bloodstream to half its original levels is on the order of 20 to 30 minutes.

By 2 to 3 hours after dose administration, blood levels fall to well less than 10% remaining as compared to almost 50% normally remaining with pertechnetate. During this time the kidney tubular system carrying the cleared chelate to the ureters has a significantly higher activity than does the surrounding tissue.

Imaging of the kidney can be performed almost immediately after injection. If using enough of the DTPA complex to yield a high enough count rate, the function of the kidney can be observed through serial images. Seconds after injection, the radioagent may be observed perfusing the kidney by the renal artery input. The agent immediately begins clearing to the tubular system and only minutes later arrives in the collecting tubules and calyxes. By about 5 minutes after dose administration, the ureters draining the complex to the bladder are visualized.

The bladder acts as a temporary storage compartment until the patient voids. Patients should be encouraged to void within the hour after the imaging procedure is complete to reduce the bladder radiation dose.

Brain imaging with the tagged DTPA complexes is successful for the same reason it is successful with pertechnetate. Initially, high concentrations of both agents infiltrate areas of the brain not protected by a blood-brain barrier and are left behind when the bloodstream clears the agent. The advantage of using the DTPA complex over pertechnetate rests with the increased clearance rate of the former, resulting in a high target-to-nontarget ratio at an earlier time after dose administration.

■ TECHNETIUM ^{99m}Tc GLUCEPTATE

Technetium ^{99m}Tc gluceptate is a linear chain molecule containing seven carbon atoms (Fig. 8-1). Its configuration is similar to glucose and other sugars. Glucose is completely metabolized by the body. Technetium ^{99m}Tc gluceptate is excreted in its entirety without modification. This latter characteristic, in addition to a structural design that allows labeling with ^{99m}Tc, makes technetium ^{99m}Tc gluceptate a useful radiopharmaceutical agent.

In the presence of stannous ion, pertechnetate is reduced, and the reduced technetium labels the gluceptate. The resulting chelate is water soluble and stable at physiologic pH.

On intravenous injection, technetium ^{99m}Tc gluceptate equilibrates rapidly within the extracellular pool with little vascular protein binding or any tissue uptake. Clearance by the kidney begins with the first pass through this organ with both filtration and tubular secretion taking part. Vascular levels fall slightly faster than that of ^{99m}Tc-DTPA, probably because of the combination in differences between protein binding and the fact that gluceptate is to a limited extent secreted by the kidney tubules. Glomerular filtration is responsible as the major mechanism of clearance for both agents, but gluceptate levels fall faster to less than 5% to 10% remaining in the blood at 1 hour after dose administration, in contrast with 10% or better at the same time with ^{99m}Tc-DTPA. Bladder retention of this agent is undesirable because radiation dose to this and adjacent structures should be minimized. Therefore prompt voiding by the patient is to be encouraged.

Brain and kidney flow studies and function studies along with imaging procedures of these organs can be performed for the same reasons given for DTPA.

■ TECHNETIUM ^{99m}Tc SUCCIMER (^{99m}Tc-DMSA)

Technetium ^{99m}Tc succimer is a simple metal chelate containing two organic acid functional groups and two mid-

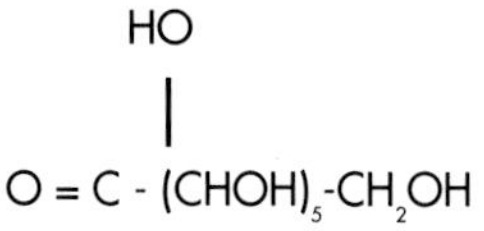

HO

|

O = C - $(CHOH)_5$-CH_2OH

Fig. 8-1. Gluceptate.

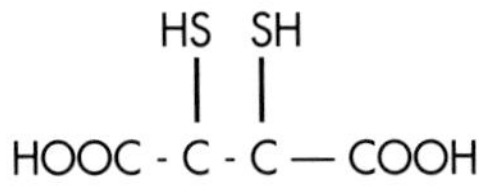

HS SH

| |

HOOC - C - C — COOH

Fig. 8-2. DMSA.

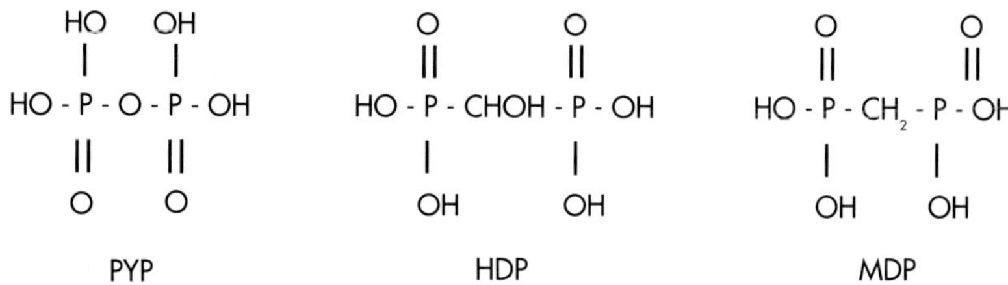

Fig. 8-3. ^{99m}Tc skeletal agents.

molecule thiol groups (Fig. 8-2). In the presence of stannous-reduced technetium, a ^{99m}Tc-DMSA chelate results. DMSA is photosensitive and therefore unstable and thus should be used promptly following preparation.

^{99m}Tc-DMSA is administered intravenously where binding of the agent to plasma proteins occurs. Delayed vascular clearance results, with half-times of 1 hour documented.

The kidney is responsible for roughly half of the blood clearance of ^{99m}Tc-DMSA within the first 2 hours. Transfer of the agent from circulating protein to renal cortex is accompanied by roughly another 20% of the agent being simultaneously excreted in the urine during this same period. Binding to renal cortex appears firm with little of the agent being retained in the medullary portion of the kidney.

Because renal accumulation and excretion are slow, function studies of the kidney using this agent are impractical. ^{99m}Tc-DMSA is best used in the morphologic evaluation of the kidney and in the identification of nonfunctioning space-occupying lesions.

■ TECHNETIUM ^{99m}Tc MERTIATIDE

Technetium ^{99m}Tc mertiatide is prepared from stannous-reduced technetium and betiatide. The resulting complex is referred to as technetium ^{99m}Tc mertiatide. The preparation procedure consists of inserting a sterile vent needle into the vial containing the lyophilized ingredients, then adding 4 to 10 ml of sodium pertechnetate containing 20 to 100 mCi. Then 2 ml of air are withdrawn from the vial, which is placed into a boiling water bath for 10 minutes. The withdrawal of air removes the inert argon gas present in the vial and replaces it with atmospheric air. Oxygen present in the air oxidizes any remaining stannous ion to prevent formation of lower valence states of technetium. The lower valence forms of technetium will form radiochemical impurities. Before reconstitution, the vials should be protected from light.

^{99m}Tc has superior physical characteristics over other radionuclides such as ^{131}I and ^{123}I. It has a short half-life, low radiation dose, and optimal gamma energy when compared to the iodine radionuclides. Technetium ^{99m}Tc mertiatide is a ^{99m}Tc-labeled renal function agent that has pharmacologic properties similar to ^{131}I- or ^{123}I-labeled hippuran. It is excreted by the kidneys by both tubular secretion and glomerular filtration. It can be used to assess renal function and renal blood flow; hence it is used for glomerular filtration rate and effective renal plasma flow studies.

Unlike other stannous-reduced radiopharmaceutical agents, the test for radiochemical purity of technetium ^{99m}Tc mertiatide does not involve thin-layer chromatography. The prepared agent is passed through a cartridge containing a material that separates the different radiochemical forms that result. Careful preparation of the cartridge must precede its use.

■ TECHNETIUM ^{99m}Tc-SKELETAL–IMAGING AGENTS

Skeletal-imaging radionuclides have undergone much improvement in recent years. Use of agents such as ^{47}Ca, ^{18}F, or strontium nuclides have been supplanted by technetium ^{99m}Tc-labeled phosphates (Fig. 8-3).

Unlike roentgenographic studies of the bone, which can detect changes in bone density only, technetium ^{99m}Tc-phosphate agents rely on changes in bone turnover rate and bone blood flow to detect lesions.

The technetium ^{99m}Tc-phosphates are comprised of two groups of compounds: (1) pyrophosphate and polyphosphate and (2) diphosphonates.

The first group, pyrophosphate and polyphosphate, was used with some success, but the images suffered from high background activity from the vasculature and soft tissue. The poor quality images were due to the in vivo instability of the agent. Once injected, the P-O-P (phosphorus-oxygen-phosphorus) bonds were broken apart as a result of enzymatic activity. As the phosphates were split into different compounds, each with its own biodistribution pattern, the images were adversely affected.

An improvement over compounds with the unstable P-O-P bond came with the introduction of the diphosphonates. Instead of a P-O-P structure, a very stable P-C-P (phosphorus-carbon-phosphorus) structure is used. The P-C-P bond is not split enzymatically in vivo.

Two diphosphonates currently in use are (1) MDP, or methylene diphosphonate and (2) HDP, or hydroxymethylene diphosphonate.

Both MDP and HDP are less protein-bound by the plasma and exhibit superior image quality, less radiation exposure to the patient, and greater diagnostic utility over pyrophosphate and polyphosphate.

Today's skeletal-imaging agents are very sensitive to changes in bone. The phosphates are absorbed to all bones, but to varying degrees. The phosphate is adsorbed to the hydroxyapatite crystal of the bone surface. In many bone diseases and injuries, the lesion will exhibit increased bone formation and repair as a result of osteoblastic activity. This area of bone formation, along with increased blood flow, results in increased uptake of the technetium phosphates. The area(s) of increased radionuclide uptake will appear as a "hot spot" on the image. Typical causes of increased uptake in bone lesions are:

1. Bone fracture
2. Arthritis
3. Metastatic disease
4. Paget's disease
5. Bone infection

In children, the epiphyseal plates at the ends of long bones will also show increased uptake of radionuclide. Conversely, diseases exist in which there is a reduction in bone formation resulting in a "cold spot" or decreased uptake of radionuclide. Osteoporosis, osteomalacia, and radiation therapy can cause reduced uptake of radionuclide in bone.

The ^{99m}Tc-labeled phosphates are available from the manufacturer as lyophilized powders. The powder is reconstituted with sodium pertechnetate to produce the radiopharmaceutical agent. The phosphates all use stannous ion to reduce technetium. The reduced technetium is complexed with the phosphate compound, and a chelate results. The ^{99m}Tc-labeled phosphate is oxygen-labile; that is, oxygen will degrade the complex. Care must be taken not to introduce air into the vial when preparing the kit or drawing a dose. This precaution should be taken with all stannous-reduced kits.

On injection, the ^{99m}Tc-labeled MDP or HDP are rapidly cleared from the plasma. Approximately 50% of the dose is retained in the skeleton, with the remainder excreted eventually in the urine. The kidney plays a major role in excretion; poor renal function will delay excretion. Because the kidney is the major route of elimination, the bladder quickly fills with radionuclide. Before imaging, the patient should empty the bladder to avoid a masking of the pelvic region.

As the ^{99m}Tc-labeled agent is cleared from the plasma and background activity is reduced, the target-to-background ratio improves. Imaging is usually performed from 1 to 3 hours after injection.

Some manufacturers add a stabilizing agent to the skeletal-imaging kit. The purpose is to counteract the effect of oxidants in the vial. Recall that oxidants render stannous ion ineffective for reducing technetium and break apart the ^{99m}Tc-drug complex. Oxidants include oxygen (which may be introduced into the vial) and peroxides, which are formed from the radiolysis of water. Oxygen is the oxidant of primary concern.

Stabilizing agents themselves are more easily oxidized than the technetium phosphate complex. Thus, the oxidant will attack the stabilizing agent instead of the radiopharmaceutical agent. Manufacturers of some MDP kits will add ascorbic acid as a stabilizing agent. HDP is manufactured with gentisic acid added as a stabilizer.

A manufacturer of a stannous-reduced kit must decide on the optimal amount of tin to add. If there is a large excess of tin, an insoluble technetium-labeled tin colloid will form. If there is too little tin, incomplete reduction of technetium may occur or instability of the agent results from oxidants being present. Using a stabilizing agent allows the manufacturer to reduce the amount of tin added to the kit without sacrificing stability and avoiding the formation of the technetium-labeled tin colloid.

■ TECHNETIUM VASCULAR AGENTS

There are several approved methods currently available to label the cardiac blood pool in evaluating cardiac and great vessel disease. The first method uses technetium ^{99m}Tc human serum albumin (HSA). ^{99m}Tc-HSA is a stannous-reduced kit which previously was used extensively. The high cost of the agent, the fact that the albumin "leaks" out of the vascular space with time, and the advent of ^{99m}Tc-labeled red blood cells (RBCs) have largely replaced it.

Labeling RBCs with ^{99m}Tc has gained widespread acceptance in recent years. By "tinning" or pretreating RBCs with stannous ion and exposing them to sodium pertechnetate, the cells become labeled with technetium ^{99m}Tc. The label appears to be irreversible for the life of the cell. There is no bladder or bowel activity outside that of unbound technetium.

In addition to evaluation of cardiac function, ^{99m}Tc-RBCs may be used to evaluate gastrointestinal bleeding. When used for this procedure, it is imperative that the technetium is completely bound to the RBCs. It is considered by many to be superior to ^{99m}Tc-sulfur colloid for these studies. Because sulfur colloid is rapidly cleared from the blood, for the detection to occur the patient must have a site of active bleeding. If the bleeding is intermittent, the ^{99m}Tc-sulfur colloid study may not detect the bleeding site. ^{99m}Tc-RBCs remain in the blood pool for hours and are able to detect these intermittent bleeding sites. Labeling efficiency must be high, however, to avoid imaging artifacts.

Three methods exist for labeling RBCs with technetium ^{99m}Tc sodium pertechnetate.

■ In vitro RBC labeling method

The in vitro labeling method required centrifugation and wash steps at one time. The in vitro labeling of red blood cells is now available in a kit form. The product comprises a vial containing lyophilized stannous chloride and two syringes, one containing sodium hypochlorite and the other a citric acid/sodium citrate mixture.

One to three milliliters of the patient's blood is added to the vial, followed by the contents of syringes I and II. When obtaining the blood from the patient, a small amount of heparin anticoagulant should be present to prevent clot formation. Gently invert the vial after each step. In order to prevent damage to the cells, a 19 to 21 gauge needle is recommended for the transfer of the blood to the vial. From 10 to 100 mCi of ^{99m}Tc-$NaTcO_4$ is added to the mixture. After a 20-minute incubation period, the labeled cells are ready for injection. A labeling efficiency of 95% or greater results from this method.

■ In vivo RBC labeling method

In this procedure, a vial of stannous pyrophosphate is reconstituted with preservative-free normal saline. The solution is injected and after a period of 30 minutes, ^{99m}Tc-$NaTcO_4$ is injected. Unlike the 95% or higher labeling efficiency of the in-vitro method, only about 75% of the radioactivity is taken up by the RBCs. The remainder will enter the extravascular space. This becomes a disadvantage in the evaluation of gastrointestinal bleeding. If $NaTcO_4$ is present in the blood, it will be secreted by the parietal cells of the stomach, causing an imaging artifact.

LABORATORY APPLICATION

MODIFIED IN VIVO RBC LABELING METHOD

Procedure

Materials

1. Twenty millicuries of technetium ^{99m}Tc sodium pertechnetate in a 10-ml syringe
2. One vial of Technescan PYP (Mallinckrodt)
3. Three milliliters normal saline solution
4. One 3-ml syringe
5. One syringe of heparin lock (100 U/ml)
6. One three-way stopcock
7. One butterfly assembly
8. One 10-ml syringe with shield

Technique

1. Reconstitute PYP solution with 3 ml of normal saline solution. Shake until dissolved. Let stand for 5 minutes.
2. Withdraw 1 to 3 ml of PYP solution and inject directly into patient. Use no heparin.
3. Allow a 10-minute mixing time.
4. Attach a three-way stopcock to the butterfly assembly.
5. Attach the heparin lock syringe to the three-way stopcock.
6. Make a venipuncture with the butterfly needle and fill the tubing with heparin lock solution.
7. Attach the 10-ml syringe with 20 mCi of ^{99m}Tc sodium pertechnetate to the three-way stopcock.
8. Turn the stopcock valve, and withdraw 4 to 5 ml of blood into the 10-ml syringe.
9. Turn the stopcock valve, and fill the tubing with heparin lock solution.
10. Disconnect the 10-ml syringe from the three-way stopcock, cap it, shield it, and gently mix by inverting the blood several times over a 4- to 5-minute period.
11. Reattach the 10-ml syringe to the three-way stopcock, turn the stopcock valve, and inject the contents of the 10-ml syringe back into the patient.
12. Optionally, the balance of the heparin lock solution can be used to flush the tubing and/or butterfly assembly can be removed from the patient and set aside to decay in storage.

■ Modified in vivo RBC labeling method

A higher labeling efficiency can be obtained over the in vivo method by modifying the procedure somewhat. As in the in vivo method, a solution of stannous pyrophosphate is injected intravenously. However, the sodium pertechnetate is not directly injected into the patient. After a 30-minute wait, the cells are drawn into a syringe containing sodium pertechnetate.

Labeling efficiencies as high as 95% can be obtained with this method.

■ TECHNETIUM HEPATOBILIARY AGENTS

For many years a search was conducted for a technetium compound that could be used as a replacement for the beta-emitting and photon-deficient ^{131}I rose bengal. The search has led to a class of substituted compounds all having iminodiacetic acid in their structure. *N*-substitution with a 2,6-dimethylacetanilide group led to formation of a compound known as HIDA or lidofenin. Research further refined the molecule by replacing the methyl groups with isopropyl groups at the 2 and 6 positions on the benzene ring. This latter compound, 2,6-di*iso*propylacetanilideiminodiacetic acid, is known as *DISIDA* or *disofenin*. A further modification of the HIDA molecule led to mebrofenin (Fig. 8-4).

Intravenous administration of these agents is followed by a rapid clearance from the vascular pool by the polygonal cells of the liver. Visualization of the liver is possible minutes after administration to a normal patient. Good target-to-nontarget ratios of the liver to surrounding tissues are normally observed within 5 minutes.

Polygonal cell secretion of these agents to the biliary tree begins immediately, and hepatic ducts and gallbladder are normally seen within 10 to 20 minutes after injection. Visualization of the cystic duct and gallbladder is normally improved as the activity accumulates in these organs at the expense of that drained from the liver. Next, the common bile duct should emerge, and the radioagent should appear in the duodenum of the normal patient.

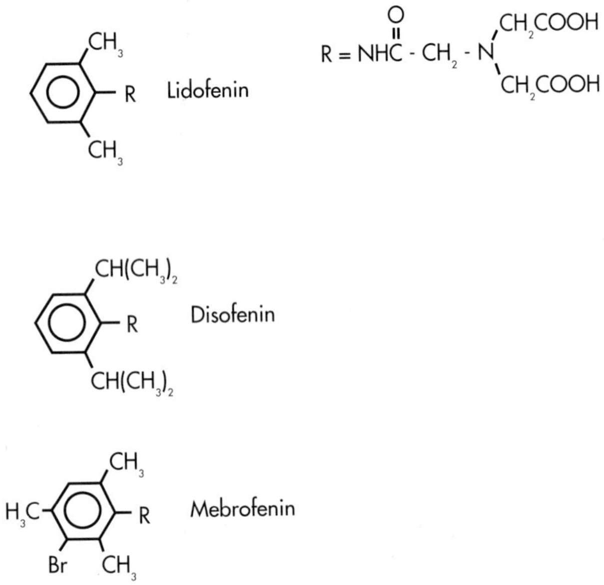

Other organ localization is not to be expected in the normal patient. However, kidney visualization does occur when there is impaired hepatocyte function as evidenced by jaundice and in cases of hepatobiliary obstruction from any cause.

Excretion of the unmetabolized agent is primarily by the fecal route.

^{99m}Tc hepatobiliary agents are valued as an aid in diagnosing acute cholecystitis and cystic and common duct obstruction.

Although all three agents have similar biodistribution routes, they differ primarily in their ability to visualize the gallbladder in elevated bilirubin states.

CH_3 — R — CH_3 Lidofenin

$R = NHC(=O) - CH_2 - N(CH_2COOH)_2$

$CH(CH_3)_2$ — R — $CH(CH_3)_2$ Disofenin

H_3C, CH_3, Br, CH_3 — R Mebrofenin

Fig. 8-4. ^{99m}Tc hepatobiliary agents.

■ LUNG VENTILATION AGENTS

Only one lung ventilation agent was available for general use until recently. This was ^{133}Xe xenon gas. There are now three agents in use (Table 8-3):

1. Xenon ^{133}Xe gas
2. Xenon ^{127}Xe gas (no longer available)
3. Krypton ^{81m}Kr gas
4. Technetium ^{99m}Tc pentetate aerosol

Agents 1 through 3 are inert gases and are chemically nonreactive. These inert gases are lipid-soluble and only slightly soluble in water. The xenons are available ready to use in glass vials from the manufacturer. Krypton ^{81m}Kr gas is available from a radionuclide generator system. The DTPA radioaerosol is produced by preparing a kit of ^{99m}Tc-DTPA in the conventional manner. Instead of administration by intravenous injection, DTPA is made into an aerosol and inhaled.

On inhalation, all four agents are for the most part subsequently exhaled. With the exception of ^{81m}Kr, the exhaled radionuclide must be collected to prevent high room air concentrations of radionuclide. The xenons are collected and

Table 8-3. Radiopharmaceutical agents used for lung ventilation studies

	^{133}Xe	^{127}Xe	^{81m}Kr	^{99m}Tc-DTPA
Energy	81 keV (35%)	203 keV (68%)	191 keV (66%)	140 keV (88%)
Half-life	5.3 days	36.4 hrs	13 sec	6 hrs
Dose (mCi)	10-20	3-5	1-6	15-25
Lung radiation dose (rad/mCi/min)	0.083	0.0048	0.0025	0.05

passed through an activated charcoal column, where they are held. The ^{99m}Tc-DTPA aerosol is simply exhaled into a filter, which traps the aerosol particles.

If a sample of xenon or krypton is made available as part of a closed system to the respiratory motions of a patient, the gas will enter the oral cavity and follow the trachea downward through its branches to the terminal alveoli. Exchange of the radioactive gas through the alveolar membranes into the bloodstream occurs but only in limited quantities. Transfer is by diffusion and is dependent on solubility and concentration. Because of their limited solubility in water and the fact that room air and blood both have some stable inert gases as normal constituents, transfer to the bloodstream is limited to that promoted by the slight shift in equilibrium pressures resulting from the additional inert gas (radioactive this time) reaching the air side of alveolar membrane.

Xenon or krypton that crosses the membrane is swept away from the lung field by blood flow and is transferred to other tissues of the body, especially those high in fat content where the additional solubility is a contributing factor. Release of this deposited gas awaits only the reduction in its bloodborne concentrations where temporary storage of xenon in fat-containing tissues has been seen during and following ventilation studies using this gas.

The result of a patient rebreathing air containing radioactive gas in a closed system is a rapid equilibrium of concentrations within the alveolar sac and the external container. Breathing in a closed system for less than 1 minute provides such an equalization of concentrations.

If valving is subsequently provided such that each patient inspiration is that of fresh room air and each exhalation is collected in a closed container or on a charcoal column, radioactive gas concentrations in the lung alveoli fall exponentially. The time required for nearly complete removal of all the tracer from the lung is on the order of only 3 to 4 minutes. Release of the gas dissolved in the vascular compartment and that temporarily deposited in fatty tissues may add 1 or 2 minutes to this time.

Using ^{99m}Tc-MAA for lung-perfusion studies, the blood flow to the lungs can be mapped. Conversely, lung ventilation studies map areas where gaseous exchange with the environment is occurring. Gaseous ventilation studies generally are divided into several phases as follows:

1. *Initial phase:* imaging the distribution of the first breath hold by the patient.
2. *Equilibrium phase:* imaging while the patient is breathing on a closed system for a 1- to 2-minute period, resulting in a high-quality image of ventilation distribution.
3. *Washout phase:* sequential imaging of the lung field during washout to identify areas of the lung where the radiogas may be trapped, thus indicating poor ventilation.

A lung ventilation study using aerosol ^{99m}Tc-DTPA is similar to gaseous studies in that special hardware is required to administer the radioactive material and to collect the exhalation waste. When a patient is breathing in a closed system where the aerosol is introduced, the radiotracer is deposited as droplets along the larger branches of the trachea and down into the prealveoli branches. Deposition at these sites is firm for a period long enough to collect images of the ventilation distribution.

The major advantage of the aerosols is the simplicity with which multiple views of the patient can be acquired. The washout phase cannot be acquired with the aerosols, however.

Lung ventilation studies with all of the agents just discussed are normally employed to complement lung perfusion studies. Correlation of the images may be helpful in characterizing chronic obstructive lung disease and pulmonary emboli from other respiratory maladies.

■ GALLIUM ^{67Ga} CITRATE

^{67}Ga is an accelerator-produced radionuclide produced through the bombardment of a zinc target with protons. This can be represented by the following reaction:

$$^{67}\text{Zn}\ (p,n)^{67}\text{Ga}$$

^{67}Ga decays with a physical half-life of 78 hours. Decay is by electron capture and results in the emission of three useful gammas. The energies and abundances are as follows:

93 keV: 36%
185 keV: 20%
300 keV: 16%

Gallium is administered intravenously and is rapidly bound to blood proteins normally transporting iron. The chemical similarity of iron and gallium may help to explain the unusual distribution patterns seen with gallium for several days following administration to a patient. However, it should be pointed out that gallium only exists in the +3 state.

When originally investigated, gallium was thought to be useful for skeletal imaging because of its uptake there. Later, this was discovered to be the result of the carrier-effect. When administered carrier-free, as it is available currently, there is no appreciable skeletal uptake.

Plotting the disappearance of gallium from the blood produces a three-phase curve. The first component, consisting of about 50% of the administered dose, disappears with a half-life of about 9 minutes. The second component disappears with a half-life of 2 hours. The remaining fraction, constituting about 10% of the administered agent, leaves the blood with a half-life of 48 hours.

Circulating gallium is transported to tissue high in iron-binding proteins where it is deposited in varying degrees. Such tissue includes, but is not limited to, the renal cortex, liver, lacrimal and salivary glands, lactating breast, bone, and lymph nodes. The agent also appears in abscesses apparently associated with invading leukocytes and the infectious bacteria. Uptake by some tumors is well established, although mechanisms of tumor uptake are not well understood.

Serial imaging of patients imaged 24 hours after dose administration reveals a great deal of the activity remaining within the kidney. Ten percent of the administered dose is excreted in the urine within the first 24 hours.

If imaging is repeated at 48 or 72 hours, kidney activity will be diminished, and bone and lymph nodes will be most apparent. A shift to liver and spleen will occur by 72 to 96 hours after dose administration. Intrabody transport from one site to another, as a result of a chemical change, is neither documented nor understood. An explanation of the shifts in maximum concentration from certain tissues to others requires investigation.

Abdominal imaging with gallium presents many problems. Gallium accumulates in fecal material and may appear as an area of abnormal uptake on an image. Most clinicians prefer several abdominal images taken over a 2- to 3-day period to see if these "lesions" move. Above 10% of gallium is excreted by the bowel route during the first week.

Gallium ^{67}Ga citrate has two major uses. One use is the identification of sites of infection, and the other is tumor localization.

In identifying sites of infection, indium ^{111}In-labeled white blood cells (WBC) may be more useful, particularly in acute infections. Chronic infections are better visualized with gallium ^{67}Ga citrate.

■ RADIONUCLIDES FOR IMAGING THE HEART

■ Thallous ^{201}Tl chloride

The use of ^{201}Tl as thallous chloride for the detection of cardiac disease has significantly increased since this agent has been made available. Following many years of research in which the members of group 1 of the periodic table of the elements were evaluated, ^{201}Tl has emerged as the radionuclide of choice for heart imaging. Because potassium is known to concentrate in normal cardiac tissue and because no suitable radionuclide of this element exists, the search for a potassium analog has led to the choice of thallium. Knowledge of the concentration of potassium by normal myocardial cells during the rest period between muscle contractions has been well established for some time. The mechanism has been described as the sodium potassium adenosine triphosphatase (ATPase) system or, more commonly, the sodium potassium pump.

During cell rest, potassium is transferred from the extracellular fluid to the intracellular contents. Thallium, having an identical charge and other similar chemical properties, appears to follow closely the biodistribution of potassium. Coupled with acceptable nuclear parameters, thallous ^{201}Tl chloride can therefore be used in the evaluation of cardiac disorders.

^{201}Tl is produced in an accelerator in which a ^{201}Tl target is bombarded by protons according to the following equation:

$$^{203}\text{Tl}\ (p,3n)^{201}\text{Pb}$$

The resulting product, ^{201}Pb, is separated from the unreacted ^{203}Tl and affixed to a column where it undergoes decay by electron capture to ^{201}Tl. The daughter is eluted as the chloride, converted to pharmaceutical grade, and distributed as thallous chloride solution.

^{201}Tl decays by electron capture with a half-life of 73.1 hours. There are two useful photons emitted during the decay process. The energies and abundances reported are 10% at 167 keV and 3% at 135 keV. Fortunately, however, ^{201}Hg daughter x-rays are also produced at 68 to 80 keV with a frequency of 94.4 photons/100 ^{201}Tl atom disintegrations. The abundance at the 68 to 80 keV level makes this portion of the spectrum most often chosen for imaging procedures. Those with cameras capable of processing multiple energies simultaneously, however, are advised to employ the higher energies as well for resolution improvement purposes.

^{201}Tl as chloride administered intravenously to a normal patient undergoing stress testing is cleared with a half-life of 3 minutes by the well-perfused myocardium. Extraction efficiencies of 85% on a single pass are reported. Within minutes after injection, total activity in the heart may approach 4% of the administered dose and can result in a target-to-nontarget ratio of 2 or better in most patients. Fasting before stressing may assist in providing even better ratios, especially at the interface of heart and liver. The balance of the injected dose is uniformly distributed throughout the musculature and several select organs such as the kidney.

Localization of ^{201}Tl in the heart appears to be the function of two interrelated physiologic entities: regional blood flow and cell viability as evidenced by its sodium potassium ATPase activity. Normal myocardium takes up ^{201}Tl uniformly throughout its mass during stress and at rest. However, maximum uptake is at peak stress.

In ischemic tissue, the reduced blood flow to the viable but poorly perfused cells can be approached on scintiphoto. The difference in uptake is better demonstrated, however, if the administration of the radionuclide is made while the patient is exercising because stress improves blood flow to normal tissue to a much greater extent than that of ischemic tissue. Nonviable tissue such as new or old infarct and scar tissue does not take up ^{201}Tl, because of a combination of possible poor blood flow and most certainly because the potassium pump is inoperable.

Approximately 10 minutes after injection, localized ^{201}Tl begins to enter what is commonly known as a "redistribution" phase. During this period, imaging of a resting patient with stress-produced ischemic defects demonstrates a "filling in" of the lesion.

Table 8-4. Systems for analyzing radiochemical purity of ^{99m}Tc-cardiac agents

Radiopharmaceutical	Support	Solvent	Compound	R_f Value
Teboroxime	Whatman 31 ET TLC	50% v/v saline/acetone	Tc (IV)	0-0.3
			Teboroxime	0.3-1
Teboroxime	Whatman 31 ET TLC	Saline	TcO_4^-	0-0.6
			Teboroxime	0.6-1
Sestamibi	Aluminum oxide TLC	Ethanol (95%-100%)	Impurity	0-0.5
			Sestamibi	0.5-1

The use of ^{201}Tl as a perfusion/uptake/redistribution agent through stress and rest-period imaging is a valuable clinical tool in detecting coronary artery disease. ^{201}Tl can provide assistance in characterizing normal, ischemic but viable, and infarcted heart muscle.

Thallium clearance from the body is mostly via the urinary route. From 4% to 8% of the substance is lost by this route in the first 24 hours. The balance is excreted with a biologic half-life of approximately 10 days. The effective half-life is about 56 hours.

■ Technetium myocardial agents

Because of ^{99m}Tc's superior imaging characteristics over thallium ^{201}Tl, as well as favorable dosimetry, a technetium ^{99m}Tc-labeled cardiac-imaging agent may have advantages. There are two FDA-approved myocardial-perfusion agents using ^{99m}Tc: technetium ^{99m}Tc-teboroxime and technetium ^{99m}Tc-sestamibi. Both are perfusion agents and their uptake into the myocardium is related to blood flow.

One potential advantage of these agents is the ability to perform a first-pass study as well as a myocardial-perfusion study using the same radiopharmaceutical agent. Another potential advantage is that higher millicurie quantities can be administered allowing sharper images to be obtained. In addition, ^{99m}Tc is more readily available than the cyclotron agent ^{201}Tl; this allows more flexible patient scheduling of the technetium ^{99m}Tc-labeled cardiac-imaging agents.

Table 8-4 provides information on radiochemical purity testing for both agents.

Technetium ^{99m}Tc-teboroxime. Technetium ^{99m}Tc-teboroxime is from the BATO (Boronic Acid Technetium diOxime) class of compounds. It is used as an intravenous injection for imaging the myocardium.

The product is supplied as a lyophilized mixture of agents. Preparation of the product consists of adding 1 ml of ^{99m}Tc-NaTcO_4 to the vial. After mixing, the vial is heated at 100° C for 15 minutes. The contents should be allowed to cool to room temperature before injection.

Following injection of 15 to 30 mCi, a rapid uptake in myocardial tissue occurs and imaging should start within 2 to 5 minutes. The agent is mostly eliminated from myocardial tissue within 20 to 30 minutes. Because of the rapid uptake and washout from the myocardium, imaging must occur immediately. Delayed images are not possible. The primary route of excretion is hepatobiliary.

Technetium ^{99m}Tc-sestamibi. Technetium ^{99m}Tc-sestamibi is from the isonitrile class of compounds. It is used as an intravenous injection for imaging the myocardium.

The product is supplied in a lyophilized form. To prepare the product, 15 to 150 mCi of ^{99m}Tc-NaTcO_4 is added in a volume of 1 to 3 ml. The vial is placed into a boiling-water bath for 10 minutes. Following heating, the vial should be cooled to room temperature before injection.

Following injection of 10 to 30 mCi, technetium ^{99m}Tc-sestamibi is cleared primarily through the hepatobiliary system, with 27% of the dose excreted via the renal route. The hepatobiliary system initially has the highest concentration of this radiopharmaceutical, followed by heart, spleen, and lungs. The start of imaging is related to heart/liver and heart/lung activity ratios. When these ratios are highest, between 1 and 2 hours postinjection, imaging is optimal. Uptake into the myocardium does not occur as rapidly as does technetium ^{99m}Tc-teboroxime. Delayed images can be obtained.

■ Positron emission tomography (PET) cardiac agents

Positron-emitting agents are produced in a cyclotron and are generally short-lived. For the most part, this characteristic limits their use to the clinical site in which the cyclotron is housed. Because of their decay scheme (emission of a positron), conventional imaging equipment cannot be used. PET cameras are specifically designed to detect the coincident 511 keV gamma rays from the annihilation of positrons. Limited availability of imaging equipment is another factor limiting the use of these agents.

PET agents for cardiac imaging can be placed into two categories: perfusion agents and metabolic agents.

Perfusion agents include rubidium ^{82}Rb (half-life = 76 seconds), available from the strontium ^{82}Sr/rubidium ^{82}Rb generator system, nitrogen ^{13}N ammonia (half-life = 9.8 minutes), and oxygen ^{15}O water (half-life = 122 seconds). The strontium ^{82}Sr/rubidium ^{82}Rb generator system can be used for up to a month (strontium ^{82}Sr half-life = 23 days), allowing facilities without a cyclotron to perform PET myocardial perfusion studies. It is also the only approved agent for PET imaging.

^{18}F-2-fluoro 2-deoxyglucose (half-life = 110 minutes) is an agent that follows some of the metabolic pathways of glucose. Myocardial muscle viability can be evaluated with this metabolic agent. The longer half-life of ^{18}F compared with other PET metabolic agents allows it to be used outside of the facility housing the cyclotron.

■ RADIONUCLIDE CISTERNOGRAPHY

Computerized axial tomography (CAT) procedures have for the most part replaced radionuclide morphologic studies of the brain. Radionuclide fluid dynamic studies, however, remain as a viable alternative to the more invasive studies such as cerebral angiography and ventriculography.

To assess fluid flow in the cerebrospinal fluid compartment of the brain and spinal column, two radionuclides are available (Table 8-5). Both have similar physical characteristics and identical kinetics, which can be used in mapping the flow of cerebrospinal fluid.

^{111}In, an accelerator-produced radionuclide, can be prepared by complexing it with DTPA, a water-soluble chelating agent. The resulting complex, indium ^{111}In-DTPA, has replaced ytterbium ^{169}Yb pentetate, which is no longer available. When injected intrathecally, ^{111}In-DTPA rises to the base in several hours. Since fluid flow is generally positive from the ventricles, the agent flows over the convexities to the parasagittal area where it is transferred unmetabolized by the arachnoid villi to the vascular compartment. Arrival at this transfer point may be 24 hours or more following injection. ^{111}In and ^{99m}Tc-DTPA have approximately the same biologic half-life in the cerebrospinal fluid compartment, that is, 10 hours.

Once in the bloodstream, the DTPA with its radiolabel is filtered by the kidney to the urine. ^{111}In-DTPA is cleared quickly with a biologic half-life on the order of 30 minutes or less, making its presence in the vascular compartment inconsequential in performing cerebrospinal fluid imaging procedures.

The radionuclide cisternogram procedure generally involves the intrathecal administration of 1 mCi or less of ^{111}In-DTPA. Imaging is begun generally within 1 to 2 hours, followed by repeat views at 4, 24, 48 and 72 hours. The latter two views are rarely performed; however, in most cases the next clinical step to be taken can be determined by viewing the 24-hour film.

Two other uses for the radionuclide cisternogram include evaluation of shunt patency and detection of rhinorrhea.

Table 8-5. Comparison of ^{169}Yb and ^{111}In

Radiopharmaceutical	Half-life	Energy	Shelf life
^{169}Yb-DTPA	31.8 days	177 keV (22%) 298 keV (35%)	long
^{111}In-DTPA	2.8 days	173 keV (89%) 247 keV (94%)	short

■ BRAIN-IMAGING AGENTS

■ Iodine ^{123}I Iofetamine

Iodine ^{123}I-Iofetamine is a lipophilic agent for brain imaging (Fig. 8-5). Because of its lipophilicity, it is able to penetrate the blood-brain barrier. This characteristic distinguishes it from previous ^{99m}Tc cerebral imaging agents such as TcO_4, technetium ^{99m}Tc-DTPA, and technetium ^{99m}Tc gluceptate. These nonlipophilic agents cannot penetrate the blood-brain barrier unless there is a breakdown as a result of disease.

On injection, iodine ^{123}I iofetamine blood levels fall rapidly. Within 10 minutes, only 2% to 8% of the dose remains in circulation. It is taken up by the brain, lungs, and liver.

Elimination of the drug is slow, with 20% excreted after 1 day. Renal excretion is the main route.

■ Technetium ^{99m}Tc exametazime

This ^{99m}Tc-labeled amine is used for evaluation of altered regional cerebral perfusion. It was formerly referred to as HM-PAO or hexamethylpropylene amine oxime.

In the preparation of this agent, stannous reduction of technetium ^{99m}Tc is used to complex it with exametazime. The complex is lipophilic, a property that permits it to penetrate the blood-brain barrier. This characteristic distinguishes it from technetium ^{99m}Tc pentetate and technetium ^{99m}Tc gluceptate, both of which cannot penetrate the barrier.

Following addition of technetium ^{99m}Tc sodium pertechnetate to the reaction vial, complexation occurs and the lipophilic technetium ^{99m}Tc exametazime is formed. This lipophilic complex undergoes a change with time, forming a less lipophilic complex. This less lipophilic complex does not appear to penetrate the blood-brain barrier and places a time limit on use of the radiopharmaceutical agent. The time period between mixing and injection should be no more than 30 minutes.

On injection, technetium ^{99m}Tc exametazime localizes in the brain, muscle, soft tissue, kidneys, lungs, and gastrointestinal tract. Approximately 5% of the injected dose localizes in the brain within 1 minute. The brain retains about

$$I-C_6H_4-CH_2-CH(CH_3)-NH-CH(CH_3)_2 \cdot HCl$$ Iofetamine

Fig. 8-5. ^{123}I-labeled brain agent.

85% of this activity for 24 hours. Excretion is through the renal route (40%) and hepatobiliary route (15%). The activity in the brain is not subject to redistribution; this permits flexibility in imaging.

■ INDIUM ^{111}In–OXINE–LABELED WHITE BLOOD CELLS

Labeling leukocytes with radionuclides has been investigated for some time, usually with phosphorus ^{32}P. In the 1970s, investigators found that by mixing ^{111}In chloride and oxine (9-hydroxyquinoline), a lipophilic complex resulted. By incubating a suspension of white cells with the ^{111}In-oxine, the white cells (WBC) became labeled.

The In^{+3} ion will not pass through the WBC membrane, because of its electronic charge. Only when it is complexed to the lipophilic agent, oxine, does it easily penetrate. On entering the white blood cell, the indium oxine complex dissociates, with indium binding to intracellular proteins. Because the In^{+3} ion binds to plasma proteins, and in particular transferrin, it is necessary to remove all traces of plasma before the WBCs are incubated with ^{111}In-oxine. The ^{111}In-labeling procedure requires aseptic technique.

■ MONOCLONAL ANTIBODIES

Monoclonal antibodies of murine origin have been developed recently for imaging various sites. Small portions of antibody molecules, such as Fab fragments, as well as whole antibodies, are labeled with various radionuclides and injected intravenously for diagnostic purposes.

Indium ^{111}In satumomab pendetide has been approved for clinical use in the imaging of extrahepatic lesions in colorectal and ovarian cancer. This murine monoclonal anti-

LABORATORY APPLICATION

5

INDIUM ^{111}In-OXINE–LABELED WHITE BLOOD CELLS

Procedure

Materials

1. 60-ml syringe with 19-gage needle
2. Ring stand and clamp
3. Butterfly infusion set
4. Three 50-ml sterile centrifuge tubes (plastic) labeled with patient ID and WBC, LPP, and WASH
5. Centrifuge
6. Normal saline solution

Technique

1. Withdraw 30 to 50 ml of blood with a 60-ml syringe fitted with a 19-gage needle and containing approximately 1000 to 1500 U of heparin. Invert gently several times to mix the heparin.
2. Remove needle from syringe and clamp in an upright position. Tilt the syringe 10 to 20 degrees.
3. Attach a butterfly infusion set to the syringe and allow the red blood cells to sediment (30 to 60 minutes).
4. Express the supernatant (leukocyte-rich plasma) into a 50-ml sterile centrifuge tube marked "WBC."
5. Centrifuge the WBC tube at 450 *g* for 5 minutes.
6. Transfer the supernatant from the WBC tube into the tube marked "LPP" (leukocyte-poor plasma).
7. Add 5 ml normal saline to the white cell button in the WBC tube. Gently resuspend the cells.
8. Add approximately 600 μCi of ^{111}In-oxine to the white-cell suspension. The ^{111}In-oxine should be added dropwise while swirling the cell suspension.
9. Allow the ^{111}In-oxine/WBC suspension to incubate for 15 to 30 minutes. Gently swirl the tube several times during the incubation.
10. Add 4 to 8 ml of the LPP to the WBC tube following incubation.
11. Centrifuge the WBC tube at 450 *g* for 5 minutes.
12. Carefully pipette the supernatant from the WBC tube into the WASH tube.
13. Resuspend the labeled cell button with 4 to 8 ml of LPP.

Continued.

14. Assay the WBC tube and WASH tube and calculate percentage labeling.
15. Check the labeled cell suspension for clumps and foreign particles.
16. Perform trypan blue exclusion test to determine cell viability.
17. Draw 200 to 500 μCi of the labeled cells into a syringe. Assay and inject.

Key points

1. Patient should not be leukopenic.
2. Foaming should be avoided because cell clumping will result.
3. Presence of plasma during incubation (step 9) will decrease percentage labeling.
4. Aseptic technique must be used throughout the procedure.
5. In any procedure in which blood is removed from a patient, manipulated, and reinjected, meticulous care must be taken to prevent the administration into the wrong patient. As the minimum precaution, all materials used—syringes, pipets, centrifuge tubes, etc.—should be labeled with the patient's name and assigned serial number. Each step in the labeling procedure should be double-checked by another individual. Detailed records of the labeling procedure should be maintained.

body, when labeled with indium ^{111}In, associates with a specific tumor associated glycoprotein: TAG-72. This particular glycoprotein is associated with adenocarcinomas. Each kit contains 1 mg of the antibody in 2 ml of a sodium phosphate buffer solution and 2 ml of sodium acetate buffer. The contents of the kit should be refrigerated between 2 and 8° C during storage. Prior to preparation of a patient dose, the kit contents should be removed from the refrigerator and allowed to reach room temperature. 0.5 ml of the sodium acetate buffer should be added to a vial of commercially available indium ^{111}In chloride. The indium ^{111}In chloride must be specifically indicated for use in labeling the antibody. After mixing the buffer with the indium, approximately 5 to 6 mCi is added to the vial containing the antibody. Gently swirl the vial to adequately mix the contents and allow to incubate for 30 minutes. Withdraw the contents through a special 0.22 μm filter, provided with the kit, into a 10-ml syringe. Use of a smaller-capacity syringe may result in incomplete filtration of the labeled antibody and a smaller patient dose. This step will remove protein particulates formed in the labeling process. The final patient dose should be 4 to 5 mCi, to be used within 8 hours of preparation. Intravenous injection should be spaced over a 5-minute period and the patient monitored for any adverse reactions.

Quality control consists of a thin-layer chromatographic procedure using ITLC-SG strips and normal saline. An aliquot of the labeled antibody should be mixed with equal parts of a 0.05 *M* solution of DTPA prepared by adding sterile water for injection to a commercially available DTPA kit. A small drop of this mixture of antibody and DTPA should be spotted onto an ITLC-SG strip and developed in normal saline. The labeled antibody remains at the origin of the strip while the radiochemical impurities migrate to the solvent front. The labeling yield should be 90% or greater.

BIBLIOGRAPHY

Adams, E.H.: Sulfur colloid flocculation due to acid leached aluminum, J Nucl Med 13:707, 1972.

Aronson, R.S.: Source of contaminants in technetium generators, J Nucl Med 12:271, 1971.

Arras, J.M., and Schadt, W.W.: Determination of radiochemical contamination on columns of Tc-99m generators, J Nucl Med 11:620, 1970.

Bardfield, P.A., and Rubin, S.: Comparative study of instant technetium from various commercial suppliers, J Nucl Med 14:880, 1973.

Berger, A., Elenbogen, G.D., and Guris, L.G.: Pyrogens, Adv Chem Ser 16:168, 1956.

Boyd, G.E.: Recent developments in generators of Tc-99m, radiopharmaceuticals and labelled compounds, vol 1, Vienna, 1973, IAEA, pp. 3-25.

Briner, W.H.: Sterile kits for the preparation of radiopharmaceuticals: some basic quality control considerations. In Subramanian, G., and others, editors: Radiopharmaceuticals, New York, 1975, Society of Nuclear Medicine, pp. 246-253.

Briner, W.H., and Harris, C.C.: Radionuclide contamination of eluates from fission product molybdenum-technetium generators, J Nucl Med 15:466, 1974.

Brucer, M.: 118 medical radioisotope cows, Isot Radiat Tec 3:1, 1965.

Brucer, M.: A herd of radioisotope cows. In Vignettes in nuclear medicine, No. 3, St. Louis, Mallinckrodt Inc., 1966.

Brucer M.: A tracer has no pharmacology. In Vignettes in nuclear medicine, No. 24, St. Louis, Mallinckrodt Inc., 1967.

Callahan, R.J.: Technetium-99m human serum albumin: evaluation of a commercially produced kit, J Nucl Med 17:47, 1976.

Chen, M., Rhodes, B.A., Larson, S.M., and others: Sterility testing of radiopharmaceuticals, J Nucl Med 15:1142-1144, 1974.

Code of federal regulations, Title 10, Chapter 1, Part 20.205, Washington D.C., 1973, United States Government Printing Office.

David, G.S.: Quality of radioiodine, Science 184:1381, 1974.

Eckelman, W., Atkins, H.L., Richards, P., and others: Visualization of the human spleen with Tc-99m-labeled red blood cells, J Nucl Med 12:310, 1971.

Gerlit, J.B.: Some chemical properties of technetium, Proceedings of the International Conference on Peaceful Uses of Atomic Energy 7:145, 1956.

Haney, T.A.: Physical and biological properties of a Tc-99m-sulfur colloid preparation containing disodium edetate, J Nucl Med 12:64, 1971.

Harper, P.V.: Technetium-99m as a scanning agent, Radiology 85:101, 1965.

Krogsgaard, O.W.: Radiochemical purity of various Tc-99m labelled bone scanning agents, Eur J Nucl Med 1:15, 1976.

Krogsgaard, O.W.: Technetium-99m sulfur colloid: in vitro studies of various commercial kits, Eur J Nucl Med 1:31, 1976.

Lathrop, K.A.: Preparation and control of Tc-99m radiopharmaceuticals: proceedings of a panel on radiopharmaceuticals from generator produced radionuclides, STI-PUB-294, Vienna, 1971, IAEA, pp. 39-52.

McKusick, K., Holman, B.L., Jones, A.G., and others: Comparison of three Tc-99m isonitriles for detection of ischemic heart disease in humans, J Nucl Med 27:878, 1986.

Phan, T., and Wasnich, R.: Practical nuclear pharmacy, ed. 2, Honolulu, Banyan Enterprises, 1981.

Physicians desk reference for radiology and nuclear medicine, ed. 30, Oradell, N.J., 1976, Medical Economics Co., pp. 92-94.

Pohost, and others: Thallium redistribution: mechanisms and clinical utility, New York, 1980, Grune & Stratton.

Rhodes, B.A., and Croft, B.Y.: Basics of radiopharmacy, St. Louis, 1978, Mosby–Year Book.

Robbins, P.J., Chromatography of Technetium-99m radiopharmaceuticals: a practical guide, SNM, 1984.

van Royen, E.A., de Bruine, J.F., and others: Cerebral blood flow imaging with thallium-201 diethlydithiocarbamate SPECT, J Nucl Med 28:178-183, 1987.

Schelbert, H.R.: Seminars in nuclear medicine, 17:145-181, 1987.

Spatz, D.D.: Reverse osmosis: the mechanism and application to dialysis, Med Instrum 8:209, 1974.

Stern, H.S.: Preparation, distribution and utilization of technetium-99m sulfur colloid, J Nucl Med 7:655, 1966.

Subramanian, G., and others: Radiopharmaceuticals, SNM, 1975.

Taylor, A., Eshima, D., Fritzberg, A.R., and others: Comparison of iodine-131 OIH and technetium-99m MAG-3 renal imaging in volunteers, J Nucl Med 27:795-806, 1986.

Wackers, F.J.T., Berman, D.S., Maddahi, J., and others: Technetium-99m hexakis 2-methoxyisobutyl isonitrile: human biodistribution, dosimetry, safety, and preliminary comparison to thallium-201 for myocardial perfusion imaging, J Nucl Med 30:301-311, 1989.

Walker, H.G.: Effect of Tc-99m on bone scan agents in subsequent pertechnetate brain scans, J Nucl Med 16:579, 1975.

Williams, S.J., Mousa, S.A., Morgan, R.A., and others: Pharmacology of Tc-99m isonitriles: agents with favorable characteristics for heart imaging, J Nucl Med 27:877, 1986.

Zimmer, A.M., and Holmes, R.A.: Radiochemical purity and stability of commercial Tc-99m-Sn-diphosphate kits using a new chromatography technique, J Nucl Med 16:584, 1975.

Package Insert, Hepatolite, DuPont, 1986.

Package Insert, Indium ^{111}In Oxyquinoline Solution, Amersham, 1985.

Package Insert, Ultra-Technekow FM, Mallinckrodt, 1985.

Package Insert, Technescan MAA, Mallinckrodt, 1986.

Package Insert, Thallous Chloride, Mallinckrodt Medical, 1985.

Package Insert, Gallium Citrate, Mallinckrodt Medical, 1984.

Package Insert, Choletec, Squibb, 1986.

Package Insert, Technescan Hida, Mallinckrodt Medical, 1986.

Package Insert, Spectamine, Medi-Physics.

Package Insert, Ceretec, Amersham Corporation, 1988.

Package Insert, Technescan MAG3, Mallinckrodt Medical, 1990.

Package Insert, Ultratag RBC, Mallinckrodt Medical, 1991.

Package Insert, Cardiotec, Squibb, 1991.

Package Insert, Cardiolite, E.I. duPont de Nemours & Co., 1991.

Package Insert, Oncoscint CR/OV, Cytogen Corporation, Knoll Pharmaceutical Company, 1992.

Chapter 9

BIOLOGICAL EFFECTS OF IONIZING RADIATION

RONALD J. SCALA

When ionizing radiation is incident on biologic systems, energy is transferred into the system according to fundamental physical principles. The effect on the biologic system often is not so predictable. This effect, or endpoint, is related to several factors, among which are total radiation dose, dose rate, radiation quality, age of the system and several other environmental factors. Also important in identifying the effect is the level of the biologic system in which the endpoint is to be investigated, be it biochemical, molecular, cellular, or at the organism level. These endpoints and the factors that affect them will be discussed in this chapter.

■ THE DOSE EFFECT RELATIONSHIP

Depending on several complex parameters, when ionizing radiation transfers energy into a biologic system, one or more endpoints result. The general incidence and/or severity of the endpoint will be related to the dose absorbed into the system. For complex organisms such as man there are two types of dose effect relationships, somatic and genetic.

■ Somatic effects

Somatic effects primarily involve diploid cells. The effect will be manifest in the individual absorbing the radiation dose. Somatic effects involve two mechanisms of action, somatic certainty (deterministic) and somatic stochastic (nondeterminant).

Somatic certainty effects. Somatic certainty effects involve high doses over large portions of the body. The effect has a certainty of expression, but only after a discrete dose level is achieved. Below this dose threshold, the effect is not seen. At the threshold dose, the incidence of the effect within a population of exposed individuals, as well as the severity of the effect within any individual, increases with dose (Fig. 9-1).

Somatic certainty effects can be influenced by fractionating or protracting the dose. Fractionation splits the total dose into smaller fractions separated by time. Protraction spreads the dose over time at a continuous, but lower dose rate.

Somatic certainty effects are further categorized into early and late effects.

Early effects manifest with the first year after the dose and are related to the number of cells killed, the repair of damage, and the turnover rate of the irradiated cell line. Examples include erythemia (skin reddening), epilation (hair loss), pulmonary pneumonitis, and radiation sickness. Somatic certainty early effects can be altered by dose fractionation and protraction. This is the basis for radiation therapy fractionation. In general, a tissue can withstand several times the dose if it is fractionated or highly protracted. Somatic certainty late effects generally occur later than 1 year after the dose. They are related to the initial dose damage and impairment due to the repair mechanisms of the body. Examples include keratosis (skin thickening), pulmonary fibrosis, cataracts, and obliterative endarteritis (thickening of the blood vessel lumen endothelium with progressive sclerosis and obstruction). Somatic certainty late effects are less influenced by dose fractionation or protraction, being proportional to total dose only. Observations of irradiated lung fields to single doses of 4500 R showed incidence of pulmonary pneumonitis, an inflammatory condition, as high as 90%. Fractionating the dose over 30 days at 150 R per day reduced the incidence dramatically. However, the incidence of pulmonary fibrosis (a fibrotic destructive condition of the lung resulting in functional impairment) after 6 months was unchanged whether the dose was fractionated or given acutely (Table 9-1).

Somatic stochastic effects. Somatic stochastic effects describe radiation effects whose incidence show no certainty of occurrence in an exposed individual, but the occurrence in an exposed population is a function of dose. They pertain exclusively to leukemia and cancers. Somatic stochastic effects are generally regarded as having no threshold and therefore any dose, however small, has some effect if the exposed population is large enough for it to be detected. Stochastic incidence involves 250 excess cancers per million Person Rems (a million persons exposed to 1 rem). By statistical laws the 250 cases will also be seen in a population of 100,000 persons exposed to 10 rems or in 10 million persons exposed to 0.1 rem. Attempts have been made to extrapolate the stochastic dose effect relationship to individuals. Because of the stochastic nature of the relationship, care must be taken in any such attempt except to describe an increased risk with dose. Because the incidence in the population appears to increase linearly with dose, the somatic stochastic dose effect is often referred to as linear nonthreshold effect (Fig. 9-2). At lower doses data are not available to substantiate the linear extrapolation; several alternate shapes have been postulated.

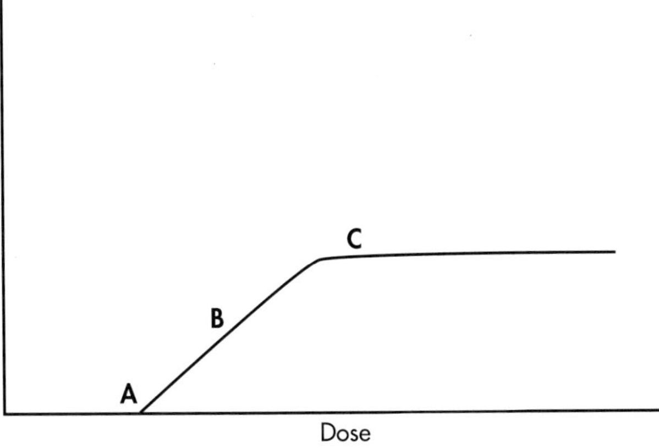

Fig. 9-1. Dose response curve for somatic certainty effects. No effect is measured until a dose threshold is reached **(A)** after which effect increases as a function of dose **(B)**. At high doses the endpoint changes as dose overkill region begins **(C)**.

Table 9-1. Effect of dose fractionation on the incidence of pulmonary pneumonitis and pulmonary fibrosis

Total exposure (R)	Rate	Effect
4500	Acute	90% pneumonitis
4500	150 R/day	<5% pneumonitis
4500	Acute	<50% fibrosis
4500	150 R/day	<50% fibrosis

■ Genetic effects

Genetic effects describe genotypical alterations in heritable traits resulting from mutations in the gene or chromosome of the germ cells. Genetic effects primarily involve haploid germinal cells. The effect is manifest not in the exposed individual but in that person's progeny. For expression of the genetic effect, the exposed cell must survive and be involved in fertilization.

Genetic effects exhibit a dose effect relationship similar to somatic stochastic effects in that describing incidence is valid in only large populations of exposed individuals. At the individual level the effect is stochastic, or uncertain, and only a risk associated with dose can be defined.

Measurement of genetic effects is difficult because of the high incidence of genetic birth defects inherent in the human population. At the cellular level, radiation-induced chromosome aberrations are detected at low doses in somatic cells. It can be concluded that similar frequencies of damage exist in germ cells exposed to radiation.

■ THE EFFECTS OF RADIATION ON THE CELL AT THE MOLECULAR LEVEL

The absorption of energy from ionizing radiation produces damage to molecules by direct and indirect actions. For direct action, damage occurs as a result of ionization of atoms on key molecules in the biologic system. This causes inactivation or functional alteration of the molecule. Indirect action involves the production of reactive free radicals whose toxic damage on the key molecule results in a biologic effect.

■ Direct action

Direct ionization of atoms in molecules is a result of absorption of energy by photoelectric and Compton interactions. Ionization occurs at all radiation qualities but is the predominant cause of damage in reactions involving high

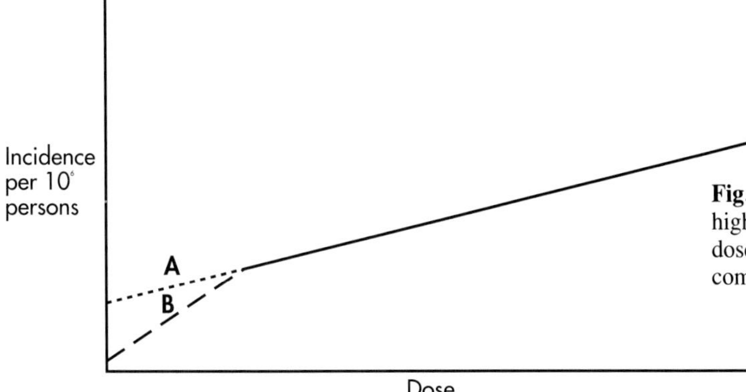

Fig. 9-2. Dose response curve for somatic stochastic effects. At high doses, incidence within the population increases linearly with dose. At lower doses the curve may continue linearly **(A)** or become a quadratic function **(B)**.

LET radiations. Absorption of energy sufficient to remove an electron can result in bond breaks.

$$\text{Ionizing radiation} + RH \rightarrow R^- + H^+$$

Excitation of atoms in key molecules can also occur resulting in bond breaks. In this case energy can be transferred along the molecule to a site of bond weakness and cause a break. Also tautomeric shifts can occur where energy of excitation can cause predominance of one molecule form.

$$\underset{\text{imidol (enol)}}{R{-}\overset{\overset{\displaystyle OH}{|}}{C}{=}NH} \leftrightarrow \underset{\text{amide (keto)}}{R{-}\overset{\overset{\displaystyle O}{\|}}{C}{=}NH_2}$$

The imidol and amide are tautomers in equilibrium with the amide (keto) predominant. In the amide form the molecule reacts in the proper biochemical chain. The introduction of excitation energy shifts the equilibrium to the imidol (enol). This causes either no reaction or a misread at the active site of an enzyme in the chain.

■ Indirect action

Indirect action of radiation involves the transfer of energy to an atom with a subsequent "decay" to a free radical species. A free radical is an electrically neutral atom with an unshared (unoccupied) electron in the orbital position. The radical is electrophilic and is highly reactive. Since the predominant molecule in biologic systems is water, it is usually the intermediary of the radical formation and propagation. The water molecule absorbs energy and disassociates into two radicals with unshared electrons in the valence shell. These are denoted by the symbols $H^\cdot$ and $OH^\cdot$ below.

$$H - O - H \rightarrow H+ + OH- \text{ (ionization)}$$
$$H - O - H \rightarrow H^\cdot + OH^\cdot \text{ (free radicals)}$$

Free radicals readily recombine to electronic and orbital neutrality. However, when many exist, as in high radiation fluence, orbital neutrality can be achieved by hydrogen radical dimerization (H_2) and the formation of toxic hydrogen peroxide (H_2O_2). The radical can also be transferred to an organic molecule in the cell.

$$H^\cdot + OH^\cdot \rightarrow HOH \text{ (recombination)}$$
$$H^\cdot + H^\cdot \rightarrow H_2 \text{ (dimer)}$$
$$OH^\cdot + OH^\cdot \rightarrow H_2O_2 \text{ (peroxide dimer)}$$
$$OH^\cdot + RH \rightarrow R\cdot + HOH \text{ (radical transfer)}$$

The presence of dissolved oxygen can modify the reaction by enabling the creation of other free radical species with greater stability and lifetimes.

$$H^\cdot + O_2 \rightarrow HO_2^\cdot \text{ (hydroperoxy free radical)}$$
$$R^\cdot + O_2 \rightarrow RO_2^\cdot \text{ (organic peroxy free radical)}$$

The lifetimes of simple free radicals ($H^\cdot$ or $OH^\cdot$) are very short, on the order of 10^{-10} seconds. While generally highly reactive they do not exist long enough to migrate from the site of formation to the cell nucleus. However, the oxygen derived species such as hydroperoxy free radical does not readily recombine into neutral forms. These more stable forms have a lifetime long enough to migrate to the nucleus where serious damage can occur. The transfer of the free radical to a biologic molecule can be sufficiently damaging to cause bond breakage or inactivation of key functions. In addition, the organic peroxy free radical can transfer the radical from molecule to molecule causing damage at each encounter. Thus a cumulative effect can occur, greater than a single ionization or broken bond.

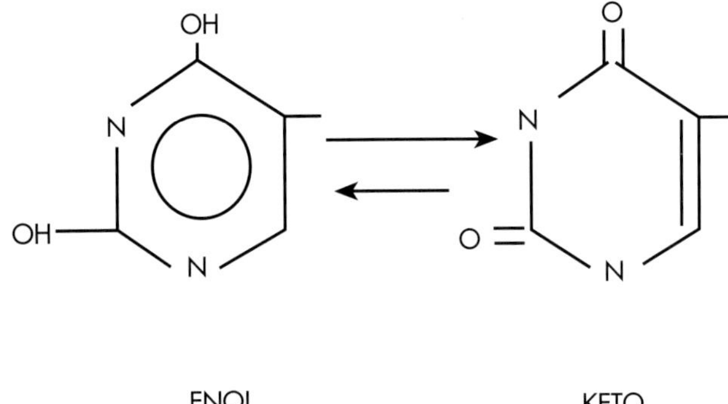

Fig. 9-3. Tautomeric equilibrium of thymine.

■ BIOCHEMICAL REACTIONS WITH IONIZING RADIATION

Nucleic acids found in living cells are of two types, deoxyribonucleic acid (DNA) and ribonucleic acid (RNA). They are complex macromolecules made of purine and pyrimidine bases on a "backbone" of alternating sugar and monophosphate molecules. The bases are nitrogen ring compounds: adenine, guanine, cytosine, thymine and uracil. The carbohydrate sugar is either deoxyribose or ribose, five carbon sugars unique to nucleic acids. The monophosphate is derived from the energy transfer molecule, adenosine triphosphate (ATP). There is considerable evidence suggesting that nucleic acids, especially DNA, are the primary target for cell damage from ionizing radiation.

Breaks in the DNA chain can disrupt function of the molecule in several ways. Transcription of the genetic code can be altered, as can synthesis of the codon strand—the duplicate, mirror image of the base sequence. In many cases breaks in the double-strand DNA can be repaired by the enzymes, DNA polymerase, and DNA ligase. These enzymes function by detecting breaks in the strand and correcting them. Before mitosis and during transcription and replication when the DNA molecule exists in a single strand, breaks are less likely to be repaired. Incorrect repair can also occur. This can result when a deletion is replaced with a different base or when a base is tautomerically shifted so repair enzymes misread the base.

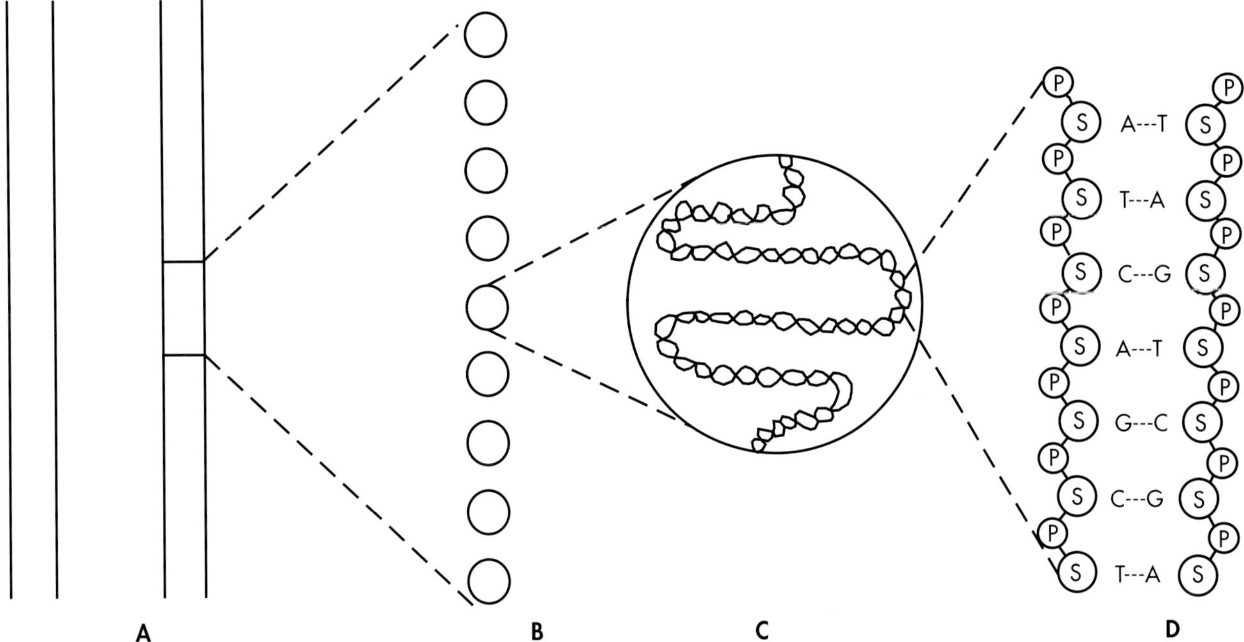

Fig. 9-4. Schematic representation of a chromosome. **A,** Alleles of the chromosome. **B,** Chromatin. **C,** 200 base pairs inside histone coat. **D,** DNA molecule.

The hydrogen bonds between adenine and thymine prefer the keto form of thymine. In the enol form, thymine will not bond to adenine and will cause a bond break or misread (Fig. 9-3).

■ Chromosomes

Chromosomes are the subcellular structures of which the genetic material, DNA, is a major component. Also contained in the chromosome structure are proteins called histones, which bind to the DNA and are responsible for the varied morphology, or shape, of the chromosome. This nucleoprotein complex is known as chromatin (Fig. 9-4). There is considerable evidence to support radiation damage to the chromatin structure as the major factor in cell reproductive death, as well as to mutations that lead to genetic and carcinogenic effects.

Chromosomes are present in pairs, and areas on pairs of chromosomes that occupy the same location are called homologous genes, or alleles. Transfer of genetic material (DNA) between alleles is considered normal to some degree and is the basis for many spontaneous mutations. Radiation can cause double-strand breaks and increase the frequency of these exchanges. In addition, radiation can cause structural aberrations with pieces of the chromosomes break free and form aberrant shapes.

■ THE EFFECT OF RADIATION ON THE CELL; CELL KINETICS

Undifferentiated cells that are growing are destined to divide. The generation time from one cell division to the next, known as the cell cycle, is dependent on species, tissue type, age, and environmental influences.

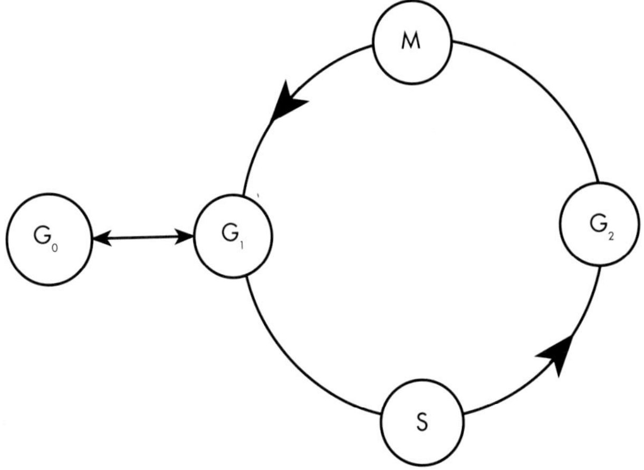

Fig. 9-5. Schematic diagram of the cell cycle: nonproliferative phase G_0, gap G_1, synthetic phase S, gap G_2, at mitosis M.

During this cycle the cell grows in volume as a result of protein, DNA, and RNA synthesis. Mitosis occurs with division of the cell. The cell cycle can be divided into phases: G_1 (gap), S (synthesis), G_2 (gap), and M (mitosis). Cells not actively growing occupy a fifth phase known as G_0. The cell in G_0 can often be stimulated to enter the active cycle by environmental stresses (Fig. 9-5).

Cells in G_0, G_1, S, and G_2 phases of the cell cycle oc-

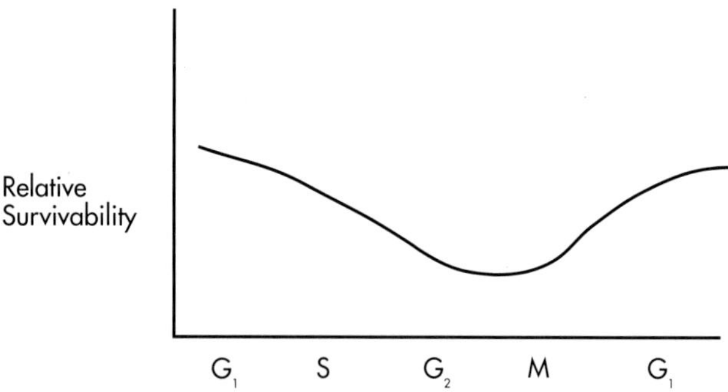

Fig. 9-6. Relative survivability of cells irradiated in different phases of the cell cycle. Synchronized cells in late G_2 and in mitosis (M) showed greatest sensitivity to cell killing.

cupy what is called the *interphase period*. During mitosis (M phase) chromosomes condense (prophase) and become aligned on the equatorial plane (metaphase). Pairs separate (anaphase) and condense at the poles of the dividing cell (telophase), and the new nucleus forms in each cell. Cells are most sensitive to cell killing during the period shortly before M phase at late interphase (G_2), and during M phase. Higher resistance is seen in cells in S phase and late G_1 phase as well as all cells in G_0 phase. Resistance in S phase may be due to the presence of synthetic enzymes capable of prompt repair of DNA breaks. However, mutation frequency increases in cells in or just before S phase (Fig. 9-6).

Irradiation of the cell causes cell death at mitosis (actually a regression of cell division) as a result of the inability to divide. RNA and protein synthesis do not halt in the sterilized cell. The result is the production of the giant cell, whose unbalanced growth eventually proves lethal to the cell.

According to the Bergonié-Tribondeau law, radiosensitivity of tissues depend on a number of factors. According to these early radiobiologists (1906), radiation response in tissue was a function of (1) a high number of undifferentiated cells in the tissue, (2) a high number of actively mitotic cells, and (3) the length of time the cells remain in active proliferation. It is not clear why lack of differentiation of the cell results in radiosensitivity. It has been shown that undifferentiated cells or cells in the process of differentiation are easily killed by radiation. The length of time that cells remain in active proliferation relates to the number of divisions between the most immature stage and the final mature stage. The longer the cell remains in active proliferation, the greater its sensitivity to radiation.

■ MODIFICATION OF RADIATION INJURY

There are several environmental factors which, in general, modify the degree of damage due to radiation. These physical factors include dose rate and fractionation, radiation quality, and temperature. In addition, several chemicals can modify the radiation effect.

■ Dose rate and fractionation

In general the lower the rate of delivery of radiation dose and the more time between radiation exposures, the more resistant the biologic system becomes. This is thought to be due to the repair of sublethal lesions before additional lesions, which cumulatively are lethal, can occur. At the cellular level this may be function of the multitarget theory. It is thought that several radiation events in close proximity, probably in the DNA or chromatin structure, must occur in a time frame short enough to cause a lethal outcome. If not in close-enough proximity, or if separated by long periods of time, natural repair can occur and the cell lives. In DNA, a single broken bond can be repaired, but a scission of both strands is often irreparable. If the two breaks occur far apart in time, repair is possible. If the breaks occur at different ends of the molecule, the DNA will not break (scission) and repair is possible.

■ Radiation quality

Because high LET radiation deposits greater amounts of energy per unit length of matter traversed, the possibility of multiple lesions in close proximity and short time frame is high. Thus high LET radiations for the same total dose are more efficient in lethality than are low LET radiations.

■ Temperature

While many cells at higher temperatures, are sensitized to radiation damage, several chromosome aberrations increase at lower temperatures. This is probably due to the suppression of the repair process at low temperatures. For cell-killing effects, tissues of higher temperatures are more radiosensitive.

■ Chemical modification

Several natural or added chemical agents, if present in the cells and tissues before the exposure, can modify sensitivity to radiation.

Oxygen. As discussed earlier, dissolved oxygen in the tissues increases the stability and toxicity of free radicals. The degree to which the effect is increased as a result of oxygenation is called the *oxygen enhancement ratio* (OER), determined by:

$$\text{OER} = \frac{\text{Dose required to cause effect without oxygen}}{\text{Dose required to cause effect with oxygen}}$$

The OER has a maximum value of 3.0. In radiation therapy normal tissue exists at about 20 to 40 mm Hg partial pressure of O_2. The maximum benefit of oxygen sensitizations at 30 mm Hg. Therefore normal tissue is not relatively effected by increasing oxygen tension. Tumor cells, however, exist in varying states of oxygenation, including a large portion of the population in hypoxia (low O_2). In addition, these cells have reduced mitosis and are highly resistant to radiation. Increasing oxygen tension will sensitive these cells. A practical problem exists in that oxygen will diffuse only 150 μm beyond the capillary wall and is ineffective in many hypoxic cells lying beyond.

Radiosensitizing agents. Several chemicals can increase the damaging effects of radiation. Analogs of purines and pyrimidines have this effect. Halogenated and substituted analogs of the DNA bases can interfere with DNA repair after radiation damages. Examples include 5-bromouracil and 6-thio-guanine. Actinomycin D inhibits nuclear RNA synthesis and potentiates radiation damage.

Nitroimidazoles are electronaffinic compounds that increase radiosensitivity of cells with a sensitization enhancement ratio (SER) of 1.2 to 2.4, where

$$\text{SER} = \frac{\text{Dose required to cause effect without agent present}}{\text{Dose required to cause effect with agent present}}$$

While SERs are lower than maximally achievable OER, these compounds diffuse farther beyond the capillary wall than does oxygen, and they can be introduced into the tumor volume via needle or catheter. They are, however, neurotoxic. They include misonidazole, desmethylmisonidazole, 5-nitroimidazole, and nitrofuran.

Inhibitors of anaerobic glycolysis such as 5-thio-D-glucose and butyric acid interfere with metabolism of hypoxic cells. This has a sensitizing effect.

Radioprotective agents. Chemicals that when present before irradiation diminish the effect of radiation are called *radioprotective agents*. The dose reduction factor (DRF) measures this protection and is derived by

$$\text{DRF} = \frac{\text{Dose to cause effect with protector present}}{\text{Dose to cause effect without protector present}}$$

Thiols are sulfur-containing reducing agents such as cysteine, 2-mercaptoethylamine, cystamine, thiourea, and AET. Thiols have a DRF ratio of 1.4 to 2.0. They are thought to protect cells by scavenging free radicals, producing hypoxia and forming disulfide bonds in proteins, thereby strengthening them. They also temporarily inhibit DNA synthesis, allowing time for the repair enzymes to complete repair of sublethal damage.

Analgesics such as alcohol, morphine and tranquilizers can reduce respiration, lowering oxygenation and increasing radioresistance. Epinephrine causes tissue hypoxia and therefore has some protective properties. Dopamine protects organisms with a DRF of 1.3. Possible actions include scavenging of free radicals and delay in DNA synthesis. Other protective agents, with varying degrees of effectiveness, include cyanide, nucleic acids, sodium fluoroacetate, melitin (free venom), bacterial endotoxin, and cyclic AMP. Cyclic AMP appears not to protect tumor cells but may be an effective prophylactic in radiation therapy.

■ THE EFFECTS OF RADIATION ON BIOLOGICAL SYSTEMS: TISSUES

As stated in the Bergonié-Tribondeau law, rapidly dividing, undifferentiated cells in tissues are the most sensitive to radiation effects. Several of the most sensitive tissues and systems follow this law.

■ Hematopoietic system

Highly sensitive to radiation killing are the cells of the hematopoietic system and the related lymphoid system. Most sensitive are the stem cells of the bone marrow, which give rise to all circulating blood cells and platelets, as well as the lymphoid tissues found in the spleen, liver, lymph nodes, and thymus. Of particular resistance are the mature circulating red blood cells and platelets; this is probably due to their lack of a nucleus. Circulating lymphocytes are quite sensitive to radiation and a measurable drop in the normal titre (about 21,000/dl) can meter radiation exposure and indicate dose levels. As little as 10 cGy can show a measurable drop in the circulating small lymphocyte population.

Within the blood-forming organs are precursor cells that are killed by radiation. The subsequent effect on circulating cell levels is not seen for days to weeks because resistant mature cells in circulation remain viable. Only after these begin to diminish by natural turnover does the decrease in cell levels become evident, because the damaged bone marrow has made no replacements. The effect is pancytopenia (depression of all cell types), resulting in hemorrhage (platelet reduction), infection (white-cell depression), and the effect of anemia from plummeting red cells.

■ Reproductive system

The cells of the reproductive system are highly sensitive to radiation effects. In the human male, stem cells and proliferating spermatogonia are highly sensitive. However, spermatids and mature sperm show considerable resistance. Also resistant are the interstitial cells of the testis, which control hormone production and secondary sexual characteristics. Therefore at sterilizing doses of 600 cGy, potency, fluid production of the prostate and seminal vesicles, as well as voice, beard and male social behavior are not affected. With a turnover time for spermatogenesis (stem cell to mature sperm) of 64 to 72 days, sterility is never seen immediately after the radiation dose, because mature sperm are resistant to the killing effects of radiation. They can sustain heritable genetic damage, however. Doses of about 600 cGy are required to permanently sterilize males (sterility occurs after several months). Although lower doses can also cause sterility after several months, the effect is temporary. Fertility and near-normal sperm counts return after 1 to 2 years.

Dose rate has an unusual effect on the incidence of sterility in males. In animals it was found that dose protraction and fractionation were more effective in causing permanent sterility. In mice a dose of 450 cGy delivered at 3 cGy per day for 150 days caused permanent sterility. An acute dose of 450 cGy caused only temporary sterility. In rats, protracting a dose of 800 cGy over a period of 5 days caused permanent sterility while the same total dose given acutely caused only temporary sterility. This may be a result of synchronizing the sperm stem cells. Proliferating stem cells in the G_2 phase or M phase of the cell cycle are killed by radiation. But since the dose is protracted at a constant low rate, resistant S and GI cells eventually progress to the sensitive phases and are killed.

In the female, radiation destroys both ovum and maturing follicles. This reduces hormone production. Therefore radiogenic sterility in females can be accompanied by artificial menopause, with significant effects on sexual characteristics and secondary genitalia.

In humans only primary and secondary oocytes are present after birth because all stem cell proliferation to oogonia has ceased. While the oocytes are moderately radiosensitive, the granulosa cells of the ovarian follicle are very sensitive, particularly during follicle maturation.

Total dose, dose rate, and age are important factors in the final effect. Younger women seem better able to recover fertility than do older women. A dose of 200 cGy permanently sterilizes women over 40 but causes temporary sterility in women age 35 and under. Menopause was caused in 50% of younger women exposed to doses of 150 to 500 cGy. Women over 40 showed 90% menopause at 150 cGy.

■ Gastrointestinal system

The gastrointestinal (GI) tract is highly sensitive to radiation. Following irradiation, the first changes seen occur in the epithelium lining of the small intestine containing millions of convolutions called *villi*. The crypt cells of the villi are highly proliferative, supplying cells that continue to differentiate and migrate to the terminal villus. There they eventually slough off into the intestinal contents. Radiation causes mitotic arrest of the crypt cells followed by eventual denudation of the villi, ulceration of the wall, and septic infiltration.

Effects on the large intestine cause functional impairment resulting in fluid and electrolyte loss, and diarrhea. Effects on the upper GI tract include vomiting, depression of acid, and pepsin secretion. Destruction of the epithelium lining of the pharynx and esophagus results in dryness, soreness, and petechia (capillary rupture).

■ Skin

Skin is relatively radiosensitive. The radiobiologic endpoints in skin are dependent on the total dose, the dose rate, and the radiation quality. Radiobiologic effects in skin include erythema (skin reddening), and temporary epilation (hair loss). At very high doses, permanent epilation and destruction of suborgans, including the vasculature, sebaceous and sweat glands, occur.

The response of the skin to ionizing radiation is called *radiation dermatitis*. This effect follows a temporal as well as dose response depending on damage to the suborgans and connective tissue. Skin responses include:

1. Initial erythema. Redness occurs within days due to capillary dilatation caused by histamine releases. Threshold dose is 200 cGy from beta radiation or 1000 R from x-ray radiation.
2. Dry desquamation. After several days the epidermis scales and peels as a result of reduction in sebaceous and sweat gland secretion, and vascular damage.
3. Erythema proper. After the third or fourth week redness with soreness and burning and edema results. This is caused by obstructive changes in the fine vasculature in the dermis.
4. Moist desquamation. At high doses of 2000 R, blisters form in the epidermis, permanent epilation results and edema with macrophage infiltration occurs. Severe damage to the vasculature and connective tissue is the cause.
5. Necrosis. At very high doses, dermal necrosis may result after erythema proper as a result of dermis destruction, or later because of obstructive changes in arterioles, infection, and subcutaneous-fat–cell destruction.
6. Late effects. After one year, at high doses dermal atrophy, deep fibrosis, hyperpigmentation and general dryness are seen. At very high doses (several thousand cGy), necrotic damage as a result of obliterative endarteritis may cause the eventual loss of limbs or large areas of the skin.

Chronic exposure at lower doses results in hyperkeratosis, characterized by thickening of the epidermis, weakening of the strata with frequent ulceration, poor healing, and decreased vascularization. Chronic exposure is also associated with radiogenic carcinoma, primarily squamous cell carcinoma.

■ Mucous membranes

Mucous membranes are also radiosensitive, particularly those in the mouth, pharynx, and esophagus. After considerable doses, dryness, soreness, and petechial ulceration of the mouth occur within 2 weeks. In the third week this progresses to swelling of the tongue with hypersecretion of the mucus, which eventually becomes a thick pseudomembrane that covers the buccal area, throat, and tongue. Later, fibrosis, ulceration, and poor vasculature accompanies skin effects.

■ Central nervous system

Generally, the central nervous system is resistant to radiation effects. Very high doses are required to cause substantial effects on the brain and nervous system. The vasculature is the limiting factor in radiation effects to the central nervous system. Effects on the vessels cause breakdown of the capillary circulation with rupture of the walls, interstitial edema, meningitis, encephalitis, and the breakdown of the blood-brain barrier. In addition, there can be infiltration of granulocytes, mast cells, and lymphocytes into the meninges. Doses of several thousand centigray are required for these effects. At higher doses, prompt killing (pynknosis) of the cerebellum has been seen. At lower doses, reversible changes in neurons can occur.

The spinal cord exhibits radiation effects including thickening of the vessels, dissolution of white matter, and myelitis after doses in the order of 5000 R. This is a delayed effect, manifesting one to several years after exposure. It is a limiting factor in radiotherapy, where the cord may receive high doses in the treatment of a nearby tumor.

Peripheral nerves are highly resistant to radiation effects. Higher doses and longer latent periods are required for expression of effects.

■ The fetus

Fetal effects are seen at relatively low doses of radiation. The fetus is a highly proliferative system with many undifferentiated cells. Therefore it is extremely sensitive to radiation effects. The effect not only depends on dose but also the gestational age at the time of irradiation. During the first trimester, damage is greatest with the resultant effect often causing spontaneous abortion (Table 9-2). During organ development and differentiation (3 to 8 weeks), irradiation results in high incidence of congenital organ anomalies—failure to develop or development with a defective deviation of structure or function. With the exception of neurons, which develop throughout gestation, differentiation does not occur after this period. Irradiation after organ development results in growth retardation or skeletal malformations. Irradiation before the fifth month was reported to cause microcephaly (small cranium) and mental retardation in children of Japanese bomb survivors. This occurred at dose levels of 10 to 19 cGy gamma with neutrons, and 150 cGy gamma only.

Table 9-2. Radiogenic effects on mouse fetus irradiated to 200 R at different gestational ages

Gestational age	Stage	Radiogenic effect
0-5 days	Embryo	Prenatal death
5-15 days	Fetus (organogenesis)	Congenital anomalies, still births, growth retardation
15-19 days	Fetus (growth)	Growth retardation, neonatal death, cancer

While data suggest nervous tissue function alterations occur at doses as low as 0.4 cGy, the measurable effect and the low incidence are not distinguishable from normal birth defect rates.

Because internally deposited radionuclides have the ability to concentrate in fetal tissue, very small amounts can have pronounced effects.

■ Lens of the eye

At doses as low as 200 to 600 cGy, damage to the lens, significant to cause eventual cataract formation, can occur. The dividing epithelium of the anterior equatorial region of the lens produces cells which migrate, elongate and organize into the transparent fibers making up the lens (Fig. 9-7). There is no mechanism for removal of cells from the system. Subsequently, radiation-damaged cells migrate to the posterior poles and centrally, as an opacity. Furthermore, disruption of the fiber organization enlarges the opacity until a cataract forms. The time from dose to formation, or latent period, is from 2 to 35 years, with a mean time of 8 years at single doses of 250 to 650 cGy.

■ Other organs

In general the viscera exhibits relative radioresistance. Usually the connective tissue and vasculature become the limiting structures, but functional damage can result from high doses.

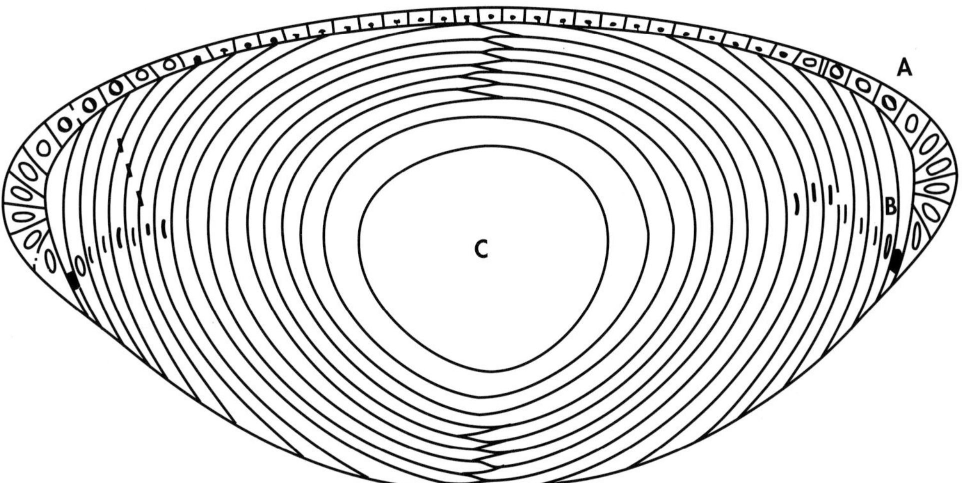

Fig. 9-7. Schematic drawing of human lens. **A,** Active epithelium gives rise to **B,** elongated cell fibers. **C,** The fibers migrate inward toward the lens nucleus. Since there is no mechanism for removal of cells, radiation-damaged cells migrate inward and form opacities and eventually cataracts.

Table 9-3. Tolerance dose ranges (cGy) for 5% to 50% pathologic findings within 5 years (TD5-50/5)

Bone marrow	200-600
Ovary	200-600
Lens of eye	500-1250
Testes	500-2000
Kidney	2100-2700
Pubic breast	1000-1250
Lung	2500-3000
Liver	3500-4500
Lymph node	4000-7000
Heart	4000-6000
Stomach	4500-5000
Colon	4500-6500
Spinal cord	5000-7000
Esophagus	600-7500
Bladder	6000-8000

Adapted from Rubin, P., and Casarett, G.W.: A direction for clinical radiation pathology: the tolerance dose. In Frontiers of radiation therapy and oncology, vol. 6, Baltimore, 1972, Karger, Basil and University Press.

Lung: Radiation pneumonitis, an acute inflammatory reaction of the functional tissue and vasculature with doses of several thousand centigray after 4 to 6 months.

Lung: Radiation fibrosis, accumulation of fibrin in alveoli and septa, 6 months to years after high doses.

Blood vessels: Hemorrhage followed by progressive thickening and proliferation of endothelial cells known as obliterative endarteritis.

Kidney: Nephrosclerosis, nephritis, hypertension, and renal failure 2 to 3 years after doses of 3000 cGy.

Liver: Hepatitis and necrosis several years after doses of 4000 cGy.

Thyroid: Hypothyroidism at doses of 100 to 4000 cGy external, after several months. Thyroid ablation at doses of 50,000 cGy internal (1 mCi ^{131}I per gram of thyroid tissue).

Table 9-3 lists tolerance doses for 5% to 50% incidence of pathologic findings within 5 years (TD5-50/5) for total doses from therapeutic radiation.

■ WHOLE BODY IRRADIATION: THE ACUTE SOMATIC SYNDROME

In humans, whole-body exposure to large acute radiation doses results in a complex of clinical symptoms collectively known as the acute radiation syndrome. The exact pathology is dose-dependent. Five dose-related clinical outcomes will be described. For each outcome a time sequence is involved.

Initial phase: "Shock" response to radiation energy deposition.

Latent period: Viable cell populations, resistant to radiation, maintain function. Normal physiology, little or no symptoms.

Manifest illness: Symptoms develop as viable cell populations decrease as a result of stem cell death and no renewal cell production.

Endpoint: Recovery with varying degrees of impairment, or death.

■ Prodromal syndrome

At sublethal doses of 25 to 150 cGy to the whole body, the prodromal syndrome, or prodrome, occurs. It manifests as "early" effects and "later" effects. Actually the prodrome occurs for all whole-body radiation outcomes, with the severity of symptoms increasing with dose. Early effects occur within hours. They include erythemia (doses > 100 cGy), fever due to vasodilatation and fluid imbalances, vomiting because of stimulation of the vomit center (as little as 25 cGy), prostration, weakness, cramps, and diarrhea.

No latent period is seen as later effects overlap the initial phase. Later effects include continuation of the early effects, as well as jaundice and scalp pain with epilation (after 3 weeks, >300 cGy). Not all symptoms appear in all cases, but higher doses result in increased incidence and severity of the prodromal effects. Recovery is complete after 48 hours within this dose range.

■ Hematopoietic or bone marrow syndrome

At high doses of about 150 to 400 cGy whole-body, the hematopoietic or bone marrow syndrome occurs. Initially a radiation prodrome occurs. This is followed after 48 hours by a latent period of up to 3 weeks, with no clinical symptoms. Laboratory analysis would show prompt depletion of small lymphocytes and progressive depletion of formed elements in the blood. Cell production in the bone marrow is halted. Due to resistant circulating mature cells and platelets, the clinical effects are not seen for several weeks after the radiation dose.

Symptoms of bone marrow syndrome include anemia, petechia, increased blood pressure, fatigue, ulcerations in the mouth, epilation, purpura, and infection. A pathologic condition results from a drop in lymphocytes, granulocytes, immunosuppression, and loss of platelets. Death due to bleeding, anemia and infection is possible in this dose range. The mean lethal dose for humans (LD50) is about 350 cGy if no medical intervention is used. If the exposed individual survives the eighth week, the manifest illness begins to subside. Laboratory results indicate slow recovery of lymphocytes and granulocytes for several months.

■ Hematopoietic/gastrointestinal syndrome

At doses in the order of 400 to 800 cGy, a modified bone marrow syndrome occurs. The initial prodrome is more severe and the latent period is shortened. The manifest illness is more severe. Contributing to the pathology and outcome are effects from gastrointestinal damage and infection. Death is more likely with these doses.

■ Gastrointestinal syndrome

Doses over 800 cGy whole-body produce the gastrointestinal or gut syndrome. Because sensitivity of the intestinal crypt cells is lower than that of bone marrow, higher doses are required to cause this radiation syndrome. However, because turnover time for the crypt cells is shorter than for bone marrow (8 days vs. months), the gut syndrome manifest illness appears sooner after dose. The latent period is 4 to 6 days after prodrome. Bone-marrow destruction is present and contributory to the outcome, but death usually occurs before the full symptomology of bone-marrow effects can manifest.

Initially, a severe prodrome occurs followed by a 2- to 4-day latent period. Manifest illness occurs at 4 to 6 days after exposure. Symptoms include hemorrhage, nausea, vomiting, diarrhea with blood, anorexia, lethargy, dehydration, and enterocolitis. The underlying pathologic condition is a result of mitotic arrest of the crypt cells followed by denudation of the villi, destruction of the capillary and lymphatic bed, plasma leakage, ulceration of the small intestine, and bacterial infiltration. The pathologic condition is complicated by platelet depletion and immune suppression. Death is likely as a result of septic infection.

■ Central nervous system syndrome

At whole-body doses on the order of several thousand cGy, an acute inflammatory and convulsive disorder of the brain and nervous system is seen. The prodrome is severe, and immediate, and it blends into the symptoms of the manifest illness. There is little or no latent period. Death is imminent within days, so the severe effects of bone marrow and gut damage will not have time to manifest.

Symptoms of the inflammatory process include apathy, somnolence and coma, headache, cramps, apprehension, shortness of breath, oliguria, diarrhea, and the regulatory failure in temperature, respiration, perspiration, and blood pressure control. The underlying pathologic condition involves the vasculature of the brain. Radiogenic damage to the vessels causes breakdown of the blood-brain barrier; vasculitis; meningitis; vasodilation; and edema within the choroid plexus, the ventricles, and the white matter. In addition, damage stimulates basophilic infiltration into the meninges and release of inflammatory agents.

Symptoms of the convulsive process include tremors, convulsions, ataxia with respiratory distress, and the loss of muscular coordination. The underlying pathologic condition is edema and brain pressure as well as pynknosis (prompt killing) of the cerebellum. Functional responses from the central nervous system (CNS) syndrome are vomiting due to vagal stimulation in the prodrome phase and later due to destruction in the vomit center and gut. A drop in blood pressure and temperature, as well as respiratory distress, are also seen. Trained performance is unaffected.

Although manifest illness is due to damage of the brain, higher doses are required to illicit the CNS syndrome if only the head is exposed.

■ SOMATIC STOCHASTIC EFFECTS: LEUKEMIA AND CANCERS

Leukemia and solid tumors, both benign and malignant, have been demonstrated in organisms exposed to ionizing radiation. The exact mechanism of radiogenic cancer, and in fact all cancers, is not well understood. It can be postulated that mutations in gene loci, deletions, or other chromosome aberrations may be involved. Several theories have been presented. There may be "cancer genes," present in all organisms, that are prevented from being expressed by suppressor genes. Damage by random radiation events to these suppressor genes would allow expression. Or, normal genes may be mutated into cancer genes by sublethal damage of radiation. The introduction of viral genetic material may stimulate or cause cancers. Contributory at higher doses is suppression of the immune system, which ordinarily neutralizes newly formed cancer cells.

Leukemia was recognized early as a chronic effect of radiation exposure in early radiologists, Japanese bomb survivors, and several other exposed populations. While it has not been demonstrated as a linear relationship at low doses, leukemia induction, like cancers, is assumed to exhibit a linear response. But unlike cancers, the latent period, or time to expression, is known to be 4 to 10 years after dose. Also, risk after 10 years decreases and in time approaches the risk of nonradiated populations.

Development of cancer following dose administration is a well-demonstrated effect. Risks of developing cancer after radiation exposure follows several "rules."

1. When compared to occupational and diagnostic levels of radiation exposure, cancer induction has been demonstrated only with high doses. The conservative view assumes that risk follows a linear relationship.
2. Cancer induction is a stochastic effect. Thus, absolute induction cannot be predicted for the individual. It can only be predicted as an excess number of cancers in an exposed population. At the individual level only an increased risk exists with increasing dose.
3. Normally cancers are of high incidence in the population. Radiogenic cancers are of low frequency. Therefore to demonstrate measurable increase above this high "background" level, large populations of exposed persons are needed.
4. Since all cancers associated with radiation occur also in the absence of radiation exposure, it is impossible to demonstrate a definite cause-effect relationship with any individual cancer.
5. Accordingly, compared to other carcinogens, radiation is weak in its carcinogenesis.

Table 9-4. Several exposed populations with radiation sources and associated cancers

Population	Radiation source	Cancers seen
1. A-bomb survivors	Gamma and neutrons, external fission by-products, internal	Leukemia, lung, liver, stomach, ovary
2. Patients receiving x-ray examination for ankylosing spondylitis	X-ray therapy	Lung, thyroid, breast, leukemia, lymphoma, stomach, pancreas
3. Tuberculosis sanatorium	Fluoroscopic x-ray examination	Breast
4. Mastitis therapy patients	X-ray therapy	Breast, thyroid
5. Tinea capitis (ringworm) radiation therapy	X-ray therapy	Thyroid
6. Thymus irradiation	X-ray therapy	Thyroid
7. Pertussis chest irradiation	X-ray therapy	Thyroid
8. Miners exposed to radon daughters	Inhaled transuranic radionuclides	Lung
9. Thorotrast contrast patients	IV thorium dioxide	Liver
10. Radium dial painters	Ingested radium series	Bone

Radiogenic cancers have been associated with several populations exposed to radiation (Table 9-4). The Committee on the Biological Effects of Ionizing Radiation (BEIR) is a component of the National Academy of Sciences/National Research Council (NAS/NRC), established in 1964 to review and evaluate data dealing with radiation exposure and protection. In the reports released by the Committee (BEIR III and BEIR V), risks associated with radiation exposure have been derived. According to the BEIR III data, cancer risks associated with radiation exposure are on the order of 250 excess cases per million-person-rems BEIR V has reported the risk could be as much as four times this. It is often assumed that the statistical nature of the absolute risk is valid for all dose rates. For instance, if a population of 1 million persons were exposed to 1 rem, the excess cancers would be about 250 (250/mill-per-rem). But a population of 100,000 exposed to 10 rems would also produce 250 excess cases. And a population of 10 million exposed to 0.1 rem would likewise produce the predicted 250 excess cancers. This implies that all radiation is potentially harmful, if a large enough population is available to measure the effect. While this rationale is used in radiation protection practices and in regulatory language, the BEIR Committee definitively states that these risks cannot be demonstrated at low doses, because of lack of data. Also, the risk numbers have been derived only from high-dose populations.

Furthermore, chronic exposure to radiation at low doses of 1 rem per year increases individual risk by about 10%. Age at exposure and at cancer expression plays a large part in the risk. Reduction in dose rate, when large total doses are considered, reduces the risk of radiogenic cancers. However, at low total doses it is assumed that dose rate is not important in assigning risk, only total dose. This implies that radiation dose is cumulative in its effect with respect to cancers.

■ GENETIC STOCHASTIC EFFECTS

In humans, natural mutation frequency, as well as mutations theoretically caused by background radiation, account for some of the defects in the present gene pool. Beneficial effects of some mutations are also present, such as the spontaneous variability that ultimately leads to species evolution.

Radiation is thought to cause additional heritable mutations in germinal cells. The mechanism, being related to radiation-induced damage to the DNA or chromosomes, is thought to be similar to cancer induction. As in cancer, genetic effects of radiation are difficult to define in the individual, particularly at low doses. The mechanism is further complicated by the fact that a mutation in a germ cell will not be expressed unless the cell is involved in fertilization. Also, mutations can cause spontaneous abortion of the fertilized embryo before pregnancy is known and measurement of the effect is possible. Many recessive mutations are never expressed because mating and conjunction of two rare recessives, required for expression, have a low probability. Lastly, measurement of genetic effects is complicated by a high natural birth defect rate.

BEIR risk data for serious genetic disorders is on the order of 100 excess defects per million live births of parents exposed to 1 rem. About 20% of the whole-body dose-equivalent from medical exposure averaged into the population is significant in the genetic dose. This is due to the use of collimation in x-ray, the major component in medical dose. Added to the whole-body component from background, at 100 mrem/year, the total genetically significant dose, or GSD, is about 0.125 rem per year. A GSD of over 250 rem per year would be required to establish and maintain the radiation-induced genetic defect rate twice that of present rates. This is known as the *doubling dose*.

In light of these data, several general statements can be made regarding radiation-induced genetic defects:

1. Assuming a linear extrapolation, any amount of radiation has the potential for mutation. Again this is not supported by human data, as no increases in human mutations have been demonstrated. Estimates rely on animal data.
2. The mutation rate is dose dependent in the population.
3. Once mutations occur, repair is unlikely.
4. Mutation damage is generally thought to be cumulative; therefore dose rate has little effect on total outcome.
5. Mutations of radiation origin are indistinguishable from those of other origins.
6. Radiation is weakly mutagenic and inherited mutations are rare, especially at low doses.

■ OTHER BIOLOGICAL EFFECTS

■ Nonspecific life-shortening effects

Animal experimentation has demonstrated clearly that a shortened life follows single or repeated doses of radiation exposure. There is not, however, conclusive evidence that this is a general manifestation of radiation exposure in humans. It is known that there is an increased incidence of leukemias and malignancies after radiation, and these are going to reduce the life span of individuals having these diseases. The problem is further complicated because it is difficult to extrapolate results of animal experimentation to humans. It is also difficult to obtain such information in human populations. Currently it can be generally stated that there is little evidence of shortened human life as a result of radiation exposure. Furthermore, there are as yet no data on humans that provide a satisfactory basis for quantitative estimation of overall life-shortening effects. The atomic bomb survivors (60,000 still living in 1950, including 7000 who demonstrated the major symptoms of acute radiation syndrome) continue to be carefully studied. Thus far there is no evidence of a higher general mortality in these groups of heavily irradiated people. There has been some controversial evidence that radiologists die 5.2 years earlier than do physicians who are not occupationally exposed to radiation. With improvements in radiation safety practices and devices in recent years, this incidence in shortened life span has been shown to decrease.

■ Early aging

The enhancement of the physiologic aging process has been associated with radiation exposure. It has been shown that fibrosis of the skin, heart muscle, lymphoid organs, and endocrine glands follows irradiation. Chronic lung inflammation has been observed. Atrophy and defective development in the skin, lymphoid organs, bone marrow, and gonads have also been seen. There have been alterations in pigment depositions in the skin and hair. These are all processes associated with aging. The whole concept of premature aging, however, is subject to controversy.

Table 9-5. Decrease in life expectancy from various causes

Cause	Days
Unmarried male	3500
Cigarette-smoking male (20 cigarettes/day)	2250
Heart disease	2100
Unmarried female	1600
Overweight 30%	1300
Coal miner	1100
Overweight 20%	900
Less than an eighth-grade education	850
Cigarette smoking-female (20 cigarettes/day)	800
Low socioeconomic status	700
Stroke	520
Pipe smoking	220
Increasing food intake 100 cal/day	210
Job with Radiation Exposure (1 rem/year for 40 years)	40
Natural radiation (BEIR)	8
Medical x-ray films	6
Coffee	6
Oral contraceptives	5
5 rem/year (occupational exposure)	5
Diet drinks	2
Reactor accidents (UCS*)	2
Reactor accidents (Rasmussen)	0.02†
Radiation from nuclear industry	0.02†
Papinlocolau test	−4
Smoke alarm in home	−10
Air bags in car	−50
Mobile coronary care unit	−125

*UCS, Union of Concerned Scientists, the most prominent group of nuclear critics.

†These items assume that all U.S. power is nuclear.

One postulated mechanism in both early aging and nonspecific life shortening is related to radiation effects on mitotic potential. It seems that a fertilized zygote has the potential for 60 cell divisions during the life span (production of 1.2E18 cells). Radiation may reduce this potential or arrest mitosis in several major cell lines prematurely.

■ Radiation enhancement

Several animal studies have demonstrated an enhancement of the immune system and life span under certain conditions in radiation exposure. The immune system in some instances has shown enhancement presumably as a result of the creation of an environment in the body (necrosis) favorable for immune reactions. The necrotic areas increase immunogenicity and stimulate certain immune cells.

Mouse studies have shown that not only does radiation not result in detrimental effects but actually increased the life span.

Low-level inconsistencies are evident in humans when considering the large range in population doses from background radiation. In areas in Colorado, background levels are over twice the U.S. average. In coastal Brazil levels are over 10 times U.S. averages, and in Madras, India, as much as 40 times. Yet, no increase in cancer rates have been observed in these areas.

■ Benefit versus risk

One would be misinformed if one assumed that radiation is unilaterally beneficial. One would be likewise misinformed if one assumed all radiation is detrimental. In fact, the beneficial outcomes of medical use of radiation (diagnostic radiology, nuclear medicine, and radiation therapy) far outweigh the theoretical risks to the individuals exposed.

Table 9-5 shows an attempted perspective of the risks associated with radiation exposure compared to other risks. It lists the life-shortening for these activities. These values seem to put radiation exposure at the occupational and diagnostic medical levels into proper perspective.

BIBLIOGRAPHY

BEIR Committee Report: The effects on populations of exposures to low levels of ionizing radiation, Washington, D.C., 1980, National Academy of Sciencies/National Research Council.

BEIR V: Health effects of exposure to low levels of ionizing radiation, Washington, D.C., 1990, National Academy Press.

Fessenden, Ralph J., and Fessenden, Joan S.: The basis of organic chemistry, Boston, 1971, Allyn & Bacon, Inc.

Geise, Arthur C.: Cell physiology, Philadelphia, 1973, W.B. Saunders Co.

Green, Jack C., and Strom, Daniel, editors: Would the insects inherit the earth? Washington, D.C., 1988, Pergamon Press, Inc.

Hall, Eric J.: Radiobiology for the radiologist, Hagerstown, Md., 1978, Harper & Row.

Levine, Louis: Biology of the gene, ed. 3, St. Louis, Mo., 1980, Mosby–Year Book.

Prasad, Kedar N.: Handbook of radiobiology, Boca Raton, Fla., 1984, CRC Press, Inc.

Rubin, P., and Casarett, G.W.: A direction for clinical radiation pathology: the tolerance dose. In Frontiers of radiation therapy and oncology, vol. 6, Baltimore, 1972, Karger, Basil and University Press.

Watson, James D., and others: Molecular biology of the gene, vol II, 4th rev ed. Reading, Mass., 1987, Benjamin-Cummings Publishing Co.

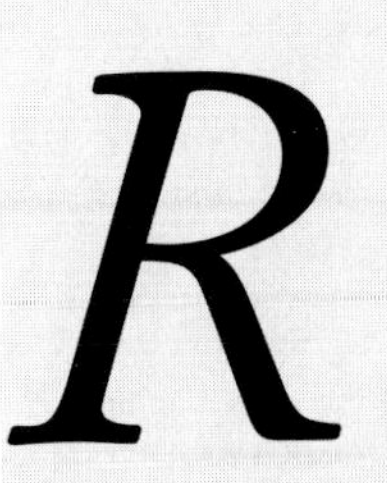

Chapter 10

ADIATION DETECTION

PAUL J. EARLY

■ PRINCIPLES OF DETECTION

Since ionizing radiations cannot be perceived by any of the human senses, it is advantageous to have some sensory device that can detect their presence. Furthermore, it is desirable to be able to quantitate the amount of ionizing radiation present, which is useful not only for radiation protection but also for diagnostic and therapeutic applications. A large number of such devices are available, and all have specific applications. These devices have been grouped into three main categories: gas detectors, scintillation detectors, and miscellaneous detectors.

■ Gas detectors

The counting function of a gas detector depends on the collection of ion pairs produced in the gas volume by the passage of radiation to the detector. These ion pairs are collected by the walls of the gas chamber, which are electrically conductive. An external circuit consists of a direct current (DC) voltage source in series with a sensitive current meter. The calibration of this current meter to read out in radiation units (mrem, rem) or radiation intensity units (mrem/hr, cpm) is necessary for the instrument to be useful for health physics applications (see Laboratory Application 4).

As ion pairs are produced by radiation passing through the enclosed volume of gas, the positive ions begin to migrate to the negative wall and the negative ions (electrons) begin to migrate to the positive wall of the detector, provided an external voltage is applied. Positive ions, which have mass many thousand times greater than that of electrons, are accelerated toward the negative electrode (cathode) at a slow rate compared to the rate at which the electron will travel to the positive electrode (anode) (Fig. 10-1).

The operation of gas detectors may best be explained through pulse heights. The number of ions collected at their respective poles is a function of voltage and is directly proportional to pulse height. A characteristic curve for gas detectors may be received by plotting pulse height versus voltage (Fig. 10-2). Figure 10-2 outlines six regions defined by changes in pulse height response to changes in voltage. These areas are called the *recombination, ionization, proportional, nonproportional, Geiger-Mueller (G-M)* and *continuous discharge regions*. The two curves, denoted by alpha and beta symbols, are typical pulse height responses to these two particles. In Fig. 10-2 the alpha curve, because the alpha particle has a greater ionizing force, corresponds to a level with 100 times the number of ion pairs initially produced by a beta particle. Each of the regions will be discussed individually. The kind of instrument used is determined by the intensity of the radiation field and whether a specific particle is responsible for the intensity.

Recombination region. If no voltage is applied between the two electrodes, no direction is given to ion pairs produced by the passing radiation. With no voltage, no ions are collected by the respective poles and no pulse is produced. This is indicated by the curve beginning at the lower left-hand corner of Fig. 10-2. The initial application of a voltage permits the collection of some ion pairs; other ion pairs recombine. The latter will not affect the current and will not be observable on the meter. As the voltage is increased, the number of ion pairs collected increases rapidly because, by increasing the voltage, the probability of an ion reaching an electrode before it combines with a positive ion also increases. This increase in pulse height continues until eventually the region of ionization is reached.

Ionization region. In the ionization region the increase in pulse height as a function of voltage no longer exists. The curve flattens out. This area is called a *plateau,* or *saturation voltage*. No increase in pulse height is seen because the voltage is sufficient to collect all ions produced by the passing radiation. There is no longer a probability of re-

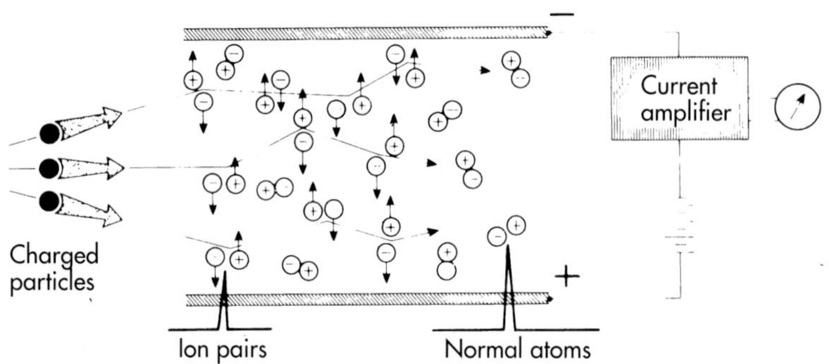

Fig. 10-1. Diagram of gas detector and its method of radiation detection by attracting the products of ionization events to oppositely charged electrodes. (Courtesy U.S. Nuclear Regulatory Commission.)

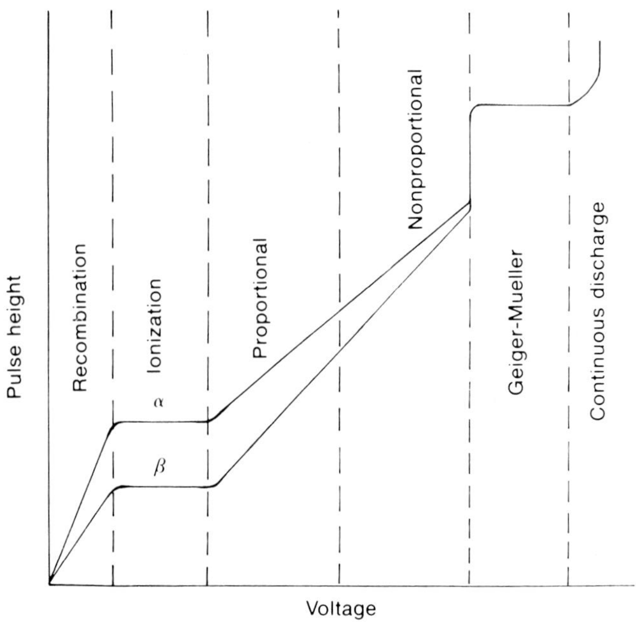

Fig. 10-2. Characteristic curve of gas detector responses to pulse height versus voltage. Curve demonstrates response expected from two different particles passing through each of three fundamental types of gas detectors: ionization, proportional, and Geiger-Mueller (G-M).

combination. Once this region is reached, further increases in voltage serve only to collect the ionized particles more rapidly.

The device used to measure radiation in this region is called an *ionization chamber*. When it is operated at the proper voltage (saturation voltage), the current (flow of electrons) going through the meter is a direct measure of the total number of ion pairs produced per unit time in the enclosed volume of gas. It is therefore a measure of the ionization produced by radiation.

The ionization chamber is used primarily in areas of high radiation intensity, such as measuring the output of an x-ray tube. Since one ion pair is produced and collected per ionization event, the pulses from single ionization events are much too small for even the most delicate electric meter to register. The proportional pulse heights of the alpha and beta curves allow differentiation between the types of emissions.

The ionization chamber may be a portable dose rate meter, such as the "Cutie Pie," which measures the intensity

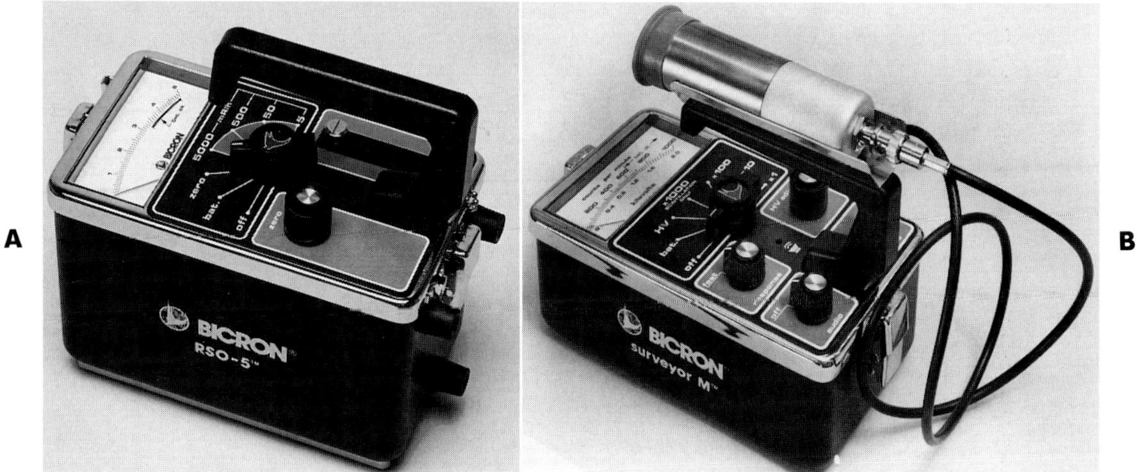

Fig. 10-3, A. Ionization-type dose rate survey meter. (Courtesy Bicron Corp., Newbury, Ohio.) **B.** Geiger-Mueller–type dose rate survey meter. (Courtesy Bicron Corp., Newbury, Ohio.)

meter, such as the "Cutie Pie," which measures the intensity of radiation per unit time (mrem/hr), or it may be a dosage measuring device such as the dose calibrator or a pocket dosimeter (a personnel monitoring device) (Figs. 10-3 and 10-4).

Dose rate meters. The portable dose rate meter is an enclosed volume of gas with a sensitive current meter and a voltage usually supplied by dry cells. The dry cells are such that a few hundred volts are supplied to the system so that the saturation voltage is reached. Although generally used in high-intensity radiation fields, dose rate ionization meters that measure very low intensities are available. These are ordinarily very expensive. An ionization-type survey meter is seen in Fig. 10-3, *A*.

Dose meters. Other ionization chambers are available that measure just the quantity (dose) of radiation rather than intensity (dose delivered over a certain unit of time), or dosage (amount of activity to be injected).

An ionization chamber can be charged to a certain voltage and the voltage source disconnected. When this chamber is exposed to ionizing radiation, the ions are collected at their respective poles, and the collection decreases the voltage (discharges) proportionally. The discharge is measured on a voltage meter that is calibrated to read in units of radiation intensity.

The dose meter must be initially charged to predetermined voltage. This is accomplished by a charger. Some chambers require a separate reader, in which case the charger and reader are in a self-contained charger-reader unit. Other chambers (dosimeters, primarily) are self-reading. In this case the chamber incorporates a quartz fiber voltage meter, which, when held up to the light, casts a shadow on a scale calibrated in units of dose (Fig. 10-4). Other self-reading dosimeters have a digital read-out for ease of reading.

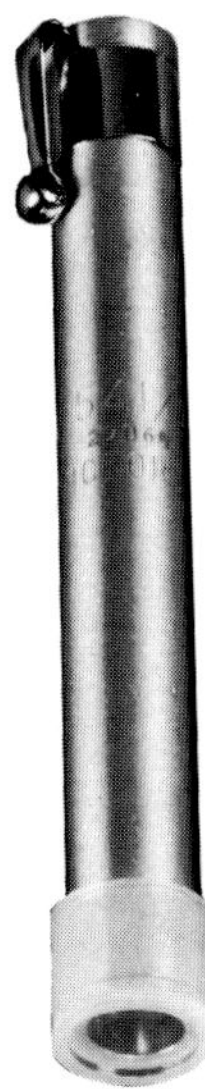

Fig. 10-4. Pen-size ionization-type self-reading dose meter, commonly called a dosimeter. (Courtesy Victoreen Instrument Co., Cleveland, Ohio.)

Proportional region. As the voltage is increased beyond the saturation voltage, another rise in the number of ion pairs collected is seen. This area is called the region of proportionality. It has already been stated that in the ionization region all ion pairs formed are collected. With additional voltage, however, there is an increase in the number of ion pairs collected (Fig. 10-2). This increase in number of ion pairs collected cannot result from increased primary ion collections, since all have been accounted for in the region of ionization. The increase is caused by the phenomenon called *gas amplification*. At higher voltages, the

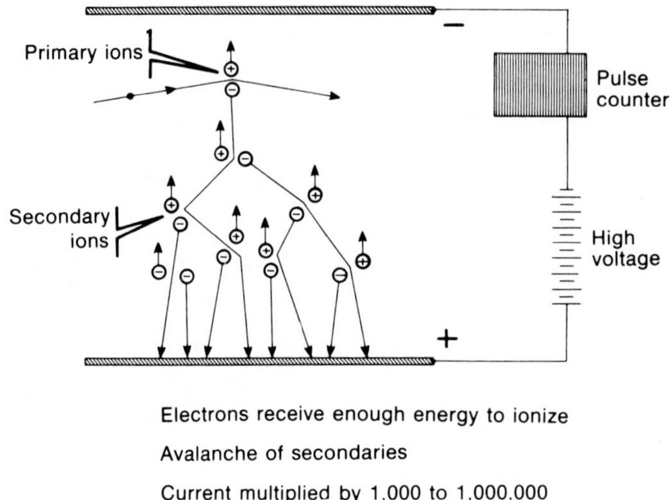

Fig. 10-5. Diagram of gas detector illustrating the phenomen of gas amplification that follows the primary ionization event. This occurs when the voltage between the electrodes is sufficiently high, which is the case in the area of proportional counting. (Courtesy U.S. Nuclear Regulatory Commission.)

increased speed or energy acquired by the ions during collection eventually gives them the capability of ionizing other gas atoms in their path to their collecting electrode (Fig. 10-5). The path of the electron as it makes its way to the positive electrode becomes tortuous, since it rebounds from one neutral molecule to another. If the electric field is sufficient, as it is in this proportional region, these electrons can obtain enough energy to ionize a neutral molecule on collision and thus create an additional ion pair, which in turn will be collected also. Because of this phenomenon, an amplification occurs whereby *more than one* ion is collected per ionizing event, in contrast to that which occurs in the ionization region. As the voltage increases in this region, the gas amplification phenomenon becomes even greater. The secondary ions also acquire enough energy to ionize other neutral atoms on their path to the positive electrode, thereby creating other secondary ion pairs. This phenomenon is called an *avalanche*.

The device used in this region is called a *proportional counter*. Many have a continuous flow of gas through the detector. This counter has a distinct advantage over the ionization chamber in that the current pulse height produced by the passage of a single charged particle is large enough to be detected. Furthermore, the pulse heights have maintained a proportionality, so that low-intensity radiation can be detected as to alpha or beta emissions by the sorting of the pulses. A problem arises because, even though the current pulses are detectable, they are so small that only the most delicate and elaborate electronic devices are used. These are generally not used in a routine nuclear medicine laboratory. They are used for detecting low-level contamination of beta particles, as in the case of contamination in a radioimmunoassay (RIA) laboratory.

Nonproportional region. Further increases in the voltage result in the two curves of Fig. 10-2 coming closer together. This region is called the region of nonproportionality. In this region true proportionality between primary ionization and the number of ions collected is no longer maintained. Instead the pulse height becomes more and more a function of the applied voltage and less and less a function of the amount of initial ionization, as the curves in Fig. 10-2 come together and lose proportionality entirely. This region is not important from the standpoint of radiation detection.

Geiger-Mueller region. Further increases in voltage result in a sharp rise in the curve in Fig. 10-2. This is called the *G-M region*. In this region the pulse height shows no difference as to primary ionization events, so there is no distinction between ionizing particles. Gas amplification is so intense in this region that a limiting value has been reached. High acceleration in this region produces a catastrophic avalanche of ions delivering a mass of electrical pulses to the collecting electrode. The avalanche of ions results from the production of high-energy electrons and low-energy photons caused by Bremsstrahlung. The voltage in the region is so high and the energy acquired by the negative member of the ion pair (electron) so great that they cause the ionization of other atoms in their path to the positive electrode (anode). To a lesser extent the high speed electrons create Bremsstrahlung photons on their path to the anode. The photons are able to strike the negative electrode (cathode) and knock electrons off its surface. They traverse the entire gas volume on their way to the anode, creating more secondary ion pairs and Bremsstrahlung. In this way, ionization is spread throughout the entire gas volume.

The size of the pulse is no longer in proportion to the initiating event. This is called the *Geiger effect*. The device for measurement of radiation in this region is called the *Geiger counter* or *G-M counter*. The voltage at which Geiger-type counting becomes established is called the *threshold*. It is followed by a *plateau,* over which the counting rate increases slowly. It is on this plateau that the proper operating voltage is selected (see Laboratory Application 7). The Geiger counter is applicable to areas of low-intensity radiation, such as determining the extent of a radioactive spill in a routine nuclear medicine laboratory, because a tremendous number of electrons are collected per single ionization event. This is in sharp contrast to the ionization chamber, where only one electron is collected per single ionization event.

The Geiger counter (Fig. 10-3, *B*) has some disadvantages. Since one ionization event spreads ionization through the entire gas volume, a second ionization event may go undetected. The time during which the counter cannot respond to another ionizing event is called its *dead time,* which makes the Geiger counter grossly inefficient (see Laboratory Application 8). Another disadvantage is that proportionality is lost. The life of a counter is the number of counts that can be accumulated before deterioration of the gas takes place. The counting life of a G-M tube is ordinarily in the range of 1 billion to 10 billion counts. This means that in the usual applications of such a counter, the shelf life would be several years. As the tube ages, the plateau of the Geiger counter becomes shorter until eventually stable operations can no longer be maintained.

Continuous discharge region. If the voltage is raised significantly beyond the G-M region, a rapid rise in numbers of ions collected is seen. This is the region of continuous discharge. Up to this point the discussion has been devoted primarily to the collection of electrons at the anode. Meanwhile, however, the positive ions, because of their mass, move slowly toward the cathode, where they are eventually neutralized.

As the positive ion approaches the negative electrode, it acquires an electron and is deionized. Since it requires energy to ionize the gas, energy must be released on deionization. This energy is released in the form of ultraviolet light, which has sufficient energy to cause another electron to be ejected from the cathode. These additional free electrons enter the gas volume and proceed toward the anode just as did the initial electrons from the primary ionization event. Furthermore, these electrons initiate avalanches on their path to the positive electrode just as did the primary ionization event. The collection of electrons from these events results in an increased number of ion collections, accounting for the sharp rise in the continuous discharge region. If this is allowed to continue, the electrode surfaces of the counter are damaged and the counter may even be destroyed. The continuous discharge can be stopped to a certain degree by a process called *quenching*. This process limits the discharge process. It can be done by momentarily reducing the voltage on the tube or by incorporating a suitable constituent into the counting gas.

■ Scintillation detectors

Certain materials have the property of emitting a flash of light or scintillation when struck by ionizing radiation. A scintillation detector is a sensitive element used to detect ionizing radiation by observing the scintillation induced in the material. When a light-sensitive device is affixed to this special material, the flash of light can be changed into small electrical impulses. The electrical impulses are then amplified so that they may be sorted and counted to determine the amount and nature of radiation striking the scintillating materials. Scintillators are used to determine the amount and/or distribution of radionuclides in one or more organs of a patient for diagnostic purposes.

The procedure of recording a scintillation involves several systems: the *detector,* the *photomultiplier,* a *high-voltage power supply,* the *preamplifier,* the *amplifier,* the *gain control,* a *pulse height analyzer,* and *display modes.* All these will be treated individually, showing the sequential stages of the detection and recording process of a disintegration.

Detector. Three major types of scintillation detectors are currently being used: organic liquid scintillation detectors, e.g., PPO (2,5-diphenyloxazole) and POPOP (1,4-*di*-2,5-diphenyloxazole benzene); inorganic crystal scintillation detectors, e.g., NaI(Tl)—thallium-activated sodium iodide; and semiconductor scintillators, e.g., Ge(Li)—lithium-drifted germanium crystals, and Si(Li)—lithium-drifted silicon crystals. BGO (bismuth germanate) and BaF_2 (barium fluoride) are also scintillators used in PET scanners (Chapter 15). The liquid scintillation detector is not as common in routine nuclear medicine laboratories and therefore will only be discussed briefly. The semiconductor type crystals are used only in research and therefore will not be discussed at all. Their value, however, is their ability to resolve the energy spectrum. Energy peaks are seen as "spikes" using these systems as opposed to curves more spread out with NaI(Tl) detectors. Their disadvantage is the complexity and cost of the equipment as well as the need for cooling agents such as liquid nitrogen to reduce the thermally induced electronic "noise."

Liquid detector. Scintillating solutions can be prepared so that when radioactive materials are added to the solution, the radiations are detected through light production. The light is detected and measured through a system of one or more photomultiplier tubes and ancillary electronic equipment to analyze and count the radiations. The liquid solution contains the material being counted, a solvent, and a scintillator. There are a variety of liquid scintillator materials, most of which are organic compounds. The solvents

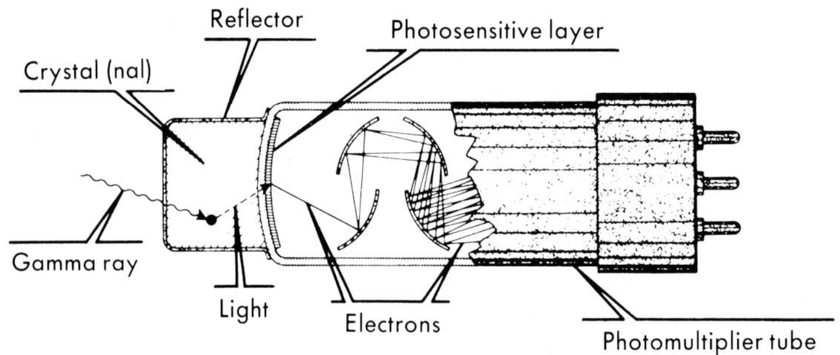

Total light to tube linearly proportional to gamma ray energy

If 1 electron ejects 5 from dynode, 11 dynodes result in 5 inches

or

about 50 million electrons output

Fig. 10-6. Crystal photomultiplier assembly illustrating the detection of a gamma ray by the crystal and its subsequent amplification through the photomultiplier tube. (Courtesy U.S. Nuclear Regulatory Commission.)

are primarily aromatic hydrocarbons, which efficiently transfer energy from the point of emission to the scintillator molecule. The use of liquid scintillation materials has its greatest advantage in its ability to detect β^- emissions or weak energy gamma rays, since the radioactive material is mixed with the scintillating material so that there is little loss of emissions by absorption before they reach the detector. Such absorption could be by the cover of the detector or by self-absorption.

Crystal detector. The most widely used scintillation detector is the solid type—a sodium iodide (NaI) crystal activated with thallium. Pure sodium iodide crystals do not scintillate at room temperature. However, if impurities such as thallium are added, centers of luminescence are produced that can be excited at room temperature by ionizing radiation.

Sodium iodide is hygroscopic (retains water) and must be kept in a moisture-free atmosphere. Consequently, the crystal is hermetically sealed. It is enclosed by an aluminum container on all sides except that side attached to the photomultiplier tube (Fig. 10-6). A glass or plastic window protects it on this end. The inside surfaces of the container have reflective capabilities. More recently, the crystal and photomultiplier have been produced as an integral assembly, eliminating the necessity for the glass or plastic shield, and the entire assembly is hermetically sealed. Should the crystal or the assembly become damaged so that there is a break in the seal and moisture enters, the crystal shows a yellow discoloration (probably caused by free iodine).

The process of detection is initiated when an incident gamma ray enters the crystal. Under ideal conditions the energy is eventually totally absorbed. This is usually accomplished through a series of Compton collisions with subsequent total absorption of the energy by a photoelectric collision. (Pair production is also possible if the incident gamma ray is greater than 1.02 MeV of energy.) Each time such a Compton collision occurs, some of the energy of the incident gamma ray is transferred to an electron that will produce luminescent light in proportion to its energy. The light is in the form of small flashes following the interactions of the ejected electrons. If the energy of the incident gamma ray is high, many Compton collisions will occur before the energy is totally absorbed. The increased number of Compton collisions will produce more secondary electrons that will, in turn, produce more flashes of light. If the energy of the gamma ray is low, fewer collisions will occur before total absorption; therefore there will be fewer flashes of light. These small flashes of light, although emitted in a sequential manner, appear to the human eye or on the photomultiplier tube as a single flash or shower of light. The intensity of the light is directly proportional to the number of flashes of light. Since the number of flashes increases with energy of the gamma ray, it can be said that the intensity of the light is proportional to the energy of the incident gamma ray. This flash of light is eventually directed to the photomultiplier tube, either by reflection from the interior surface of the aluminum housing or by the direction in which it was emitted.

Photomultiplier. The photomultiplier is a light-sensitive device that is optically connected to the sodium iodide crystal. Its purpose is to convert the light energy from the crystal to electrical energy and amplify the resultant pulse of electricity. The photomultiplier tube consists of a photocathode and usually a series of 10 dynodes. The photocathode receives the flash of light from the crystal. The photocathode consists of a material that responds to waves of light energy, much like any atom responds to waves of gamma energy in the Compton effect; the incident light wave hits the atoms of the photocathode and causes electrons to be ejected. This is called *photoemission*. The principle of this operation is not unlike that which occurs in "electric eye" applications. The number of electrons released from the photocathode is directly proportional to the intensity of the light from the crystal.

As the electrons are emitted from the photocathode, they are drawn to the first of the 10 dynodes in the photomultiplier tube (Fig. 10-6). They are drawn to the dynode because of an applied voltage between the photocathode and that dynode. This voltage accelerates the electron, impinging it on the dynode with such force that more than one electron is released from the dynode. This is called *secondary emission*. These electrons are then drawn to the second dynode by a similar increase in applied voltage, whereupon secondary emission occurs again. This process continues throughout the entire photomultiplier tube. By the time the electrons have left the tenth dynode, the number of electrons released may be on the order of millions. The photomultiplier tube therefore possesses the ability to convert one flash of light to a burst of millions of electrons—hence the name photomultiplier. The usual terminology to describe this burst of electrons is a voltage pulse, and the number of electrons collected at the last dynode is proportional to the voltage pulse height.

A system of proportionality exists throughout the entire crystal photomultiplier assembly. This can be summarized by the following:

1. The pulse height is proportional to the number of electrons received at the last dynode, which is in turn dependent on the number of electrons released by the photocathode.
2. The number of electrons released by the photocathode is directly proportional to the intensity of the light received from the crystal.
3. The intensity of the light received from the crystal is directly proportional to the energy of the incident gamma ray.
4. *The pulse height is directly proportional to the energy of the incident gamma ray.*

High-voltage power supply. In any standard counting device (scaler or rate meter) almost invariably there is a separate voltage supply unit to provide high voltage to the photomultiplier tube. The total high voltage applied to the tube is divided among the various dynodes. For instance, if the voltage is 500 V, a 50 V potential difference exists between successive dynodes (voltage and potential difference are synonymous). If 1000 V were applied to the photomultiplier tube, a potential difference of 100 V would exist between successive dynodes. The purpose of the high-voltage power supply is to provide enough "attraction" of the electrode that secondary emission will occur each time an electron hits a dynode. It is important that this high-voltage power supply be very stable. Instability of this voltage power supply is called *drift*. It may be caused by temperature change, change in line voltage, and so on. The reason for being concerned with drift, or rather the lack of it, is its effects on secondary emission. The number of secondary electrons produced by each electron that strikes a dynode is directly dependent on the voltage that exists between the two dynodes. Should the voltage at time of calibration be such that 5 electrons are released by secondary emission for each electron striking the dynode, then a drift in the voltage might cause only 4 electrons to be given off by secondary emission. This would alter the clinical results considerably. (This will become clearer during the discussion of pulse height analysis and the completion of Laboratory Application 9.)

The drift may occur upward as well. If it is sufficient, the voltage becomes so great that electrons are pulled off the dynodes without other electrons striking the dynode. This is referred to as *thermal emission,* or "noise." This phenomenon is easily demonstrated by increasing the voltage without a source of radioactivity. Eventually a high count rate is received, caused by thermal emission.

Preamplifier. The preamplifier is generally found at the rear of the detector assembly. Its purpose is to amplify the voltage pulse by a factor of 4 to 5 and then to match the impedance of the systems. The latter is a fairly complicated principle, the definition of which is not of particular importance to nuclear medicine personnel. Impedances between the photomultiplier tube and amplifier must be matched so that there is no loss of power. For this reason, a reduction in pulse height is sometimes necessary. The preamplifier also provides a driving force, characteristics of which are such that the pulse will not be lost in the several feet of cable connecting the detector to the main scaler chassis. The pulse is then fed into the amplifier.

Amplifier. The pulses that are fed into the amplifier have a wide variation in pulse height because there is a wide variation in energies of gamma rays striking the scintillation crystal. All of these pulses must be increased in amplitude by a constant factor so that the final pulse is still proportional to the energy lost by the gamma ray in the crystal. This is called *linear amplification*. Nonlinear amplification would defeat the purpose of pulse height analyzers because all pulses, regardless of their size, would be amplified to the same height. The amplifier consists of four tubes or transistors in two successive sections. The voltage gains for the two sections are approximately 70 to 120, so that the overall amplification is something more than 8000. The amplifier receives pulses on the order of millivolts. If 1 mV were sent through this amplifier, it would be increased to 8 V. The amplifier is capable of amplifying to 100 V or more with negligible distortion.

Pulse shapers. Another function of amplifiers is pulse shaping. A pulse shaper is defined as a charge-to-voltage converter that increases the signal-to-noise ratio, which would enhance the validity of recording a detected event.

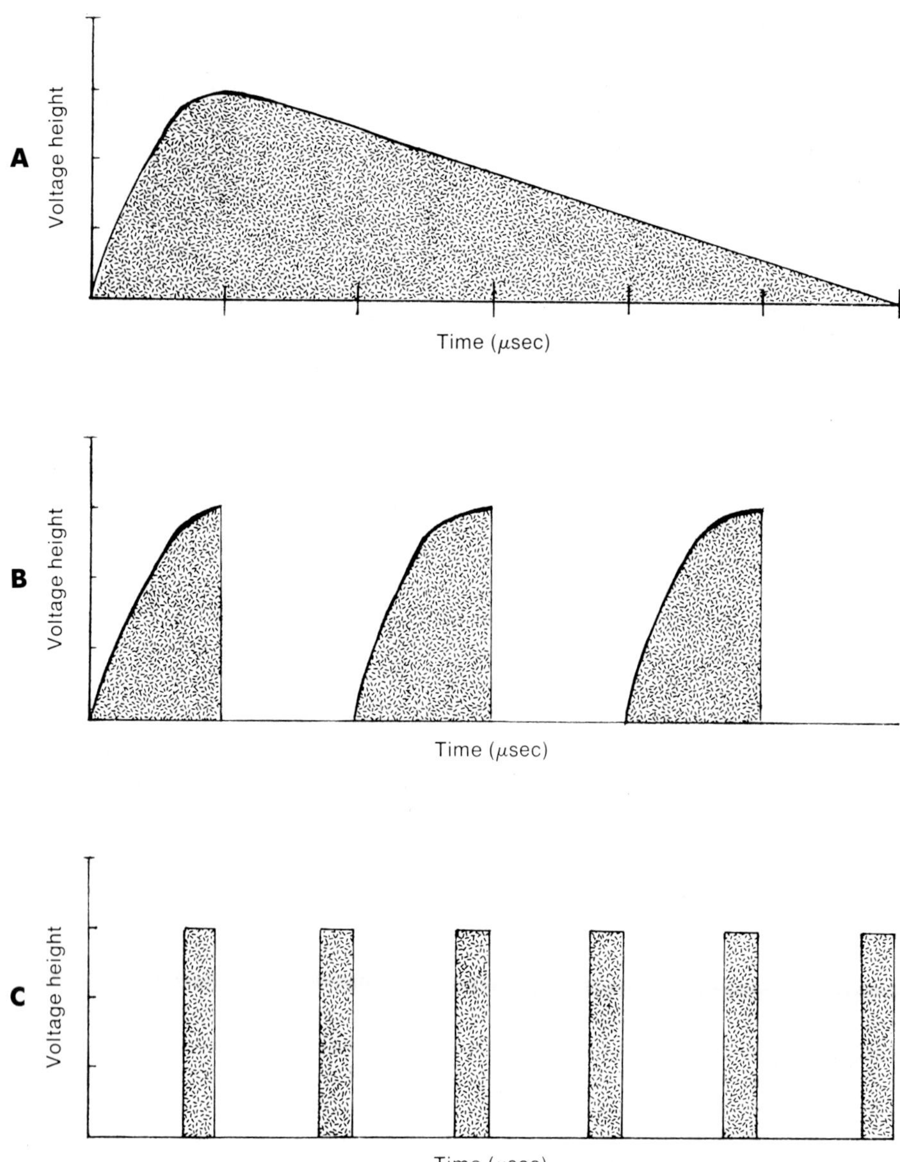

Fig. 10-7. Effects of pulse shaping through a charge-to-voltage converter. **A,** Integrated voltage waveform. **B,** Same voltage waveform terminated at its maximum voltage height, allowing for more events to be processed during the "decay time" of the waveform in **A. C,** Same waveform shaped differently, allowing for even more events to be processed during the decay time of the waveform in **A.**

In so doing, count rate capability is usually increased.

One of the most effective areas in which pulse shapers can be used in nuclear medicine equipment is following the use of a charge-to-voltage converter in which the current generated by the detector is changed to a voltage pulse. The electronic components are better able to use the information in this form. During the detection of a single photon event, the largest number of electrons from the photomultiplier tube arrives at the anode of the tube at approximately the same time, and the rest of the electrons generated by that same detection event arrive at a decreasing rate with time. The conversion of this current information to voltage results in a characteristic curve (Fig. 10-7, *A*). This curve is referred to as an *integrated voltage waveform*. The most important part of the waveform is its maximum height. Therefore if it were electronically possible to terminate the waveform at its maximum height, more time would be available to process a subsequent event (Fig. 10-7, *B*). Further refinements could result in a square waveform (Fig. 10-7, *C*).

There are many techniques used to perform these corrections and pulse manipulations, the description of which is felt to be beyond the scope of this book. Needless to say, this concept of pulse shaping is much more complicated

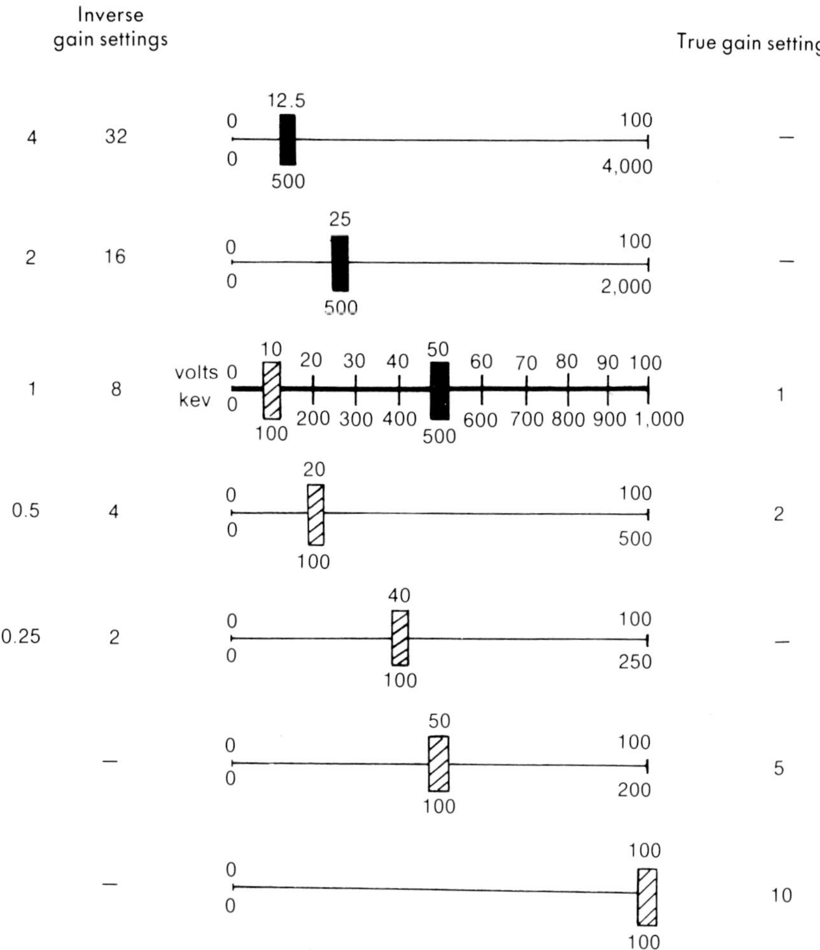

Fig. 10-8. Principle of gain control, using various settings. Values to the left of the diagram represent the principle of inverse gain as seen on most scalers. Values to the right of the diagram represent the principle of true gain as seen on most scanners and other electronic equipment.

than as presented here. There are an infinite number of waveforms possible, and these have to be matched to a particular component for proper efficiency and function. The time for integration of the voltage waveform must be adequate to ensure statistical accuracy. If the waveform being shaped is that of the X or Y position signal, the integration time must be adequate for proper positioning of the cathode ray tube (CRT) electron beam or the resolution of the clinical image would be poor. These decisions are the job of the electrical engineer designing the instrument. Suffice it to say that this concept of pulse shaping has allowed the count rate capabilities of these imaging devices to increase by at least one order of magnitude since the development of the original commercially available instrument.

Gain control. Between the two sections of the amplifier there is a stepped gain control. This allows the operator to increase or decrease the amplification as desired. In scalers there are usually five such positions represented in a variety of ways, depending on the manufacturer of the detector. Gain control values are usually represented by the numbers 32, 16, 8, 4, and 2 or 4, 2, 1, 0.5, and 0.25. Regardless of their value, they do the same thing. The five steps on the gain control represent full gain, one half, one fourth, one eighth, and one sixteenth of the maximum gain; at each step the amplification is one-half that of the next higher step. This type of gain is called an *inverse gain.* Other numerical sequences are also possible, not always representing the halving process. Equipment manuals should be consulted.

Sometimes the exact opposite is true in the use of gain settings. These settings may be represented by the numbers 1, 2, 5, and 10, which, rather than decreasing the amplification by factors of one half, actually increase the amplification by the factor indicated by the number. Therefore a pulse of a certain height on a gain of 1 would be increased to twice the height on the gain of 2, five times the height on the gain of 5, and ten times the height on the gain of 10. This is called a *true gain.*

A simplified explanation of gain settings is shown in Fig. 10-8. The dark line (third from the top) represents the actual settings on the gain control. This is expressed as a range of 0 to 100 V, equivalent to 0 to 1000 keV on that gain setting. The usual procedure is to calibrate on midgain (a value of 8 or 1, depending on the settings available). By calibrating on this gain, the operator has essentially set each small division on the discriminator dials (which have 1000 small divisions) to be equal to that number in kiloelectron volts. The gain setting essentially expands or contracts that scale, depending on the gain settings used. If the operator has amplified the pulse to 50 V (500 keV), by changing the gain setting to 16 (or 2) that same pulse would no longer be found at the 500 units setting, but would be found at approximately the 250 setting. If the settings are changed to 32 (or 4), that same pulse will now be found at a 125 value. The converse is also true. If, going back to the gain settings of 8 (or 1), the operator is analyzing a 10 V pulse (100 keV), the pulse would be found at 100 keV. If the gain settings are changed to 4 (or 0.5), the pulse will now be seen at a setting of 200 keV, or if the gain setting is changed to 2 (or 0.25), that same pulse will be seen at 400 keV units. By the increasing of the numerical value of the gain setting, the pulse height has actually been decreased, and therefore the operator must go down the scale to receive it; conversely, by decreasing the gain settings, the pulse height has actually been increased, and the operator must go up the scale to receive the pulse.

In using the *true gain* settings as found on some units, the figures to the right in Fig. 10-8 apply. As the gain setting is increased, the pulse amplitude is also increased; therefore the operator must go up in analyzer units to receive the pulse. A 100 keV pulse on range 1 would be found at 100 keV units; however, on range 2 the same pulse would be found at 200 keV units, on range 5 at 500 keV units, and on range 10 at 1000 keV units.

Most linear amplifiers will only analyze pulses from 0 to 100 V high. This ability to analyze is most accurate from 10 to 100 V. If low-energy pulses are to be amplified correctly and subsequently analyzed, they must be amplified further by the gain settings. For example, if an operator were using ^{125}I which has 35 keV (3.5 V), inaccuracies would result if it were to be analyzed on gain settings of 8 (or 1), since the pulse is not high enough to be analyzed

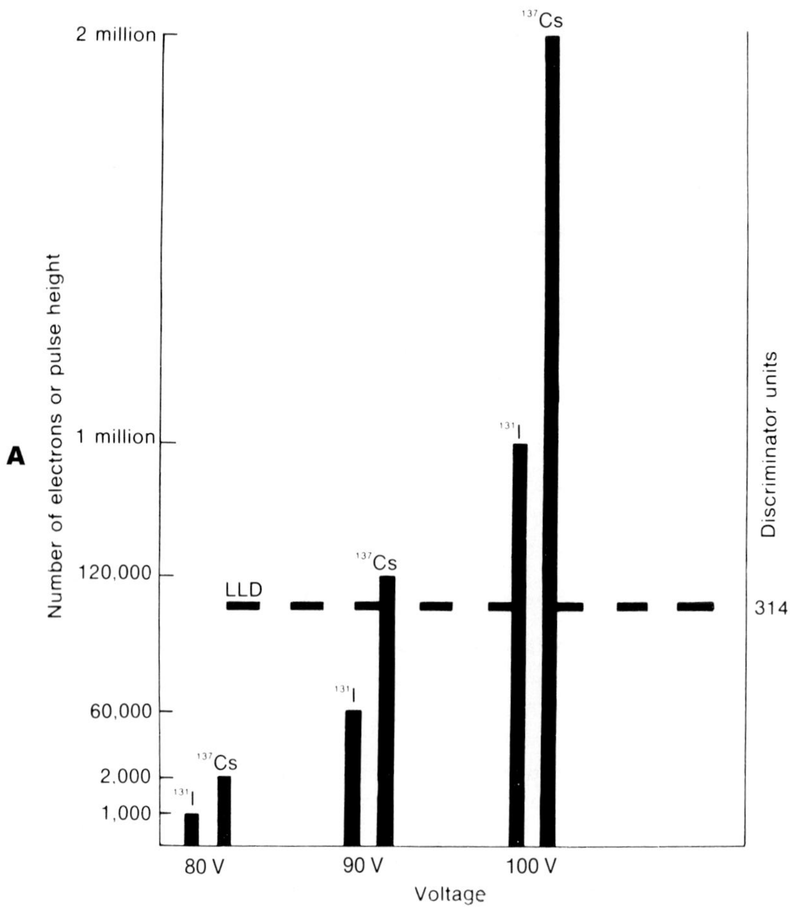

Fig. 10-9. Principle of pulse height analysis. **A,** Lower level discrimination only. Only pulses rising above the LLD setting are accepted and counted. **B,** Spectrometer. Only pulses rising above the LLD and falling below the ULD are accepted and counted.

correctly. The alternative is to change the gain settings to 4 (or 0.5), at which point the pulse would be seen at 70 keV units (7.0 V). For the 80 keV (8.0 V) of ^{201}Tl gammas a gain setting of 1 would be inadequate; however, a gain setting of 10 would be more accurate. By the judicious use of gain settings, low-energy electromagnetic radiations would not be all squeezed down into a range of a few volts where they are not discernible. The same is true of energy radiations greater than 1000 keV. For example, ^{60}Co decays with a gamma emission having an energy of 1.17 and 1.33 MeV. This is representative of 117 V and 133 V and is greater than the range of the analyzer. In this case the pulse height will have to be decreased so that it will fall within the analyzer's capabilities. This could be accomplished on a scaler by changing the gain settings to 16 (or 2) or 32 (or 4). In this way the pulse height would be halved or quartered, respectively, for correct analysis. (See Laboratory Application 14 for further discussion.)

It becomes clear that each spectrum to be investigated must be treated individually, and the operator must choose the most advantageous gain setting for the radionuclide to be used to its fullest advantage. After the appropriate gain settings and voltage settings have been chosen, the pulse is now capable of being correctly analyzed.

Pulse height analyzer. The pulse height analyzer is an electronic device that enables the operator to select pulses of a certain height and to reject all pulses of a different height. There are two types of pulse height analyzers: lower level discriminators and spectrometers. The former do not recognize any pulse height below a predetermined level. The spectrometers do not recognize any pulse heights below one level and above another level; they recognize only those which fall between the two settings. A device that isolates only one set of pulses is called a *single-channel analyzer*. Most analyzers on instrumentation used in a routine nuclear medicine department are single-channel analyzers. (A multichannel analyzer is a circuit combining two or more single-channel analyzers to provide simultaneous and sequential counting of radioactivity in more than one energy range or more than one pulse height.)

Since pulse heights are directly proportional to the number of electrons collected at the last dynode, a pulse height analyzer might best be described by comparing that number of electrons to the energy of incident gamma as a function of voltage (Fig. 10-9). Suppose a sample of activity is being used that contains two isotopes of varying energies, for example, ^{131}I (364 keV) and ^{137}Cs (662 keV). Assume total absorption in the crystal and that the intensity of the

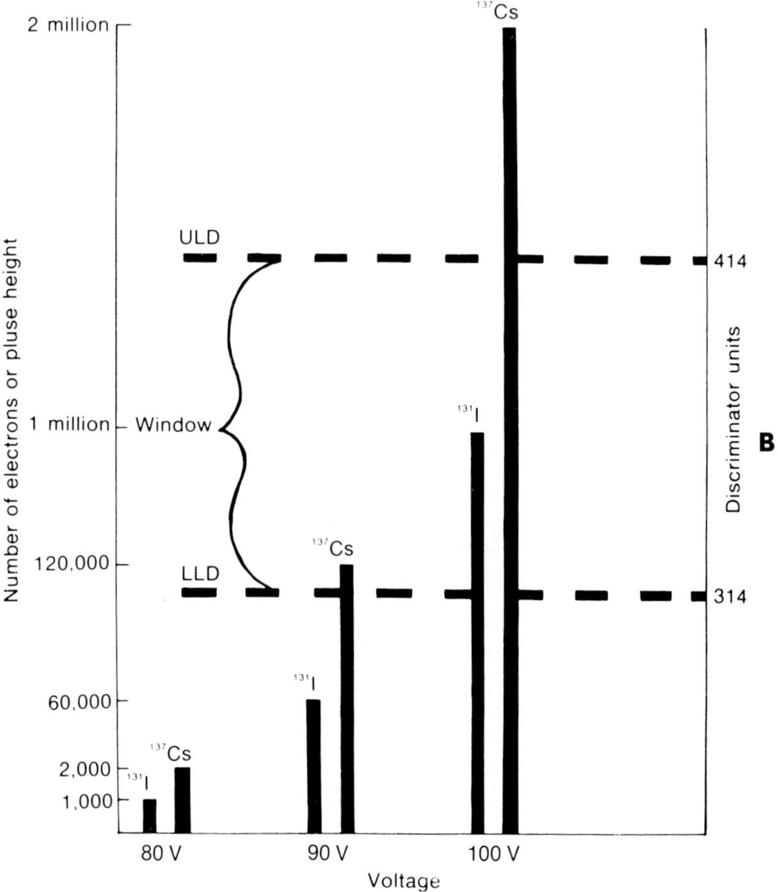

Fig. 10-9, cont'd. For legend see opposite page.

light was such that 1 photoelectron was emitted from the photocathode for ^{131}I and that 2 photoelectrons were emitted for ^{137}Cs. If a potential difference existed between each dynode of 80 V (800 V to the entire system), the attraction force of the dynode to the electron might provide sufficient energy to release 2 secondary electrons for each primary electron striking each dynode. Since there are 10 dynodes, the number of electrons accumulated at the end of the photomultiplier tube would be 2^{10}, or approximately 1000 electrons. Similarly, if each of the 2 ^{137}Cs photoelectrons releases 2 electrons by secondary emission, the end result would be 2×2^{10} electrons, or 2000 electrons accumulated at the end of the photomultiplier tube. The pulse heights are represented in Fig. 10-9 above the units 80 V.

Should the voltage to the dynodes be increased so that a potential difference of 90 V exists between each dynode, the attraction force would be greater and the number of electrons released by secondary emission might increase to 3 electrons for each electron striking the dynode. The ^{131}I single electron from the photocathode would be multiplied to a factor of 3^{10}, or 60,000 electrons, and the ^{137}Cs would be 120,000, as seen in Fig. 10-9, above 90 V. Should the voltage be increased to 100 V per dynode, the number of electrons produced by secondary emission might increase to 4, therefore 4^{10} or approximately 1,000,000 electrons for the ^{131}I absorption and 2,000,000 electrons for the ^{137}Cs absorption, as in Fig. 10-9 above 100 V.

Lower level discriminator. By the arbitrary setting of a threshold that a pulse must rise to or exceed in height to be counted, a lower level discriminator (LLD) has been established. In Fig. 10-9, *A,* at 80 V, neither ^{131}I nor ^{137}Cs would have been counted because neither pulse height attains the lower level discriminator setting. At 90 V, however, the ^{137}Cs pulse rises higher than the LLD setting, and therefore it would be counted; the ^{131}I pulse would not. At 100 V, both the ^{131}I and the ^{137}Cs would be counted because both rise above this LLD setting.

It is important to note that the use of an LLD allows the separation of a higher energy radionuclide from a lower energy radionuclide, but the reverse is not true. At 90 V, only the pulses from ^{137}Cs are seen and counted and therefore discriminated from ^{131}I pulses. There is no voltage setting, however, that will separate ^{131}I from ^{137}Cs. Any setting that includes the lower energy radionuclide must necessarily include the higher energy radionuclide too. This is termed *integral counting*.

Spectrometer. The spectrometer is an electronic device that enables the operator to reject any pulse whose height falls below one analyzer setting or above another. Should an upper level discriminator (ULD) be introduced, as in Fig. 10-9, *B,* placed at a level higher than the lower setting, such a device has been electronically arranged. The LLD continues to reject any pulses that do not rise to that level, and the ULD will reject any pulses rising higher than this level. This is called *differential counting*. By using this two-level arrangement, both high-energy radionuclides and low-energy radionuclides can be separated from each other by varying the voltage. If 90 V are applied to each dynode, only the higher energy ^{137}Cs will be detected and recorded. If 100 V are applied, ^{131}I would be the only radionuclide to be counted. The area between the upper level and the lower level discriminators is called a *window*. Accordingly, pulse height analysis can be a function of voltage. This is not the general use of a pulse height analyzer; however, in some instruments this is the case. The windows are automatically preselected, and the voltage is varied to accommodate the window (see Laboratory Application 9).

The usual method of describing an ULD is to say that it discriminates against all pulses above a certain pulse height. This approach to an explanation is simply describing an effect. A spectrometer is actually two LLDs acting in combination with an anticoincidence circuit. Figures 10-10 and 10-11 will help explain their operation.

Figure 10-10 illustrates schematically the pathway that a pulse travels after the absorption of a photon by a sodium iodide crystal. It passes the preamplifier at the end of the photomultiplier tube and goes through the cable to the amplifier, where it is further amplified. The pulse is then divided and sent to LLD No. 1 and LLD No. 2. If the pulse(s) is not rejected by either one of the LLDs, it will pass to the anticoincidence circuit for acceptance or rejection. If it is accepted by the anticoincidence circuit, it will go on to the read-out system, where one event (count) will be recorded.

Figure 10-11 displays a gamma spectrum of two radionuclides. The placement of the LLDs indicates a desire to count only ^{131}I photons. Such will be the case because of the following: If a Compton event is "seen" by the detector, both LLDs will reject the pulse because the pulse is lower than either LLD setting. If a ^{137}Cs gamma ray is detected, both LLDs will accept the pulse because the pulse is higher than either LLD setting; however, since both pulses will arrive into the anticoincidence circuit in coincidence, they are rejected at that stage. If an ^{131}I gamma ray is absorbed by the crystal, the pulse is accepted by LLD No. 1 but rejected by LLD No. 2. By this electronic technique, only pulses from ^{131}I pass the anticoincidence circuit. Therefore only pulses from ^{131}I will activate the read-out mechanism, where one event will be recorded.

The normal use of a pulse height analyzer is to predetermine the voltage setting and change the window to see the different pulses. This is accomplished by presetting the LLD and ULD, placing a source near the crystal, and adjusting the voltage until the highest count is reached. The dials governing the settings of LLDs and the ULDs are usually 10-turn, 1000-unit potentiometers. These are two main control dials listed as the lower level setting, or base (E dial), and the window, or upper level setting (ΔE dial). Both dials are usually calibrated to read from 0 to 100 V

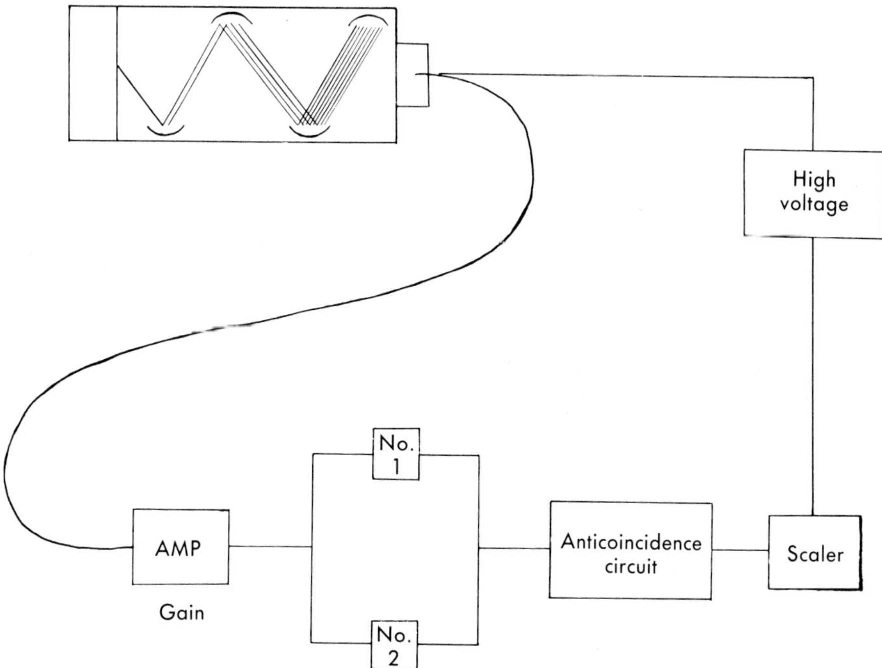

Fig. 10-10. Schematic of a scintillation detection system.

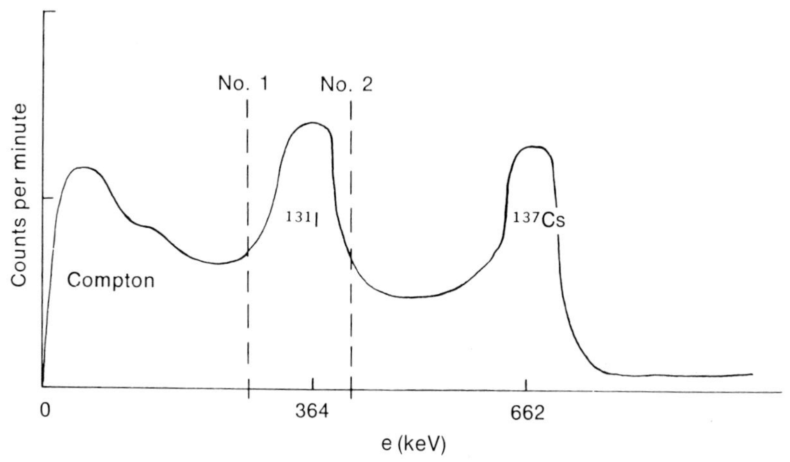

Fig. 10-11. Spectrum of a mixed gamma sample.

(0 to 1000 keV).* The upper level dial, if designated as window, is usually calibrated to read from 0 to 30 V (0 to 300 keV).* There are two different types of ULDs, since on scalers the ULD is dependent on the LLD and exists as a window riding on top of the lower level discriminator setting. For instance, it is known that ^{137}Cs (actually, ^{137m}Ba) has a gamma energy of 662 keV. If the machine were to be properly calibrated using this source, a suggested lower level discriminator setting would be 652 units on the 1000 unit potentiometer and the window would be set at 20 units, meaning that the window would be from 652 to 672 units. On some instruments the ULD is completely independent of the LLD, in which case the LLD would read 652 units and the ULD would read 672 units to calibrate the same source.

*This is true only with proper gain settings.

It can be seen from Fig. 10-9 that by increasing the high voltage, the pulse height of any event that occurs in the sodium iodide crystal can also be increased. Rather than setting the window at arbitrary settings and varying the voltage, the usual procedure is to calibrate the voltage setting so that the 1000 units on the 10-turn potentiometer become equivalent to keV units (Laboratory Application 9). ^{137}Cs is the usual standardizing source because of its monoenergetic gamma at 662 keV. The procedure of calibration is to set the arbitrary units on the analyzer to 652 units and 672 units. If a ^{137}Cs source is placed near the crystal and the voltage is increased, eventually the pulse will be built up to such a point that it will be received by the preset window. The voltage at which the maximum count is received would be equivalent to seeing all energies between 652 and 672 keV. If the voltage is increased any further, the pulse heights will be driven above the upper level discriminator setting and rejected. That point at which the highest count is received is the proper operating voltage, for it has essentially calibrated the arbitrary units on the analyzer control dials to read in terms of keV and no longer in arbitrary units. It is important to point out that this is true only at the gain setting used at the time of calibration. Should the gain be changed, these units will have a new meaning in energy units dependent on that gain control.

After the usual calibration procedure, each unit on the potentiometer is equal to 1 keV. Since the voltage has produced pulse heights proportional to the energy of the incident gamma ray, it is now possible to slide the window upscale or downscale to accept pulses from other radionuclides of different energies. By calibration, 662 potentiometer units have become 662 keV units; therefore 364 potentiometer units are now 364 keV, and pulses from ^{131}I will be recorded. Similarly, ^{99m}Tc will be recorded at 140 units, and so on. This suggests a linearity between pulse height and voltage. This is generally true for all energies above 100 keV (10 V). Below that level, adjustments must be made in gain, voltage, or window settings. This is often a cause of decreased count rate in the use of ^{125}I (35 keV). The voltage determined for counting ^{137}Cs and all energies above 100 keV often does not apply to ^{125}I. Either the voltage must be redetermined for this radionuclide using the ^{137}Cs voltage as a base (the voltage, although representative of many lost counts, should only be slightly deviated from the value found for ^{137}Cs), or the window must be changed (see Laboratory Application 13). Which of these procedures should be used is the subject of much controversy. Whatever the procedure, it should include gain, since its use would be most advantageous in this situation.

Most commercially available pulse height analyzers provide the flexibility of using just the LLD or the spectrometer. These may be simply an "in-out" switch. The "out" position signifies just the LLD; the "in" position signifies a window. It may also be listed as "integral" and "differential," respectively. When the switch is in the "integral" or "out" position, it essentially cuts out the operation of the ULD.

Gamma spectrum. A gamma spectrum is a linear graph of the number of counts received per unit(s) of kiloelectron volts (see Laboratory Application 10). Another way of expressing a gamma spectrum is the number of times a pulse of a certain height occurs per unit of time. In Fig. 10-9, *B*, LLD may be designated as having units of 314 keV and the ULD as having units of 414 keV. At a voltage setting of 100 volts per dynode the ^{131}I pulse height is exactly in the center of the window. Although this is theoretically correct, not all pulses of ^{131}I are represented by exactly 364 keV energy. Since the highest percentage of ^{131}I decays by the emission of a gamma ray of 364 keV, this should be the case. The fact is that most of these pulses are near the 364 keV energy peak but do not always reach it exactly. Actually, they extend from approximately 314 to 414 keV (see Laboratory Applications 11 and 12).

The reasons for this are several. If the gamma ray was not totally absorbed in the crystal, which is possible, the intensity of the light emitted in the crystal and the pulse height would indicate this. These pulses would probably not occur anywhere near the main peak of ^{131}I. They are referred to as *scatter*. Those that occur near the main peak but represent a slight increase or a slight decrease in energy are primarily those that have been totally absorbed but that for some reason have not been faithfully reproduced by the instrumentation. A gamma ray that was totally absorbed near the outside edge of the crystal, for example, would have to pass its light all the way through the crystal for it to be seen by the photocathode. Consequently, some of the intensity of the light would be lost through transmission. This would appear to be slightly lower in energy than one that was totally absorbed in an area of the crystal immediately adjacent to the photocathode.

Another reason for pulse variation are the dynodes. It is impossible to expect each dynode to faithfully multiply the number of electrons each time an electron strikes it. In some cases, if the voltage was such that 4 secondary electrons were supposed to be released and only 3 were, the pulse height would actually be lower, giving the illusion that the energy of the incident gamma ray was less. In other cases the number of secondary electrons released from the dynode may be 5 instead of 4, at which point the pulse height would be increased, giving the illusion that the energy of the incident gamma ray was greater than 364 keV. If one more or one less electron were released at the first dynode, it would have considerably more effect than if this discrepancy existed on the last dynode; the deficiency or abundance of electrons is changed by a power of 10 if it occurs on the first dynode, a power of nine on the second, and so on. For this reason, the end result is a variety of slightly different pulse heights; all represent valid counts from ^{131}I and should be used in the analysis of the radionuclide.

A sample of the variety of pulse heights is seen in Fig. 10-12. If the number of times a pulse height occurs were counted and plotted versus the representative energy of that pulse height, a graph would be produced similar to that shown in Fig. 10-13. This is exactly the case of the gamma spectrum. Rather than showing the gamma spectrum as just

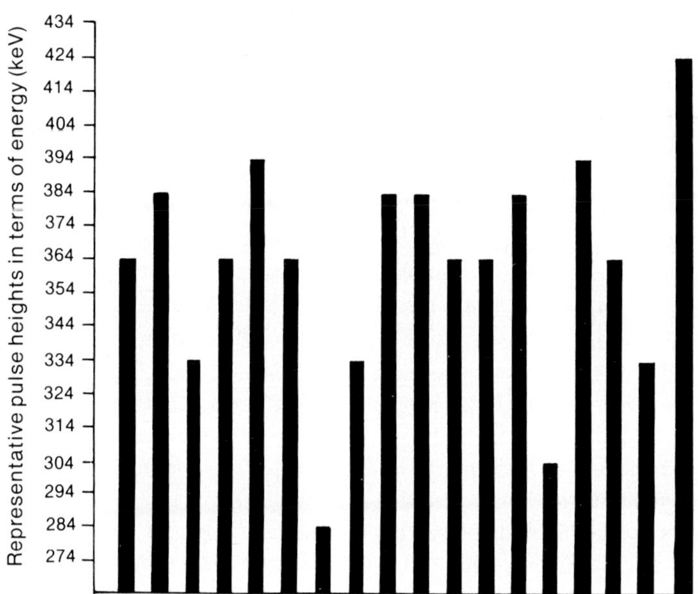

Fig. 10-12. Representative pulse heights in terms of energy. Variety of pulse heights that might be received from the interaction and complete absorption of 18 ^{131}I gamma photons with a crystal detector. Their absorption and subsequent amplification represent energies other than 364 keV even though every one of these pulses is from a 364 keV ^{131}I gamma photon.

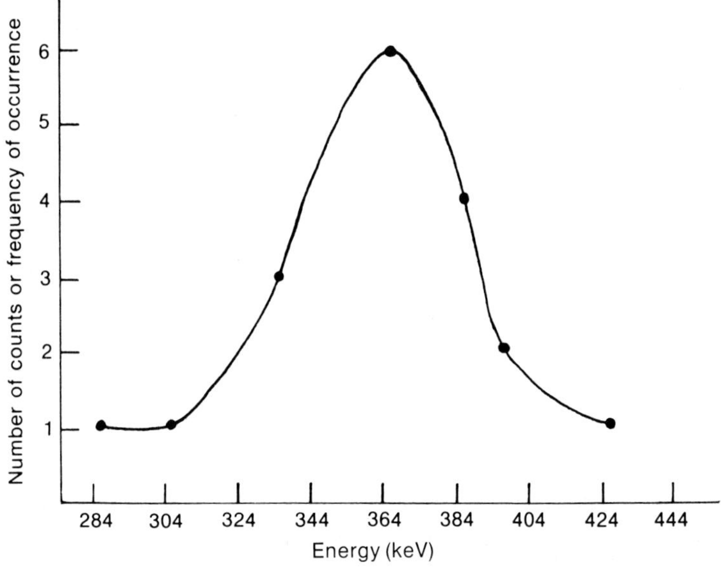

Fig. 10-13. Plot of number of pulses (counts) versus the representative energy of each pulse from Fig. 10-12.

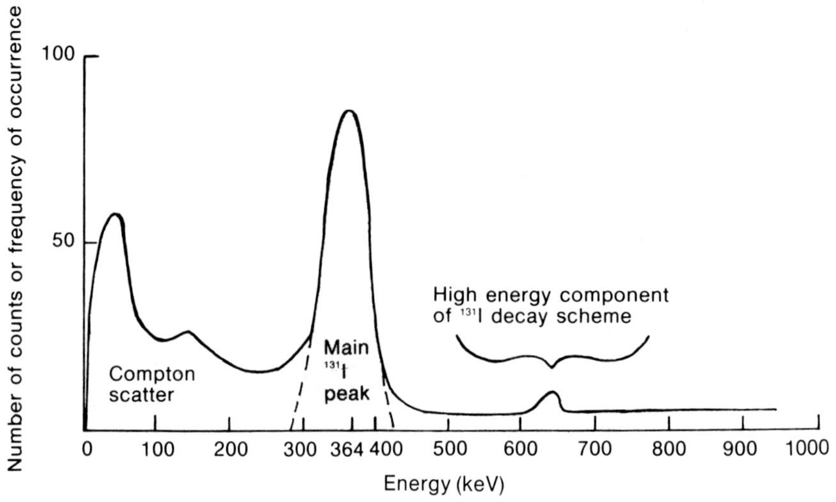

Fig. 10-14. Gamma spectrum of ^{131}I.

the main energy peak, it shows the numbers of pulses of energy from 0 to 1000 keV, as seen in Fig. 10-14.

Plotting a gamma spectrum. An analogy may be made between plotting a gamma spectrum and plotting the heights of a random sampling of 50 men. Of the 50 men, the heights may be as follows:

Height	Number of people
6′4″	1
6′2″	2
6′1″	6
6′	9
5′11″	13
5′10″	9
5′9″	7
5′8″	2
5′6″	1

By plotting number versus height, a curve would be received (as in Fig. 10-15) similar to the ^{131}I main energy peak.

The gamma spectrum can be plotted much like counting the number of men in the example just given. The men would have been asked to line up according to increasing height and then counted according to height. The same principle is applied in plotting a gamma spectrum. With the proper voltage, a narrow window is set. Only those gammas within the narrow window would have been counted for a predetermined period of time. The process is repeated changing only the window until the entire spectrum is displayed. With Figs. 10-12 and 10-13, a window could have been set with an LLD at 324 and the window set at 20, therefore counting a window of 324 to 344. In a preset period of time three counts would have registered, and the number would be plotted in the center of the window (334). If the same window is retained but the LLD is increased to 354, the window would be reading all pulses having the

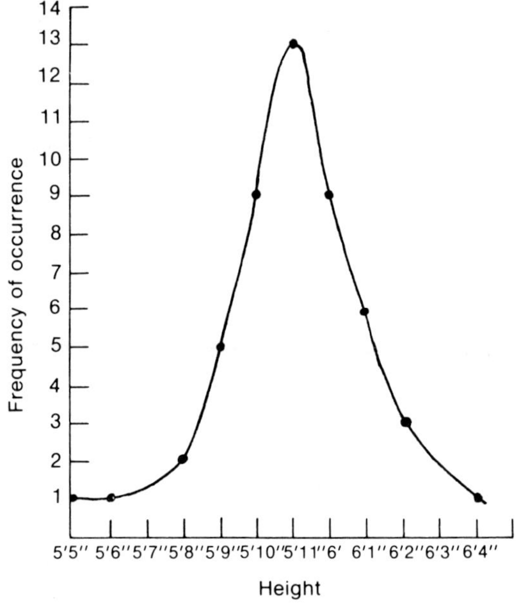

Fig. 10-15. Heights of a sampling of the population versus frequency of occurrence. A graph of this nature is analogous to a gamma spectrum in which pulse heights (representative of different energy levels) are plotted against frequency of occurrence.

height representative of 354 keV to 374 keV, at which point six counts would have registered and that number would be plotted in the middle of the spectrum (364). This would be continued until the entire spectrum is displayed. In actual practice a smaller window is usually preferred, and the LLD is usually increased in smaller increments than has been shown in this example. A typical peak may be run with a 10 keV window and increases in increments of two units.

Narrow windows used for calibration purposes are *not*

the windows used for routine nuclear medicine procedures. Routine studies require a larger window. The reason for using a larger window is the stability of the LLD and the window width. This is important for the accurate performance of the system. Narrow window counting requires the ultimate in stability. By increasing the window width to include most of the peak, two purposes are served—to increase the counting rate and therefore obtain better statistics and to reduce the effect of possible analyzer instability. According to the graph in Fig. 10-13, appropriate analyzer settings would be an LLD of 324 and a window of 80 (or a ULD of 404). This determination of working window width should be performed on all scintillation detectors for each radionuclide and checked periodically. Although this is a relatively long procedure with a standard single-channel analyzer, a gamma spectrum can be accomplished rapidly by using a single-channel analyzer in series with a count-rate meter or by using a multichannel analyzer.

Multichannel analyzers (MCA). An MCA is a circuit that combines two or more single channel analyzers to provide simultaneous or sequential counting of radioactivity in more than one energy range. The number of channels can be as many as there are numbers of picture elements (pixels) in the computer in one direction, for example, 64, 128, 256, 512, and so on. The MCAs have a multitude of uses in clinical applications of nuclear medicine. Gamma spectra can be performed quickly on the MCA because each channel is analyzed individually but is recorded at the same time. Most commercially available camera systems are capable of doing this now. It is used effectively and efficiently to set and to check proper window settings. MCAs are used effectively in radionuclides with more than one energy peak (such as ^{67}Ga and ^{111}In) to bracket each peak and enhance image quality. Before this use of MCAs, the image was received by accepting all peaks in one large window, which meant accepting large amounts of background and scatter counts to degrade the image, or, in the case of multipeak radionuclides, accepting counts from only one peak and therefore accepting fewer counts, which also meant degrading the image or accumulating counts for a much longer period of time. With the advent of triple peak capabilities, an optimum window could be set for each peak, reducing the background and increasing count rate. Radionuclide identification or, even more significant, determination of radionuclide contamination by way of gamma spectrum is another excellent use of this multichannel capability.

Display modes. There are two types of display modes, the scaler and the count rate meter.

Scaler. A scaler is an electronic circuit that accepts signal pulses from a radiation detector and counts them. Scalers provide a unit for rapid counting of electrical pulses that result from light flashes from ionizing radiations interacting in the crystal. This method of counting is far superior to the dark-adapted eye. The scaler is usually electronically devised so that the operator has a choice between accepting a certain number of counts (preset count) or a predetermined period of time over which counts can be accumulated (preset time). With preset time, the scaling device will count the number of events that occur during a set interim of time and will then shut off automatically; the number of counts becomes the variable. With preset count, the predetermined number of counts are accumulated, after which the scaler is automatically shut off; time becomes the variable.

Count rate meter. Another type of display mode is the count rate meter. This is a radiation detector connected to an indicator that continuously shows the average rate of counts coming from the detector per preselected time periods. Count rate meters have wide usage in survey meters and laboratory monitors, since their usual purpose is to promptly indicate increases in activity.

There are two types of rate meters currently in use: the analog rate meter and the digital rate meter. The fundamental difference between the two types is in the kind of memory used to store information from the incoming pulses. The analog rate meter stores a *charge* that is proportional to the number of pulses received per unit time. A digital rate meter stores the *count* in digital form much like the scaler. Since rate meters are so dependent on time constants, a discussion of time constants is warranted.

The *time constant* is an electronic averaging property of the circuit for determining the time interval over which the summation of the incoming pulses is taken. Since the nature of radioactive decay is one of random events, fluctuations will be seen in the count rate meter. The degree of fluctuation is dependent on the time constant or the count rate or both. It is similar to taking subsequent counts on a scaler and plotting them. If a radioactive source counted 10,000 cpm, variations between readings would not be appreciable; the counts will not vary by much more than 2% from the true count rate. Plotting the results of subsequent 1-minute counts would yield almost a straight line. The count rate meter with the time constant set for 1 minute performs this accumulation and averaging automatically. When the meter is connected to a stripchart recorder, the results are graphed as in Fig. 10-16, *A*. Note that there is a delay in reaching the true count rate. Actually, the rise in count rate is an exponential function of time. For this reason, the rate meter reads only approximately 50%* of the true count rate value at the time indicated by the time constant; that is, the time constant is 1 minute, but at 1 minute only a count rate of 5000 cpm is indicated. The true count rate (10,000 cpm) is not realized until after approximately 4 minutes (four times the time indicated by the time constant). With such a long time constant in this count-rate situation, statistical variations are not a factor.

By using the same source of radioactive material but reducing the time constant to 0.01 minute (100 counts per

*If this were a true exponential function, it would read 69.3% of the true count rate at 1 minute if the time constant were set at 1 minute.

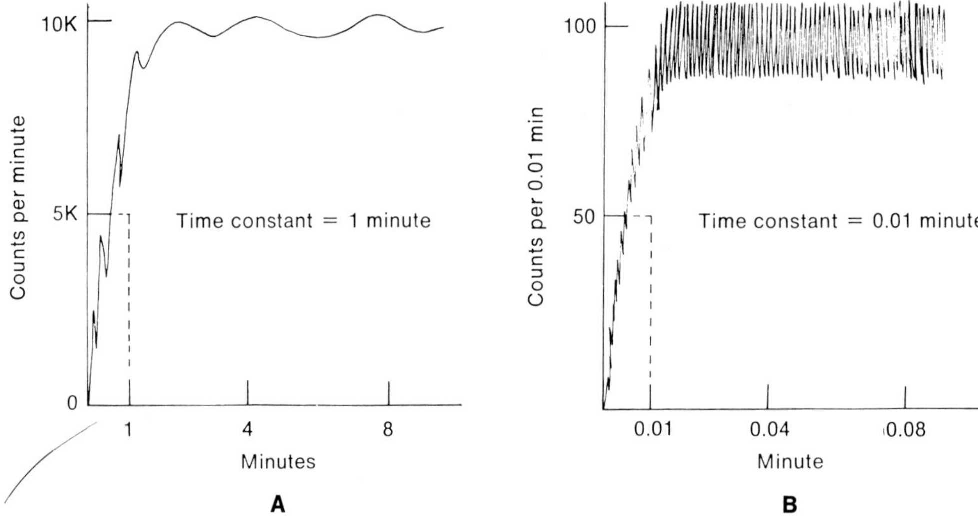

Fig. 10-16. A, Effect of a time constant on the response of a count rate meter. Long constant of 1 minute at the indicated count rate allows only slight deflection of the needle, but it requires four times the time constant setting to achieve 100% value. **B,** Effect of a much shorter time constant but the same count rate. Vascillation of the needle is greater, but four times the time constant is still necessary to achieve the 100% value.

0.01 minute), a stripchart record similar to that in Fig. 10-16, *B,* will be obtained. The statistical fluctuation now becomes a real factor. Counts may vary from one averaging period to another by as much as 20% from the true count rate. Note that it still requires four times the time constant value to achieve the true reading, that only 50% of this value is received by the time indicated on the time constant setting, but that at this setting the true value is required in one-hundredth the time.

Based on this discussion, the setting of the time constant must be a compromise—a compromise between the response required of the particular study and the statistical accuracy of the resultant data. Longer time constants and higher count rates produce relatively less statistical uncertainty and therefore result in a more stable meter reading. If the time constant is too long, the response to sudden increases or sudden decreases in count rate (both are exponential functions) will be too slow, and the true clinical situation will perhaps be overlooked. If the time constant is too short, the statistical variations in count rate may present erroneous information.

Analog rate meters. Analog rate meters used to be the most common type of count rate meter. This rate meter allows a response that is directly proportional to the count rate. A delay is required, however, before an equilibrium state is reached, and this delay is a function of the time constant. This delay suggests a lag of the rate meter, therefore the shape of curves is distorted, especially with dynamic function studies. Techniques are available to correct this, but in routine clinical studies such techniques are not warranted. This type of rate meter is usually associated with a continuously moving graph paper (stripchart recorder) that plots the changes in activity (renograms).

Digital rate meters. The digital rate meter is becoming more and more the rate meter of choice in nuclear medicine instrumentation because of the present clamor for digital information as well as the present trend for computer analysis of data. The use of a digital rate meter makes both of these possible.

The digital rate meter may be thought of as an automatic reset scaling device in which the number of counts per unit time is continuously recorded. A standard scaler can be thought of as a simple digital rate meter. If the scaler continuously counted for a specified period, automatically recorded the count, and was then reset and allowed to count again, this would be the essence of a digital rate meter. On the digital rate meter, each time the entire process is recycled the counts received during this predetermined counting period (which is adjustable) can be recorded on a visual display of numbers, printed or punched on tape, or graphed on a stripchart recorder as in the analog rate meter. There is a difference, however, in the appearance of the graph. It does not have a smooth curve as does the classic renogram, for example; it has a "stepped" appearance. This graph is called a *histogram.*

Modifications of scintillation detectors. The basic process of detecting and recording gamma rays is the same in all scintillation detectors, but there are modifications based on use and the nuclear medicine procedure. Following is a discussion of the most common modifications.

Probe. The scintillation detector in probe form is the common method of performing thyroid radioiodine uptake measurements. The present recommendations are that ^{123}I be used for this purpose on a routine basis because of the radiation dose given to the thyroid tissue. However, choice of an uptake probe should consider ^{131}I because occasionally ^{131}I is used and in therapeutic applications, bioassays must be performed. To detect the ^{131}I, it is necessary that the NaI crystal be not less than 1 inch in diameter with a thickness of not less than 1 inch, since about 70% of the ^{131}I gamma rays that enter the crystal are absorbed by 1 inch of sodium iodide. It has been determined that a thicker crystal would increase the counting efficiency, but the increase would be less than the increase in background count. The standard ^{131}I uptake probe contains a 1½-inch diameter by 1-inch thick crystal. By increasing the diameter from 1 inch to 1½ inches, both the background and the ^{131}I counting efficiencies are doubled. This becomes important from the standpoint of statistics in short counting periods. Currently the larger diameter crystal seems preferred. Collimators* for an uptake probe are such that the entire thyroid gland is seen. This distance is usually between 20 to 30 cm for an adult thyroid gland (Laboratory Application 21). It should be emphasized that it is essential to see the entire gland. Since distance is constant to all patients, that distance must be such that all of the largest thyroid is included even if that would include great amounts of nonthyroid tissue in patients with smaller thyroids. One exception to the constant distance might be in studies of children. In these cases the distance may be shortened.

Well counter. A well counter is a scintillation crystal detector formed with a central well into which biologic samples (blood, urine, tissue) can be inserted and their radioactive emissions counted. The major advantage of this arrangement is the increased counting efficiency that results from surrounding the sample with the detector (Fig. 10-17). The diameter and depth of the well is a variable, and the thickness of the crystal immediately surrounding the counting sample is a variable. For these reasons, the ability to count higher-energy radionuclides varies considerably and the efficiency with which lower energy radionuclides are counted varies, but to a lesser degree. Other sizes of crystals are available that accommodate larger volumes or have a greater thickness of sodium iodide for greater counting efficiencies. The detection of pulses from this type of scintillation detector is the same as with any scintillation detector.

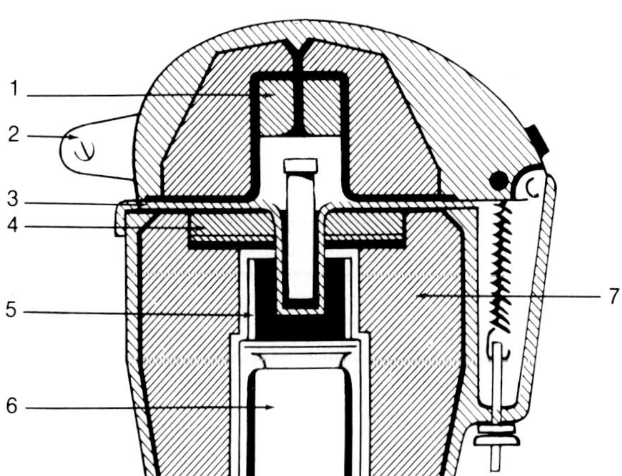

Fig. 10-17. Cross-sectional view of scintillation well detector. *1,* Removable lid plug; *2,* handle; *3,* splash guard; *4,* lead beaker plate; *5,* large well crystal; *6,* photomultiplier tube (6292); *7,* lead shield. (Courtesy Picker International, Inc., Highland Heights, Ohio.)

■ Miscellaneous detectors

In addition to the gas detectors and the scintillation detectors, there are other detectors that use neither of these operating principles. Film badges and thermoluminescent dosimetry are two other possibilities.

Film badges. The film badge is probably the most commonly used radiation detection device today. It provides a reasonably accurate means of determining doses from neutron, beta, gamma, and x-radiation. Most film badges consist of a plastic holder containing radiation-sensitive film, usually of dental film size or 35-mm photographic film. The film badge also contains a variety of filters used to absorb certain radiations of varying energies. The variety of filters placed at different points on the film badge allows identification of a specified type of radiation. The use of these absorbers gives an indication of the penetration and energy of the radiation producing the exposure. There is also an area on the film badge that has no filter and is not covered by even the plastic holder. Beta as well as very weak energy gamma radiation can be detected in this area.

Films are developed and then evaluated by measuring the density of the blackening on the film. These measurements are compared to standard films that have been exposed to known radiation doses. Generally, film badges are capable of measuring doses from 50 mrem to 500 mrem.

The film badges are worn on the pocket or the belt of nuclear medicine personnel. The same film may be worn for a week to a month, usually. The length of time depends on the sensitivity of the film and the amount of radiation to which the radiation worker is exposed. Since nuclear medicine personnel are usually exposed to very low levels of radiation, the longer the film is worn, the greater will be the accuracy of the measurement. The film badge is not sensitive to radiation exposures much below 50 mrem. It is suggested that nuclear medicine personnel wear their film badge for periods of 1 month at a time so that the radiation level will fall more nearly into the sensitive area. With the

*A collimator is a device placed in front of a sodium iodide crystal for purposes of defining a region from which radiations are emitted to the exclusion of all other regions. A region could be as large as an entire organ (thyroid, kidney) or as small as a lesion within an organ (brain tumor). Many collimators are available for different purposes.

advent of radionuclide generator systems the Nuclear Regulatory Commission has suggested that the radiation worker use finger badges as well. These are usually of the thermoluminescent variety, however.

Film badges have an advantage over other types of monitoring devices in that they provide a reasonably accurate record at a low cost. Furthermore, since the film badges are not developed, evaluated, or recorded in the nuclear medicine laboratory, the film badges provide a permanent unbiased record of exposure. The disadvantage of a film badge is that, because the mailing, evaluation, and return of the report requires approximately 3 weeks, an immediate record of exposure is not available. Other disadvantages include the fact that film badges may become darkened if improperly handled, such as when left on a radiator or on clothes that are sent to the laundry.

Thermoluminescent dosimetry. Thermoluminescent dosimetry (TLD) is a method of radiation detection that is rapidly gaining acceptance as a personnel monitoring device. Materials used for thermoluminescence are primarily calcium fluoride and lithium fluoride. When exposed to ionizing radiation, these materials absorb the energies released in the material. This energy is liberated only on subsequent heating of the material. As the temperature reaches a characteristic value, the energy is released in the form of light, which is analyzed for exposure intensities—hence the name thermoluminescence.

TLD offers a variety of uses in radiation medicine. In addition to personnel monitoring applications, it is used in the measurement of doses in tissues surrounding a therapeutic tissue implant source. The thermoluminescent method appears to be much more sensitive than the film badge.

Radiation detection laboratory applications

LABORATORY APPLICATION 6

CALIBRATION OF A SURVEY METER

Purpose

The survey meters used routinely in nuclear medicine are of two basic types: the ionization type, commonly called the *Cutie Pie,* and the Geiger-Mueller (G-M) type. There is a basic difference between the two types in that the response of the "Cutie Pie" depends on the nature and energy of the radiations, whereas that of the G-M does not. This means that values indicated by the G-M survey meter hold true only if the radiation to which it is exposed is the same as that used for calibration. The "Cutie Pie," however, will indicate a true value regardless of the type of energy of radiation. With the advent of energy-compensated G-M meters, this difference between G-Ms and "Cutie Pies" is no longer valid. Energy response curves (Fig. 10-18) show these differences.

In either case, however, the values indicated by the survey meter when exposed to a radiation field have no meaning unless the instrument is calibrated and is known to function properly.

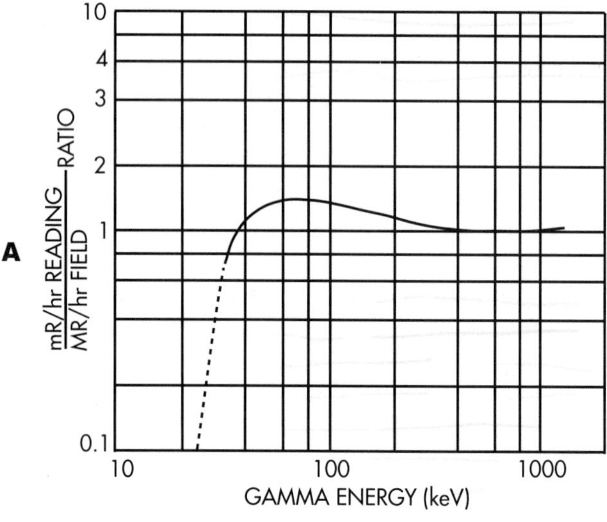

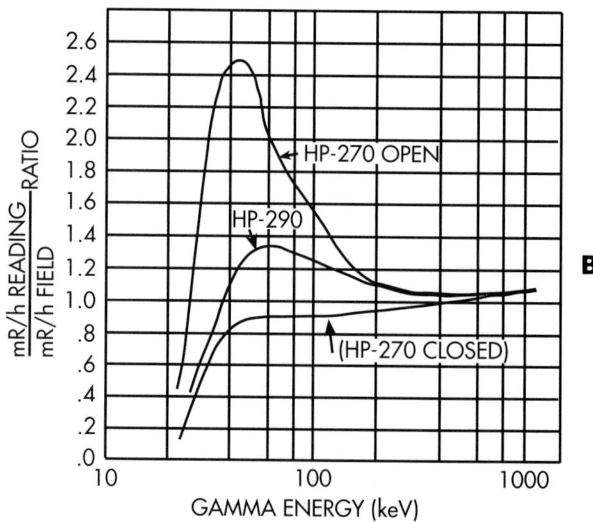

Fig. 10-18. Energy response of an energy-compensated G-M survey meter **(A)** versus one that is not **(B).** (Courtesy Eberline.)

The purpose of this exercise is to calibrate a survey meter so that the radiation intensity units have meaning. The following formula expresses the relationship between radiation intensity with regard to energy, activity, and distance:

$$\text{mrem/hr} = \frac{n \times I_\gamma}{S^2}$$

mrem/hr = Radiation intensity (in mrem per hour)
n = Activity in millicuries (mCi)
I_γ* = mrem/hr/mCi at 1 meter
S = Distance from source in meters

A similar formula is available for radium as the calibration source:

$$\text{mrem/hr} = \frac{\text{Number of milligrams of radium}}{S^2}$$

S = Distance from source in yards

These formulas can be used to calibrate survey meters, as is indicated in the procedure section.

Procedure

Materials

1. Survey meter (to be calibrated).
2. Radioactive point source. The activity of the point source should be traceable by documented measurements to a standard certified within 5% accuracy by the U.S. National Institute of Standards and Technology (NIST). One such source is a lead-shielded device containing up to 165 mCi of ^{137}Cs (Fig. 10-19) containing moveable attenuation filters (see Technique 1). If a shielded device is not available, "bare" sources may be used (see Technique 2) with obvious personnel exposure drawbacks. Thirty mrem/hr will be received at 1 meter from 85 mCi (3145 MBq or 3.145 GBq) of ^{137}Cs or 21 mCi (777 MBq) of ^{60}C.
3. Meter stick.
4. Logarithmic graph paper.

*I_γ values for some common radionuclides are as follows: ^{60}Co = 1.32; ^{226}Ra = 0.825; ^{131}I = 0.22; ^{99m}Tc = 0.072; ^{57}Co = 0.09; ^{137}Cs = 0.33.

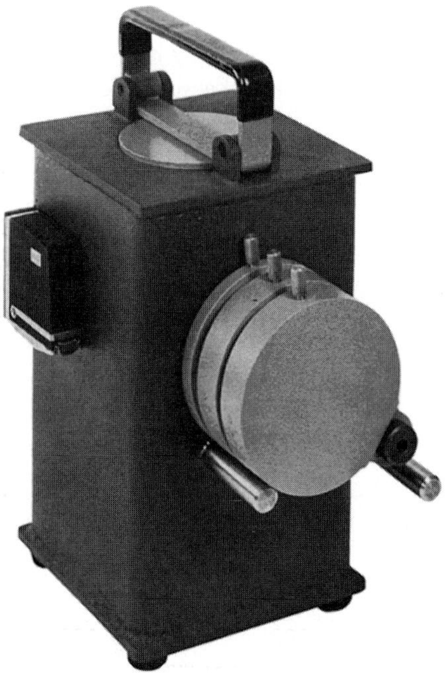

Fig. 10-19. Lead-shielded survey meter calibration device equipped with three moveable filters. The operator interposes different combinations of the attenuators between the radioactive source and the detector, reducing the radiation intensity by a known quantity. (Courtesy Victoreen, Inc., Cleveland, Ohio.)

Continued.

Technique 1

1. Check batteries on survey meter by turning indicator to appropriate position.
2. Zero survey meter by turning indicator to appropriate position (if any) and turning the zero adjust knob. Some survey meters can be zeroed in a radiation field; others cannot. Refer to instrument instruction manual.
3. Calculate the distance for 80% of the maximum range of the instrument, with no filtration, using the appropriate formula in this exercise (e.g., ×100 range representing 0 to 1000 mrem/hr = 800 mrem/hr).
4. Place survey meter at calculated distance.
5. Remove all filters and move ^{137}Cs source to the calibration position.
6. Take reading. Adjust the meter (if necessary) to read the calculated value (800 mR/hr).
7. Insert filter that will decrease the value by approximately 20% to 30%. (With a 0.25 filter, dose rate should reduce to 200 mrem/hr, or 800 mrem/hr × 0.25.) Adjustments may be necessary to the control potentiometer. Consult instrument procedure manual. Some survey meters do not allow this manipulation.
8. Change scales to ×10, remove the 0.25 filter, and insert a filter that will reduce the value of the source by about 10%. (Using a 0.1 filter, dose rate will reduce to 80 mrem/hr, or 800 × 0.1.) Adjust if necessary.
9. Leaving the 0.1 filter in place, insert the 0.25 filter. Dose rate should reduce to 20 mrem/hr (800 × 0.1 × 0.25). Adjust if necessary.
10. Change scales to ×10, remove the 0.25 filter, and insert a filter(s) that will reduce the value of the source to about 1%. (Using 2 − 0.1 filters, the dose rate will reduce to 8 mrem/hr [or 800 × 0.1 × 0.1].) Adjust if necessary.
11. Leaving both 0.1 filters in place, insert the 0.25 filter. The dose rate should reduce to 2.0 mrem/hr (800 × 0.1 × 0.1 × 0.25). Adjust if necessary.
12. Such a calibration technique results in the survey meter being calibrated on 3 ranges at two well-spaced points on the scale.

Technique 2

1. Place source on a plastic foam block on the table, with the source at one end and the survey meter at the other. The foam block is used to reduce scatter. (CAUTION: Continual awareness of and therefore protection from an exposed source of radiation cannot be emphasized enough during this exercise.)
2. Check batteries on survey meter by turning indicator to appropriate position.
3. Zero survey meter by turning indicator to appropriate position (if any) and turning the zero adjust knob. Some survey meters can be zeroed in a radiation field; others cannot. Refer to instrument instruction manual.
4. Begin taking readings at 1 meter, 0.9 meter, 0.8 meter, and so on, until one entire range has been completely covered. Be sure that the distance indicator on the meter stick and the gamma point source bisect the active part of the chamber at right angles to each other. Record distance and radiation intensity in milliroentgens per hour.
5. The readings must be such that each scale is calibrated at approximately one third and two thirds of full scale.
6. Calculate the radiation intensity. Calculations should be made after the recordings on the survey meter so as to allow unbiased readings. Nuclear Regulatory Commission requirements can be found in 10 CFR 35.51 with technical assistance in Appendix B of *Regulatory Guide* 10.8, Revision 2, August 1987.

Data treatment

1. Plot the actual readings versus the calculated results on logarithmic graph paper. Actual readings are recorded on the ordinate (vertical axis), calculated readings on the abscissa (horizontal axis).
2. Connect the points with the best straight line. *This is the calibration graph of the instrument.*

3. To use the graph, find the point of your actual reading, follow it to the right until the calibration line is intersected, and read down and report the calculated (or true) exposure dose rate. Only the true exposure rate, not actual readings, should appear on radiation surveys.
4. Repeat for as many ranges as possible.
5. For uncalibrated ranges, place the meter to effect maximum deflection of the needle and switch to the next highest range. Observe the dose rate. If it is not the same as on the calibrated range, determine a correction factor.
6. Once calibrated, a long-lived radioactive source should be measured and recorded. This source should be used as a check source to verify instrument calibration before each use (see Key point 3).

Example

See Fig. 10-20.

Key points

1. Readings within ±20% will be considered acceptable if a correction chart or graph as shown in Fig. 10-20 is attached to the instrument; greater than 20% indicates a need for repair or replacement.
2. Readings above 1000 mrem/hr need not be calibrated. However, such scales should be checked for operation and approximate correct response.
3. A dedicated check source shall be used as a calibration check source. This is usually a long-lived beta emitter that can serve as a calibration check. If its value is the same from time to time, then the calibration chart is valid. Any time the value changes, recalibration is necessary. Be sure to arrange the probe shield the same for each reading. Read before each use, after each maintenance and/or battery change, or at least quarterly. No record is required.
4. If the check source is a beta emitter, the physical barrier must be removed. This varies from instrument to instrument. Refer to instrument operational manual.

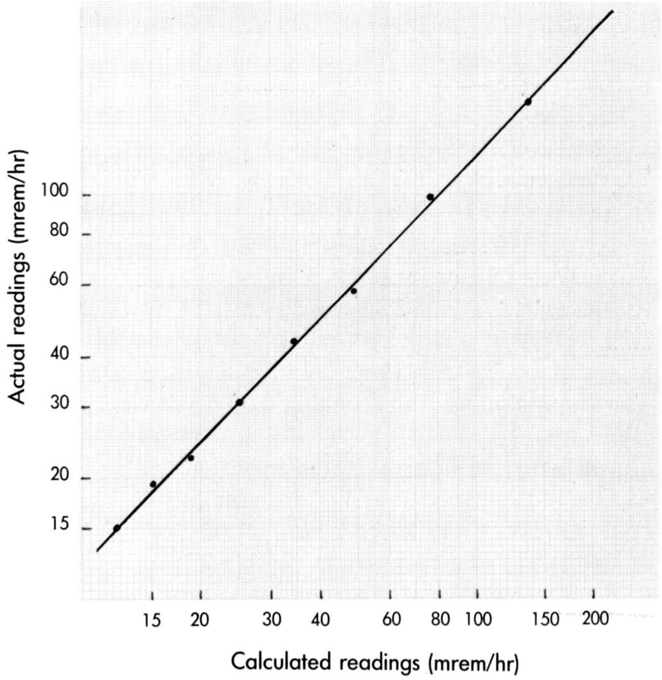

Fig. 10-20. Calibration graph of a radiation survey instrument. This graph was calibrated using a 10-mCi ^{60}Co point source with readings taken at 0.1 m intervals ranging from 0.3 to 1 m from the source.

Continued.

5. The inverse square law can be demonstrated in this exercise. With a gamma point source, the dose rate value at 0.5 m should be approximately four times the dose rate at 1 m because the distance was halved.
6. The information on the calibration graph or chart should be transposed to a smaller graph that can be taped to the bottom of the survey meter.
7. Some survey meters have calibration adjust dials that eliminate the need for a graph. Some survey meters have just one such dial; others have dials for each range. Sometimes the meter with just one adjust dial adjusts *only* for one range, whereas the others remain uncalibrated. Refer to instruction manual.
8. Some survey meters have screws on the dial itself. This is *not* a calibration dial, even though turning it will move the needle indicator. This is also true for count rate meters.
9. Earphones should be used (if available) for area surveys because they have an immediate response to radiation, whereas the meter itself is fed electronically through a slow time constant. Relying solely on the needle deflection of the meter may cause areas of contamination to be missed.
10. Survey meters should be recalibrated annually. A record must be maintained for 3 years.
11. The fact that calibrated ionization chambers give true dose rate readings regardless of the radionuclide being measured (termed *energy independent*), whereas most* G-M survey meters give true dose rate readings only on the radionuclide of calibrations (termed *energy dependent*), has various applications, as follows:
    a. The G-M survey meter is used for low-level area surveys because of its sensitivity to low-level radiation. However, if it is calibrated with high-energy radionuclides such as ^{60}Co, its values for lesser-energy radionuclides such as ^{99m}Tc are too high. This represents a safety factor for all other radionuclides.
    b. The "Cutie Pie" survey meter will give a more exact radiation dose rate because it produces pulses proportional to energy; however, it cannot be used in low-intensity radiation fields, because of its insensitivity to low intensities.
    c. The G-M survey meter would be the instrument of choice for measuring activity of any number of different radionuclides because approximately the same value would be received for each source of equal activity regardless of the energy of the radionuclide (10 mCi of ^{131}I would give the same reading as 10 mCi of ^{99m}Tc on a G-M survey meter, whereas that value for ^{99m}Tc would be less on a "Cutie Pie," although it would be a truer value).
12. Three kinds of scales are frequently used on survey meters:
    a. Meters on which the user selects a linear scale must be calibrated at no less than two points on each scale. The points should be at approximately ⅓ and ⅔ of full scale.
    b. Meters that have a multidecade logarithmic scale must be calibrated at no less than one point on each decade and no less than two points on one of the decades. Those points should be at approximately ⅓ and ⅔ of the decade.
    c. Meters that have an automatically ranging digital display device for indicating rates must be calibrated at no less than one point on each decade and at no less than two points on one of the decades. Those points should be at approximately ⅓ and ⅔ of the decade.
13. The record of calibration should be kept for at least 3 years and should include the following:
    a. A description of the calibration procedure
    b. Date of calibration
    c. Description of the source used
    d. Certified exposure rates from the source
    e. Rates indicated by the instrument being calibrated
    f. Correction factors deduced from the calibration data
    g. Signature of the individual performing the calibration
14. The same procedure can be repeated with dosimeters. This will provide a calibration graph applicable only to the dosimeter used in the determination. Each dosimeter used should be

*Energy-compensated G-M survey meters are now available which can respond as though they were energy-independent. (See Fig. 10-18.)

calibrated the same way and a calibration graph kept of each one. Dosimeters are also subject to "leakage" (a reduction in the charge resulting in an elevated exposure rate) just by sitting and not being exposed to ionizing radiation. The amount of leakage and a correction factor can be found simply by allowing the dosimeter to remain over the weekend far removed from the nuclear medicine or radiology departments and observing the radiation dose.

LABORATORY APPLICATION

7

VOLTAGE CALIBRATION OF A GEIGER-MUELLER TUBE

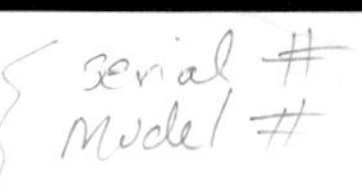

Purpose

It is important that each instrument used in the detection of radiation be calibrated properly to ensure accurate readings and therefore proper radiation protection practices. The G-M survey meter is no exception to this principle.

If a sample is placed beneath a tube and the voltage applied to the tube slowly increased, a voltage will be reached at which the G-M tube just begins to perceive a few counts, as indicated by the readout system. This is the *starting potential*. As the voltage is increased slightly a rapid increase in counting rate is observed. This voltage is known as the *threshold*. Beyond the threshold, further increases in the voltage over quite a range will produce little effect on the counting rate. This region is known as the *plateau*. Within this plateau range, the proper operating voltage is selected. The *operating voltage* should be selected relatively close to the threshold voltage (within the lower 25% of the plateau) to help preserve the life of the tube. If the voltage is increased indiscriminately beyond the plateau region, the region of continuous discharge is reached and the tube may be seriously damaged.

Procedure

Materials

1. G-M detector unit
2. Readout system (count rate meter with a variable high-voltage selector is adequate)
3. Radionuclide
4. Linear graph paper

Technique

1. Reduce high voltage to its lowest setting. This avoids running the G-M tube.
2. Turn on detection unit. Allow for warm-up as indicated in instruction manual.
3. Place radionuclide in a counting position as close to G-M tube as possible.
4. Increase high-voltage adjustment controls until counts are perceived. If ranges and high-voltage indicators are all on the same selector, be sure to have selector on lowest range.
5. Record voltage setting at which counts are initially received. This is termed the *starting potential*.
6. Begin to increase the voltage in consistent increments and observe the count rate. Record voltage and counts per minute.
7. Continue in this manner only until the entire length of the plateau is reached. This requires that the area of continuous discharge be reached, but *do not allow the tube to remain with this voltage applied to it*.

Data treatment

1. Plot counts per minute versus voltage on linear graph paper [counts per minute on ordinate (vertical axis), voltage on abscissa (horizontal axis)]. The graph paper has three components—a steep rise, a plateau, and a second steep rise.
2. Identify the following on the graph:
   a. Starting potential
   b. Threshold
   c. Plateau
   d. Region of continuous discharge
3. Explain why a plateau exists.

Continued.

4. What phenomenon causes the continuous discharge?
5. Why is it necessary to determine the proper operating voltage?
6. Why is a midplateau voltage not used?
7. What is meant by a "quenching" gas?

Example

See Fig. 10-21.

Key points

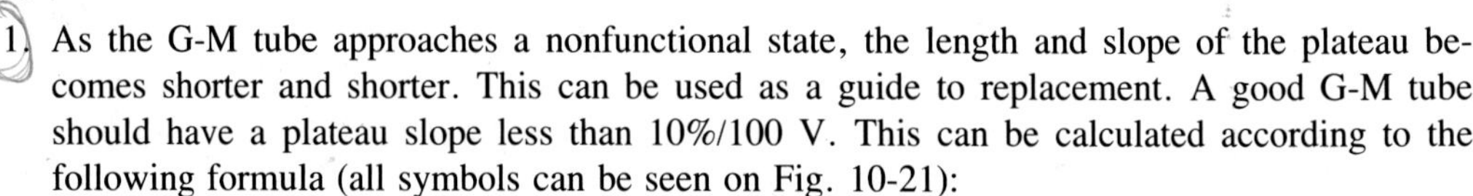

1. As the G-M tube approaches a nonfunctional state, the length and slope of the plateau becomes shorter and shorter. This can be used as a guide to replacement. A good G-M tube should have a plateau slope less than 10%/100 V. This can be calculated according to the following formula (all symbols can be seen on Fig. 10-21):

$$\text{Percentage/100 V} = \frac{100\ (R_2 - R_1)/R_1}{V_2 - V_1} \times 100$$

R_1 = cpm at initial part of plateau
R_2 = cpm at final part of plateau
V_1 = Voltage at initial part of plateau
V_2 = Voltage at final part of plateau

Applying this formula to Fig. 10-21, the percent per 100 V would be as follows:

$$\%/100\text{ V} = \frac{100(7600 - 6400)/6400}{1120 - 960} \times 100 = 11.7\%/100\text{ V}$$

2. The G-M tube can become seriously impaired if allowed to remain in the continuous discharge region.
3. G-M tube saturation is a phenomenon known to exist when the survey meter is brought into contact with a high-activity radiation source. In this instance, the survey meter will not respond at all to the radiation. Moving the survey meter away from the source will cause it to respond again.

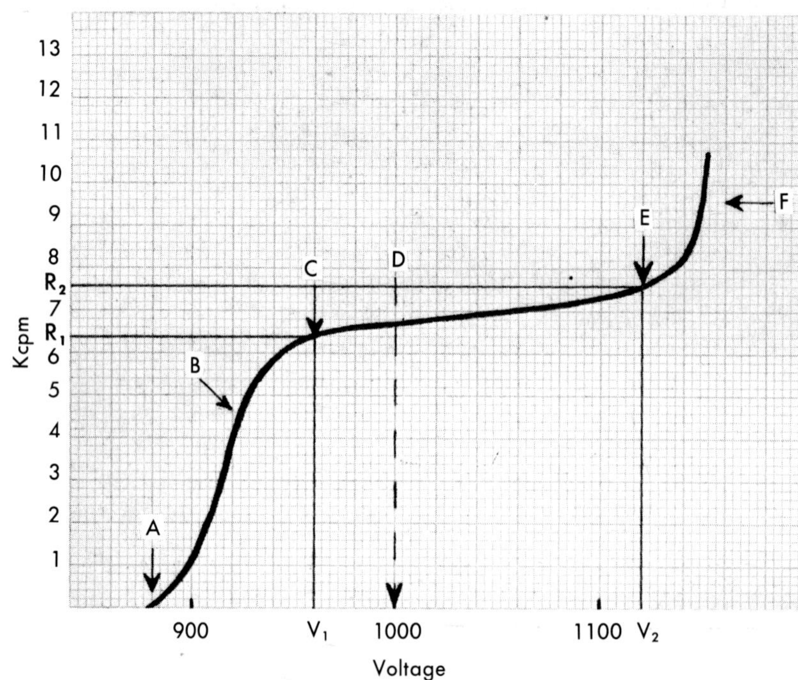

Fig. 10-21. Characteristic calibration curve of a G-M tube. This curve was received by plotting the count rate on the ordinate and voltage on the abscissa. As voltage increased, the count rate increased. Significant areas on this characteristic curve are identified as follows: **A,** starting potential; **B,** knee (lower threshold); **C** to **E,** plateau; **D,** proper operating voltage; and **F,** region of continuous discharge.

LABORATORY APPLICATION

8

DEAD TIME

Purpose

Dead time is the interval immediately following the observance of an ionizing event. During this time a G-M counter is insensitive and does not respond to another ionizing event. This is also known as *resolving time*. In G-M tubes the occurrence of a dead time is the result of the inability of the already ionized gas molecules to produce a separate pulse until after they recombine. If an incoming ionizing event occurs during this time, it will simply occur unrecorded. Resolving time in a G-M survey meter can run as high as 200 μsec.

Scintillation counters also have an analogous dead time.* This time is much shorter than that in a gas detector and results primarily from the duration of the pulse produced by the photomultiplier tube. A second event occurring before the completion of the pulse from the first event results in a mere lengthening of the pulse produced by the photomultiplier tube. Thus two or more absorbed events may record only one discrete pulse and therefore one count. This time for scintillation detectors, however, is so short (2 to 5 μsec) that accurate counting is often limited to the response speed of the electrical or electromechanical counting mechanisms. In any event, whatever the cause may be of the overall dead time of a counting setup, it will put an upper limit on the counting rate that can be measured accurately. Because the dead time of an instrument influences the observed count rate, it is advantageous to determine its resolving time occasionally. Any drastic changes may lead one to suspect component failure. Subtle changes may result in a loss of efficiency at higher count rates, thus suggesting that the user perform tests within the count rate area of linear response (Laboratory Application 18).

The purpose of this exercise is to determine the dead time of a G-M detector system. This is most easily done with a paired source. These are commercially available, or one can be prepared with a small piece of filter paper. Preparation simply involves placing several drops of dilute ^{99m}Tc (enough for good statistics—from 2 to 10 μCi) on the center of a piece of filter paper, allowing it to dry, and then cutting the filter paper into two equal parts.

A refinement of this technique and the mathematical formula as applied to scintillation cameras used in quantitative nuclear cardiology studies can be found elsewhere in this text. The principle is introduced here to make the student aware of changes in the observed count rate versus the true count rate and the amount of count loss accounted for by this parameter.

Procedure

Materials

1. G-M detection unit
2. Readout system, preferably a scaler as opposed to a count rate meter
3. Paired source

Technique

1. Turn on scaler main power and high voltage.
2. Adjust detector to proper operating voltage. This was determined in Laboratory Application 7.
3. Place both halves of source as close to the G-M tube as possible. A planchet should be used to prevent combination.
4. Count sample for 20,000 counts.
5. Record count and time. This value becomes R_{12} in the formula.
6. Count half of the source for the same amount of time.
7. Record count and time. This value becomes R_1 in the formula.
8. Count the other half of the source for the same amount of time.
9. Record count and time. This value becomes R_2 in the formula.

*This form of dead time is described as *nonparalyzable dead time*. This is in contrast to *paralyzable dead time*, a constant time interval during which a system is unable to record a second event.

Continued.

Data treatment

1. Calculate dead time as follows:

$$T = \frac{R_1 + R_2 - R_{12}}{2(R_1 \times R_2)}$$

T = Resolving time (in seconds)
R_1 = Count rate of one-half source (counts per second)
R_2 = Count rate of other one-half source (counts per second)
R_{12} = Count rate of whole source (counts per second)

(Be sure to convert time to seconds.)

2. What is the resolving time for this instrument?
3. If a sample counted 10,000 cpm, what is the actual count? (See Key point.)
4. Why would you expect a lower value if a scintillation detector were used?

Key point

1. The true count rate can be determined by the following formula:

$$R_t = R_o \left(\frac{R_o T}{1 - R_o T}\right) + R_o$$

R_t = True count rate
R_o = Observed count rate (10,000 cpm in this instance)
T = Resolving time

LABORATORY APPLICATION

9

CALIBRATION OF A SPECTROMETER

Purpose

The spectrometer is a form of pulse height analyzer that enables the rejection of pulses with heights below one level and above another. The purpose of this exercise is to calibrate the spectrometer. This is accomplished by determining the proper operating voltage applied to the dynodes of the photomultiplier tube that will convert the arbitrary units of the spectrometer potentiometer to meaningful units expressed in energy units. The pulse height analyzer is set with a window spaced equally below and above the energy of a radionuclide of known energy (preferably monoenergetic), using the potentiometer units that express this energy. (For example, ^{137}Cs has a monoenergetic gamma of 662 keV, so that an LLD setting of 652 and ULD setting of 672 will result in a 10-unit window above *and* below the representative peak energy.) Increases in voltage as applied to the photomultiplier tube will result in the pulse heights being raised to greater and greater heights. Eventually, the pulse will be perceived by the preset window and be counted. The point at which the highest count is received is considered the calibration voltage (or proper operating voltage) because at this point pulse heights of the primary gamma photons have been positioned centrally in the preset window. Also at this point the arbitrary units of the spectrometer potentiometer have assumed meaning in keV units of energy or voltage units (662 units = 662 keV, or 66.2 volt pulse; therefore 364 units = 364 keV, or 36.4 volt pulse, and so on). These primary gamma photons could have been received by a preset window of 300 to 320 just as well, with a much lower voltage to the photomultiplier tube, but then these arbitrary units would not be so easily converted to kiloelectron volt units.

Another method of explaining this calibration procedure is from the standpoint of a gamma spectrum. Increases in voltage cause the gamma spectrum to shift to the right. As voltage is increased, the primary energy peak moves toward the preset window. Eventually more and more of the peak enters the window, resulting in an increased count rate from the perception of "high-energy" components of the peak. As the proper operating voltage is approached, the primary energy peak becomes centrally located in the window, resulting in the highest count rate. As voltage increases further, the primary energy peak moves out of the window with a resultant decrease in count rate from the perception of the "low-energy" components of the peak (Fig. 10-22). Further increases in voltage would move the Compton component of the gamma spectrum into "view." This explanation will become more meaningful in the next laboratory application.

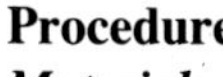

Procedure

Materials

1. Scintillation detector
2. Spectrometer with the capacity to set both upper and lower level discriminators
3. Readout system, such as a scaler or count rate meter
4. Calibration standard, such as a ^{137}Cs source of 0.8 to 1.0 μCi
5. Linear graph paper

Technique

1. Turn voltage control to its lowest point. This prevents damage to the photomultiplier tube.
2. Turn on main power and high voltage of the instrument. The main power is usually kept on at all times to prevent damage to the electronic components resulting from sudden surges of power.

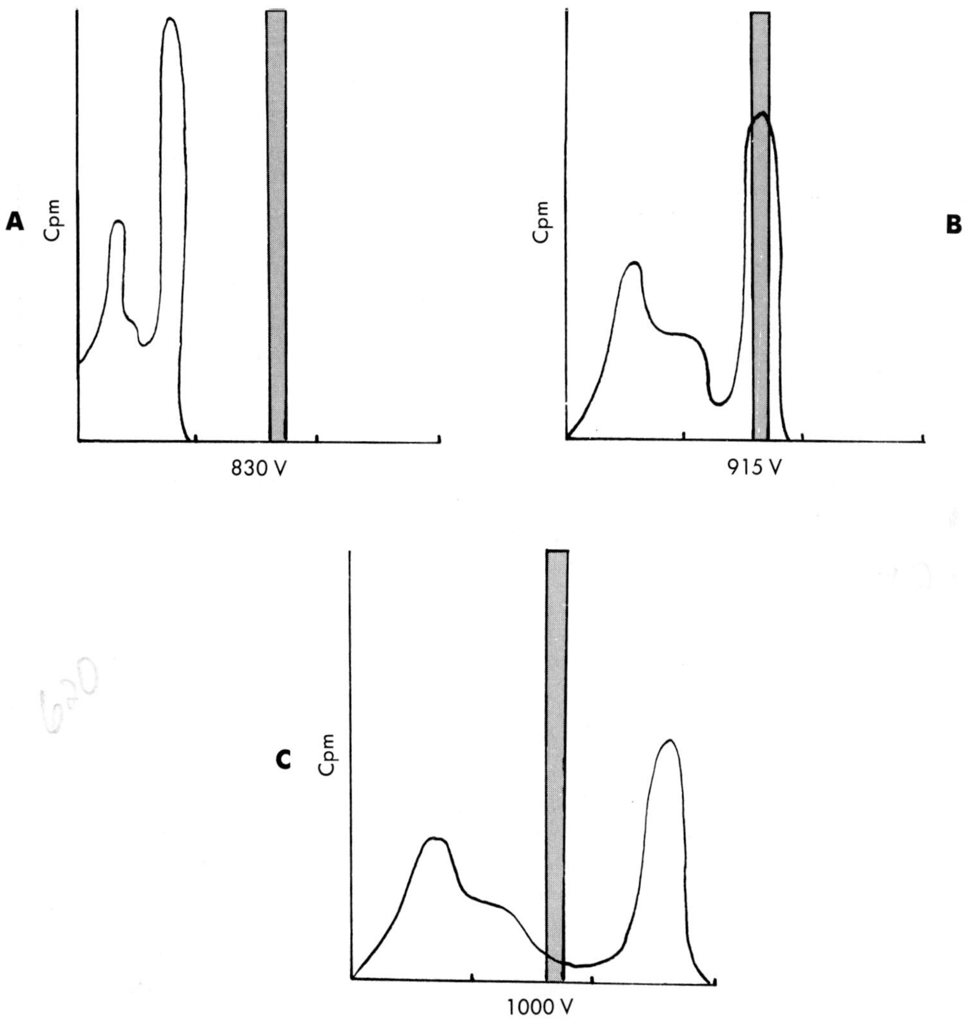

Fig. 10-22. Effect of changing voltages on gamma spectrum shifts. As voltage is increased, the gamma spectrum shifts to the right. The gray region represents the window. **A,** Not enough voltage has been applied to the photomultiplier tube, and the window is only counting the cosmic radiation or background. **B,** Enough voltage has been applied that the entire spectrum is shifted to the right and into the preset window. A portion of the primary energy peak of this radionuclide is now being counted at these window and voltage settings. **C,** Primary peak being shifted to the right and beyond the preset window so that counts now being received are from Compton scatter.

Continued.

3. Note gain* settings (if any). Calibration results are valid only on that gain setting.
4. Set spectrometer to receive pulses from ^{137}Cs standard. Be sure that other parameters are set for using the unit's spectrometer capabilities (See Key Point 10). A 3% window is considered adequate for ^{137}Cs. This is equal to 20 units on the potentiometer, which on calibration is equal to 20 keV (See Key Point 10).
5. Place calibration standard (^{137}Cs or ^{133}Ba) in counting position. Position inside the well or on the probe crystal or on the scanner crystal with the multihole collimator removed.
6. Start readout system counting and increase voltage until counts begin to be received by the readout system. If a scaler is used, set a long preset time or preset count but only for this portion of the exercise.
7. Record voltage setting at which counts are initially received. Voltage may be recorded either in actual voltage units or in potentiometer units, whichever is available.
8. Begin at this voltage setting and take 1-minute counts, recording counts per minute versus voltage. Continue to increase voltage in two-unit increments, counting each time for 1 minute. Record counts per minute and voltage. Determination may be refined by recording in one-unit increments (if equipment allows) as the peak is approached. Continue until count rate decreases to at least 75% of the highest count rate received.
9. Repeat the laboratory application on each of the available gain settings. Use the same 20-unit window on the potentiometer.

Data treatment

1. Plot counts per minute versus voltage on linear graph paper for all gain settings. Counts per minute is plotted on the ordinate (vertical axis), voltage on the abscissa (horizontal axis).
2. Determine proper operating voltage as the voltage used to receive the highest cpm for all gain settings. This voltage is accurate for ^{137}Cs and *usually* for all other radionuclides above 100 keV, provided the window is varied to accommodate the different-size pulses from the primary gamma peaks of other radionuclides. However, this must be similarly checked for each radionuclide (Laboratory Application 11).
3. Explain why the count rate decreases after reaching the proper operating voltage.
4. Could a count rate meter and/or a count rate recorder be used more effectively in this determination? Explain.
5. What is the effect on the proper operating voltage as the gain settings are increased? Decreased? Inversely related or directly related? (Refer to Laboratory Application 12.)

Example

See Fig. 10-23.

Key points

1. Through selection of the proper operating voltage in the prescribed manner, each potentiometer unit is now equal to 1 keV, assuming 1000 units represents 1000 keV.
2. Temperature, both external and internal, is critical to the calibration of the instrument.
3. Room temperature should be kept constant.
4. The instrument should not be near a window, an air conditioner, or a heat outlet.
5. Instruments with the main power turned off require at least 30 minutes warm-up time, especially tube models.
6. Instruments with standby capabilities should be left in this position when not in use.
7. Instruments using the standby position require only 2 minutes for warm-up.
8. Crystals using multihole collimators should have the collimator in place when not in use for insulation purposes.
9. *Recalibrations should be performed at least daily* as a continuous check for voltage drift. This may be done simply, with a minimum of expended time, by observing the count rate at three voltage settings: (1) at the most recent acceptable voltage setting, (2) at a voltage setting 1 potentiometer unit less than the most recent setting, and (3) at a voltage setting 1

*Other names include attenuator range and multiplier.

potentiometer unit greater than the most recent setting. In each of the latter two cases, the count rate should decrease, ensuring against voltage drift. Should the count rate increase, voltage should be changed until the maximum count rate is reached. This becomes the new voltage setting.

10. There are two types of spectrometers, one with the ULD set independently of the LLD and one with the ULD dependent on or "riding on top of" the LLD. In the former, the ULD is set at the desired keV level (it can actually be set lower than the LLD, in which instance no pulses from the amplifier are accepted for counting); in the latter, the window is set as to how many units above the LLD is desired. In this spectrometer calibration determination, a 3% window encompassing the primary energy peak of ^{137}Cs would be as follows: independent window—LLD = 652, ULD = 672; dependent window—LLD = 652, ULD = 20.

    Some instruments have the capacity to expand the analyzer section so as to better define the sizes of the various pulses. In these instruments, each unit on the ULD is one-tenth the value it has on any other setting, so that in setting a 3% window around the primary energy peak of ^{137}Cs, the LLD setting would still read 652 but the ULD setting would read 200. Refer to instrument manual for proper usage of these parameters.
11. ^{137}Cs is used for this determination because it has a monoenergetic (one energy) gamma emission. (Actually, the gamma being "seen" here is not ^{137}Cs at all, but the isometric transitional state of ^{137}Ba, ^{137m}Ba; but for years the 662-keV gamma has been attributed to ^{137}Cs and it is still referred to as a ^{137}Cs gamma.) ^{129}I could also be used for calibrations for the same reason and is preferred by many, especially radioimmunoassay laboratories, because its gamma emission has a more realistic energy, 39 keV. If the calibration source were not monoenergetic, it would be possible to "calibrate" on a lesser gamma peak, and the kiloelectron volt values assigned to the spectrometer potentiometer units would be erroneous.
12. Voltage should not fluctuate appreciably from day to day, If it does, service is indicated.

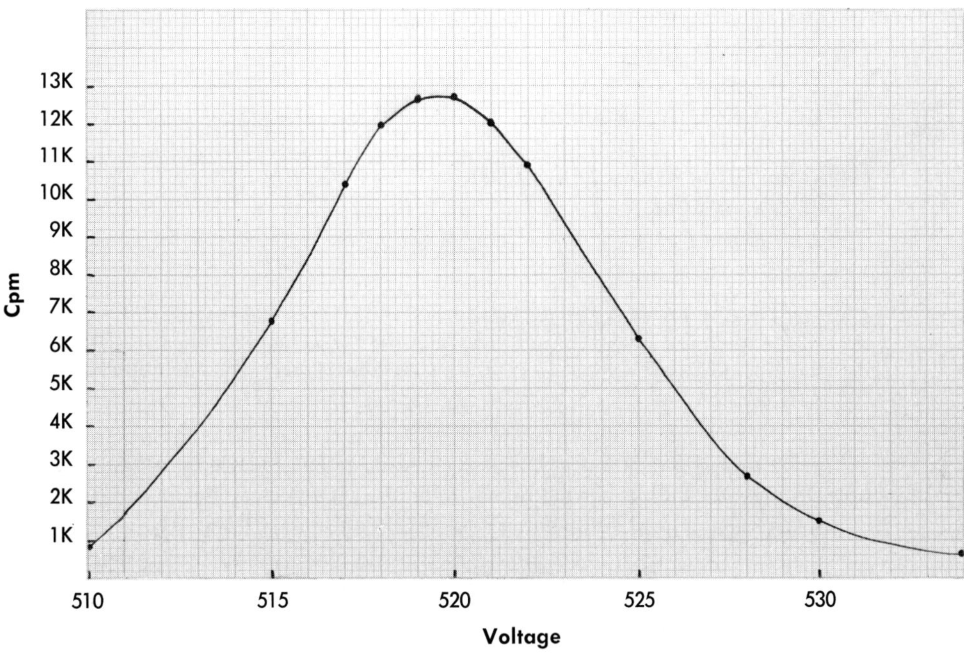

Fig. 10-23. Spectrometer calibration curve. Calibration voltage is determined as that voltage setting which results in the largest number of counts. In this case, the unit would be considered calibrated with a voltage setting of 520.

Continued.

13. Records should be kept daily on the following parameters:
    a. Test cycle (should be 3600 cpm)
    b. Background (should not fluctuate appreciably from time to time)
    c. Voltage applied to photomultiplier tube after calibration
    d. Counts per minute received on a long-lived radionuclide standard (such as ^{137}Cs)
14. After calibration, regardless of the change in voltage, all the same settings can be used as previously determined because calibration constitutes the shifting of the spectrum back to its original position.

LABORATORY APPLICATION 10

DETERMINATION OF A GAMMA ENERGY SPECTRUM

Purpose

This exercise is designed to observe the complete energy spectrum of a radionuclide. In Laboratory Application 7 the potentiometer units were calibrated to read in kiloelectron volt units by adjusting the voltage to its proper operating setting. It is now possible to run a differential spectrum by using the scaler as a single-channel analyzer. Three purposes are served in such a determination: (1) observation is made of all contributions to the gamma spectrum as to their energies and the relative amount of each; (2) the correct settings of the upper and lower level discriminators can be determined (Laboratory Application 12); and (3) the resolution of the crystal can be determined (Laboratory Application 11).

Two procedures are described—one using a single-channel analyzer and one using a multichannel analyzer (MCA).

Procedure

Materials

1. Scintillation detector
2. Spectrometer with the capacity to set both upper and lower level discriminators
3. Scaler or count rate meter
4. Six samples of radioactivity as follows:
    a. 0.5 μCi ^{131}I only
    b. 0.5 μCi ^{137}Cs only
    c. 0.5 μCi ^{131}I *plus* 0.5 μCi ^{137}Cs
    d. 5.0 μCi ^{51}Cr only
    e. 0.5 μCi ^{131}I *plus* 5.0 μCi ^{51}Cr
    f. 100 μCi ^{131}I
5. Linear graph paper
6. Lead filters

Technique for single-channel analyzer

1. Adjust detector voltage to proper operating voltage (see Laboratory Application 7) and lock (if possible) at that setting. Do not change gain setting.
2. Turn LLD (or *E*) to its lowest setting.
3. Turn ULD (or ΔE) or window to read 20 potentiometer units above the LLD setting. This represents a 20 keV window. Be sure other parameters are set for using the unit's spectrometer capabilities (see Laboratory Application 9, Key Point 10).
4. Place ^{137}Cs source in counting position and observe a 60-second count or count rate, depending on instrument capabilities. A 0.5- to 1.0-μCi source or a source counting 100,000 cpm in a window encompassing its primary energy peak is considered adequate for this purpose.
5. Record count or count rate as a function of the window setting. (If LLD = 50 and ULD = 70, record counts as representative of a midwindow setting, or 60.)
6. Advance both the LLD and ULD 10 potentiometer units (10 keV). Observe and record the 60-second count or count rate at this new window setting. If a dependent window is used (as in most scalers), a change in the LLD automatically increases the ULD by the same units. In these units the ULD is "reading on the top" of the LLD.

7. Continue in this fashion, advancing in increments of 10 units, recording counts at the mid-window setting until the entire gamma spectrum is complete. Refinements, particularly at the primary energy peak, can be achieved by reducing the 10-unit increases to 1 unit on both the LLD and the ULD.
8. Repeat the exercise with the lower energy radionuclide. ^{131}I is used here as an example.
9. Repeat the exercise with the two radionuclides in combination. Any other two radionuclides with a wide separation of energies could be used.
10. Repeat the exercise with two radionuclides having principal gamma energies close to one another, for example, use ^{131}I and ^{51}Cr.
11. Plot counts per minute versus window setting on linear graph paper. Counts per minute are usually plotted on the ordinate (vertical axis), keV units on the abscissa (horizontal axis).

Technique for multichannel analyzer*

1. Remove collimator from camera and invert detector. Be careful to avoid stress on cables. Cover crystal with plastic-backed absorbent paper.
2. Place test-tube holder on face of crystal.
3. Place ^{137}Cs source in holder, select 20% window, and adjust voltage or window until window is centered on photopeak.
4. Accumulate 1-minute spectrum. Note counts accumulated. Identify parts of spectrum.
5. Place ^{131}I in test-tube holder without removing ^{137}Cs source or changing its window and accumulate 1-minute spectrum. Note counts in ^{137}Cs window.
6. Remove ^{137}Cs source; using 20% window, adjust voltage or window until window is centered on ^{131}I photopeak.
7. Accumulate 1-minute spectrum. Note counts accumulated in ^{131}I window.
8. Place ^{137}Cs in test-tube holder and, without removing ^{131}I source or changing its window, accumulate spectrum; note counts.
9. Repeat the exercise with two radionuclides having principal gamma energies close to one another, for example, ^{131}I and ^{51}Cr.

Data treatment

1. At what energy does the most prominent peak occur? (Use ^{131}I data for this purpose.)
2. What could you do to correct the situation if the highest count received represented an energy less than the primary energy peak of the radionuclide?
3. What could you do to correct the situation if the highest count received represented an energy greater than the primary energy peak of the radionuclide?
4. Does the energy of your prominent peak correspond with the information about this radionuclide on the trilinear chart of nuclides?
5. Are there any other less prominent peaks? What energies are they?
6. Do the relative percentages of the less prominent peaks concur with the trilinear chart of the nuclides? Explain.
7. Label your graph or photograph as to the following (see Fig. 10-24):
   a. Compton area
   b. Primary peak
   c. Peaks of lesser importance (minor peaks)
8. Are all peaks indicated in the trilinear chart observable on the graph? Explain
9. Repeat steps 3 and 4 with 1 mm of lead between the source and the detector. Does this change the nature of the spectrum? Explain (see Key Point 1).
10. Repeat the determination with a 1 to 2 mCi source. Does this change the nature of the spectrum? Explain (see Key Point 1).
11. Repeat the determination, using the 1 to 2 mCi source with lead filtration. Does this reestablish the first gamma spectrum? Explain.
12. Continued increases in the voltage, as in Laboratory Application 9, will result in a reverse gamma spectrum. Explain.

*Most departments now have MCA capability on their scintillation cameras.

Continued.

13. Plot the data from ^{137}Cs.
14. Plot the data from ^{131}I *plus* ^{137}Cs in the same sample. Use different colors for each set of data points so that the three different gamma spectra can be easily identified.
    a. What has happened to the primary energy peak of the lower energy radionuclide? Explain.
    b. What has happened to the primary energy peak of the higher energy radionuclide? Explain.
15. Without further consideration, can a valid count be received by counting a high-energy radionuclide in the presence of a low-energy radionuclide? Explain.
16. Without further consideration, can a valid count be received by counting a low-energy radionuclide in the presence of a high-energy radionuclide? Explain.
17. Plot the data from ^{131}I, ^{51}Cr, and these two radionuclides in combination on the same sheet of graph paper. Use different colors for each set of data points for ease of identification.
18. How are the results from step 17 similar to the results from step 14?
19. How are the results from step 17 different from the results from step 14 with respect to the separation of the two radionuclides?
20. Name a clinical situation in which ^{131}I may be a contaminant of ^{57}Co; in which ^{131}I may be a contaminant of ^{51}Cr.

Example

See Fig. 10-24.

Key points

1. A source of radioactivity must be used for this determination that is not so low in activity as to alter results statistically or so high as to introduce artifacts caused by coincidence counting. Usually a 1.0 μCi source is sufficient. Coincidence counting in scintillation crystals can occur when a sodium iodide crystal "sees" two gamma rays of the same energy at the same time and records it as one gamma ray of twice the energy. For example, *two* gamma rays of ^{99m}Tc,

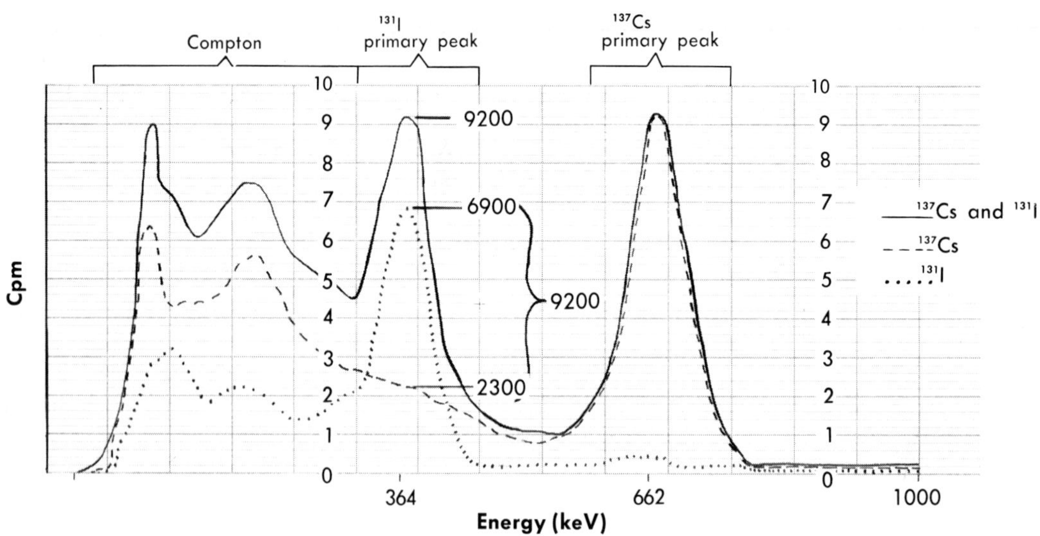

Fig. 10-24. Gamma spectra and effects of dual nuclide studies. Graph illustrates results of two radionuclides used simultaneously and their effects on each other. ^{137}Cs in the presence of a lower energy radionuclide (^{131}I) has no effect on the count rate. (Count rate for ^{137}Cs, both alone and combined with ^{131}I, is the same.) The reverse is not true, however. Count rate for ^{131}I alone is considerably lower than that for ^{131}I combined with ^{137}Cs. This is because Compton for higher energy ^{137}Cs falls into the ^{131}I window and therefore is counted with the primary peak of ^{131}I. The result is that the combined count rate of ^{131}I and ^{137}Cs is the same as counts received from ^{131}I alone added to counts received from Compton of ^{137}Cs at the same point on the spectrum. The same is true for any other point on the spectrum.

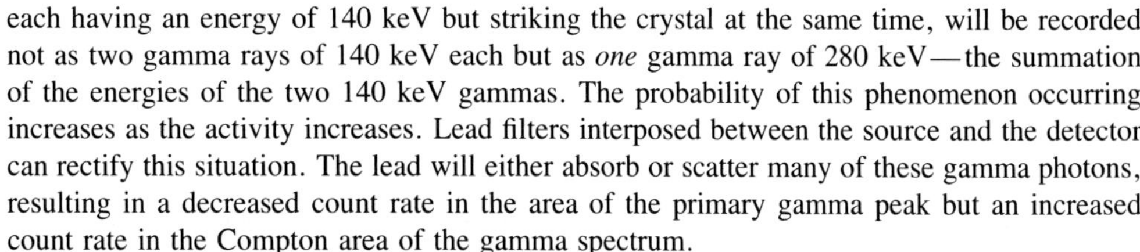

each having an energy of 140 keV but striking the crystal at the same time, will be recorded not as two gamma rays of 140 keV each but as *one* gamma ray of 280 keV—the summation of the energies of the two 140 keV gammas. The probability of this phenomenon occurring increases as the activity increases. Lead filters interposed between the source and the detector can rectify this situation. The lead will either absorb or scatter many of these gamma photons, resulting in a decreased count rate in the area of the primary gamma peak but an increased count rate in the Compton area of the gamma spectrum.

2. Considerations of statistical fluctuations in the low count rate areas of this determination can be disregarded. Counts lasting 60 seconds will suffice if the count rate is at least 10,000 counts per 60 seconds in the area of the primary gamma peak.
3. The use of a count rate meter or an MCA greatly increases the speed with which these determinations can be performed because of the almost instantaneous recording or count rate in the first instance, or the simultaneous but individual recording of events occurring in many windows (channels) in the case of the MCA.
4. Percentages of contributions from various gamma peaks can be qualitatively determined by simply observing the size of primary versus minor peaks. ^{131}I is a good example: 83% of all gamma contribution results from the 364 keV gammas, whereas 7% of all gamma contributions results from the 637 keV gamma. Note the size of these two peaks.
5. Further consideration is given to data treatment in Laboratory Application 16. Laboratory application, however, applies only to two radionuclides having widely separated primary gamma peaks.

LABORATORY APPLICATION 11

DETERMINATION OF THE ENERGY RESOLUTION OF A GAMMA SPECTROSCOPY SYSTEM

Purpose

Theoretically, since all gamma rays emitted from a monoenergetic gamma-emitting radionuclide such as ^{137}Cs have exactly the same energy, all pulses resulting from their detection would have the same amplitude. Furthermore, having the same amplitude, they should all appear at exactly the same point on a gamma spectrum. As has been seen in the preceding determinations, this is not true. The display of gamma photons on a gamma spectrum more closely resembles a bell-shaped curve, representing gamma photons of many energies, rather than a "spike," representing gamma photons of a single energy. Although a "spike" is what should be displayed, this could happen only if the entire system of scintillation detection were perfect. Such is not the case. *Apparent* increases and decreases in pulse amplitude occur as a result of incomplete gamma absorptions in the crystal, losses of light intensity during crystal transmission, nonproportional release of electrons at the photocathode, infidelity of electron multiplication at the dynodes, and imperfections in the linearity of pulses in the amplifier. Defects in any of these components causes a widening in this bell-shaped curve, an undesirable effect that, if serious enough, makes continued use impossible.

Energy resolution is the term describing the limitations of such a spread of the primary photopeak. It is calculated as the ratio of the width of a photopeak (measured at a point equal to one half the amplitude of the peak) to its energy. The usual acceptable limit for a ^{137}Cs standard is from 8% to 12%. The purpose of this exercise is to determine the percent resolution on a gamma scintillation detection system.

Procedure

Materials

1. Scintillation crystal detector unit
2. Spectrometer
3. Readout system, either scaler or count rate meter
4. Various sources of radioactivity (1 μCi of ^{137}Cs is generally used for this purpose)
5. Linear graph paper

Continued.

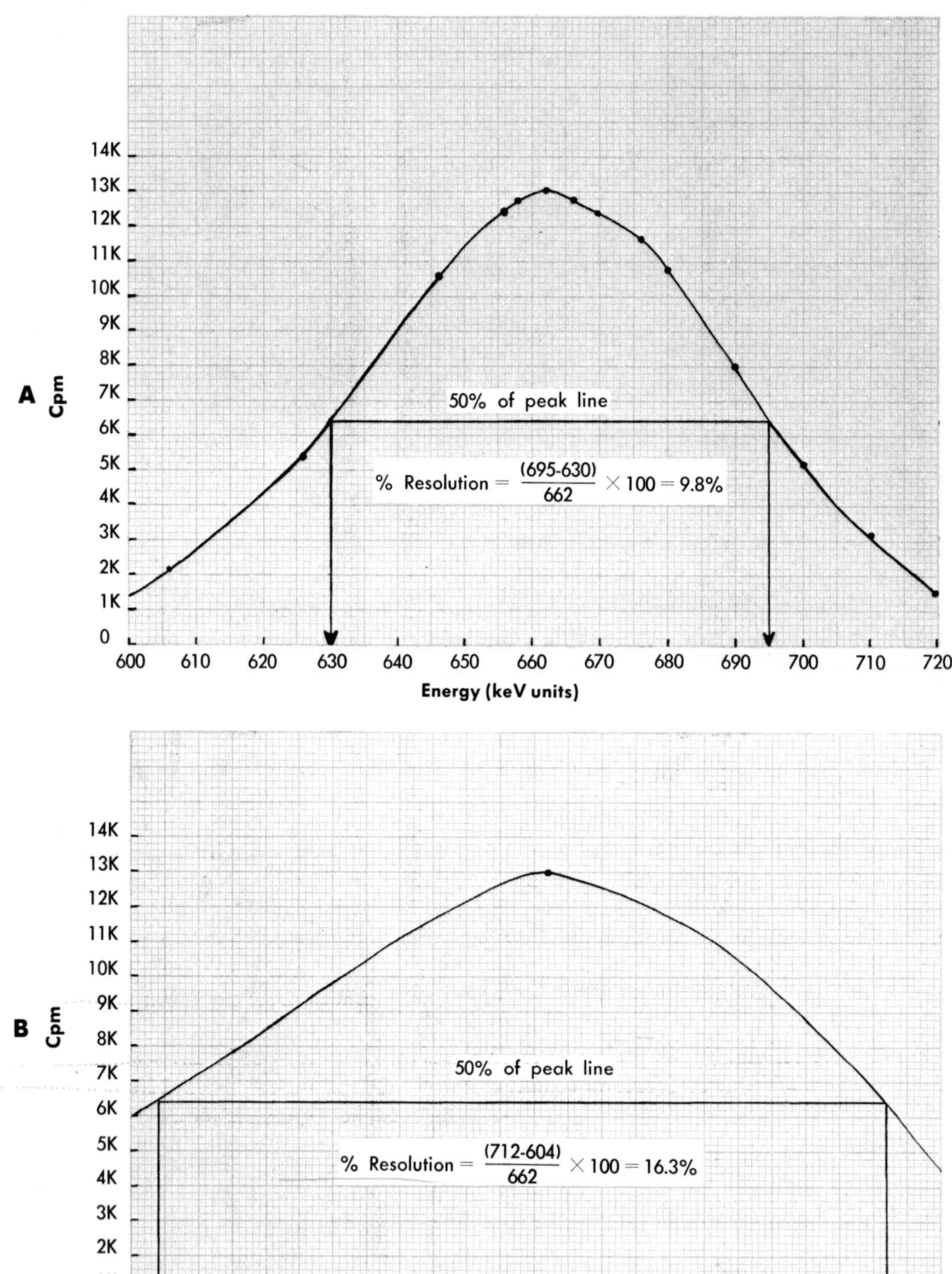

Fig. 10-25. Two different gamma peaks showing resolution determinations. **A,** Gamma energy peak of ^{137}Cs having a percent resolution of 9.8%. This is an acceptable value for crystal resolution, and the unit is functioning properly. **B,** Gamma energy peak on a cracked crystal where ^{137}Cs has a percent resolution of 16.3% and is therefore unacceptable for continued use.

Technique

1. Turn on scaler main power and high voltage.
2. Adjust detector voltage to proper operating voltage and lock (if possible) at that setting.
3. Turn LLD to approximately 100 units below the primary energy peak of the radionuclide in use. This does not require an entire gamma spectrum, only the part displaying the primary gamma peak in its entirety.
4. Turn the ULD (or ΔE) or window to read 20 potentiometer units above the LLD setting. This represents a 20 keV window. Be sure other parameters are set for using the unit's spectrometer capabilities (see Laboratory Application 9, Key Point 10).
5. Place radionuclide in counting position.
6. Observe a 60-second count or count rate, depending on instrument.
7. Record count or count rate as a function of a midwindow setting (if LLD = 270 and ULD = 20, plot as 280).
8. Advance both the LLD and ULD 10 potentiometer units (10 keV). Observe and record the 60-second count or count rate at this new window setting.
9. Continue in this fashion, advancing in increments of 10 units and recording counts at the midwindow setting, until the entire primary gamma peak is displayed. Refinements, particularly at the primary energy peak, can be achieved by reducing the 10-unit increases to 1 unit on both the LLD and the ULD.

Data treatment

1. Plot counts per minute versus window settings on linear graph paper (see Fig. 10-25).
2. Determine the point in energy units where the highest count was received. This should correspond with the energy of the principal gamma emission.
3. Determine the point on the graph on both sides of the primary peak that represents 50% of the highest count received. Draw a vertical line from each of these two points until it intersects with the abscissa. What are these two points in kiloelectron volt units?
4. Subtract the smaller value from the larger value. This is defined as the *full width half maximum* (FWHM). What is this value in kiloelectron volt units?
5. Calculate the resolution by the following formula:

$$\text{Percentage resolution} = \frac{\text{FWHM (in keV units)}}{\text{Energy of peak (in keV units)}} \times 100$$

   What is the resolution for ^{137}Cs? (Resolution for ^{137}Cs usually falls between 8% and 12%; see Fig. 10-25.)
6. Repeat this determination with other radionuclides. Does resolution improve or worsen with increasing energy?
7. Assuming that 8% to 12% resolution is adequate for ^{137}Cs on any scintillation crystal system, would it be proper to contact a service repairman if resolution were determined to be 5%? 25%? Both? Give an example of what could be responsible for a resolution value of 25%.

LABORATORY APPLICATION

12

DETERMINATION OF PROPER WINDOW SETTINGS

Purpose

This exercise will help determine the proper window settings on the spectrometer so that as many acceptable pulses as possible will be received and counted by the analyzer system. Acceptability, theoretically, would be any pulse having a height representative of exactly the primary energy peak of the radionuclide. Practically, however, many other pulse heights occur that are both higher and lower than that of the primary energy peak, which cannot be construed as anything other than complete unadulterated gamma absorptions in the scintillation crystal.

The purpose of this determination is to ascertain which pulses are acceptable and which are questionable and therefore not acceptable. In this way, through the acceptance of more counts, statistical error will be improved and/or counting times will be reduced. Window settings encompassing 75% of the entire energy peak are usually considered to be appropriate. With the use of a 75% window,

Continued.

pulses arising from background radiation and scattered radiation falling into this energy range will not alter the results. Furthermore, with the use of a 75% window, only approximately 10% of the counts (most of which are questionable) are lost.

The use of a 75% window is not always permissible, such as in the case of very low energy gamma rays or when an attenuating medium like lead is interposed between the source and the detector. Then different values must be used, usually resulting in an asymmetric window. (A 75% window usually results in a symmetric window having just as many units on each side of the primary energy peak.)

Procedure

Materials

1. Scintillation crystal detector unit
2. Spectrometer
3. Readout system, either scaler or count rate meter
4. Various sources of radioactivity
5. Linear graph paper
6. Lead filters

Technique

1. Turn on scaler main power and high voltage.
2. Adjust detector voltage to proper operating voltage and lock (if possible) at that setting.
3. Turn LLD to approximately 100 units below the primary energy peak of the radionuclide in use. This does not require an entire gamma spectrum, only the part displaying the primary gamma peak in its entirety.
4. Turn the ULD (or ΔE) or window to read 20 potentiometer units above the LLD setting. This represents a 20 keV window.
5. Place radionuclide in counting position. A 1.0 μCi source or a source counting 100,000 cpm in a window encompassing its primary energy peak is considered adequate for this purpose.
6. Observe a 60-second count or count rate, depending on instrument capabilities.
7. Record count or count rate as a function of the midwindow setting (if LLD = 270 and ULD = 20, plot as 280).
8. Advance both the LLD and ULD 10 potentiometer units (10 keV). Observe and record the 60-second count or count rate at this new window setting.
9. Continue in this fashion, advancing in increments of 10 units, recording counts at the midwindow setting until the entire primary gamma peak is displayed. Refinements, particularly at the primary energy peak, can be achieved by reducing the 10-unit increases to 1 unit on both the LLD and the ULD.

Data treatment

1. Plot counts per minute on the ordinate (vertical axis) versus energy units on the abscissa (horizontal axis) on linear graph paper.
2. Determine the point in energy units where the highest count was received. This should correspond with the energy of the principal gamma emission.
3. Determine the point on the graph on both sides of the primary peak that represents 25% of the highest count received. Draw a vertical line from each of these two points until it intersects with the abscissa. The units on the abscissa are expressed in kiloelectron volt units. These represent optimum LLD and ULD settings. What are they?
4. What settings would be used on a dependent window?
5. What settings would be used on an independent window?

Example

See Fig. 10-26.

Key points

1. This determination should be performed on all radionuclides and on every piece of equipment with which these radionuclides are used. A record should be kept of these partial gamma spectra.
2. This determination should be performed before any calibration techniques, such as the technetium generator, if the assay technique using the attenuation medium is used. Window settings here are extremely critical for correct assay of ^{99m}Tc.
3. Once performed, window settings will not alter appreciably (provided the spectrometer is calibrated routinely) until major repairs of the instrument are required. Following the repairs, these determinations should be run again.
4. Note that narrow windows (10 to 20 keV) are used for calibration purposes, but that windows used for routine nuclear medicine procedures are much wider, sometimes as large as 100 keV or more.
5. It is often advisable when using lower energy radionuclides to use an eccentrically placed window. The classic example of this is ^{99m}Tc. An optimum window setting for this radionuclide in performing imaging procedures is to set the LLD at a point representing 75% of the highest count received (on the low-energy side of the peak) and to set the ULD at a point representing 25% of the highest count received (on the high-energy side of the peak). This eccentrically placed window effectually increases the target-to-background (primarily scatter) ratio, since scatter is so prevalent in studies such as brain images with this radionuclide. Others have suggested that an optimum window for ^{99m}Tc is a 25% window (25% of the energy), with the LLD being placed 5% below the primary energy (at 133 keV) and the ULD being placed at 20% above the primary energy (at 168 keV). This can be effected on a system that does not have independent window settings by "peaking in" on a 10% window selection and switching to a 25% window for the clinical study. To use an eccentric window, however, it is necessary to have the camera tuned to accept this window arrangement, or nonuniform floods will occur. The advent of nonuniformity correction circuits have corrected this problem.

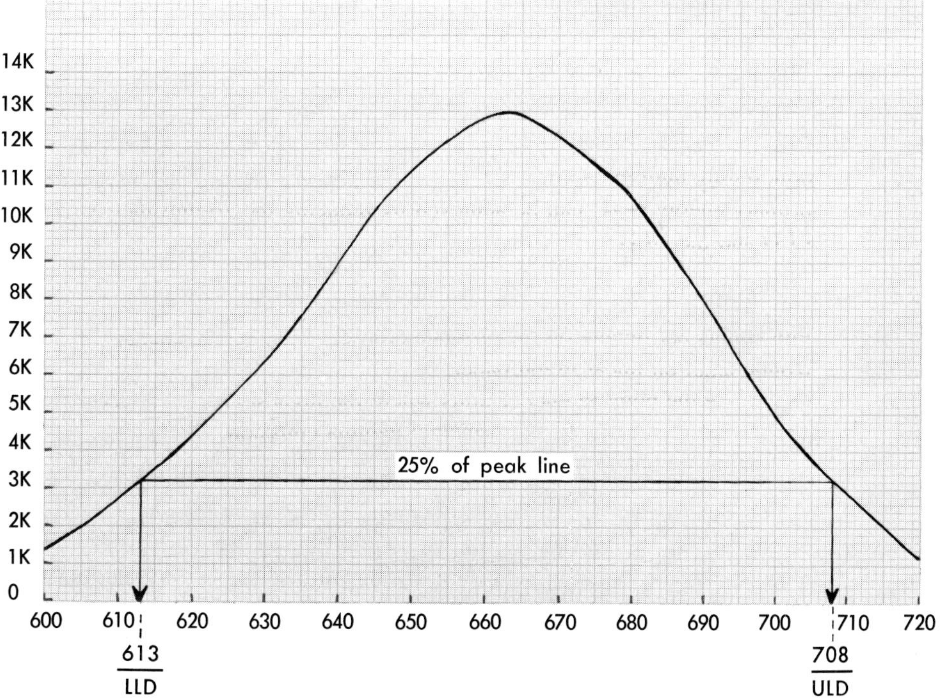

Fig. 10-26. Gamma energy peak of ^{137}Cs, showing proper placement of upper and lower level discriminators. If the instrument had independent window settings, proper window settings would be LLD = 613, ULD = 708. If the instrument had dependent windows, proper window settings would be LLS = 613, window = 95.

LABORATORY APPLICATION 13

LINEARITY OF CALIBRATION RESPONSE

Purpose

In Laboratory Application 9 the proper operating voltage was determined so that the arbitrary unit on the pulse height analyzer potentiometers (usually 1000 units on each) would have meaning in energy units. It is most practical to make each unit equal to 1.0 keV, since few of our routine radionuclides exceed 1000 keV (1.0 meV). For this reason, the LLD was set at 652 and the ULD at 672, so that when the highest count rate was achieved, these units no longer were arbitrary units but took on values in energy units. Unit 652 now represents 652 keV, and unit 672 now represents 672 keV. Likewise, because pulse heights are proportional to energy and linearly amplified, unit 364 now represents the primary energy peak of ^{131}I, unit 320 now represents the primary energy peak of ^{51}Cr, and so on. The ultimate value of this information is that, with the voltage remaining unchanged, the window can be moved up or down to receive and count whatever pulse height is desired, this being dependent on the energy of the radionuclide under scrutiny.

This rationale usually holds true for all the higher energy radionuclides (above 150 keV) but does not apply to the radionuclides of lesser energy (below 150 keV). The voltage found to "peak" in ^{137}Cs may not "peak" in ^{99m}Tc, for instance, assuming a 20 keV spread centered around 140 units on the pulse height analyzer potentiometers (LLD = 130, ULD = 150). It may be that the voltage would have to be increased or decreased to receive the highest count rate from a ^{99m}Tc source. An increase in voltage would result in the entire gamma energy spectrum being shifted to the right; a decrease in voltage would result in the entire gamma energy spectrum being shifted to the left. Either case is an example of *nonlinearity*. In almost every type of nuclear instrumentation, nonlinearity exists for ^{125}I (35 keV), but this radionuclide becomes involved in another parameter of nuclear instrumentation, gain control. This is treated in Laboratory Application 14.

The purpose of this laboratory application is to determine whether such nonlinearity exists in any of the available nuclear instruments and to present methods necessary to correct this defect.

Procedure

Materials

1. Scintillation crystal detector unit
2. Spectrometer
3. Readout system, either scaler or count rate meter
4. Following sources of radioactivity:
   a. 1.0 μCi ^{137}Cs
   b. 1.0 μCi ^{51}Cr
   c. 1.0 μCi ^{131}I
   d. 1.0 μCi ^{201}Te
   e. 1.0 μCi ^{99m}Tc
   f. 1.0 μCi ^{57}Co
   g. 1.0 μCi ^{125}I
5. Linear graph paper

Technique

1. Turn on scaler main power and high voltage.
2. Adjust detector voltage to proper operating voltage with the ^{137}Cs standard.
3. Record voltage and primary gamma energy of the radionuclide used.
4. Repeat this determination with each of the radionuclides listed under materials using a 20 keV window for the determination of the proper operating voltage of each radionuclide. Record the optimum voltage and energy of each, making sure to adjust the window to accommodate the energy in each instance.

Data treatment

1. Plot proper operating voltage on the ordinate (vertical axis) versus energy on the abscissa (horizontal axis) on linear graph paper.

2. Is your instrument nonlinear for some radionuclides?
3. List the radionuclides that exhibit nonlinearity.
4. Are these nonlinear radionuclides low energy or high energy?
5. List the various radionuclides used and their optimum voltage settings.

Example

See Fig. 10-27.

Key points

1. Radionuclides lower than 100 keV in energy are expected to exhibit the nonlinearity phenomenon when compared with ^{137}Cs on the same gain setting. This is one of the reasons for understanding the proper operation of gain (Laboratory Application 12).
2. This determination should be performed on all instruments in the nuclear medicine laboratory.
3. Linearity can be corrected by two methods:
   a. The voltage may be adjusted to accommodate the window and thereby compensate for nonlinearity. This is what actually was done in this determination when the nonlinearity phenomenon was exhibited.
   b. The window may be adjusted to accommodate the voltage. This method is actually thought by most to be the best. In this method the voltage found to be optimum for ^{137}Cs is also used for the low-energy radionuclides. However, when this voltage is used, another spectrum involving just the gamma energy peak is run to establish new window settings. This procedure may result in a window that appears to be asymmetric or even off the peak but in reality is not. Its effect is to shift the window to the right or to the left to compensate for the primary gamma energy peak being shifted also to the right or to the left, respectively, because of this nonlinear problem.

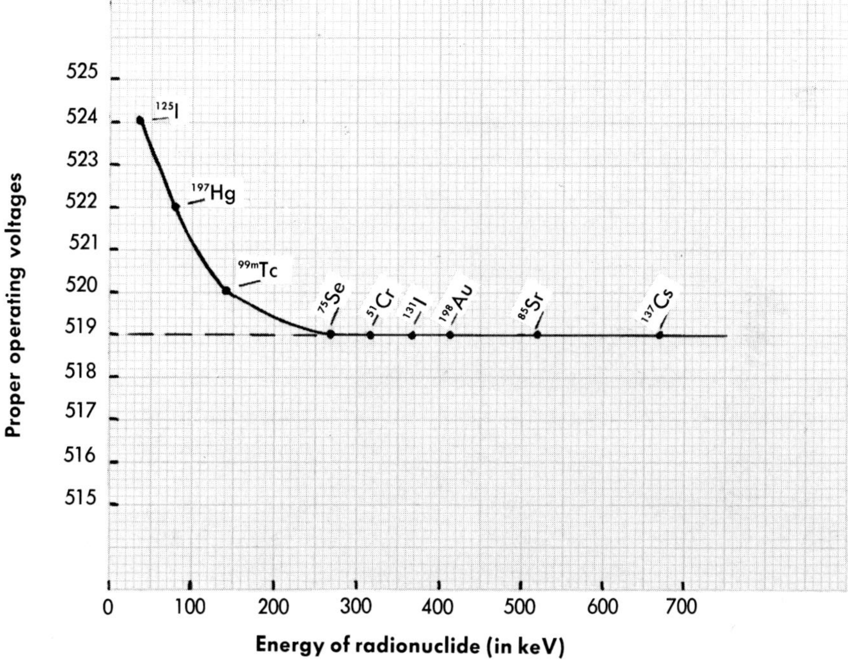

Fig. 10-27. Characteristic graph depicting nonlinearity of calibration response. Solid line, slight nonlinearity in voltage calibration response, beginning with ^{99m}Tc and progressively deteriorating as the energy of the radionuclide becomes less, as with ^{197}Hg (77 keV) and ^{125}I (35 keV). Completely linear response would appear as a dotted line. On this graph, voltage must be increased with lower energy radionuclides. Some instruments might be represented by a decrease in voltage with lower energy radionuclides.

LABORATORY APPLICATION

14

EFFECTS OF GAIN

Purpose

It has already been demonstrated in previous exercises that the height of any pulse resulting from the absorption of a gamma photon in the scintillation crystal can be altered by variations in the voltage applied to the photomultiplier tube. An increase in the voltage causes an increase in the pulse height; a decrease in the voltage causes a decrease in the pulse height. This is a variable control. The alteration in the pulse height is a result of increases or decreases in secondary emission at the dynode section of the counting system.

The same effect can be demonstrated by the use of gain. However, this is usually a stepped control (increments of 2×), and the alteration in the pulse height is a result of changes in the amplifier section of the counting system. This method of altering pulse heights has as its advantage the ability to keep voltages applied to the photomultiplier tube at a low level, thereby increasing the life span of the photomultiplier tube. In fact, many technologists prefer to use gain and voltage in this fashion—keeping gain high and voltage low—for all radionuclides. This method of calibration means the changing of *gain and voltage* as well as the window for each radionuclide. This also means rejection of the concept of calibrating so that each arbitrary unit on the spectrometer potentiometer is equal to 1 keV. The result is that all the values of the gain, voltage, and especially spectrometer would appear to be meaningless to the person knowledgeable only in the calibration technique, but it carries with it the economy of longer use of the same photomultiplier tube. This method will not be discussed here.

Although almost all radionuclides can be counted on the same gain setting if the unit is calibrated in the manner specified in this procedure manual, there are notable exceptions, such as ^{125}I and ^{60}Co. Pulses can be thought of as bursts of electrons or voltages. The calibration of a spectrometer not only makes it possible to convert the 1000 units on the spectrometer potentiometer to 1000 keV units, it also makes it possible to express the pulse in units of voltage from 0 to 10 or from 0 to 100. For purposes of this discussion, voltages of 0 to 100 will be used. Therefore after calibration a pulse as a result of the total crystal absorption of a ^{137}Cs gamma could be expressed accurately as equal to (1) 662 potentiometer units, (2) 662 keV, or (3) 66.2 V. The voltage value can be increased either by increasing the gain or the voltage applied to the photomultiplier tube or both. Since gain is usually a stepped control, voltages are increased or decreased by a factor of 2, depending on the direction of each turn of the gain control.

Another way of looking at the principle of gain is to relate it to the gamma spectrum. Just as increases and decreases in the high voltage cause shifts of the gamma spectrum to the right and to the left, respectively, so also do increases and decreases in gain cause shifts to the right and to the left, respectively.

Table 10-1. Voltage equivalents at various gain* settings

		Gain settings				
Radionuclide	**Energy (keV)**	**1†**	**2**	**4**	**8**	**16**
^{125}I	35			3.5	7.0	14.0
^{133}Xe	80			8.0	16.0	
^{99m}Tc	140			14.0		
^{51}Cr	320			32.0		
^{131}I	364			36.4		
^{137}Cs	662			66.2		
^{59}Fe	1,095; 1,292		54.8; 64.6	109.5; 129.2		
^{60}Co	1,173; 1,332		58.7; 66.6	117.3; 133.2		

*This table is valid only with *true* gain settings in a calibrated, completely linear counting system.

In *inverse* gain systems (most scalers) the voltage values are the reverse. Refer to instrument instruction manual.

†These numbers are used only as examples. These values change, depending on the instrument. Refer to instrument instruction manual.

Most pulse height analyzers are capable of correctly analyzing only pulses from 10 to 100. Table 10-1 (underlined numbers) shows several radionuclides that do not fall into this category. Those with not enough voltage include ^{125}I and ^{133}Xe. To increase the voltage of each of these pulses to an acceptable level, true gain must be increased. When such pulses are altered in voltage, their pulse heights are also altered proportionally. Therefore to accept and count the pulses from one of these radionuclides to which gain has been applied, the window must be raised or lowered, depending on the gain setting. For instance, according to Table 10-1, ^{125}I on a gain of 16 will produce its energy peak at 140 potentiometer units, ^{133}Xe at 16 units on a gain of 8, and ^{60}Co at 587 and/or 666 units on a gain of 2. This is true only if voltage is linear between various gain settings.

The purposes of this exercise are manifold: to determine the type of gain (inverse* or true); to determine whether voltage is linear between various gain settings; if not linear, to determine the proper operating voltage of each gain setting or to determine the proper window setting of each radionuclide to which gain must be applied; and to determine the effect of gain on window values.

Procedure

Materials

1. Scintillation crystal detector unit
2. Spectrometer with gain controls
3. Readout system
4. The following radionuclides:
   a. 1.0 μCi ^{125}I
   b. 1.0 μCi ^{99m}Tc
   c. 1.0 μCi ^{51}Cr
   d. 1.0 μCi ^{137}Cs
   e. 1.0 μCi ^{60}Co
5. Linear graph paper

Technique

1. Turn on main power and high voltage of the instrument.
2. Place gain control on a setting midway between the maximum and minimum settings. These numerical values change from instrument to instrument.
3. Calibrate the instrument, using a ^{137}Cs standard with a 3% window centered around the primary gamma energy.
4. What is the proper operating voltage on this gain setting?
5. What is the count rate of the ^{137}Cs source at the calibration voltage expressed in counts per minute?
6. Remove the ^{137}Cs source, take a background count, and express in counts per minute.
7. Replace ^{137}Cs source, turn gain to the next highest dial value from the calibration gain setting, and take a 1-minute count. What is the count per minute?
8. Keeping ^{137}Cs source in place, turn gain to the next lowest dial value from the calibration gain setting and take a 1-minute count. What is the count per minute?
9. If the counts received in step 7 are closer to background (step 6), the instrument has an *inverse gain* (decreases in the value of the gain setting indicate increases in gain). If the counts received in step 8 are closer to background, the instrument has a *true gain* (increases in the value of the gain setting indicate increases in gain). In either case, the pulse height and/or pulse voltage would have been reduced by half, and, since the spectrometer was not changed, the window would only be counting background. The background being counted, however, would have twice the energy.
10. What type of gain is on this instrument?
11. Either step 7 or step 8 resulted in a count rate considerably higher than background. This is because the gamma spectrum has been shifted to the right, causing Compton to be seen by the unchanged window. Does this fit your answer to step 10?

*Inverse gain is found on most scalers.

Continued.

12. Using the ^{137}Cs standard, turn gain to half the calibration gain setting and reduce the spectrometer values by half. For example, if calibration values of an independent window* were true gain = 4, spectrometer = 652 to 672, change to read true gain = 2, spectrometer = 326 to 336. If the calibration values for a dependent window* were true gain = 4, LLD = 652, window = 20, change to read true gain = 2, LLD = 326, window = 10.†
13. Check voltage linearity between these two gain settings by recalibrating the voltage.
    a. Does the proper operating voltage of this range agree with step 4? If not, what is the voltage for this range? (Disagreement reflects nonlinearity.)
    b. Counts should closely agree with results of step 5. Do they?
14. It is considered better to adjust the window to accommodate the voltage rather than vice versa. Reset the voltage determined in step 4 and determine the proper window setting to receive the same count. What are the new window settings?
15. Your count rate should closely agree with the count rate received in step 5. Does it? What is this count rate?
16. Repeat step 14 on the following radionuclides at the appropriate gain settings.

Radionuclides (energy)	Gain	LLD	ULD or window
^{125}I (35 keV)			
^{133}Xe (80 keV)			
^{99m}Tc (140 keV)			
^{137}Cs (662 keV)			
^{59}Fe (1095; 1292 keV)			
^{60}Co (1173; 1332 keV)			

17. With a 20 keV window calibrated at midgain (for example, 8), what size would the window be (in kiloelectron volt units) at the following gain settings?

Gain setting	True gain	Inverse gain
2		
4		
8	20 keV	20 keV
16		
32		

18. With a 20 keV window calibrated at midgain (for example, 8), what would the window be changed to (in kiloelectron volt units) to maintain the same count rate at the following gain settings?

Gain setting	True gain	Inverse gain
2		
4		
8	20 keV	20 keV
16		
32		

*See Laboratory Application 9, Key Point 10.
†See Key Point 1.

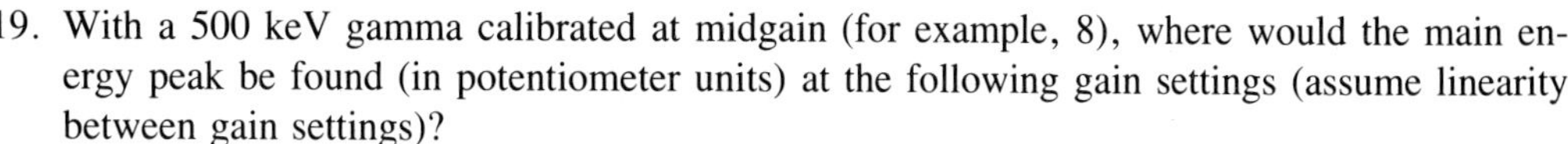

19. With a 500 keV gamma calibrated at midgain (for example, 8), where would the main energy peak be found (in potentiometer units) at the following gain settings (assume linearity between gain settings)?

Gain setting	True gain	Inverse gain
2		
4		
8	500 keV	500 keV
16		
32		

20. Assume a true gain and ^{137}Cs calibrated on a gain of 1. With a change of gain to 2, are there any window settings that will receive the peak energy using a 1000-unit potentiometer?
21. In the example in step 20, can the peak be counted if the integral counting mode is used? Explain.
22. Is there a variation in count rate from ^{137}Cs counted on a calibrated gain setting of 1 versus ^{137}Cs integrally counted on a gain setting of 2? Explain.

Key points

1. As gain is decreased to produce half the pulse height, the pulse height analyzer must be lowered to half the original value to receive and count the pulses. This means that a spectrometer set at 662 potentiometer units to receive 662 keV must be reduced to 331 potentiometer units. Each of these units is now equal to 2 keV in value. *The same effect is seen on the values given to the dependent window,* so that a 20 keV window on full gain is increased to 40 keV on one-half gain on most units.* This necessitates reducing the window value to 10 to maintain a 20 keV window. This is true for an increase or true gain.
2. If proper operating voltage fluctuates, window settings determined in this exercise are worthless. However, recalibration can restore these values.
3. Some units have fine-gain accommodations that allow even more refined "peaking" of the primary gamma peak to the selected voltage and gain settings. The fine gain is a variable-type control, whereas the coarse gain is usually a stepped-type control.
4. Gain controls are sometimes on the back of the instrument.
5. Note on step 16 under Procedure that *if the system is linear between ranges,* approximately the same windows and voltage can be used for ^{125}I, ^{197}Hg, and ^{99m}Tc. Only gain has to be changed. It is understood, however, that the size of the window will change with respect to the change in gain.
6. In determining the proper windows for ^{125}I and ^{197}Hg, one is advised to use a 20-unit window, regardless of the value in kiloelectron volt units. The result is a much better defined gamma peak.
7. The manipulation of gain and voltage can be used to advantage when lower energy radionuclides are being counted in the presence of "after photomultiplier tube" noise, such as in electronic noise from the cable. Because it falls into the lower portion of the energy spectrum, it often interferes in the accurate counting of ^{125}I. In this case, it is often possible to separate the noise from the primary energy peak of ^{125}I by increasing the voltage and decreasing the gain. The increased voltage amplifies the pulses from the photomultiplier tube while the decreased gain reduces the pulses from any electronic component after the photomultiplier tube.

*Refer to instrument instruction manual.

BIBLIOGRAPHY

Bogardus, C.R., Jr.: Clinical applications of physics of radiology and nuclear medicine, St. Louis, 1969, Warren H. Green, Inc.

Chandra, R.: Introductory physics of nuclear medicine, ed. 4, Philadelphia, 1992, Lea & Febiger.

Chase, G.D., and Rabinowitz, J.L.: Principles of radioisotope methodology, ed. 3, Minneapolis, 1967, Burgess Publishing Co.

Goodwin, P.N., and Rao, D.V.: An introduction to the physics of nuclear medicine, Springfield, Ill., 1977, Charles C Thomas, Publisher.

Goodwin, P.N.: Recent developments in instrumentation for emission tomography, Sem. Nucl. Med. 10(4):322-334, Oct. 1980.

Gottschalk, A., and Potchen, E.J.: Diagnostic nuclear medicine, Baltimore, 1976, The Williams & Wilkins Co.

Greer, K.L., Jaszczak, R.J., and Coleman, R.E.: An overview of a camera-based SPECT system, Med. Phys. 9(4), July/Aug. 1982.

Hendee, W.R.: Medical radiation physics, ed. 2, Chicago, 1979, Mosby–Year Book.

Hine, G.J.: Instrumentation in nuclear medicine, vol. 1, New York, 1967, Academic Press, Inc.

Hine, G.J., and Sorenson, J.A.: Instrumentation in nuclear medicine, vol. 2, New York, 1974, Academic Press, Inc.

Johns, H.E. and Cunningham, J.R.: The physics of radiology, ed. 4, rev. ed., Springfield, Ill., 1983, Charles C Thomas, Publisher.

Quimby, E.H. and Feitelberg, S.: Radioactive isotopes in medicine and biology, ed. 2, Philadelphia, 1963, Lea & Febiger.

Rhodes, B.A.: Quality control in nuclear medicine, St. Louis, 1977, Mosby–Year Book.

Rocha, A.F.G. and Harbert, J.C.: Textbook of nuclear medicine: basic science, Philadelphia, 1978, Lea & Febiger.

Rollo, F.D.: Nuclear medicine physics, instrumentation, and agents, St. Louis, 1977, Mosby–Year Book.

Shilling, C.W.: Atomic energy encyclopedia in the life sciences, Philadelphia, 1964, W.B. Saunders Co.

Sorenson, J.A. and Phelps, M.E.: Physics in nuclear medicine, ed. 2, New York, 1987, Grune & Stratton, Inc.

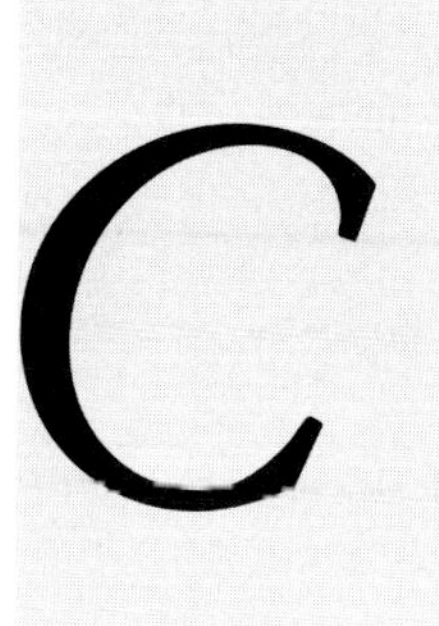

Chapter 11

ONSIDERATIONS OF COUNTING AND IMAGING

PAUL J. EARLY
WILLIAM H. MILLER

The detection and subsequent count rate obtained from a radioactive source is governed by many factors. These factors include the operating voltage, resolving time, geometry, scatter, energy resolution, absorption, background, efficiency of counting, collimation, and statistics. All of these factors depend on the detector itself, the counter, the source of radiation, and the material surrounding the source.

■ OPERATING VOLTAGE

The count rate obtained from a given source with a Geiger or scintillation detector is highly dependent on the voltage applied to the detector. This has already been discussed at great length, and in this chapter it is assumed that the proper operating voltage has been determined.

■ RESOLVING TIME

Every counting system, whether ionization or crystal, requires a certain recovery period after the detection of a pulse before the system is capable of counting a second pulse. In the discussion of Geiger-Mueller (G-M) tubes it is stated that after an ionization event the electrons travel quickly to the anode, but the positive ions travel at a much slower rate to the cathode. During the travel time of the positive ions, no other ionization events are seen by the detector. This description of a G-M counter helps to distinguish the fine differences between dead time, resolving time, and recovery time. The time period during which ions are traveling to their respective poles and during which therefore no pulse of any kind can be generated is called *dead time*. The time period during which sufficient numbers of gas atoms have recombined and therefore partially restored the gas (at least sufficiently to record an event) is called *resolving time*. The time period required for all atoms to recombine and therefore the detector to return to its full potential (actually, potential difference) is *recovery time*.

Scintillation detectors have resolving times from 10^{-6} to 10^{-7} seconds, and the scaler has a resolving time of 10^{-5} seconds. In the case of a scintillation crystal, it is often the scaler that is the limiting component in the system, rather than the detector.

As a result of the phenomenon of dead time, the observed counting rate is always less than the true counting rate (see Laboratory Application 8). There is a certain probability that one or more pulses follow a detected event within the interval of the resolving time and are not counted. As the counting rate increases or the resolving time increases, this probability becomes greater. If the counting rate and resolving time are known, the number of events that are lost can be predicted, and the observed counting rate can be corrected (see Laboratory Application 18).

In these days of high count-rate imaging techniques, the way that these systems handle this problem of resolving time becomes important. Some early G-M counters and scintillation cameras were such that if the count rate was high, the events would be recorded for awhile, then the system would shut down and no events would be recorded. This was disastrous for a cardiac flow study. The reason for this phenomenon was that the events were being seen by the detector, but the associated electronic component was not having sufficient time to recover from each recording. If the system cannot recover from one event, it cannot record another. These systems are said to be *paralyzable*.

These paralyzable systems are such that each event resets the recovery process before it has had sufficient time to recover to the point that another event can be recorded. With no events being recorded, the system shuts down. Advanced electronics in cameras and self-quenching G-M survey meters have improved this situation. They allow the recording of only those events that occur after the system has had sufficient time to recover. These systems are called *nonparalyzable*. In these systems, if the count rate exceeds the saturation point of the system, there will be a reduction in count rate/unit activity but not a shutdown of the system.

■ GEOMETRY

The geometric relationship between source and counter has a profound influence on the count rate obtained for a given activity. The count rate is particularly sensitive to the size and shape of the source and detector and to the distance between the source and detector.

The inverse square law (discussed in detail in Chapter 6 has a profound influence on count rate. Using a point source, the counting rate is decreased by one fourth if the distance is doubled; it is increased by a factor of 4 if the distance is halved. In the case of a source of activity that is not a point source, this relationship does not hold exactly, but the relationship between count rate and distance is still profound.

This principle is important in routine nuclear medicine procedures such as the thyroid uptake study and the renogram. For instance, an uptake study that does not use the same distance between detector and thyroid as between the detector and the standard represents a gross change in count rate, and therefore the results are erroneous.

Perhaps the greatest disregard for proper geometry considerations is not in the correct use of a probe but in counting samples in a well detector. Distance and inverse square are not so readily recognized in this type of detection procedure. A common problem is comparing the counts from a 4-ml standard to a 2-ml unknown, where it is possible to collect only 2 ml of serum. To obtain a correct count, the *geometry must be identical,* unless a correction factor is known. This means that the technologist cannot compare the two samples by counting the 2-ml sample and multiplying by 2. The 2-ml sample must be diluted with an activity-free solution to 4 ml, then the count multiplied by 2, since more of the emissions from the 2-ml sample are being exposed to the detector than from the 4-ml sample (Fig. 11-1). The gray area in Fig. 11-1 represents percentage of counts that are not exposed to the detector from the 4-ml sample but are exposed from the 2-ml sample. Since more of the emissions are allowed to go undetected by the 4-ml sample, the count could not be accurately compared to a 2-ml count (see Laboratory Application 19).

The size and shape of the detector also influence the count rate. For example, some counters, called 4π counters, completely surround the source and are geometrically able to count all radiations emitted. Two π counters detect only 50% of the radiation emitted, because they surround only half of the source. Probe-type detectors count only a small fraction of the emitted radiations, and well-type detectors, by partially surrounding the source, can detect 50% or more.

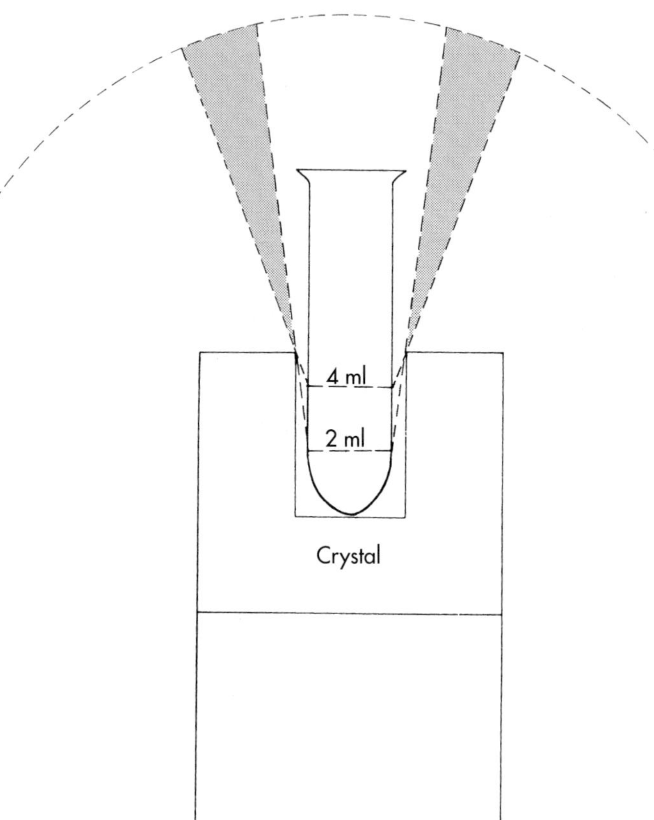

Fig. 11-1. Diagram illustrating the importance of geometry considerations in well counting. A 2-ml sample has greater than one half the count rate of a 4-ml sample of the same material because a greater number of photons go undetected (gray area) from the 4-ml specimen.

■ SCATTER

Scatter is the term applied to radiation that is diverted from its original path by some type of collision. Radiation is emitted in all directions from its source. Those radiations emitted directly toward the detector may be counted. Those radiations emitted in any direction other than into the detector may be deflected in such a way that they eventually strike the detector and also are counted. Since a collision of some kind is necessary, these emissions are reduced in energy. Barring pulse-height analysis, this type of scatter would *increase* the count rate. The degree of scatter is influenced by the atomic number and the thickness of the backing material. Scatter increases as either of these factors increases. Beta particles can be deflected by heavy nuclei through angles greater than 90 degrees and therefore can increase the count rate. Gamma ray back-scatter is caused either by Compton collision, resulting in a photon of lower energy traveling in a different direction from the primary gamma, or by pair production, wherein two 0.511 MeV photons are ultimately produced. This scatter phenomenon is extremely important in understanding the principles of collimators. Scatter can reduce the count rate if it occurs in the material between the source and detector when gamma rays or charged particles are deflected out of the beam.

■ ENERGY RESOLUTION

Theoretically, since all gamma rays emitted from a monoenergetic gamma-emitting radionuclide such as ^{137}Cs have exactly the same energy, all pulses resulting from their detection would have the same amplitude. Furthermore, having the same amplitude, they should appear at exactly the same point on a gamma spectrum. As has been seen in the section entitled "Gamma spectrum" in Chapter 10 and Laboratory Application 10, this is not true. The display of gamma photons on a gamma spectrum resembles more a bell-shaped curve, representing gamma photons of many energies, than a "spike," representing gamma photons of a single energy. Although a spike is what should be displayed, this could happen only if the entire system of scintillation detection were perfect. Such is not the case. *Apparent* increases and decreases in pulse amplitude occur as a result of incomplete gamma absorptions in the crystal, losses of light intensity during crystal transmission, nonproportional release of electrons at the photocathode, infidelity of electron multiplication at the dynodes, and imperfections in the linearity of pulses in the amplifier. Defects in any of these components causes a widening in this bell-shaped curve, an undesirable effect that, if serious enough, is incompatible with continued use. *Resolution* is the term describing the limitations of such a spread of the primary photopeak. It is calculated as the ratio of the width of a photopeak (measured at a point equal to one-half the amplitude of the peak) to its energy. This value varies depending on the energy of the radionuclide (see Laboratory Application 11).

■ ABSORPTION

Absorption of radiation differs from scatter in that the total energy of the radiation is dissipated in the absorbing material. Three sites of absorption exist in any counting situation: the source itself, the media between the source and detector, and the detector. All influence the resultant count rate.

Absorption occurring in the source, called *self-absorption,* reduces the count rate. This can be significant in particle counting. In some cases self-absorption limits the number of counts that can be detected from a source material. As more radioactive material is added, it absorbs as many radiations as it emits. Gamma ray detection does not usually involve problems with self-absorption. However, if the gamma ray energy is less than 0.1 MeV or if the source is large, such as a human body or an organ, then self-absorption must be considered.

Absorption of radiation occurring in the media between the source and detector also reduces the count rate. An example would be the air and the window of the detector in beta or alpha particle detection. For gamma ray detection it is usually unnecessary to take into account those gamma rays absorbed by the air or the detector window. However, a material of high density may absorb many of the gamma rays.

The final site of absorption occurs in the detecting medium. The detection of radiation depends on the absorption or transfer of energy from the radiations to the detector. Particulate radiations in general are absorbed by the detector if they have sufficient energy to penetrate the detecting medium. Therefore precautions must be taken to prevent the particles from being absorbed before they reach the sensitive volume of the detector. This is the rationale behind liquid scintillation counting. With gamma rays the problem is different. It is possible for a gamma ray to travel through a detector without interacting with complete absorption and therefore, using correct pulse-height analysis, go undetected. The chance of this happening decreases as the mass or the density of the detector increases. Therefore gaseous detectors such as Geiger tubes stop only a few gamma rays, whereas scintillation detectors stop many more gamma rays.

■ BACKGROUND

All counters record some activity with a source present. This activity is known as *room background activity.* It is caused by radiation from natural radionuclides and cosmic rays entering the detector and by instrument noise. The *gross count* of a source also includes background counts. Thus to obtain the *net count* from the source alone, the background count rate must be determined and subtracted from the gross count rate.

Many times the room background activity does not represent a significant change in the count, in which case it is a waste of time to consider it at all. In most of the recently developed instruments, background count rate never exceeds 100 counts/minute. Generally, any background count less than the square root of the total count can be disregarded because it does not introduce a significant amount of error into the procedure. For example, if the count rate were 10,000 cpm, a background count rate less than 100 dpm would be considered insignificant ($\sqrt{10,000} = 100$).

The primary purpose of a background determination is assurance that the instrument is operating properly. A room background count is performed *each day of use* by determining the proper operating voltage and allowing the unit to count for a predetermined unit of time without a source of activity near or in the detector. Background counts should be taken in the approximate clinical situation. For instance, the background count for the thyroid uptake probe should be taken with the probe pointing in the same direction as it would if it were being used for a patient count; the room background count of a well detector should be taken with the lid closed if this is the way it is being used with patient samples, or with the lid of the well open if the clinical use of the unit dictates this procedure.

EFFICIENCY OF COUNTING

The factors just discussed are all a part of counting efficiency. The efficiency of any system is loosely defined as that which is obtained from the system divided by that which is put into the system. It can also be expressed as a formula:

$$\text{Efficiency} = \frac{\text{Counts/unit time}}{\text{Disintegrations/unit time} \times \text{Mean number/disintegration}} \times 100$$

To determine the efficiency of a well counter, it is possible to purchase a calibrated solution (^{131}I, for example) in which the disintegrations per second are known. For example, 1.0 μCi (0.037 MBq) of a calibrated solution of ^{131}I can be used to determine the efficiency of counting. A microcurie has already been defined as 2.22×10^6 dpm, but this sample has been counted using the 364 keV gamma, which is 83.8% abundant, and determined to be only 222,000 (2.22×10^5) cpm. The efficiency can be determined as follows:

$$\text{Efficiency} = \frac{2.22 \times 10^5}{2.22 \times 10^6 \times 0.838} \times 100 = 11.9\%$$

This result would indicate that the unit is capable of counting only 11.9% of all disintegrations and therefore is only 11.9% efficient. The measurement of any radionuclide in a biologic sample need not be determined for its absolute value of disintegrations per unit time. In a routine nuclear medicine department the only concern is usually for relative values—the relative comparison of the activity in one sample with the relative value of the activity in another sample. The physician need not have the absolute value to make a valid diagnosis (see Laboratory application 17). However, absolute values are necessary in some areas of a good health physics program. The Nuclear Regulatory Commission states that a proper action level for decontamination of ^{131}I is when removable contamination reaches 200 net dpm/100 cm^2 or greater. To convert counts per minute (cpm) to disintegrations per minute (dpm), efficiency factors must be determined.

Coincidence counting

Once efficiency has been established for a certain set of circumstances, this percentile remains fairly constant as long as these parameters do not change or until some major repair is indicated on the detector-readout assembly. There is one exception to this statement, however. It is possible to exceed the capabilities of the detection system by increasing the radioactivity in the source being counted. Count rates may continue to increase with each subsequent increase in radioactivity but not in proportion to the increase in activity (see Laboratory Application 18, Part I). This phenomenon may better be explained by simply stating that two highly radioactive but equal sources placed simultaneously near a scintillation crystal result in a count rate less than both samples placed in identical geometrics but counted separately and then summed. The reason is that as the radioactivity increases, the probability of simultaneous gamma interactions in the crystal increases. When this occurs, a coincident pulse is registered as only one event by the recorder, or if the magnitude of the coincidence pulse height exceeds the upper-level discriminator setting, there is no registry of the interaction at all. As a result, the efficiency of the scintillation detector decreases as the activity increases. In fact, at the point where coincidence loss begins, a second energy peak of twice the energy of the incident photons begins to develop and continues to build as activity increases. As suggested, 2 primary energy photons interacting with the scintillation crystal at the same time are being seen as 1 photon of twice the energy (for example, ^{99m}Tc at 140 keV also have a second peak at 280 keV) (see Laboratory Application 18, Part II). In fact, if the increases in activity continue, the actual count rate will also decrease. In some of the older paralyzable type imaging systems this would result in complete electronic shutdown of the instrument. In most of the new nonparalyzable types of imaging systems this point is reached with significant loss in resolution. Therefore it is important to know these capabilities of the equipment and not the exceed them.

COLLIMATION

Electromagnetic radiation of longer wavelengths, such as light, can be focused by bending rays through lenses or by reflection from polished surfaces. Electromagnetic radiations of shorter wavelengths, however, do not respond to such mechanical manipulations. The only way a gamma ray can be removed from its path is by absorption or scatter of the ray. Therefore a device must be used that can eliminate from detection all gamma rays except those of interest. This device is called a *collimator*. The collimator is generally constructed of lead and extends in front of the scintillation detector. The lead is arranged in a configuration that allows it to perform the desired function. In the usual nuclear medicine laboratory two types of collimators are used, the flat-field collimator (a modification is the straight-bore collimator) and the multihole collimator. There are three types of multihole collimators: parallel-hole, diverging, and converging (focused). Each of these types of collimators has different characteristics, since each is used for a different purpose. In addition, there are pinhole collimators.

Perhaps the most informative method of demonstrating the characteristics of these collimators is by the use of isocount lines (Fig. 11-2).

Flat-field collimators

In the event that a whole organ such as a thyroid or kidney is to be seen by the detector, the collimators must be designed to eliminate not only a portion of the background radiation but also radiation coming from other parts of the patient's body. The collimator chosen for this use must be able to detect radiations coming from any part of the organ

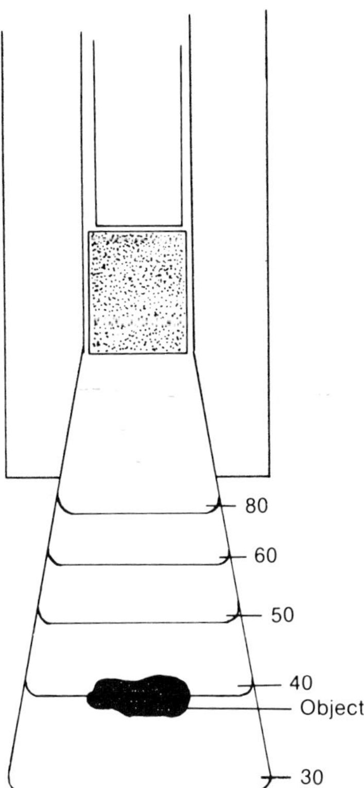

Fig. 11-2. Flat-field collimator whose characteristic is demonstrated by construction of isocount lines, indicating uniform "vision" through organ under investigation.

of interest. A flat-field collimator would be used, since a flat response is received at a certain distance from the face of the collimator (Fig. 11-2). In Fig. 11-2 the isocount (same count) or isoresponse is demonstrated as having a flat portion, which increases in diameter as the distance from the face of the collimator is increased. A point source lying anywhere along such a line would result in the same number of counts. A line drawn directly across the face of the collimator with the point source centrally placed would represent 100%, the maximum count detectable. The same source located anywhere on the 80% isocount line would give a count equal to 80% of the maximum count (see Laboratory Application 21).

When the collimator is used to visualize a whole organ, the distance that the collimator is placed away from the organ must be great enough to enable the detector to see the whole organ and to have a relatively uniform sensitivity to the entire organ. The flat-field collimator serves the uniform sensitivity criterion well because of its flat response. The distance required to see the entire organ depends on the collimator and the diameter of the detector. For example, a 1½-inch diameter detector requires a 36-degree collimator to include a large thyroid at a distance of 20 cm. At a distance of 35 cm the same detector requires a 20-degree collimator.

■ Straight-bore collimator

In other nuclear medicine applications it is more desirable not to view the entire organ as a whole but to study particular segments of an organ independently from the rest of it. This requires a detector that views only a small area at a time—a special collimator.

The collimator used to view small areas of an organ is one that can also distinguish between small areas of differing count rates. Such a collimator is rated by *resolution*. Resolution is the minimum distance between two radioactive objects that can still be distinguished as two distinct sources by the collimator. The degree of resolution varies with the physical design and material of the collimator, as well as with the energy of the gamma rays being counted. A collimator is chosen according to the requirements of a specific application. In general, a collimator with good resolution should be used for studies of small organs, and a collimator with poorer resolution can be used for larger organs.

One of the first collimators used for viewing small areas of an organ was the straight-bore collimator (Fig. 11-3), which is nothing more than a large piece of lead with a small hole bored through it. The piece of lead is attached to the face of the scintillation detector. The resolution of the collimator is influenced by the diameter and the length of the hole; the smaller the bore and the longer the collimator, the greater its resolution. Figure 11-3 displays in a simple manner the effect of collimator length and bore size to resolution. All radiations emitted in the direction of the crystal and within the dotted lines are detected in their pure energy state. Both detectors are aimed at two ⅝-inch areas of activity situated ⅝ inch apart and at a depth of 3 inches from the face of the collimator. The first detector, which has a shorter collimator with a larger bore size, is unable to differentiate between the two lesions because the *solid angle of inclusion* encompasses both lesions. This detector would have poor resolution. The second detector has a collimator that is increased in length and decreased in bore size. The same two areas of activity, situated identically in respect to each other and to the collimator, are resolved as the detector unit passes over them. Emissions from the two areas of activity are not detected in their pure energy state if the detector is situated as depicted. As the detector moves to the right or to the left, pure emissions are seen only from the right or left areas of activity, respectively. Resolution is then greatly enhanced, and the system could be expressed as having a resolution of ⅝ inch. Another important fact regarding resolution is that as resolution increases, sensitivity suffers. The collimator sees fewer and fewer events as resolution increases.

These principles of resolution are basic to understanding the influencing factors of any collimator, be it single-bore, focused, or parallel-hole. These principles are easy to understand in the straight-bore collimator, but they often seem more complex when extended to the multibore or multichannel type collimator. However, there is no differ-

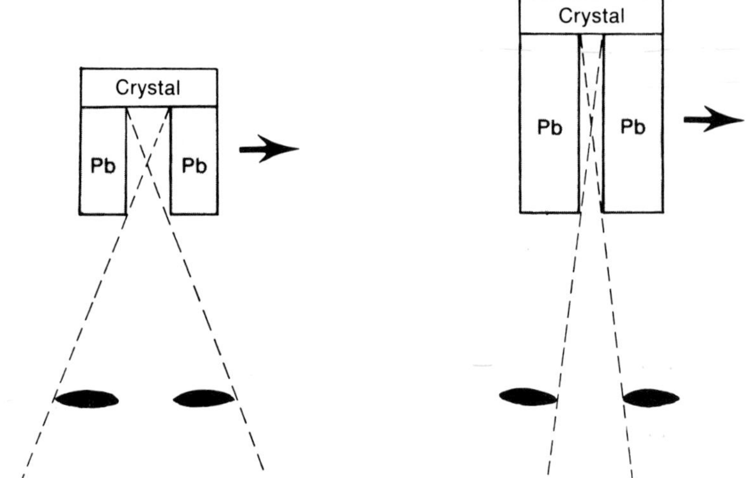

Fig. 11-3. Straight-bore (single-hole, single-channel) collimator illustrating effects of size and depth of hole on resolution. Dotted lines indicate the solid angle of inclusion. These same limits are analogous to penumbral limit lines in radiation therapy.

ence. The principles are the same, only the number of holes has changed.

■ Multihole collimators

Characteristics. The *number of holes* in a collimator is determined by the crystal size of the detector and the required septal thickness. In general, it can be stated that the number of holes for any given size crystal increases as the resolution increases. A decrease in number of holes suggests either nonuse of the entire crystal, larger holes, or thicker septa.

There are both low-energy collimators and medium-energy collimators available today. As gamma rays increase in energy, the ability of the collimator to absorb or deflect them becomes less. Medium-energy gamma rays require greater septal thickness than do low-energy gamma rays. This reduces sensitivity because the greater the thickness of lead, the smaller the area of crystal used. Consequently, two types of collimators are available based solely on their septal thicknesses: (1) a low-energy collimator, which is designed for all radionuclides having gamma energies less than 150 keV, and (2) a medium-energy collimator for all radionuclides having energies greater than 150 keV and less than 300 keV. Medium-energy collimators can be used for imaging an organ containing a low-energy radionuclide, but the reverse is not true. Sensitivity is much less with the medium-energy collimator and a low-energy radionuclide than with a low-energy collimator and a low-energy radionuclide.

Parallel-hole collimators. A multichannel parallel-hole collimator, as is used in a stationary imaging device (camera), consists of a lead plate with thousands of channels parallel to one another. Each channel accepts only vertically oriented gamma rays from one specific area. A gamma-ray image of the subject is then projected onto the scintillation crystal detector.

With normal use of this collimator, the subject is positioned as close as possible to the face of the collimator. The reason for this practice is that the resolution of the collimator, termed *extrinsic resolution,* is best for organs or parts of organs closest to the collimator. Sensitivity is not a factor. Resolution decreases with increasing distance from the collimator for the reasons depicted in Fig. 11-4. It is curious that with parallel-hole collimators there is only little loss in count rate as the organ is moved farther away from the face of the collimator. This curiosity can be explained by the fact that although radioactivity *decreases* by the inverse square of the distance, the area "seen" by each individual hole *increases* by approximately the square of the distance. These two opposing phenomena tend to cancel each other out, resulting in only a slight loss in sensitivity with increased distance.

The factors affecting resolution in parallel-hole collimators are exactly the same as those affecting resolution in all collimators, that is, the length and size of the hole. The technologist only has to be sure to have the patient as close to the face of the collimator as possible (Fig. 11-5).

Diverging collimators. Scintillation camera systems that have 9- or 10-inch effective viewing areas present a problem for many patients requiring pulmonary studies or studies in which it is desirable for both liver and spleen to be viewed on the same image. The problem is that many patients are larger than the 9- to 10-inch effective crystal area. The problem can be resolved by going to a larger crystal camera or by the use of diverging collimator (Fig. 11-6). This collimator is the opposite of focused collimators

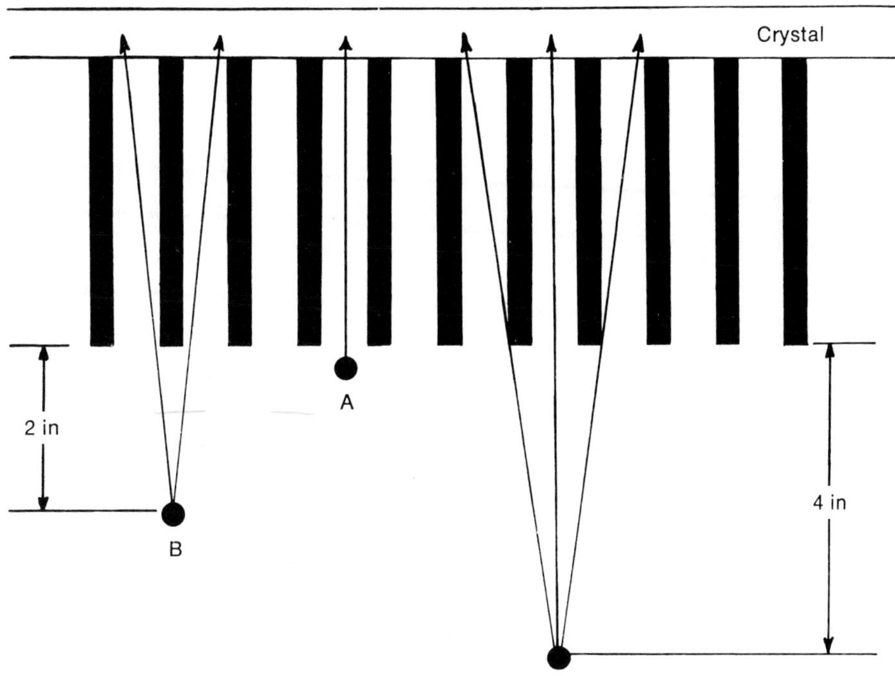

Fig. 11-4. Parallel-hole collimator illustrating loss of resolution with depth.

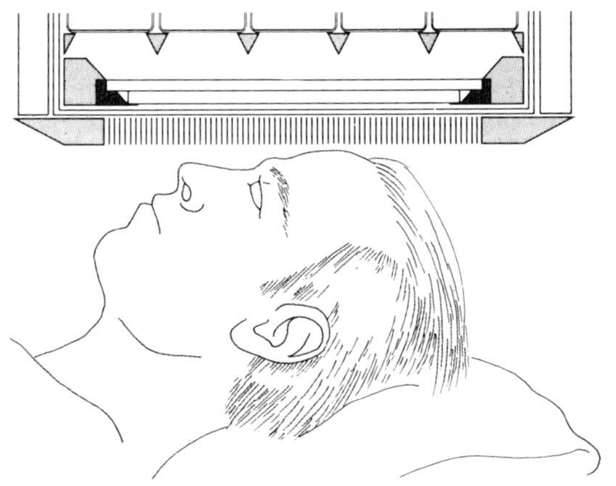

Fig. 11-5. Multichannel parallel-hole collimators as used with brain images. (From Anger, H.O.: In Wagner, H.M., Jr., editor: Nuclear medicine, New York, 1975, HP Publishing Co. Originally published in *Hospital Practice*.)

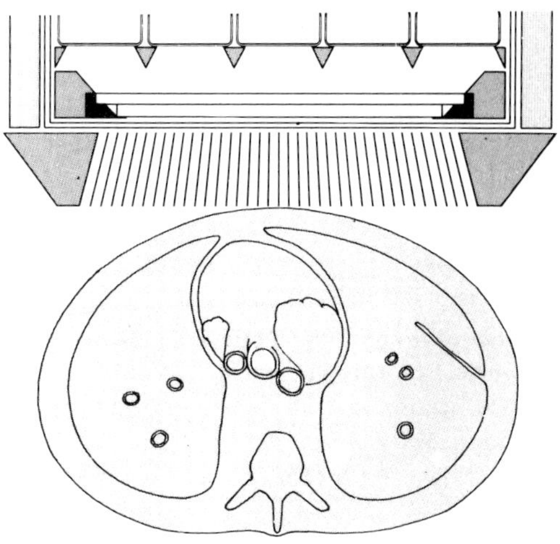

Fig. 11-6. Multichannel diverging collimator as used with lung images. (From Anger, H.O.: In Wagner, H.M., Jr., editor: Nuclear medicine, New York, 1975, HP Publishing Co. Originally published in *Hospital Practice*.)

as used in rectilinear scanners, in that the center hole is perpendicular to the crystal and the holes begin to diverge at an increasingly greater angle. In this way a greater field of view is possible. Unlike parallel-hole collimators, the image gets smaller as its distance increases from the face of the collimator. Furthermore, the resolution decreases at a more rapid rate as the organ moves away from the detector. It is apparent by the construction of the diverging collimator that the center of the collimator has the best resolution with depth because it approximates the parallel-hole collimator. Furthermore, the resolution of the crystal itself (termed *intrinsic resolution*) is better in the center; there-

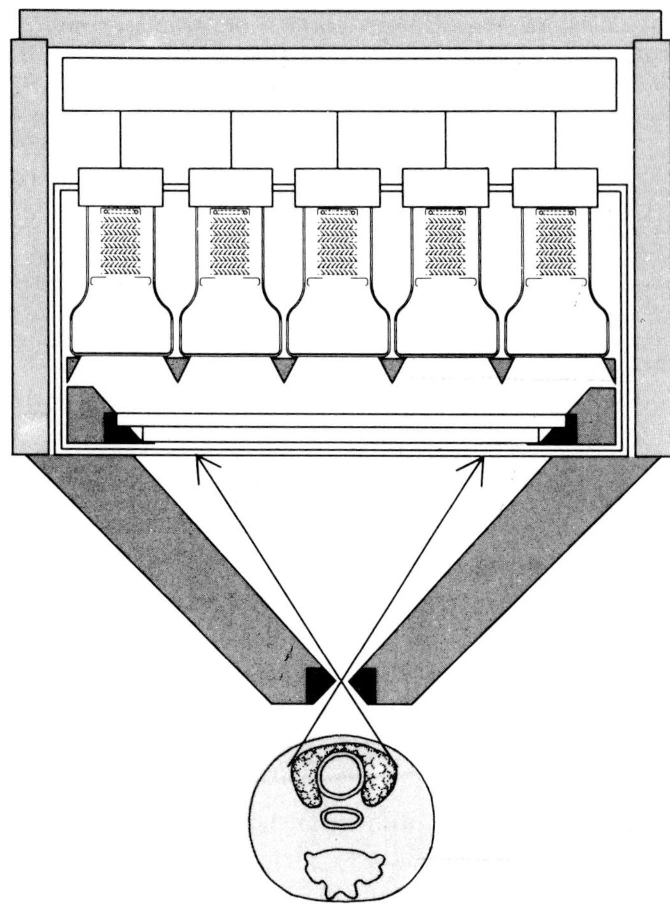

Fig. 11-7. Pinhole collimator as used with thyroid images. (From Anger, H.O.: In Wagner, H.M., Jr., editor: Nuclear medicine, New York, 1975, HP Publishing Co. Originally published in *Hospital Practice*.)

fore the total resolution of the camera is better in the center. (This fact is useful with camera systems larger than 11 to 13 inches, where for better resolution the image can be visualized by using only the center section of the system.) Both intrinsic and extrinsic resolution (and therefore total resolution) deteriorate as information gets farther and farther away from the center of the crystal.

Converging collimators. Some manufacturers of diverging collimators have arranged it so that this collimator can be reversed to create a converging collimator. When the collimator is inverted, it takes on the resemblance of a focused collimator. On a scintillation camera, however, it is used to magnify and increase the resolution of small objects, as does the pinhole collimator (Fig. 11-7). The converging collimator solves the problems of the diverging collimator: poor intrinsic and extrinsic resolution away from the center of the crystal. The inversion of the diverging collimator to create a converging collimator allows the technologist to restrict information to the center of the crystal, thereby enhancing intrinsic resolution, and to use the tapered hole to its best advantage, increasing extrinsic resolution. This collimator has been used to advantage for imaging of the thyroid, imaging of posterior fossa tumors, and pediatric studies.

■ Pinhole collimator

The pinhole collimator operates on the old-fashioned box camera principle (Fig. 11-7). It consists of a single small aperture at the end of a lead shield. The collimator is so designed that x rays entering at any angle through the pinhole are seen by the scintillation detector. This is unlike the single-bore collimator, in which the gamma ray must enter at an angle perpendicular to the face of the crystal to be detected. This principle does not involve the refraction and convergence of rays; therefore focusing is not a problem. Regardless of its distance from the camera, a source appears on the image with as much sharpness as the aperture size and the distances involved permit. It is also apparent that when the distance of the subject to the pinhole is equal to that of the pinhole to the detector, a 1:1 relationship of size exists. When the subject is moved farther from the pinhole, a reduction of size occurs; and when the subject is moved closer, magnification occurs. In a comparison of a pinhole collimator to a converging collimator, the pinhole collimator provides the best resolution for small subjects positioned a short distance from the aperture; however, the pinhole collimator does this at the expense of sensitivity. The converging collimator has greater sensitivity. Pinhole collimators have been used to take pictures of large organs but much less effectively. This is accomplished by positioning the subject at great distances from the aperture. This principle has been used for entire lung fields, liver imaging, and so on. Pinhole collimators have greater resolution than do parallel-hole collimators, but sensitivity is decreased. Another disadvantage of the pinhole collimator is that it falls off in efficiency at the edges of the image.

■ STATISTICS

When a source of radioactivity is designated as having a certain activity, it is in effect designated as having a certain number of disintegrations per unit time taking place, since units of activity are defined as the number of disintegrations per unit time (Table 4-1). When such a source is designated as having a certain number of disintegrations per unit time, it is only an average, not a constantly reproducible number. The disintegration of a radioactive atom is a *random* event; therefore the number of disintegrations is a random variable. It is impossible to predict exactly which atom is going to decay next and exactly how many will disintegrate per unit time; it is possible only to determine an average.

For this reason a basic knowledge of statistics is indispensable to the technologist and the physician for correct use of radionuclides and interpretation of the results of counting or imaging procedures. The physician must use statistical knowledge in evaluating the precision and accuracy* of the counting data. Decisions must be made as to the number of counts to be accumulated (preset count) or the time necessary to accumulate a certain number of counts (preset time), the minimum dose that should be administered, and the travel speed of a rectilinear imaging device. The likelihood that a difference between counts of two different samples or two different areas on an organ image represents a significant difference rather than the random variability between two identical samples or areas must also be determined.

This discussion of statistics treats the statistics of sample counting and imaging as two separate entities because they are not easily related to one another. However, in both cases the number of events recorded (counts) must be *adequate* to be certain that major differences in the results are not a function of poor statistics.

■ Statistics of sample counting

Since the number of disintegrations per unit time is a variable, it is to be expected that the counts from the same sample for the same period of time will not be identical. In fact, they can vary considerably, depending on the number of counts accumulated. *As the number of counts increases, the variation between subsequent counts on the same sample also increases, but the percent error between subsequent counts decreases.*

An explanation of this statement requires a discussion of the Poisson distribution principle. This principle, applicable to the observation of random events, states that the standard deviation is proportional to the square root of the number of observed events. This can be expressed as a formula as follows:

$$\sigma = \sqrt{N}$$

σ = Standard deviation or standard error
N = Number of observed events (counts)

If the number of counts is 100, one standard deviation is $\sqrt{100}$, or 10 counts. (The 100 counts is a quantity, not intensity. It makes no difference as to the length of time required to accumulate that 100 counts.) This is usually expressed as plus or minus one standard deviation, or ± 10 counts from the true count of 100. Furthermore, it is an accepted principle from the Poisson distribution that 68% of all counts fall within this range of 90 to 110 counts (Fig. 11-8). In other words, if a count were taken 100 times on a sample that emitted 100 counts, 68 of the counts would fall somewhere within a range of 90 to 110 counts, and 32 of those counts would fall outside that range. Another way of expressing this relationship is that if a sample were counted only long enough to accumulate 100 counts, the observer could be confident that 68% of the time (approximately two thirds of the time) that count would be within ± 10 counts.

Furthermore, if $1\sigma = \pm 10$ counts, then $2\sigma = \pm 20$ counts, and $3\sigma = \pm 30$ counts. The Poisson distribution principle also states that 95% of all counts fall within $\pm 2\sigma$, and 99% of all counts fall within $\pm 3\sigma$. In this case, 95 of the 100 counts would fall within a range of 80 to 120 counts, and only one of the counts would fall outside the range of 70 to 130 counts. Accordingly, the observer could be 95% confident that any count on a 100-count sample would be within ± 20 counts of the true value and 99% confident that it would be within ± 30 counts. These relationships are depicted in Fig. 11-8, in which $\pm 1\sigma$ is the 68% level, $\pm 2\sigma$ is the 95% confidence level, and $\pm 3\sigma$ is the 99% confidence level.

The value of the material just presented lies in the percent error that a certain number of counts is likely to intro-

*Precision and accuracy are two entirely different entities. A practiced rifleman can shoot a target four times in a row in almost the exact spot but outside the bull's-eye—precise but not accurate. Another rifleman may possess enough experience to have all four shots hit the bull's-eye—precise and accurate.

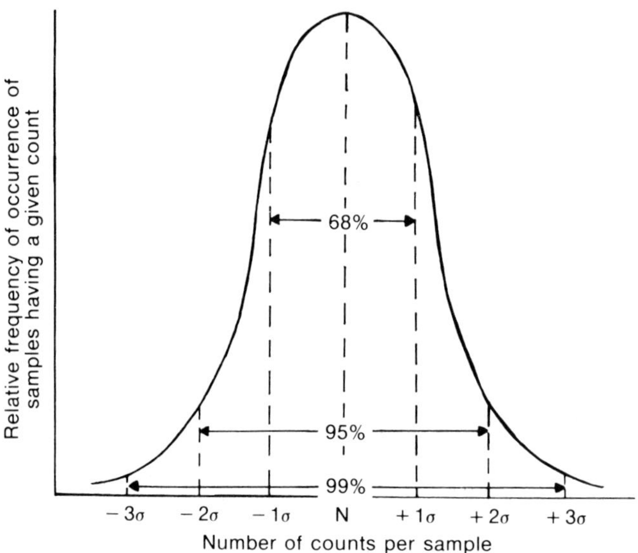

Fig. 11-8. Poisson distribution curve. Curve is plotted as number of counts per sample versus number of times that sample count occurs. In a series of 100 like samples (or the same sample counted 100 times), a 10,000-count sample would result in the largest percentage of counts having a value of 10,000 per predetermined time period. However, not all counts in this time period would be 10,000 because of the phenomenon of random decay. Some are larger, some smaller. The above figure predicts that 68 of the 100 counts will fall within $\pm$ 1σ (9,900 to 10,000), 95 within $\pm$ 2σ, and 99 within $\pm$ 3σ.

duce into the study. For instance, the 100 counts used in the example just given shows that the observer is only 68% sure that the count received is within ±10 counts of the true value. This is not many counts per se, but it represents a ±10% error. This is completely unacceptable as far as the results are concerned. To go to the higher confidence levels of 95% or 99% introduces an error of ±20% and ±30%, respectively, which is even worse.

To correct this problem and since the whole area of statistics is based on the number of counts, the situation could be helped by counting 1000 events instead of 100. In this situation, $\sigma = \sqrt{1000}$, or 32. Therefore 68% of all counts would be within a range of 968 to 1032, which represents an error of ±3.2%. By increasing the number of counts, the range has increased (from 20 to 64 for ±1σ), but the percent error has decreased. Furthermore, a count of 10,000 would present a standard deviation of ±100 but would represent a percent error of only ±1%. These relationships are summarized in Table 11-1 and the following:

50% of all counts fall within ±0.675σ
68.3% of all counts fall within ±1.0σ
90.0% of all counts fall within ±1.65σ
95.4% of all counts fall within ±2.00σ
99.7% of all counts fall within ±3.00σ
Probable error = ±0.675σ(50%)
Standard error = ±1.000σ(68.3%)
Reliable error = ±1.650σ(90%)

Table 11-1. Summary of relationship of counts to percent error

Number of counts	1 σ (68%)	Range	Percent error
100	± 10	90 to 110	±10.0
1,000	± 32	968 to 1,032	± 3.2
10,000	±100	9,900 to 10,100	± 1.0
100,000	±317	99,683 to 100,317	± 0.3

In routine nuclear medicine work the decision must be made by the observer as to how many counts must be accumulated to have reasonable confidence that the count is within an acceptable degree of error. A common solution to the problem is to accumulate enough counts that the observer is 95% confident that the count received is within ±2% error. Table 11-1 shows that a count of 10,000 represents a 68% chance of being within ±1% error. Since 2σ represents the 95% confidence level, the continuation of the table would read as follows:

Number of counts	2 σ (95%)	Range	Percent error
10,000	±200	9800 to 10,200	±2

Accordingly, if the operator accumulated 10,000 counts, he or she would be 95% certain that any such count would be within ±2% of the true value. These are reasonably good statistics for routine nuclear medicine procedures and provide the rationale behind the rule of thumb that *regardless of the time required, 10,000 counts should always be accumulated.*

The relationships between the number of counts and percent error, as related to the desired confidence level, can be expressed mathematically as follows:

$$\text{For 68\% confidence level } N = \frac{10{,}000}{V^2}$$

$$\text{For 95\% confidence level } N = \frac{40{,}000}{V^2}$$

$$\text{For 99\% confidence level } N = \frac{90{,}000}{V^2}$$

N = Number of counts
V = % error

The 68% confidence level is generally used for preliminary studies when an approximate statistical evaluation is warranted. The 95% confidence level is used for routine work, and the 99% confidence level is used for research work.

A research project might require the best statistics possible without sacrificing too much time in counting. This would generally mean a statistical accuracy of ±1% error 99% of the time (99% confidence level). The question of how many counts must be accumulated would be solved as follows:

$$N = \frac{90{,}000}{V^2} = \frac{90{,}000}{(1)^2} = \frac{90{,}000}{1} = 90{,}000 \text{ counts}$$

This formula could also be used to substantiate the 10,000 counts rule of thumb, which states that by accumulating 10,000 counts, the result has a 95% chance of being within ±2% of the true value. Using the 95% confidence level formula and substituting 2% for the percent error, the number of counts to be accumulated is as follows:

$$N = \frac{40{,}000}{V^2} = \frac{40{,}000}{(2)^2} = \frac{40{,}000}{4} = 10{,}000 \text{ counts}$$

In some studies, such as the Schilling test, it may take as long as 25 to 30 minutes to accumulate 10,000 counts.

Background counts must also be considered when making the final decision of how much time to allow for the count or how many counts must be accumulated for a statistically valid result. There are methods to mathematically calculate the background count value, but they are not practical to use. As mentioned previously, if the total count is at least the square of the background count, background need not be considered statistically (background must be considered when using net counts per minute). In most clinical situations the background is never that high. If it is, the background count is subtracted from the gross counts and counting is continued until 10,000 *net* counts are received.

■ Statistics of imaging

Statistics also play a major role in imaging techniques with stationary cameras. The importance of statistics in imaging techniques is similar to their importance in sample counting, since an adequate number of events must be recorded to be certain that the lack of a statistical count does not influence the results (diagnosis). The exact number of counts varies from the rule-of-thumb value of 10,000 used in sample counting. The purpose of stationary imaging is to detect and record a certain number of events for an entire organ.

In older instrumentation a predetermined number of counts (thousands or hundreds of thousands of counts) is agreed on before a study. Each type of organ study varies as to the number of counts necessary to be accumulated to effect a study of diagnostic value. In addition to the preceding, many new scintillation cameras now offer the capability of using information density (ID)* to ensure the acquisition of a statistically significant image. This new capability consists of a 1 cm^2 area of interest that can be moved to any portion of the image with a joystick. A number is then selected to represent the desired ID, and only those counts originating in that 1-cm^2 area are registered. The acquisition of image information automatically terminates when the proper ID is reached.

Three different parameters are of concern is establishing such a value: saturation effects, background cutoff, and dot size. The saturation effects come into play when two flashes of light occur at the same place. If the detection device has reached a state of saturation, the second event, which becomes superimposed on the first, is not displayed as a change in the intensity of the dot. Since under usual conditions the intensity would become brighter if two flashes occurred at the same place (suggesting a greater concentration in that area), information is lost if the saturation point has been reached.

Background erase (cutoff or suppression) also affects the image quality. This parameter is generally used to intentionally prevent recording from areas of an organ in which the concentrations of activity are no more than background level. This device is generally used to reduce the interpretive complications of background radiation. However, if the setting of the background erase is too high, more counts than desired are lost.

The size of the dot on the image is also important and is directly dependent on the set intensity, which is a function of the number of counts to be accumulated. As the accumulation increases, the intensity must be set lower; therefore the size of the dot decreases and vice versa. Small density differences in the dots become more difficult to detect if the dots are small with large spaces between them. Conversely, large dots result in the loss of resolution. Out-of-focus dots also result in loss of resolution.

*Usually expressed in counts per square centimeter.

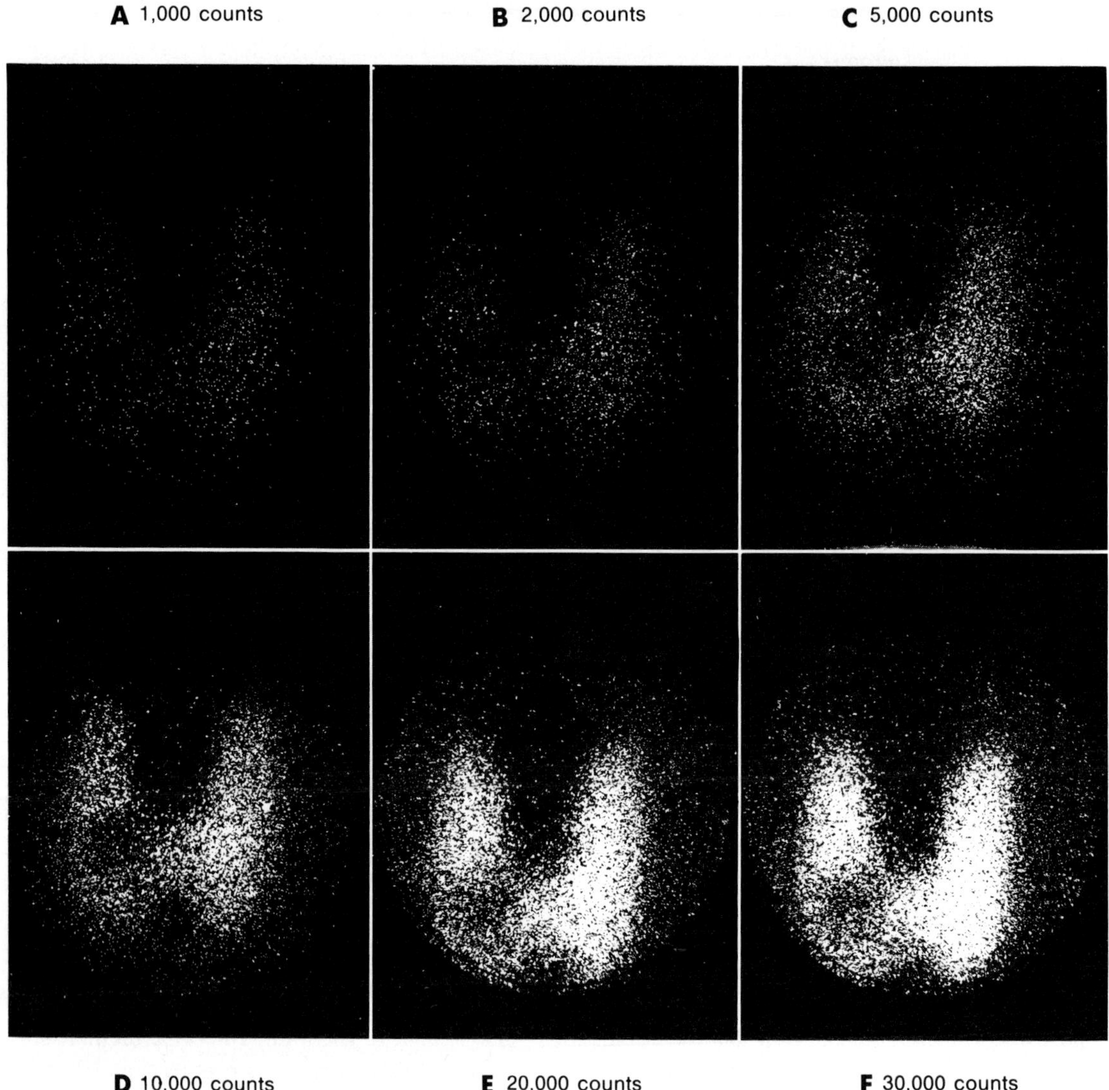

Fig. 11-9. Effect of statistics using a stationary imaging device. As the number of accumulated counts increases, the image becomes more formative, and diagnosis is easier. A point can be reached, as evidenced by views **E** and **F,** where too many counts are accumulated, the detection device becomes saturated, and information is lost.

These three factors must be taken into consideration when arriving at a statistical value. It has been stressed throughout this discussion of statistics that statistical accuracy increases with increased number of observed events. This is true only to a point with a stationary imaging device. Eventually, principles such as saturation and coincidence loss reduce the image quality and efficiency of detection, and as a result, the study suffers.

Figure 11-9 is a study with a thyroid phantom showing how too few or too many counts affect the image. Too few counts result in a poor image, if any at all. As the counts are increased, the quality of the image also increases. Eventually saturation occurs, and image quality is lost. This could be corrected by reducing the intensity.

■ Statistics of computers

Another dimension of statistics is how they apply to computers. Each pixel is only able to acquire a certain amount of information before it saturates and image information is lost. Conversely, if each pixel does not receive enough information, the study will suffer from a lack of statistical information. (See Chapter 12 for details.)

LABORATORY APPLICATION

15

STATISTICS

Purpose

The understanding and application of the principles of statistics have become some of the most important aspects of nuclear medicine. By the misuse of statistics, lesions can be eliminated, or they can be produced when there are none; a patient can be reported as abnormal when he or she is normal or vice versa. Almost any value or image can be produced because of a lack of good statistics.

The goal for good statistical information in sample counting is considered to be 10,000 counts. It makes no difference whether the sample is counted for 10 minutes or 1 minute as long as a total of 10,000 counts above background has been accumulated. The purpose of the first part of this laboratory application is to demonstrate the effects of statistics on percent error, confidence levels, and the Poisson distribution.

A procedure used to evaluate detector reliability from a statistical point of view is called the *chi-square test*. Its basis is the Poisson distribution. If all count rates fall within an expected deviation from a mean value (as evidenced in the first part of Laboratory Application 15), there should be some way to evaluate whether a limited number of count-rate values fall within an expected deviation from the mean. This would assure the radiation worker, without taking a large series of counts, of the probability that the individual variation of each of the measurements from their average value conforms to what is predicted by the laws of nuclear radiation statistics. This is the purpose of the chi-square test. Deviations outside the expected variation may indicate faulty performance of the equipment. The purpose of the second part of this laboratory application is to demonstrate this useful evaluation technique.

In the chi-square test several counts are taken for a predetermined amount of time, their means are found, and the squares of the differences of each individual count from that mean are added and then divided by the mean. It can be expressed mathematically as follows:

$$\chi^2 = \frac{\Sigma(\eta_i - \bar{\eta})^2}{\bar{\eta}}$$

η_i = Individual count rate values
$\bar{\eta}$ = Mean value of all counts

The distribution of chi-square is known, and values are given in Table 11-2 on p. 190.

The goal for good statistical information in scintillation cameras is at least an ID of 2000 events/cm^2. The purpose of the third and fourth parts of this laboratory application is to demonstrate the effects of statistics on imaging procedures.

Procedure

Materials

1. Well and scaler unit for the first and second parts of the exercise
2. Gamma camera for the third part of the exercise
3. 1 mCi (37 MBq) of ^{137}Cs
4. Thyroid phantom filled with 25 to 50 μCi (1-2 MBq) ^{131}I
5. Thyroid phantom filled with 1 to 2 mCi (37-74 MBq) ^{99m}Tc
6. Linear graph paper
7. Cylindrical phantom with "hot" and "cold" spots for the evaluation of SPECT performance parameters

Technique 1

1. Use the ^{137}Cs standard with its active end pointed away from the well; determine the approximate time required to count 100 counts. Using a preset count of 100, count 10 to 20 times, note the time, and use the average.
2. Using the time determined in step 1, count the sample 100 times, and record each count. Do not change any parameter. After recording each count, reset and count again.

Continued.

Table 11-2. Table of chi-square

Degrees of freedom* (N-1)	There is a probability of 0.99	0.95	0.90	0.50	0.10	0.05	0.01
	that the calculated value of chi-square will be equal to or greater than						
2	0.020	0.103	0.211	1.386	4.605	5.991	9.210
3	0.115	0.352	0.584	2.366	6.251	7.815	11.345
4	0.297	0.711	1.064	3.357	7.779	9.488	13.277
5	0.554	1.145	1.610	4.351	9.236	11.070	15.086
6	0.872	1.635	2.204	5.348	10.645	12.592	16.812
7	1.239	2.167	2.833	6.346	12.017	14.067	18.475
8	1.646	2.733	3.490	7.344	13.362	15.507	20.090
9	2.088	3.325	4.168	8.343	14.684	16.919	21.666
10	2.558	3.940	4.865	9.342	15.987	18.307	23.209
11	3.053	4.575	5.578	10.341	17.275	19.675	24.725
12	3.571	5.226	6.304	11.340	18.549	21.026	26.217
13	4.107	5.892	7.042	12.340	19.812	22.362	27.688
14	4.660	6.571	7.790	13.339	21.064	23.685	29.141
15	5.229	7.261	8.547	14.339	22.307	24.996	30.578
16	5.812	7.962	9.312	15.338	23.542	26.296	32.000
17	6.408	8.672	10.085	16.338	24.769	27.587	33.409
18	7.015	9.390	10.865	17.338	25.989	28.869	34.805
19	7.633	10.117	11.651	18.338	27.204	30.144	36.191
20	8.260	10.851	12.443	19.337	28.412	31.410	37.566
21	8.897	11.591	13.240	20.337	29.615	32.671	38.932
22	9.542	12.338	14.041	21.337	30.813	33.924	40.289
23	10.196	13.091	14.848	22.337	32.007	35.172	41.638
24	10.856	13.848	15.659	23.337	33.196	36.415	42.980
25	11.534	14.611	16.473	24.337	34.382	37.382	44.314
26	12.198	15.379	17.292	25.336	35.563	38.885	45.642
27	12.879	16.151	18.114	26.336	36.741	40.113	46.963
28	13.565	16.928	18.939	27.336	37.916	41.337	48.278
29	14.256	17.708	19.768	28.336	39.087	42.557	49.588

*The number of degrees of freedom is usually one less than the number of observations N.

Data treatment

1. Find the average (η). (Add all counts and divide by 100.) Assume this to be the true value.
2. What is the range for $\pm 1\sigma$, assuming $\sigma = \sqrt{\eta}$?
3. Determine the number of times the count fell in this range.
4. Does this correlate with the Poisson distribution?
5. What is the range for $\pm 2\sigma$?
6. Determine the number of times the count fell in this range.
7. Does this correlate with the Poisson distribution?
8. What is the range for $\pm 3\sigma$?
9. Determine the number of times the count fell in this range.
10. Does this correlate with the Poisson distribution?
11. Explain the reason for the variations between the percentile received (number of counts) and the percent confidence levels.
12. What was the lowest count?
13. What was the highest count?
14. Assume an unknown and a standard, both having the same count, as the value received in step 1. The unknown actually displayed the lowest number of counts (step 12), and the standard displayed the highest number of counts (step 13). What percentage of error or standard error (SE) was introduced into the study just because of randomness of decay?

$$SE = 100\frac{\theta}{\eta}$$

θ = Difference between highest and lowest count

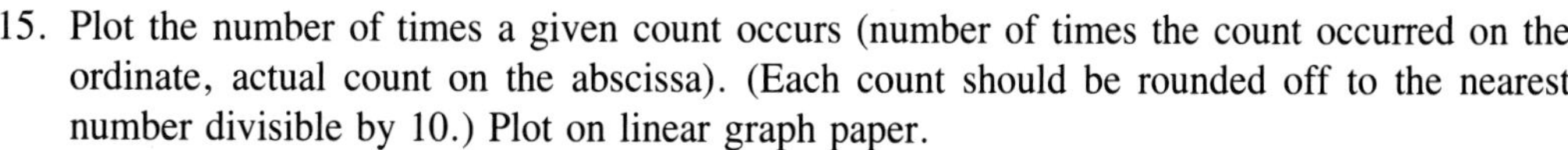

15. Plot the number of times a given count occurs (number of times the count occurred on the ordinate, actual count on the abscissa). (Each count should be rounded off to the nearest number divisible by 10.) Plot on linear graph paper.
16. Although step 15 does not display a perfect Poisson distribution, a little imagination will approximate it. What could be done to make it a better representation?
17. Reverse the ^{137}Cs standard so that the active end is pointed toward the well. Repeat the procedure, using 10,000 counts instead of 100 (indicate the following under remarks):
    a. Average count (true count).
    b. Range for $\pm 1\sigma$.
    c. Number of times the count fell in this range.
    d. Does this correlate with Poisson distribution?
    e. Range for $\pm 2\sigma$.
    f. Number of times count fell in this range.
    g. Does this correlate with Poisson distribution?
    h. Range for $\pm 3\sigma$.
    i. Number of times the count fell in this range.
    j. Does this correlate with Poisson distribution?
    k. What was the lowest count?
    l. What was the highest count?
    m. If the unknown displayed the lowest and the standard displayed the highest count, what percentage of error was introduced into the study?
    n. Compare percentage error obtained from 10,000 counts with that obtained from accepting only 100 counts (step 14).
18. Plot the number of times that a given count occurs. (Each count should be rounded off to a number divisible by 100.)

Technique 2

1. Using the ^{137}Cs standard, determine the approximate time required to count 10,000 counts.
2. Using the time determined in step 1, count the sample for 10 times. Any number of times is permissible as long as the correct values from Table 11-2 are used.

Data treatment

1. Find the average ($\bar{\eta}$).
2. Subtract each of the 10 individual values from the mean. Record the positive *and negative* values.
3. Square the differences. This step makes all negative values positive.
4. Add the squares, and divide by the mean. Use the blank form below.

Chi-square test

	η	$\bar{\eta} - \eta$	$(\bar{\eta} - \eta)^2$
1			
2			
3			
4			
5			
6			
7			
8			
9			
10			

$\Sigma\eta_i$ = ______ $\Sigma(\bar{\eta} - \eta)^2$ =

$\div N$ = 10 $\div \eta$ = ______

$\bar{\eta}$ = ______ χ^2 = ______

Continued.

5. Correlate the value received in step 4 with Table 11-2. The value should fall between 0.90 and 0.10. Note definition of "degrees of freedom" in Table 11-2.
6. If the chi-square value is abnormal, it implies that the unit is not able to reproduce an identical counting situation within an acceptable degree of error. One such measurement is not adequate to call for a service check because the chi-square values represent a range of 80% of all possibilities (that is, 10% of all chi-square values should be less than 4.168, and 10% of all chi-square values should be greater than 14.684). To prove malfunction based on chi-square values, it would be necessary to repeat the study several times and receive abnormal values more than 20% of the time.

Technique (part 3)

1. Fill thyroid phantom with 25 to 50 μCi (1-2 MBq) ^{131}I, and image at the following ID values: 200, 250, 400, 800, 1100, 1600, 2000, 4000.
2. Does perception of lesions become more readily discernible as ID is increased?
3. Image thyroid phantom, using ID 2000 values six times on the same film. Comment on the results.
4. Fill thyroid phantom with 1 to 2 mCi (37-74 MBq) ^{99m}Tc, and position before the gamma camera, as close to the collimator as possible. Take a series of pictures with a low-intensity setting, accumulating the following number of counts: 50,000, 100,000, 200,000, 500,000. Are any lesions missed? Are any lesions filled in? Comment on your results.
5. Repeat step 3 with a high-intensity setting.
6. Repeat step 3, varying the intensity inversely proportional to the counts accumulated.
7. Comment on your results.

Technique for SPECT (part 4)

1. Fill cylindrical "hot"- and "cold"-spot phantom with water and introduce 10 mCi (370 MBq) ^{99m}Tc. Mix thoroughly.
2. Image phantom by varying:
   a. Degrees of rotation: 180° vs. 360°.
   b. Accumulation time per stop: 5 sec, 10 sec, etc.
   c. Number of stops.
   d. Filters
      (1) Full slice through "hot" spots. Evaluate using all available filters.
      (2) Full slice through "cold" spots. Evaluate using all available filters.

Example of chi-square test

η	$\bar{\eta} - \eta$	$(\bar{\eta} - \eta)^2$
1 9231	119	14161
2 9294	56	3136
3 9288	62	3844
4 9331	19	361
5 9443	−93	8649
6 9470	−120	14400
7 9450	−100	10000
8 9281	69	4761
9 9295	55	3025
10 9412	−62	3844
$\Sigma\eta_i = 93495$ $\div N = 10$ $\bar{\eta} = 9350$		$\Sigma(\bar{\eta} - \eta)^2 = 66181$ $\div \eta = 9350$ $\chi^2 = 7.078$*

*For 9 degrees of freedom (10-1) the value of chi-square should fall between 4.168 (0.90) and 14.684 (0.10). Therefore, the counting unit can reproduce a series of subsequent counts within an expected deviation from the mean.

3. Do different filters work better on high-count studies?
4. Do the same filters work best on low-count studies?
5. Comment on the role of statistics to resolution and choice of filters.

LABORATORY APPLICATION 16

ASSAY OF MIXED GAMMA SAMPLE

Purpose

As indicated in Laboratory Application 10, a lower-energy radionuclide cannot be counted in the presence of a higher-energy radionuclide without some further considerations. The Compton contribution from the higher-energy radionuclide is counted in the window encompassing the lower-energy radionuclide, invalidating the data. An increased count rate of the lower-energy radionuclide results.

However, there are methods to correct such interference, since a situation in which a patient or a patient sample contains more than one radionuclide presents itself routinely in a busy nuclear medicine department. Often it is considered desirable to perform dual nuclide studies on the same patient. The purpose of this exercise is to determine the amount of interference of the higher-energy radionuclide and by calculation determine the count rate resulting only from the primary gamma peak of the lower-energy radionuclide.

Procedure

Materials

1. Scintillation crystal detector unit with spectrometer
2. Any two radionuclides having widely separated primary gamma peaks (for example, ^{131}I and ^{99m}Tc); prepare two samples as follows:
   a. 0.5 μCi (0.0185 MBq) ^{131}I
   b. 0.5 μCi (0.0185 MBq) ^{131}I plus 0.5 μCi (0.0185 MBq) ^{99m}Tc
   (The volume of each sample must be the same to rule out geometry differences.)

Technique

1. Turn on scaler main power and high voltage.
2. Adjust detector to proper operating voltage.
3. Determine proper window settings for ^{131}I and ^{99m}Tc.
4. Set spectrometer for ^{99m}Tc, and take a background count. This value becomes B_1.
5. Without changing the window, count the sample containing only ^{131}I. This value becomes S_1 (the contribution of ^{131}I Compton plus background in the ^{99m}Tc window).
6. Without changing the window, count the sample containing both nuclides. This value becomes P_1 (background + ^{131}I Compton + primary gamma of ^{99m}Tc).
7. Change spectrometer to ^{131}I window, and take a background count. This value becomes B_2.
8. Without changing the window, count the sample containing only ^{131}I. This value becomes S_2.
9. Without changing the window, count the sample containing both nuclides. This value becomes P_2.

Data treatment

1. Calculate ^{131}I contribution factor in ^{99m}Tc window as F.

$$F = \frac{S_1 - B_1}{S_2 - B_2}$$

2. Calculate *actual* contribution of ^{131}I in ^{99m}Tc window as C.

$$C = F(P_2 - B_2)$$

3. Calculate *net* count rate of ^{99m}Tc from ^{99m}Tc activity in the mixed sample.

$$\text{Net } ^{99m}\text{Tc} = P_1 - B_1 - C$$

Continued.

4. If all background counts are low, the formula can be simplified.

$$\text{Net } ^{99m}\text{Tc} = P_1 - \frac{P_2 S_1}{S_2}$$

See Key Point 2.

Key points

1. In most clinical situations in which a lower energy radionuclide study has been requested following another of higher energy, it is often easiest to determine the amount of Compton interference by simply taking a background sample before performing the second study. This assay of mixed gamma technique is generally used when two studies are being performed simultaneously.
2. Although the rationale may seem unclear and the mathematics perhaps cluttered by symbols, etc., the student of nuclear medicine technology is urged not to lose sight of the purpose of this experiment. Since the amount of Compton scatter always remains in fixed percentage of the counts in the primary energy peak (assuming all conditions such as window sizes, scatter media, etc., are constant), then all that is necessary is to count any sample containing only the high-energy radionuclide twice: (1) in its proper window *and* (2) in the window that is going to be used to count the lower energy radionuclide. Simply, then, express the latter as a percentage of the former. When presented with the mixed gamma source, count the source in both windows, but reduce the counts received from the low-energy window by that percentage of the counts received from the high-energy window.

LABORATORY APPLICATION

17

EFFICIENCY

William H. Miller

Purpose

The term *efficiency,* as used in nuclear measurement, is often misunderstood. Two definitions are used. Some uses of the term refer to the ratio of actually observed counts to the total number of gamma photons reaching the detector. This use has been referred to as *geometric efficiency*. The term is generally used in describing the efficiency of imaging equipment. Another use of the term relates to the ratio of observed events to the total number of disintegrations occurring within the radioactive sample. This use has been called *intrinsic efficiency*. It refers to the overall ability of a radiation counting device to detect and record the radioactivity of the sample. This experiment is designed to investigate intrinsic efficiency.

Several variables can affect intrinsic efficiency. These include high voltage, resolution, resolving time, self-absorption, nature of the radiation and its detector, and geometry. The purpose of this exercise is to demonstrate how some of these variables can affect efficiency and introduce errors into a study.

Absolute activities of samples are required only in certain kinds of work, rarely in routine nuclear medicine. Usually it is necessary only to know the relative activities from which usable calculations can be made. An example can be used to illustrate the point.

CASE 1

A patient who was given an oral dose of ^{131}I has a 24-hour thyroid uptake of 4000 cpm. A standard representing the dose given to the patient and counted immediately after the patient count yields 20,000 cpm.

$$\text{24-hour percentage uptake} = \frac{4000}{20{,}000} \times 100 = 20\%$$

CASE 2

The physician does not believe that the results of Case 1 correlate with the clinical impression and asks to have the study recounted. This time another machine is used that is 50% as efficient as the one used in Case 1. The results this time yield only 2000 cpm from the patient and 10,000 cpm from the standard.

$$\text{24-hour percentage uptake} = \frac{2000}{10{,}000} \times 100 = 20\%$$

The results are identical, even though the efficiency is different, because the relative values of each count are unchanged.

This would not be true, however, if the results from the standard counted on the instrument used in Case 1 were compared with the patient count used in Case 2. In this case considerable error would be introduced into the study, as follows:

$$\text{24-hour percentage uptake} = \frac{2000}{20{,}000} \times 100 = 10\%$$

This would also hold true if a standard were counted on one day and an unknown were counted days to weeks later. If during this interval of time the efficiency of the equipment had changed, the results would be erroneous. This is one reason a long-lived monoenergetic gamma emitter (such as ^{137}Cs) should be counted daily. The same count rate indicates no change in efficiency.

Procedure

Materials

1. Two scintillation detectors and readout systems
2. ^{137}Cs calibration standard

Technique 1: intrinsic efficiency

1. Calibrate the high voltage on each of two scintillation detectors.
2. Set appropriate windows for a reference standard.
3. Count the same standard in each instrument, accumulating at least 10,000 counts.
4. Express the two values in counts per minute.
5. Determine percentage efficiency by the following:

$$\frac{N \times 100}{C \times \eta_i \times 2.22 \times 10^6}$$

where:

N = Counts per minute from source
C = μCi in source
η_i = mean number of radiations per disintegration (from MIRD)
2.22×10^6 = Conversion of μCi to disintegrations per minute
100 = Percent

6. Which instrument has the greatest efficiency, assuming an identical source to crystal orientation?
7. List some factors to explain this difference.
8. Can any of these factors be controlled by the operator?

Effect of voltage on efficiency

Technique 2:

1. Calibrate the high voltage on a scintillation detector unit.
2. Set proper windows.
3. Count ^{137}Cs source in normal position for 10,000 counts.
4. Record value in counts per minute.
5. Invert ^{137}Cs source, and count for 10,000 counts.
6. Record value in counts per minute.

Continued.

7. Calculate the following:

$$\text{Percentage "uptake"} = \frac{\text{Net cpm inverted}}{\text{Net cpm normal}} \times 100$$

8. Change high voltage setting up or down by just 5 units, and recount source in inverted position only.
9. Record value in counts per minute.
10. Calculate:

$$\text{Percentage "uptake"} = \frac{\text{Net cpm inverted}}{\text{Net cpm normal}} \times 100$$

11. Explain the difference in values between steps 7 and 10.
12. Would this explain why the same efficiency must be maintained for comparative counts, such as the preceding?
13. Suppose a Monday count at a high-voltage setting of 1000 is compared against a Tuesday count at a high-voltage setting of 1020. Will the comparison be valid? How could validity be determined?

Effect of window settings on efficiency
Technique 3:

1. Calibrate the high voltage on the detector unit.
2. Set a window of 652 to 672.
3. Count ^{137}Cs source in normal position for 10,000 counts.
4. Record value in counts per minute.
5. Invert ^{137}Cs source, and count for 10,000 counts.
6. Record value in counts per minute.
7. Calculate:

$$\text{Percentage "uptake"} = \frac{\text{Net cpm inverted}}{\text{Net cpm normal}} \times 100$$

8. Change windows to 632 to 692, and recount source in inverted position only.
9. Record value in counts per minute.
10. Calculate the following:

$$\text{Percentage "uptake"} = \frac{\text{Net cpm inverted}}{\text{Net cpm normal*}} \times 100$$

11. Explain why establishing consistent window settings for all comparative counts is necessary.

CONCLUSIONS

The foregoing should have revealed some of the gross errors that can be introduced into nuclear medicine calculations. Questions that should be continually asked by all nuclear medicine personnel are: (1) What windows were used? (2) What instrument was used on the first count? (3) Has the high voltage changed? If so, has the efficiency been restored?

*Use same values as in step 4.

LABORATORY APPLICATION

18

COINCIDENCE LOSS

Purpose

As determined in Laboratory Application 17, the efficiency of a scintillation crystal can be affected by many different parameters. One of the most easily demonstrated parameters is that of coincidence loss. The efficiency of any scintillation detector eventually reaches a point where it decreases as the activity increases. At that point the system begins to demonstrate coincidence loss. The purpose of this laboratory application is to determine that point so that all activities can be kept under that level, thereby ensuring more accurate results. A case to illustrate the effects of a loss of linearity is one in which a nuclear medicine department uses 400 μCi (15 MBq) of ^{123}I for radioiodine uptakes. It may be that such a technique results in a standard count rate of 800,000 net cpm, whereas the 24-hour patient uptake results in a count rate of 200,000 net cpm. The results would be calculated as follows:

$$\text{24-hour percentage uptake} = \frac{\text{Net patient count}}{\text{Net standard count}} \times 100 = \frac{200{,}000}{800{,}000} \times 100 = 25\%$$

If, however, the count-rate response was not linear at the 800,000 cpm count-rate level, it may well be that counts were lost because of coincident gamma interactions in the crystal. Had the count rate been linear, the standard count may have netted 1 million cpm. In this case, the true 24-hour ^{131}I uptake should have been 20%, according to the following:

$$\text{24-hour percentage uptake} = \frac{200{,}000}{1{,}000{,}000} \times 100 = 20\%$$

The disregard for coincident losses in these cases introduced an error of 20% into the study. One way to compensate for such a problem is to count a diluted standard of the administered source.

As an example, had a standard consisting of one fifth of the administered dose been counted and multiplied by 5 (dilution factor), the test result would have been accurate, as seen below:

$$\text{24-hour percentage uptake} = \frac{200{,}000}{200{,}000 \times 5} \times 100 = \frac{200{,}000}{1{,}000{,}000} \times 100 = 20\%$$

Disregard for this phenomenon of coincident losses is another method whereby introduced errors can alter the test results and consequently the medical management of the patient. Had these percentages represented values between a normal and a hypothyroid patient or a normal and a hyperthyroid patient, the patient may have been subjected to a course of therapy that not only would have been unnecessary had the test been performed correctly but may actually have caused harm.

Procedure

Materials

1. Scintillation well detector and readout assembly
2. Radioactive sources (^{131}I)
3. Test tubes (approximately 25 tubes)
4. Pipettes
5. Remote pipetting device
6. Disposable gloves

Technique (part 1)

1. Determine proper operating voltage of system.
2. Determine proper windows for radionuclide to be counted.
3. Pipette the following activities into each of 24 test tubes and dilute to 2.5 ml. (See key point 1 for preparation of the following activities.)

Continued.

4. Complete the following table (see key point 2):

Activity		cpm source on top of well (with window)	cpm source in well (with window)	cpm source in well (integral counting)
0.1μCi	(3.7 kBq)			
0.2μCi	(7.4 kBq)			
0.3μCi	(11 kBq)			
0.4μCi	(15 kBq)			
0.5μCi	(18.5 kBq)			
0.7μCi	(26 kBq)			
0.8μCi	(30 kBq)			

Activity		cpm source on top of well (with window)	cpm source in well (with window)	cpm source in well (integral counting)
1.0μCi	(37 kBq)			
1.2μCi	(44.4 kBq)			
1.5μCi	(55.5 kBq)			
1.7μCi	(62.9 kBq)			
2.0μCi	(74 kBq)			
2.2μCi	(81.4 kBq)			
2.5μCi	(92.5 kBq)			
3.0μCi	(0.10 MBq)			
4.0μCi	(0.15 MBq)			
5.0μCi	(0.185 MBq)			
6.0μCi	(0.22 MBq)			
7.0μCi	(0.26 MBq)			
8.0μCi	(0.30 MBq)			
9.0μCi	(0.33 MBq)			
10.0μCi	(0.37 MBq)			
11.0μCi	(0.41 MBq)			
12.0μCi	(0.44 MBq)			

Data treatment

1. Plot activity versus count rate on linear graph paper (three curves). (See Fig. 11-10.)
2. Label curves "on well," "well window," and "well integral."
3. Why, in one word, was it necessary to raise each sample to an equal volume?
4. At what activity in the well (with a window) does your instrument begin to give nonlinear results?
5. At what activity on the well does your instrument begin to give nonlinear results?
6. How could you count a source whose activity yields a count rate in the nonlinear portion of your in-the-well curve?
7. At what activity in the well with an integral window does the instrument begin to give nonlinear results?
8. Can reliable information be derived from excessive activities by narrowing the window, thus lowering the count rate to within the linear range? Why?
9. Is the scaling mechanism or the PMT of your instrument responsible for the nonlinearity at higher activities? How can you tell?
10. What is the most practical method of reducing activity as far as the crystal is concerned?

Coincidence counting (part 2)

1. Select three activities from the previous part that show a linear increase in count rate while in the well, plus all those that are too radioactive to provide linearity.
2. Double the primary gamma energy of the source, and set the spectrometer to receive that energy.
3. Count each sample for 1 minute.
4. Plot count rate versus activity.
5. Explain why your graph looks as it does.

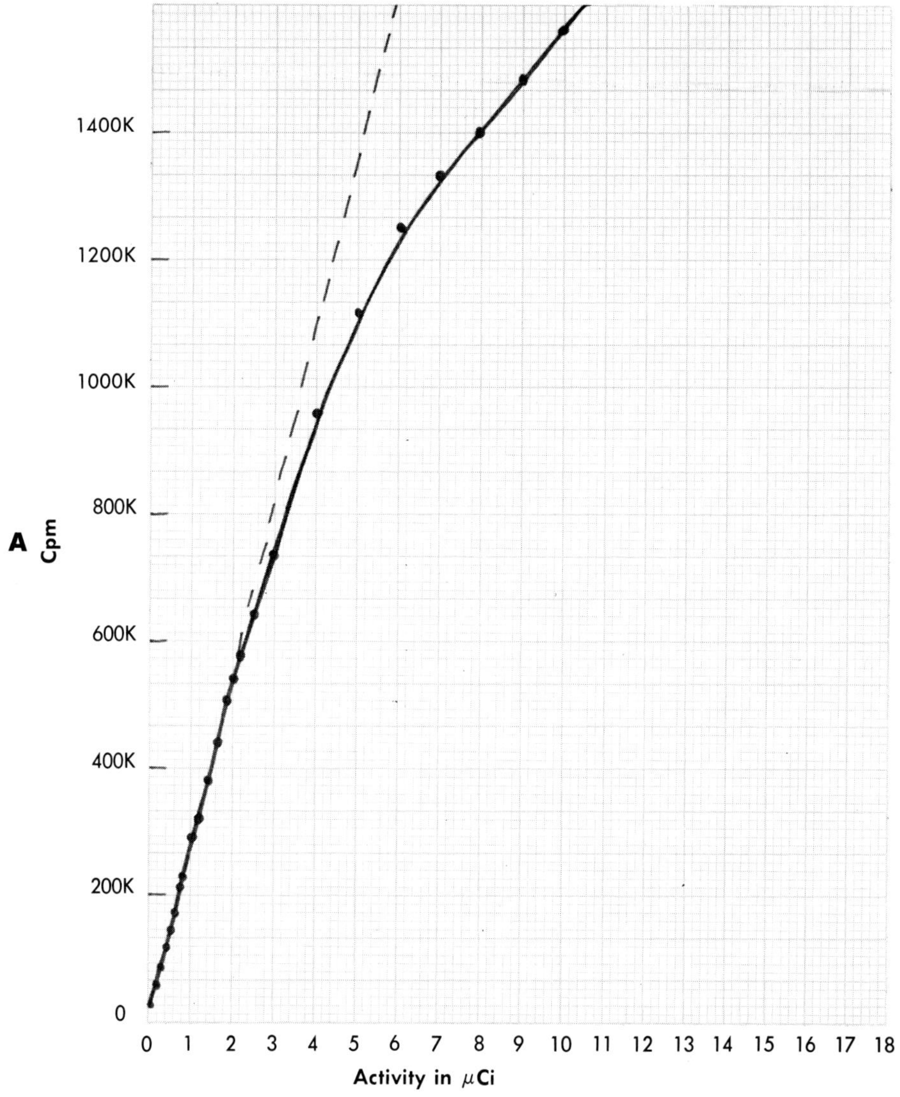

Fig. 11-10. Determination of linearity of detector efficiency. Detector is only capable of "seeing" and counting a certain number of events per unit time before it starts to lose efficiency. In modern equipment this loss of efficiency is primarily caused by the inability of the detector to distinguish between two closely timed crystal events (coincidence counting). All three graphs were determined using ^{99m}Tc. **A,** Nonlinearity beginning at approximately 2 μCi (using 5-keV window), receiving 600,000 cpm.

Continued.

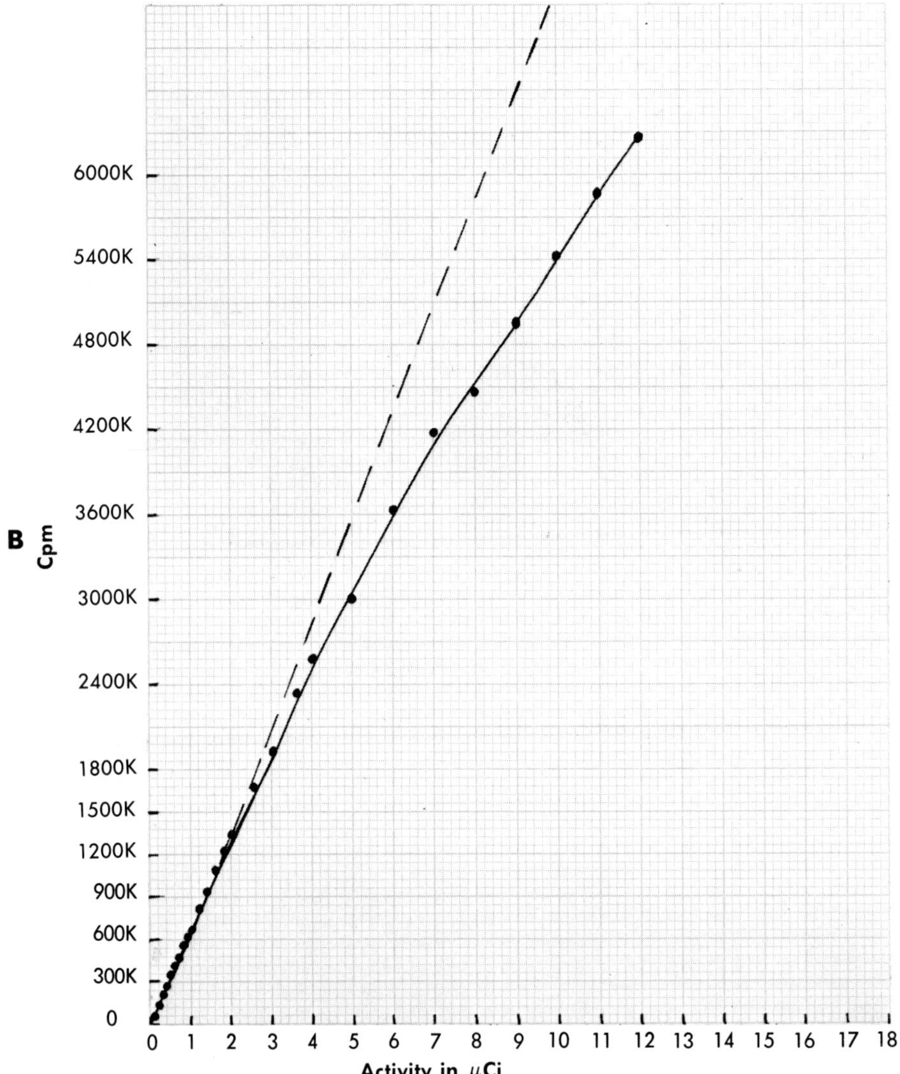

Fig. 11-10, cont'd. B, Nonlinearity beginning at approximately 2 μCi (using integral mode) but receiving 1,500,000 cpm. This demonstrates that linearity is a function of the detector, not of the window settings. **C,** Uses a source counted outside the well with a 50-keV window (same window setting as graph **A**). Nonlinearity does not begin until a source of approximately 20 μCi is reached, but that count rate (600,000 cpm) correlates exactly with that of graph **A,** demonstrating again that nonlinearity is a function of the detector.

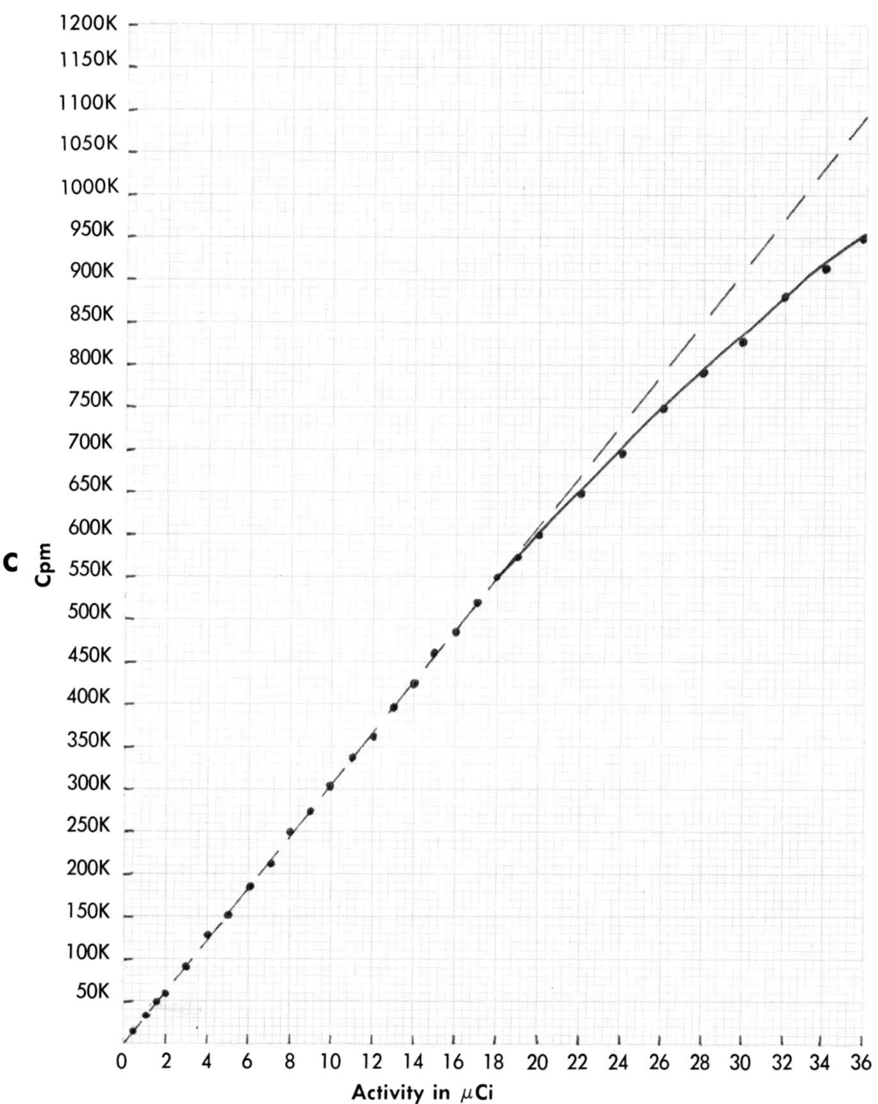

Fig. 11-10, cont'd. For legend see opposite page.

Continued.

Key points

1. The various activities can be prepared from the following two stock solutions:
   a. Accurately measure 150 μCi (5.5 MBq) into a 25 ml volumetric flask.
   b. Raise the volume to 25 ml to make the first stock (concentration 6 μCi/ml).
   c. Make up activities from 3 to 12 μCi (0.1 to 0.5 MBq).
   d. Accurately transfer 4.16 ml from the first stock into a second 25 ml volumetric flask.
   e. Raise the volume to 25 ml to make the second stock (concentration of 1 μCi/ml).
   f. Make up activities from 0.1 to 2.5 μCi (3.7 to 92.5 kBq)
2. Each source should be counted three times:
   a. The first count should be made with the activity in the most proximate location to the crystal as possible. The windows should be set according to the nuclide being counted.
   b. The second count should be made with the same window settings but with the source placed at a more distant point to the crystal.
   c. The third count should be made with the source in the same position as in step 1 but with the upper level discriminator switched off or set at its maximum opening and the lower level discriminator as low as possible without introducing machine noise to the count.

LABORATORY APPLICATION

19

GEOMETRY

William H. Miller

Purpose

Geometry as related to nuclear medicine may be defined as the spatial relationship of the activity to the detector. Any changes in this relationship affect the counting efficiency. As an example, a source counted inside a well yields a higher efficiency than a source counted on top of the same well or a syringe measured in a dose calibrator compared against the same activity in a capsule. Other examples less obvious but capable of introducing gross errors into numeric results are uptake probe positioning over the thyroid versus dissimilar positioning over the standard or counting a patient sample inside a scintillation well versus counting its standard contained in a syringe on top of the well. Any nuclear medicine procedure involving the comparison of count rates of unknowns to that of a standard must be made with the consideration of the effects of geometry on efficiency.

Equally important to the understanding of the influence of geometry on efficiency is the understanding of when two sources to be compared are not in the same geometry. Source *distance* from the crystal and its effect on efficiency were just cited. Less apparent but no less important is the *shape* of the source. If 1 ml of a solution of activity is placed in a 1-ml syringe and counted, and another milliliter of the same solution is placed in a 5-ml syringe and counted, the counts recorded from each may be significantly different. This is because of the change in the shape of the sources being counted. Finally, if an equal activity is distributed in two dissimilar *volumes,* even though the shapes are the same, the counts produced may vary.

In instances when two sources are to be compared but their geometry differs, factors can be used to correct the count recorded from one of the sources, thus enabling a valid comparison. *Conversion factors* are specific mathematic figures that can be applied to an observed count rate to convert it to a figure usable in a calculation. These conversion factors can be used any time a valid relationship is desired between two sources whose geometries vary.

Suppose it was desirable to count the actual source to be administered to a patient. Such a source, regardless of its intended use, usually contains more radioactivity than can be counted inside the well (see Laboratory Application 18). The source may be counted outside the well, using distance or shielding (such as the lid of the well detector), as long as a conversion factor has been predetermined. The predetermined conversion factor can only be applied to counts recorded from sources in geometries identical to those used in determining the conversion factor. The purpose of this factor is to convert the counts recorded from a source outside the well to counts that *would have been* received had the source been counted inside the well. The following case illustrates this point.

A capsule is counted on top of the well (used as a standard) and yields 100,000 net cpm. The capsule is administered to a patient with an estimated blood volume of 5000 ml. Some time later a 5-ml sample of blood is drawn and counted down in the well, yielding 100 net cpm/ml. If the percentage uptake to the blood is calculated

$$\text{Percentage uptake to whole blood volume} = \frac{\text{Net blood cpm/ml} \times \text{Estimated blood volume} \times 100}{\text{Net capsule cpm}}$$
$$= \frac{100 \times 5000 \times 100}{100{,}000} = 500\%$$

an error becomes apparent because it is not possible to have an uptake greater than 100%. The calculation is erroneous because of the comparison of two counts received from dissimilar geometries. It could be corrected by the use of a conversion factor, however, duplicating the same changes in geometry.

The conversion factor can be determined by taking a similar capsule, counting it on top of the well, dissolving it in 1000 ml (a 1:1000 dilution), and counting a 5-ml sample of the diluted source inside the well, dividing by 5 to achieve counts per minute per milliliter, and multiplying the results by 1000 (the dilution factor). This value is what the capsule would have counted if it were possible to count it inside the well. The geometry correction factor is calculated as follows:

$$\text{CF} = \frac{R_d \times \text{DF}}{R_o}$$

CF = Conversion factor (capsule on well to 5 ml in well)
R_d = Net counts per minute per milliliter in desired geometry (5 ml in well)
R_o = Net counts per minute in observed geometry (capsule on well)
DF = Dilution factor

Suppose it has been ascertained that a similar capsule (counted outside the well) yielded 80,000 net cpm. Suppose a 5-ml diluted source, prepared as stated, yielded 6000 cpm, which, when divided by 5 ml, equals 1200 cpm/ml. Then the conversion factor for this particular set of geometric relationships would be 15.0, according to the following:

$$\text{CF} = \frac{1200 \times 1000}{80{,}000} = 15.0$$

Any time this set of geometric circumstances is repeated, the observed count rate from the capsule counted on top of the well can be multiplied by this conversion factor (15.0) to determine the count rate that the capsule would have yielded had it been possible to count it inside the well.

Returning now to the original problem of a 500% uptake to the blood, the calculations can be corrected to read as follows:

$$\text{Percentage uptake to whole blood volume} = \frac{\text{Net blood cpm/ml} \times \text{Estimated blood volume} \times 100}{\text{Net capsule cpm (on top of well)} \times \text{CF}}$$
$$= \frac{100 \times 5000 \times 100}{100{,}000 \times 15}$$
$$= 33\%$$

This is a more realistic answer.

Similar geometry problems can exist in comparing dissimilar volumes. A count rate received from a 2-ml source counted inside the well cannot be simply multiplied by a factor of 2 to receive the count rate of a 4-ml sample. It must be diluted up to 4 ml, counted, and then multiplied by 2; or a conversion factor must be determined. Conversion factors are also necessary for comparing dissimilarly shaped counting vials.

The problem of geometry is perhaps one of the most abused areas of nuclear medicine techniques. Many errors in past nuclear medicine procedures can be traced to a lack of consideration for geometric relationships. The purpose of this exercise is to expose the technologist to some of these geometry variables and to determine how to compensate for them.

Continued.

Procedure

Materials

1. Scintillation detector and readout system
2. Radioactive sources (^{131}I is adequate)
   a. Stock solution (20 ml); 40,000 to 50,000 cpm/ml
   b. Capsule (50 μCi [2.0 MBq]) is adequate)
3. Two different-diameter test tubes; both must fit into well detector
   a. Large diameter, referred to as a counting vial
   b. Small diameter, referred to as a test tube
4. Syringe, 2.5 ml
5. Syringe holder; any type of holder that accommodates a syringe at a reproducible constant distance from the well

Technique

1. Determine proper operating voltage.
2. Set proper window.
3. Complete the following table:

Same activity, decreased concentration*

Volume (stock)	*Vial count in well*	*Same vial count on well*	*Test tube count in well*	*Same test tube count on well*
1 ml	______	______	______	______
2 ml	______	______	______	______
3 ml	______	______	______	______
4 ml	______	______	______	______
5 ml	______	______	______	______
6 ml	______	______	______	______
7 ml	______	______	______	______
8 ml	______	______		
9 ml	______	______		
10 ml	______	______		

*See Key Point 1.

Miscellaneous conversion factors

Volume and shape†	*2.5-ml syringe count on top of well*	*Volume and shape*	*Vial count in well*
1 ml in 2.5 ml syringe	______	5 ml in counting vial	______
Shape‡	*Capsule count on top of well*	*Volume and shape*	*Vial count in well*
Capsule	______	5 ml in counting vial	______

†See Key Point 2.
‡See Key Point 3.

Data treatment

1. Using the preceding data, determine the conversion factor that will convert the following:
   a. A 1-ml in-well vial count to a 3-ml in-well vial count
   b. A 1-ml in-well vial count to a 5-ml in-well vial count
   c. A 5-ml in-well vial count to a 1-ml in-well vial count
   d. A 10-ml in-well vial count to a 4-ml in-well vial count
   e. A 2-ml in-well vial count to a 2-ml top-of-well count
   f. A 4-ml in-well vial count to a 4-ml top-of-well vial count
   g. A 10-ml top-of-well vial count to a 10-ml in-well vial count
   h. A 5-ml top-of-well vial count to a 5-ml in-well vial count
   Are the values for *e* and *f* the same?
   Are the values for *g* and *h* the same?
   Why?

2. Using the preceding data, determine a conversion factor that will convert the following:
   a. A 1-ml in-well vial count to a 1-ml in-well test-tube count
   b. A 5-ml in-well vial count to a 5-ml in-well test-tube count
   c. A 7-ml in-well test tube count to a 7-ml in-well vial count
3. Using the preceding data, determine a conversion factor that will convert (may be two or more steps) the following:
   a. A 1-ml on-well vial count to a 1-ml in-well test-tube count
   b. A capsule on-well count to a 5-ml in-well vial count
   c. A capsule on-well count to a 10-ml in-well vial count
   d. A syringe on-well count to a 3-ml in-well vial count
   e. A syringe on-well count to a 4-ml in-well test-tube count
   f. Arrive at 3*e* by another route.
4. Assume your supervising physician asks you to prepare a chart of conversion factors to be applied to count rates obtained from the same activity in liquid sources of volumes from 1 to 7 ml in test tubes counted in the well. Furthermore, assume that he or she asks that the correction factors be relative to a 5-ml volume; that is, a count rate from any volume within the indicated limits, when multiplied by the correction factor, would equal that of the same activity in a 5 ml volume. From your data, prepare the chart by graphing the conversion factor on the vertical axis versus the corresponding volume on the horizontal axis.
5. A patient was given 0.5 μCi (18.5 kBq) of ^{57}Co-tagged vitamin B_{12}. The capsule was counted on top of the well before administration, and the count rate was 10,000 cpm. The 24-hour urine sample was 2000 ml, of which 4 ml was counted in the well and yielded 150 cpm. Compute the percentage excreted by this patient as follows:

$$\text{Percentage excreted} = \frac{\text{Net urine cpm/ml} \times \text{Urine volume} \times 100}{\text{Net capsule cpm} \times \text{CF}}$$

6. A patient with an estimated blood volume of 4000 ml received 54 μCi (2.0 MBq) of ^{131}I-tagged triolein. A 54-μCi (2.0 MBq) 10-ml vial standard was counted on top of the well and yielded 140,000 cpm. Because of the patient's extremely poor veins and low blood pressure, you were able to obtain only 2 ml of blood from the patient, who became unreasonably indignant after the fourteenth stick. The 2 ml of blood was counted and showed a count rate of 175 cpm. Calculate the percentage uptake of the patient. As follows:

$$\text{Percentage uptake} = \frac{\text{Net blood cpm/ml} \times \text{Estimated blood volume (ml)} \times 100}{\text{Net standard cpm} \times \text{CF}}$$

7. Explain why, in the first table, the addition of nonradioactive water decreased the observed count rate.

Key points

1. Pipette 1 ml of the stock solution into a vial and a test tube. Count each in and on the well. Then add 1 ml of tap water to each and recount in and on the well. Continue adding water in 1 ml aliquots and counting until the table is filled in.
2. Using a 2.5-ml syringe, draw up 1 ml of stock solution. Expel air and install a clean needle and needle cover; do not refill the needle. Count in an appropriate syringe holder on top of the well. Record the count in the table. Remove the needle and cover and expel the contents of the syringe into a vial. Refill the syringe with 1 ml of water (do not flush). Reinstall the needle and cover and recount on top of the well. Subtract the second count from the first and enter the total in the table. Add tap water to the vial until the volume is 5 ml. Mix gently and count down in the well. Enter data in the table.
3. Count the capsule in a reproducible geometry on top of the well. Enter the count in the table. Dissolve the capsule in warm water, raise the volume to exactly 1000 ml (do not lose activity in unnecessary transfers). Mix gently. Pipette exactly 5 ml into a vial and count down in the well. Divide the in-well count by the volume (5) and multiply by the dilution factor (1000). Enter the result in the table.

Continued.

LABORATORY APPLICATION

20

MINIMUM DETECTABLE ACTIVITY (MDA)

Purpose

As demonstrated in Laboratory Applications 18 and 19, there is a limit as to the number of events that a counting system can handle within an acceptable degree of error. Conversely, there is a minimum number of counts that can be considered statistically significant for any counting system. In a low-count situation, the counts obtained must always be compared to the background counts expected during the same measuring time. One approach is to identify that net count-rate above background that can reasonably be expected to be more than a statistical fluctuation in background. This net count-rate is often set at three times the standard deviation of the background count. This relationship is called the *Mininum Detectable Activity* (MDA) and can be expressed as:

$$\text{MDA (cpm)} = 3\sqrt{R_b/t}$$

where:

R_b = background count rate
t = counting time

Procedure

Materials

1. Scintillation well detector and spectrometer
2. 0.5 μCi (18.5 kBq) ^{137}Cs (NBS traceable)
   0.5 μCi (18.5 kBq) any other nuclide desired

Technique

1. Turn on scaler main power and high voltage.
2. Set window for ^{137}Cs with a 20-keV window.
3. Adjust detector to proper operating voltage.
4. Adjust window to a clinical window.
5. Determine a 10-minute background
6. Count ^{137}Cs standard for 1 minute.
7. Determine % efficiency (Laboratory Application #17).
8. Count wipe test for 10 minutes.

Data treatment

1. Calculate MDA for this system in counts per minute (cpm).
2. Calculate MDA for this system in disintegrations per minute (dpm).
3. Given the example:
   Three wipe tests from three ^{137}Cs sealed sources result in total counts of 30, 50, and 5500 cpm.
   Background counts are 200 counts/10 min or 20 cpm. (Assume detector to be 35% efficient for ^{137}Cs.)
   Q. What is the MDA in cpm?
   A. MDA = $3\sqrt{(200 \div 10)} = 3 \times 4.47 = 13.5$cpm
   Q. What is the MDA in dpm (μCi or Bq)?
   MDA = $13.5 \text{ cpm} \div 0.35 = 3.0 \times 10^7$ dpm
   A. $\frac{3.0 \times 10^7}{2.2 \times 10^6} = 1.8 \times 10^{-5}$ μCi (0.6 Bq)
   Q. For 30-cpm wipe test, what is the removable activity in μCi (Bq)?
   A. Net cpm = 30 − 20 = 10 (<MDA and acceptable)
   (Report as "<MDA, which is 1.8×10^{-5} μCi")
   Since 10 net cpm is less than what would be expected from the statistical fluctuation of background, it is not clear if the counts received are anything more than background. However, it clear that since the MDA is much less than 0.005 μCi, there is insignificant contamination. This source can remain in service.

Q. For 50-cpm wipe test, what is the removable activity in μCi (Bq)?
A. Net cpm = 50 − 20 = 30 cpm (>MDA)

$$\frac{30 \text{ cpm}}{2.2 \times 10^6(.35)} = 4 \times 10^{-5} \ \mu\text{Ci (1.5 Bq)—acceptable}$$

Since 30 net cpm is greater than what would be expected from background, it is clear that there is contamination on the wipe. However, the amount is far less than 0.005 μCi and no further action is required.

This source can remain in service.

Q. For 5500 cpm wipe test, what is removable activity in μCi (Bq)?
A. Net cpm = 5500 − 20 = 5480 (>MDA)

$$\frac{5480}{2.2 \times 10^6(.35)} = 0.007 \ \mu\text{Ci (250 Bq)—unacceptable}$$

Since this value is far greater than the MDA, it is clear that this value could not have been generated by statistical fluctuations.

This source must be removed from service because it has >0.005 μCi removable radioactivity. Furthermore, in accordance with 10CFR35.59(e) (21), a report must be filed within 5 days to the appropriate NRC Regional Compliance Office with a copy to the Director, Office of Nuclear Safety and Safeguards, U.S. Nuclear Regulatory Commission, Washington, D.C., describing the equipment involved, the test results, and the action taken.

LABORATORY APPLICATION

21

COLLIMATORS

Purpose

Collimators are devices that define the area from which the nonscattered gamma rays come. They perform this function by either absorbing unwanted gamma rays or scattering them. The latter results in gamma rays of reduced energy so that the pulse height analyzer rejects them. Collimators are usually constructed of lead and extend out from the crystal of the detection unit.

There are several types of collimators, varying according to desired function. Some collimators allow gamma rays from the entire gland or organ to be detected (flat-field collimators), whereas others limit the area of detection to a small portion of the gland (focused collimators). Others consist of thousands of holes that accept only vertically oriented gamma rays (parallel-hole collimator) or gamma rays converging on the crystal from the organs (diverging collimator).

The characteristics of a collimator are best demonstrated by the construction of isoresponse curves (isocount lines), especially for the flat-field and focused varieties. For the flat-field collimator, isoresponse curves indicate the area of inclusion so that the correct distance (from collimator to organ) is used to perceive gamma rays from the largest of organs. It also indicates the distance at which the collimator must be set so that small variations in organ depth do not appreciably alter the results of the test statistically.

For the focused collimator, isoresponse curves determine the sensitivity of the collimation system, focal depth, focal length, focal width, and, to a certain extent, degree of resolution.

The purpose of this laboratory application is to determine these characteristics in an effort to better understand the function of a collimator.

FLAT-FIELD COLLIMATOR

Procedure

Materials

1. Uptake probe
2. Flat-field collimator
3. Readout system
4. Rectilinear scanner
5. Scanner collimators
6. Radionuclide sources: ^{99m}Tc and ^{131}I

Continued.

7. Capillary hematocrit tube to prepare point source
8. Sealing clay for item 7
9. Linear graph paper
10. Isoresponse plotter, easily constructed by taping a piece of linear graph paper to a piece of cardboard and punching holes at every major intersection of the graph paper with a sharp-pointed instrument to hold the capillary hematocrit tube upright (each major intersection is equal to 1 cm)

Technique for isoresponse determination

1. Calibrate counting device, and set appropriate window.
2. Place capillary hematocrit tube in concentrated ^{99m}Tc or ^{131}I source of radioactivity. Capillary tube fills by capillary action, so the tube needs only to be touched to the surface of the radioactive source.
3. Seal both ends following the filling process. ^{131}I is preferred because the exercise is long, and ^{131}I has a long half-life. If ^{99m}Tc is used, correction should be made periodically for decay.
4. Place board so that the entire capillary tube is seen by the crystal (Fig. 11-11).
5. Place source as close as possible to the face of the collimator and in the centermost position. Take a 1-minute count. This should be at least 40,000 to 50,000 cpm, ideally 100,000 cpm.
6. Use another piece of graph paper identical to the plotter and record cpm at the intersection where the capillary tube was placed. It is easier to record this point as 100% and, using the scaler as a calculator, record all other points as a percentage of the 100% isocount point.
7. Move capillary tube to all other points on the graph paper, and record counts per minute or percent. As the source is moved farther away from the crystal, the distance between each consecutive 10% level gets larger. Of what principle is this an example?
8. Continue in this manner in all directions until counts fall to 10% of the initial count (100% isocount point). Place capillary tube at various places to the rear of the probe. Is a statistical number of counts received? If so, what danger does this represent as to doing a thyroid uptake and thigh count with the patient in the sitting position? How can this danger be averted?
9. Connect all points with the same counts (or percentage) to form the isoresponse pattern (Fig. 11-12). Connecting points with values of 90%, 80%, 70%, 60%, 50%, 40%, 30%, 20%, and 10% is adequate.
10. Determine the distance that would encompass the largest of thyroid glands and yet represent no greater than a 5% variation in isocount lines throughout a distance of 2 inches (see key point 5). What is this distance?

Key points

1. An isocount line implies that a point source placed anywhere on that line will give the same result.
2. In the early years of radionuclide imaging, a manual scan was performed by moving the probe over the organ, plotting such counts, and drawing isocount lines between points of similar count rate. The same thing can be done now by feeding all of the information into a computer and receiving isoresponse data back on a variety of readout instruments.
3. The low-energy collimators are designed to absorb or scatter all unwanted gamma photons from 150 keV or below, whereas medium-energy collimators are designed to absorb or scatter all photons between 150 and 300 keV.
4. The resolution of scanning or the smallest lesion able to be differentiated by a particular scanning system is usually determined by the 50% isocount line. It is referred to as the *full width at half max (FWHM)*. This is to indicate that the count rate must fall at least to 50% in the area between two lesions for a distinction between the two lesions to be displayed on the printout system. This is because if the count rate is greater than 50%, the overlapping parts of the two curves, when partially superimposed (because of the proximity of the two lesions to each other), result in a higher count rate than when the probe is just over one lesion (Fig. 11-13).

Continued.

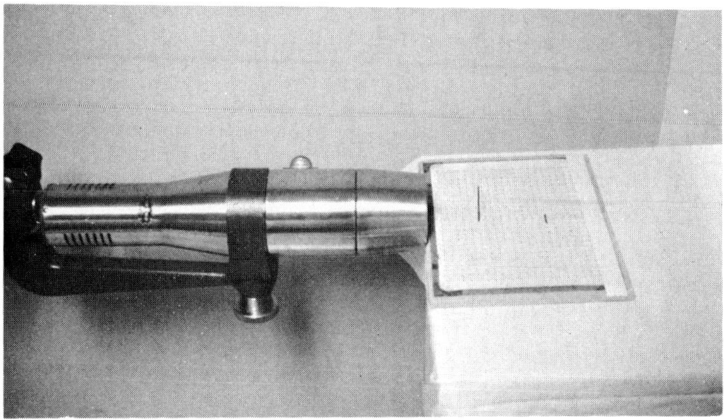

Fig. 11-11. Demonstration of technique used to plot isoresponse curves of flat-field collimator. Dark line situated about one-third of the distance across the graph paper is a darkened capillary tube (for ease of visualization) rising vertically from the horizontal plane of the piece of graph paper. Capillary tube containing radioactivity serves as point source for this study.

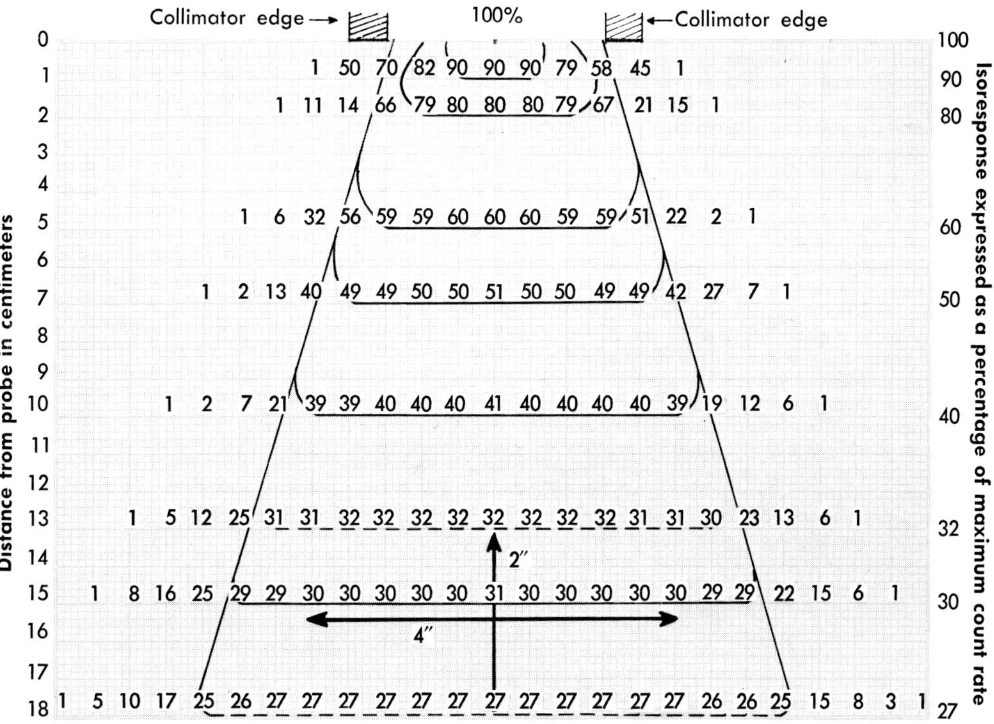

Fig. 11-12. Isoresponse curve of flat-field collimator, indicating an optimum distance bar setting of 15 cm from leading edge of collimator. At this distance the flat-field response is at least 4 inches wide, and a distance of 2 inches between the isoresponse lines represents a 5% variation in the percentage of isoresponse. This should accommodate the largest of thyroid glands.

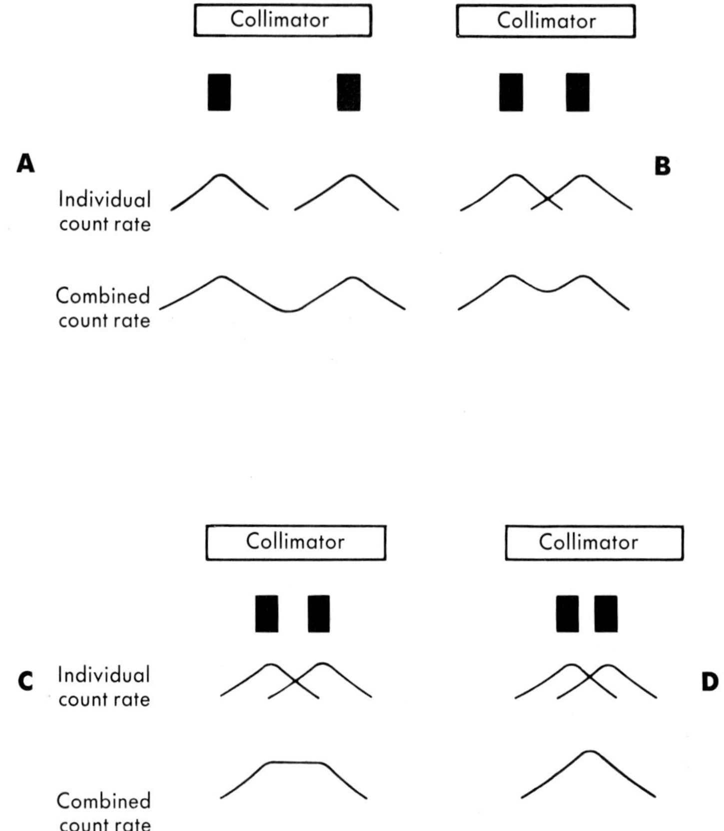

Fig. 11-13. Effects of collimator on resolution. Note decreasing ability of focused collimator to resolve two "hot" lesions as they are moved closer and closer together. **A,** Lesions are sufficiently far apart that complete resolution of the two lesions is accomplished. Individual count rates do not overlap; therefore combined count rates and images would show two distinct lesions. As lesions are moved closer together, as in **B,** there is some overlap of individual count rates, and the combined count rate reflects this. Collimator is still able to resolve the two lesions, although not as completely as in **A. C,** If these same two lesions are near enough that 50% (full width at half maximum [FWHM]) of one peak overlaps 50% of the other peak, all resolution is lost. Combined count rate and subsequent images would not distinguish between the two lesions. They would appear as one large lesion. This fact is further emphasized in **D.**

5. The largest of thyroid glands is generally considered to be no greater than 4 inches wide and 2 inches deep. The appropriate distance from the edge of the uptake probe to the thyroid gland is that distance that permits a flat response through a distance of 4 inches and represents no greater than a 5% isoresponse between two isoresponse lines 2 inches apart (see Fig. 11-11).
6. Be aware that distance marking on commercially available distance probes (used on thyroid uptake systems) usually measure from the crystal and not from the face of the collimator, as performed in this exercise.
7. Recent studies in which isoresponse curves were plotted in tissue-equivalent material show that the focal depth is shortened by about 25% relative to the in-air focal depth.
8. Camera collimators and their resolution measurements are discussed in Chapter 13.

■ QUALITY CONTROL OF A DOSE CALIBRATOR

Probably the most often used major piece of instrumentation in the nuclear medicine department is the dose calibrator. With few exceptions,* the Nuclear Regulatory Commission's regulations have made it mandatory that nuclear medicine departments have the capability of assaying each radiopharmaceutical dose before its administration. The most convenient way of complying with these regulations is through the use of one of the commercially available ionization well dose calibrators. Regulatory agencies are also requiring that more quality control evaluations be performed on dose calibrator instrumentation than on any other instruments in the nuclear medicine department. The following discussion and procedures for quality control evaluation of a commercial dose calibrator are followed by a brief description of assaying for ^{99m}Tc and ^{99}Mo via other instrumentation routinely found in nuclear medicine departments.

Most dose calibrator designs use sealed gamma-ray ionization chambers with associated electronics measuring their DC output current and converting it to direct digital readout in millicuries or a multiple thereof. The reentrance well design may be as large as 2.5 inches inside diameter and 11 inches in depth, allowing for use of a wide variety of syringes and vials of different shapes and sizes. Although the use of sealed ionization chambers essentially eliminates the need for temperature and pressure corrections, numerous variables can affect the accuracy of the activity reading displayed by the dose calibrator. These include the size and shape of the container in which the activity is measured, the density and thickness of the container material, the position of the activity within the ionization chamber, and the energy range of the photons associated with the nuclide being assayed.

*P-32.

In part, because of the necessity to compensate for the many variables that can affect dose calibrator accuracy and the need for delivery of good patient care by ensuring reliable and accurate measurements of the radiopharmaceutical doses before administration, the following quality-control evaluations are required for the dose calibrator.

■ Instrument activity linearity

This evaluation determines the activity linearity of a dose calibrator over the entire range of activities used; that is, it ensures that the dose calibrator reads accurately at activity levels such as 200 mCi (14.8 GBq) as well as levels such as 10 μCi (370 kBq). This evaluation must be performed at the time of installation of the dose calibrator and quarterly thereafter.

LABORATORY APPLICATION

22

TESTING INSTRUMENT LINEARITY

Procedure

Testing instrument linearity requires a source of ^{99m}Tc containing the highest dosage administered to a patient.

Assay the source containing ^{99m}Tc in the dose calibrator. Be sure to subtract background levels of activity to obtain the activity in millicuries. Repeat the assay at various time intervals throughout the day (for example, every 1 to 2 hours). The procedure should continue to 10 μCi (370 kBq). Calculate the predicted activities at each time interval for which a reading is taken, and plot the calculated activity versus time on semilogarithmic graph paper. Plot activity on the vertical logarithmic scale and time on the horizontal linear scale. Plot the measured net activity for each time interval versus the predicted curve as plotted previously. The measured activity as plotted should not exceed 10% of the calculated activity if the instrument is functioning properly. If disagreement exceeds 10%, the instrument is in need of repair or replacement.

Alternative method

A method that has the potential for reducing personnel exposure as well as achieving additional benefits has been introduced. The procedure uses a test kit called *Calicheck*™.*

The Calicheck™ kit consists of six lead-covered tubes that are designed to attenuate ^{99m}Tc gamma radiation by known values (Fig. 11-14). When the tubes are sequentially placed over a source of activity in the dose calibrator, the readings obtained simulate the natural decay process. Within minutes seven successive measurements that represent values that would have been obtained at known times, hours after the initial assay, are acquired. Data sheets and operator's instructions are provided by the manufacturer. Handling of radioactive material is reduced, thereby maintaining exposures

*Calicheck™, P.O. Box 25589, Cleveland, OH 44125.

Continued.

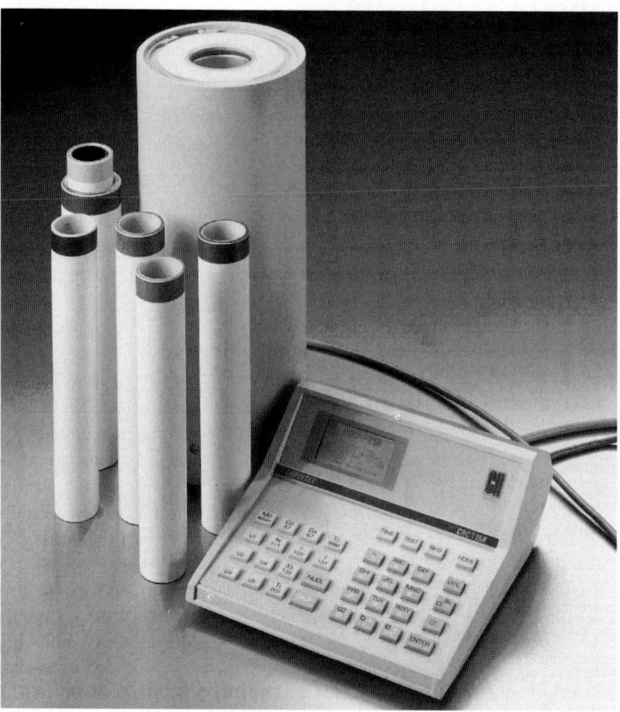

Fig. 11-14. Calicheck™ kit showing six tubes of different lead thicknesses to simulate decay of a radionuclide as a substitute for the activity linearity test.

"As Low As Reasonably Achieveable" (ALARA). A significant savings in time is realized because the entire test can be conducted within a matter of minutes. There may also be a monetary savings when using this procedure, because the activity needed for the activity linearity evaluation can subsequently be used for radiopharmaceutical kit preparation or patient dose administration.

Note that the procedures just discussed, or any others not specifically approved by your governing regulatory agencies, may need to be approved by those agencies through license amendment before the procedures can be implemented.

■ Geometric evaluation

Depending on the volume size of the ionization chamber used, there may be a significant variation in activity measured as a function of the sample volume or configuration. The extent to which these geometric variations affect the activity reading are determined and correction factors applied if these variations are greater than ±10%. For example, if 10 mCi of technetium as assayed in a 30-ml vial is displayed as only 9 mCi when all the activity is transferred to and measured in a syringe, we have a discrepancy of 1 mCi. Therefore a correction factor of 1.1 must be applied to the activity reading from the syringe. Geometric variation evaluations need be determined only at installation. Licensees shall mathematically correct dosage readings for geometry error that exceeds 10%.

LABORATORY APPLICATION 23

TESTING GEOMETRIC VARIATION

To measure the variation with volume of liquid, a 30-ml vial containing 2 mCi (74 MBq) of ^{99m}Tc in a minimal volume such as 1 or 2 drops can be used.

1. Assay the vial containing 2 mCi (74 MBq) of ^{99m}Tc at the appropriate instrument setting. Be sure to subtract background levels to obtain the net activity.
2. Increase the volume of liquid in the vial in stepwise fashion, such as 2, 4, 8, 10, 20, and 25 ml, by adding the necessary amount of water or saline solution. After each increase in volume, gently swirl the vial to ensure uniform distribution of the activity and then assay as above.
3. Select one volume as a standard and calculate the ratio of measured activities for each volume to the reference volume activity. The standard volume selected might be the volume of the reference standard used in performing the test for instrument accuracy. The ratio represents the volume correction factor (CF). For example, if activities of 2.02 and 2 mCi are measured for 4 and 8 ml volumes and 8 ml is the reference volume selected, then the 4 ml volume CF would be calculated as follows:

$$4 \text{ ml volume CF} = \frac{2}{2.04} = 0.98$$

4. Plot the CFs against the volume on linear graph paper. This graph can then be used to select the proper volume CFs for routine assays.
5. Calculate the true activity of a sample as follows:

$$\text{True activity} = \text{Measured activity} \times \text{CF}$$

   Be sure that the CF used is for the same volume and geometric configuration as the sample measured.
6. Repeat procedure using each commonly used syringe.

■ Instrument accuracy (energy linearity)

The dose calibrator should be evaluated to determine its accuracy in reading the activity of several radionuclides at various energy levels. The evaluation should be performed with at least two radionuclides such as ^{137}Cs and ^{57}Co in the form of reference standards whose activity is traceable to NIST standards. The activity levels of the reference sources used should approximate those levels normally encountered in the nuclear medicine department and should have roughly the same geometric configuration. For best accuracy, low-energy reference standards such as ^{125}I and ^{133}Xe should be in vials of the same composition and wall thickness as the actual samples to be measured. Instrument accuracy evaluations should be performed at installation and annually thereafter. Licensees shall repair or replace dose calibrators if inaccuracy exceeds 10%.

Documentation showing the results of these evaluations should be maintained on file for review by the appropriate regulatory agencies. Also note that documentation must be obtained verifying that these evaluations have been performed on "loaner" dose calibrators that may be used while the department's dose calibrator is out for repair. Documentation should be obtained from the organization supplying the loaner or by performing the evaluation in your department before clinical use of the loaner unit.

LABORATORY APPLICATION 24

TESTING INSTRUMENT ACCURACY

The test for instrument accuracy involves the assay of two NIST traceable references.

1. Assay one of the reference standards in the dose calibrator at the appropriate nuclide setting. Be sure to subtract background levels to obtain a net activity.
2. Repeat the assay for a total of three determinations and average the results. The average activity determined should not exceed 10% of the certified activity of the reference standard after decay corrections.
3. Repeat the above steps for the other reference standard selected.

■ Instrument constancy

In this evaluation, a reference source of a long-lived radionuclide, such as ^{137}Cs, should be assayed at all commonly used radionuclide settings. Although the readings obtained do not display a true activity measurement (with the exception of the ^{137}Cs setting), these readings should be consistently reproducible on a day-to-day basis. The instrument constancy evaluation should be performed daily.

The reference standards mentioned earlier should be calibrated as traceable to NIST standards. Calibration accuracy of the calibration sources will generally have error limits less than ±5%. Most manufacturers have standardized a calibration geometry of a nominal 30-ml multidose vial with 20 ml of contents. Two commonly used radionuclide standards are ^{137}Cs and ^{57}Co.

To perform geometric variation evaluations, all configurations and sizes of vials and syringes in which activity might be contained and assayed in the dose calibrator should be available.

LABORATORY APPLICATION 25

TESTING INSTRUMENT CONSTANCY

A long-lived radionuclide reference standard will be checked at each of the dose calibrator settings corresponding to radionuclides to be used each day.

1. Assay the reference standard (for example, ^{137}Cs) in the dose calibrator at the appropriate setting. Be sure to subtract background levels to obtain the net activity. The activity displayed, with background and decay considered, must not exceed 10% of the predicted activity based on the value obtained at the time of the original accuracy test.
2. With the same reference standard still in place, repeat the assay for all of the commonly used radionuclide settings. With background and decay considered, variations in displayed activities must not exceed 10% of the most recent reading at that setting. If variations greater than ±10% are noted, arrangements should be made for immediate repair or adjustment of the instrument.

From another point of view, the following indicates the frequency at which quality control examinations should be performed:

1. *Daily:* Test for instrument constancy.
2. *Quarterly:* Test for instrument linearity (activity linearity).
3. *At installation and annually thereafter:* Test for instrument accuracy (energy linearity).
4. *At installation:* Test for geometric variation.

■ Quality-control program

Having completed all of the system checks described in the first 25 exercises of this book, one needs to devise a quality-control program to serve as a satisfactory check on all systems. The following program for a routine nuclear medicine department is suggested:

A. Daily
   1. Well detector
      a. Calibrate spectrometer and record voltage.
      b. Measure and record sensitivity, using calibration standard. Use the same pulse-height analyzer parameter each day. Look for any abnormal variances.
      c. Measure background activity and record.
      d. Record date and technologist performing the quality control procedure.
   2. Uptake probe
      a. Calibrate spectrometer and record voltage.
      b. Measure sensitivity, using calibration standard. Use same pulse height analyzer parameter each day.
      c. Measure background activity and record.
      d. Record date and technologist performing the quality control procedure.
   3. Camera
      a. Calibrate system for ^{99m}Tc. Record settings for voltage window and intensity.
      b. Perform flood study with correction. Save flood.
   4. Dose calibrator
      a. Perform constancy check.
   5. Surveys/wipe tests
      a. Perform area survey of all generator elution, kit preparation, and/or dose-preparation areas at end of working day.
      b. Survey all new shipments of radiopharmaceuticals. Record.
      c. Perform wipe test applicable to new shipments of radiopharmaceuticals. Record.

B. Weekly
   1. Surveys/wipe tests
      a. Perform area survey of all areas where radionuclides are used and/or stored. Record.
      b. Perform wipe test of all areas where radionuclides are used and/or stored. Record.

C. Quarterly
   1. Well detector
      a. Determine crystal energy resolution or whenever nonreproducibility is suspected.
      b. Perform a chi-square test for reproducibility.
      c. Confirm that calibration is linear by comparison with one or more (preferably more) radionuclides of different energy.*
      d. Confirm proper window settings on all radionuclides used.
   2. Uptake probe
      a. Determine crystal energy resolution.
      b. Perform a chi-square test for reproducibility.
      c. Confirm that calibration is linear by comparison with one or more (preferably more) radionuclides of different energy.*
      d. Confirm proper window settings on all radionuclides used.
   3. Camera
      a. Perform resolution studies, both intrinsic and total system resolution.
      b. Confirm sensitivity stability.
      c. Check for deterioration in saturation capabilities.
      d. Measure dead time, if applicable.
   4. Take inventory of all sealed sources.
   5. Survey storage area(s) of all sealed sources (include brachy therapy).

D. Semiannually
   1. Surveys/wipe tests
      a. Perform wipe test on all sealed sources greater than 100 μCi.

E. Annually
   1. Dose calibrator
      a. Perform accuracy check.
   2. Surveys
      a. Calibrate survey meters.

*Necessary only if other-energy radionuclides are used clinically and the calibration voltage is assumed to be the same for all. If the patient or patient sample is "peaked" each time, this quality-control procedure is not necessary.

BIBLIOGRAPHY

Blahd, W.H.: Nuclear medicine, New York, 1965, McGraw-Hill Book Co.

Chandra, R.: Introductory physics of nuclear medicine, ed. 4, Philadelphia, 1992, Lea & Febiger.

Chase, G.D., and Rabinowitz, J.L.: Principles of radioisotope methodology, ed. 3, Minneapolis, 1967, Burgess Publishing Co.

Conway, T.T., and Weiss, S.: Polaroid film artifacts, J. Nucl. Med. Tech. 4(4):183-188, 1976.

Fundamentals of instrumentation and imaging in nuclear medicine, copyright Eastman Kodak.

Gottschalk, A., and Potchen, E.J.: Diagnostic nuclear medicine, Baltimore, 1976, The Williams & Wilkins Co.

Hendee, W.R.: Medical radiation physics, ed. 2, Chicago, 1979, Year Book Medical Publishers, Inc.

Hine, G.J.: Instrumentation in nuclear medicine, vol. 1, New York, 1967, Academic Press, Inc.

Hine, G.J., and Sorenson, J.A.: Instrumentation in nuclear medicine, vol. 2, New York, 1974, Academic Press, Inc.

Johns, H.E., and Cunningham, J.R.: The physics of radiology, ed. 4, revised edition, Springfield, Ill., 1983, Charles C Thomas, Publisher.

King, E.R., and Mitchell, T.G.: A manual for nuclear medicine, Springfield, Ill., 1961, Charles C Thomas, Publisher.

Merrigan, J.A., Sanderson, G.K., and Miale, A.: Selection of film for imaging in nuclear medicine, Med. Radiogr. Photogr. 53(2):22, 1977.

Quimby, E.H., and Feitelberg, S.: Radioactive isotopes in medicine and biology, ed. 2, Philadelphia, 1963, Lea & Febiger.

Rhodes, B.A.: Quality control in nuclear medicine: radiopharmaceuticals, instrumentation, and in-vitro assays, St. Louis, 1977, Mosby–Year Book.

Rollo, F.D.: Nuclear medicine physics, instrumentation, and agents, St. Louis, 1977, Mosby–Year Book.

Shilling, C.W.: Atomic energy encyclopedia in the life sciences, Philadelphia, 1964, W.B. Saunders Co.

Shapiro, J.: Radiation protection: a guide for scientists and physicians, ed. 2, Cambridge, Mass., 1972, Harvard University Press.

Strauss, H.W., and Pitt, B.: Cardiovascular nuclear medicine, ed. 2, St. Louis, 1979, Mosby–Year Book.

Wagner, H.N.: Principles of nuclear medicine, Philadelphia, 1968, W.B. Saunders Co.

Wagner, H.R.: Medical radiation physics, Chicago, 1970, Year Book Medical Publishers, Inc.

Chapter 12

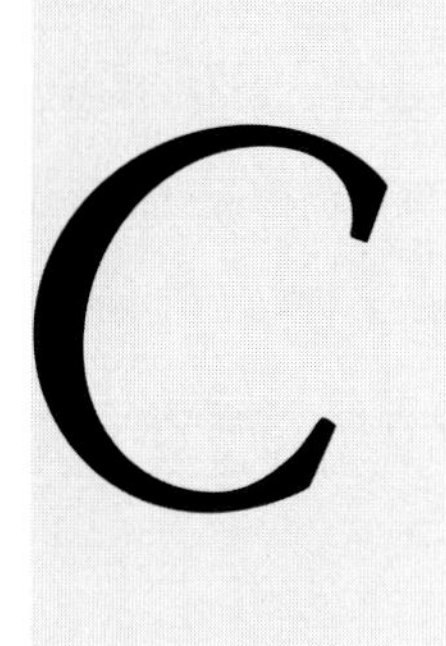

OMPUTER FUNDAMENTALS

PAUL J. EARLY
DAVID P. MIHALIC

Paul J. Early

Computers have not been a staple of the nuclear medicine department until the advent and subsequent tremendous success of nuclear cardiology. Before this time, computers were physically large, electronically overpowered, difficult to use, and seen in only the largest of nuclear medicine departments. Because of their high price tag, when they were available, they were usually cost-justified by time-sharing them with other departments within the hospital. In so doing, the exact functions and tasks required of a dedicated computer for a nuclear medicine department were determined and produced, resulting in a discouragement of the time-sharing concept. This natural evolution of dedicated nuclear medicine mini-computers gained quick acceptance by the nuclear medicine community. Nuclear cardiology procedures cost-justified their purchase for even the smallest of nuclear medicine departments. These tremendous developments have taken only a couple of decades and are responsible for the recent surge in renewed excitement in nuclear medicine procedures.

■ BASIC COMPUTER CONCEPTS

A computer with the ability to handle a large number of electronic signals quickly and accurately finds a logical application when *interfaced* (connected) with a scintillation camera during the visualization of organs. This logic becomes apparent if nuclear medicine procedures are considered electronically speaking as (1) accumulation, (2) processing, and (3) presentation of data. Simply restating these steps in computer terminology describes the operational sections of a modern digital computer (Fig. 12-1).

Every modern digital computer contains the same five basic sections, which are as follows:

1. Input
2. Memory
3. Control } CPU
4. Arithmetic/logic
5. Output

The middle three sections, memory, control, and arithmetic/logic, are usually termed the *central processing unit (CPU)*.

The general flow of data begins with the input section. This section accepts the raw data (analog electronic signals from the detector) and converts them into a form (digital) that can be readily used by the CPU. The data are then stored in the memory section until such time as the CPU directs their processing. The CPU, always acting under a specific set of instructions called a *computer program,* directs the appropriate raw data from the memory section to the arithmetic/logic section (ALU). Here the data may be added, subtracted, multiplied, divided, or otherwise acted on in the manner prescribed by the computer program. The CPU then directs the return of the processed data to the memory section, where depending on the program they may temporarily remain or be transferred to bulk storage. However, eventually this information continues to the output section where it is translated from the machine language of the computer to the language of its human operator.

The performance of a CPU is rated according to clock speed in megaherz (MHz), or how many million instructions per second (Mips) the CPU can handle. In all CPUs there is a clock that sends out precisely timed pulses. The CPU uses these pulses to synchronize the CPU operation. Speeds of these pulses are available up to 50 MHz or 50 million ticks per second. The higher the MHz number, the shorter the time required for the pulse to travel the longest path in the CPU. Therefore, miniaturization enhances speed by reducing pulse travel distance. The higher the MHz number, the faster the CPU and the quicker the results.

Mips is the other method for calculating computer speed. The greater the number of instructions the CPU can finish per second, the more powerful the computer. This statement must be modified depending on the complexity of the instructions. At a minimum, computers should be compared with the Mips method by using similar sets of instructions.

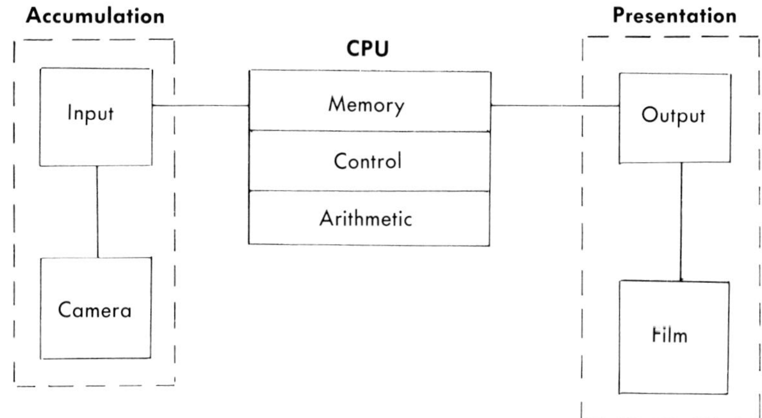

Fig. 12-1. Digital computer interfaced with scintillation camera.

Other techniques are emerging to make computers even faster.

■ Hardware versus software

Computer hardware may be defined as all of the electronic or electromechanical devices, components, and gadgetry that comprise the physical makeup of the computer. *Software* is a term to describe all the programs and routines used with the computer hardware.

Computers vary in their method and ability to handle words of information fed to them. These differences are purposely built into the computer to provide a more efficient or better suited approach to a particular application. Regardless of these differences, some underlying principles of hardware are common for all computers.

Bytes and bits. In a computer information is conveyed by means of electric pulses. As an example, the 10 digits of the decimal system can be represented by electronic pulses of equivalent voltage levels. Computation may then be performed in the manner familiar in decimal mathematics. For example, if the digit 5 is represented by a pulse of 5 V and the digit 6 by a pulse of 6 V, then the sum of these two digits may be obtained by simply adding their voltages and measuring the result as 11. This is descriptive of an *analog* method of addition; computers that employ this technique are *analog computers*.

One difficulty with such a method is that the computer must be able to transfer its data from one section to another. This results in complicated electronics in the analog computer and permits the possible introduction of errors induced by noise or other variations in voltage levels.

Although the analog computation as just discussed uses a continuously variable physical quantity, a *digital computer* is designed to use pulses having only *two* discrete voltage levels. This is similar to Morse code. The Morse code reduces all information to dots and dashes. With computers a *code* is developed that also uses only two values (0 and 1) and is termed a *binary* system (Fig. 12-2).

For example, two commonly used voltage states in the digital computer are 0 V (no pulse) and +5 V (pulse). The 0 V pulse may represent the binary 0, and the +5 V pulse may represent the binary digit 1. The term *BInary digiT* indicates a single character of the binary system and is referred to by the computer term *bit*. It can have a value of only 1 or 0. By the use of the binary system any number of the familiar decimal system may be converted easily for use by the computer. The decimal value in column one of Fig. 12-2 is represented by an equivalent binary number as shown in column three. Each bit signifies a power of two, so that 11 is represented by 1011 or ($2^3 + 2^1 + 2^0$).

Binary counting can be simulated by counting in the binary system shown in column two. A bank of lights is electrically connected in such a manner that an incoming pulse causes a change of status. That is, if the light is off, it will be lighted, and if it already is lighted, it will go out, with the pulse continuing to the left. Each possible combination of lights and no lights (pulse and no pulse) is then generated and corresponds to a number in the decimal system.

It is apparent that large numbers in the decimal system would be even larger numbers in the binary system. However, the computer easily compensates for this apparent unwieldiness because of its ability to handle the binary numbers with incredible speed.

To follow the digital computer's method of addition, the reader should return to the mathematic problem given previously—the addition of 5 and 6. To perform this operation in the binary mathematic system, one first substitutes the decimal numbers with the binary numbers and completes the addition by following the appropriate rules.

Binary mathematic rules of addition
$0 + 0 = 0$ with no carry
$0 + 1 = 1$ with no carry
$1 + 0 = 1$ with no carry
$1 + 1 = 0$ with a carry of 1

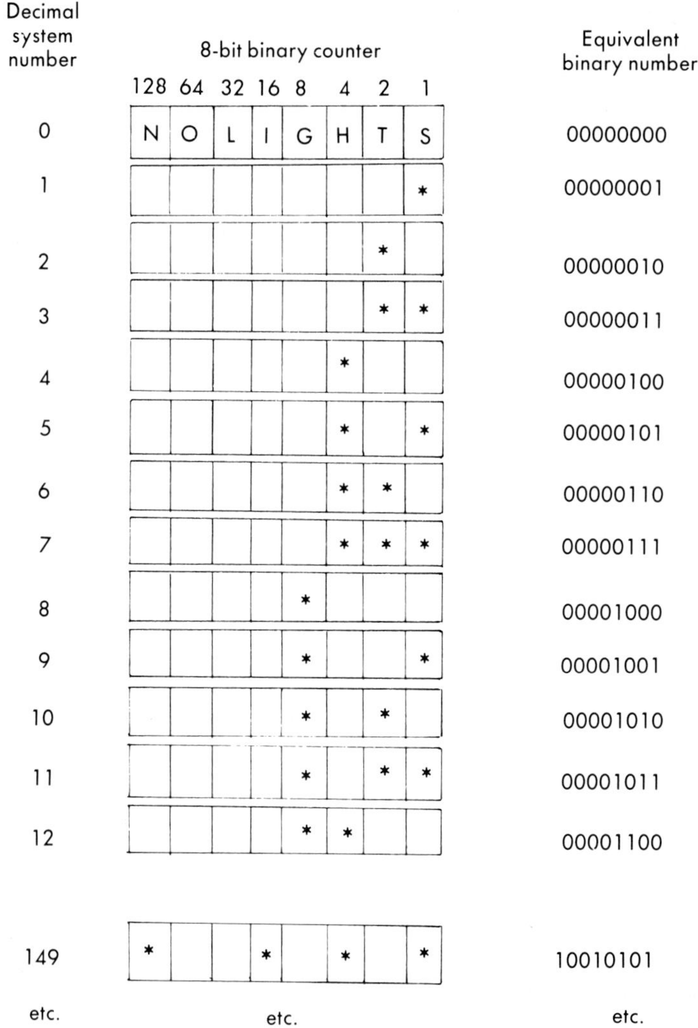

Fig. 12-2. Eight-bit binary counter showing how each bit responds with light or no light, depending on how many counts have been received. First count lights up the first light. Second count turns off the first light and turns on the second light. Third count turns on lights one and two. Fourth count turns off lights one and two and turns on light three, etc. Computer counts in identical fashion (see Fig. 12-9).

Substituting,

Decimal	Binary
5	101
6	110
11	1011

The equivalent of the decimal 11 is the 4-bit answer, *1011*.

All other problems in mathematics are simply treated by the digital computer in the same manner by following the other rules of the binary number system.

The binary answer obtained from the problem just given (1011) can be treated by the computer as one piece of information. This is a definition of the computer term *word,* which is the basic unit of information in the computer. In this case it is a *data word*. The term *word* can also be used to describe an *instruction* or an *address* (location). Each word consists of a certain number of bits processed together by the CPU (usually 16). Specifications for the computer's memory can be expressed in terms of numbers of words that it can accommodate.

Word length can be increased to 32 and 64 bits in modern computers. Computers with the ability to handle larger word lengths allow for increased data storage in a given computer location. Perhaps more important, however, these computers require fewer steps to process the same amount of data stored in 16-bit word length computers and are therefore hundreds of times faster. The instruction word, as its name implies, contains bits of information indicative of the particular procedure to be carried out. The address word, on the other hand, contains bits of information indicating the location of the data word(s) that are to be processed.

In the example of a computer interfaced to a scintillation camera the data word can be composed of bits indicating the number of counts obtained at a specific location by the crystal. The address word contains information indicating the location of these counts, whereas the instruction word can contain the directive to add to this data word any future counts occurring in the same area of the crystal.

Generally speaking, the data words of information are stored in the memory section of the computer, whereas the instruction and address bytes are associated with the arithmetic and control sections.

Byte is another basic component of computer terminology that describes one half of a word, usually 8 bits in length. Computer memory can also be described in terms of number of bytes such as 16K (16,384 or 2^{14}), 32K (32,768), or 64K (65,536) into the megabyte range. Other terms no longer useful are the *nibble* and the *crumb*. A *nibble* has also been described as 4 bits in length with a *crumb* being only 2 bits in length, according to the following chart:

	Bit	Info	Powers
Bit	1	1	2^0
Byte	8	256	2^3
Word	16	65,536	2^{14}
Nibble	4	16	2^2
Crumb	2	4	2^1

The American Standard Code for Information Interchange (ASCII) is subscribed to by all computer languages. It translates input information into machine language based on what keys on the keyboard are punched. According to ASCII each word is 8 bits in length divided up into two 4-bit sections. The first 4 bits identify the input as being a number, a letter, or a symbol. A number is identified by the prefix 1011, a letter by 1100 or 1101, depending on whether it is in the first or last half of the alphabet. The last 4 bits define the actual number or letter depending on the prefix. For instance, if the last four letters were 1010, it could mean the number 10 or the letters J or Z depending on the prefix. The following material lists the ASCII code for some numbers and letters.

1=10110001	A=11000001	Q=11010001
2=10110010	B=11000010	R=11010010
3=10110011	C=11000011	S=11010011
4=10110100	D=11000100	T=11010100
5=10110101	E=11000101	U=11010101
6=10110110	F=11000110	V=11010110
7=10110111	G=11000111	W=11010111
8=10111000	H=11001000	X=11011000
9=10111001	I=11001001	Y=11011001
10=10111010	J=11001010	Z=11011010
	K=11001011	
	L=11001100	
	M=11001101	
	N=11001110	
	O=11001111	
	P=11010000	

■ Analog scintillation cameras

Most cameras used in nuclear medicine departments today are of the analog type. The signal coming from the scintillation detector is as a result of a single discrete photon interacting with the crystal. This is true whether it is a well, an uptake probe, an Anger scintillation camera, or a rectilinear scanner. However, by the time the light produced in the sodium iodide crystal is collected by the photocathode and amplified by the dynodes of the photomultiplier tube (PMT), the resultant electric signal is not a discrete electric "spike" but more of an electric "peak," its highest point representing some value in voltage (Fig. 12-3, *A* and *B*). This is an *analog signal* and can be defined as *any signal in which voltage changes with time*. Pulses from an Anger camera can also be displayed on an oscilloscope as signals whose voltage value changes as a function of time.

Camera/computer interface. The first device that is encountered by the electronic signals generated by a scintillation camera is its interface to the computer, analog-to-digital converter (ADC). This circuitry converts the analog voltages of the camera to the digital needs of the computer. Since a scintillation camera produces two signals for a gamma event (*X* and *Y* coordinates), the interface between the camera and the nuclear medicine computers is supplied with two ADCs, one for each signal.

Converters: ADC or DAC. Any of these analog signals can be converted to digital signals through the use of an *analog-to-digital converter* (ADC). This is performed through the use of a ramp converter that causes a capacitor to be charged by the incoming signal. The time required to discharge is measured by an internal clock. This time is recorded as a digital signal characterized by the count of pulses from the internal clock, which would be proportional to the magnitude of the input signal. Although there are many ADC techniques, the most usual in nuclear medicine because of the importance of pulse height analysis is through a pulse height to time conversion. Digital pulses are given the same voltage value regardless of the pulse height. Variations in pulse height are expressed as variations in the length of time that the pulse is allowed to exist (Fig. 12-3, *C*). In this form the information is easily stored and retrieved in computer systems. By reversing the process, it is easy to see that information in digital form can also be changed to an analog signal. The systems that perform this function are called *digital-to-analog converters (DAC* or *D/A)*.

■ Digital scintillation cameras

Until recently, only the analog type of camera was available. The conversion of the analog signal to a digital signal takes time, thereby reducing the capacity to handle counts. With the advances of microprocessor technology, it is now possible to use digital signal processing starting with the analog pulses from the base of each PMT. Other suggestions for improvement include taking the electrons

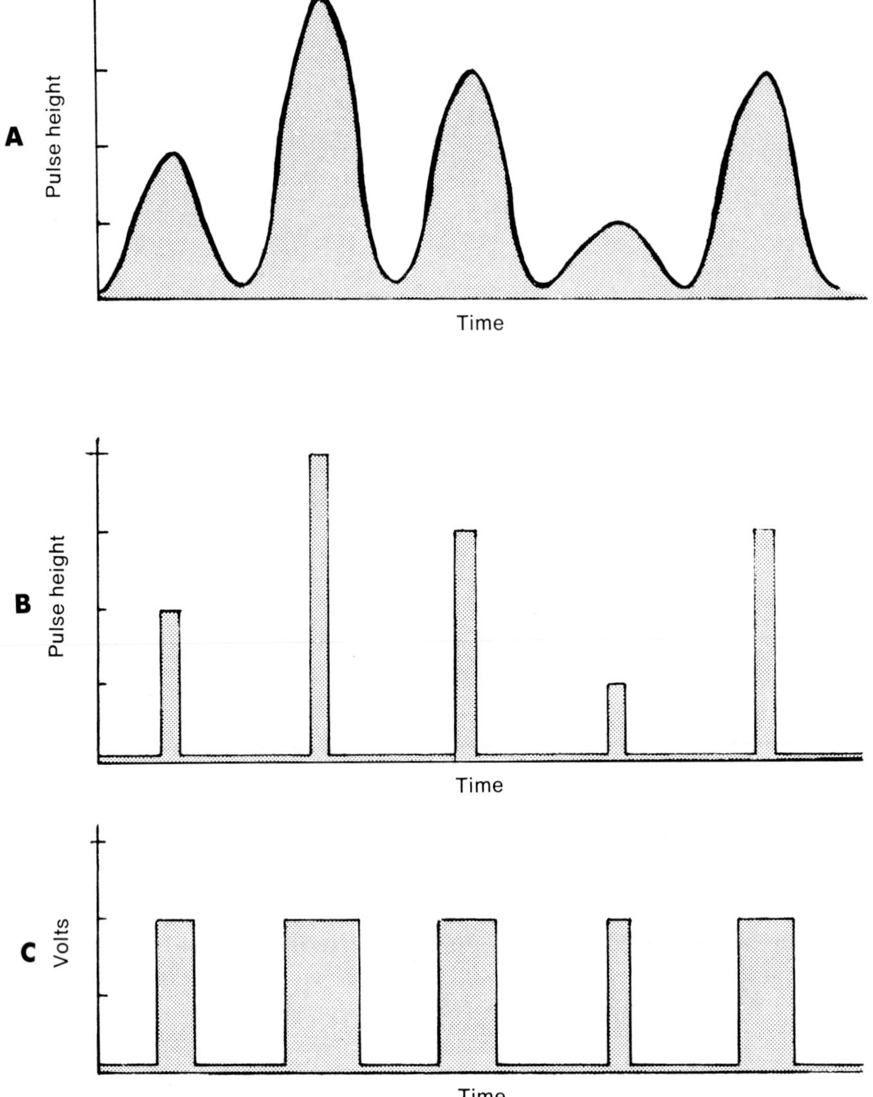

Fig. 12-3. **A** and **B,** Representative pulses from detector in analog form. **C,** Same pulses in digital form as seen following a conversion by way of ADC. Variations in pulse height are reflected as a difference in time. Most ADCs currently used in nuclear medicine use this pulse height-to-time conversion technique.

directly from the phosphor and processing them through solid-state multiplier tubes. By using a series of microprocessors, a digital camera can greatly accelerate acquisition and provide capabilities for data storage analysis and display. Other capabilities performed during data acquisition are energy correction, spatial resolution correction, and automatic recalibration of the system for circuit imbalance and detector drift. Count-rate capabilities are said to be 200,000 cps with a 10% count-rate loss and as high as 500,000 cps with some resolution loss.

■ INPUT/OUTPUT

Magnetic media is a general term used to classify any of the forms of information storage or transfer that incorporate the magnetic properties of iron or ferrous material. This includes the use of magnetic tape, diskettes, and core.

Paramount to a discussion of the uses of these types of devices is an understanding of some basic properties of magnetism. These properties may be demonstrated by collecting two ordinary sewing needles and a bar magnet. The two needles when placed together initially show no attraction for each other. Stroking one of the needles with the bar magnet in a continuous fashion induces this needle to become magnetized, and it is then able to attract the other needle. The needle that is magnetized exhibits the common property of having one end, perhaps the point of the needle, become the "north" pole, whereas the "eye" of the needle becomes the "south" pole. Striking or dropping the nee-

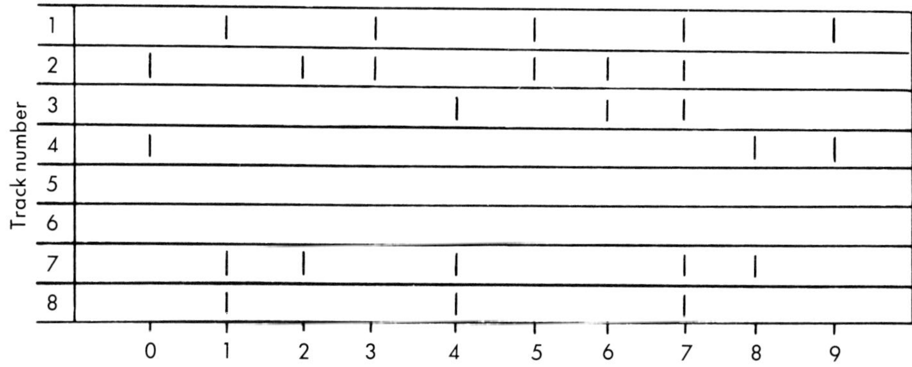

Fig. 12-4. Magnetic tape.

dle results in a loss of its induced magnetic properties. If desired, the needle may be remagnetized in the opposite direction. That is, the point of the needle becomes the south pole and vice versa.

This simple experiment describes the properties inherent in magnetic media that are incorporated by the input/output (I/O) section for use with a digital computer. Specifically, these properties are as follows:

1. The ability to have two distinct states (magnetized and nonmagnetized or north and south poles), the "code" of the binary numbers 0 and 1
2. The ability to magnetize or demagnetize (or change the direction of the magnetic field) with enormous speed
3. The ability of one piece of ferrous material to determine (sense) the magnetic state or field direction of another, which permits the transferring of information from one section to another

■ Magnetic tape

Magnetic tape can be used as an I/O device. Its use is similar to the familiar tape recording systems of home entertainment units. Both systems have tape transports, recording heads, and playback heads. Information is placed on the tape in a digital form. This is performed by recording on a present or absent basis with regard to its magnetic state.

The tape is made of plastic and coated on one side with a ferrous oxide. It is often 1 inch wide, with common lengths of 2400 or 3600 feet. Spaced across the tape width and running the entire length are tracks. These tracks simply serve as designated areas for locating the magnetized spots and typically are six or eight in number. A six-track tape has six possible locations for writing information, whereas an eight-track tape has eight such areas. The tracks are arranged in random order simply to increase the overall wear of the tape (Fig. 12-4).

The pattern of the magnetized ferrous oxide spots (represented by dashes) across the width of the tape and along its length is a coded representation of the data stored on it. As may be seen, many possible different combinations of "spots" (bit) and "no-spots" (another bit) are available. On a section of tape that has been used to record a nuclear medicine study, one may find the pattern of magnetized spots to be the binary equivalent of the number of counts (gamma events) that occurred in a certain portion of the detector.

In computer terminology the recording of information on magnetic media is called *writing,* whereas the playing back of any of the magnetic media to retrieve information is called *reading*. Both these functions are carried out by a system that is appropriately called the *read/write head.* Read/write heads perform their function by making use of the magnetic properties as discussed. The write head records its information by inducing specific locations of tape to become magnetized, whereas the read head performs the reverse of this operation by sensing which of the spots are magnetized.

A concern when using any magnetic materials is the extreme care required to keep the heads and tapes clean. Particles such as lint, dust, hair, and fingerprints can interfere with the read/write head, since the head actually flies above the surface of the ferrous oxide but at a distance less than the thickness of any of them (Fig. 12-5).

Reliability of magnetic materials is a problem. These materials cannot be used indefinitely, repeatedly reading and writing, without distortion and loss of data. The more use, the greater the possibility of dirt, smudges, etc., resulting in loss of data.

■ Magnetic diskettes

Magnetic diskette devices have become the standard of the industry as a general purpose acquisition and storage unit. They usually take two forms: a hard diskette and a soft ("floppy") diskette. These diskettes take the physical form of conventional phonograph records except that instead of grooves on both sides, they have magnetic recording tracks on a coating of ferrous oxide.

The hard diskette is a fixed diskette, capable of storing and rapidly processing millions of bytes of information. The information usually cannot be removed, although some computers can use diskette cartridges (Fig. 12-6) that are removable. Usually the fixed hard diskette stores all the pro-

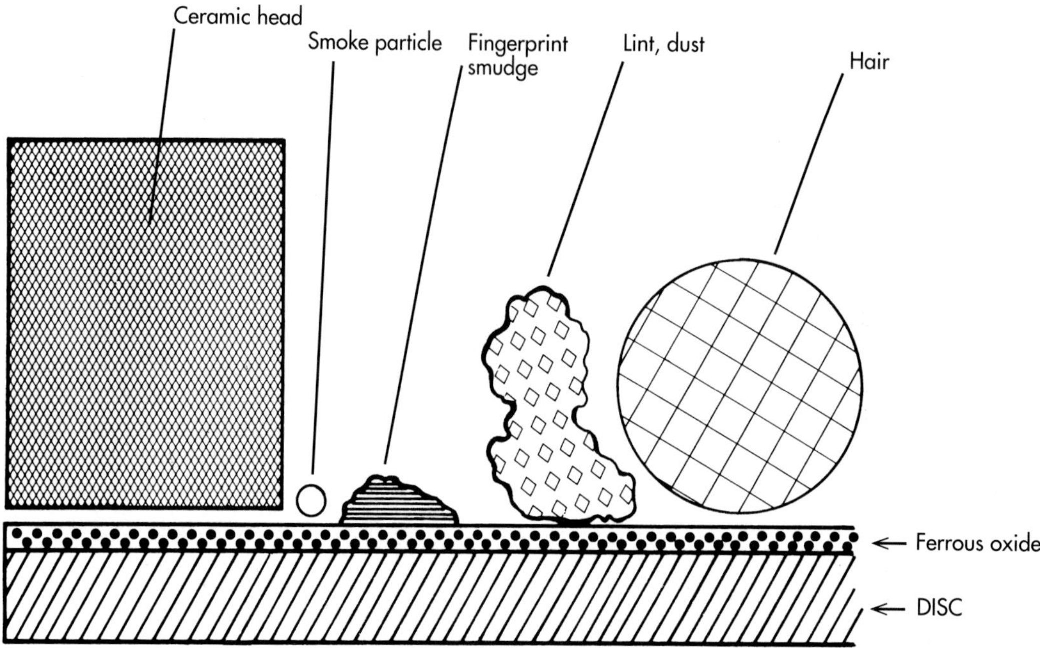

Fig. 12-5. Relative sizes of various materials that can cause a diskette to "crash."

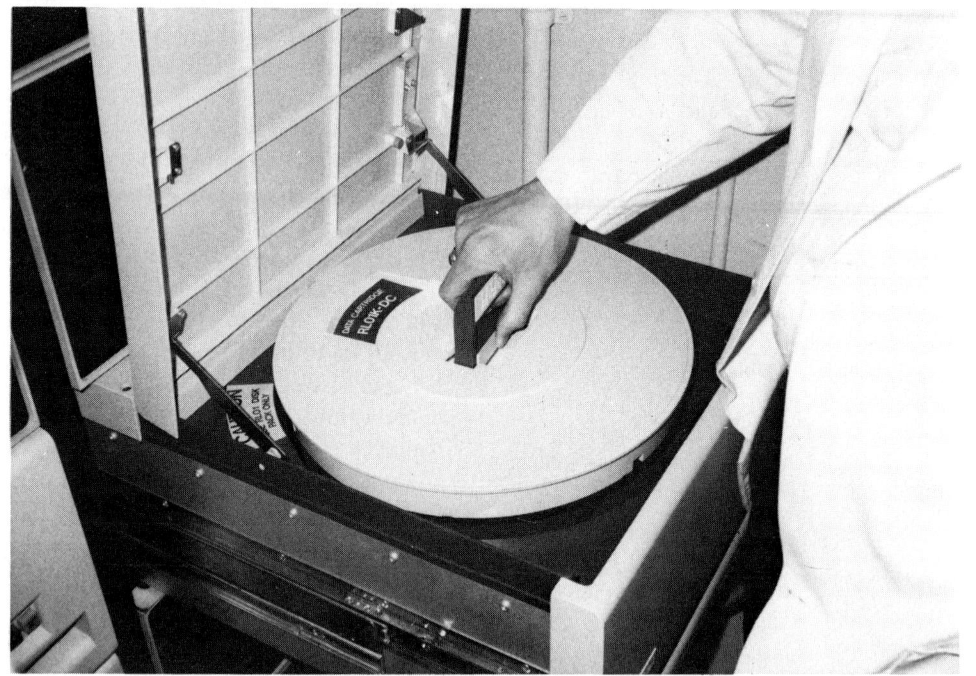

Fig. 12-6. Diskette cartridge.

grams but can be used as a data store as well, but only temporarily. If diskette cartridges are used, a certain type of program (for example, kidney flow study) is generally stored on the cartridge with space for storage of a large number of patient studies. They measure as large as 15 inches in diameter and are approximately 1 inch thick, requiring a fairly large storage cabinet if all patient studies are to be kept.

A floppy diskette (Fig. 12-7) takes its name from the fact that it is made of soft pliable plastic, coated with ferrous

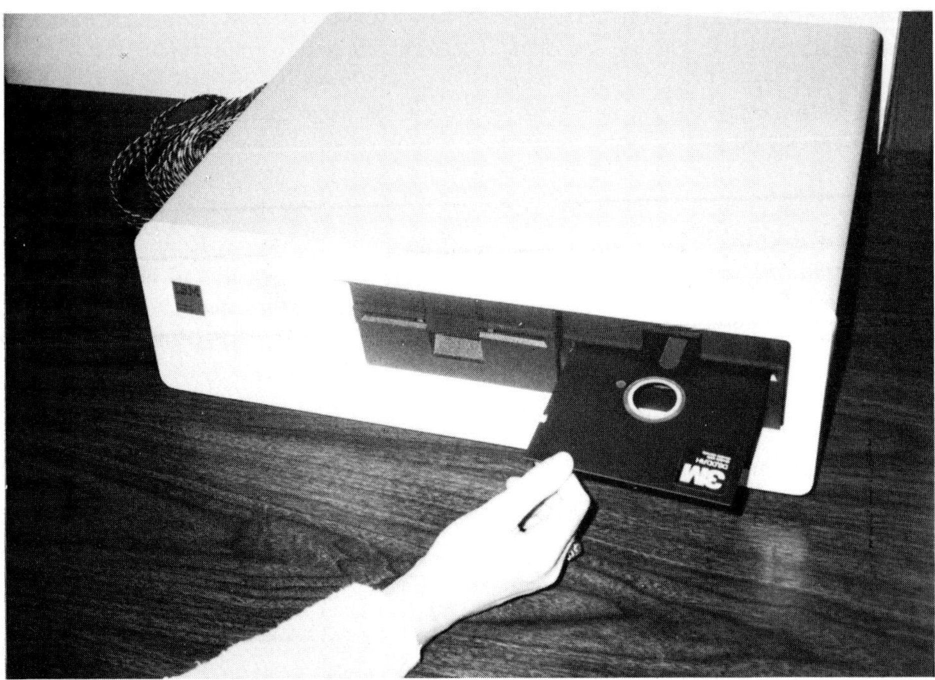

Fig. 12-7. Floppy diskette.

oxide and therefore flexible. These diskettes cannot store as much information as can the hard diskette or the diskette cartridge. However, one advantage of floppies is that they are inexpensive, although they have a finite lifetime. Because they are small (3 to 8 inches in diameter) and thin (1/8 inch), physical storage is not a consideration. They are much slower for search and transfer of information than are the fixed diskette or diskette cartridges but not nearly as slow as magnetic tape.

Winchester disk. One of the recent advances in disk design is the Winchester disk. This is a nonremovable disk consisting of a hermetically sealed unit containing both the rotating disk and the read/write mechanism. It has a storage capacity of approximately 100 times that of the floppy. Another feature of the Winchester disk is that the read/write heads rest on the disk, since it is never removed, whereas with floppies the heads are compressed onto the surface of the diskette when in use and relaxed when not. This allows for damage to develop in the heads. It becomes even a greater problem in a mobile system, since the heads in a floppy system are not pressed against the diskette during motion and therefore are subject to damage.

Many other forms of I/O devices are in great use. Included among these are the familiar punched card and paper tape, both of which use a series of punched holes to code information for digital use. The operation of these and the other I/O devices is not within the scope of this discussion. Regardless of the type of input, however, once the information has been coded in the proper form, it is transferred to the memory section to begin the desired manipulation.

Tape cartridge. Another type of bulk storage device is the tape cartridge. This is beginning to be more popular than conventional storage devices discussed above. These tape cartridges are about the size of tapes used on stereo cassette players. They comprise 600 feet of quarter- or half-inch–wide tape inside a sealed plastic container. The tapes have up to 24 tracks across their width and up to 12,000 bpi (bytes per inch) along their length providing up to 80 megabytes (MB) of storage capacity. Compare this to the large reels of 2400 feet of magnetic tape which record at 1600 bpi or approximately 40 MB. There seems to be good reason for their increasing popularity.

■ COMPUTER MEMORY

The heart of any computer is the memory. It is just so many thousands of microscopic electronic switches, known as *gates,* printed on a tiny silicon board known as a *chip*. An electric charge is routed through these gates, opening some and closing others to create patterns that can be made to approximate the patterns of human logic.

■ Core memory

Until fairly recently, the main memory in most computers was referred to as *core* memory. Core memory is described as nonvolatile because data cannot be destroyed when the power is off. The alternative type of memory is the *semiconductor* or *solid state* variety. These lose stored data when the power is turned off and therefore are termed *volatile;* however, methods are available to prevent semiconductors from being volatile (see ROM). Because semiconductors are the most common form of memory in nuclear medicine, this section will discuss only this type of memory.

Image matrix. Figure 12-8 shows several matrix formats. In reality, a more common matrix size is 64 × 64 bits or a total of 4096 separate addresses up to as large as 512 × 512 (262K addresses) for high resolution images. Memory is built of many such matrices stacked one on top of another. Often 8 such matrices stacked on one another constitute the memory section; each of the 4096 addresses now referencing 8 bits. In this example each location is known as an *address* or *pixel* (a contraction of the two words *pic*ture *el*ement) and each group of 8 bits can be referred to as a *byte,* or an 8-bit word.

Figure 12-9 is a simplified illustration of building up counts in memory as radionuclide activity is absorbed in a scintillation crystal. The accumulation of counts is achieved by alternating the direction of magnetization on the core to indicate the appropriate binary values (1 and 0) of decimal

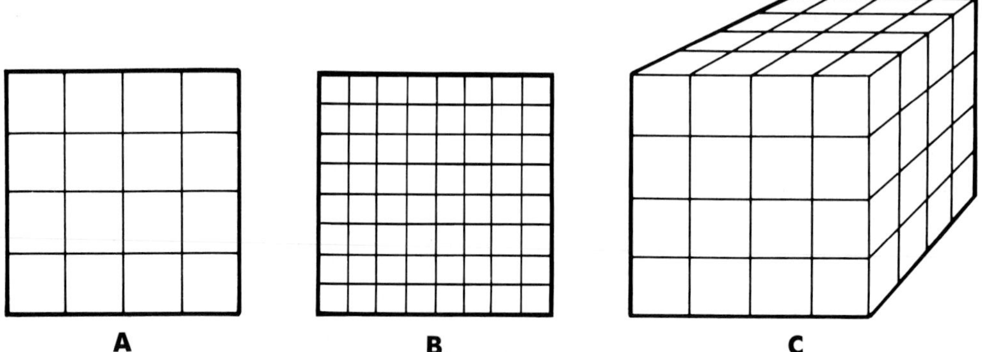

Fig. 12-8. **A** and **B,** Two different matrix sizes. Number of image points (pixels) increases with larger matrices. Resolution increases with the number of pixels. **C,** Matrix, 4 × 4, with a 4-bit length.

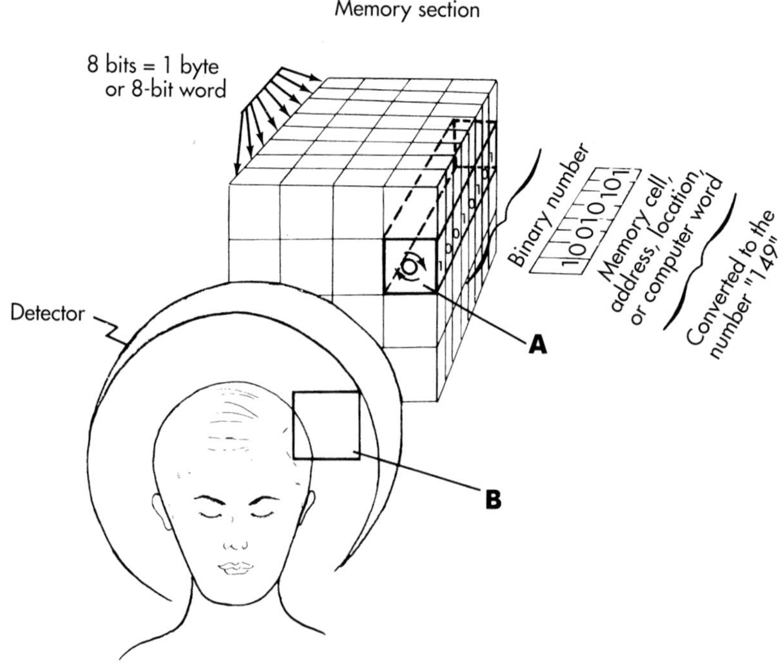

Fig. 12-9. Computer memory. **A,** Zero or one can be written in core. **B,** 149 gamma events occur within this area. For a memory section of 4096 addresses, this area would measure 4.4 by 4.4 mm on a 10-inch crystal.

equivalents (A). Thus the 149 gamma events that occur at area B are represented in memory as the 8-bit computer data word 10010101. The entire organ image is simply the extension of this simple principle to the other addresses in computer memory. The greatest number of total counts that can be written in a single memory cell is simply the largest number that can be presented with eight characters of the binary system (in this case 2^8-1 or 255). For a memory of 4096 separate cells or addresses (64 × 64 matrix) each would reference an area of approximately 4.4 by 4.4 mm on a scintillation camera having a 10-inch field of view.

In expressing the storage capacity of a computer memory, both the number of addresses (rounded to the nearest thousand) and the word length (number of bits per word) are given. For example, the memory unit just described is referred to as a 4K (4000 but actually 4096) 8-bit word computer.

The matrix sizes available for use with any camera system are of great importance to the accuracy of a nuclear medicine study from two different standpoints: (1) image resolution and (2) statistical reliability of the results. In addition, there are two matrixes with which to be concerned: acquisition matrix and display matrix.

Image resolution. In general, the larger the matrix size, the smaller the pixel and the better the resolution; that is, a 256 × 256 image or display matrix has better resolution than a 64 × 64 matrix. However, much depends on the size of both matrixes. If the acquisition matrix is 64 × 64 and the display matrix is 128 × 128, the resolution is as good as the 64 × 64 acquisition matrix capabilities. The image has been interpolated to make it more pleasing to the eye.

Statistical reliability. Just as in any image, the technical aspect of acquiring a good image depends on proper statistics.

In a 128 × 128 memory on a 10-inch field of view camera, each pixel represents 1⁄12 inch, or on a 15-inch camera, each pixel represents 1⁄8 inch. With a 64 × 64 memory matrix on a 10-inch field of view camera, each pixel is 1⁄16 inch, or on a 15-inch field it is slightly larger than 1⁄5 inch. In a 10-inch camera, 32 by 32 equals 1⁄3 inch, or in a 15-inch camera it equals smaller than 1⁄2 inch/pixel. With a 2× zoom the pixel sizes for each matrix are reduced by 50% (Table 12-1).

Following a study of Table 12-1, it can be seen that the solution to resolution is to use as large a memory matrix as possible and on "zoom" when conceivable. However, the one consideration not discussed is statistics. If it is assumed that the average nuclear medicine study contains approximately 1.5 million counts and about two thirds of the pixels are viewing the organ, then a 128 × 128 matrix (or 17K pixels) will display 1.5 million counts in 10,600 memory locations. This is equal to an average of 141 counts/pixel. The statistical accuracy of the counts in each pixel (±10) is approximately equal to 12 counts. It was decided that the resolution was marginal, and mistakenly a 256 × 256 matrix (or 65K pixels) was chosen on a repeat study so that the same two thirds of the crystal represented 43.7K pixels. With this arrangement each pixel received 35 counts/pixel with a statistical accuracy of ± 6 counts. To acquire this study on a 256 × 256 matrix is poor technique.

■ Semiconductor memory

Memory of the solid state variety came on the computer scene with the advances in integrated circuits (IC). Basically an IC is a highly miniaturized printed circuit (PC) board with all of the components required of a memory circuit already built in (that is, transistor, capacitors, etc.). These tiny PC boards, referred to as *chips,* are as small as a fingernail and are getting smaller. The chip is a small rectangular block with a small hole in the middle of its top and metallic pins from its bottom (Fig. 12-10). Inside the hole rests a tiny and extremely thin piece of silicon or germanium. Each piece of silicon has had as many as hundreds of thousands of pathways burned into its surface with a strong ultraviolet light.

A semiconductor memory relies on the function of storing electron charges rather than on the absence or presence of a magnetized area and therefore requires a very stable power supply. Using the same concept of the binary system, the binary values of 1 and 0 are represented by a simple on or off state. Shut off the power and this on-off pattern is destroyed ("erased"). The semiconductor memory is arranged the same way as core memory, having pixel matrixes of 64 × 64, 128 × 128, 256 × 256, etc., with the ability to expand the memory by adding more ICs. Since the rationale of operation is stored charges (or lack thereof), it is easy to understand why data are lost when the current is turned off.

RAMS, ROMS, and PROMS. The memories discussed so far are all capable of being written or erased.

Table 12-1. Crystal area represented by each pixel for different matrix sizes

Matrix	Pixel size 10 inches	Pixel size 15 inches	Zoom (2×) pixel size 10 inches	Zoom (2×) pixel size 15 inches
128×128	0.078	0.117	0.04	0.058
64× 64	0.156	0.234	0.078	0.117
32× 32	0.312	0.468	0.156	0.234

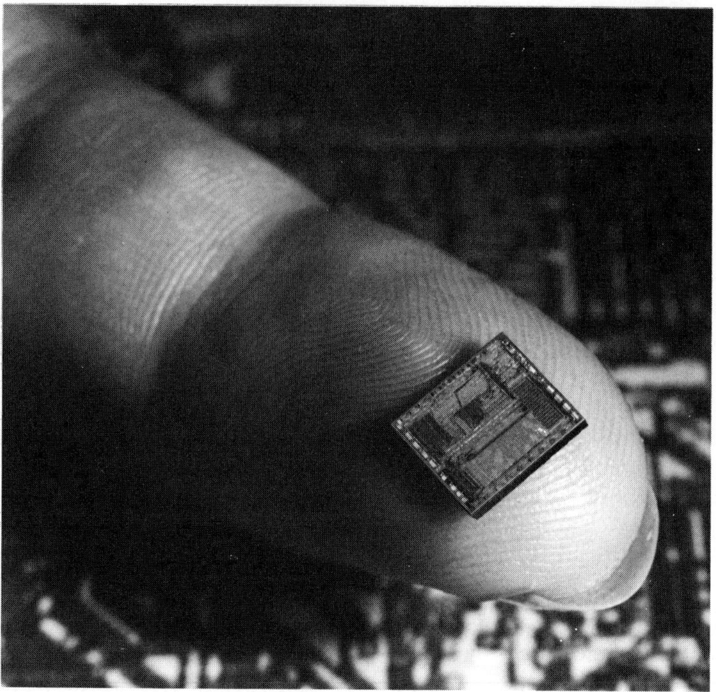

Fig. 12-10. Microprocessor chip. (From Bushong, S.C.: Radiologic science for technologists, ed. 5, St. Louis, 1993, Mosby–Year Book, Courtesy Intel Corp.)

These are called *RAMs* (an acronym for *R*andom *A*ccess *M*emory). It is the portion of the memory to which the computer user or a program can gain direct access at any time. As already described, RAM is temporary; it loses its programs, instructions, or information when power is interrupted. (A camera flood correction is a good example of a RAM. If power is interrupted, another flood for correction purposes must be acquired.)

When a computer runs a program using a semiconductor-type memory, it is often necessary to have part or all of the program reside permanently in memory, unchanged, and able to be addressed whenever required. It is also necessary when using a high-level computer language (Fortran, BASIC, etc.) that the compiler (a language translator that converts programs and commands from a high-level language into machine language) be placed permanently in memory. To do this, *ROMs* (an acronym for *R*ead *O*nly *M*emory) were developed. Their purpose is to make the normally volatile semiconductor memory nonvolatile. Many techniques have been developed to perform this capability. They range from programming the memory to simply blowing the appropriate fuses to the appropriate bits to hold the desired program (similar to blowing household fuses) to the use of voltage high enough to overcome the insulation around leak-minimized capacitors and force a charge into them. Once in the capacitor, the charge is trapped by the surrounding insulation and remains indefinitely. (A program for camera flood correction is a good example of a ROM. If power is interrupted, the program does not disappear, since it is in ROM, but the corrected flood does, since it is in RAM.)

There is a form of ROM in which the program can be altered called *PROM* (*P*rogrammable *R*ead *O*nly *M*emory). It can be reprogrammed by the user only under special conditions. The PROM data are erased by intense ultraviolet light in at least one instance and reprogrammed by the application of a predetermined current through the PROM.

■ Buffer memory

Buffer memory is a special kind of RAM to compensate for differences in the speed with which information can be handled between the CPU and peripheral devices (e.g., paper printer). The printer is much slower than the CPU. Therefore, the buffer memory is an intermediate holding area located outside the CPU for temporarily storing data from the CPU until such time as the printer (in this case) is able to accept it. The CPU can transfer at rates of thousands to millions of characters or instructions per second (Mips), whereas the printer can accept only several hundred; the printer, then, is the limiting factor. Once transferred, the CPU is free to be used for another operation.

■ CONTROL SECTION

The most important component of the control section is an electronic oscillator, commonly referred to as the *clock*. The clock generates a stream of pulses on a regularly timed basis that open and close all the other circuits in the computer. In this manner the control section is able to regulate the external and internal operations of all the sections. Since it initiates and synchronizes everything in the computer, the clock is sometimes likened to a heartbeat. Another portion of the control section is the control panel or console for direct human to machine communication. This contains a number of "start" and "stop" buttons, as well as the individual controls for the various I/O devices and displays. For a scintillation camera interfaced with a dedicated computer, some common control would be available for (1) cathode ray tube (CRT) display, (2) image orientation (X, Y, and Z planes), (3) region of interest (ROI), (4) uniform field correction, (5) addition and subtraction, (6) smoothing, (7) interpolation, and (8) histogram generation. In addition, there are the usual controls to display or indicate the number of the study, patient identification, time of the study, and counts obtained.

Although the control section directs the implementation of instructions, the actual performance of nuclear medicine data manipulation is carried out in the arithmetic section of the computer.

■ ARITHMETIC/LOGIC SECTION

The various electronics circuits of the arithmetic/logic section are scattered throughout the computer. This section performs all of the addition, subtraction, multiplication, and division functions of the computer.

There are *registers* used as temporary storage locations, *comparers* used in mathematic operations, *counters* to tally items of information such as instructions, and *flip-flops* used to perform logic statements (for example, comparing numbers). Interconnecting all of these elements is a network of other electronic and logic circuits that directs the signals along their appropriate paths.

■ NUCLEAR MEDICINE APPLICATIONS

Although many applications of the digital processing of images are currently being developed, several uses are common. The important applications are treated separately.

■ Nonuniformity correction techniques

Uniformity, or rather the lack of it, has been a constant problem since the advent of the scintillation camera (Anger type). The cause of this nonuniformity is largely twofold: (1) the variations in sensitivity across the face of the crystal and (2) nonlinearities in the position signals, resulting in spatial distortions caused by generation of an area of apparently decreased radioactivity surrounded by a ring of apparently increased radioactivity. The latter defect causes bar phantoms to "barrel" and data from linearity phantoms to be malpositioned, to say nothing of the effects on clinical results. This can be true in a uniform flood system and often is the case in a nonuniform flood situation. The reverse is even more often the case; that is, a nonuniform flood study with no appreciable spatial distortions.

The enigma of the design engineer regarding this problem is that uniformity has always been a compromise with resolution; as resolution is increased, uniformity decreases and vice versa. It becomes the job of the engineer to decide at what point both facets will be compromised to give an acceptable clinical result. With the advent of nonuniformity correction techniques, this dilemma has been solved with a design for resolution and a correction for nonuniformity.

There appear to be at least five different techniques of correcting for nonuniformity. These techniques can apply correction to areas as great as 20% deviation from the average and are as follows:

1. Matrix division, using the computer to either subtract counts from the "hot" areas of a stored image or add counts to the "cold" areas of a stored image
2. Count skimming (also known as count skipping)
3. Z pulse modulation (rarely used)
4. Sliding energy window (also known as micro-Z processing)
5. Spatial distortion correction

Matrix division. This nonuniformity correction technique divides the camera face into squares. Each square corresponds to a location in the computer memory (Fig 12-8). This location should be no smaller than a 64 × 64 matrix or a total of 4096 pixels. Each detected event (a bit) from a flood is recorded in its corresponding pixel location in the computer memory. The collection continues until there is a statistically significant number of counts in each memory location or until such time as a preselected number has been recorded. Then the recording of events stops. The computer is then capable of searching each location and determining the total number of counts stored in each location. If all locations have the same number of stored events, nonuniformity correction is unnecessary. This is rarely the case. In the usual situation, computers identify the magnitude of the deficiency in each location and correct for it by equalizing all points to no greater than ±5%, either by the addition of counts or the deletion of counts. Suppose that the computer program was such that in a 64 × 64 matrix the program would turn off whenever a single pixel received 500 counts (64 × 64 × 500 = 2 million total counts in the flood). Further, suppose that the computer in its systematic search of each pixel notes that some pixels have accumulated only 450 counts; the computer calculates the deficiency to be a 10% reduction from the maximum counts. The computer records that and will in future studies (either floods or clinical images) correct those locations by either randomly adding 10% more counts to each of them (termed *matrix addition,* which decreases the time of the study) or randomly rejecting 10% of the counts in each of them (termed *matrix subtraction,* which increases the time of the study). This procedure is carried out for all memory loca-

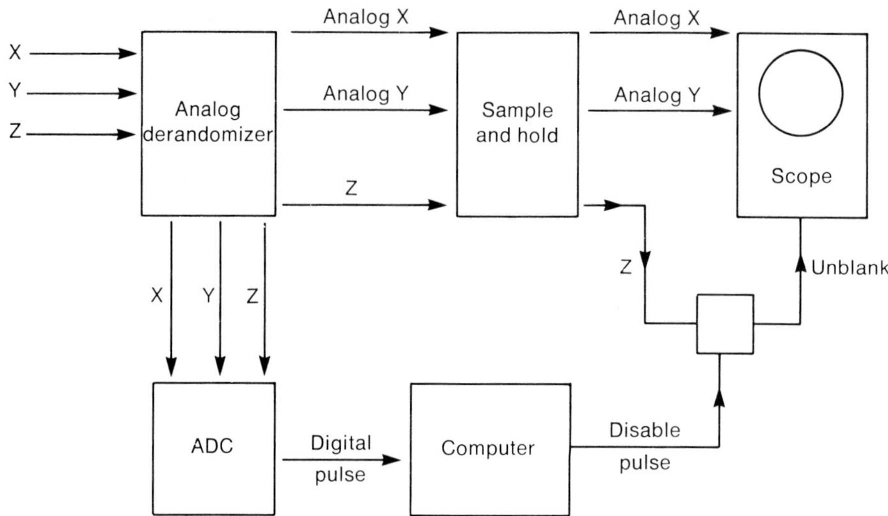

Fig. 12-11. Modified version of schematic of count-skimming circuit.

tions, with appropriate correction techniques generated for each.

Count skimming. This nonuniformity correction technique is an attempt to avoid the long dead time necessary in the matrix division-rejection technique. This system uses an *analog derandomizer circuit* in conjunction with a *sample and hold circuit* and a minicomputer. The *X* and *Y* position signals and the unblank pulses go directly to an analog derandomizer (Fig. 12-11) rather than to the CRT. This derandomizer is capable of storing up to eight random events from the camera and releasing them at a rate of 200,000 counts/sec. In this way the events are derandomized and put into a form that the ADC and the computer can handle easier and faster. The other advantage is that since pulses (counts) from the camera are random, sometimes a second pulse arrives during the dead time of the system (called *pulse pileup*) and is not counted. The derandomizer is able to count these pulses; therefore the count rate capabilities of the system are increased. The signals are then sent out of the derandomizer and divided—one set going to the ADC, the other to a sample and hold circuit. The latter is composed of two capacitor memories that serve to delay the analog signal from reaching the CRT. During the delay period, the second set of signals is being sent to the ADC, digitized, and made accessible for the computer to either store as a flood or allow for correction from the stored flood by rejection of counts in "hot" areas. If the event is to be rejected, the correction circuit will release a signal to disable the unblank pulse that is being released at the same time (along with the *X* and *Y* position signals) by the sample and hold circuit; therefore no event is recorded on the CRT. If the computer accepts the event, no disable pulse is generated, and the event is allowed to record on the CRT.

***Z* pulse modulation.** Another rarely used technique for nonuniformity correction is that of *Z* pulse modulation. The *Z* pulse or unblank pulse is typically of a uniform width (Fig. 12-12, *A*). This allows the response of the electron gun in the CRT to be the same for each event and therefore to be displayed with the same intensity on film. The approach to *Z* pulse modulation is to vary the pulse width of the *Z* signal (Fig. 12-12, *B*), thereby varying the response of the electron gun in the CRT. The resultant film then appears uniform because *Z* signals from hot areas are shorter and displayed with less intensity than those from cold areas, whereas *Z* signals from cold areas are longer and therefore displayed with increased intensity on film. This system also uses an analog delay system to allow the memory to develop a correction factor for the event and modulate the *Z* pulse. This technique does not involve either addition or rejection of counts; therefore the time for individual clinical studies has not changed whether on or off correction. Since the correction occurs at the CRT on the analog signal, this approach would not allow for correction of a computer-generated image. Another program, such as matrix division, would be required for the computer itself.

Sliding energy window. Another approach to correction circuits is that of a sliding energy window. This approach is based on the belief that the major contributors to nonuniformities in the flood study are the crystal, the PMTs, the "light pipes," and the interfaces among them. The variations in light distribution relating to these factors result in a slight shift of the photopeak on each of the PMTs. The spectrum seen in "peaking in" the instrument is a composite of all of these individual peaks (Fig. 12-13). Since each peak varies slightly, the composite peak is a broader one. To accept a clinical window based on this composite image is to accept more scatter and a degraded image. A better solution would be to set a window for each energy peak of each PMT. Ideally, since a computer is used, a win-

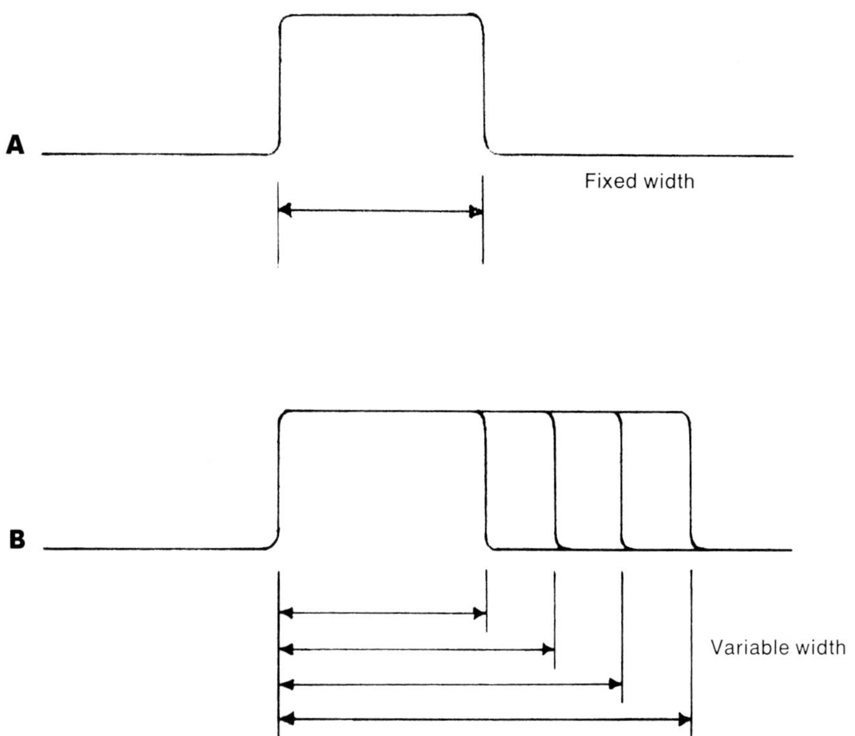

Fig. 12-12. A, Typical *Z*-pulse width. **B,** Pulses of various widths as result of *Z*-pulse modulation.

dow could be set for the energy peak received by each pixel. Therefore a 64 × 64 matrix computer would be likened to 4096 individual pulse-height analyzers, each setting its own optimum window. This is the case with the sliding energy window technique. In this way uniformity is improved and energy resolution is optimized because each window is treated separately rather than in common. Any causes for nonuniformity not related to energy are corrected by any of the other correction techniques already mentioned.

Techniques have recently been developed to make these corrections "on the fly." Since this technique is designed to correct for variations in point source sensitivity (count rate) by shifts in the average photopeak pulse height, the energy window can be adjusted on an event-by-event basis.

Spatial distortion correction. Another technique that can be performed on the fly is that of spatial distortion correction. In this cause for nonuniformity, local counts are compressed or expanded to provoke the nonlinearities. Such distortions are caused by nonlinear changes in light distribution within the scintillator. These spatial distortions can be corrected by removing the distortion and recording the detected event in its appropriate spatial location.

This is performed by using a precisely known pattern (bar phantom, hole phantom, or a regular array of point sources). Since the true location is known, the distorted location is measured, and a correction displacement factor is calculated and applied to the *X* and *Y* coordinates and stored in memory. With these correction factors in memory, each event can be adjusted "on-line." The technique repositions each event in real time without introducing additional dead time.

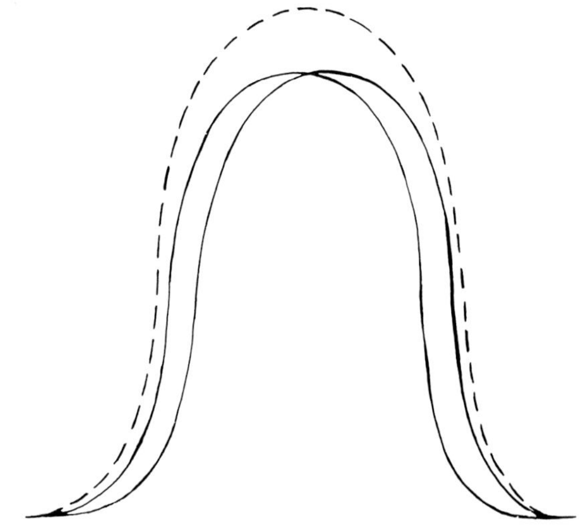

Fig. 12-13. Solid lines, energy peaks from two separate photomultiplier tubes (PMTs); dotted line, composite energy peak. To encompass both energy peaks from these two separate PMTs, a larger window would be necessary, resulting in reduced resolution of a clinical image.

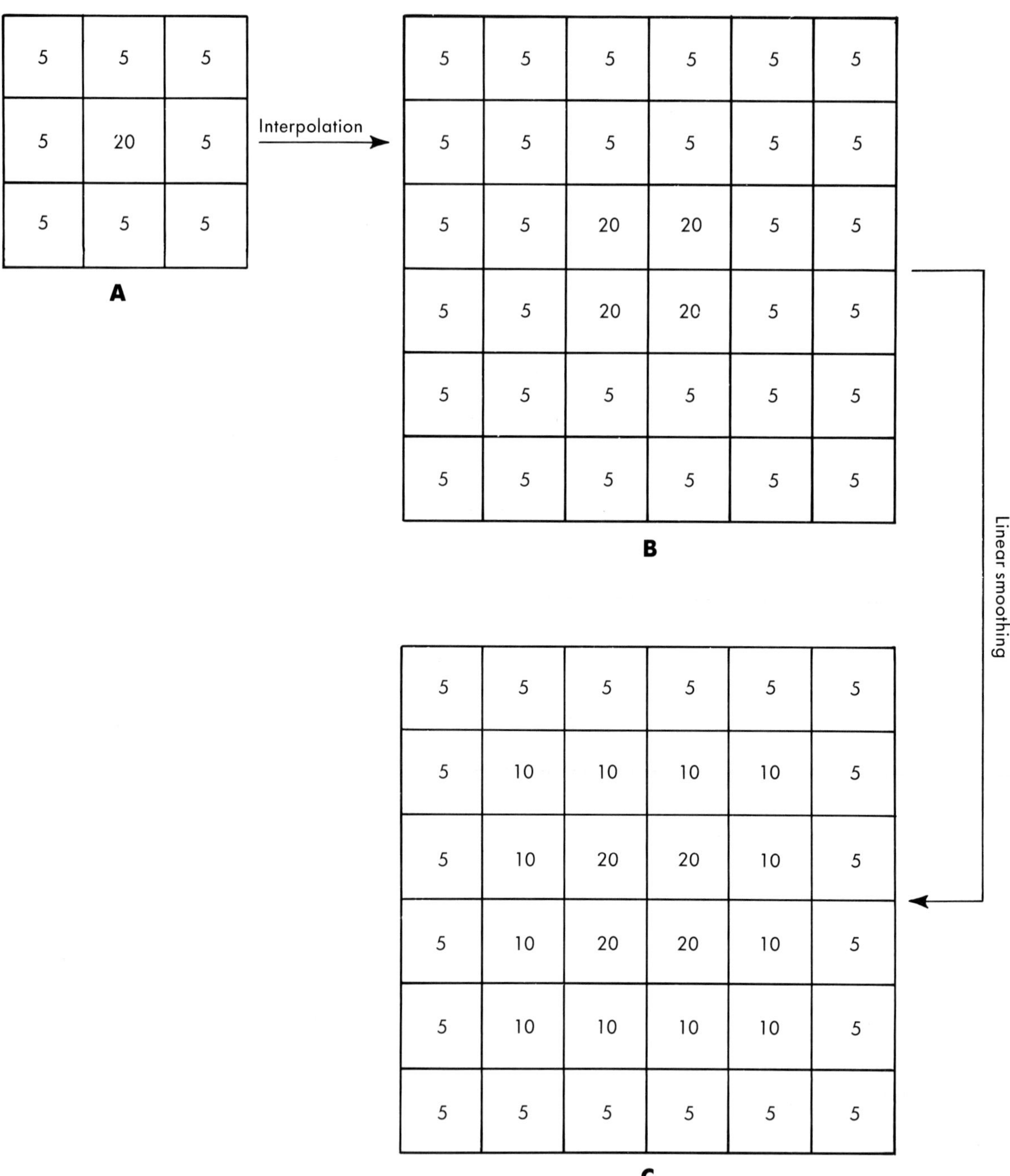

Fig. 12-14. Example of interpolation in which a 3 × 3 matrix, 1-bit deep, has been changed to a 6 × 6 matrix, 1-bit deep through interpolation. For each pixel in **A,** there are four pixels in **B,** and their values have been averaged in **C** to achieve a linear smoothing effect. In this way the image seems to have a more analog appearance by diminishing the distracting feature of the discrete pixel (raster effect) of the digital image.

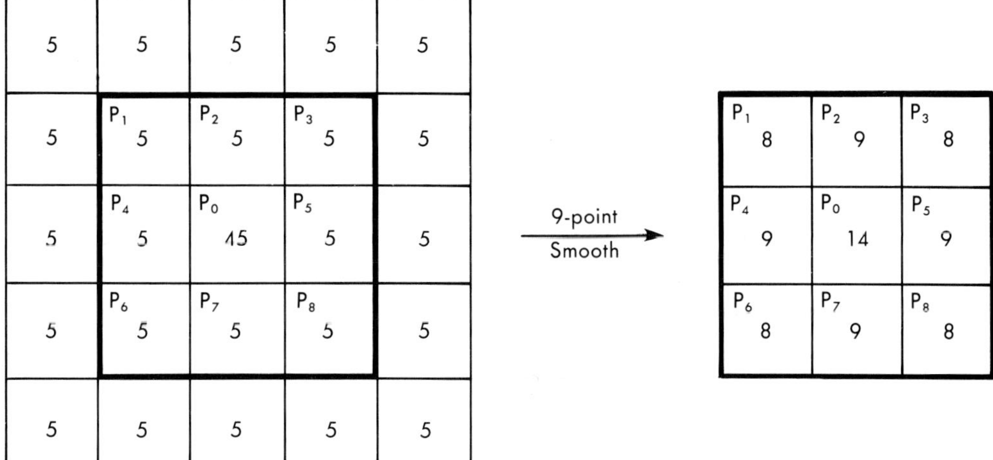

Fig. 12-15. Nine-point smoothing algorithm has been applied to the area inscribed by solid lines. Smoothing process continues by incrementing that 9-point area, 1 pixel to the right, so that P_5 is now in the center pixel and reapplying the algorithm, then moving it diagonally so that P_3 occupies the center point, etc.

■ Acquisition techniques

There are several techniques to acquire and record information from a scintillation camera. They are static, dynamic, list, and gated.

Static acquisition mode. In the static mode a preset number of counts or a preset time determines the length of time for the study. The single image is recorded one frame at a time and placed in a matrix so that events from an organ are recorded in the pixel represented by the area from where the counts come. This can be modified slightly with a special program for whole-body images, using whole-body tables.

Interpolation. Interpolation is a feature sometimes used to reduce the digital raster effect on a static (and dynamic) image. It does not improve the accuracy of the image, but it gives it a more pleasing appearance. There is no loss of data, and raw data are left unaltered. The idea is to replace the smaller acquisition matrix with a larger matrix. Sometimes an interpolation program calls for a linear smoothing (Fig. 12-14). This linear smoothing can occasionally assist the interpreter at the time of reading in removing a bothersome artifact.

Smoothing. Smoothing is usually reserved for a weighted interpolation. These are often called *filters*. There are two types of filters that have been useful in nuclear medicine: spatial and temporal. Temporal filters are discussed in the section under dynamic acquisition.

Spatial filters. Spatial filters are usually used on static images to attempt to remove statistical fluctuations in the image. This is accomplished by modifying the values of the data points within the image. A two-dimensional 9-point smoothing program is the standard of the industry. An algorithm (formula) for such a filter is as follows:

$$P_0 = \frac{1}{36}\,[8\,P_0 + 4\,(P_2 + P_4 + P_5 + P_7) + 3\,(P_1 + P_3 + P_6 + P_8)]$$

where

P_0 = Center pixel
$P_{1,3,6,8}$ = Corner pixels
$P_{2,4,5,7}$ = Remaining pixels

This formula gives weighted values to the pixels in the 9-pixel field by placing most emphasis to the center pixel with the least emphasis to the corners. In an image the 9-pixel bracket would be incremented to the next pixel and recomputed, and then to each pixel in the image, etc. Figure 12-15 illustrates one such 9-point smoothing algorithm. Figure 12-16, *C,* illustrates the results of this 9-point spatial filter of the original image, Fig. 12-16, *A*. Sometimes an image may go through three or four such smoothing procedures before the image is acceptable to the interpreter. Other smoothing techniques are also available, such as the one-dimensional, five-point smoothing program or different weightings applied to the 9-point program.

Background correction. One of the simplest forms of background correction is to continuously subtract one count from each pixel in the image until the desired image is achieved. Other techniques use linear interpolation techniques, and others even resort to weighted averages. Figure 12-16, *B,* is the result of a background subtract/smoothing technique. These results clearly show the value of reducing the background as an aid to interpretation.

Slice profiles. Profiles are attempts to quantify a static image. A row of data points are moved through the area on the image involved. Those values are then plotted to show a profile (Fig. 12-17).

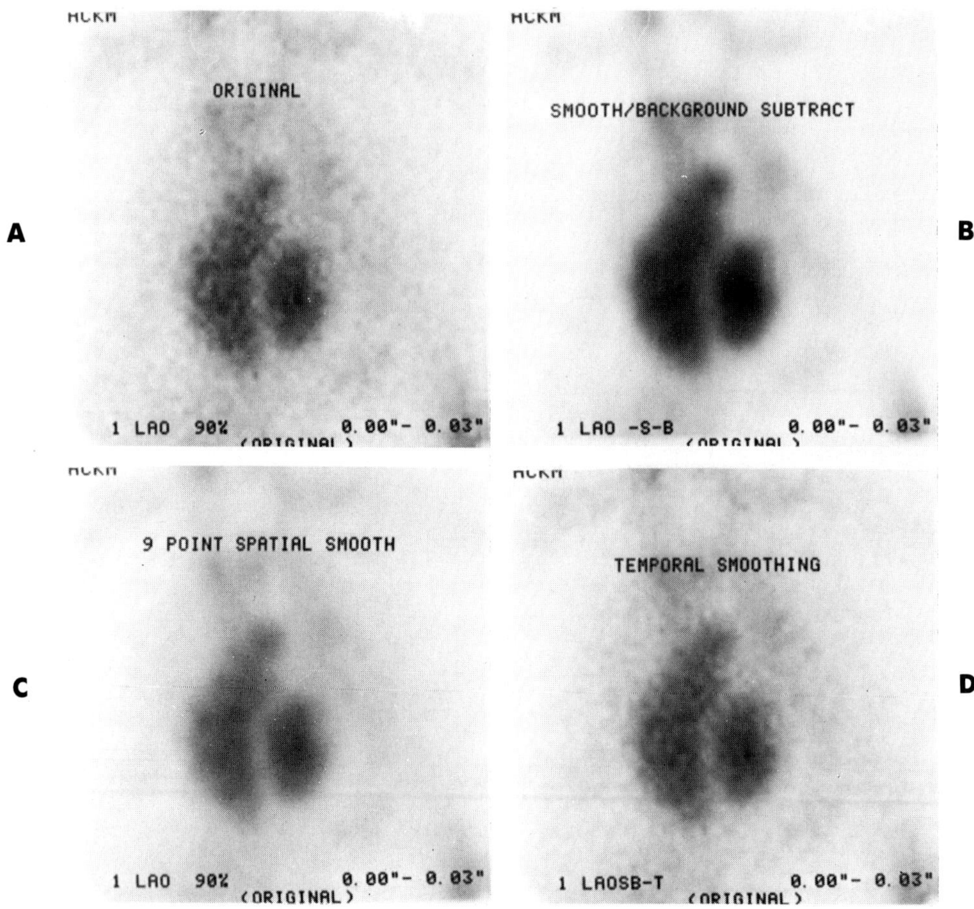

Fig. 12-16. **A,** Original cardiac image with **B, C,** and **D** demonstrating several types of smoothing techniques. (Courtesy Galesburg Cottage Hospital, Galesburg, Ill.)

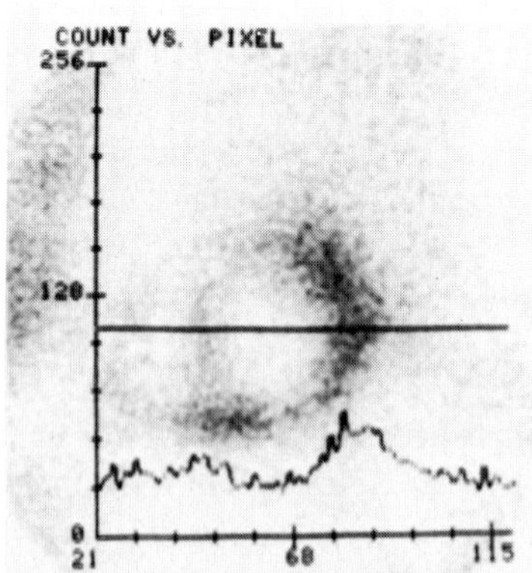

Fig. 12-17. Slice profile of ^{201}Tl heart image. Collected an optimum resolution matrix and evaluated by taking a row of pixels through area of interest and plotting each pixel to generate the histogram. (Courtesy St. John's Hospital, Springfield, Ill.)

Zoom mode. Sometimes it is important to make use of only a small portion of the camera field of view. This is particularly applicable to cardiac images. All state-of-the-art camera/computer devices are capable of magnifying the image so that the desired area displays as a full-screen image. This program is called *zoom mode*.

There are two types of magnification. One type is applied *following* the study in which the size of the pixels in the center field of view is magnified by some factor. In this approach to magnification the number of pixels representing the ROI remains unchanged. There is no loss or gain in resolution—simply magnification of the central field of view of the camera (called *post-process zoom*).

The other form of magnification is one in which an a priori decision is made so that the smaller image is collected on the entire matrix. In this version of magnification (called *pre-process zoom*) the small ROI is represented by the number of pixels that it would have in the large image times the magnification factor. In this form resolution increases (Fig. 12-18).

Dynamic acquisition modes. There are two techniques used to acquire dynamic nuclear medicine studies such as

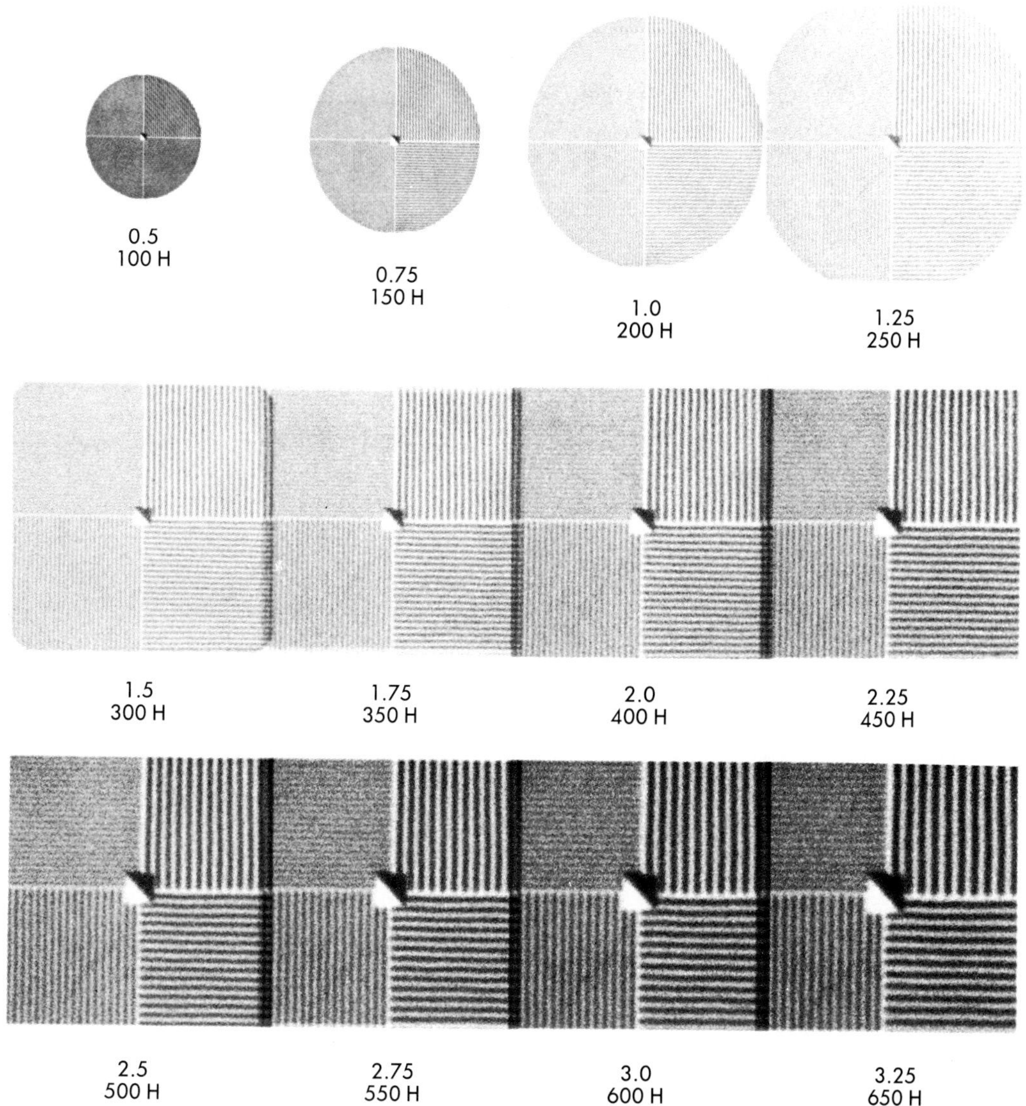

Fig. 12-18. Zoom mode demonstrating increased resolution as image is magnified. (Courtesy St. John's Hospital, Springfield, Ill.)

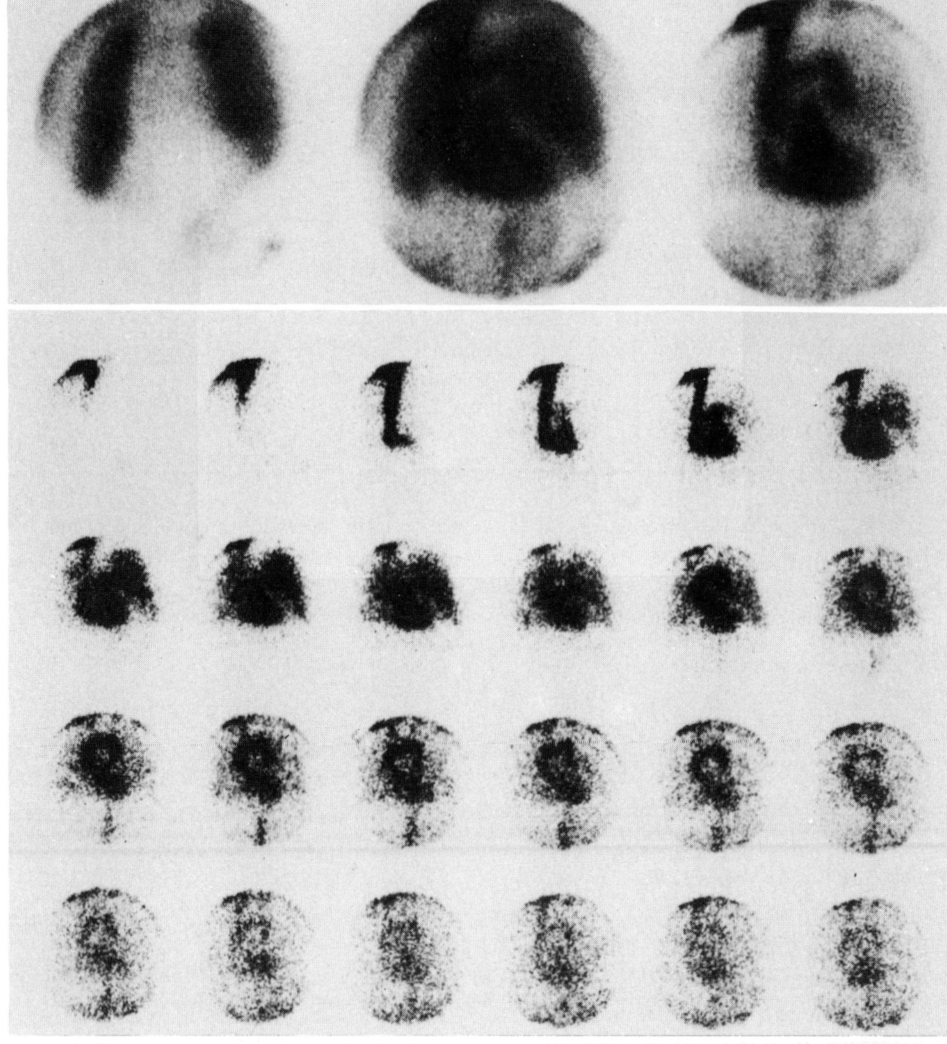

Fig. 12-19. Varied format as presented on 8 × 10 x-ray film using multiformat programmer. Large image in upper left is a transmission image of the lungs. Large image in middle is a transmission image combined with a static flow image through the heart. Large image in upper right is just the static flow image. The 24 smaller images represent a cardiac flow, reading from left to right. (Courtesy Holy Family Hospital, Des Plaines, Ill.)

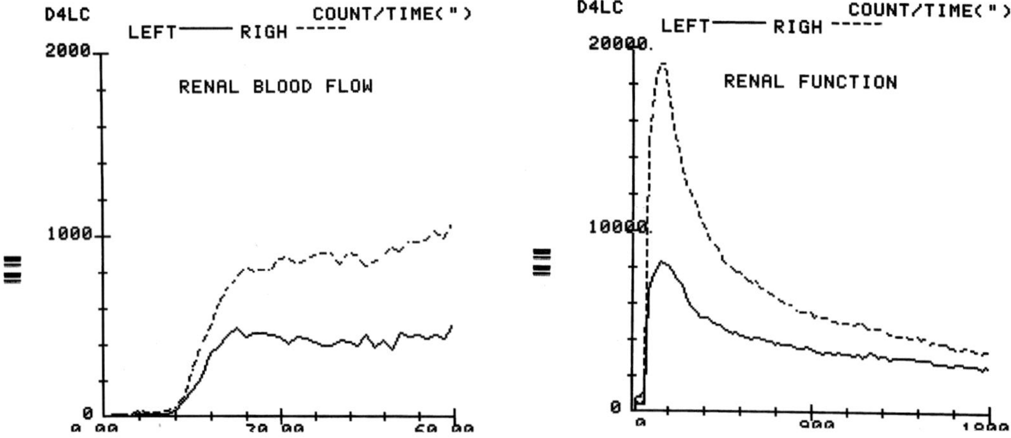

Fig. 12-20. Renal histograms of blood flow and renal function generated by a computer plot of data over time using ROIs around kidneys in Fig. 12-22. (Courtesy Memorial Medical Center, Jacksonville, Fla.)

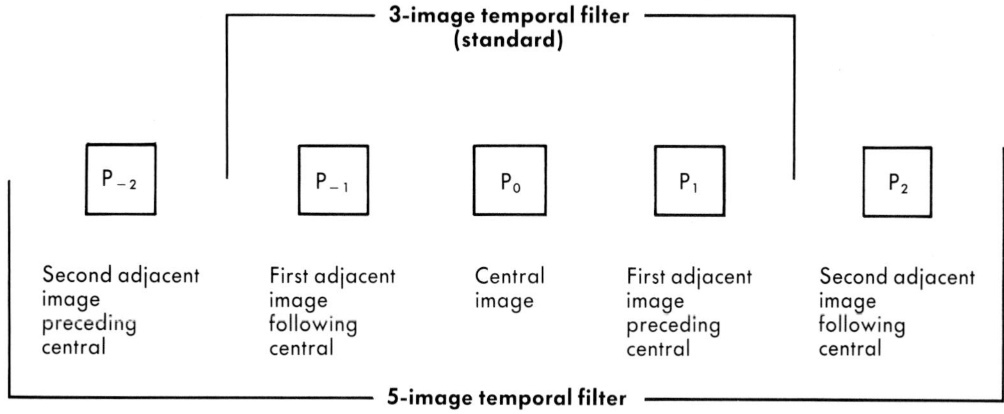

Fig. 12-21. Schema for three-image and five-image temporal filter (Refer to clinical results in Fig. 12-16, *D*.)

cardiac flow studies. They are frame mode and list mode. Frame mode requires less computer space and irreversible a priori decisions. List mode usually requires a tremendous amount of computer space, but data are easier to modify to get the desired results.

Frame mode. In frame mode, images are built and stored in computer memory for a preset period of time or preset count just as in static mode. However, as soon as the acquisition is complete, it immediately begins to collect a second image on the next frame. While the second image is being stored on another portion of the memory, the first image is being transferred to the diskette. (This is called *buffering* and explains why twice as much memory is required for dynamic studies as in static imaging.) Images in the frame mode can be replayed in rapid sequence in a cinema format in order to provide a motion picture of the organs, or each frame can be recorded on film (Fig. 12-19).

If counts in these various images were plotted (or portions of the image, using ROIs), the curve will not be smooth but can be used to adequately display such dynamics as blood flow or organ function. These plots are called *histograms* and are seen often to demonstrate renal physiology (Fig. 12-20).

Smoothing

Temporal filters. Temporal filters can be performed only on dynamic images, since they involve a weighted averaging technique between each pixel in one image and the same pixel in the frame immediately preceding and following the image (a standard three-image temporal filter), or between a pixel in one image and the same pixel in the two frames immediately preceding and following the image (a five-image temporal filter) (Fig. 12-21). These values are added together to develop a weighted average that replaces the original pixel value of the central image. The filter then moves to another image, and the procedure is repeated until all images are smoothed and a filtered dynamic study is created. An algorithm for such a filter is as follows:

$$P_0 = 0.5P_0 + 0.25\,(P_1 + P_{-1})$$

where:

P_1 = Counts in pixel following the central image
P_{-1} = Counts in pixel preceding the central image
P_0 = Counts in pixels of central image

A five-image filter might carry the following algorithm:

$$P_0 = 0.5\,P_0 + 0.25\,(P_{-1} + P_1) + 0.125\,(P_{-2} + P_2)$$

Figure 12-16, *D*, displays such a temporal filter.

There is some loss of spatial resolution using this technique because the heart is changing positions during this summing process. However, the ability to view the cinema image without flicker, using this technique, more than compensates for the small loss in resolution.

Regions of interest. One of the features of using computers for dynamic images (and some static images) is the ability to select small portions of the image and evaluate the area for count content, reflecting either concentration or flow of radionuclide to that area. The areas are called *regions of interest (ROIs)* (Fig. 12-22). This can be performed with the use of joysticks, cursor lines, or light pens.

Joysticks. Joysticks are small rods that can be moved back and forth and up and down to delineate an area on the screen. The joystick is fitted with two variable resistors that reflect the position of the *X* and *Y* axes via the production of 2 −V output. These voltages are converted to digital signals received by the display screen where corresponding points are addressed and flagged.

Cursor lines. Cursor lines can be used when the exact shape of the ROI is not important. Cursor lines are simply two horizontal lines and two vertical lines that can define any size square or rectangular area when the distance between both sets of parallel lines is changed. The area inside the rectangle (or square) area is the ROI.

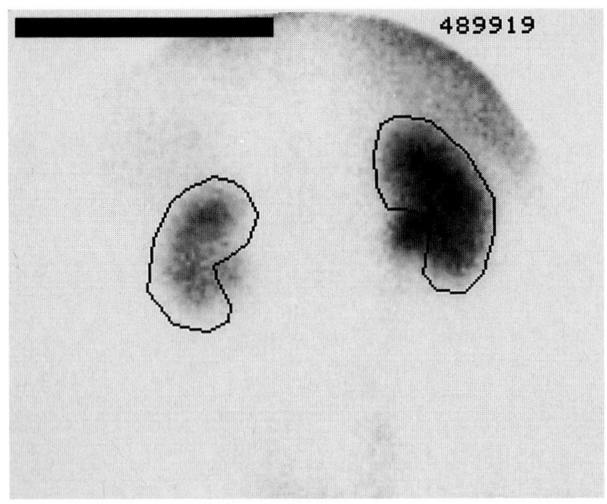

Fig. 12-22. Regions of interest (ROI) as drawn manually with a joy stick. Histograms generated from these ROIs can be seen in Fig. 12-20. Note reduced activity in left kidney is reflected in reduced flow and function. (Courtesy Memorial Medical Center, Jacksonville, Fla.)

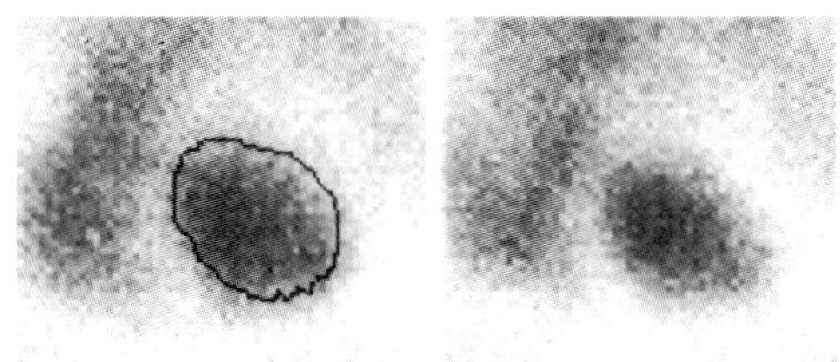

Fig. 12-23. ROI drawn with light pen around left ventricle in diastole. (Courtesy Marymount Hospital, Cleveland, Ohio.)

Light pens. Light pens can also be used to define ROIs. The light pen is aimed at the display screen where the computer senses its position by intensifying the pixel(s) representing that position (Fig. 12-23). Not all display screens are capable of using this technique, since the light output of the screen in the ROI must be sufficient to trigger the light pen. In areas of low count rate, that aspect is particularly troublesome.

Phase analysis. Phase analysis is a relatively new technique that calls for collecting cardiac images at high frame rates (<20 msec/frame). At these high frame rates the sequence (or phase) of ventricular contraction can be determined. These frames are evaluated for time and activity and compared, pixel for pixel, against a sinusoidal curve. With this technique, abnormalities in the sequence of electric conduction through the heart can be studied. Two images are obtained with this technique: an amplitude image and a phase image.

The amplitude image provides an image of the heart based on the values of the maximum count changes at each pixel with no regard to phase. This image is used to describe the magnitude of cardiac contraction.

The phase image provides information on when the maximum counts occur in each pixel with respect to the phases of the sinusoid. This represents the volumetric changes in each pixel and can be related to the electric stimulation of that portion of the heart that initiated the action. A phase image demonstrates which areas of the heart beat in phase, with the atria, with the ventricles, and out of phase, such as in arrhythmias. Phase images have been used to demonstrate the waves of contraction in a heart study by using a program that calls for the pixel to turn black at the maximum count rate for one frame only. Foci of arrhythmic activity can be detected in this way. Phase analysis has also been used to study the sequence of contraction generated by pacemakers implanted at various sites in the heart, patients with left bundle branch block, and those with ventricular tachycardia.

List acquisition mode. In list mode each event is recorded by its existence and location directly into memory. List mode does not provide any readily available information at the completion of the study. It is simply a list of events and where they occurred (its X and Y coordinates). Each event is recorded in its own frame.

On completion of the study an image can be constructed from list mode. No a priori decisions are required with list mode. Once recorded, decisions can be made (and changed) as to matrix size, frame rate, etc., and all from the original data. This is a distinct advantage. The disadvantage is that relatively fast disk drives are required for data collection.

This is also a buffered system, since information is being transferred to diskette while more information is being recorded. List mode can use less diskette space than frame acquisition, but there is "break even" point depending on count rate, matrix size, and frame rate. A renal study and right ventricular ejection fraction (first pass) are good examples of recording in list mode.

Multigated acquisition mode. Organ motion in nuclear medicine studies has long been a distressing problem for the interpreter of nuclear medicine procedures. Liver and lung motions have been irresolvable problems since the advent of the rectilinear scan. Scintillation cameras have helped but not solved the problem. Early attempts to limit liver motion during a scanning procedure ranged from strapping the patient across the diaphragm and to the cart so tightly that diaphragmatic breathing (the cause of liver motion) was discouraged to "freezing" the phrenic nerve, which innervates the diaphragm. Attempts were made to image lungs with the camera only during the short pauses of inhalation or exhalation. Composite images were formed by manually turning on the camera each time the patient inhaled and held the breath, and manually turning off the camera during exhalation. A statistically valid image was achieved by repeating the process many times. This on-off procedure is referred to as *gating*. All of these attempts met

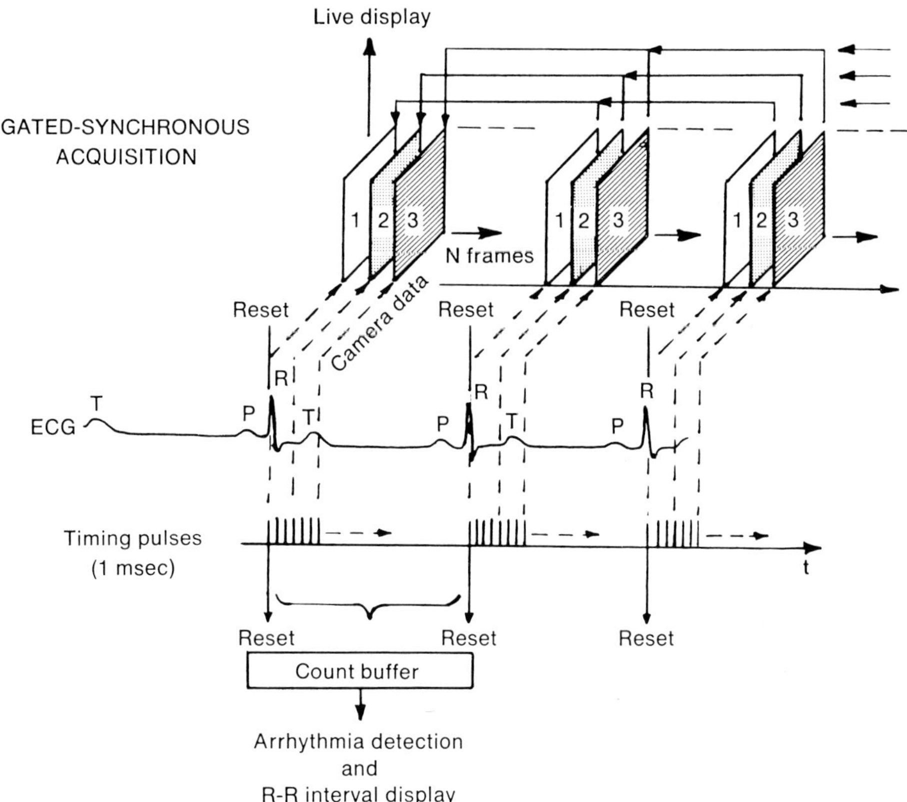

Fig. 12-24. Gated frame mode data acquisition for cardiac studies. Data from gamma camera are in *N* frames between each *R* wave with the *R* wave causing reset to frame one. *N* may be up to 48 in 32 × 32 acquisition or up to 12 in 64 × 64 acquisition. Data collected during each heartbeat are added to those from previous beats so that valid statistical images result. A continually updated display of the first frame together with *R-R* interval, number of cycles collected, and number of cycles rejected is displayed on computer display screen. (From Cradduck, T.D., and MacIntyre, W.J.: Semin. Nucl. Med. **7**(4):323-336, Oct. 1977.)

with little success because there was no easy way to signal the imager to automatically turn on at any specific time and turn off at some other preordained time.

Another organ that would require some sort of gating mechanism to be visualized is the heart. The acquisition of a composite camera image of the heart at end systole (end of the contracting and pumping phase) or end diastole (end of the relaxing and filling phase) or both was considered unattainable by most. The reason is that it was humanly impossible to gate the heart manually. Counts were recordable at the various stages of action, using something as simple as an external probe and a strip chart recording device but not images.

The first significant change was the advent of the Brattle Physiological Synchronizer. This device accepted the leads from an electrocardiogram (ECG) machine and used the ECG signals, such as the R or T wave, to automatically signal the camera to turn on at the beginning of a wave and off at its end. In this way a composite image could be made of the heart in the same stage of contraction or relaxation. Clinically significant images were formed by accumulating counts during that short portion of the cardiac cycle over several hundred heartbeats. Similar leads were used to signal inspiration or expiration cycles for automatic gating of lung images.

The computer extended the capabilities of the Brattle gater even further. With the computer, in combination with the ECG and the internal clock (see section on control), the cardiac cycle can be framed into many segments (for example, 48), each segment representing a different position of the heart during one complete cycle (Fig. 12-24). A composite image of each position is possible when interfaced with a multiformat programmer (Fig. 12-25). This is accomplished by preselecting the number of frames desired, which sets up the 1 msec clock to allow for a certain number of pulses to occur before moving the image to another computer frame or another position on the CRT or television. The imaging is triggered by the first R wave after the system is started. Each subsequent frame is opened for collection under the control of the internal clock until another R wave causes data collection to reset and begin again with the first frame. This is multigated acquisition (MUGA). The

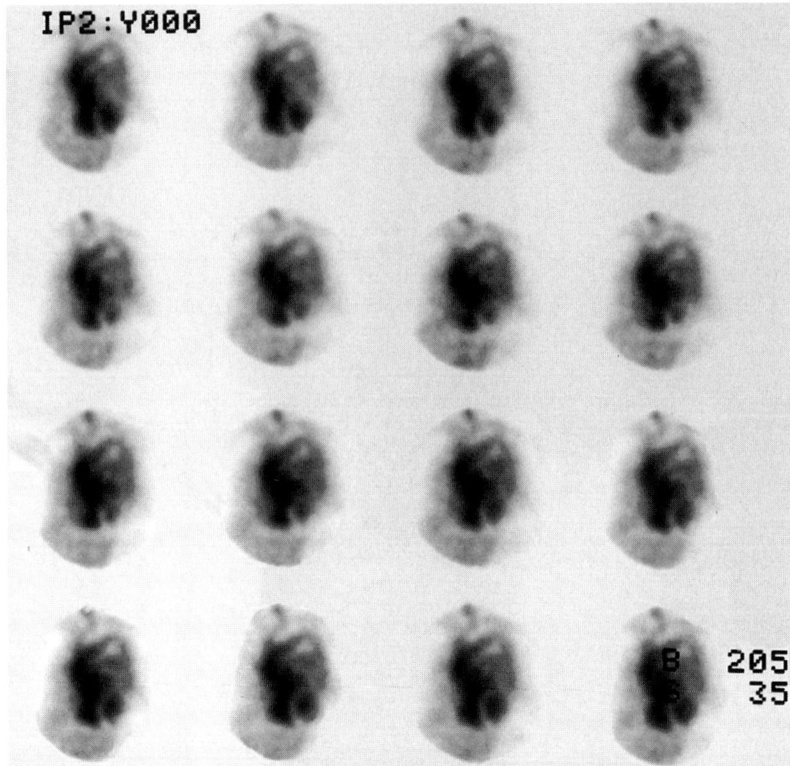

Fig. 12-25. MUGA clinical study showing 16 phases of the heart cycle from diastole through systole and back to diastole. (Courtesy Memorial Medical Center, Jacksonville, Fla.)

procedure continues for 300 to 500 heartbeats, with each frame of each heart cycle adding to its previous counterpart to provide a series of clinically significant images of the heart in each position of the cardiac cycle. Rejection circuits are available to disallow the recording of information from arrhythmic heartbeats.

From this recorded information several determinations can be made. Since the computer image is based on numbers, it is easy to recall numbers for the determination of ejection fraction and stroke volume. The computer can generate left ventricular volume curves of counts versus time. Single-pass calculations as well as multigated calculations can be used. Wall motion studies can be performed by recalling all frames of data sequentially at a rate of speed that is variable, termed *ciné mode*. With all these data on the computer, many more studies will be available in the future. Especially significant is that with the advent of mobile cameras and minicomputers, entire cardiovascular recording capabilities can be arranged on a mobile unit to bring modern, state-of-the-art nuclear medicine to the bedside of the critically ill patient.

Wall motion. The evaluation of the degree of motion of the heart wall (especially that of the left ventricle) can be of value to the nuclear cardiologist. This is easily done by superimposing the frames showing end systole and end diastole, outlining the edges of the heart in each and measuring the degree of motion between the two walls (Fig. 12-26). Many programs from different manufacturers are available to accentuate and quantify these differences.

Edge detection. To perform the wall motion procedure, a program must be available for "edge detection." In this situation the operator is allowed to choose a threshold level of counts (sometimes the program includes this selection). The computer then searches the area of the ventricle for that count and "flags" it by accentuating the pixel to white or black. From the enclosed area, total counts are recorded for ejection fractions, and cardiac output determinations. Walls so outlined can be superimposed for wall motion evaluations.

Edge detection can also be performed manually, using a joystick or a light pen (Fig. 12-27). To perform these edge detection procedures with any degree of reproducibility, it is necessary that the image be of the highest resolution possible. To calculate reasonably accurate ejection fractions, it is necessary to be able to "draw" a good ROI. It is important that if a ventricular ejection fraction is desired, the ROI does not include other cardiac chambers or paracardiac organs. Absolute attention to technique and details such as the following are essential: high resolution collimators, enough counts for good resolution, a frame time

A

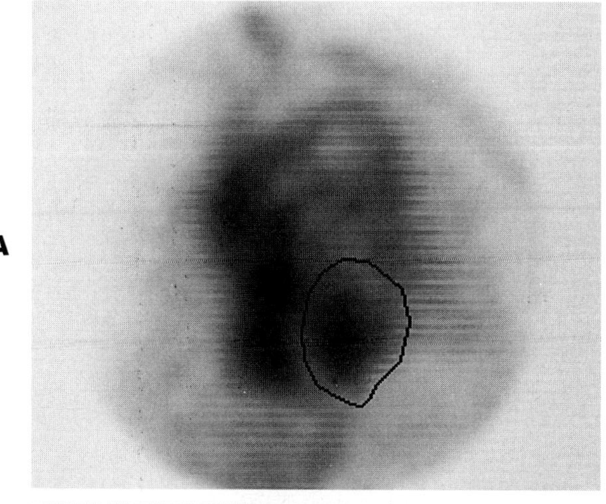

B

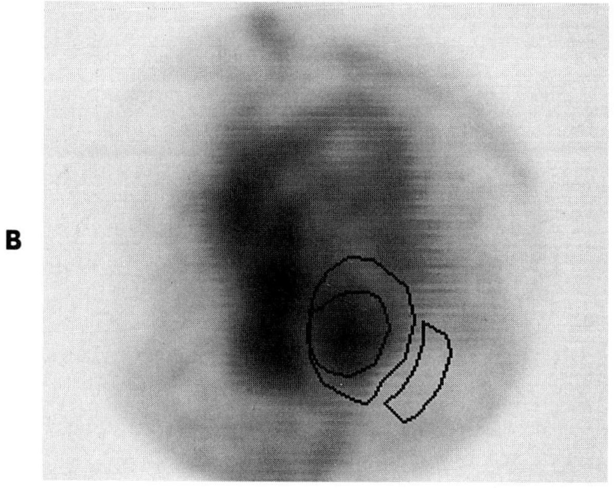

Fig. 12-26. **A,** ROI outlining the left ventricle in diastole. **B,** Superimposing an ROI outlining the left ventricle in systole. An incomplete circle is also seen to show background in the ejection fraction computation. (Courtesy Memorial Medical Center, Jacksonville, Fla.)

short enough to minimize any recording of cardiac motion, correct selection of filters during processing, and good patient positioning. With these points reproducibility is improved and proper interpretation is ensured.

■ Image reconstruction techniques

With the advent of Single Photon Emission Computerized Tomography (SPECT) (Chapter 14), computers have become indispensable in reconstructing images so obtained. With SPECT imaging techniques, the responsibility of the system is to generate a third dimension from a series of two-dimensional images. This process requires a scintillation camera that will rotate around the organ of interest, stopping at selected intervals and generating images at each stop. These images are then stored in a computer until the entire organ has been viewed from a multitude of angles. Reconstruction algorithms (computer programs) are then

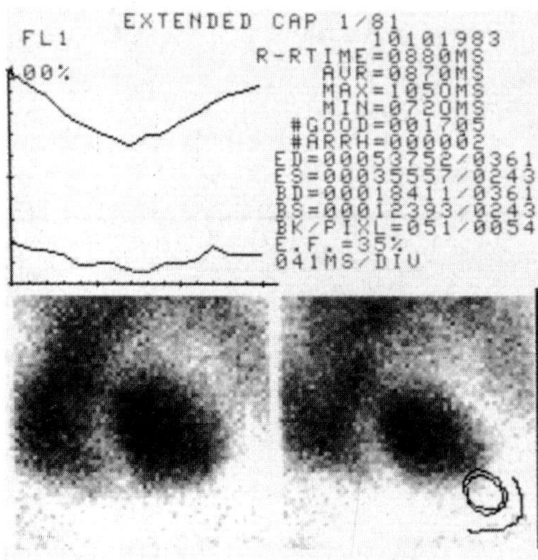

Fig. 12-27. Edge detection of left ventricle for calculation of ejection fraction (EF = 35% in this case). (Courtesy Marymount Hospital, Cleveland, Ohio.)

used to assimilate all these images and reconstruct them into three-dimensional images from which tomographic slices can be made at any level and in any direction (Fig. 12-28).

■ Back projection reconstruction techniques

The method of reconstruction by way of back projection is perhaps the simplest of all reconstruction techniques. It is a composite of all the planar images at each of the stops around the body. When sectioned, these will provide data that can be manipulated and massaged. Most SPECT systems use back projection techniques. There are two types of back projection: simple and filtered.

Simple back projection. In the case of simple back projection, as in any reconstruction technique, photon information received from one pixel is translated to all other pixels perpendicular to the detector. This is called a *ray sum*. The translation results in a star-like projection around each lesion, as point sources (Figs. 12-29 *B* and 12-30, *A*). The result is a reconstructed image that gives the correct location but is intolerably blurred unless additional techniques are used. It would be possible to enhance this image by simply subtracting counts from each pixel in the image until a tolerable image is received (Fig. 12-30, *B*). Just as in any subtraction technique, however, such manipulations can lead to overcompensation, with the resultant exaggeration of count density fluctuations (especially in low-count density studies) and clinically false studies. Therefore, more comprehensive techniques for suppression of background is necessary.

Filtered back projection. Perhaps the most commonly used technique for back projection is that of using filters. This becomes an easy and effective way to remove the star-like pattern around each photon source. Rather than back-project the unprocessed image data, the images are first fil-

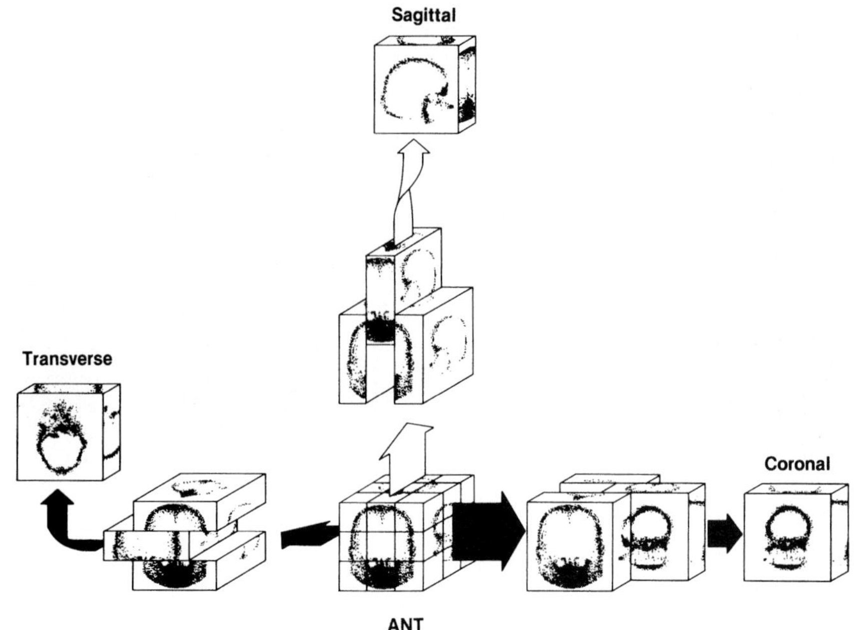

Fig. 12-28. Image orientation of transverse, sagittal, and coronal slices. (Courtesy Nuclear Medicine Group, Siemens Medical Systems, Inc., Hoffman Estates, Ill.)

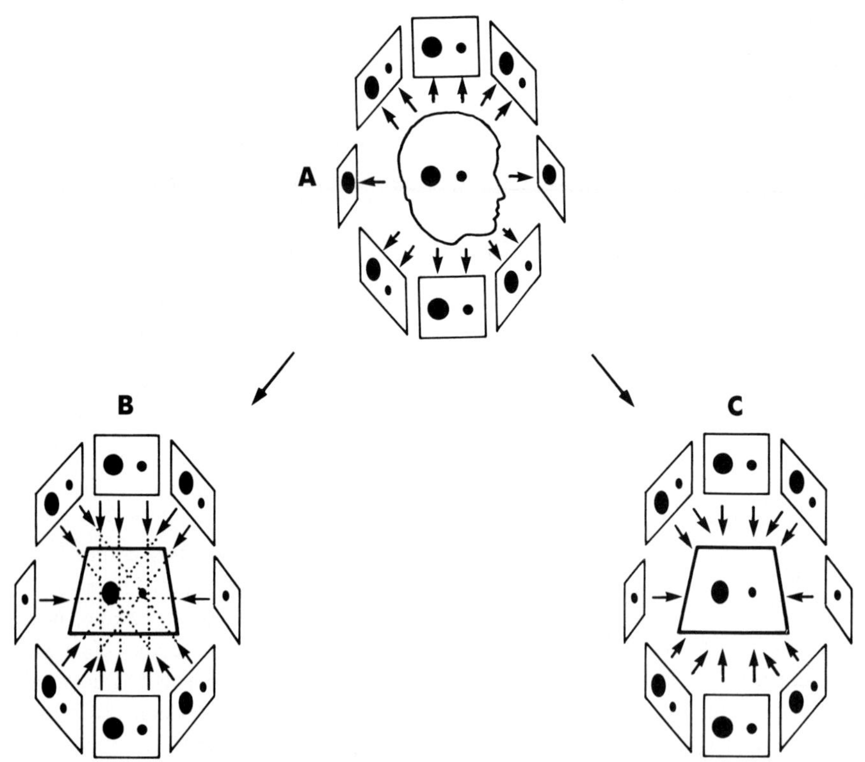

Fig. 12-29. Reconstruction techniques showing original set of acquired images from eight different locations, **A,** and reconstructed via simple back projection, **B,** and filtered back projection, **C.**

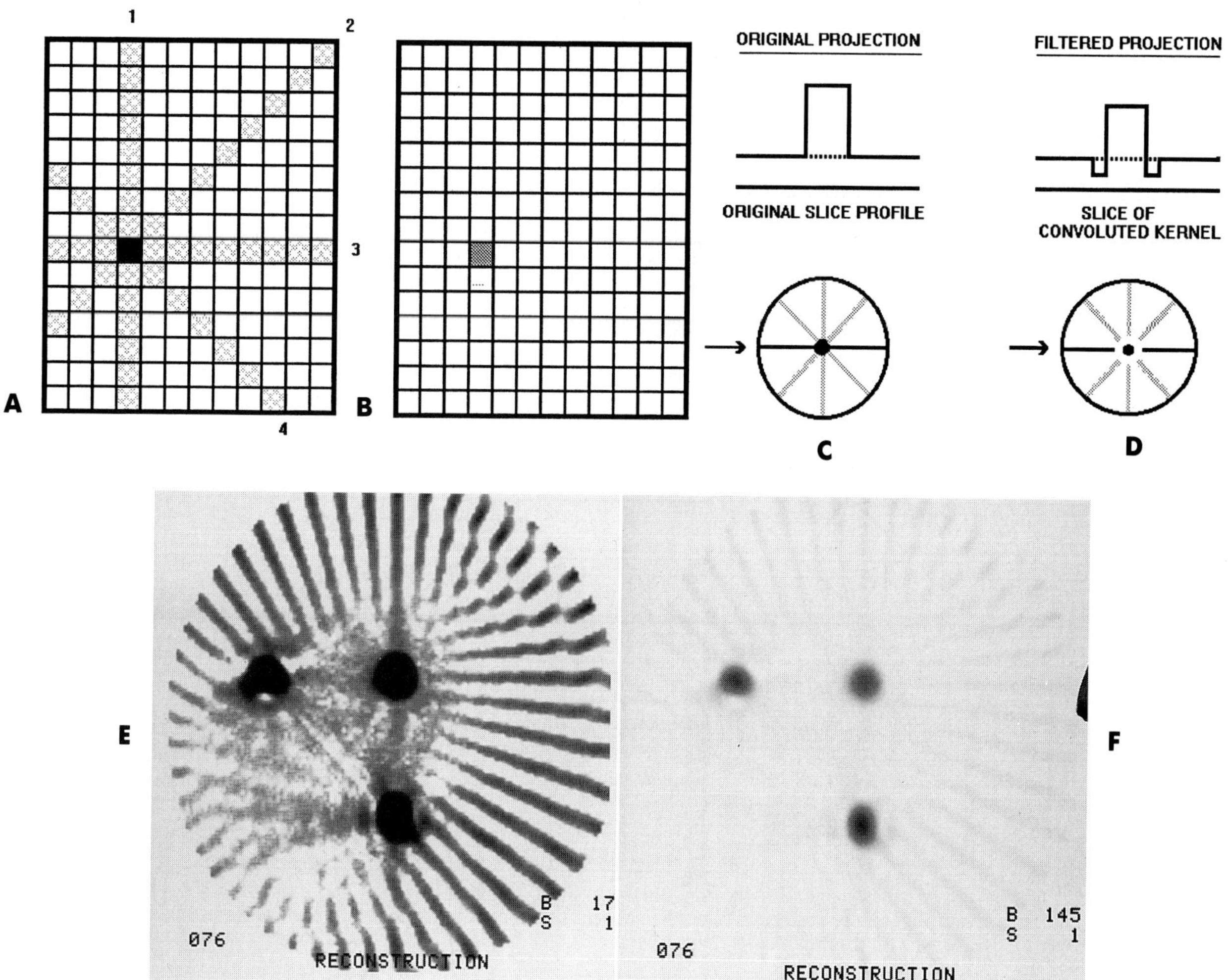

Fig. 12-30. A, The original image in simple projection showing individual pixels arranged in a star-like pattern. Star pattern is due to the ray sums of four camera positions around the point source. **B,** Resultant subtracted image after subtracting one count from each pixel of Fig. 12-30, *A*. The exact location of the point source in this simplistic explanation is identified. **C,** Schematic diagram showing a slice profile *(arrow)* along a horizontal ray sum *(dark line)* and through the centrally placed point source. **D,** Same slice profile through the convolved filtered image showing the negative areas around the point source to enhance contrast. **E,** Actual image of three point sources before filtering and, **F,** after filtering. Note resolution of point sources and reduction in intensity of the ray sums on the last image.

tered. (Filters may be applied before or after back projection; however, prefiltered data are unretrievable.) Another term used for filtered is *convolved;* therefore the filter function is often called the *convolution kernel* or *filter function*. Such a covolution kernel is designed by viewing the source from each gantry angle as a count profile (Fig. 12-30, *C*). Then negative values are applied to the count profile (Fig. 12-30, *D*). These negative components from one projection tend to partially cancel the positive components from other projections. In so doing, the star pattern is reduced and the fidelity of the resultant image is enhanced (Fig. 12-30, *C*). A further in-depth discussion of filters can be found on page 245.

■ Iterative reconstruction technique

The iterative technique (sometimes called *algebraic*) for reconstruction was one of the first applied to nuclear medicine. This has been largely replaced by the filtered technique, but some algorithms are returning to this approach to reconstruction because quantitation is more accurate.

Figure 12-31 displays a 2 × 2 matrix with a different number of counts from each pixel. If this source were imaged with a planar scintillation camera, the resultant image would reflect the ray sums in each pixel, not the true value of counts in each pixel of the original source. To determine their true value, iterative reconstruction techniques can be applied.

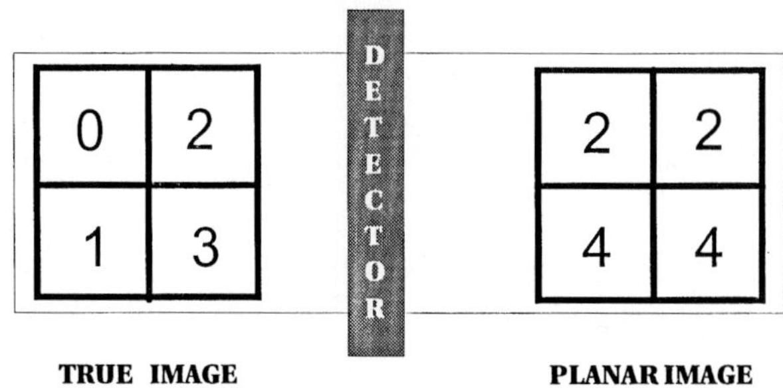

Fig. 12-31. Planar image of counts received from a 2 × 2 matrix source. Note that the true value of each pixel on the planar image is not accurate. Compare with Fig. 12-32.

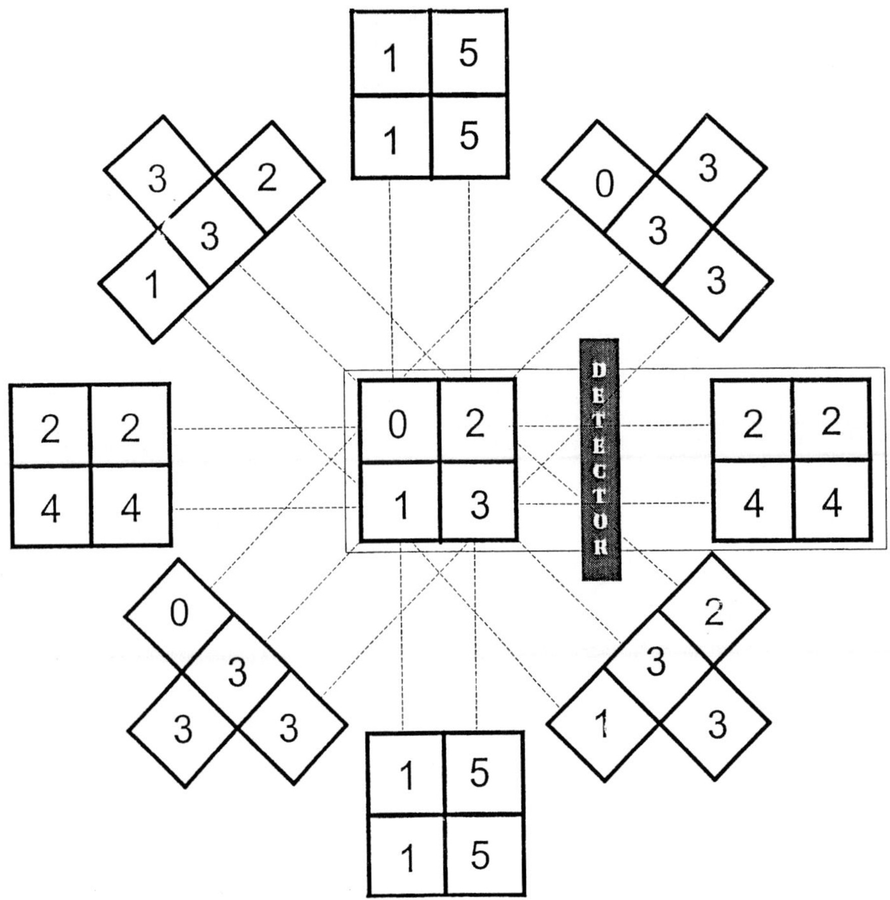

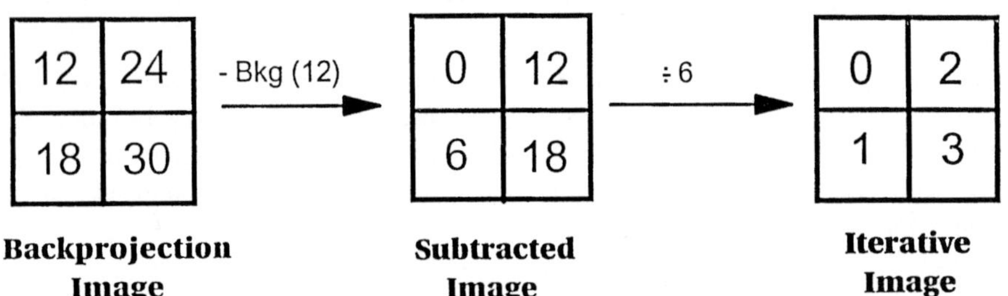

Fig. 12-32. SPECT image of the same source as in Fig. 12-31 demonstrating the same problem (i.e., the true value of each pixel at each position of the detector as it rotates around the source is not known. However, through iterative reconstruction techniques and appropriate algorithms as demonstrated, the true values of each pixel in the first 2 × 2 matrix can be determined).

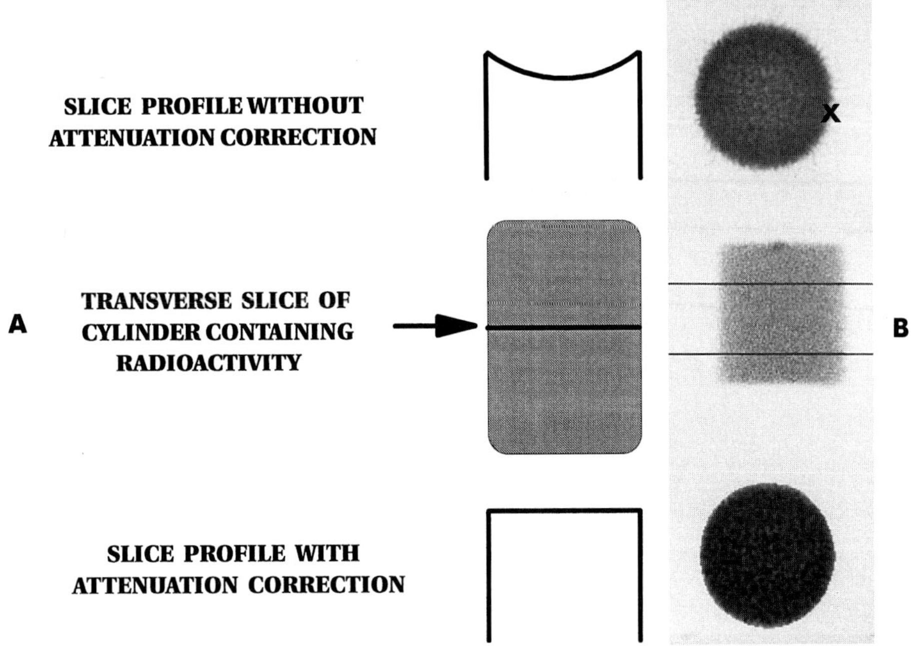

Fig. 12-33. A, Schematic showing via a slice profile *(arrow)* through the transverse slice of a cylinder containing evenly dispersed radioactivity with and without attenuation correction techniques applied. **B,** Illustration of the same concept. Note that without attenuation corrections, the reconstructed slice looks as though there is less activity in the center of the cylinder than on the edges.

Figure 12-32 displays the same 2 × 2 matrix but this time viewed by a SPECT camera at eight different positions, with each of the eight images displaying ray sums in each pixel for that particular projection. However, when all ray sums for each pixel in all eight images are added (back projected) and then submitted to the iterative reconstruction algorithm of subtraction and division, the true value of each pixel is received.

While this is a simplistic approach to explaining iterative techniques, it becomes extremely complicated when applied to a 512 × 512 matrix. Nonetheless, the same principle applies, but computers become a necessity.

■ Attenuation correction

One fact that bears special consideration in any evaluation of a SPECT image is that of photon attenuation in the organ under study. This is particularly true in the use of low-energy radionuclides like ^{99m}Tc. This radionuclide has a linear attenuation coefficient (μ) of 15%/cm (0.15 cm^{-1}) in water. Some investigators have found the use of an empirical ^{99m}Tc linear attenuation coefficient of 10% (0.10 cm^{-1}) to be better than the theoretical value of 0.15 cm^{-1}. Radionuclides such as ^{201}T1 present an even greater problem. The problem is that photons emerging from the center of the organ are more attenuated than those arising from the edge. This is easily exemplified using a cylinder filled with a uniform source of ^{99m}Tc (Fig. 12-33). Without applying attenuation correction techniques, a slice profile through the cylinder will yield a "dish" pattern indicating a higher peripheral activity than that occurring centrally. With attenuation correction techniques, the same slice profile will yield a flat response through its volume, indicating uniformity.

A simplistic attenuation correction formula can be expressed as:

$$I = I_0 \, e^{-\mu x}$$

where

I = Intensity at the surface of the cylinder (skin)
I_0 = Original intensity
μ = Linear attenuation coefficient (^{99m}Tc = 0.15 cm^{-1})
x = Distance in centimeters from point of photon emmission to the surface of the cylinder (skin)

This formula has been refined by Chang, Slaboda, and others to make it more applicable to whole-body situations involving more than a uniform source of water. An in-depth discussion of these vector algorithms is beyond the scope of this discussion. Suffice it to say that the computer is capable of calculating these corrections and making the necessary adjustments for each photon detected. The correction factors can be applied pre- or post-reconstruction.

■ Frequency

Frequency has been defined in the section on Electromagnetic Spectrum as number of cycles per second. In computer terms, frequency is defined as number of peaks per unit distance with peaks and valleys (sine wave) being represented by high-frequency noise (primarily statistical fluctuations) and low-frequency background, respectively. Somewhere between these two extremes lies the true frequency response of counts from the image. Consider for the moment a computerized image of a bar phantom study. A histogram of the counts across the image would produce a continuous sine wave (Fig. 12-34). Extend that image to a computer bar pattern of 32 bars per 64 pixels or a frequency of 0.5 cycles/pixel. This is the highest frequency and therefore the highest resolution possible; it is referred to as the *Nyquist frequency*. Another camera system might be only able to resolve 16 bars per 64 pixels (0.25 cycles/pixel) while another's resolution might be 8 bars per 64 pixels (0.125 cycles/pixel); the last quandrant being 4 bars/pixel (0.0625 cycles/pixel). Since the Nyquist frequency is the highest frequency possible, an image with greater frequency will not be faithfully reproduced, and some of the high-frequency information will be lost. This is termed *aliasing*. The same phenomenon occurs in movies and explains the appearance that stagecoach wheels rotate backwards. The frequency of the spokes changing their position is greater than the sampling rate of the video. Similarly, frequencies from an image that would be greater than the Nyquist frequency would not accurately reflect the distribution of the radioactivity. This is highly evident in the low–count-rate studies in which statistical fluctuations play havoc on a valid image.

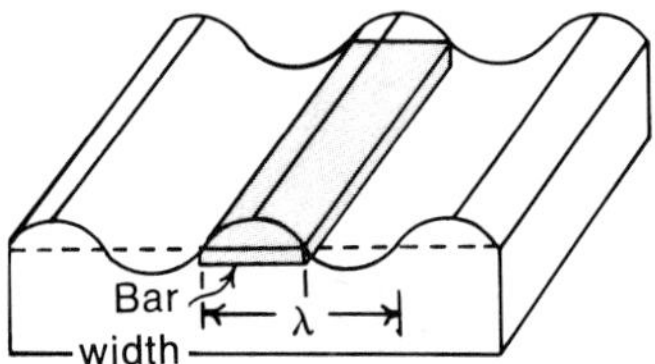

Fig. 12-34. Typical bar phantom showing the sinusoidal function of the counts received from its image. Each bar width of the bar phantom corresponds to a particular frequency.

The three components of any image can be displayed as shown in Fig. 12-35, *A*. The use of a Ramp filter will rule out much of the low-frequency background but will accept the high-frequency noise. This may be acceptable in high count rate studies where noise is statistically insignificant. Conversely, the Hamming filter is used to reject the high frequency noise and accept background. Combinations of these two filters (Fig. 12-35, *B*) are often used to offer compromises in resolution and smoothing.

This section has included important information in preparation for understanding the next section on Processing Techniques.

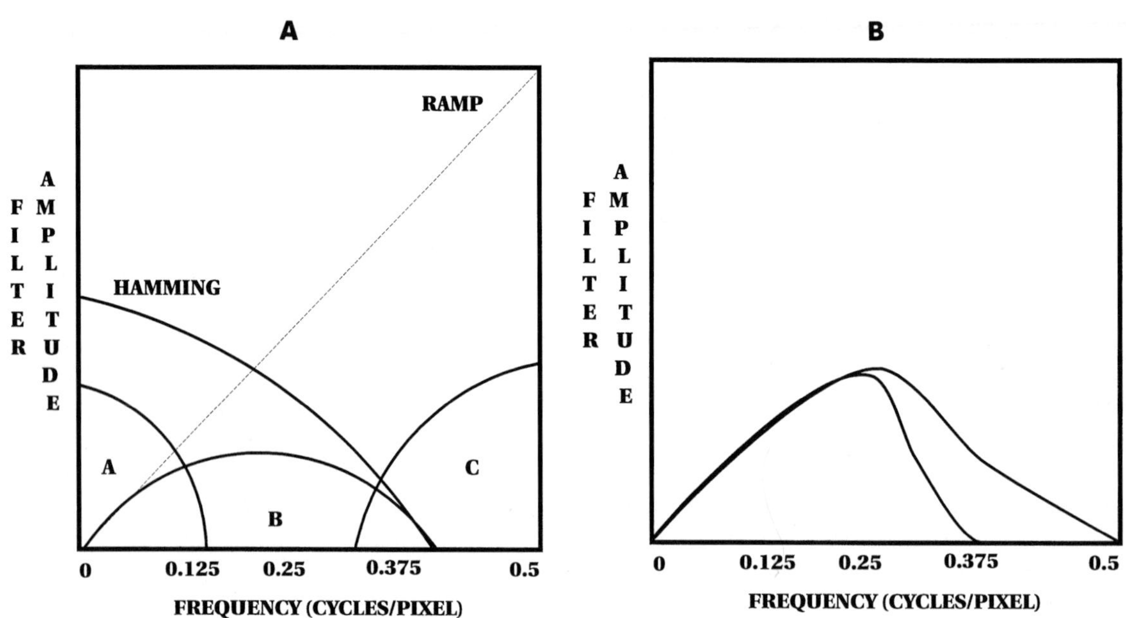

Fig. 12-35. A, Graph showing the gross relationship of the three components of any computer image including low frequency background information *(A)*, source information *(B)*, and high frequency noise *(C)*. Use of the Ramp filter or Hamming filter or preferably a combination of the two filters would reduce the undesirable high and low frequencies, resulting in a better image. **B,** The Hamming filter (with a cutoff of 0.5 cycles/pixel and 0.375 cycles/pixel filter windows) have been multiplied by a Ramp filter and plotted as filter amplitude versus frequency.

Processing techniques

David P. Mihalic

■ TIME, SPACE, AND FREQUENCIES

In the everyday world we are used to dealing in what is termed the *spatial domain*. This means simply that the "things" we deal with (including nuclear medicine images) can be looked at or mapped somewhere in space. Normally this is a three-dimensional space (x-y-z planes) with some reference to time (fourth dimension). However, when looking at medical images we are viewing a two-dimensional representation of a three-dimensional object. Additional information is supplied by the image intensity (the brightness of each dot in the picture) or by the number of counts in each pixel in the computer image. These dimensions of the medical image represent its spatial domain.

Besides the spatial domain of an image, there may be a temporal domain as well. In a dynamic study, a number of image frames are acquired over a time interval. The data for any given point in an image matrix may change over time. The temporal domain, therefore, represents either the change in data content for each pixel from frame to frame or the change that occurs per unit of time.

In addition to representing image data in the space/time domain, we may analyze the same data in the "frequency domain," or "Fourier space." The frequency domain exists only in the mathematical realm. As such it cannot be fully explained without reference to mathematical functions. The frequency domain represents the image data (distribution of the counts in the image) as a sinusoidal function of their position in the image. This functional count distribution can be expressed as a sum of sine and cosine functions. That is to say that the image data can be represented as an amplitude distribution of discrete sine and/or cosine function elements.

Analysis of images reveals that useful information is represented as the mid- to low-frequency components of the image data. The higher frequency components are usually noise and the very low frequencies correspond to background counts.

Noise is a generic term referring to any type of unwanted signal in the data. Noise can show up as statistical fluctuations in the signal (image data) or it can be generated by electronic components within the camera/computer system itself. In addition, noise can be generated from the external world through power supplies, magnetic influences, electrostatic causes, etc.

In SPECT clinical procedures, therefore, we have information we want to keep (signal) and information we wish to get rid of (noise). It is the aim of the filtering process to optimize the ratio between signal and noise or signal-to-noise ratio (SNR). Whenever noise is filtered from data, there will always be a loss of some desirable information as well. There is always a trade-off between the amount of signal one can keep and the noise one can eliminate. This is why there exist a number of filters from which to choose, allowing one to optimize the signal-to-noise ratio. In addition, each filter has parameters associated with it that can be tailored to facilitate the best SNR.

■ SPECT DATA ACQUISITION AND RECONSTRUCTION

As the SPECT camera rotates about the patient, projection data is gathered from each angle in a series of parallel rays forming a planar image. Each ray in the image frame is a summation of information collected along that projected line. The summed value is assigned to every pixel in the ray projection.

During SPECT reconstruction, as data from each angle overlap the data from other angles, a summation occurs that results in a smeared or blurred image. Each ray is back projected into an empty image matrix in the array processor. Before back projection each ray is filtered to deblur the effects of adjacent ray contributions.

During the back projection process, the reconstruction of any point in the image matrix is affected by *all* surrounding points. That is, each point of activity "bleeds" into the other points and consequently affects the data content of those points. The amount of contribution of one point to another follows a definite mathematical expression as a function of the distance between points. The farther away the point from the point being reconstructed, the smaller the effect. We can, therefore, compute the amount of each adjacent ray that must be back projected along with the intersecting ray to construct a given point. This is done by adding a negative ray (according to the spatial filter function) to each of the adjacent rays. The equation that defines the percentage of each ray to be back projected is called the *filter function*.

■ SPECT FILTERS

The purpose of the SPECT filter is to preserve as much signal as possible and to reduce noise. The filter determines which frequencies from the projection data are passed and used in the reconstruction of the nuclear medicine image. It removes artifacts from reconstructed images and corrects for blurring that results naturally from the summation of the projection data.

In the reconstruction matrix, the effect of a single point in that matrix on another point is mathematically predictable. Therefore, filters can be constructed in such a way that their behavior is also predictable. Thus, a basis is formed for selecting filters according to how they affect the final image reconstruction.

In actual practice, SPECT filters are empirically chosen for the type of study being reconstructed, based largely on the data density of the acquired raw data. In general, the more data collected, the greater will be the SNR ratio that will result in a better image. What this means is that as count density increases there is less need to filter out noise. Conversely, low-count studies contain more noise in relation to signal and therefore require more careful processing (filtration) to obtain the sharp boundary differences between the useful data and the noise content.

Table 12-2 lists a choice of five filter types. These filters are arranged according to their relative abilities to preserve resolution and suppress noise. Figure 12-36 shows a filter spectrum of these same filters.

The Ramp filter demonstrates the highest image resolution and consequently the highest amount of noise. This results in sharp areas of contrast in the image that after reconstruction may yield ring artifacts. A high count rate is required to use this filter effectively. As such, the Ramp filter is not suitable for routine SPECT image reconstruction.

Table 12-2. Five different SPECT filters arranged according to imaging parameters

Parzen	Bartlett	Hamming	Butterworth	Ramp
Low noise ⟶ High noise				
Low resolution ⟶ High resolution				
Smooth image ⟶ Digital image				

Other filters (e.g., Parzen) are at the other end of the filter spectrum (Fig. 12-36). They are just the opposite of the Ramp filter, yielding the lowest image resolution and consequently the lowest amount of noise. As such, the image appears very smooth—to the point at which it may actually mask lesions within the reconstructed image. Then it too becomes unproductive for SPECT reconstruction.

The Bartlett and Hamming filters are used primarily to reconstruct SPECT images that contain low-count statistics and require a fair amount of smoothing to reduce the statistical fluctuations from the noise content in the raw data. The Bartlett and Hamming filters are most frequently used to reconstruct thallium, bone, and gallium images.

The Butterworth filter is perhaps the most frequently used filter in SPECT reconstruction. It offers the best trade-off between smoothness and sharpness of edge. It is most frequently used in the reconstruction of brain, liver, and lung images. The Butterworth filter is the most versatile of the currently used SPECT filters because it has several pa-

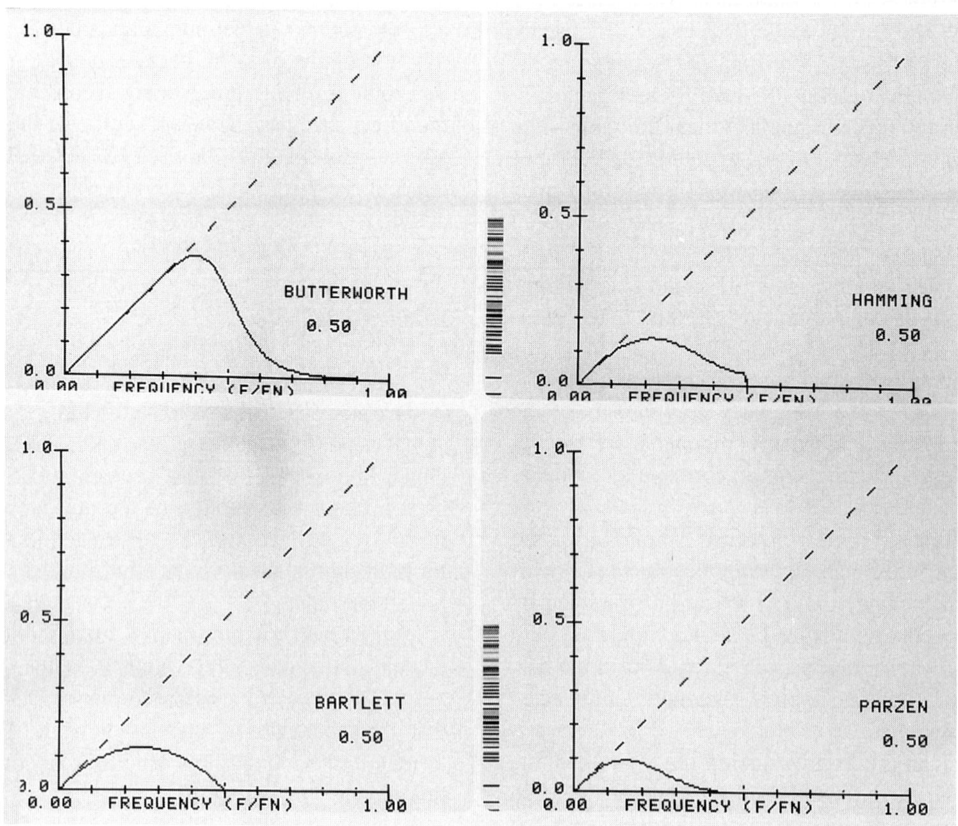

Fig. 12-36. Comparison of various SPECT filters in frequency space. All are set at 0.5 cutoff. Note that the most filtering will be provided by the Parzen filter. The dotted line represents the RAMP filter. (Courtesy Memorial Medical Center, Jacksonville, Fla.)

rameters that can be specified to determine the final filter function.

All SPECT filters are specified by cutoff frequency. The Butterworth filter is further modified by the parameter known as ORDER.

■ CUTOFF FREQUENCY

The cutoff frequency (CO) is used to specify the bandwidth of the filter. That is, the cutoff frequency determines which frequencies in the image data are passed and which are suppressed.

The spatial filter controls how much of the collected data is allowed to influence the reconstruction of any given point in the image matrix. The lower the cutoff frequency, the more influence there is from surrounding data points in the final reconstruction of the given matrix point. Therefore, lowering the cutoff frequency degrades the image resolution, creating a smoother display. Conversely, raising the cutoff frequency improves image resolution.

In the case of Butterworth filters, a further modification to the filter function occurs with the parameter of ORDER. The ORDER modifies the filter by varying the slope of the filter function (Fig. 12-37). That is, the ORDER parameter can be used to shape the filter function so that the trade between smoothness and sharpness of edge is optimized.

In the ideal camera system, noise would not be produced and the image data would only have to be filtered to deblur the effects of the back projection process. In such a case, the Ramp filter would be the ideal choice since it can be constructed to equally pass all frequencies up to a specified cutoff and will deblur the back projected image data. In reality, however, image data always contain noise. Therefore, a "window function" must be constructed to determine which frequencies will be passed and which will be suppressed by the final reconstruction filter.

To derive the reconstruction filter, the window function must be multiplied by the Ramp function in frequency space. This will create a filter that has the noise suppression and resolution characteristics of the window function and the deblurring effect of the Ramp (Fig. 12-35, *B*). The inverse Fourier transform is performed on the final filter to obtain the filter function in the spatial domain. This then is

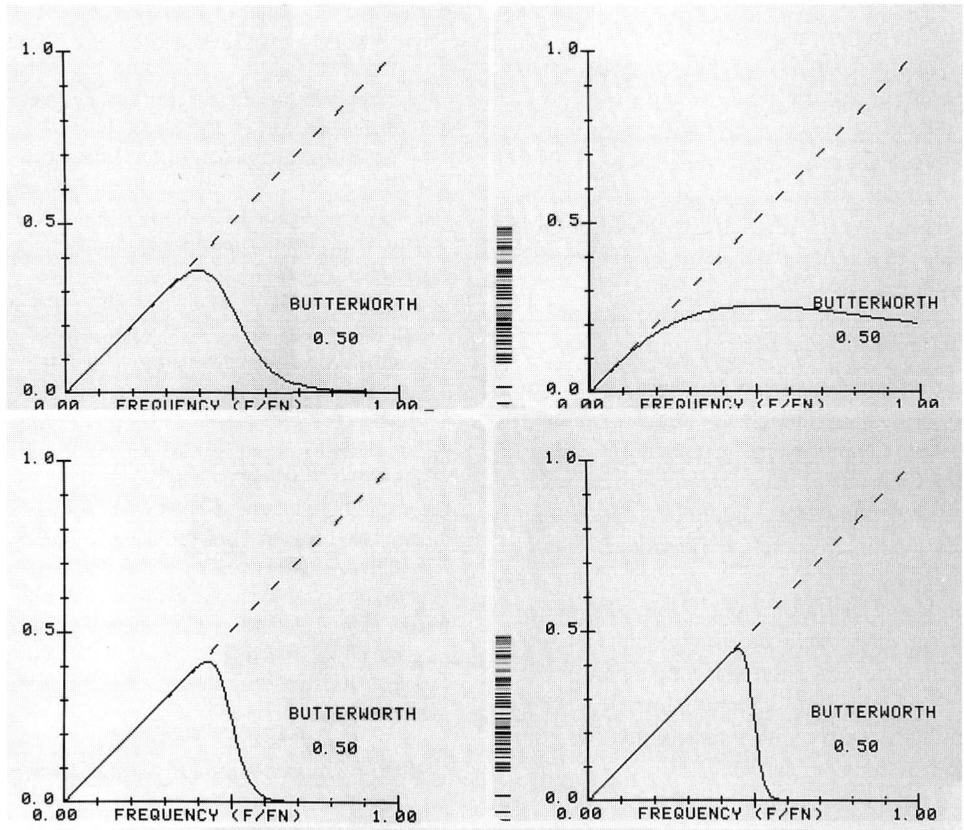

Fig. 12-37. Filter spectrum (frequency vs. amplitude) of four Butterworth filters, all having the same cutoff value of 0.5 but a varying order as follows: A = 5, B = 1, C = 10, and D = 20. (Courtesy Memorial Medical Center, Jacksonville, Fla.)

Table 12-3. Suggested SPECT filters

Study	Filter	Cutoff	Order
Bone scan (Low statistics)	Butterworth	0.2	3
Bone scan (High statistics)	Butterworth	0.3	4
Brain scan	Butterworth	0.2	3
Gallium scan (Low statistics)	Butterworth or	0.2	3
	Hamming	0.3	—
Gallium scan (High statistics)	Butterworth	0.3	4
Thallium scan	Hamming	0.3	—
Liver scan	Butterworth	0.3	4
Lung scan	Butterworth	0.3	3

convolved with the raw-image data, and then back projected to produce the reconstruction image.

In the final analysis, the selection of SPECT filters for image reconstruction is an empirically determined practice. Since the selection of filters is based considerably on the data density of the acquired image, we find that for any given study type (e.g., lung, liver, brain), a filter with a specific cutoff frequency and/or ORDER can be used repeatedly to reconstruct the same type of study. This is because the data density from one liver scan to another, for example, will not vary significantly from one patient to another. Therefore, one type of SPECT filter may be specified for each type of clinical study that is performed.

Listed on Table 12-3 are the commonly performed SPECT imaging procedures and recommendations for filters that can be used for image reconstruction. This list is not to be seen as absolute. The filters listed should be considered as guidelines to determine which filters appear most appropriate for each type of imaging procedure.

■ ENVIRONMENTAL FACTORS

Because of the sensitivity of the read/write heads on computer systems, it is clear that cleanliness is paramount in maintaining any computer system. Temperatures and humidity are also important. High temperatures can cause severe damage to the electronics resulting in intermittent failures and generally unreliable operation. Variations in temperature allow magnetic tape to stretch, thereby distorting and perhaps even losing the information.

Low humidity can cause static electricity that can cause the computer to fail. An ideal value for temperature is 70° F ± 2° F with a relative humidity of approximately 45% ± 5%. Humidity of this value prevents condensation from occurring on the diskette memory surface. It is suggested that all diskettes be stored in the room where they are used to prevent formation of condensation when moving them through different levels of humidity.

Glossary

adder digital circuitry to add binary code

address name, label, or number that identifies the storage location of a piece of information

ALGOL (algorithmic language) computer language that expresses computer programs by algorithms and thus simplifies programming

alphanumeric all letters of the alphabet, numbers, and special characters

analog representation or measurement of a system by continuously variable physical entities (for example, continuously changing voltage)

analog computer computer that operates on analog signals

arithmetic unit part of the central processor of a computer that performs the arithmetic and logic operations

ASCII (American Standard Code for Information Interchange) standard set of 128 codes for upper and lower case letters, numbers, punctuation, and special communication control characters (see p 219)

assembler internal program containing the assembly language translation code

assembly language symbolic programming language that can be translated directly into machine language instructions and is usually computer specific

binary code uses two distinct characters, 0 and 1, to designate numbers and letters (see bits)

binary digit in binary notation either 0 or 1 (see bits)

binary number expressed in binary fashion (as a string of bits)

bits (binary digits) binary code in which numbers are translated into powers of 2 and are counted from 0 to 1

buffer storage area that can temporarily hold data input or output to match the speed differences (in data flow) between devices

bug error in a program or operation

byte group of bits (usually eight) handled together and treated as a unit by a computer

COBOL (COmmon Business Oriented Language) business language for computers

compiler set of programs that converts a program into the machine language instructions of a particular computer

control unit portion of the CPU involved with the transfer of instructions, information, and the organization of sequence of operations

core memory most common form of main memory, in which binary data are presented by the switching of the polarity of magnetic cores (see magnetic core memory)

CPU (central processing unit) portion of a computer system that controls the interpretation and execution of computer instructions; includes an instruction control unit, a memory unit, and the arithmetic/logic unit

data acquisition unit peripheral device that acquires signals from equipment and transmits them to a computer

data base file of data organized in such a way that information can be accessed and used for one or more applications without regard to physical storage location

data processing general name for all functions (procedures) carried out on data by computers

debug isolate and remove all errors from programs

diagnostics series of programs that test program instructions during compiling and printout messages to isolate problems with program code; also test hardware functioning

diskette disk-shaped magnetic storage device

diskette pack fixed or movable storage unit consisting of one or more magnetic diskettes mounted on a spindle and used on a disk drive, where it spins continuously

downtime time (usually expressed as a percentage) computer system or device is out of operation during the period of its scheduled use

file collection of related information kept as a unit

FORTRAN (FORmula TRANslation) computer language suited for scientific and mathematic work

hardware physical equipment of a computer system

high-level language language in which each instruction corresponds to multiple instructions when written in machine code; for example, FORTRAN, BASIC, ALGOL, COBOL

interface translation device to modify external signals into computer-compatible input (see data acquisition unit); connection between two pieces of computer hardware or software

internal memory see magnetic core memory

I/O (input/output) terminal device capable of feeding information into and retrieving it from a computer

language coding system used to write instructions for a computer (see ALGOL, assembly language, COBOL, high-level language, machine language)

machine language language used by computer hardware

magnetic core memory common form of internal memory device using magnetic material (cores), with each core able to store the electric equivalent of 1 bit because it can be magnetized in one of two directions (see core memory)

magnetic diskette random access storage device consisting of plates coated with a magnetic surface on which data can be stored and retrieved

magnetic tape bulk storage device in which data are stored on the magnetic surface of tape; a slow-access storage medium compared to a magnetic diskette

MODEM (MOdulator/DEModulator) device that enables data to be transmitted over long distances by way of telephone lines

off-line portions of a computer not under control of the CPU

on-line portions of a computer that operate directly under control of the CPU

peripherals any piece of equipment physically separated from the CPU but under its control

RAM (Random Access Memory) memory constructed to reduce the access time on location of stored data; can be written and read

read/write head compartment of a magnetic storage device that can write (send) data to storage and read (retrieve) them from storage

real time computer operations that occur fast enough to be analyzed and used at that moment for decision making

register device in the CPU that stores data for future use

ROM (Read Only Memory) memory capable of being read but not rewritten

software all programs and routines used with computer hardware

storage capacity quantity of data that can be stored in memory

time sharing process by which programs are interleaved with or without a priority basis to ensure the most efficient system performance

word collection of bits treated as a single entity

word length number of bits composing a word; different for various model computers; there are 8-bit words, 12-bit words, 16-bit words, and even 32-bit words

BIBLIOGRAPHY

Bernier, D.R., Christian, P.E., and Langan, J.K.: Nuclear medicine technology and techniques, St. Louis, 1993, Mosby–Year Book.

Cradduck, T.D., and MacIntyre, W.J.: Camera-computer systems for rapid dynamic imaging studies, Semin. Nucl. Med. 7(4):323-336, Oct. 1977.

Enlander, D.: Computers in medicine: an introduction. St. Louis, 1980, Mosby–Year Book.

Erickson, J.J., and Rollo, F.D.: Digital nuclear medicine, Philadelphia, 1983, J.B. Lippincott Co.

Gottschalk, A., and Potchen, E.J.: Diagnostic nuclear medicine, Baltimore, 1976, The Williams & Wilkins Co.

Hine, G.J., and Sorenson, J.A.: Instrumentation in nuclear medicine, vol. 2, New York, 1974, Academic Press, Inc.

Hughes, E.M.: A beginner's guide to memory: on computing, Inc., 1981.

Lapidus, S.N.: A new method of correction for detection of nonuniformity in gamma cancers, Stamford, Conn., Raytheon Medical Electronics.

Lee, Kai H.: Computers in nuclear medicine: a practical approach, New York, 1991, Society of Nuclear Medicine.

Lieberman, D.E.: Computer methods: the fundamentals of digital nuclear medicine, St. Louis, 1977, Mosby–Year Book.

Muehllehner, G., Colsher, J.G., and Stoub, E.W.: Correction for nonuniformity in scintillation cameras through removal of spatial distortion. J. Nucl. Med. 21:771-776, 1980.

Perry, J.R., and Mosher, C.E.: Factors influencing the choice of a nuclear medicine computing system, Clin. Nucl. Med., 6(105):19-26, 1981.

Rhodes, B.A.: Quality control in nuclear medicine: radiopharmaceuticals, instrumentation and in-vitro assays, St. Louis, 1977, Mosby–Year Book.

Rollo, F.D.: Nuclear medicine physics, instrumentation, and agents, St. Louis, 1977, The C.V. Mosby Co.

Strauss, H.W., Pitt, B., and James, A.E., Jr.: Cardiovascular nuclear medicine, St. Louis, 1974, Mosby–Year Book.

Technical Data Sheet NTD-002 and NTD-004: Solon, Ohio, Ohio Nuclear, Inc., 1980.

Todd-Pokropek, A.E., Erbsmann, F., Soussaline, F.: The non-uniformity of imaging devices and its impact in quantitative studies, IAEA-SM-210/154, 1983.

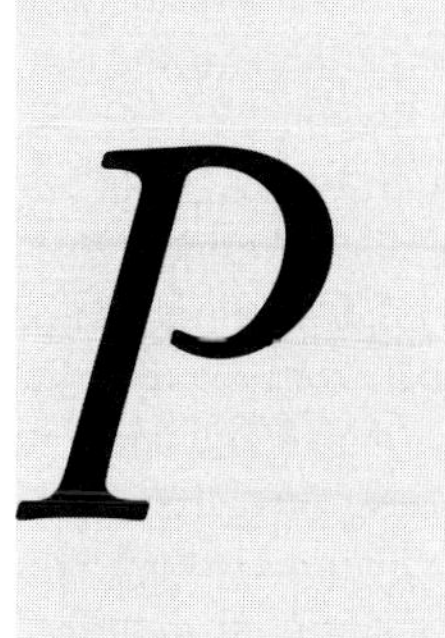

Chapter 13

LANAR IMAGING

PAUL J. EARLY

All the detection devices described in previous chapters deal with the simple counting of radioactivity in a sample or in an organ as an indicator of function or concentration. By modifying these same principles of detection, the scintillation detector can be used to show radionuclide distribution in the body and in its organs, both as a planar imaging system and a tomographic system. Both types of systems can be performed with stationary or moving detectors. With the exception of positron emission tomography (PET) scanners (see Chapter 15 for a full discussion of this topic), all imaging devices require collimators. All use a crystal-photomultiplier assembly. This section deals only with planar imaging systems.

■ PLANAR IMAGING SYSTEMS

Planar systems are all conventional imaging systems that collect and present all data as though they were coming from a single plane. There is no tomographic effect. These systems include the rectilinear scanner and stationary cameras.

■ Rectilinear scanners

Rectilinear scanners are of two types: single detector assembly and multiple detector assembly. Both types have fallen into limited use with the advent of scintillation cameras because of the latter's ability to perform a clinical study quickly. The development of the multiple detector assembly was an attempt to speed up the imaging process while using the principle of rectilinear scanning. This system also has not been widely accepted in the nuclear medicine community.

Single detector assembly. In 1950 Benedict Cassen and associates found that by using the newly developed scintillation counter mounted on an automatically moved carriage and attached to a dot-producing mechanism that responds to the electrical impulses from a scintillation counter, the spatial distribution of radioactive iodine in the thyroid gland could be printed mechanically. As a result, Cassen opened up a whole new area of radioisotope use in medicine.

These automatic scanners, called rectilinear scanners, make a map of the location of radioactive materials in a patient's body. The scanner moves across the organ in one or more planes until the organ or the area in question has been completely surveyed by the scintillation counter. As it moves back and forth across the organ containing radioactivity, the scanning mechanism produces electrical impulses proportional to the amount of activity present in the area that, at that instant, is covered by the scintillation probe. It creates a picture on x-ray film. A small cathode tube moves synchronously with the scintillation detector over x-ray film. As scintillations are received, a collimated cathode light source flashes for a preset length of time, producing a spot on the film. The developed x-ray film demonstrates the organ and its concentrations of radioactivity as dots or squares of darkening on the film. Variations in concentrations of activity can be seen as dots ranging from white (not seen on film) through shades of gray to black. The black areas represent high concentrations of radioactivity, and the varied gray areas represent lesser concentrations of radioactivity. These systems, primarily used for thyroid imaging, are being manufactured only on a limited basis.

Multiple detector assemblies. This rectilinear imaging device consists of two opposing detector heads, each head consisting of multiple NaI crystals and multiple associated photomultiplier tubes, each crystal with a focused collimator. The action of the heads is to move in synchrony along the entire body while the crystals, moving as a unit in each head, move back and forth across the body. The images generated by the upper and lower detector heads are displayed simultaneously on a CRT. The obvious advantage of this unit is speed and, with its thick crystals and high-energy collimation, better efficiency and resolution with higher energy radionuclides such as ^{67}Ga. This system is not seen often in nuclear medicine departments today.

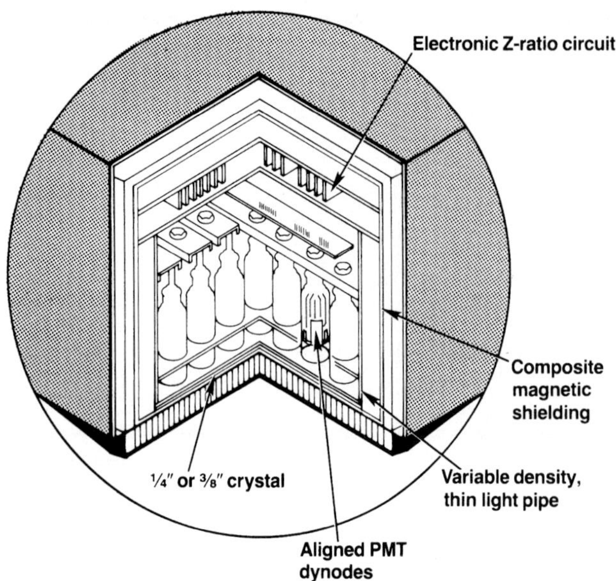

Fig. 13-1. Cut-away diagram of single crystal stationary imaging device. (Courtesy Picker International, Cleveland, Ohio.)

■ Single crystal camera

The single crystal camera, commonly called the *scintillation camera,* or *Anger camera,** is a device that views all parts of the radiation field continuously, rather than scanning the subject point by point. Today, commercially available scintillation cameras employ a single sodium iodide crystal measuring from 11 inches to 20 inches in diameter and from ¼ to ½ inch in thickness as the detector unit. This crystal is viewed by a bank of photomultiplier tubes (from 19 to 91 and more) usually arranged in a hexagonal array. In some systems the photomultiplier tubes are separated from the crystal by a transparent optical "lightpipe." This lightpipe is critical to the resolution of the entire system. The thinner the lightpipe and the closer the material to the index of refraction of the crystal, the better the resolution. In both instances the light collection from the scintillation crystal is enhanced, contributing statistically to the ease with which the position and pulse-height information can be processed.

In the Anger camera, gamma rays pass through the holes of the collimator and are completely absorbed in the scintillation crystal. Those incompletely absorbed are perceived by the system as being of lower energy and are therefore rejected by proper pulse-height analysis, resulting in the photon not being counted. The light that is produced is emitted in all directions and is received by many of the photomultiplier tubes (Fig. 13-1). The closest photomultiplier tube to any given scintillation event receives the most light. Since it receives the most light, that photomultiplier tube also produces the largest pulse in comparison to the surrounding photomultiplier tubes, which also produce a pulse but of decreasing height. The digitization of the event can occur as early as this point; hence the name "digital camera" even though the detection event is strictly an analog event (see Fig. 12-3). The output signal from each of the phototubes goes directly to a resistor or capacitor network (electronic Z-ratio circuit) where impulses from all the phototubes are modified, processed, and converted to four output signals that carry all the necessary position information, as well as the pulse-height information. The position information is obtained from four of the output signals, called the X^+, X^-, Y^+, and Y^- signals. A fifth signal, the Z signal, is the pulse-height signal. It is proportional only to the brightness of the sum of the scintillations from all the involved photomultiplier tubes, with no regard whatsoever as to where the scintillation occurred in the scintillation crystal. This Z signal is obtained by adding the pulses from all the photomultiplier tubes involved in the detection of the event to determine, after all the processing of the position signals has taken place, whether the spectrometer is going to accept or reject the event.

H.O. Anger used seven photomultiplier tubes in his initial camera design, as shown in Fig. 13-2. Each of the phototubes contributed to each of the four position signals via the capacitor network. A fixed portion of the output signal from each of the phototubes is distributed to the four position signals. Note that tube 7 contributes the same proportion of the signal to all four position signals, therefore indicating that the event occurred directly under tube 7. An event that occurred directly under tube 3 would be distributed only to three position signals (X^+, X^-, and Y^-) with the X^+ receiving three times as much signal as X^-. These signals are then sent to ancillary data display equipment such as CRTs. (These will be discussed later in this chapter.)

*Camera concept was proposed by H.O. Anger in 1956 and the basic principle has not changed substantially since that time, although other techniques are being introduced in recent production models.

■ Multicrystal camera

The multicrystal stationary imaging device* is an instrument with multiple crystals on the detector assembly. The detector head is made up of a matrix, measuring 6 by 9 inches and consisting of 294 separate scintillation crystals that form a grid of 14 by 21 crystals. Each crystal is 7⁄16 inches wide and 1½ inches thick. These crystals are mounted in a mosaic pattern and are separated from one another by lead. These lead separators help stop gamma and light rays from crossing into adjacent crystals. This "cross

*An updated version is the *Scinticor*. This system uses a single NaI (Tl) crystal, 20- by 20-inch square and 1-inch thick, slotted so as to effectively create 400 (20 × 20) individual detector elements coupled to 115 photomultiplier tubes. A method similar to the Anger method of position analysis of each detection event is now being used (Fig. 13-3).

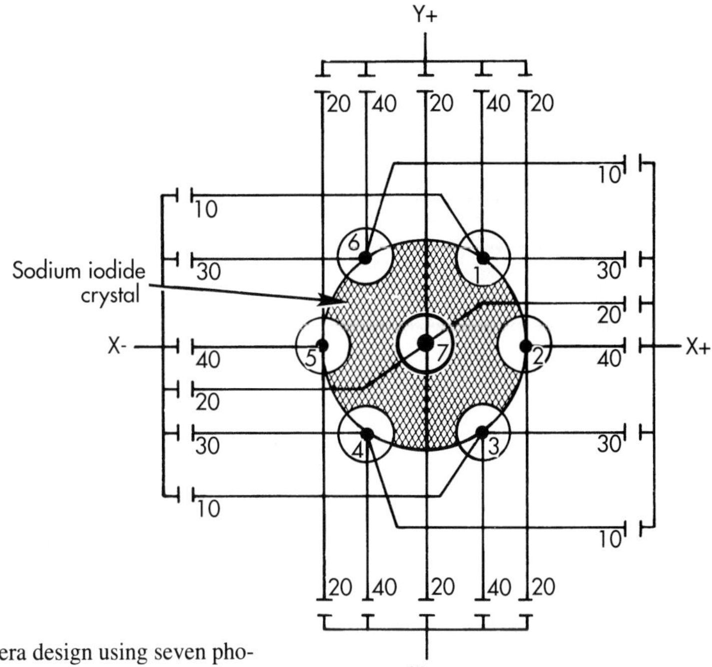

Fig. 13-2. H.O. Anger's original camera design using seven photomultiplier tubes.

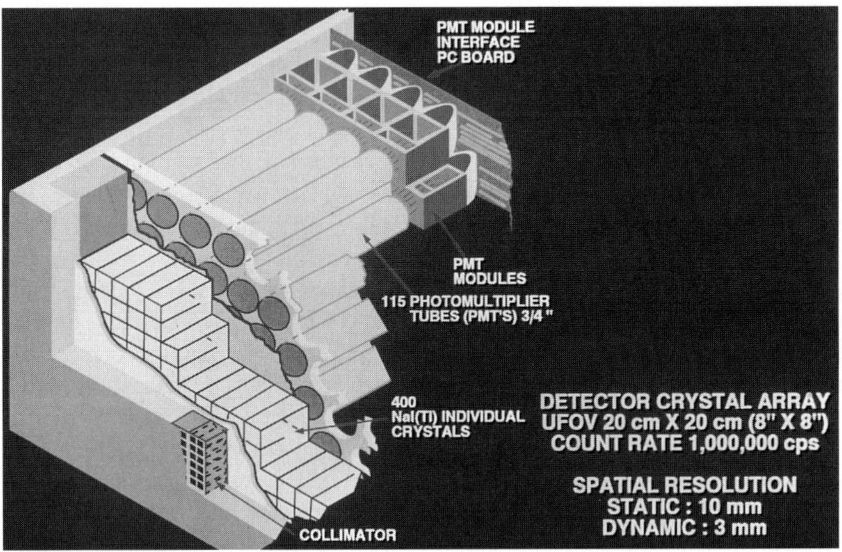

Fig. 13-3. Detector head of multicrystal stationary imaging device. (Courtesy Scinticor, Inc., Milwaukee, Wisc.)

talk" is further reduced by the use of a multihole collimator having 294 tapered holes. Each hole corresponds to each crystal element in the mosaic. The purpose of the thick mosaic scintillator is to obtain high detection efficiency for medium- and high-energy gamma rays, which is not possible with the scintillation camera.

Each of the 294 crystals in the 9- by 6-inch mosaic is optically connected by a pair of Lucite lightpipes to two of the bank of 35 photomultiplier tubes (see Fig. 13-4). One lightpipe goes to the X axis, and the other lightpipe goes to the Y axis. In this way simultaneous pulses from the two photomultiplier tubes identify the crystal element in which

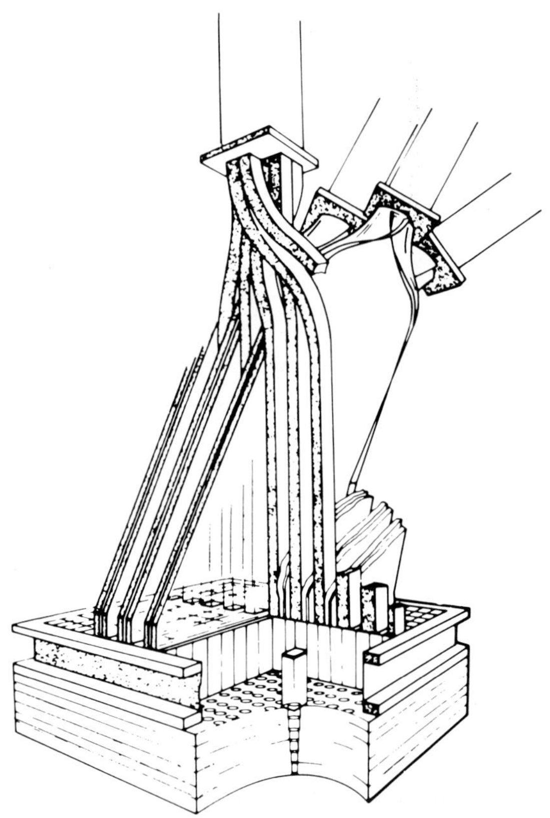

Fig. 13-4. Cut-away diagram of lightpipe assembly.

the scintillation occurred. A light is then produced on the recording oscilloscope face corresponding to the original location of a gamma ray or scintillation of light resulting from the gamma ray. With this arrangement, only 294 discrete storage locations for gamma quanta are available. Position of these gamma quanta therefore takes place in a digital fashion. The information is registered on a two-dimensional core memory conforming to the detector matrix. The contents of the core memory can then be transferred to magnetic tape diskettes. An anticoincidence circuit eliminates gamma rays scattered between one crystal and another in the mosaic. This technique eliminates scintillations caused by both the original gamma ray and the scattered gamma ray. As in the Anger camera, the signals from the two photomultiplier tubes are summed and fed to a pulse-height analyzer for acceptance or rejection.

Since this instrument has only 294 storage locations, the original instrument was such that each image was composed of 294 units of information. This camera now is used in conjunction with a programmed bed that moves 16 times within each individual crystal, yielding 4704 independent data points that are used for image construction. Each move is equal to 2.78 mm per move. This bed motion allows each detector crystal to scan a square area with 1.11-cm sides. Bed motion is visibly undetectable.

■ CAMERA DATA DISPLAY EQUIPMENT

Scintillation cameras yield X and Y position signals that must be used by some ancillary data presentation equipment. Four such ancillary pieces of equipment are (1) a cathode ray tube oscilloscope, (2) a multiformat programmer, (3) a variable persistence scope, and (4) a whole-body imaging table.

■ Cathode ray tube oscilloscope

X and Y position signals generated by the scintillation camera can be sent to the cathode ray oscilloscope to direct the beam of the oscilloscope to the position of the original scintillation in the crystal. As with the scintillation camera, the oscilloscope can also be thought of as a pie cut into four pieces, with the cuts serving as *x* and *y* coordinates. The normal position of the electron beam of the oscilloscope is in the center of the phosphor (Fig. 13-5, *dotted line*). When in this "resting" position, the electron gun is not activated (called *blank*); therefore no electrons strike the phosphor of the oscilloscope face. The activation of the electron gun requires an accepted Z pulse from the pulseheight analyzer, now called the *unblank* pulse. This unblank pulse will turn the electron beam on for a short period of time (a function of the unblank pulse width), only after the X and Y position signals have been allowed to stabilize. This ensures that the electron beam will strike at the point on the phosphor representative of the point on the detector crystal. Should that event be in the exact center of the crystal, then the electron beam is not moved and the unblank pulse turns on the electron beam. However, if the event occurred anywhere other than in dead center, the electron beam will require a change in direction. This is the purpose of the horizontal (X) and vertical (Y) deflector plates.

Since electrons will change their directions slightly in an electric or magnetic field, the magnitude of the position signals will change the course of the electron beam. This is accomplished by making the poles within the oscilloscope either more positive with respect to one another or more negative with respect to one another in all four directions. This affords an infinite number of positions on the oscilloscope face for the electron beam to be directed. The total resolution of the scintillation camera system depends on the collimation (extrinsic resolution) and the crystal and its associated electronics (intrinsic resolution) to properly adjust the polarity of these signals to the oscilloscope. By so doing, it correctly directs the electron beam to a position on the oscilloscope that corresponds with the position of the original scintillation in the crystal. The electrons striking the phosphor on the oscilloscope will excite the atom comprising the phosphor, which produces a flash of light. This flash of light can then be recorded on film. Each dot on the oscilloscope is a result of that electron beam being directed to a new location on the oscilloscope screen. Each change

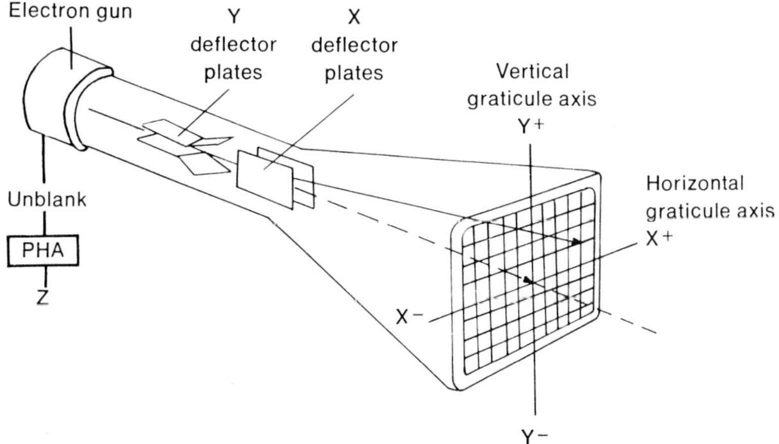

Fig. 13-5. Schematic of an oscilloscope.

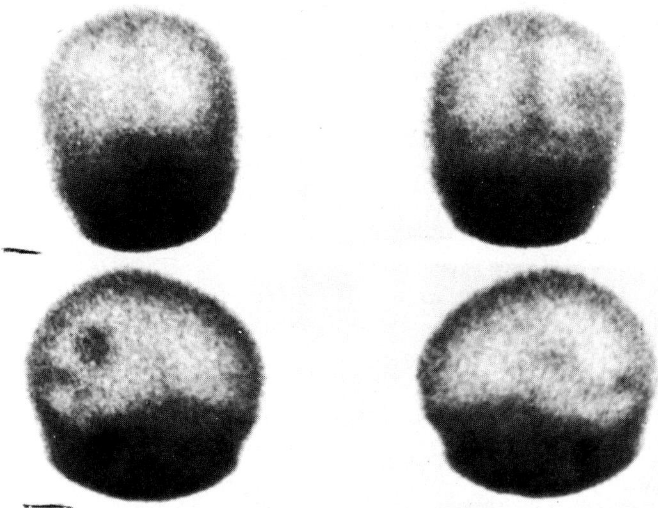

Fig. 13-6. Multiple views of brain image displayed on one piece of standard size x-ray film using multiformat programmer.

in location is produced by another event that occurred in the detector. The recording of these events over a period of time results in an image on film that displays the distribution of the radionuclide within an organ.

■ Multiformat programmer

An adaptation of this process of placing one whole image on one piece of film is to place more than one image on a single film (Fig. 13-6). A unit that allows this is termed a *multiformat programmer*. The concept of this system is to apply a constant gain to each signal that enters the oscilloscope. This changes the magnitude of the position signal so that in effect the center of the electron beam has been changed. Furthermore, its movement will be restricted to one section of the oscilloscope face and therefore to one section of the film. This gain change also minifies the image. During a second exposure the position of the image can be changed automatically or by manually pressing a position button. This automatically sets another gain, allowing the second exposure to be restricted to another portion of the oscilloscope face. In this way many smaller views can be placed on one piece of film. This has been found to be particularly useful with dynamic flow images, in which less information is lost by the electronic change in position than by the automatic mechanical advancement of photographic film.

■ Variable persistence scope

Oscilloscopes, as generally used in medicine, have phosphors that stay excited for a known amount of time; therefore light is emitted by this phosphor for a predetermined length of time. There was no way in which this "persistence" time could be varied. Since different phosphors persist for different amounts of time, an oscilloscope was selected for a particular use by the persistence time of the phosphor. Phosphors having a short persistence are commonly selected for general use because most signals are repetitive and occur at a rate fast enough that flicker is not bothersome. However, long persistence is often sought to display slowly moving biomedical phenomena and applications in which the traces must persist after the moving spot. Although many long-persistence phosphors are available, most do not properly accommodate the signal and are easily burned. Other applications could take advantage of the ability to vary the persistence so as to have a phosphor that would persist for a long period of time when needed and then alternately persist for a very short period of time. Since persistence is an inherent property of the phosphor, this is not possible except by artificial means.

The ability to vary the persistence is achieved by what is now called a *variable persistence scope* (p-scope) (Fig. 13-7). This type of scope consists of three surfaces and two electron guns. The three surfaces are (1) a collector mesh that acts as a device to orient electrons so that they travel perpendicular to the phosphor and parallel to the CRTs longitudinal axis, (2) an electron storage mesh that is an electrostatic surface on which an image is written or generated, and (3) the phosphor itself. The two electron guns are the writing gun, which writes with a focused high-energy beam, and a flood gun, which continually sends a cloud of electrons toward the three plates.

The writing gun produces a focused stream of high-energy electrons that passes through the collector mesh (some are collected) and "writes" a channel of positive charges on the electron storage mesh. This is accomplished by the high-energy electron beam knocking off electrons from the storage screen by secondary emission similar to that which happens on the dynodes of the photomultiplier tube. The absence of these electrons makes the area where the electron beam struck positive with respect to the other areas of the screen. The electrons produced by secondary emission are accelerated toward the phosphor, where they strike and excite their atoms with the subsequent release of energy in the form of visible light. The degree of brightness of the recorded event on the phosphor is a function of the voltage *(growth rate)* applied to the cathode of the CRT. As this voltage is increased, the energy of the "writing" electrons is increased. As these higher energy electrons strike the electron storage mesh, a greater number of secondary electrons are emitted from its surface. These are then accelerated to the phosphor, creating an increasingly larger and increasingly brighter spot on the oscilloscope phosphor.

Persistence is a function of the flood gun. This electron gun continually sends a cloud of electrons toward the phosphor. Since the electron storage mesh is usually negatively charged in its entirety, the cloud of electrons is prevented from getting to the phosphor and being collected by the collector mesh. It is only when the writing gun generates its relative positive charge on the electron storage mesh that these electrons from the electron cloud are attracted to it and through it. These electrons then are accelerated to the phosphor to persist the image by continuing to excite the phosphor. The usual length of time that light is visible on a cathode ray tube oscilloscope screen (that is, from the time that the light is first seen through the inherent decay time of the phosphor) is 0.2 second. The variable persistence scope allows one to extend that time up to 60 seconds. *Variable persistence* is achieved by varying the rate of erasure of the electron storage mesh. This erasure is controlled by varying the rate of discharge of the electron storage mesh, thereby making the area that possessed a relative positive charge more negative. The rate at which this discharge occurs is the variable. As the positive area be-

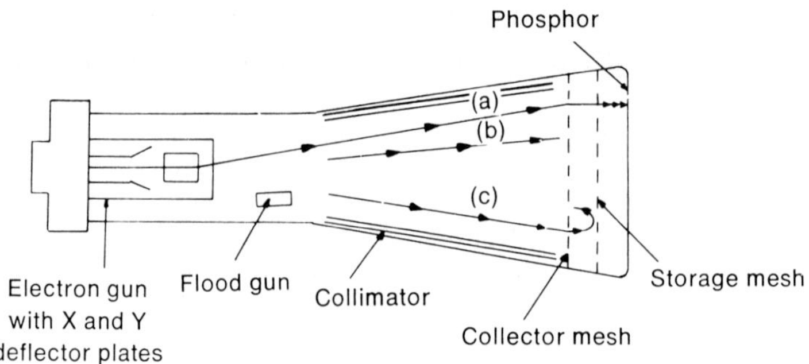

Fig. 13-7. Schematic of variable persistence scope. **(a),** High-energy "writing" beam of electrons being oriented by the collector mesh and knocking off several secondary electrons from the storage mesh. **(b),** Electrons being absorbed by the collector mesh. **(c),** Electrons passing through the collector mesh but being repelled by the negative charge on the storage mesh, to finally be absorbed by the collector mesh.

comes less positive, fewer electrons from the flood gun are allowed through to the phosphor, and the dot gets lighter and lighter. Eventually the positive area is completely discharged, and the dot of light disappears. In reality, then, increased persistence is a result of decreasing the erasure rate. "Blooming," or phosphor flare-up, occurs in variable persistence scope when the erasure time is faster than the inherent decay time of the phosphor. When these conditions exist, the phosphor responds by a flare-up caused by the overwhelming number of events striking the phosphor. A recent development as a replacement for the p-scope is the digital CRT scope. This instrument digitizes the display into a 64 × 64 matrix. The scope continually "refreshes" itself at a predetermined count accumulation. It is an excellent tool in high count-rate situations, but since there is no way to adjust the sensitivity on most models, it loses utility in low count-rate situations.

■ Whole-body imager

Another adaptation to electronically manipulating position information is the *whole-body imaging table* (Fig. 13-8). With this system the patient, the detector, or both are moved lengthwise on a specially designed scanning platform past the scintillation detector. The detector "sees" one longitudinal section of patient anatomy as defined by the limiting edges of the detector field of view. Integrated data from the longitudinal section is presented to the cathode ray tube as a "minified" display to accommodate the total body image. An indexing mechanism within the table allows for subsequent longitudinal sections, dependent on patient width. One, two, or three passes are electronically selected. The electronics keeps the image from overlapping, which would result in a blurring of the image. Consequently, these lines represent a displacement rather than a loss of information. "Single pass" whole-body cameras are also available. These cameras view the whole body in one pass by the detector as opposed to a composite image made by three passes over the whole body. Altered electronics and special fanshaped collimators make this technique possible.

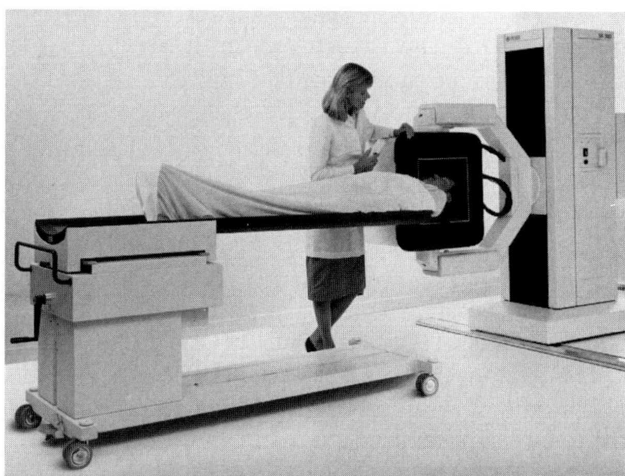

Fig. 13-8. Scintillation camera with whole-body imaging table. To perform whole-body imaging, the table would require rearranging so as to be parallel with the track on the floor. (Courtesy Picker International, Cleveland, Ohio.)

To ensure high sensitivity and constant uniformity over the entire scan area, it is necessary that each portion of the body appear in the detector's field of view for the same amount of time. This depends on three essential factors that are automatically controlled. First, the crystal must be electronically masked to restrict the area of sensitivity to a rectangular format, which eliminates the integration of counts from the otherwise overlapping edges of a circular aperture detection system. Second, the patient must be "overscanned" at the head and feet to ensure uniform exposure of these areas to the detector. Third, the speed of the platform or crystal and movement must be kept constant and smooth, regardless of the patient's weight and the position of the scanning platform.

As the drive mechanism moves the scanning platform or the detector head in a continuous motion, a digital shaft encoder electronically transmits to the oscilloscope the platform positive relative to the detector. The information is then recorded on film relative to the position of the detector at the time that the event occurred.

■ QUALITY ASSURANCE AND CONTROL

Quality assurance and control procedures are necessary in every department of the hospital to maintain standards and to ensure reproducibility of tests. This is especially true of the nuclear medicine department where radioactive drugs are being introduced into patients and expensive sophisticated equipment is being used. General quality assurance and instrument quality control are essential.

■ General quality assurance

Quality assurance starts when a study is ordered by a physician and continues through the final report being typed and placed on the patient's chart. It encompasses many areas of the hospital and many policies and procedures before the final product is achieved.

The first area of quality assurance is the physician's order for the study. The requisition must be sent to the department with the correct patient name, room number, age, requesting physician, identification numbers, and study to be performed with a pertinent diagnosis.

The study must then be scheduled. In the past there have been many difficulties in scheduling multiple nuclide studies on the same patient because of the many radionuclides employed. With the advent of ^{99m}Tc compounds, there is no longer a great problem. However, there are still some general rules that should be followed:

1. Laboratory studies should be performed before imaging studies. The Schilling test should always be the

first laboratory study performed if more than one in vivo study is ordered on the patient. Thyroid uptake studies should be performed before ^{67}Ga images.
2. High-energy nuclide studies, such as gallium images, can usually be performed before or after a ^{99m}Tc compound image because of the energy differences and the microcurie quantities, compared with the millicurie quantities of ^{99m}Tc. However, they should not be performed on the same day unless the high-energy study is done first.
3. Most technetium compound images do not interfere with each other because of their short half-lives, but the biodistribution of the tracer must be kept in mind when one is scheduling sequential studies. For example, a liver scan should be performed before ^{99m}Tc pertechnetate images to avoid bowel activity, which would be seen overlying the liver if the studies were performed in the reverse order, assuming that the studies were to be completed in 2 days.
4. ^{99m}Tc pertechnetate brain images should be performed before polyphosphate and pyrophosphate bone images. It has been demonstrated that following a polyphosphate or pyrophosphate bone image with a pertechnetate brain image causes plexus, leading to false positive results. Apparently, the increased activity in the superior sagittal sinus, transverse sinuses, and choroid plexus leads to false positive results. Apparently the tin labels the erythrocytes following bone imaging, and the pertechnetate attaches to the tin-labeled red blood cells. A wait of as long as 6 days may be necessary if the bone image is performed first.

Another area of importance in scheduling the patient is preparation requirements. This information should be made available to the hospital personnel involved. Abdominal images such as liver, pancreas, and Meckel's diverticulum should be performed before colon or upper gastrointestinal x-ray examination, because the barium will attenuate the radionuclides and can lead to false-positive results. Thyroid studies should be performed before the patient's having any studies done with contrast media, such as IVP, gallbladder, or CT studies with contrast media. Each patient area should have a list of nuclear medicine procedures stating the preparation for the study and other tests that may interfere with that study, as well as whether the patient is to have oral intake restricted. The patient must then be transported to the department for the study. On the patient's arrival, the technologist is responsible for checking patient identification (usually a wrist band) and for injecting the correct dose of radiopharmaceutical into the correct patient. In the case of in vitro studies, samples must be drawn on the correct patient, labeled appropriately, and stored until the assay is performed.

Whether multiformat imaging or a computer-assisted study is used, the technologist must process the images after they are performed. Knowledge of proper use and handling of these is essential to produce a diagnostic image. The most sophisticated imaging systems must rely on some type of photographic processing. If film quality is not good or the film processor is not performing properly, all of the technologist's experience and the expensive equipment will not produce a high-quality diagnostic image. Departments that have their own processors should take the following steps to ensure that the equipment is functioning properly:

1. Follow manufacturer's start-up procedure.
2. Allow sufficient time for temperature to stabilize.
3. Check solution temperature, water temperature, drier temperature, and replenishment rates.
4. Run exposed, but unprocessed, film through the processor each morning to clean residue from racks and to check for scratches.
5. Clean crossover racks at the end of each work day.

A preventive maintenance program with a local processor or chemical company ensures routine cleaning, maintenance, and a constant supply of fresh chemicals.

After processing of a study is complete, the study should be checked for quality by the technologist before it is presented to the department physician for interpretation. All studies should be labeled correctly with patient identification data and date of study. The technologist should check for correct placement of radioactive markers. Any unusual views, patient position, artifacts, or patient condition should be noted for the physician to avoid errors in diagnosis. A pertinent patient history is also of great importance as an aid to interpretation of the study. Previous studies on the same patient should be indicated with films for interpretation. Following interpretation, the report is ready to be transcribed by clerical personnel and placed on the patient's chart. The radiopharmaceutical used and the activity administered must be on the report. If it is not, this information must be handwritten on the patient's chart. Copies of the report are placed on the chart, sent to the referring physician, and maintained in the department with the patient studies.

At this time the study is complete and the patient study is filed according to the department's filing system.

A breakdown in any of the areas mentioned can cause an error to be introduced that often cannot be corrected without additional time and cost to the department, patient, and hospital. Interdepartmental and intradepartmental communications, as well as written policies and procedures, will aid in eliminating quality assurance breakdowns.

■ Instrument quality control

Quality control of instruments includes all equipment in the nuclear medicine department, such as uptake probes, well detectors, scintillation cameras, and dose calibrators. All of the quality control procedures for uptake probes and well detectors have been addressed in the Laboratory applications preceding this section. Laboratory applications such as the calibration of a spectrometer (5), the determination of a gamma energy spectrum (6), energy resolution (7), proper window settings (8), and proper gain setting (10) apply to all equipment. Laboratory applications such as assay of a mixed gamma sample (12), efficiency (13), coincidence loss (14), and geometry (15) apply primarily to uptake probes and well detectors. Since all of these quality-control procedures have been discussed already and constitute all of the procedures required of uptake probes and well detectors, the following section on instrument quality assurance will restrict its discussion to the scintillation camera, with a special section dedicated to the dose calibrator. A suggested quality control program for all nuclear medicine equipment is included at the conclusion of Chapter 14.

The acquisition and installation of a new scintillation camera represents, in most cases, a tremendous amount of time on the part of all persons concerned. Representatives from each manufacturer spend a great deal of time discussing the merits of their respective systems. They spend time with technical as well as administrative personnel. Visits are made to various institutions that already have the units as an integral part of their nuclear medicine department. Opinions of other associated personnel, consultants, and financial officers are weighed. Manufacturer's specifications are compared, and finally a decision is made and the unit installed.

It is necessary at this point to spend some time examining the unit before using it on patients to determine if the manufacturer's specifications are met. The following pages include procedures for such an evaluation.

The quality assurance of a scintillation camera has been the subject of the National Electrical Manufacturers Association (NEMA) and its Diagnostic Imaging and Therapy Systems Division. NEMA represents manufacturers of nuclear medicine equipment who devise and agree on standards that all manufacturers must meet. Each camera must meet these standards before it leaves the factory. The ideal situation then is to apply these same standards to the camera once it is installed in the hospital. Unfortunately, some of the procedures require complicated programming skills and a much larger computer than the usual nuclear medicine computer. In addition, implementing NEMA standards requires an MCA such that each channel is equal to or less than 0.3 mm in width (1000 channels or more). To complicate the situation, invasive testing is required, since it will be necessary to tie the MCA into the X and Y leads in the head of the camera. This maneuver often voids the warranty of the manufacturer unless performed in cooperation with the manufacturer's service representatives. For these reasons, not all of the NEMA standards are applicable in a hospital situation. We present the NEMA standards to the user for the purpose of background knowledge.

LABORATORY APPLICATION

26

QUALITY CONTROL
Testing parameters for a scintillation camera

The crystal of the scintillation camera has characteristics that are of paramount importance. For instance, if variations in response exist between areas of the same crystal, an artifact may be presented on the image that may be erroneously interpreted as a lesion. Such variations can be eliminated by proper calibration ("tuning") of the photomultiplier tube servicing the area of the defect or by applying the nonuniformity correction circuit. These are characteristics that should be determined and known before using a scintillation camera on any patient. The purpose of the following exercises is to point out some of these characteristics and how they can be determined and routinely monitored.

Purpose of proper intensity settings

The determination of appropriate intensity settings is an important aspect of technology in the use of a scintillation camera, especially with an analog readout. The intensity defines the size and brightness of the dot placed on the film, whether it be 35 mm or single-emulsion x-ray film.* The proper intensity settings are determined by using a bar phantom, setting the instrument for the predetermined number of counts or ID, and taking pictures each time the intensity is changed. If the intensity is too low, the picture becomes underexposed and detail is lost because of lack of information. If the intensity is too high, the picture becomes overexposed and detail is again lost; but this time it is lost because the capabilities of the display system have been exceeded and saturation has resulted. The proper intensity setting for a variety of counts to be used on various clinical studies is desired.

*This is not a problem with computer-assisted images since modifications are made on the computer image and then photographed.

Continued

Procedure for proper intensity settings

Materials

1. ^{99m}Tc point source of 100 to 200 μCi (3.7 to 7.4 MBq) is adequate
2. 3-mm–thick lead ring (if available) to mask "edge packing" artifact
3. Bar phantom

Technique

1. Remove collimator and invert.
2. Place lead ring on detector.
3. Place bar phantom on detector.
4. Arrange point source at a distance of 5 UFOV* diameters.
5. Set appropriate pulse-height analyzer setting using a 20% window.
6. Adjust intensity until dots are barely visualized on the scope.
7. Begin accumulating pictures at various intensities and various predetermined counts or IDs. Procedures to follow call for images with total counts of 1×10^6 or 2×10^6, and 8×10^6.

Data treatment

1. Select intensity setting providing the best resolution for the various counts or IDs.
2. Make a record for future reference.

Key points

1. Perform at installation and after a voltage change.
2. Older units have phosphors on the CRT, which exhibit an afterglow phenomenon following the recording of an event (Fig. 13-9). This creates a situation in which the rate of accumulation must be considered in the selection of a proper intensity setting. If the count rate is high, the afterglow is significant and requires a slight reduction of the intensity setting. The same count at a lower rate requires a higher intensity setting because of reduced afterglow effects.
3. Since the UFOV can be defined as a circular area within a diameter that is the largest in-

*UFOV, Useful field of view of the camera (the collimated field of view). See Key point 3.

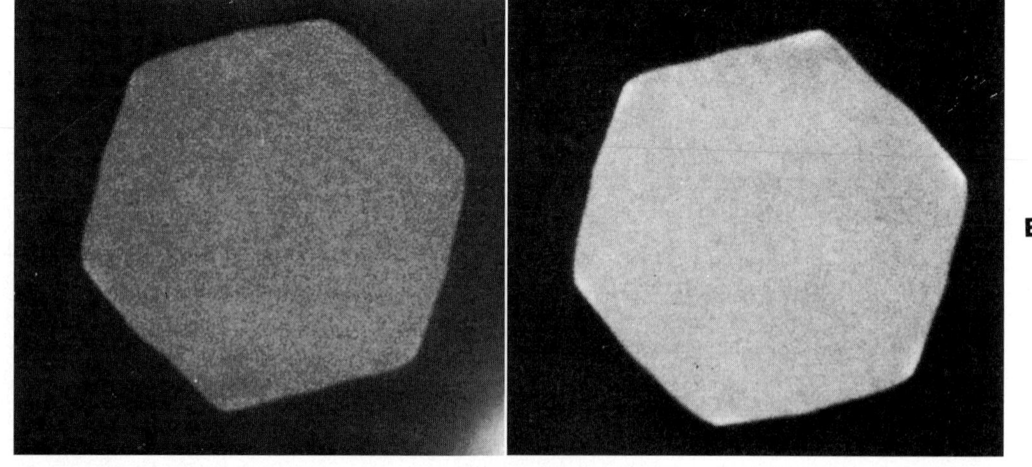

Fig. 13-9. Effect of "afterglow" on a cathode ray tube (CRT) phosphor. **A,** Flood study collecting 2 million counts in 66 seconds. **B,** Another flood study collecting the same number of counts, but in 46 seconds, with all other parameters remaining the same. Note the increased intensity on the study in **B,** accumulated over a shorter period of time. This phenomenon does not exist in digital displays.

scribed circle within the collimated field of view, the UFOV can be determined as follows:

a. Place four ^{57}Co point sources at the farthest points in both the X and Y directions as seen on the monitor.
b. Measure the distance in both directions.*
c. Express as UFOV.
d. CFOV (central field of view) = UFOV × 0.75.

Purpose of flood field uniformity

Flood field uniformity is defined as the parameter of a scintillation camera's ability to present a uniform count density image. It is absolutely essential to good diagnostic technique. A nonuniform area may be visualized as a "hot" spot or a "cold" spot. These areas may be diffuse patterns throughout the field of view, or they may be perceived as discrete areas approximating the size of the photomultiplier tube serving that area of the crystal. Any of these nonuniformities could be detrimental to accurate diagnosis. "Cold" areas could be read as tumors in the liver (Fig. 13-10) or infarcts in the lung, while a "hot" area could be read as a brain tumor. A flood study would rule out such nonuniformities. A cracked crystal (Fig. 13-11), a weak or nonfunctioning photomultiplier (Figs. 13-12 and 13-13), a defective collimator (Fig. 13-14), or a defective CRT (Fig. 13-15, *A*) can be detected by this technique.

*Both X and Y directions should have equal values if X and Y gains are correct.

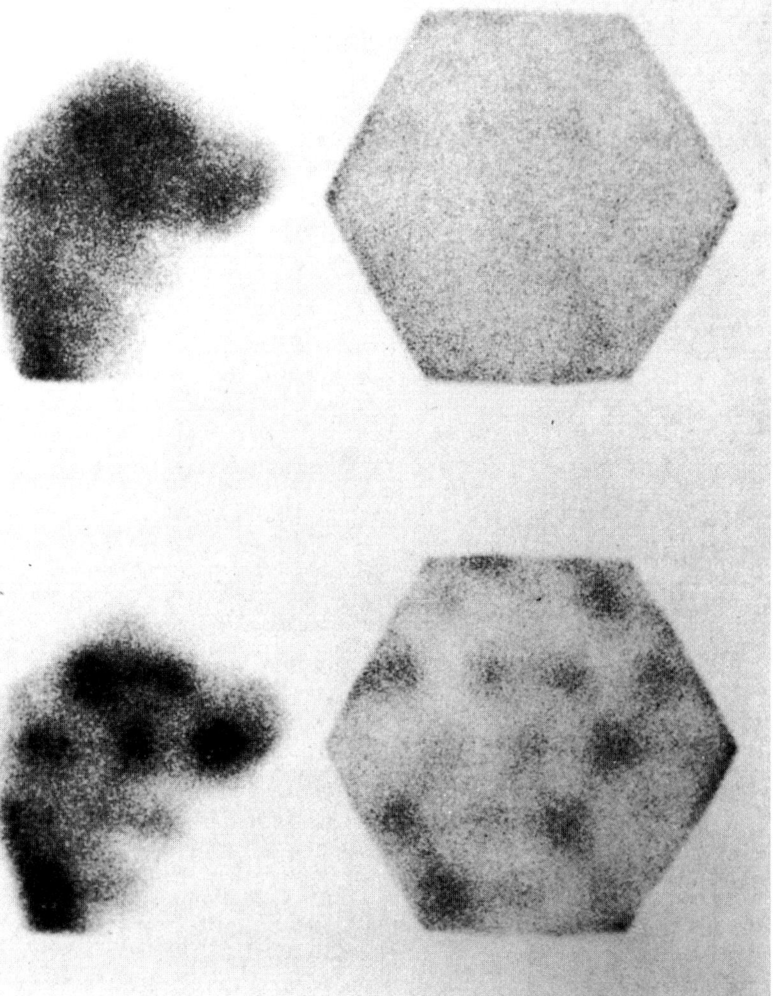

Fig. 13-10. *Above,* Liver image compared with daily field flood image for control. *Below,* Same lines imaged with an asymmetric window enhancing artifactual lesions. Corresponding field–flood-control image shows that lesions correspond to field nonuniformities. (From Paras, P., Van Tuinen, R.J., and Hamilton, D.R.: In Rhodes, B.A., editor: Quality control in nuclear medicine; radiopharmaceuticals, instrumentation, and in vitro assays, St. Louis, 1977, Mosby–Year Book.)

Continued.

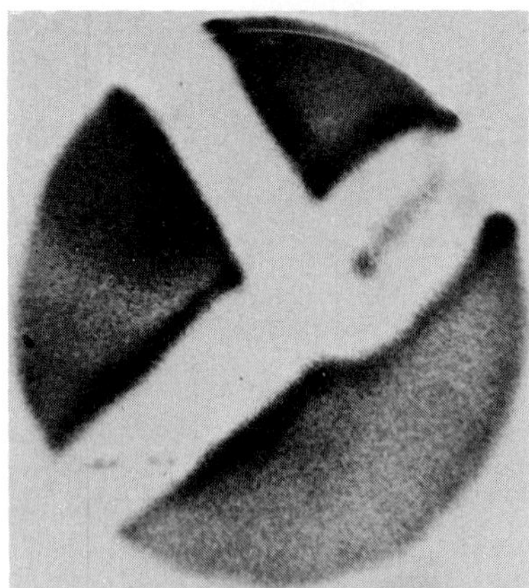

Fig. 13-11. Cracked crystal.

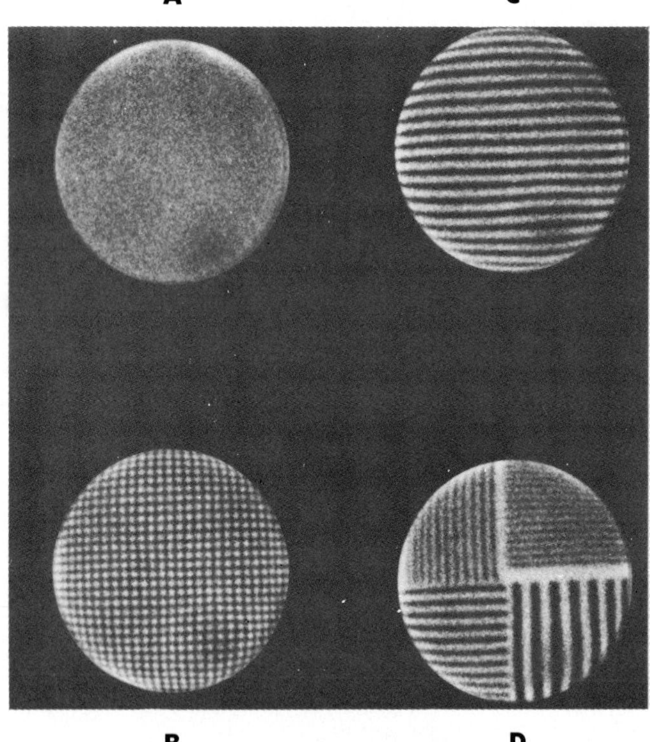

Fig. 13-12. Images showing characteristic findings associated with a photomultiplier tube not properly balanced. **A,** Flood field. **B,** Orthogonal-hole phantom. **C,** PLES phantom. **D,** Four-quadrant bar phantom images. (From Rollo, F.D.: Nuclear medicine physics, instrumentation, and agents, St. Louis, 1977, Mosby–Year Book.)

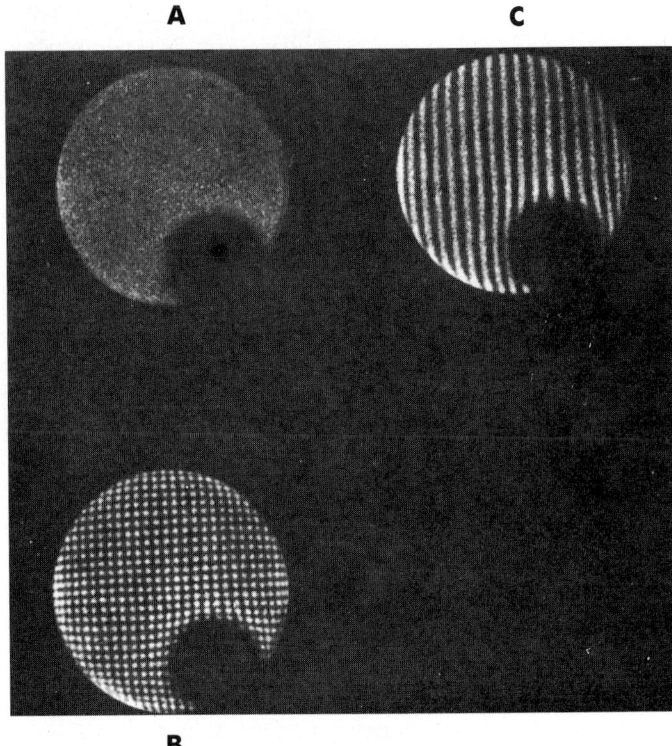

Fig. 13-13. Images characteristic of a photomultiplier tube not functioning. **A,** Flood field. **B,** Orthogonal-hole phantom. **C,** PLES phantom. (From Rollo, F.D.: Nuclear medicine physics, instrumentation, and agents, St. Louis, 1977, Mosby–Year Book.)

Fig. 13-14. Line artifact in collimator realized only with an 8- to 10-million–count acquisition.

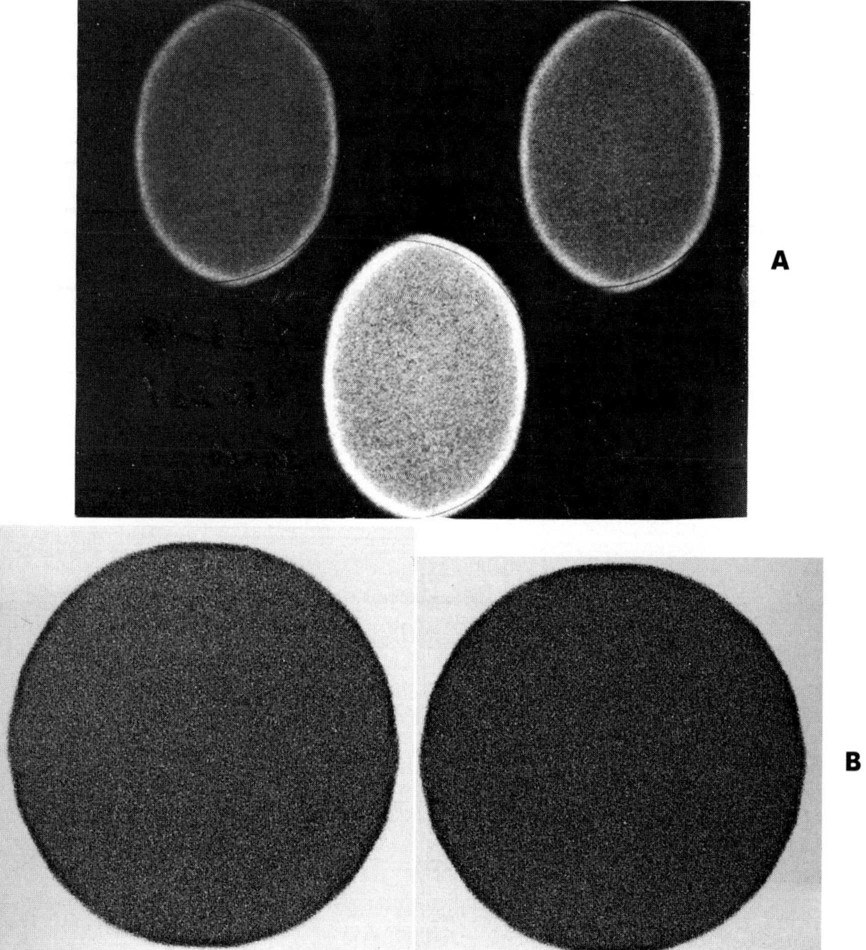

Fig. 13-15. A, Oval flood caused by improper adjustment of X and Y deflector plates in the CRT and demonstrating edge-packing. **B,** Uniform crystal response with masking of edge-packing effect.

Procedure for total system uniformity

Materials

1. ^{57}Co flood source of 1 to 5 mCi (37 to 185 MBq) is adequate; radionuclide is uniformly plated on one side of diskette; count rate should be less than or equal to 20,000 cps
2. Flood phantom; fill with water and add 1 to 5 mCi (37 to 185 MBq) of ^{99m}Tc; this is a suitable alternative to step 1; count rate should be less than 20,000 cps
3. ^{99m}Tc point source of 100 to 200 μCi (3.7 to 7.4 MBq) is adequate; count rate of no greater than 20,000 cps is desirable
4. ^{99m}Tc point source of 20 mCi (740 MBq) for collimator integrity.
5. 3 mm thick lead ring (if available) to mask "edge packing" artifact on intrinsic studies (Fig. 13-15, *B*)
6. All collimators

User's technique for total system uniformity

1. Place collimator on detector and invert detector head. Some systems must be inverted to change the collimator. In those systems, leave detector inverted.
2. Place ^{57}Co flood source with ±1% uniformity or ^{99m}Tc-loaded flood phantom on collimator (Fig. 13-16). If a flood phantom is used, protect against contamination by interposing plastic-backed absorbent paper between the phantom and the detector.

Continued.

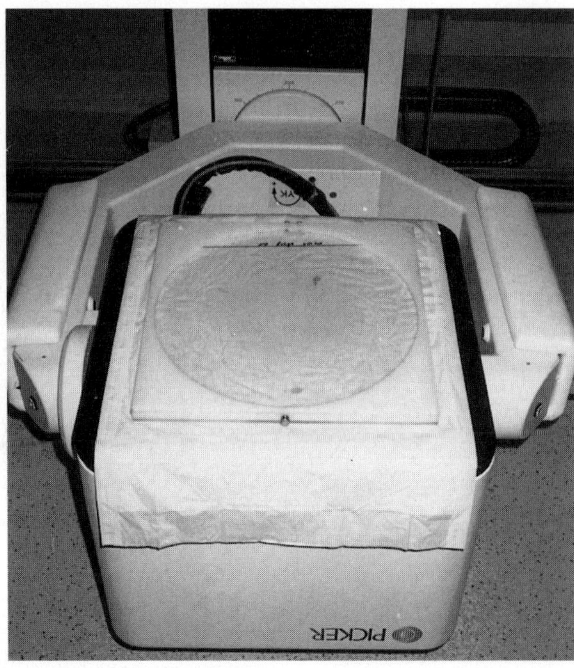

Fig. 13-16. Setup on inverted scintillation camera head for uniform field flood determination with a collimator, using a flood source.

3. Set and visually verify appropriate pulse height analyzer setting with a 20% window.
4. Set appropriate intensity, if required.
5. Collect 1 million uncorrected counts* if a camera with a standard field of view is used; collect 2 million uncorrected counts for a camera with a large field of view. (Larger numbers of counts are required for SPECT, i.e., 60 to 120 million.)
6. Collect a corrected flood.
7. Repeat with the window placed on the high side of the energy peak and again on the low side of the energy peak (Figs. 13-17 and 13-18).
8. Repeat flood with collimator rotated (Fig. 13-19).†
9. Repeat using all available collimators.
10. Store corrected floods.

User's technique for collimator integrity (nonparallelism) of parallel-hole collimators

1. With collimator on detector, turn collimator perpendicular to the floor with detector facing into the room.
2. Place 20 mCi (740 MBq) point source of ^{99m}Tc 15 to 20 feet away and aligned with the center hole.
3. Set and verify appropriate pulse-height analyzer setting with a 20% window.
4. Set appropriate intensity, if required.
5. Collect 100 to 500k count image. In the case of large detectors, repeat, aligning source with various locations on the detector.
6. Repeat on all parallel-hole collimators.
7. All images should be round (Fig. 13-20, *top;* rationale shown in Fig. 13-20, *bottom*).

*Acceptance testing requires 8-10 million counts also. Not all cameras allow uncorrected floods.
†Not all cameras will allow this technique due to collimator interlock system.

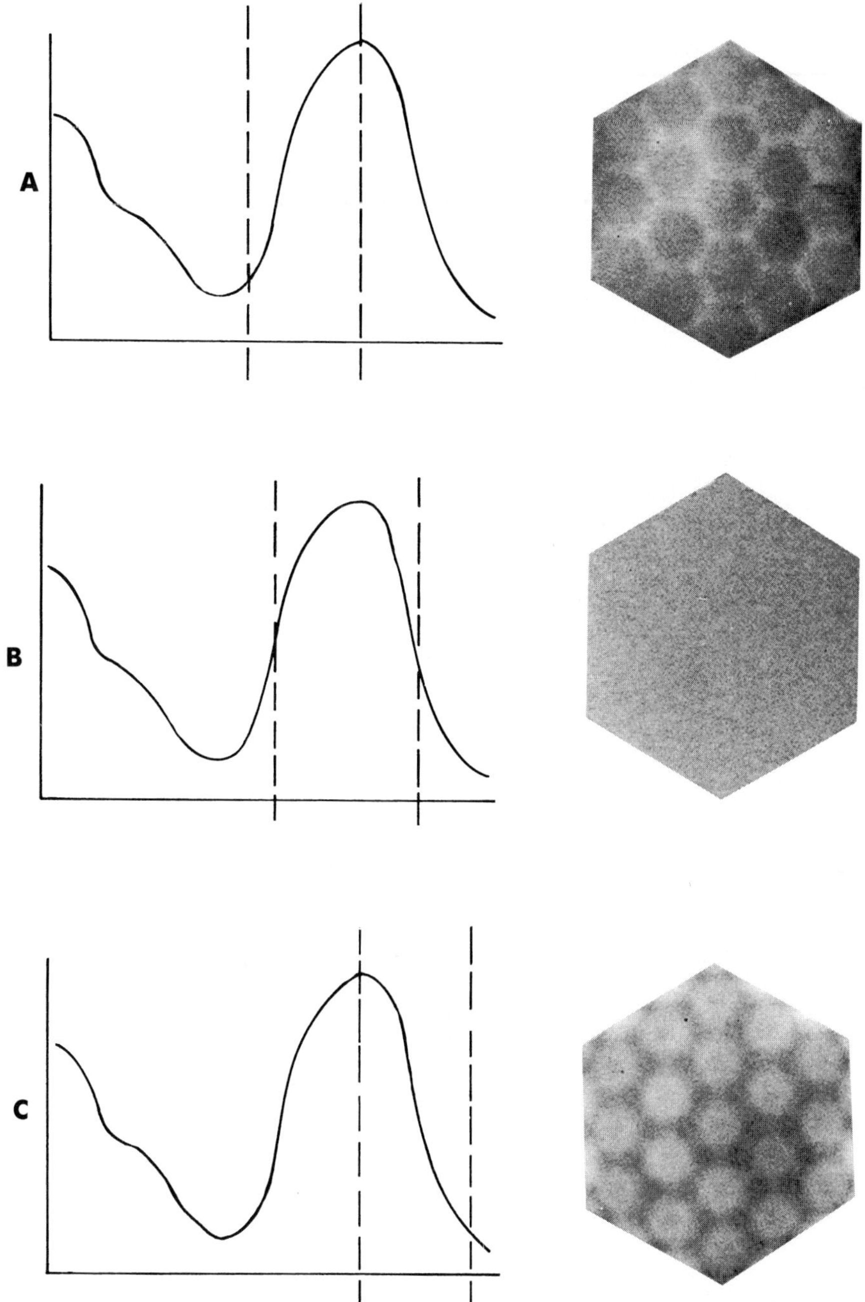

Fig. 13-17. Effects of window settings on flood results. **A,** Flood study taken with the window set to the low-energy side of the primary energy peak, showing "hot" spots over each phototube. **B,** Same flood study taken with the window centrally set on the primary energy peak. **C,** Flood study repeated, only this time with the window set to the high-energy side of the primary energy peak, showing "cold" spots over each phototube.

Continued.

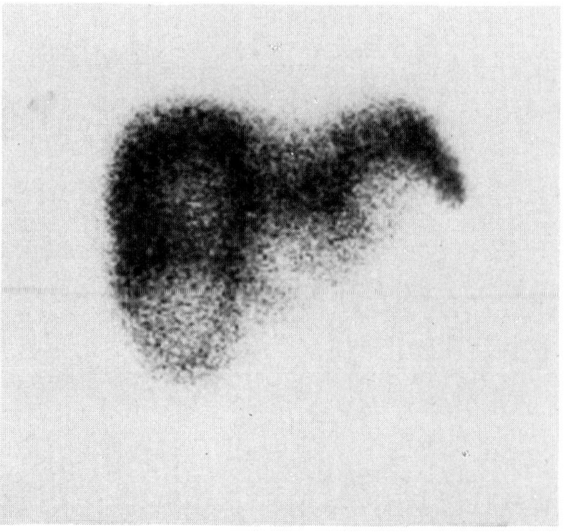

Fig. 13-18. Normal liver study performed with ^{99m}Tc-labeled sulfur colloid; however, the window used was that of ^{57}Co from the morning flood study, resulting in an "off-peak" window for ^{99m}Tc.

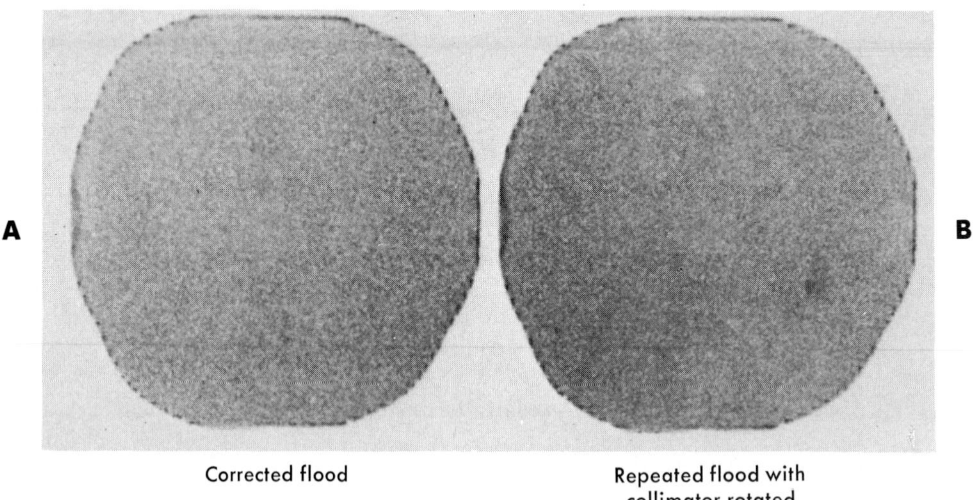

Fig. 13-19. Technique for checking collimator integrity by using the matrix addition nonuniformity correction capability. **A,** Normal corrected flood study using a collimator. **B,** Flood study repeated with the collimator slightly rotated. Areas that were once corrected now show "cold" areas and defects have been rotated to show "hot" areas, as in the defect shown in Fig. 13-14.

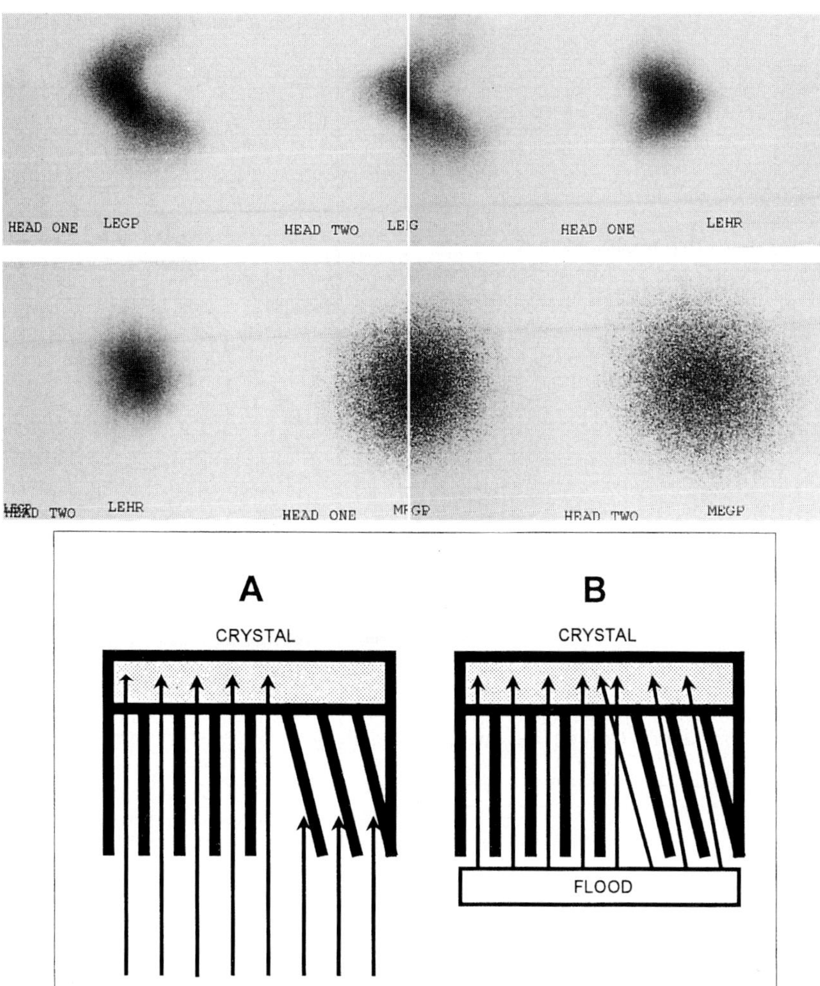

Fig. 13-20. *Top,* Collimator integrity study checking for collimator hole parallelism showing three acceptable collimators *(bottom row),* one marginal *(top, right),* and two *(top, left),* unacceptable. *Bottom,* Schematic demonstrating the rational behind checking parallelism of parallel-hole collimators with a distant point source. Crystals A and B both have parallel hole collimators, some of which have been caused to be nonparallel on the right side of each crystal. Crystal A is being evaluated with a 20 mCi point from 20 feet away. By so doing, all the gamma rays are almost parallel, not allowing the gamma rays to enter the crystal through the nonparallel holes. Crystal B demonstrates why a flood source will not identify the problem. The nonparallel holes will accept angled gamma rays and result in a uniform flood.

Procedure for intrinsic uniformity

Manufacturer's (NEMA) procedure for intrinsic uniformity (Fig. 13-21)

Remove the collimator and, using a 20% window centrally positioned around the ^{99m}Tc energy peak, and a 3 mm thick lead ring (to identify the UFOV), place a ^{99m}Tc source 5 UFOV diameters away (Fig. 13-21, *A*). Accumulate a flood on a 64 × 64 matrix at a rate not greater than 20,000 cps, such that the center pixel receives a minimum of 4000 counts (or 16 million counts per flood study). Perform a 9-point smoothing maneuver on the accumulated counts. Express both integral uniformity (a maximum deviation) and differential uniformity (a maximum change of counts over a range of any 5 pixels in all rows and in all columns) for both UFOV and CFOV* according to the following formulae:

$$\text{Integral uniformity} = \pm 100\,\frac{(\text{max} - \text{min})}{(\text{max} + \text{min})}$$

$$\text{Differential uniformity} = \pm 100\left[\frac{\text{Largest slice deviation (Hi} - \text{Low)}}{\text{Hi} + \text{Low}}\right]$$

*CFOV, Central Field of View, or 75% of the diameter of the UFOV.

Continued.

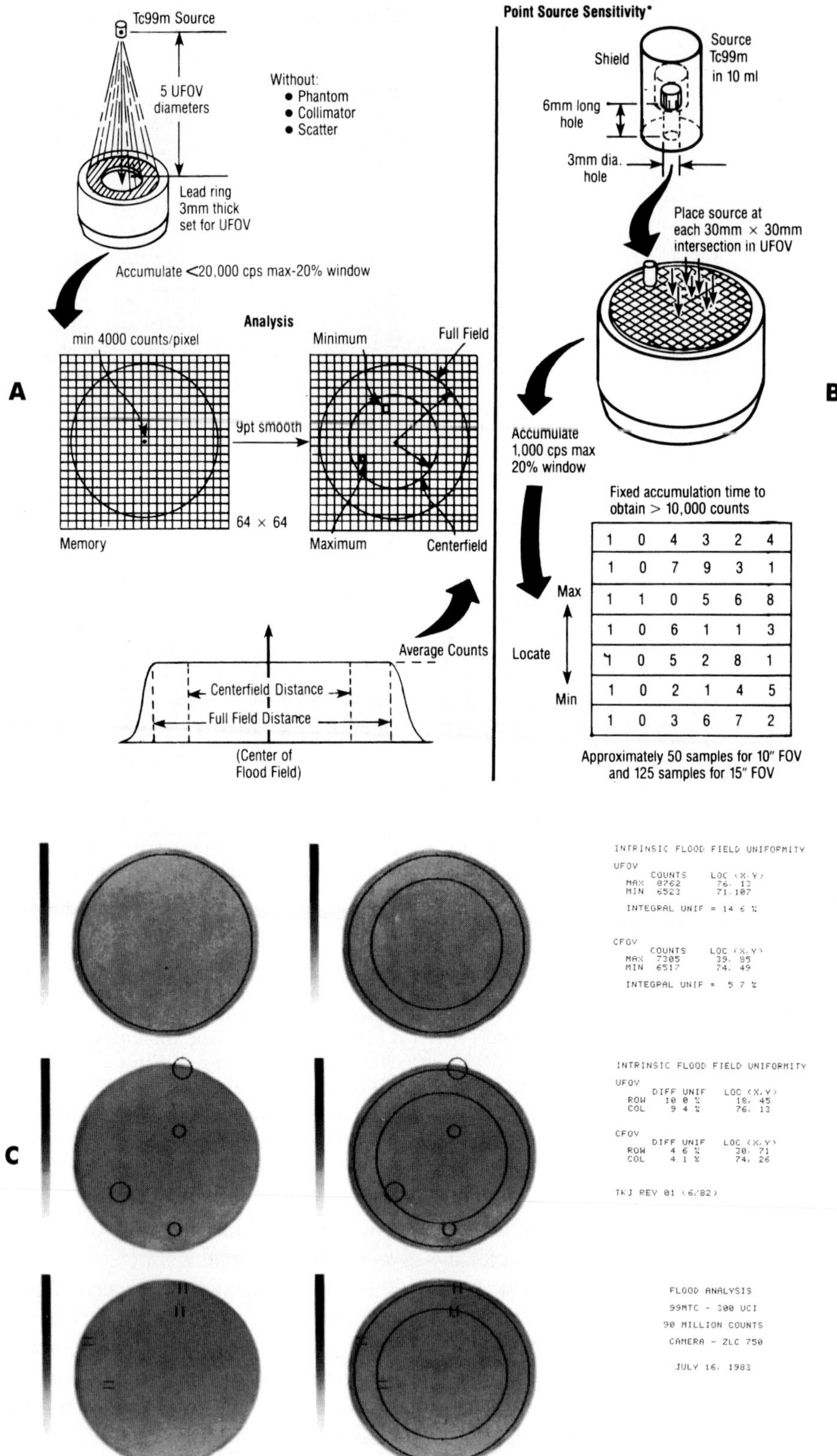

Fig. 13-21. **A** and **B,** NEMA procedure for intrinsic flood field uniformity. **C,** Program for a clinical nuclear medicine computer to evaluate intrinsic flood field uniformity. (**A** and **B,** From NEMA standards for performance measurements of scintillation cameras, Pub. No. NU 1-1980, National Electrical Manufacturers' Association, Copyright 1980, Medical Multimedia Corp. Courtesy Picker International, Cleveland, Ohio. **C,** Courtesy St. John's Hospital, Springfield, Ill.)

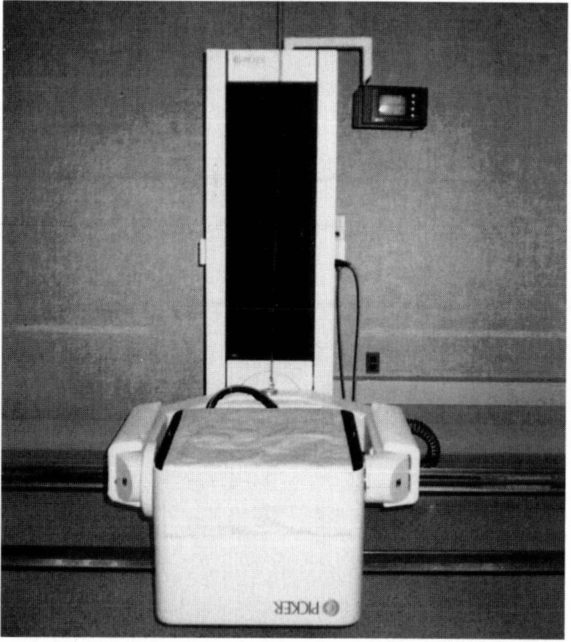

Fig. 13-22. Setup on an inverted scintillation camera head for uniform field flood determination without a collimator, using a syringe at a distance as point source. Syringe taped to the rod at the top of the photograph contains 100 to 200 μCi of ^{99m}Tc. By placing a bar phantom or Hines-Duley phantom on top of the crystal, a study of intrinsic resolution also can be determined.

An alternative procedure is called *point source sensitivity.** A shielded source of ^{99m}Tc (Fig. 13-21, *B*) is placed on the surface of the uncollimated detector at each 30 × 30 mm intersection in the UFOV. Determine a time to accumulate more than 100,000 counts at a rate of 10,000 cps maximum, with a 20% window. Record counts at each intersection and apply results to formulas above. Approximately 125 samples are required for a 15-inch FOV.

The manufacturer's procedure for NEMA's "measured standard" requires a sophisticated software program and a fairly powerful computer to perform this "number crunching." Programs are available, however, for some clinical units (Fig. 13-21, *C*). In addition, the "class standard" procedure is time-consuming. Neither procedure can be performed easily at the user level if a program such as in Fig. 13-21, *C*, is not available.

User's procedure for intrinsic uniformity

1. Remove collimator.
2. Place lead ring (if available) on detector.
3. Arrange point source at 5 UFOV diameters (See Fig. 13-22).
4. Set and visually verify appropriate pulse-height analyzer setting with a 20% window.
5. Set appropriate intensity if applicable.
6. Collect 1 million uncorrected counts if a camera with a standard field of view is used; collect 2 million uncorrected counts for a camera with a large field of view. Collect at two different count rates; 20,000 cps and 75,000 cps (see key point 16). Note time.
7. Collect a corrected flood for the same number of counts as in step 6. Note time.
8. Repeat the flood with the window placed on the high side of the energy peak (Fig. 13-17, *C*) and on the low side of the energy peak (Fig. 13-17, *A*).

Data treatment

1. Visually inspect films for nonuniformities. If acceptable, file as daily record (Fig. 13-23).
2. Calculate the uniformity correction factor (UCF) as follows:

$$\text{UCF} = \left[\frac{\text{Time for corrected flood} - \text{Time for uncorrected flood}}{\text{Time for correction flood}}\right] \times 100$$

*This procedure is considered by NEMA to be a "class standard" that characterizes a specific performance parameter typical of the given model number or series of scintillation cameras for which it applies. Usually the parameter is of auxiliary interest and is a subset of a "measured standard."

Continued.

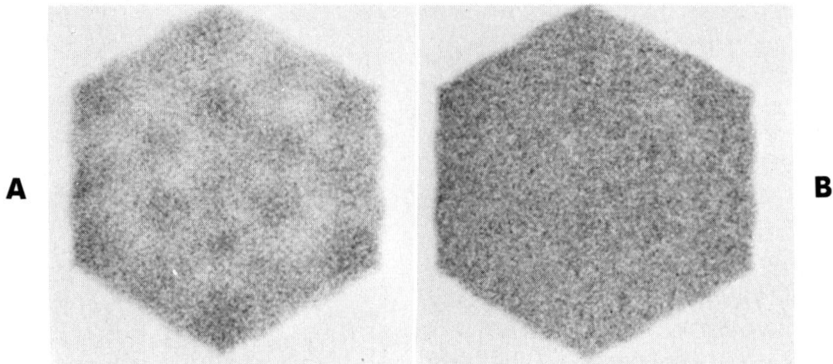

Fig. 13-23. Effects of nonuniform correction techniques. **A,** Abnormal flood study. **B,** Flood study repeated with correction techniques applied.

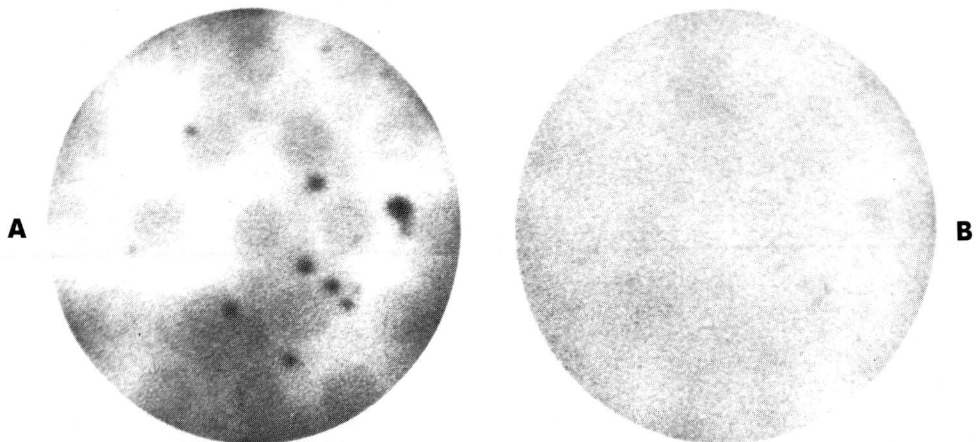

Fig. 13-24. A, Measles as evidenced on "off-peak" flood study. **B,** Measles severe enough to be seen in the "on-peak" flood and therefore on clinical studies.

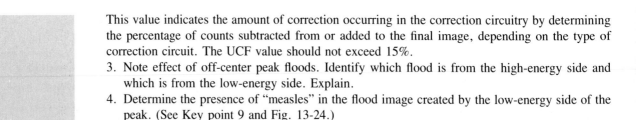

This value indicates the amount of correction occurring in the correction circuitry by determining the percentage of counts subtracted from or added to the final image, depending on the type of correction circuit. The UCF value should not exceed 15%.

3. Note effect of off-center peak floods. Identify which flood is from the high-energy side and which is from the low-energy side. Explain.
4. Determine the presence of "measles" in the flood image created by the low-energy side of the peak. (See Key point 9 and Fig. 13-24.)

Key points

1. A flood study should be performed daily, or at any time during the day that suspicions are aroused that uniformity has been degraded. This is usually based on similar abnormal clinical results on sequential patients.
2. To ensure uniformity with radionuclides of other energies, it is recommended that floods be performed with 100- to 200-μCi point sources of those radionuclides in question.
3. Nonuniformity correction circuits are currently available by all camera manufacturers. Variations by as much as 25% to 30% are claimed to be correctable by some manufacturers.
4. Computer programs are available or can be generated to evaluate, to a lesser degree than NEMA, the amount of nonuniformity with respect to the other areas on the flood study. An-

other technique, although crude, is to use a pinpoint densitometer and move the film from area to area, checking for unacceptable variations in the density of the film.

5. Variations between the corrected and the uncorrected image should be no greater than 15%.
6. Tolerances on nonuniformity variations should be checked just before the warranty on a new system expires to take full advantage of the warranty.
7. Nonuniformities visualized using the intrinsic method are generally exacerbated with collimation, rather than improved.
8. Floods should be performed with and without correction on a weekly basis to anticipate the need for a tune-up before that time when correction cannot be made by the system. In this way, delays incurred in getting service can be averted. A visual inspection of both films should be adequate. Off-peak floods are particularly useful in accentuating areas of nonuniformity.
9. "Measles" is a phenomenon caused by either the loss of the hermetic seal on the crystal or a defective sealing agent between the crystal and the light pipe. In the case of the hermetic seal, moisture enters the crystal-lightpipe interface and migrates across the crystal until it is trapped by a tiny imperfection in the crystal surface. As more moisture enters, the imperfection increases in size because the moisture dissolves the crystal. This process continues until the pool of water is visible on an off-peak flood study and eventually a corrected clinical study.

   In the case of the sealant between the crystal-lightpipe interface, the byproduct of the epoxy-hardening process will dissolve the crystal to the point where it is seen on floods and clinical images.

   In either case, the imperfections serve as a scattering medium (having a different index of refraction) or as an absorption medium for the light produced in the scintillation crystal, such that the event that the light represents will appear reduced in energy. When the flood is taken on the low-energy side of the spectrum, these areas are accentuated.
10. In the presence of serious nonuniformities and lack of service personnel, the interpretation of an emergency study may be assisted by comparing the clinical study to the flood for that day.
11. Floods should be performed on all collimators periodically to check for defective collimators.
12. To avoid cracked crystals, it is imperative that the camera always be left protected by a collimator. The collimator acts as a protector of crystal, as well as a dissipator of sudden changes of heat or cold.
13. Camera crystals have been known to crack with temperature changes as small as 8° F per hour. This should preclude the location of a camera near a window air conditioner. Furthermore, it is recommended that room temperatures not be lower than 40° F or greater than 110° F.
14. Flood images should be evaluated under the same energy conditions used for patient imaging. If off-peak ^{99m}Tc imaging techniques are used, the flood studies should be checked for uniformity at this pulse-height setting.
15. Verify that floods obtained with gamma-ray energies other than those used for uniformity correction are acceptably uniform for clinical studies, especially ^{201}Tl, ^{67}Ga and ^{131}I. If these are not uniform, a correction flood for each of these is warranted.
16. Intrinsic uniformity studies are performed at two different count rates: 20,000 cps and 75,000 cps. It is important to know if the uniformity holds true for image acquisitions at both high and low count rates.

LABORATORY APPLICATION

27

SYSTEM SENSITIVITY

System sensitivity is the parameter of a scintillation camera with its collimator in place that characterizes its ability to efficiently detect incident gamma rays.

Purpose

A constant awareness of the sensitivity of a camera system is helpful in predicting trouble with the system. Changes in the sensitivity can occur for a variety of reasons, including the following: (1) nonuniformities in the crystal response, (2) decreased energy resolution, (3) incorrect collimation, and (4) improper selection of settings that control pulse-height analysis and/or voltage/gain. A sensitivity check serves as an easily reproducible procedure for verifying that, in general, the response of the entire system is adequate. Sensitivity checks could be performed every day using the data from the generation of a field flood. Consideration must be given to using a ^{57}Co or ^{99m}Tc flood source or a ^{99m}Tc point source on a total-system determination.

Manufacturer's (NEMA) procedure for system sensitivity

Using a collimated detector and a 20% window centrally positioned around the ^{99m}Tc energy peak, invert the detector and place a standard 100-mm diameter petri dish on the protected collimator (Fig. 13-25). Place 1 to 2 mCi (37-74 MBq) of ^{99m}Tc in enough solution that it fills 3 mm of the petri dish. Counts should be less than 10,000 cps. A dose calibration should be used to measure the source and the empty syringe to receive the exact amount of activity used. Results are to be expressed as counts per minute per microcurie.

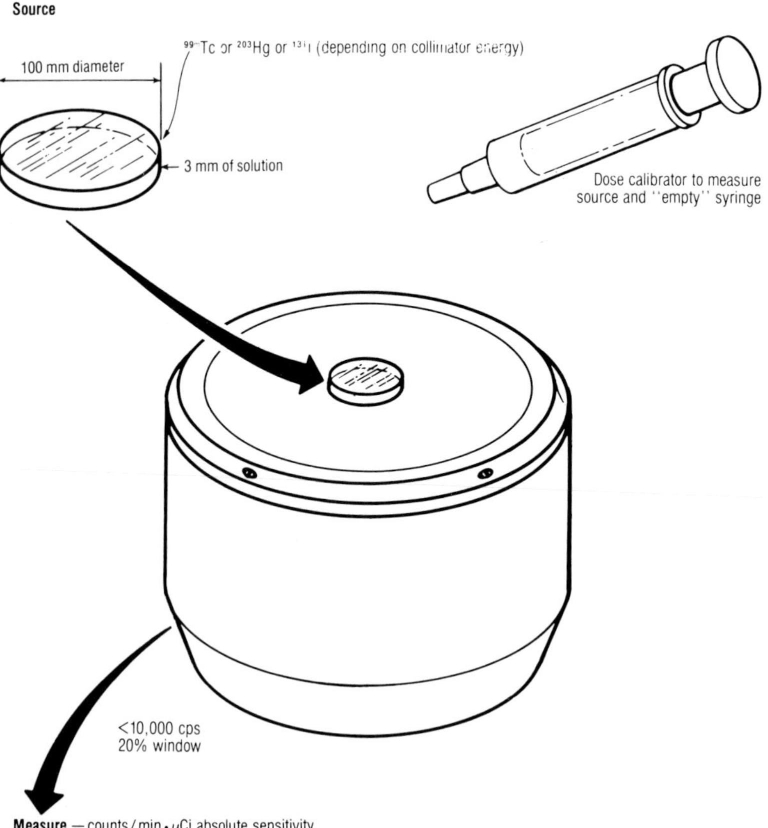

Fig. 13-25. NEMA procedure for system sensitivity. (From NEMA standards for performance measurements of scintillation cameras, Pub. No. NU 1-1986, National Electrical Manufacturers' Association, 1986, NEMA. Courtesy Picker International, Cleveland, Ohio.)

Materials

1. Place approximately 100 to 200 μCi (3.7 to 7.4 MBq) in a 100-mm petri dish; count rate should be <10,000 cps.
2. Parallel-hole collimator *only,* since diverging or converging collimators are too sensitive to the source-detection distance.

User's procedure for system sensitivity

1. Place collimator on detector.
2. Place source on detector with spill protector.
3. Set and visually verify appropriate pulse height analyzer setting with a 20% window.
4. Collect 10 1-minute counts.

Data treatment

1. Determine mean counts per minute.
2. Remove source and count background.
3. Express sensitivity as net counts per minute per microcurie.
4. Perform chi-square test (see Laboratory application 15 and Key point 4 below).

Key points

1. It is important that activities of the various sources used are close to those suggested in the exercises because at these levels the sensitivity response is quite linear. However, to exceed these levels is to decrease the sensitivity because of problems of coincidence counting, dead times, and so on.
2. Be sure that all sources are centered to the detector at the time of the determination. The persistence scope readily identifies the limits of the source.
3. Repeat with all parallel-hole collimators and confirm labels via efficiency factors from the manufacturer.
4. Chi-square test is invalid if displayed counts are rounded off to the nearest thousand or if "sample-and-hold" circuits are used. Most new cameras use these electronic devices.

LABORATORY APPLICATION

28

INTRINSIC SPATIAL RESOLUTION

Purpose

The ability of a scintillation camera system to resolve clinical lesions and therefore assist the physician in an early diagnosis is the objective. All improvements in electronics, collimators, crystal, and so on, have this as the end point. This ability is termed *resolution* and is a function of both the collimator (collimator resolution) and the crystal and its associated electronics (intrinsic resolution). The relationship is expressed as follows:

$$R_s = \sqrt{R_i^2 + R_c^2}$$

R_s = Total-system resolution
R_i = Intrinsic resolution
R_c = Collimator resolution

It is obvious that any improvements in collimator design or electronic components are going to increase total-system resolution.

Intrinsic spatial resolution is defined as the parameter of a scintillation camera that characterizes its ability to accurately determine the original location of a gamma ray on an X-Y plane without collimator. It has seen improvement with the replacement of round photomultiplier tubes with hexagonal tubes, the use of thinner ("shaved") crystals, improved interfaces between crystal and photomultiplier tube, the use of threshold amplifiers, and other new electronic techniques. It is proper to periodically check this parameter to determine deterioration in resolution capabilities. It also is necessary to check this parameter on installation of a new unit or on repair or upgrade to the detector head of an older unit. This is one of the parameters given on instrument price quotations. The resolution value is expressed in terms of full width at half maximum (FWHM) and full width at tenth maximum (FWTM) for UFOV and CFOV.

Continued.

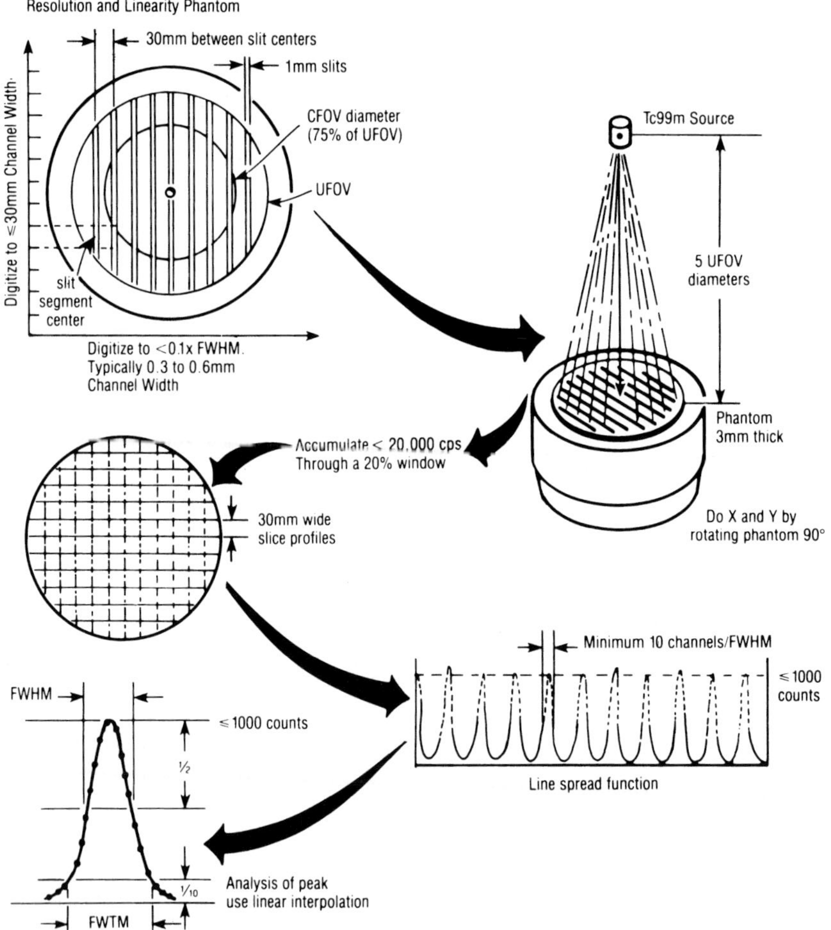

Fig. 13-26. NEMA procedure for intrinsic spatial resolution. (From NEMA standards for performance measurements of scintillation cameras, Pub. No. NU 1-1980, National Electrical Manufacturers' Association, Copyright 1980, Medical Multimedia Corp. Courtesy Picker International, Cleveland, Ohio.)

Manufacturer's (NEMA) procedure for intrinsic spatial resolution

Remove the collimator and, using a 20% window centrally positioned around the ^{99m}Tc peak, place the *Resolution and Linearity Phantom** on the detector with a ^{99m}Tc point source of 100 to 200 μCi (3.7-7.4 MBq) at a distance of 5 UFOV diameters (Fig. 13-26). Arrange a 30-mm–wide slice profile across the slits and accumulate counts at a rate less than 20,000 cps on an MCA (minimum 10 channels/FWHM) such that the peak channel in each line spread function (LSF) receives less than 1000 counts. The LSF of each slit is analyzed for FWHM and FWTM on UFOV and CFOV. Move the 30 mm slice to the adjacent 30 mm section and repeat. Continue until UFOV is analyzed. Rotate phantom 90 degrees and repeat in both directions for CFOV.

Materials

1. 100 to 200 μCi (3.7 to 7.4 MBq) point source of ^{99m}Tc
2. 100 to 200 μCi (3.7 to 7.4 MBq) point source of ^{131}I (or any higher energy radionuclide)
3. 100 to 200 μCi (3.7 to 7.4 MBq) point source of ^{123}I (or any lower energy radionuclide)
4. Lead ring (if available) to mask edge artifacts
5. Bar phantom (The best phantom is one in which the smallest set of bars cannot be visualized.)

*3 mm thick lead phantom covering the UFOV with a 2 mm slit on 30 mm slit centers.

User's procedure for intrinsic spatial resolution

Without special material, a sophisticated pulse-height analyzer, and computer capabilities, the NEMA procedure cannot be performed. However, the standard bar phantoms can be used to confirm these specifications, with the recognition that FWHM is a unit describing the resolution of a line pair (the lead bar plus the space between that bar and the next bar); therefore the smallest bar able to be resolved should equal one half the FWHM. As earlier, consideration must also be given to pulse-height–analyzer settings, window width, and the energy of the radionuclide used. The usual technique is to use ^{99m}Tc on a centered 20% window. A larger window, an eccentrically placed window (to the scatter side of the peak), or a lower energy radionuclide will all decrease resolution. An eccentrically placed window to the high-energy side of the peak should enhance resolution.

1. Remove collimator and invert detector head.
2. Arrange ^{99m}Tc point source at 5 UFOV diameters.
3. Place bar phantom on detector.
4. Set and visually verify appropriate pulse height analyzer setting using a 20% window.
5. Set appropriate intensity.
6. Collect 1 million counts if a camera with a standard field of view is used; collect 2 million counts for a camera with a large field of view.
7. Repeat, rotating each time, until the smallest set of bars appears in all four quadrants. (See Key point 2.)
8. Repeat, rotating so that bars run at 45-degree angles to the normal X and Y axes. This technique stresses the positioning system to its maximum. (Do not use electronic rotation circuits for this procedure.)
9. Repeat step 6, reducing window to 10%; to 5%.
10. Repeat step 6, widening window to 35%; to 50%; to 100%.
11. Repeat step 6, placing 20% window to the scatter side of the energy peak. A corrected flood study may be required first.
12. Repeat step 6, placing 20% window to the high side of the energy peak. A corrected flood study may be required first.
13. Repeat step 6, using the higher-energy radionuclide; using the lower-energy radionuclide.
14. Repeat step 6 with centered ^{99m}Tc source at 2 feet; at 1 foot. Note times required for each image.
15. Repeat step 6 at 1-foot distance with ^{99m}Tc source off center.
16. Repeat step 6, changing bar-detector distance by 2 inches; 4 inches.
17. Repeat resolution study at 75,000 cps count rate.

Data treatment

1. Visually inspect films for degree of resolution. Does it agree with manufacturer's specifications? (See Key point 3.)
2. Is resolution the same in all quadrants?
3. Are bars straight (no wavy lines, no "barreling") regardless of orientation of bars to camera? Straight bars mean good intrinsic spatial linearity. (See NEMA procedure on p. 274.)
4. What are the resolution effects with the following?
   a. Reduced window width
   b. Increased window width
   c. Eccentrically placed window to the low-energy side
   d. Eccentrically placed window to the high-energy side
   e. High-energy radionuclide
   f. Low-energy radionuclide
   g. Source at different distances, centered to camera
   h. Source at different distances, off-center
   i. Changing bar-detector distance
5. What is resolution at 75,000 cps count rate?
6. Did the time required to obtain images at different source-detector distances vary? Did it approximate the inverse square? Should it?

Continued.

Key points

1. Intrinsic resolution studies should be performed at the time of installation or detector head repair and at regular intervals (monthly or quarterly) following installation.
2. Variations in resolution have been observed from one quadrant to another. It has been noted that when two quadrants exhibit decreased resolution, these quadrants are usually diagonal to each other, rather than on the same side of the crystal, as one might expect.
3. FWHM = 1.75 × bar-phantom resolution.

LABORATORY APPLICATION

29

SYSTEM SPATIAL RESOLUTION

Purpose

System spatial resolution is defined as the parameter of a scintillation camera and collimator that characterizes its ability to accurately determine the original location of a gamma ray on an X-Y plane. Since collimator resolution is difficult to determine, the logical parameter to be tested routinely is the system-spatial resolution (detector with collimator). Collimators have seen improvement in recent years in better design, more uniform septal thicknesses, and improved manufacturing techniques. All these changes have been made with improved system spatial resolution as the end product.

Figure 13-27 demonstrates the effects of distance on resolution by using a liver slice phantom at varying distances from the face of the collimator. Two different collimators were used for this study: a parallel-hole collimator and a diverging collimator. In such a comparison, it is apparent that the resolution of the parallel-hole collimator is much better than that of the diverging collimator at any of the same distances. It is also apparent that both images deteriorate as the object is moved farther away from the face of the collimator, the image deteriorating more quickly with the diverging collimator.

It should be apparent from these images that the detector head of any scintillation camera should always be placed as close as possible to the organ being studied, that is, touching the patient's skin. Contamination of the collimator (especially using ^{99m}Tc, since it is secreted in perspiration) should be prevented by using some disposable material, such as thin celluloid film (Saran Wrap) or its equivalent.

Since most users have neither access to the special materials required for the manufacturer's procedure nor an adequate pulse-height analyzer, the NEMA procedure cannot be performed. However, see Key points 5 and 6.

Materials

1. ^{57}Co flood source of 1 to 5 mCi (37 to 185 MBq)
2. Flood phantom (fill with H_2O and 1 to 5 mCi (37 to 185 MBq) ^{99m}Tc)
3. Bar phantom (the best phantom is one in which the smallest set of bars cannot be visualized)

Manufacturer's (NEMA) procedure for systems spatial resolution

With collimator in place, using a 20% window centrally positioned around the ^{99m}Tc energy peak, arrange two capillary tubes (ID = 1 mm) that run the length of the UFOV such that they are 50 mm apart and 100 mm from the collimator face (Fig. 13-28). Fill tubes with ^{99m}Tc. Arrange a 30-mm slice profile across the capillary tubes and accumulate counts at a rate less than 10,000 cps in an MCA (minimum 10 channels per FWHM) such that the peak channel in each LSF receives more than 10,000 counts. Determine FWHM and FWTM* averages for the CFOV. Repeat using 100 mm Lucite forward scatter medium and 50 mm Lucite backward scatter medium. This scatter arrangement simulates scatter conditions of ^{99m}Tc in the heart.

*Millimeters per channel is calibrated by number of channels peak to peak divided by 50 mm.

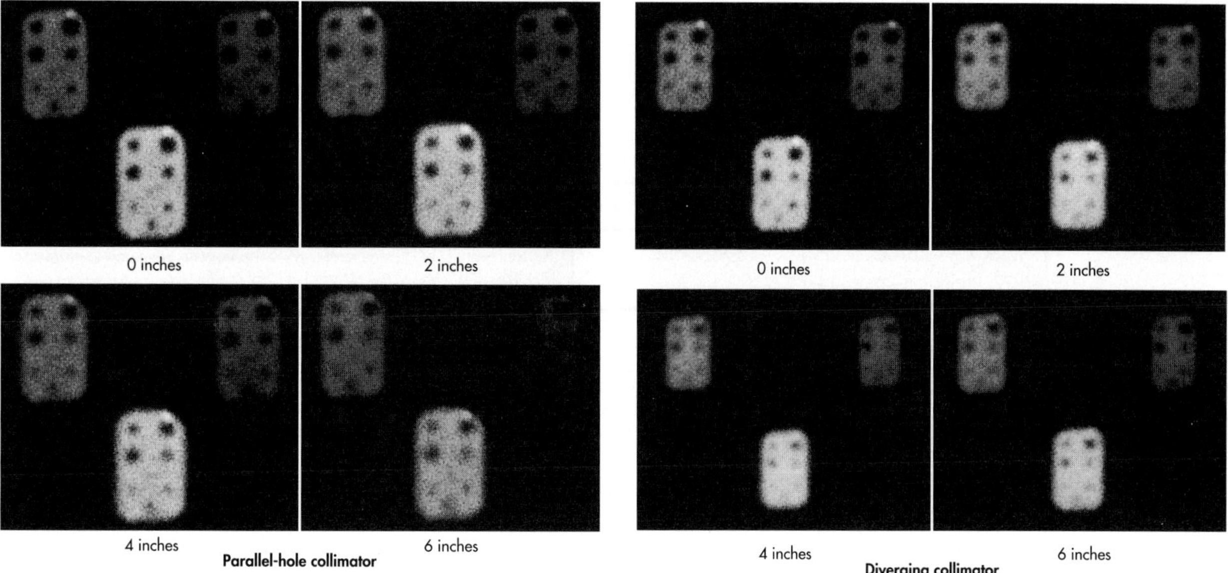

Fig. 13-27. Effects on resolution using a parallel-hole collimator as a liver slice phantom is moved from the face of the collimator to 6 inches from the face at 2-inch increments. Compare with the diverging collimator study performed in the same manner. The image is smaller (and gets smaller with increasing distance), and resolution deteriorates faster with the diverging collimator.

User's procedure for system spatial resolution

1. Attach parallel-hole collimator and invert detector.
2. Arrange bar phantom and ^{99m}Tc flood source on face of detector (Fig. 13-29).
3. Set and visually verify appropriate PHA setting using a 20% window.
4. Set appropriate intensity.
5. Collect 1 million counts if a camera with a standard field of view is used; collect 2 million counts for a camera with a large field of view.
6. Repeat at 2 inches, 4 inches, and 6 inches on all collimators. Note the time required to collect each image.
7. Repeat, using ^{57}Co flood source.
8. Repeat steps 5 and 6 with all available collimators.

Data treatment

1. Visually inspect films for degree of resolution. Do they agree with the manufacturer's specifications? (See Key point 3.)
2. Are bars straight? Did collimation correct "barreling" or wavy lines noted in intrinsic resolution studies (if available)?
3. Which collimator has the best resolution at the face of the collimator? Which collimator has the best resolution at a distance from the face of the collimator? Do these determinations agree with those of the manufacturer?
4. Is it possible for two different collimators, rated at different resolution capabilities at depth, to have the same resolving capability at the face of the collimator? Explain.

Continued.

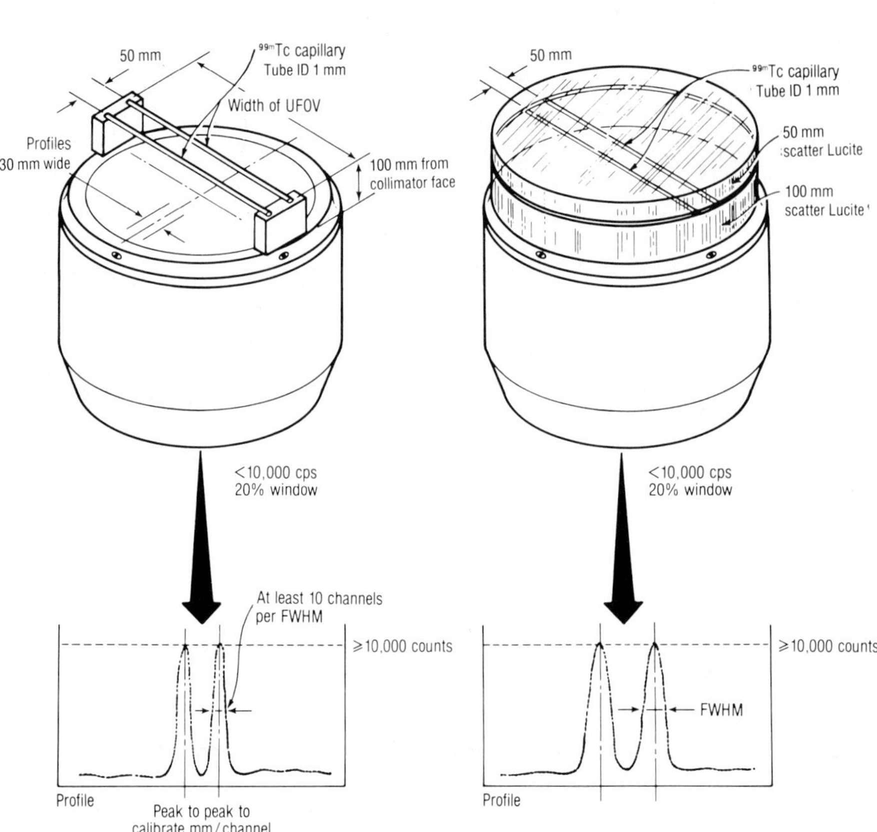

Fig. 13-28. NEMA procedure for systems spatial resolution with and without scatter. (From NEMA standards for performance measurements of scintillation cameras, Pub. No. NU 1-1986, National Electrical Manufacturers' Association, Copyright 1986, NEMA. Courtesy Picker International, Cleveland, Ohio.)

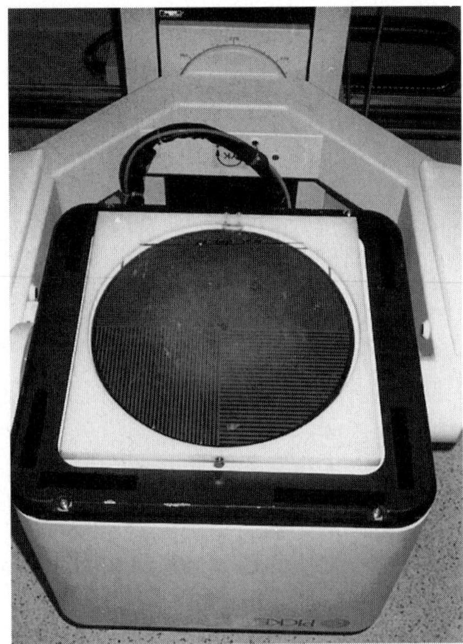

Fig. 13-29. Setup on an inverted scintillation camera head for determination of total-system resolution. Bar phantom is sandwiched between the uniform flood source (filled with 1 to 2 mCi of ^{99m}Tc) and the camera collimator. Spatial volume resolution can be determined by replacing the bar and flood phantom with Hine's phantom.

5. Is there any appreciable difference in the time required to collect the predetermined number of counts as the bar-detector distance is changed? Repeat with a point source at different distances. Do these times change? Explain.
6. List the difference in the time required to collect the predetermined counts for each collimator. Do these agree with the sensitivity values of the manufacturer?
7. Using a pinhole collimator, determine the distance from the face of the collimator where a 1:1 relationship exists (providing a 1:1 display capability is possible). One-centimeter markers are available or can be made for this purpose. Does magnification occur closer to or farther away from that point?
8. Describe resolution changes (if any) between ^{99m}Tc and ^{57}Co. Explain.

Key points

1. Total-system resolution studies should be performed at the time of installation or detector head repair and at regular intervals (monthly or quarterly) following installation.
2. If the bar phantom is perfectly oriented to the direction of the holes in the collimator, so that the septa between the holes cover one whole row of holes, the resultant image may be misinterpreted to suggest an erroneously high resolving capability.
3. If the bar phantom is imperfectly oriented to the direction of the holes in the collimator, so

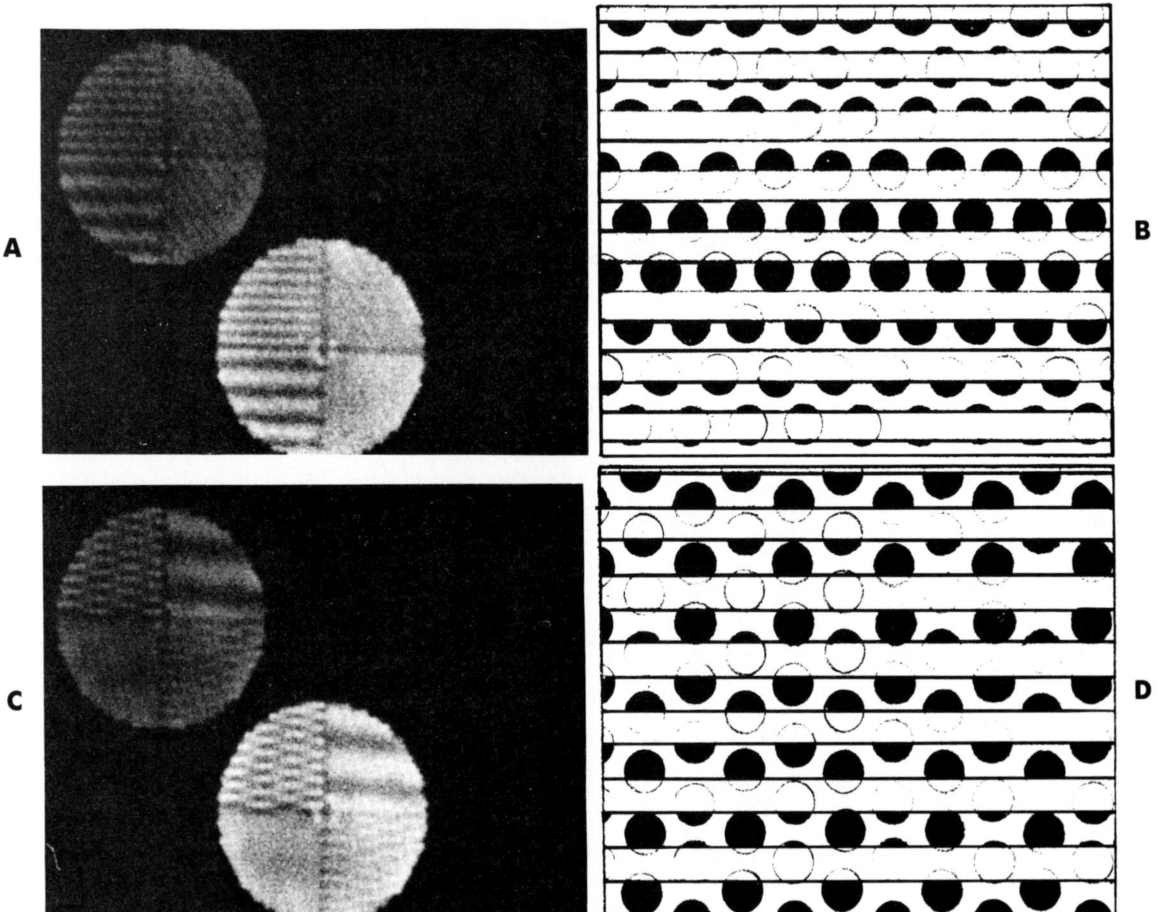

Fig. 13-30. Moiré patterns. Large-bar pattern seen in the lower left quadrant of **A** is graphically demonstrated in **B;** discontinuous bands seen in the upper-left quadrant of **C** are graphically demonstrated in **D;** dark bands perpendicular to the direction of the bars seen in the upper-left quadrant of **A** are demonstrated in **E;** and diagonal bands (the result of bars not parallel to holes) seen in **F** are demonstrated in **G.** (From Maguire, W.J.: J. Nucl. Med. Tech. 7(2):81, 1979.)

Continued.

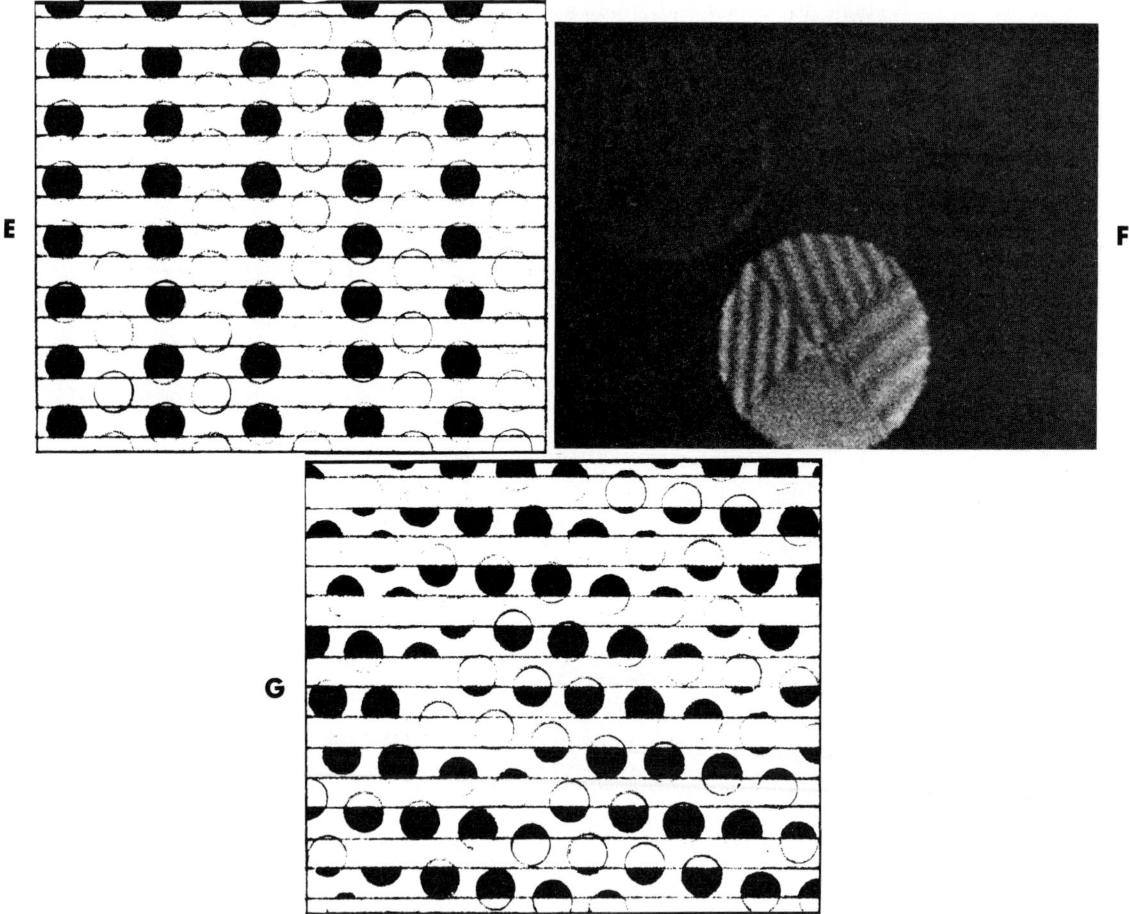

Fig. 13-30, cont'd. For legend see page 279.

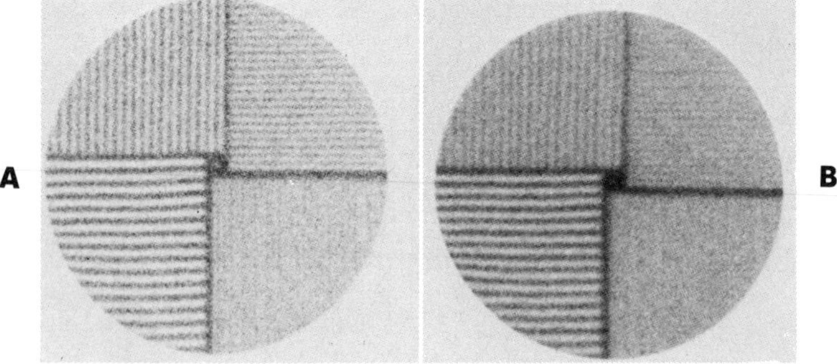

Fig. 13-31. Resolution comparison. **A,** Bar phantom study performed using a high-resolution collimator, collecting 1 million counts in 42.7 seconds. **B,** Same bar phantom performed using a high-sensitivity collimator, collecting 3 million counts in 49.4 seconds. Note the increased resolution with the high-resolution phantom (using approximately the same amount of time); yet only one third of the counts were accumulated.

that the bars travel at an angle to the line of holes in the collimator, then a moiré pattern* develops, visualized as lines running at angles to the direction of the bars (Fig. 13-30).

4. There is not a single bar phantom available to test all cameras by the technique just described. However, a bar phantom can be used for all systems by placing the phantom at a 45° angle and using markers to indicate distances along the bars. As the bars diverge away from the detector, the camera loses its ability to resolve them.
5. The NEMA procedure can be used if the camera has computer capabilities, provided the pixel size is determined. The pixel size is determined using manufacturer's protocol or as follows:
   a. Place two point sources (such as ^{57}Co sources) on the X axis exactly 100 mm apart in the center of a parallel-hole collimated detector. Collect a 100,000-count image (corrected) using a 20% window on a 512 × 512 matrix (or a 256 × 256 matrix with a ×2 preprocess zoom). A slice profile is drawn through these two points. Display counts/pixel (see Fig. 14-24.) Determine the number of pixels between two pixels with maximum counts. Repeat on the Y axis.
   b. Pixel size (mm/pixel) = 100 ÷ number of pixels between 2 pixels with the maximum count The pixel size variation between the X and Y axis should not exceed 2.0 mm.
6. Knowing the pixel size in millimeters, the NEMA procedure can now be determined via capillary tubes filled with ^{99m}Tc, using slice profiles and a display of counts per pixel.
7. A complete resolution study of each of the collimator varying times, rather than counts, may reveal that given the same amount of time, a high-resolution collimator may produce an image with better resolution than a collimator with a lower resolution rating, even though the count rate is significantly reduced (Fig. 13-31).

*A pattern of lines that result when two regular patterns overlap. The same pattern on silk produces a *watered* appearance, which is the meaning of the French word *moiré*.

LABORATORY APPLICATION

30

SATURATION

Purpose

With the advent of nuclear cardiology, a tremendous amount of emphasis has been placed on the ability of a system to handle high count rates. It is possible to provide more events per unit of time than the system is capable of detecting and processing in the same amount of time, at which point *saturation* of the system is achieved. To increase the count rate beyond this point is to lose resolution, to lose count rate, and therefore to expose a patient to more radiation than is necessary. The higher the count rate that the system can handle, the better the statistics of the cardiac study. Therefore it is important that this parameter be checked at the time of installation of the system and periodically thereafter.

NEMA standards for this procedure can be performed by the user (Fig. 13-32).

The results of this study vary in accordance with the size of the pulse-height–analyzer window and the degree of scatter. Some systems have a selector that activates a high–count-rate handling capability with a resultant decrease in resolution. Operation manuals should be consulted.

Procedure

Materials

1. ^{99m}Tc point source of 500 μCi (18.5 MBq)
2. 3-mm–thick UFOV lead ring (if available)

Technique

1. Remove collimator. Place lead ring on detector and rotate detector 90°.
2. Arrange point source 1 m from detector.
3. Set and visually verify appropriate pulse-height analyzer setting for ^{99m}Tc with a 20% window, in a corrected mode.
4. Set times for 1-second intervals. Set "hi" count rate mode, if applicable.
5. Begin to move source in small increments, each time recycling the 1-second times and making a mental note of increasing count rates.

Continued.

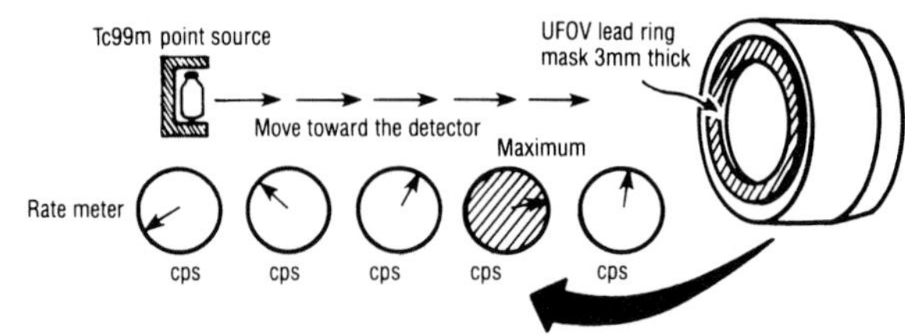

Fig. 13-32. NEMA procedure for maximum count-rate test (saturation). (From NEMA standards for performance measurements of scintillation cameras, Pub. No. NU 1-1980, National Electrical Manufacturers' Association, Copyright 1980, Medical Multimedia Corp. Courtesy Picker International, Cleveland, Ohio.)

6. Continue until the highest count rate is reached, and record.
7. Repeat with a 35% window; a 50% window; a 100% window (if possible).
8. Redetermine the saturation point using the bar phantom at a 20% window.
9. Photograph bars at saturation.

Data treatment

1. Does the saturation point agree with the manufacturer's specifications at 20%? At 35%? At 50%? At 100%?
2. Does resolution of the bar phantom change at the saturation point?
3. At what percentage of saturation count rate does resolution deteriorate?
4. Repeat, using "normal" count rate mode, if applicable. Is there any difference in the saturation point? In resolution?

LABORATORY APPLICATION 31

INTRINSIC DEAD TIME MEASUREMENTS (TEMPORAL RESOLUTION)

Purpose

Dead time was defined in Laboratory application 8 with respect to an ionization-type survey meter. It is the minimum time interval following a nuclear event after which another nuclear event can be accepted. (Another term used to describe this relationship is *pulse pair resolution*. For all practical purposes, at low count rates, dead time and pulse pair resolution can be used interchangeably.) It has special application in scintillation cameras. It would have better application in a nonparalyzable system that would allow the detection and processing of all events regardless of their frequency. This is not the case with the scintillation camera. However, because state-of-the-art camera systems respond as though they are nonparalyzable in a clinical situation (using ^{99m}Tc with a 20% window under proper scatter conditions) over a clinically useful range of count rates, the measurement may have application. The rationale for measuring dead time is to determine at what observed count rate the data loss will be approximately 20%. Using the activities greater than that amount that produces that observed count rate causes no appreciable increase in statistical information. It merely increases the radiation dose to the patient.

The application of dead time corrections is most applicable to the scintillation camera that is being used for quantitative nuclear cardiology. In this instance there can be significant counting losses and therefore significant degradation of statistics with higher count rates. It presents little problem to the imaging portion of nuclear cardiology (or the imaging of any other organs for that matter), just the ability to quantitate events for such calculations as firstpass ejection fractions. There is a point that can be reached, however (probably not clinically), where resolution will (especially in newer systems) deteriorate as the system approaches count saturation.

Procedure for 20% count-rate loss curve

The generation of a count-rate curve is the test of the camera to maintain count rate fidelity with increasing radioactivity. It is a more definitive test than that of saturation. Further, all camera manufacturers quote its value on their specifications sheet. This procedure follows NEMA protocol (Fig. 13-33).

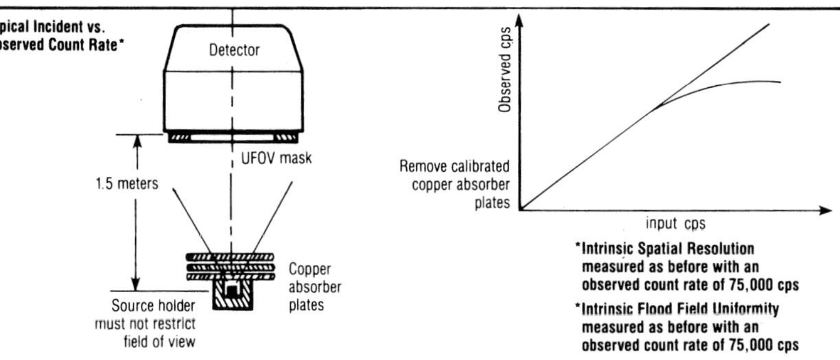

Fig. 13-33. NEMA procedure for 20% count-rate loss curve (From NEMA standards for performance measurements of scintillation cameras, Pub. No. NU 1-1986, National Electrical Manufacturers' Association, Copyright 1986, NEMA. Courtesy Picker International, Cleveland, Ohio.)

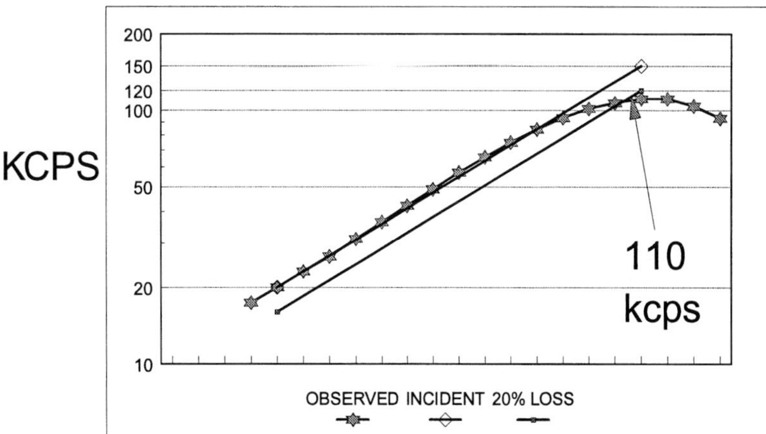

Fig. 13-34. 20% count-rate–loss curve plotting actual counts received versus calibrated Cu absorber plates (21.23% count-rate increase per plate) as plates are removed from a radioactive source. Note that the actual counts received *(curved line)* become less than the theoretical count *(straight solid line)* as the count rate increases. A 20% count rate loss is seen at 110 kcps. One could also plot theoretical versus actual counts on log-log paper.

Materials

1. 20 mCi (740 MBq) ^{99m}Tc in 5-ml vial (in Pb source holder)
2. 20 to 30 copper filters 2 to 3 mm thick (each calibrated to known attenuation factors; see Key point 1).

Technique

1. Attach UFOV mask on uncollimated camera.
2. Raise camera 1.5 m from the source holder such that the source holder does not restrict the field of view.
3. Place source in source holder and all Cu absorber plate on source holder.
4. Note count rate (Kcps).
5. Begin removing Cu absorber plate sequentially, recording increase in count rate each time until all Cu plates are removed.

Data treatment

1. Plot count rates received versus count rates expected on log-log paper.
2. Determine count rate at which the camera system loses 20% of the expected counts (Fig. 13-34).
3. Compare with the manufacturer's specifications.

Key points

1. Percent (%) attenuation of each Cu absorber plate can be calibrated individually using a smaller source of ^{99m}Tc and a thyroid uptake probe.
2. If all Cu absorber plates provide the same attenuation, the plot of expected vs. received should be a straight line on log-log paper.

Continued.

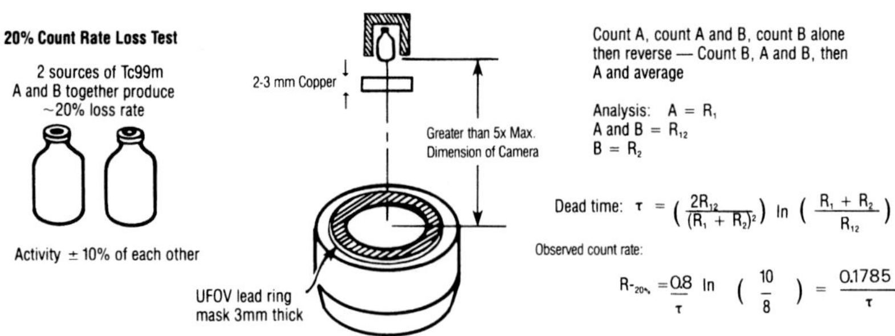

Fig. 13-35. NEMA procedure for dead-time measurement. (From NEMA standards for performance measurements of scintillation cameras, Pub. No. NU 1-1980, National Electrical Manufacturers' Association, Copyright 1980, Medical Multimedia Corp. Courtesy Picker International, Cleveland, Ohio.)

3. The 20% count-rate loss point can be easily determined by drawing a second straight line, parallel to the theoretical (0° count-rate loss) line, but at 20% of the theoretical line. At low count rates, the data points will follow the theoretical lines. As it approaches 20% count loss rates, it will begin to stray from the theoretical. When the data points cross the 20% line, the test is complete.
4. The count rate reflecting a 20% loss as determined above is used for both intrinsic and total system dead-time measurements to follow.

Purpose of dead-time measurement

Calculation of dead-time is accomplished through a dual source technique. Sources are matched (±10% of each other) and contain activity that when counted together approximate the 20% count-rate loss as determined above. To account for decay, two series of data are collected and averaged. The series should be counted as follows: R_1, R_{12}, R_2 followed by R_2, R_{12}, R_1. NEMA protocol can be used for this procedure.

Manufacturer's (NEMA) procedure for dead-time measurement

Prepare two sources of ^{99m}Tc that together produce approximately a 20% count-rate loss and are each within ±10% of each other. Since it is necessary to determine the dead time (τ) to know this value (unless the dead time quoted on the manufacturer's specifications is used), it is safe to start with two sources whose total activity at 1 m from the uncollimated detector (containing a 3-mm–thick UFOV lead ring) is less than 20,000 cps (Fig. 13-35). The NEMA procedure is to count source A alone (R_1) in a source holder as shown, then source A + B (R_{12}), then source B alone (R_2). Next reverse the order, counting source B alone (R_2), source A + B (R_{12}) and source A alone (R_1); then average. Compute dead time as follows:

$$\text{Dead time: } \tau\ (\mu\text{sec}) = \left(\frac{2R_{12}}{(R_1 + R_2)^2}\right) \ln \left(\frac{R_1 + R_2}{R_{12}}\right)$$

Using the dead-time results, compute the input count rate at which 20% of the counts are lost because of dead time, according to the following:

$$\text{with source holder } R_{-20\%} = \left(\frac{0.8}{\tau}\right) \ln \left(\frac{10}{8}\right) = \frac{0.1785}{\tau}$$

$$\text{without source holder } R_{-20\%} = \left(\frac{1}{\tau}\right) \ln \left(\frac{10}{8}\right) = \frac{0.2231}{\tau}$$

User's procedure for dead-time measurements

Dead-time measurements are affected by scatter conditions and analyzer window width. As scatter conditions increase, dead time increases; conversely, as window width increases, dead time decreases. For this reason, Adams and others (1978), addressing the subject of nuclear cardiology, suggest that dead-time measurements on a scintillation camera be performed with a 20% window width, centered on the ^{99m}Tc photopeak, using a two-source phantom designed to simulate scatter conditions of ^{99m}Tc in the heart (Fig. 13-36).

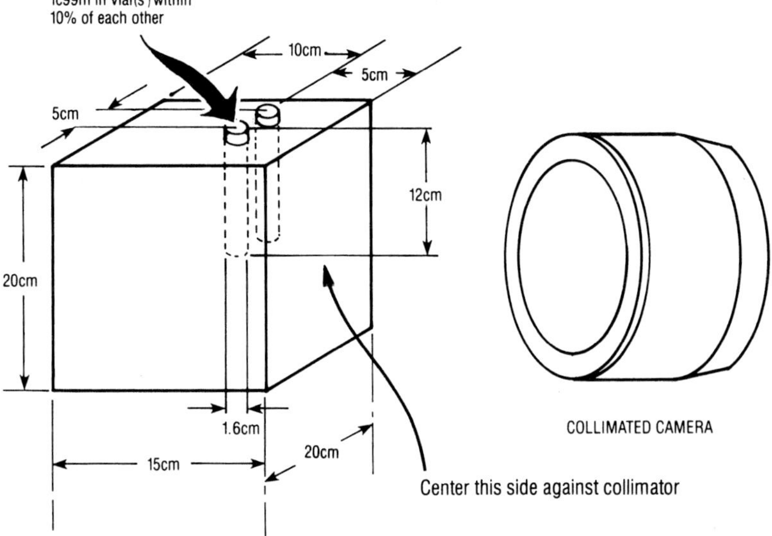

Fig. 13-36. Two-source phantom for dead-time measurements under simulated clinical conditions. (From measurements of the performance parameters of gamma cameras, HEW Pub. No. (FDA) 78-8049, Rockville, Md., 1977, U.S. Department of Health, Education and Welfare.)

Materials required for alternative procedure

1. Adams dead-time phantom
2. Two ^{99m}Tc sources of approximately 20,000 cps total, using 3 to 7 mCi (100 to 250 MBq) in a scatter phantom
3. High-resolution collimator

Technique

1. Place collimator on detector and direct horizontally.
2. Place phantom with the surface nearest the test tube at the collimator face.
3. Set and visually verify 20% window.
4. Count all times for 100 seconds.
5. Determine background in counts per second (cps).
6. Count source A in phantom (R_1).
7. Count sources A and B in phantom (R_{12}).
8. Remove source A and count source B in phantom (R_2).
9. Repeat count in reverse order. Use average for following computation.

Data treatment

1. Compute dead time as follows:

$$\tau(\mu\text{sec}) = \left[\frac{2\,R_{12}}{(R_1 + R_2)^2}\right] \ln\left[\frac{(R_1 + R_2)}{R_{12}}\right] \times 10^6$$

2. Determine from Fig. 13-34 the maximum observed count rate that can be handled by your camera to result in a loss no greater than 20% of the expected count rate.
3. Compute count rate at which 20% of the count rate is lost by the following:

$$R_{-20\%} = \frac{0.1785}{\tau}$$

4. Repeat in the uncorrected mode. Any difference? Why?

Key point

1. Some camera systems can switch into a special electronic mode to handle high count rates to reduce this dead time, sometimes at the expense of resolution. Since resolution is not a factor in dynamic studies, this high-count–rate mode should be used to its intended advantage.

LABORATORY APPLICATION

32

MULTIPLE-WINDOW SPATIAL REGISTRATION

Purpose

Multiple-window spatial registration is defined as the parameter of a scintillation camera that characterizes positional deviations in the image at different energies. It is disastrous to a ^{67}Ga study when three ^{67}Ga photons, each of a different energy but all from the same organ location, are received by their respective energy windows but are positioned on the CRT in different locations. Obviously resolution suffers greatly. It is important to determine if this is a problem with all scintillation detectors.

As usual, invasive testing, sophisticated MCAs, and special equipment (collimated point source) make this procedure difficult to perform at the user end, and therefore it is impossible to confirm manufacturers' specifications. Because the parameter is so important, two procedures may be followed by the user, depending on whether the user's camera is computer-assisted or not.

User's procedure for multiple-window spatial registration (with no computer)

Materials

1. Approximately 100 μCi (3.7 MBq) ^{67}Ga
2. Bar phantom

Technique

1. Remove collimator, insert lead collar, and invert.
2. Set a window for each of the three energies of ^{67}Ga (93, 184 and 296 keV).
3. Place bar phantom on detector; place source at 5 UFOV diameters.
4. Accumulate images, using all three peaks. Note times.
5. Accumulate images, using each peak individually.
6. Accumulate images, using the three different combinations of two peaks.
7. Perform three floods, using each of the three windows, superimposing all three images on the same film.

Data treatment

1. Evaluate for best resolution.
2. Evaluate for best time.
3. Evaluate combinations from step 6 for best clinical results.
4. Determine if all three bar phantom images from step 4 superimpose perfectly.
5. Determine if all three floods from step 7 superimpose perfectly.

NEMA procedure for multiple-window spatial registration (with computer)

The NEMA procedure for multiple-window spatial registration can be performed with a computer without acquiring a high-performance MCA as suggested by NEMA. The technique uses the information already ascertained for pixel sizing (see Key point 5 on page 281).

Materials

1. 1 mCi ^{67}Ga. Dilute to 10 ml. Place 2.5 ml aliquots into each of 4 to 5 ml vials. Place each vial in a small Pb source container (6 mm thick) with a 3-mm hole drilled into the bottom.

Technique

1. Place medium energy collimator on detector and invert detector.
2. Place four ^{67}Ga sources at two places on the X and two places on the Y coordinates at 75% of the UFOV.
3. Acquire *and process* 100,000 count images on a 512 × 512 (or 256 × 256 at × 2 zoom) matrix at:
   a. 93 keV; 20% window, centrally placed
   b. 184 keV; 20% window, centrally placed
   c. 296 keV; 20% window, centrally placed

Data treatment

1. Generate slice profiles of each point source in both the X and Y directions (see Key point 3).
2. Print out counts/pixel.
3. Determine X and Y positions of each point source at each energy level via analysis of maximum pixel count (see Fig. 14-24).
4. Calculate maximum displacement in pixels. See Table 13-1.
5. Determine maximum displacement in millimeters according to the following formula:

$$\text{Maximum displacement (mm)} = \text{Maximum displacement (pixels)} \times \text{pixel size (mm)}$$

Key points

1. This information should be included in the manufacturer's specifications.
2. If a different size matrix is used, pixel sizing will require recalculation.
3. Some manufacturers provide for a 1-pixel ROI, which can be moved to each point source until maximum count is reached, at which time the X and Y coordinates are noted on the screen. This saves much time in obviating the need for slice profiles, etc.

Table 13-1. Data for multiple-window spatial registration

Position / Energy	12:00		3:00		6:00		9:00	
	x	*y*	*x*	*y*	*x*	*y*	*x*	*y*
93 keV 194 keV 296 keV								
Maximum displacement (pixels)								

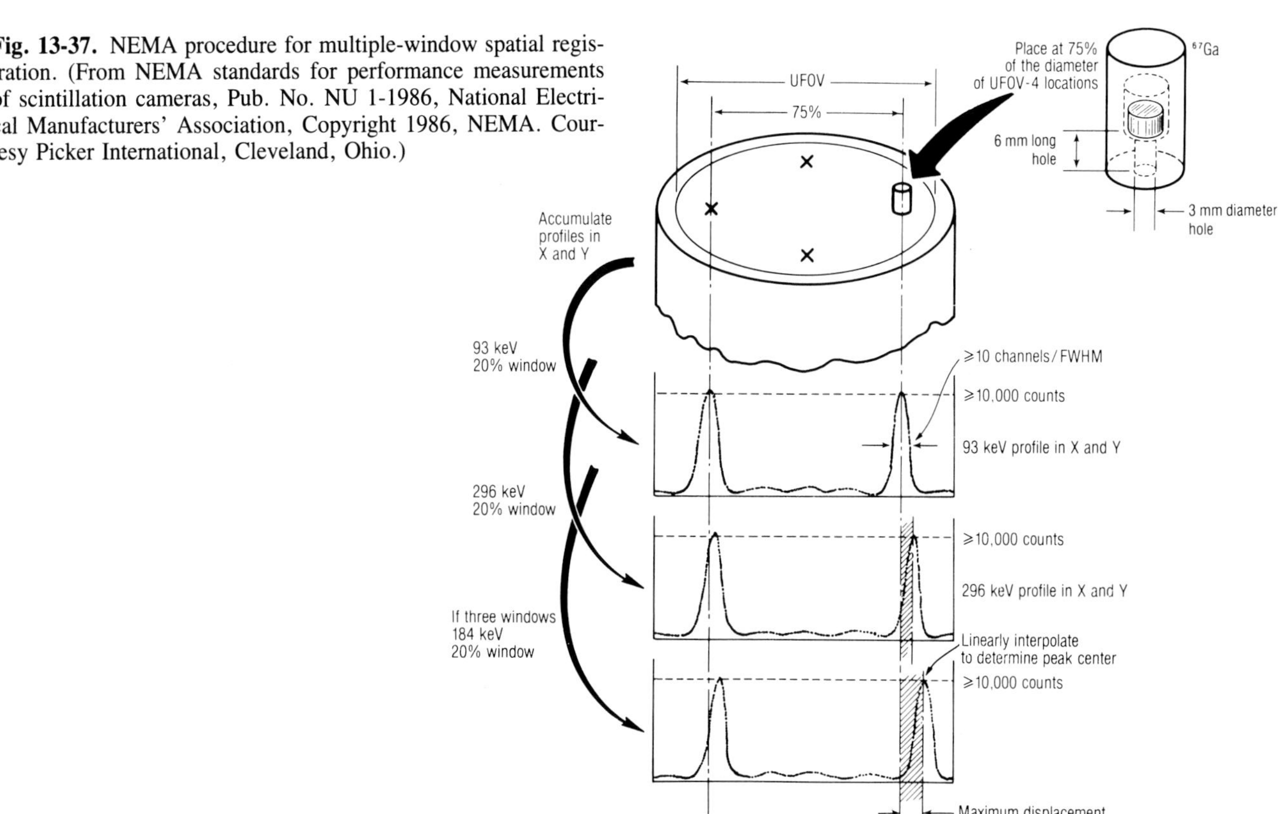

Fig. 13-37. NEMA procedure for multiple-window spatial registration. (From NEMA standards for performance measurements of scintillation cameras, Pub. No. NU 1-1986, National Electrical Manufacturers' Association, Copyright 1986, NEMA. Courtesy Picker International, Cleveland, Ohio.)

Continued.

Manufacturer's (NEMA) procedure for multiple-window spatial registration

Prepare a ^{67}Ga source as a collimated point source (Fig. 13-37) and place source at a well-identified place on the uncollimated detector at 75% of the UFOV. Place the source at two places in the X coordinate and two places in the Y coordinate. Accumulate slice profiles in both X and Y directions at all three peak energies (93, 184, and 296 keV) using 20% windows. The LSF should be evaluated on an MCA (more than 10 channels per FWHM) such that the peak channel in each LSF receives more than 10,000 counts. The results are reported in millimeters of maximum displacement. (Known distances between the two points of the slice profile are used to calibrate millimeters per channel.)

LABORATORY APPLICATION

33

INTRINSIC SPATIAL LINEARITY

Spatial linearity is defined as the parameter of a scintillation camera that characterizes the amount of positional distortion caused by the camera with respect to incident gamma events entering the detector. The user can test for spatial linearity by looking for wavy lines or "barreling" on the bar-phantom studies received during the resolution studies. NEMA, however, has rigorous requirements for spatial linearity.

Manufacturer's (NEMA) procedure for intrinsic spatial linearity

Remove the collimators and, using a 20% window centrally positioned around the ^{99m}Tc energy peak, place the *Resolution and Linearity Phantom* on the detector (Fig. 13-38) with a ^{99m}Tc point source of 100 to 200 μCi (3.7-7.4 MBq) at a distance of 5 UFOV diameters. Arrange a 30-mm–wide slice profile across the slits, and accumulate counts at a rate less than 20,000 cps on an MCA

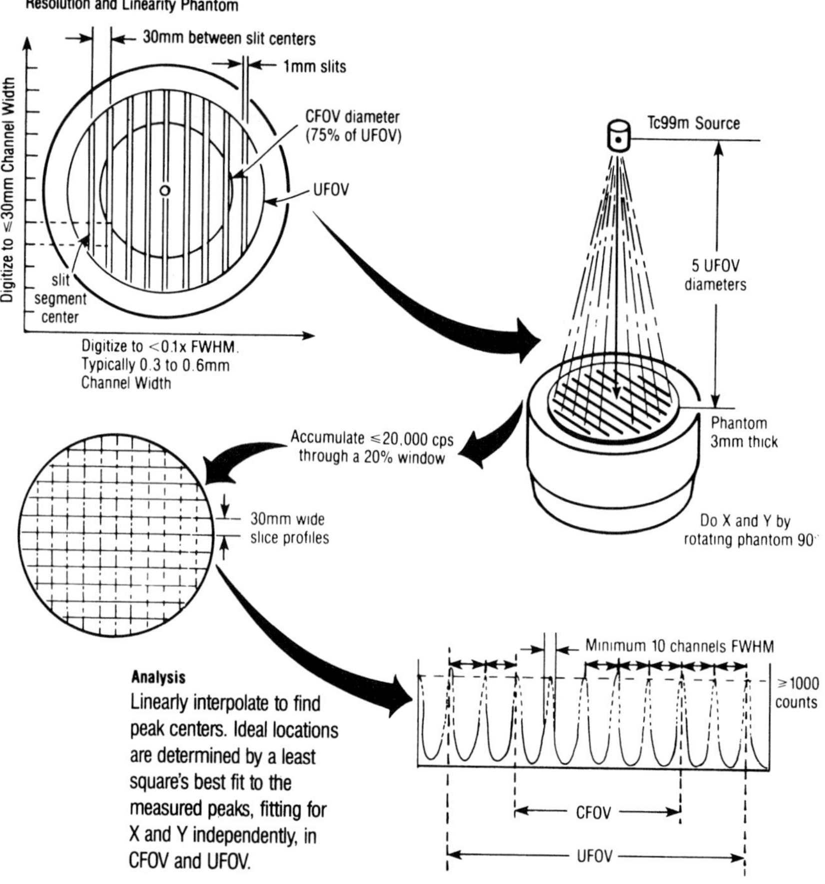

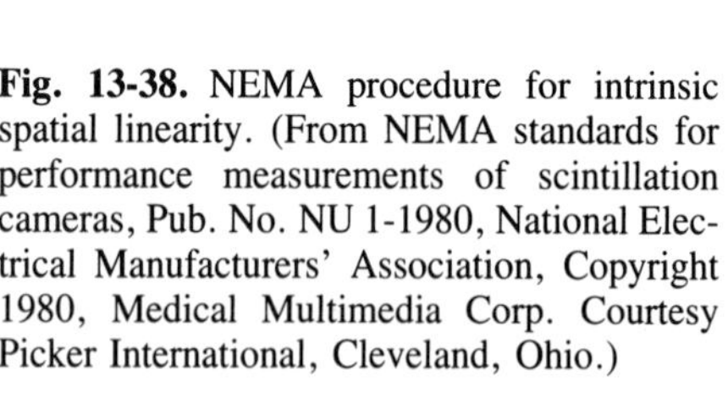

Fig. 13-38. NEMA procedure for intrinsic spatial linearity. (From NEMA standards for performance measurements of scintillation cameras, Pub. No. NU 1-1980, National Electrical Manufacturers' Association, Copyright 1980, Medical Multimedia Corp. Courtesy Picker International, Cleveland, Ohio.)

(minimum 10 channels per FWHM) such that the peak channel in each LSF receives more than 1000 counts. Analyze the LSF of each slit to determine the amount of peak shift from the ideal peak location (in millimeters) as both a standard deviation of LSF peak separation and as the maximum amount of spatial displacement for both CFOV and UFOV. The 30-mm slice is then moved to the next 30-mm section and repeated. This continues until the UFOV is analyzed. The phantom is then rotated 90° and repeated.

LABORATORY APPLICATION

34

INTRINSIC ENERGY RESOLUTION

Energy resolution is defined as the parameter of a scintillation camera that characterizes its ability to accurately identify the photopeak events. It determines the camera's ability to distinguish between primary gamma events and scattered events. This is impossible for the user to do without a refined MCA and invasive testing techniques. NEMA has developed a technique for the manufacturer, however.

Manufacturer's (NEMA) procedure for intrinsic energy resolution

Remove the collimator and, using a 20% window centrally positioned around the ^{99m}Tc energy peak and a 3-mm–thick lead ring (to identify the UFOV), place a ^{99m}Tc source 5 UFOV diameters away (Fig. 13-39). Flood the camera with ^{99m}Tc at a rate of less than 20,000 cps so that a pulse-height analyzer possessing a minimum of 50 channels/FWHM will display an energy spectrum with

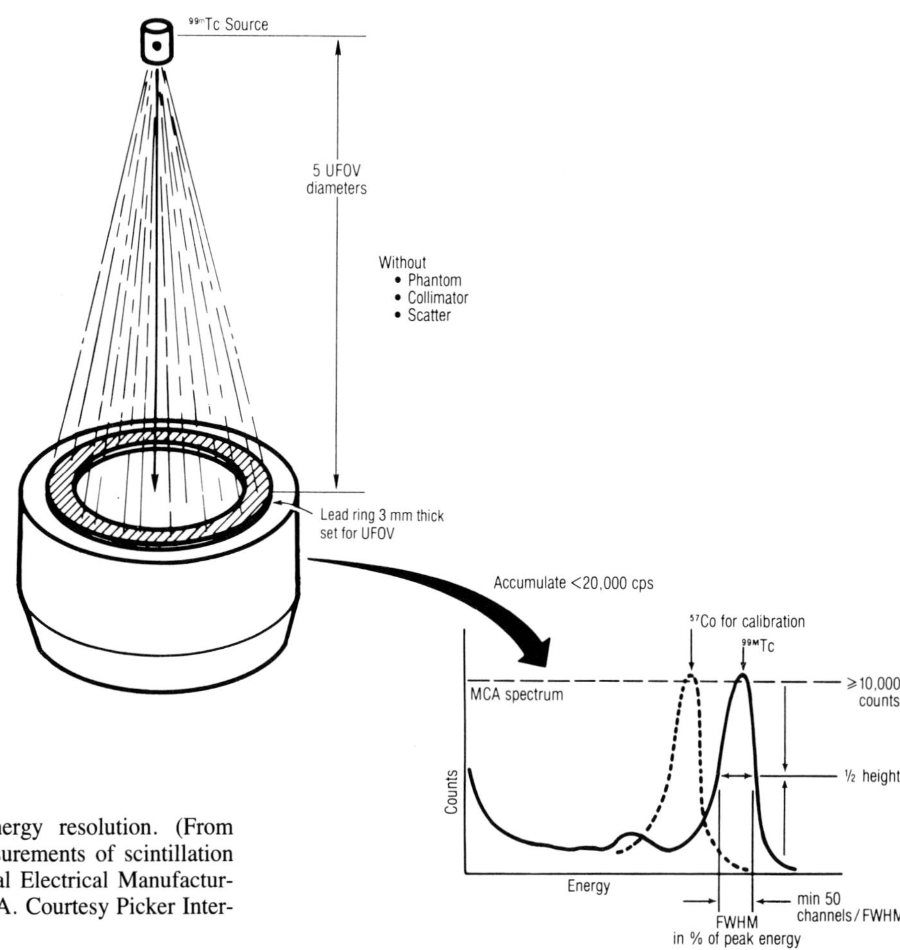

Fig. 13-39. NEMA procedure for energy resolution. (From NEMA standards for performance measurements of scintillation cameras, Pub. No. NU 1-1986, National Electrical Manufacturers' Association, Copyright 1986, NEMA. Courtesy Picker International, Cleveland, Ohio.)

Continued

greater than 10,000 counts in the peak channel. Repeat with ^{57}Co so that the channels can be calibrated in kiloelectron volts according to the following:

$$\text{keV/channel} = \frac{\text{No. of channels between peaks of } ^{99m}\text{Tc and } ^{57}\text{Co}}{\text{Energy difference between 140 and 122}}$$

Energy resolution is expressed as the ratio of FWHM to photopeak energy expressed as a percentage (see Laboratory application 11).

BIBLIOGRAPHY

Scintillation camera acceptance testing and performance evaluation, AAPM Report No. 6, New York, 1980, Amer. Inst. of Physics.

Computer-aided scintillation camera acceptance testing, AAPM Report No. 9, New York, 1982, Amer. Inst. of Physics.

Rotating scintillation camera SPECT acceptance testing and quality control, AAPM Report No. 22, New York, 1987, Amer. Inst. of Physics.

Adams, Ralph: Suggested revision of NEMA standards, J. Nucl. Med. **25:**814-816, 1984.

Adams, R.J., and others: Dead time measurements in scintillation cameras under scatter conditions simulating quantitative nuclear cardiology, J. Nucl. Med. 19:538, 1978.

Chandra, R.: Introductory physics of nuclear medicine, ed. 4, Philadelphia, 1992, Lea & Febiger.

Croft, Barbara Y.: Single photon emission computed tomography, Chicago, 1986, Year Book Medical Publishers, Inc.

English, R.J., and Brown, S.E.: Single photon emission computed tomography: a primer, New York, 1990, Society of Nuclear Medicine.

Heyda, B.W., Croteau, F.R., and Govaert, J.A.: A third generation digital camera, SPIE 454:478-484, 1984.

Emission computed tomography: the single photon approach, HHS Publication FDA 81-8177, Washington, D.C., Aug. 1981, Health and Human Services.

Hughes, A., and Sharp, P.F.: Factors affecting gamma camera nonuniformity, Phys. Med. Biol. 33(2):259-269, 1988.

Maguire, W.J.: Special effects due to bar phantoms, J. Nucl. Med., 7(2):81, 1979.

Murphy, P.H.: Acceptance testing and quality control of gamma cameras including SPECT, J. Nucl. Med., 28:1221-1227, 1987.

Myers, M.J., and Fazio, F.: The case for emission computed tomography with a rotating gamma camera, Appl. Radiol. 10(4): July/Aug. 1981.

NEMA standards for performance measurements of scintillation cameras, Pub. No. NU1-1986, National Electrical Manufacturers Association, NEMA, 1986.

Rao, D.V., Early, P.J., Chu, R.Y., Goodwin, P.N., and Graham, L.S.: Radiation control and quality assurance surveys—nuclear medicine a suggested protocol, ACMP Report No. 3, 1986.

Sorenson, J.A., and Phelps, M.E.: Physics in nuclear medicine, New York, 1987, Grune & Stratton, Inc.

Tuscan, M.J., Rogers, W.L., Juni, J.E., and Clinthorne, N.H.: Analysis of gamma camera detector stability and its effect on uniformity correction for SPECT, J. Nucl. Med. Technol. 13(1), March 1985.

Woronowicz, E.M., Eisner, G.T., Gullberg, G.T., Nowak, D.J., and Mulko, J.A.: Factors affecting single photon emission computed tomography image quality and recommended QC procedures. Milwaukee, Wis., General Electric Medical Systems Operations.

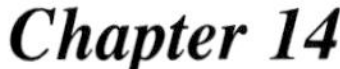

Chapter 14

SPECT IMAGING: SINGLE PHOTON EMISSION COMPUTED TOMOGRAPHY

PAUL J. EARLY

■ DISCUSSION

The concept of tomography is not new to the nuclear medicine community. In fact it precedes x-ray computed tomography (CT) both for single photon sources and positron emitters. It was, however, confined to a few prestigious health-care centers. It was not until the development of CT that tremendous strides were made with single photon emission computed tomography (SPECT). Its rapid growth and development can also be attributed to the availability of small dedicated computers that have a high capacity for the acquisition of data, and to the many sophisticated computer software programs—all at a price consistent with the budget guidelines of most hospitals. Improved clinical results are the end-product to this nuclear medicine modality.

Improved clinical results are due to improved target (T) to nontarget (NT) ratios (Fig. 14-1). Planar images record and therefore visualize all radioactivity from the surface of the detector head to infinity (Fig. 14-1, *A*) This results in a large contribution to the image from areas that are of no interest and thus degrade the image. SPECT, however, eliminates unnecessary information, both foreground and background (Fig 14-1, *B*), improving the T:NT ratios and resulting in a more direct image. Currently, there are two types of SPECT devices in use in nuclear medicine. They are termed *longitudinal* and *transaxial*. Longitudinal devices image in one plane, not unlike the old rectilinear scanner, but carry with them the associated electronics to simultaneously image separate planes. Transaxial devices allow the detector to rotate around the patient, collecting information in a single slice through the body.

Longitudinal devices dealing with SPECT are those of multiplane tomographic scanners and stationary cameras using multipinhole collimators or rotating slant-hole collimators. All three are approaches to tomography but have been superceded by the transaxial devices. The multipinhole collimators suffered from reduced angular sampling and therefore superimposition of information. The rotating slant-hole collimator provided a large area of view, more uniformity of sensitivity, and resolution with depth; however, software was primitive and the unit was mechanically complex. For these reasons, the discussion here will be limited to transaxial devices.

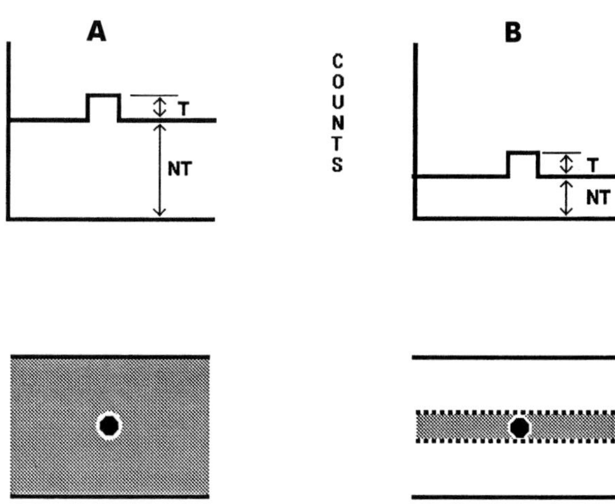

Fig. 14-1. Schematic showing the value of SPECT **(B)** versus planar **(A)** in improving target to nontarget ratios (T:NT) by removing background and foreground information and thus improving the image.

Transaxial devices include any tomographic camera that rotates around the patient collecting information so that a slice through the body can be reconstructed. Devices included in this category are the multicrystal transaxial tomographic camera (few in number) and the rotating Anger gamma camera. This discussion will be restricted to the latter.

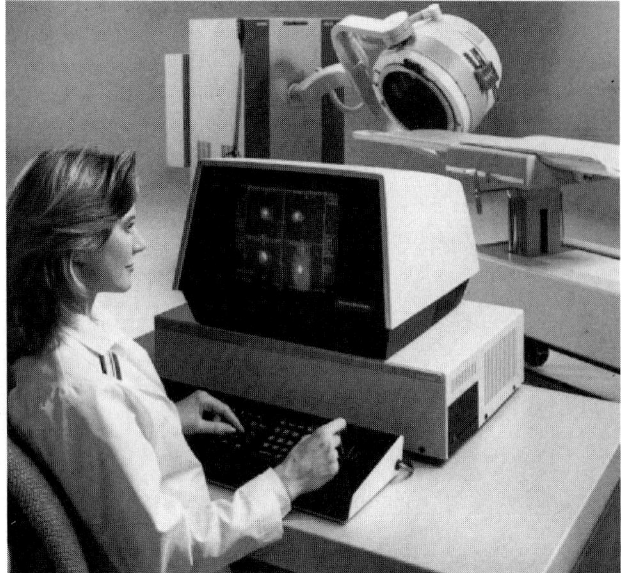

Fig. 14-2. Rotating Anger camera. (Courtesy Nuclear Medicine Group, Siemens Medical Systems, Inc., Hoffman Estates, Ill.)

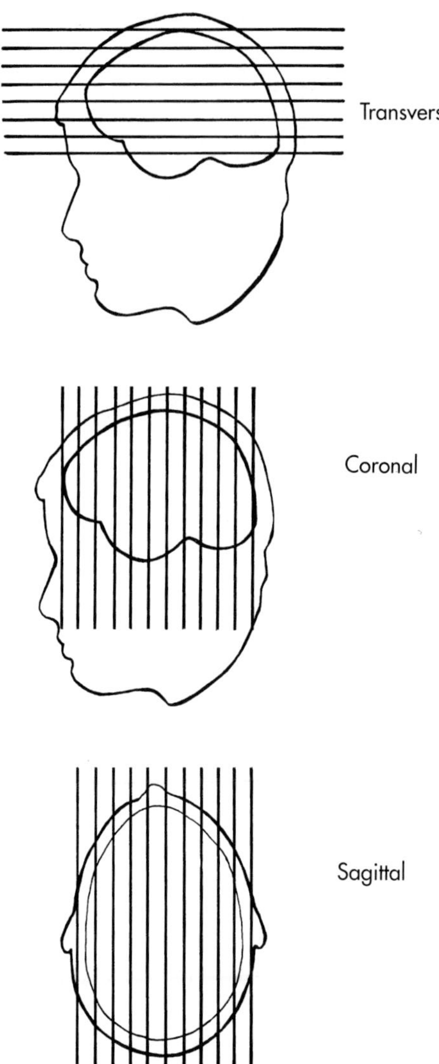

Fig. 14-3. Tomographic orientations.

■ ROTATING GAMMA CAMERA

In the case of the rotating gamma camera (Fig. 14-2), one or more scintillation detector heads are mounted in a ring gantry which, when positioned properly, will cause the detector(s) to rotate around the body at the level of the organ under investigation. These systems are designed to rotate up to 360°, and then stopping, collecting and recording an image at multiple equal angles through the total angle of rotation ("stepped" rotation). Some systems are capable of collecting a sample for every one degree of rotation (or 360 images). Selections are made also for image-collection times, which determine how long the detector stops at a certain location before proceeding to the next location. Some systems employ continuous rotation, while others allow a choice between continuous and stepped. When continuous rotation is chosen, the number of images is usually preselected. Therefore, the continuous mode is usually designed for high statistical studies. Some believe that this is the only way in which SPECT should be employed.

Instruments vary, but images may be acquired on matrix sizes from 64 × 64 up to 512 × 512; however, SPECT reconstruction is usually at lesser matrix sizes, usually not more than 128 × 128. The number of stops and the accumulation time per stop provide a large variation in number of counts per image. Once the images are acquired and stored, the computer assimilates the data and reconstructs slices of the image using conventional reconstruction techniques. These systems allow for the generation of slices as low as one pixel thick to slices composed of multiple pixels in thickness.

■ Reconstruction techniques

Reconstruction techniques are similar to those used in CT reconstruction except that SPECT information comes from radionuclides inside the body and therefore *emitted* radiation as opposed to, CT information coming from radiation *transmitted* through the body from an external x-ray source. Techniques used for SPECT image reconstruction are discussed in Chapter 12. The time required for this reconstruction is of a wide range based on such variables as number of detectors, concentration of radionuclides in the organ, number of images stored, number of counts per image, reconstruction formula (or algorithm) used, and capability of the computer. The speed of the reconstruction process is greatly increased through the use of an array processor, which is basically a "number cruncher" that can re-

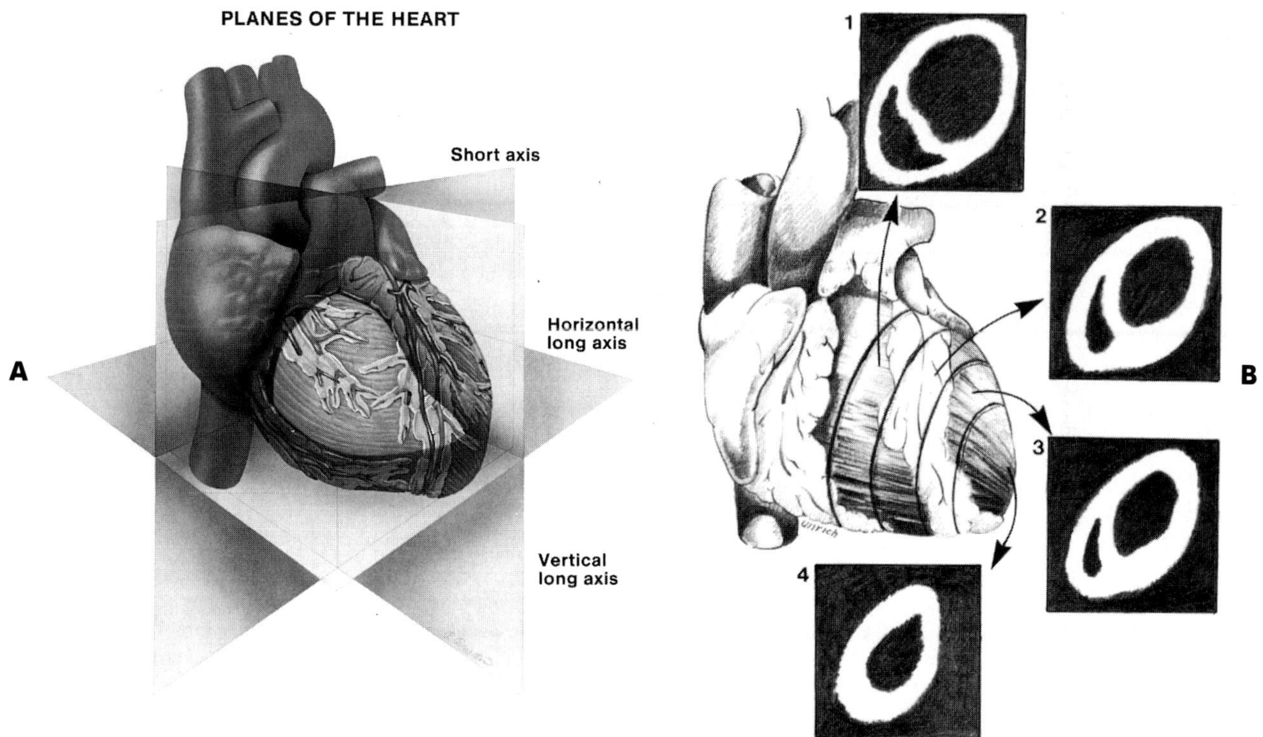

Fig. 14-4. **A,** Tomographic planes of the heart. **B,** Apex to base slices of the myocardium. (**A,** From Folks, R., and others: Cardiovascular SPECT, JNMT 13:3, Sept. 1985. **B,** From English, R.J., and Brown, S.E.: SPECT—a primer, Soc. of Nuc. Med., 1990.)

duce the reconstruction time from as long as 30 or 40 minutes to 3 or 4 seconds. An array processor is absolutely essential to effectively make use of state-of-the-art computers and their algorithms. Once the data for image reconstruction are obtained, the SPECT system is capable of orienting and processing the data to acquire transverse, coronal, and/or sagittal slices (Fig. 14-3) without further data acquisition. As the field becomes more complex and the needs of the nuclear medicine practitioner better defined, the reconstruction programs become more sophisticated. The limitless possibilities are becoming more evident in the field of nuclear cardiology. The heart, unlike other organs, normally is oriented in such a way that it lies neither entirely within one plane nor entirely parallel or perpendicular to any of the anatomic planes of the body (Fig. 14-4). This oblique orientation causes many difficulties in interpretation. Techniques and reconstruction algorithms are now available, however, to reorient the heart such that the reconstructed slices, (termed *short axis slices*) are perpendicular to the long axis of the heart. This orientation reduces interpretative errors caused by reduced perfusion at the base of the heart in the region of the valve plane.

Another reconstruction program with unique application in nuclear cardiology is the "bull's-eye" profile (Fig. 14-5, *A*). This reconstruction program uses the short axis slices and plots the maximum counts per pixel along a radius originating from the center of the left ventricle through the myocardium. About 40 radii are used to perform the evaluation, which is displayed as concentric rings with the smaller apical slices in the center proceeding out to the larger basal slices on the periphery, each divided into quadrants as shown. These profiles are generated for each tomographic slice at stress and redistribution. Blood supply to the various portions of the reconstructed "bull's-eye" image is known (Fig. 14-5, *B*). Once the data are reconstructed, these bull's-eye plots can be compared to "normal" files stored in the computer to assist in analysis of both phases Displays can take a variety of forms to include raw and blackened pixel plots, raw and standard deviation plots, blackened pixel and standard deviation plots, and standard deviation plots and color map. Planar images (single-organ as well as whole-body) can also be acquired from the system. In fact, if it were not for this, many hospitals would not be able to justify the purchase of a SPECT system, because not all patients require tomography studies. Since the system uses standard parallel-hole collimators, the rotational head becomes a valuable asset for positioning the detector for planar images of an immobile or restrained patient.

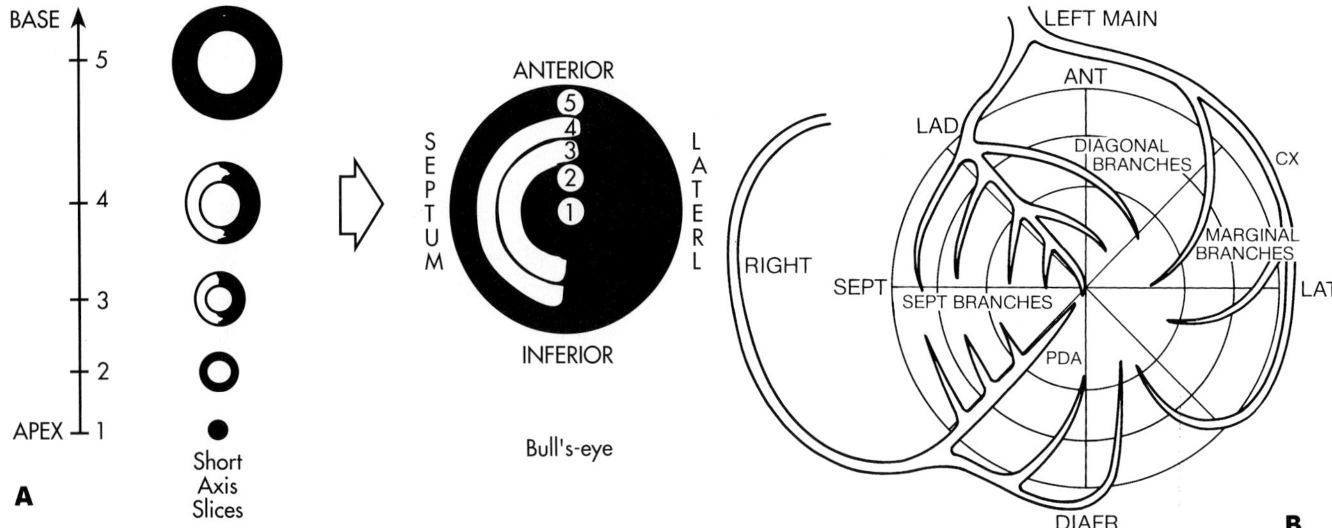

Fig. 14-5. A, Schematic of a "bull's-eye" profile of a thallium-201 heart study. (From Folks, R., and others: Cardiovascular SPECT, JNMT 13:3, Sept. 1985). **B,** Normal "bull's-eye" plot of artery distribution. (Courtesy Picker International, Cleveland, Ohio.)

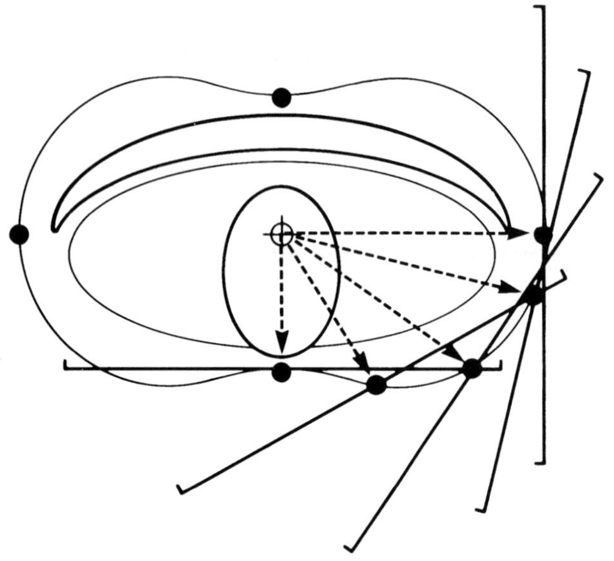

Fig. 14-6. Peanut orbit. (Courtesy Picker International, Cleveland, Ohio.)

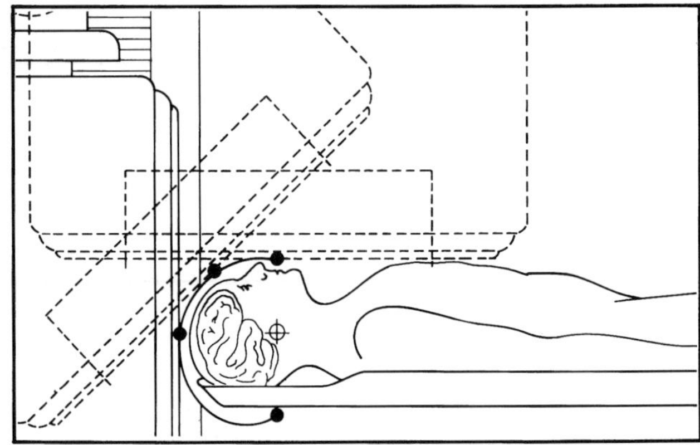

Fig. 14-7. A technique for high resolution SPECT brain scan. (Courtesy Picker International, Cleveland, Ohio.)

■ Resolution aspects of SPECT

One item of concern regarding SPECT resolution is that the rotation of the tomography unit is in a large circle so as to clear the shoulders of the patient. In circling, the detector is closest to the body laterally, but at great distance from the surface of the body (and therefore even farther from its organs) both anteriorly and posteriorly. Since collimators are used and images degrade in resolution, the farther away these collimators are from the organ under study, the more raw data collected both anteriorly and posteriorly are necessarily degraded. Some manufacturers have introduced an oval pattern, sometimes referred to as "peanut orbit" (Fig. 14-6), to attempt to minimize this deficiency. Another approach to increased resolution in SPECT is the issue of 180° acquisitions versus 360° acquisitions. This issue, which may always be controversial, is most obvious when organs are not centrally located in the body (heart, liver, spleen) where it might seem logical that a 180° acquisition might be best. Conversely, centrally located organs such as lungs, kidneys, and brain might benefit from 360° acquisitions. The controversy centers on issues of spatial resolution, geometrical distortion, and attenuation correction. In heart

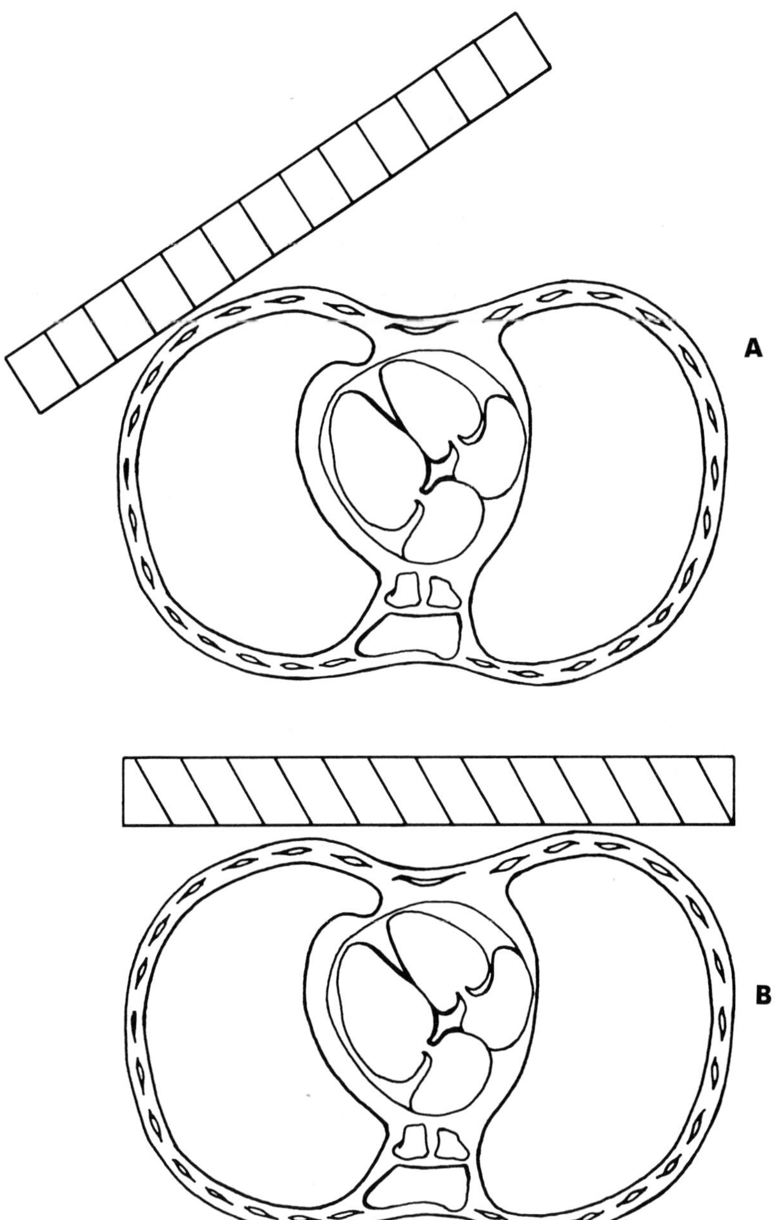

Fig. 14-8. Cross-sectional diagram showing disadvantages of parallel-hole collimator (**A**) versus slant-hole collimator (**B**) in position for an LAO view of the heart. Parallel-hole collimator must be positioned about twice as far from the heart as slant-hole collimator, causing losses in resolution and sensitivity.

studies, for instance, some clinicians feel that a 360° acquisition is inferior because data acquired while the detector is on the right side of the patient suffer from lack of spatial resolution and proper attenuation correction, while others feel the 180° acquisition suffers from geometric distortion. The same could be said for liver and spleen studies from the left and right sides of the body, respectively.

Brain studies can also be imaged by 180° acquisition (provided the software is available), by moving the detector in a cephalad direction from under the table up over the vertex of the brain and down toward the caudad position (Fig. 14-7). This acquisition mode allows closer proximity to the brain and thus, favorable count rate and resolution. A unique aspect of this approach for the neurologic patient is that the procedure is almost complete before the anxious patient is aware of the procedure. Many of the drawbacks of a 360° acquisition of the brain can be overcome by using special collimators (long-bore or slant-hole). A modification of the multichannel parallel-hole collimator is the slant-hole collimator. The 30° slant-hole collimator is used (both in planar and SPECT imaging) for superior images of the heart; it has also been proposed for the brain. Figure 14-8 illustrates how the collimator placed flat against the chest (B), will provide a perfect 30° LAO view of the heart. This collimator will provide better resolution of the left ventricle than will a conventional parallel-hole collimator (A), because the camera is positioned at a greater distance from the ventricle. Similarly, a long-bore collimator will be effective in brain studies because of its ease of placement in close proximity to the brain as it rotates 360° around the head. This collimator affords increased resolution, but at the sacrifice of count rate.

LABORATORY APPLICATION

35

Quality assurance of a SPECT system

CENTER OF ROTATION (COR)

Any evaluation of a SPECT system begins with the satisfactory completion of all procedures involved in the acceptance and evaluation of a planar system. Any defect that is present in a planar image is magnified in a SPECT evaluation. Any defect in the planar studies should be corrected before continuing with this exercise.

Purpose

Since tomographic images from SPECT are reconstructed from data acquired as the detector head(s) move in a circular (or elliptical) orbit around the object, it is important to the reconstruction process that the computer is able to "fix" on a center point. This point falls on a line fixed in space that is parallel to the scan table and perpendicular to the plane of the gantry (Fig. 14-9). This point is called the center of rotation (COR). It is important that all information is referenced to this point at each position throughout the rotation of the detector head. With parallel-hole collimators, the mechanical alignment is very important. The plane of the detector must be parallel to the axis of rotation. For this to be the case, the detector head must be horizontal with the floor at 0° and 180°, and vertical to the floor at 90° and 270° rotation (see Key point 10). The basic purpose of the procedure is to confirm a mirror image at 0° and 180° to determine if the detector can observe the same set of parallel lines at 0 and 180°.

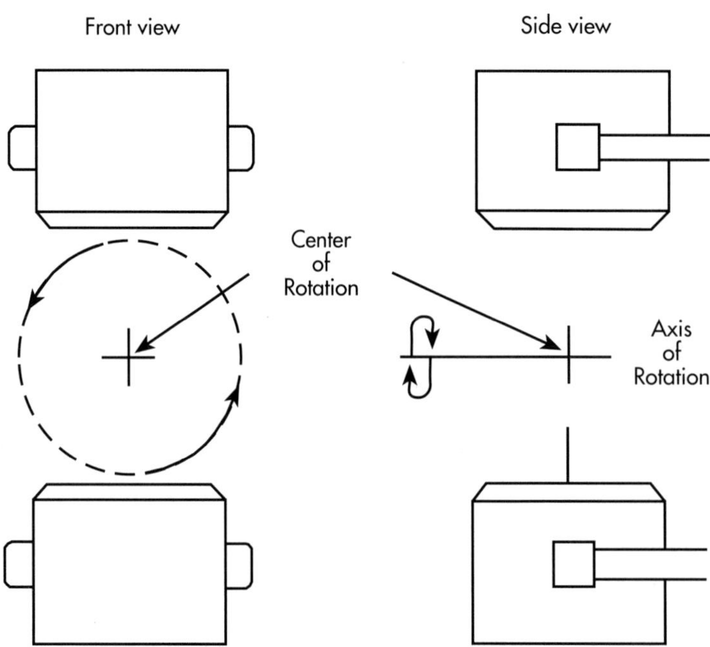

Fig. 14-9. Schematic of a SPECT system illustrating the center of rotation (COR) and the axis of rotation.

Procedure

Materials

1. ^{99m}Tc point source prepared according to manufacturer's instructions.
2. Collimator (one of routine use)

Technique

(Refer to manufacturer's procedure. Below is a typical procedure.)

1. Arrange a 20% symmetrical window.
2. Position source slightly off-center approximately 5 cm from approximate COR, or refer to manufacturer's procedure manual.
3. Arrange a 15-cm circular orbit. (This may require a special device extending over the edge of the imaging table.)
4. Acquire a 360° image on the computer matrix to be used for imaging. No greater than 32 projections are required, with not less than 20,000 counts per projection.

Data treatment

1. Compute COR using algorithm of manufacturer.
2. Generate a sinogram image using algorithm of the manufacturer (see Key Point 1).

Key points

1. As the detector moves around the source, a sinusoidal curve represents the location of the point source as seen by the detector at each of the 32 stops. The location changes based on the detector's orientation with the point source (Fig. 14-10). A plot of these various locations produces the sinusoidal curve as viewed in the transverse direction (Fig. 14-11, *A*). In the axial direction, it should produce a straight line (Fig. 14-11, *B*).
2. The COR correction corresponds to the pixel (more precisely, to the portion of the pixel) midway between the maximum and the minimum deviation of the point source. That location should be determined by the computer to be ±1 mm. The exact location of the COR on a 64 × 64 matrix is 32.5.

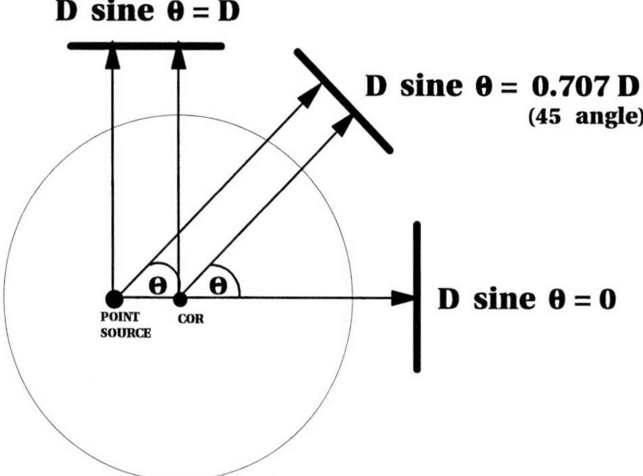

Fig. 14-10. Projection geometry of a point source placed off the COR at two camera positions. When the detector is parallel to two lines, one passing through the COR and the other passing through the axis of rotation (position *A*), the projected point is recorded at a distance, *D*. When the detector moves by some angle theta (position B), the projected point is now at a distance *D* cosine theta from the COR. A plot of this apparent movement of the point is seen on Fig. 14-11.

Continued.

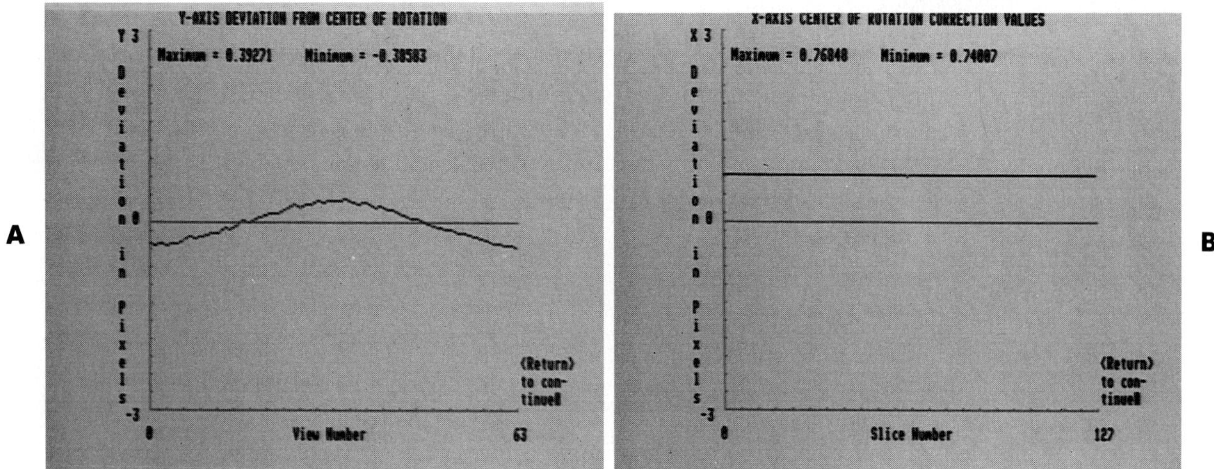

Fig. 14-11. Sinograms of an off-center point source with its location plotted as a function of the gantry angle, resulting in a sinusoid in the transverse direction **(A)** and a straight line in the axial direction **(B).**

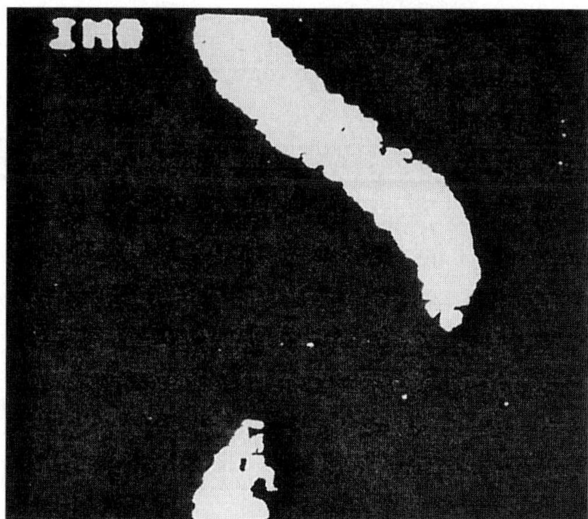

Fig. 14-12. Normal display of a sinogram. (Courtesy G.E. Medical Systems.)

3. If there is any deviation in the perfect sine wave result of the COR determination, the change could be a result of: *(a)* the detector not completing a true circular path, *(b)* the wrong collimator (although this is a problem on very few cameras and should be confirmed on acceptance), or *(c)* the weight of detector, which can cause the detector to go "out of circle" in certain positions as it rotates. This may also be a function of the collimator weight. In these cases, a "second order" COR correction is possible. The latter, of course, would absolutely preclude the use of any other collimator with this COR correction.
4. A cine of the COR study might also be revealing. Motion of the point source is only expected along the *X*-axis. Motion along the *Y*-axis could be a result of *(a)* mechanical alignment of the detector, *(b)* rotation of the detector within the gantry, or *(c)* angulation of the collimator holes in a slant-hole collimator.
5. A sinogram display of the organ studied is often useful in evaluating the fidelity of a clinical study. A normal display is seen in Figure 14-12. In a minimal amount of time, other problems, if present, could be identified (Figs. 14-13 to 14-15).
6. Computer programs are also available to automatically measure pixel size (important for attenuation correction) and X- and Y-gain determinations. These values should be checked rou-

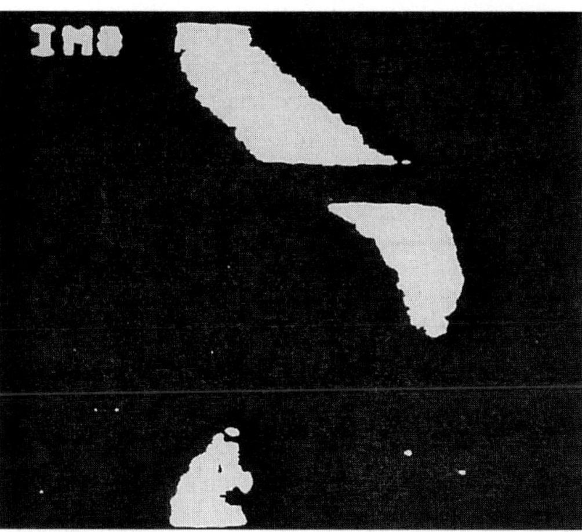

Fig. 14-13. Missed planar views during acquisition. (Courtesy G.E. Medical Systems.)

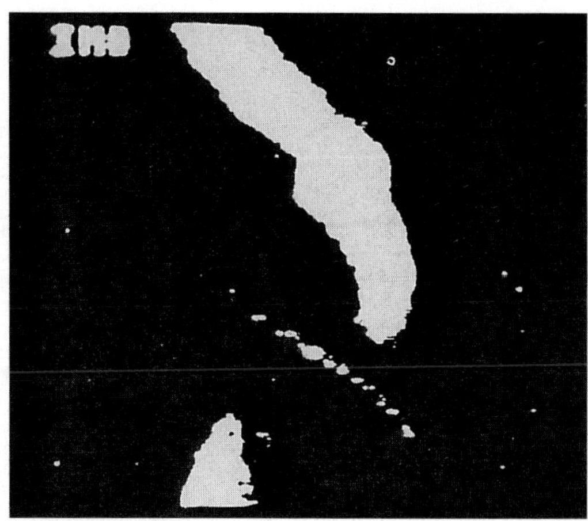

Fig. 14-14. Repeated planar views during acquisition. (Courtesy G.E. Medical Systems.)

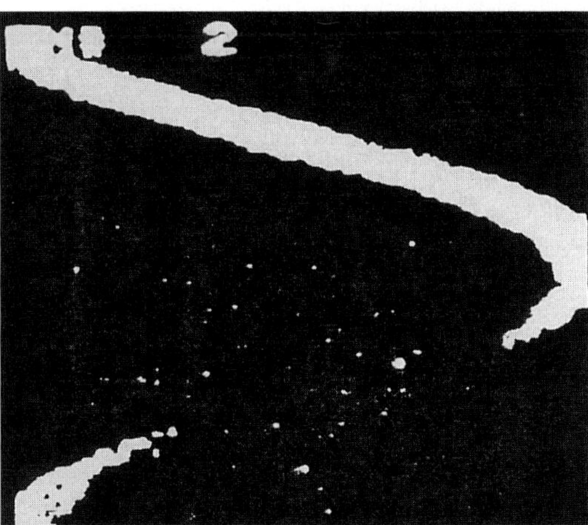

Fig. 14-15. Intended organ of study is placed outside the field of view. (Courtesy G.E. Medical Systems.)

tinely if they are not already part of the analysis package. Pixel size is easily performed manually by measuring two point sources placed at known intervals from each other. Pixel size is determined as follows:

$$\frac{\text{Distance of point source (millimeters)}}{\text{Number of pixels between point sources}}$$

This procedure should be performed both in the *X* and *Y* directions. Their values should be equal and unchanged with time.

7. Mechanical alignment can be checked with a "jig" that allows a point source to be exactly positioned at two different distances from the collimator (Fig. 14-16). In the case of the mechanical alignment problem, the images of the two sources should not perfectly superimpose.
8. Misalignments are always worse in elliptical orbits than in circular ones. Furthermore, defects are magnified even more in elliptical than in circular orbits. It is therefore recommended that these studies be performed on circular orbits first.
9. Mechanical alignment should be measured with a carpenter's level because of the infidelity

Continued.

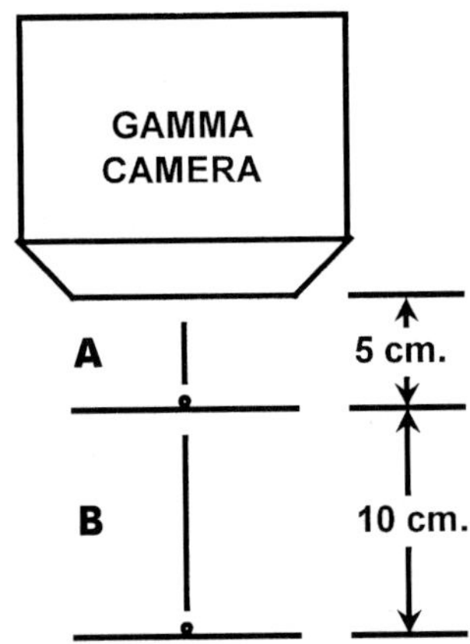

Fig. 14-16. "Jig" for the collimator hole angulation test. An image is made at source location **A.** The source is then moved to location **B,** where a second image is made. These two images should perfectly superimpose.

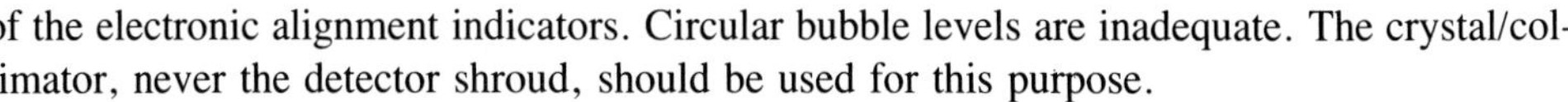

of the electronic alignment indicators. Circular bubble levels are inadequate. The crystal/collimator, never the detector shroud, should be used for this purpose.

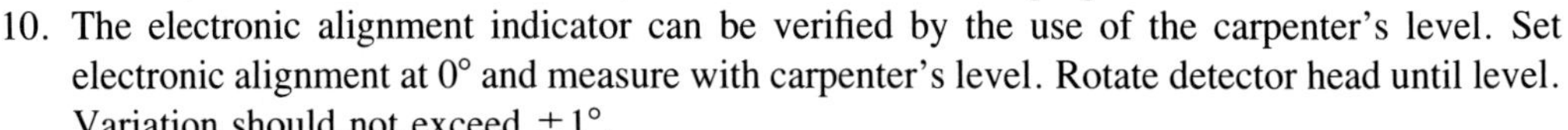

10. The electronic alignment indicator can be verified by the use of the carpenter's level. Set electronic alignment at 0° and measure with carpenter's level. Rotate detector head until level. Variation should not exceed ±1°.

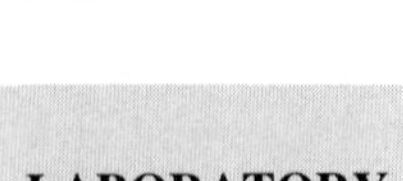

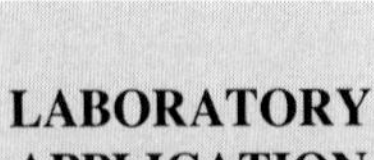

LABORATORY APPLICATION

36

UNIFORMITY

The merits of uniformity have been well documented in Chapter 13. Although uniformity is important in planar images, it is essential to tomographic images. Any borderline nonuniformity in a planar image is magnified many times in the SPECT image. The reason is that a small area of nonuniformity (which may be out of an area of involvement in a planar image) will move around the image as the detector moves around the organ, creating a circular defect (a bull's-eye pattern [Fig. 14-17]). The bull's-eye pattern can also be seen extrinsically in collimator defects, poor statistics, and incomplete mixing of flood phantom. While the above problems are generated by the camera and its accessories, other factors extraneous to the equipment itself create special problems to the uniformity study as the detector makes its circular path around the object. These problems are gravitational; magnetic field (earth, motor, or magnetic resonance) and areas of increased background are due to the presence of radioactive sources (hot labs, the patient, etc.). All these parameters can be evaluated in situ during acceptance and routinely thereafter.

Procedure

Materials

1. ^{57}Co flood disc (uniform to ±1%), *or*
2. 10 mCi (370 MBq) ^{99m}Tc in water-filled *flat* disc flood phantom (see Key point 9). Mix thoroughly.
3. 20 mCi (740 MBq) ^{99m}Tc in water-filled, cylindrical phantom*
4. Collimators

Technique 1

1. Attach collimator.
2. Arrange a 20% symmetrical window.

*NEMA, Fig. 14-18, Nuclear Associates, Fig. 14-19; or Jasczczak phantom.

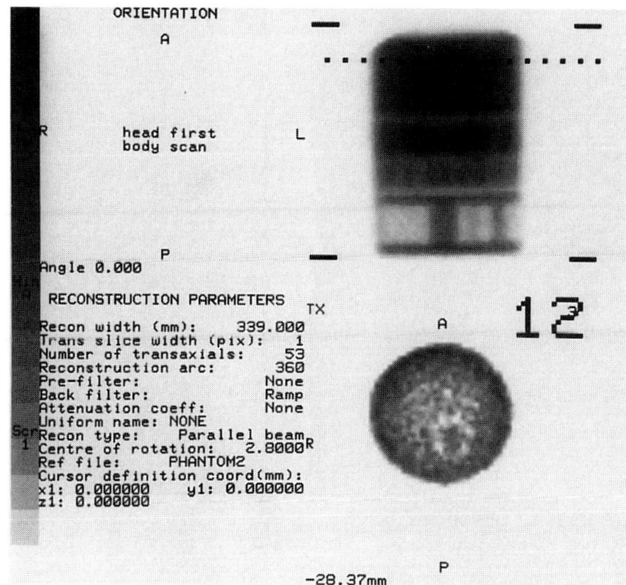

Fig. 14-17. Bull's-eye artifact following SPECT reconstruction as a result of a non-uniformity.

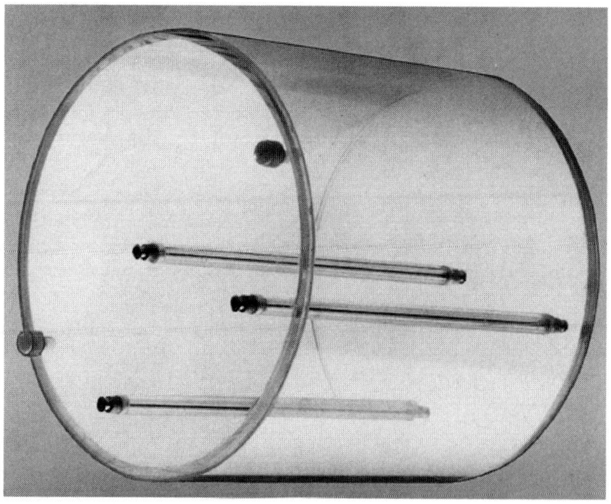

Fig. 14-18. NEMA phantom. (Courtesy Nuclear Associates, Carle Place, N.Y.)

3. At a rate not greater than 30,000 cps, acquire and store in computer memory a 30-million–count uniformity correction flood* on a 64 × 64 matrix (or 120-million–count uniformity correction flood on a 128 × 128 matrix), using the flood disc or the water-filled disc phantom.
4. Correct for nonuniformities and produce hard-copy image for records.
5. Repeat for all collimators (see Key point 6).

Technique 2

1. Arrange the cylindrical phantom such that the long axis is parallel to the axis of rotation. Acquire a 360° tomographic study on a 128 × 128 matrix using the largest number of angular samplings and a circular orbit with a radius of rotation of 15 cm. See Key point 4. Acquisition time should be such that a four-pixel–thick slice from the reconstruction image will yield 2 million counts.
2. Correct each image for nonuniformities.
3. Reconstruct images using 4-mm–slice thicknesses, a ramp filter, and attenuation correction (see Key point 5).
4. Repeat on all collimators.

Data treatment

1. Determine nonuniformity by:
   a. Visual inspection. *Procedure 1:* Are the images visually acceptable? Are there any noticeable defects on any of the projections? *Procedure 2:* Are there any bull's-eyes artifacts visible?
   b. Evaluate integral and differential uniformity by a computer program similar to NEMA seen in Fig. 13-21, *C*.

*NEMA suggests 50,000 counts per pixel, but the capability of some computers does not allow this collection of counts in the routine nuclear medicine department.

Continued.

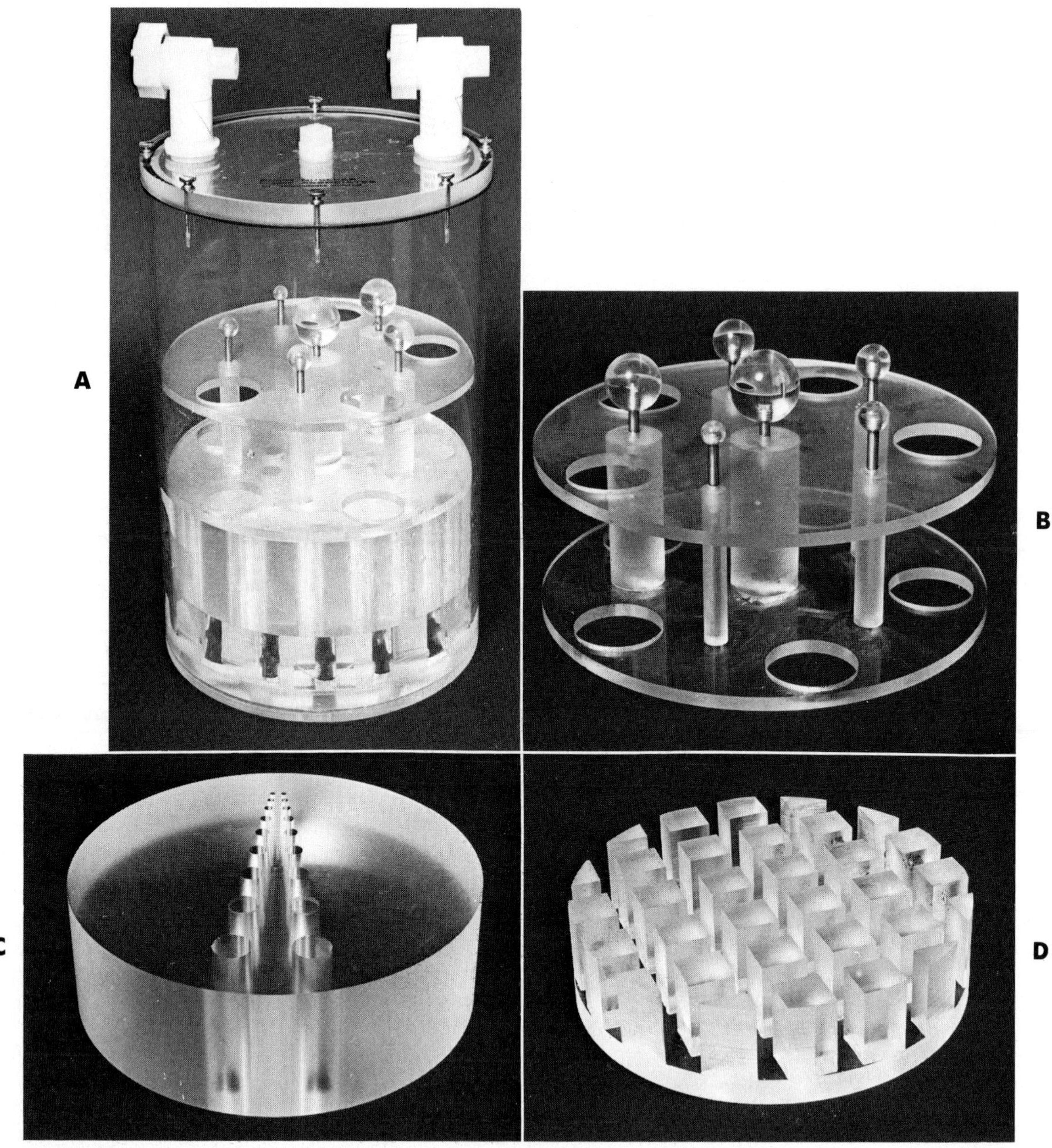

Fig. 14-19. A, SPECT phantom. **B,** Solid plastic spheres and rods of SPECT phantom. **C,** Solid plastic with cylindric-hole pairs of SPECT phantom. **D,** Grid pattern of SPECT phantom. (Courtesy Nuclear Associates, Carle Place, N.Y.).

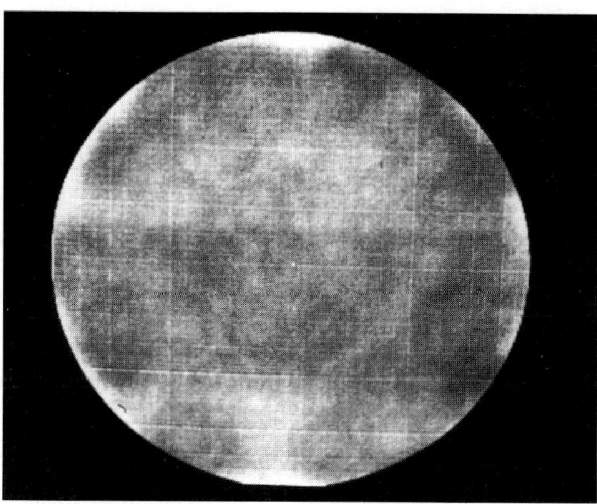

Fig. 14-20. Inadequate differential linearity within the ADC, resulting in horizontal and vertical bunching of counts. (From English, R.J., and Brown, S.E., SPECT—a primer, Society of Nuclear Medicine, 1980).

Key points

1. A flood image of 30 million counts provides about 10,000 counts per pixel in the useful field of view (UFOV) on a 64 × 64 matrix collection or a statistical accuracy of ±1% accuracy 68% of the time.
2. A flood image of 30 million counts is also adequate for a 128 × 128 matrix image, provided the flood image is smoothed. Some feel that flood images should not be smoothed to reduce statistical variations because collimator defects will not be visualized. However, if this same smoothing process is used in the preprocessing of clinical images, it may be appropriate to smooth, depending on how correction factors are generated.
3. Correction floods should be obtained for all collimators and all commonly used radionuclides.
4. A radius of rotation of 15 cm may require a special holding device, made of a rigid material yet low in attenuation, that extends from the end of the imaging bed.
5. Attenuation correction factor for ^{99m}Tc is 0.15 cm^{-1} (15% per cm) in H_2O. Empirically, this value has been reduced for clinical studies to 12%. Other radionuclides use other values. Consult the manufacturer's recommendations.
6. Line artifacts in collimators (Fig. 13-14) are often created at the time of manufacturing as a result of *(a)* improper alignment of the lead foil, *b)* lead foil separation because of improper handling of the collimator, or *(c)* twisting of the lead foil as the collimator is lifted in a twisting motion out of its jig (see Fig. 13-20, *A* and *B*). These are often only seen in an 8- to 10-million–count flood. Denting, which causes the lead foil to fold over the hole(s) and thereby attenuate the photons, will also cause regional changes in sensitivity (see Fig. 13-19).
7. One component often overlooked is the analog-to-digital converter (ADC). This device may create as many problems as any other single component in the camera system. Their fidelity (gain changes and matrix offset drift) and their speed are always in question. Nonlinearities can also be introduced by the ADC (Fig. 14-20). Because of these differential nonlinearities, counts become "bunched" at certain pixels, producing linear defects in the *X* and *Y* directions only. If present, service is indicated.
8. Flood image collected at a rate of 30,000 counts per second ensures a dead time of less than 10%. To exceed this dead time rate is not advised.
9. Water-filled phantoms have a tendency to bulge in the center; however, specially designed phantoms are now available to reduce this problem. A ½ -inch thick phantom will require less than a 0.005-inch bulge to generate a uniformity of ±1%. Commercially available ^{57}Co flood discs are preferred, if not essential.

LABORATORY APPLICATION

37

ANGULAR VARIATION OF FLOOD FIELD UNIFORMITY AND SENSITIVITY

Purpose

This test is one which checks the camera's ability to maintain uniformity and sensitivity as a function of its angular position. Stray magnetic fields as well as stray radiation can cause such changes. Magnetic fields have taken on new meaning with the advent of magnetic resonance; however, the earth's magnetic field as well as that of motors in the vicinity play a role. (See Key point 3 after "uniformity"). Stray radiation fields can be exhibited through radioactive patients, or hot labs and dosing areas in the vicinity.

Procedure

Materials

1. ^{57}Co flood disc (uniform to ±1%), *or*
2. 10 mCi (370 MBq) ^{99m}Tc in water-filled flat disc flood phantom (see Key point 9 after "Uniformity")
3. Low-energy, general-purpose collimator

Technique

1. Secure ^{57}Co or ^{99m}Tc liquid flood phantom to collimated detector.
2. Set appropriate 20% central window.
3. Acquire a 2 × 10^6 count flood at 0° position and record time.
4. Repeat the process *using the same time* (accounting for decay, if appropriate) at 90°, 180°, 270°, and 360° (same as 0°) camera rotational positions (see Fig. 14-21).

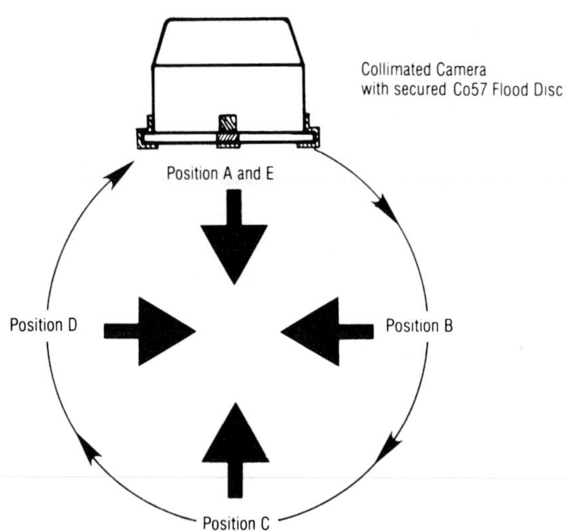

Accumulate 50,000 ± 10% counts per pixel at 10,000 - 30,000 cps through 20% window for each position, using fixed acquisition time.

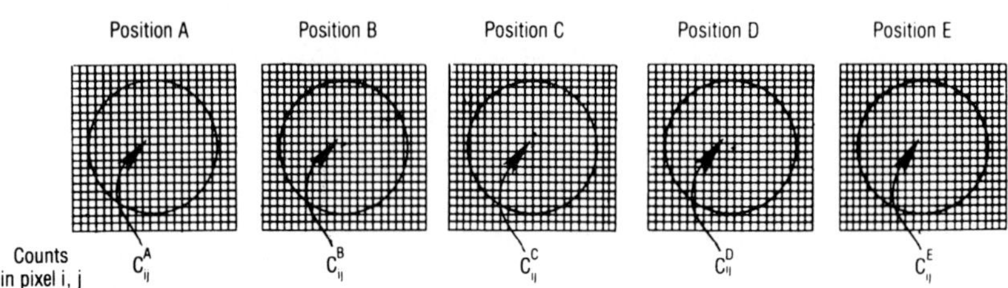

Fig. 14-21. Angular variation of flood field uniformity and sensitivity. (Courtesy Picker International, Inc., Cleveland, Ohio.)

Data treatment

1. Subjectively review each flood study for nonuniformities. Are any unacceptable or do any differ appreciably from the other (see Key point 4)?
2. Calculate maximum sensitivity variation (MSV) as follows:

Angle	Counts	Uniformity (subjective) Acceptable	Unacceptable
0°	____	____	____
90°	____	____	____
180°	____	____	____
270°	____	____	____
360° (or 0°)	____	____	____

$$\%\ \text{MSV} = \frac{\text{Maximum counts} - \text{minimum counts}}{\text{Maximum counts} + \text{minimum counts}} \times 100$$

Normal: <1% MSV

Key points

1. NEMA procedures for angular variation of uniformity suggest the reporting of the maximum percentage of pixels whose difference in counts recorded between two angular positions exceed 1, 2, or 3 standard deviations.
2. It is known that phototubes may pull away from their crystal interface in the 180° orientation.

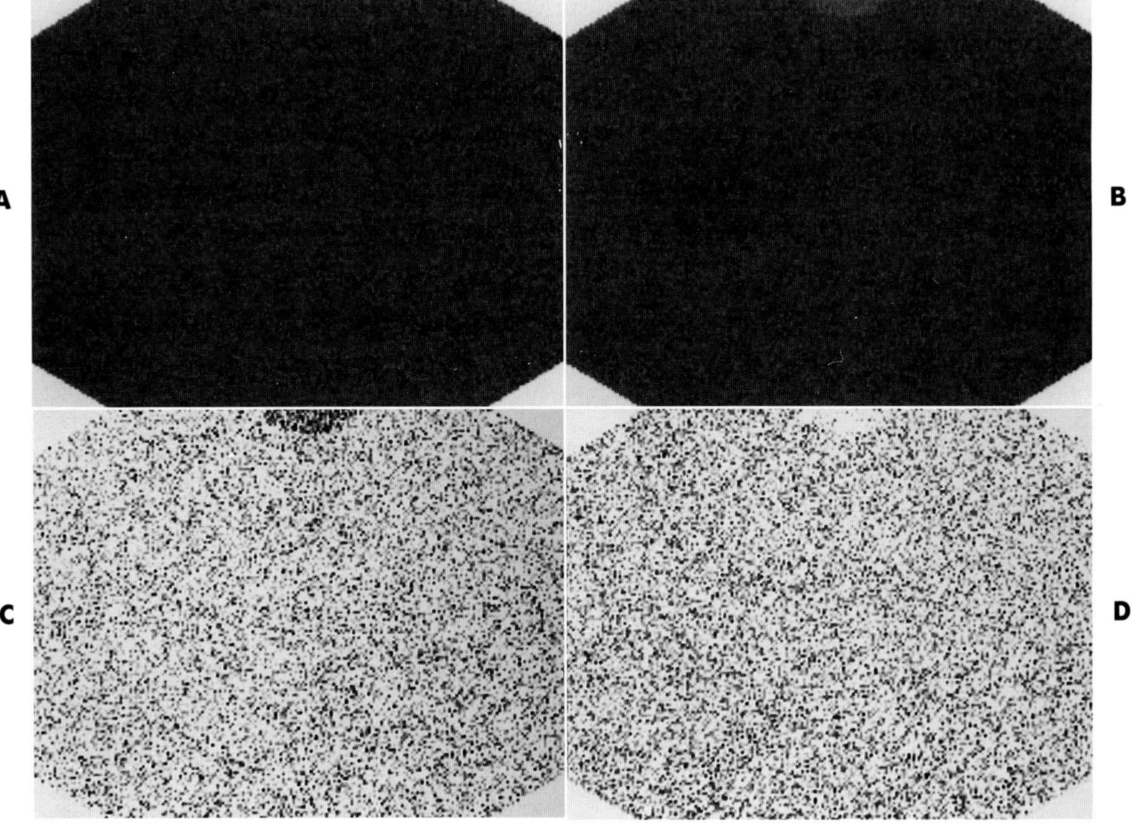

Fig. 14-22. Technique to subjectively evaluate angular variation using subtraction. Flood A (taken at 0°) minus flood B (taken at 90° and showing an area of count paucity) = subtracted flood C (showing random differences throughout the image except for an accentuated area of nonuniformity). Subtraction of flood B from flood A yields a reverse image (subtracted flood D). The latter is not always that obvious in situations of lesser dissimilarities.

Continued.

3. Magnetic fields are less of a problem in state-of-the-art cameras because phototubes are now being protected against stray magnetic field of low intensity.
4. An easy technique to evaluate angular variations in uniformity is to subtract the floods after they are acquired at different angles from each other. The result should be background. However, the 0° flood should be subtracted from the 90° flood and vice versa, and similarly with other angles to fully evaluate uniformity in this manner (see Fig. 14-22).

LABORATORY APPLICATION

38

ANGULAR VARIATION OF SPATIAL POSITION

Purpose

As seen in the exercise on uniformity, there is cause for concern regarding changes in uniformity and sensitivity as the detector assumes different angles in its path around the organ. There is no less concern for displacement of information as the detector maneuvers through these same angular variations. To have identical information in different pixel locations as the detector encircles its object would cause a loss of resolution. This procedure is to confirm that such displacement of information does not occur.

Procedure

Materials

1. Five ^{57}Co point sources, nominally 1 mm in diameter. Activity should be within ±20% of each other.
2. Plastic spacers 1 to 2 cm thick to which ^{57}Co sources are attached.

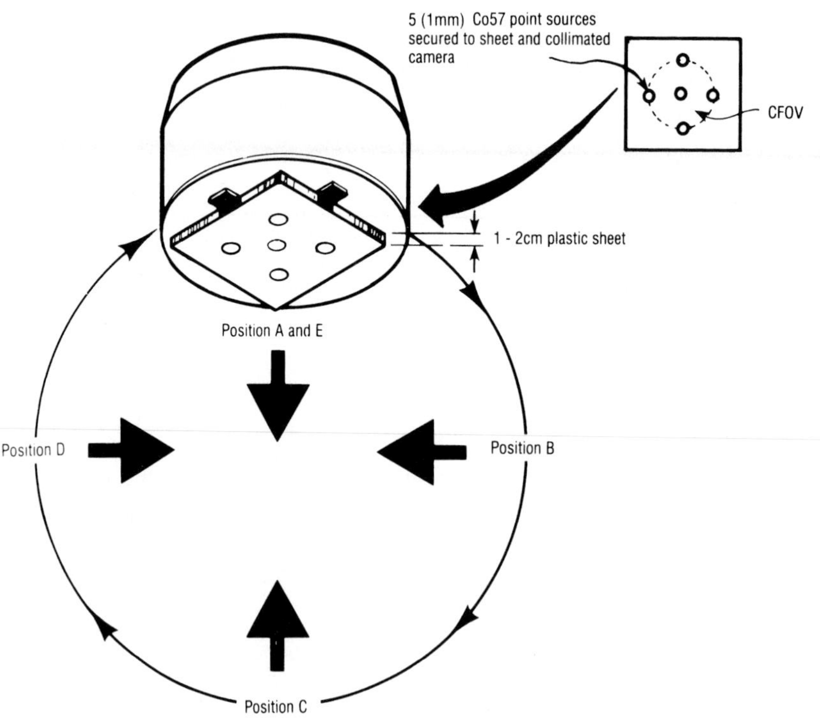

Fig. 14-23. Angular variation of spatial position. (Courtesy Picker International, Cleveland, Ohio.)

Technique

1. Peak camera with high resolution collimator using a 20% symmetrical window.
2. Arrange and secure to the collimator five ^{57}Co point sources with one in the center and the other four outlining the approximate central field of view (CFOV) in an *X, Y,* orientation (see Fig. 14-23).
3. Collect a 100,000-count planar image at each of the following detector angular orientations: 0°, 90°, 180°, 270°, and 360° (a repeat of 0°). The count rate should not exceed 20,000 cps, acquired into a 256 × 256 matrix, or largest matrix size available.

Data treatment

1. Arrange a slice profile through all point sources in both the *X* and *Y* directions of each of the five images.
2. Determine the pixel location of each point source (i.e., pixel receiving maximum count*) in each image in both the *X* and *Y* directions by evaluating the count printout of the slice profile (Fig. 14-24).
3. Calculate the largest displacement of the five sources in both the *X* and *Y* directions between any two of the five angular positions acquisition (10 combinations); convert to millimeters and calculate maximum displacement where:

$$\text{Maximum displacement (in millimeters)} = \sqrt{(X_1 - X_2)^2 + (Y_1 - Y_2)^2}$$

(See data collection sheet, Table 14-1)

*If computer displays only channels of the multichannel analyzer (MCA) and not pixels, then the MCA must be calibrated by measuring the distance between two of the sources, as follows:

$$\text{millimeter/channel} = \frac{\text{Millimeters between sources}}{\text{Number of channels between peaks}}$$

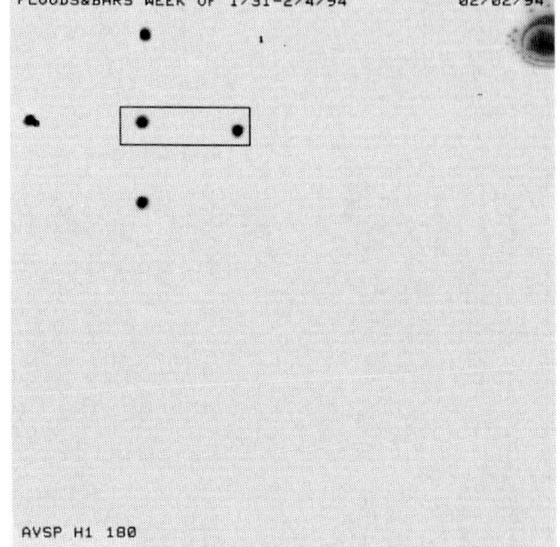

Fig. 14-24. Image and ROI profile with accompanying counts/pixel printout showing the maximum count/pixel location of a point source. Other ROIs must be generated on other points of interest.

	56	57	58	59	60	61	62	63	64	65	66	67	68	69	70	71	72	73	74	75
56	27	46	53	71	54	47	53	50	48	44	49	57	33	107	125	46	39	39	48	21
57	41	64	254	820	329	83	67	44	49	49	37	54	86	210	293	94	50	45	37	26
58	51	117	2075	6527	2812	203	76	40	42	38	47	53	140	997	1822	363	73	49	45	36
59	41	211	5300	16430	7069	423	69	48	48	44	36	92	413	5195	8849	2039	108	51	37	31
60	57	285	6617	20586	8975	496	77	40	52	52	48	82	810	10529	17327	3924	139	57	42	27
61	59	282	6548	21016	9146	539	76	56	56	62	54	104	883	11805	19780	4407	178	73	29	32
62	65	324	6568	20126	8782	534	110	72	71	77	97	131	829	10958	18242	4601	212	75	39	35
63	95	330	5462	16499	7194	542	222	162	159	140	166	197	780	9194	16364	4119	324	99	52	28
64	86	415	6074	17505	7780	530	178	107	94	100	122	147	764	9752	19017	5055	333	100	34	37
65	98	476	6434	19180	8443	540	128	82	68	92	100	115	639	9270	19876	5831	334	131	35	27
66	96	422	5663	17715	7907	534	155	126	123	123	154	163	604	7672	17158	5512	384	125	37	35
67	85	330	6110	18273	8078	540	158	117	88	102	122	143	530	7696	18878	6671	402	92	48	28
68	77	329	6823	20506	9140	563	104	75	49	43	66	62	402	7685	20863	7674	389	65	38	43
69	58	287	6822	20751	8956	513	91	61	43	59	42	72	348	7348	20636	8085	400	85	47	37
70	54	284	6847	20719	8838	475	74	75	50	51	73	67	277	6322	19024	8064	381	54	50	41
71	48	268	6169	18120	7409	391	57	45	63	61	56	89	213	4260	13418	6154	332	46	37	38
72	70	181	3479	10751	4447	277	73	52	52	36	42	48	107	1538	4814	2163	181	46	39	28
73	55	117	1451	4838	2007	166	60	58	52	41	44	58	57	204	523	256	71	45	33	36
74	45	61	341	1078	488	88	55	55	46	33	52	47	45	54	48	38	38	25	34	36

Continued.

Table 14-1. Data collection table for angular variation of spatial position

Source orientation / Camera orientation	12:00		3:00		6:00		9:00		Center	
	X	Y	X	Y	X	Y	X	Y	X	Y
0°										
90°										
180°										
270°										
360°										
Maximum displacement										

Data treatment:
1. Determine maximum displacement for each source orientation in both the X and Y directions and record.
2. Choose the largest displacement value from the five X maximum displacement values (X_D) and from the five Y maximum displacement values (Y_D).
3. Convert each of these two values to millimeters (Key point 5, pp 13-39).
4. Calculate displacement:

$$\text{Displacement (millimeters)} = (X_D^2 + Y_D^2)^{1/2}$$

4. The above calculation could also have been figured by using the region of interest (ROI) capability around each point (Fig 14-23). In the interest of speed, file all five images through the ROI before moving to another ROI.

Key points

1. When using the ^{57}Co point sources, the plastic sheet may have a hole at the location of the radioactivity for increased sensitivity. The only purpose of the sheet is to move the sources back far enough to allow greater interaction with more PMTs. Hollow spacers would serve the same purpose.
2. An acceptable calculation of the displacement of information from the outer source through all five camera orientations reaffirms a correct COR.

LABORATORY APPLICATION

39

RECONSTRUCTED SYSTEM SPATIAL RESOLUTION

Purpose

System spatial resolution is the culmination of all the studies that have preceded this exercise. All previous exercises play a role in what size lesions can be visualized by the SPECT system. This is, after all, the "name of the game"—resolution.

Currently, there are two methods to evaluate resolution. One is the NEMA approach using the NEMA phantom (Fig. 14-18), which determines resolution of an imaging system with the classical expression of resolution—line-spread function (LSF) and the subsequent determination of full width, half maximum (FWHM). The other approach is a more subjective evaluation using a phantom containing a variety of hot and cold lesions in an environment of radioactivity (Fig. 14-19). The latter phantom may well satisfy the age-old concern of physicians who are less interested in FWHM measurements but more inclined to ask the question "What size lesion can I see with this system?"

Procedure 1 (NEMA)

Materials

1. NEMA phantom
2. Six syringes (2.5 ml) containing the following:
   a. 4 mCi (150 MBq)/1.0 ml in one syringe
   b. 2.5 mCi (100 MBq) 1.0 ml in each of two syringes
   c. Three empty syringes

This should ensure an accumulation count rate of <20,000 cps.

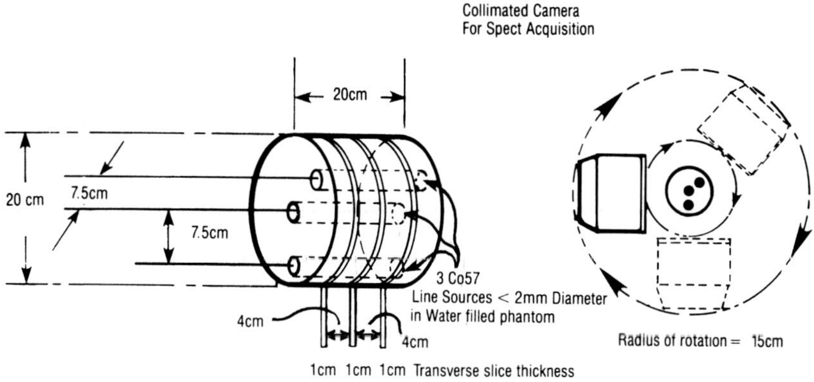

Accumulate projections into 256 × 256 matrices or 128 × 128 (zoomed × 2) matrices at < 20,000 cps through 20% window

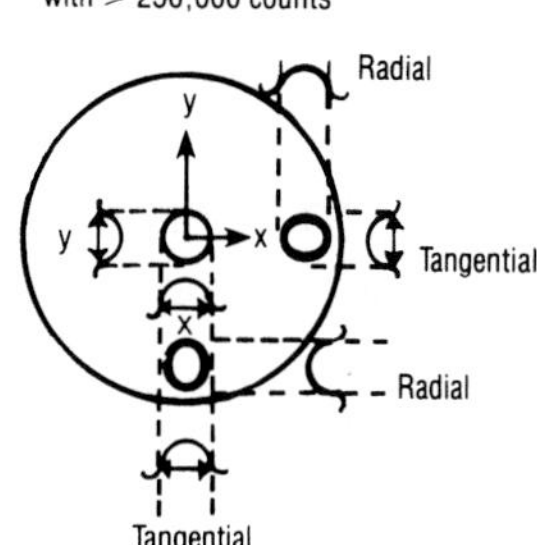

Fig. 14-25. Reconstructed system spatial resolution. (Courtesy Picker International, Cleveland, Ohio.)

Technique

1. Attach an LEHR collimator and confirm an acceptable COR and mechanical alignment.
2. Arrange a 20% window for ^{99m}Tc.
3. Accumulate a correction flood acquired into a:
   a. 256 × 256 matrix (no zoom), *or*
   b. 128 × 128 matrix with a ×2 preprocess zoom.
4. Fill NEMA phantom with tap water.
5. Remove needle and lock the three syringes containing radioactivity into the LEHR; lock devices on phantom according to the following arrangement:
   a. 4 mCi source in center line source
   b. 2.5 mCi sources in each peripheral line source
6. Attach empty syringes to the opposite side of each line source and draw contents into the line source. Leave all six syringes locked in place throughout the entire procedure.
7. Arrange the phantom such that the long axis is parallel to the axis of rotation and that the two off-center line sources will lie along the *X* and *Y* axis.
8. Set ideal radius of rotation of 150 mm (15 cm) around a 360° circle.
9. Set time per stop so that each slice = >250,000 counts according to:

$$\text{Total Counts/Stop} = \frac{\text{Phantom length (millimeters)}}{\text{Slice thickness (millimeters)}} \times \frac{\text{Desired counts/slice}}{\text{Number of stops}}$$

10. Begin SPECT study.

Data treatment

1. Reconstruct the images with a Ramp filter using appropriate attenuation correction and uniformity correction factors.
2. Reconstruct three slices transverse to the line source, each slice 10 mm ±3 mm at:
   a. Center of phantom
   b. 40 mm on each side of center (Fig. 14-25)

Continued.

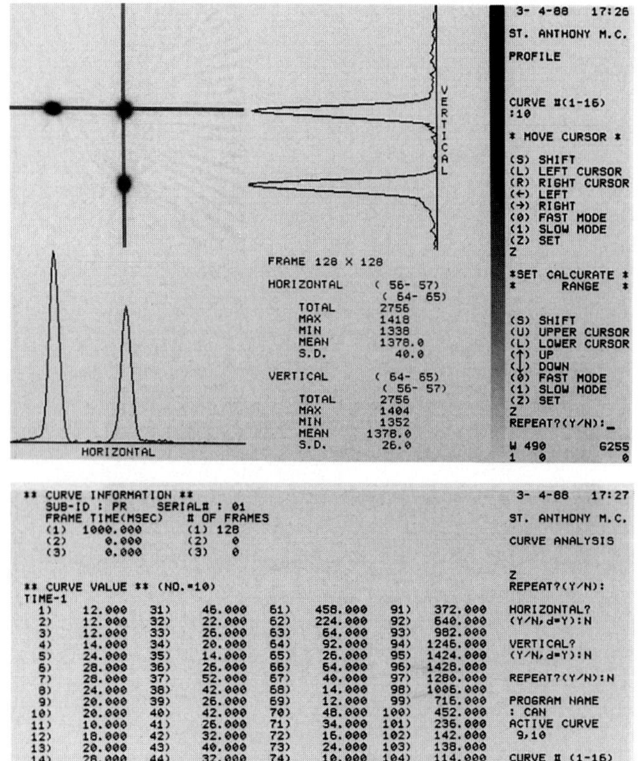


```
** CURVE INFORMATION **                                          3- 4-88   17:26
   SUB-ID : PR    SERIAL# : 01
   FRAME TIME(MSEC)    # OF FRAMES                              ST. ANTHONY M.C.
   (1)  1000.000       (1) 128
   (2)     0.000       (2)   0                                  CURVE ANALYSIS
   (3)     0.000       (3)   0

** CURVE VALUE ** (NO.= 9)                                      (S) SHIFT
TIME-1                                                          (U) UPPER CURSOR
  1)     6.000   31)   392.000   61)   478.000   91)    4.000   (L) LOWER CURSOR
  2)     6.000   32)   164.000   62)   752.000   92)    4.000   (↑) UP
  3)     6.000   33)    60.000   63)  1118.000   93)    0.000   (↓) DOWN
  4)    12.000   34)    28.000   64)  1338.000   94)    0.000   (0) FAST MODE
  5)    12.000   35)    16.000   65)  1418.000   95)    2.000   (1) SLOW MODE
  6)    22.000   36)     4.000   66)  1280.000   96)    6.000   (Z) SET
  7)    18.000   37)    14.000   67)  1002.000   97)    0.000   Z
  8)    22.000   38)    20.000   68)   702.000   98)    0.000   REPEAT?(Y/N):
  9)    36.000   39)     6.000   69)   438.000   99)    6.000
 10)    36.000   40)     2.000   70)   234.000  100)    4.000   HORIZONTAL?
 11)    32.000   41)     2.000   71)    90.000  101)    0.000   (Y/N,d=Y):N
 12)    32.000   42)     0.000   72)    48.000  102)    2.000
 13)    48.000   43)     8.000   73)    38.000  103)    0.000   VERTICAL?
 14)    44.000   44)    20.000   74)    30.000  104)    4.000   (Y/N,d=Y):N
 15)    42.000   45)    20.000   75)    28.000  105)    0.000
 16)    52.000   46)     6.000   76)    36.000  106)    8.000   REPEAT?(Y/N):N
 17)    60.000   47)     6.000   77)    28.000  107)   10.000
 18)    60.000   48)     0.000   78)    28.000  108)    8.000   PROGRAM NAME
 19)    82.000   49)     4.000   79)    28.000  109)    2.000   : CAN
 20)   152.000   50)    18.000   80)    22.000  110)    0.000   ACTIVE CURVE
 21)   306.000   51)    10.000   81)    14.000  111)    2.000    9,10
 22)   586.000   52)     8.000   82)    32.000  112)    4.000
 23)   968.000   53)     2.000   83)    36.000  113)    0.000   CURVE # (1-16)
 24)  1352.000   54)     0.000   84)    24.000  114)    0.000   : 9
 25)  1758.000   55)    10.000   85)    28.000  115)    0.000
 26)  1974.000   56)    24.000   86)    30.000  116)    0.000   CONTINUE?
 27)  1860.000   57)    50.000   87)    10.000  117)    0.000   (Y/N:d=Y):_
 28)  1534.000   58)   112.000   88)    18.000  118)    0.000
 29)  1128.000   59)   160.000   89)    24.000  119)    0.000   W 490      6255
 30)   728.000   60)   266.000   90)    14.000  120)    0.000   1   0         0
```

```
** CURVE INFORMATION **                                          3- 4-88   17:27
   SUB-ID : PR    SERIAL# : 01
   FRAME TIME(MSEC)    # OF FRAMES                              ST. ANTHONY M.C.
   (1)  1000.000       (1) 128
   (2)     0.000       (2)   0                                  CURVE ANALYSIS
   (3)     0.000       (3)   0
                                                                Z
** CURVE VALUE ** (NO.=10)                                      REPEAT?(Y/N):
TIME-1
  1)    12.000   31)    46.000   61)   458.000   91)   372.000   HORIZONTAL?
  2)    12.000   32)    22.000   62)   224.000   92)   640.000   (Y/N,d=Y):N
  3)    12.000   33)    26.000   63)    64.000   93)   982.000
  4)    14.000   34)    20.000   64)    92.000   94)  1246.000   VERTICAL?
  5)    24.000   35)    14.000   65)    26.000   95)  1424.000   (Y/N,d=Y):N
  6)    28.000   36)    26.000   66)    64.000   96)  1428.000
  7)    28.000   37)    52.000   67)    40.000   97)  1280.000   REPEAT?(Y/N):N
  8)    24.000   38)    42.000   68)    14.000   98)  1006.000
  9)    20.000   39)    26.000   69)    12.000   99)   716.000   PROGRAM NAME
 10)    20.000   40)    42.000   70)    48.000  100)   452.000   : CAN
 11)    10.000   41)    26.000   71)    34.000  101)   236.000   ACTIVE CURVE
 12)    18.000   42)    32.000   72)    16.000  102)   142.000    9,10
 13)    20.000   43)    40.000   73)    24.000  103)   138.000
 14)    28.000   44)    32.000   74)    10.000  104)   114.000   CURVE # (1-16)
 15)    36.000   45)    30.000   75)    10.000  105)   108.000   : 9
 16)    28.000   46)    38.000   76)     6.000  106)   104.000
 17)    30.000   47)    58.000   77)    10.000  107)    76.000   CONTINUE?
 18)    20.000   48)    52.000   78)    14.000  108)    58.000   (Y/N:d=Y):
 19)    16.000   49)    56.000   79)    26.000  109)    52.000
 20)    16.000   50)    88.000   80)    24.000  110)    58.000   STRIKE CR KEY !
 21)    22.000   51)   148.000   81)    16.000  111)    54.000
 22)    40.000   52)   290.000   82)     2.000  112)    44.000   CMND : N,10
 23)    30.000   53)   548.000   83)     4.000  113)    36.000   ACTIVE CURVE
 24)    34.000   54)   820.000   84)    14.000  114)    34.000    9,10
 25)    38.000   55)  1124.000   85)    22.000  115)    18.000
 26)    50.000   56)  1352.000   86)    12.000  116)    26.000   CONTINUE?
 27)    36.000   57)  1404.000   87)    12.000  117)    28.000   (Y/N:d=Y):_
 28)    24.000   58)  1300.000   88)    50.000  118)    48.000
 29)    32.000   59)  1010.000   89)    96.000  119)    50.000   W 490      6255
 30)    44.000   60)   730.000   90)   194.000  120)    30.000   1   0         0
```

Fig. 14-26. Image and slice profiles with accompanying counts/pixel printout showing line spread functions of each point source in the X and Y directions, FWHM values are calculated from these numerical printouts. (Note: Image processed on 128 × 128 matrix. Better FWHM Values could be achieved on 128 × 128 on a x2 zoom or on a 256 × 256 matrix size.)

Table 14-2. Data collection table for reconstructed system spatial resolution

Slice \ Point source	Tangential		Radial		Center	
	3:00	6:00	3:00	6:00	X	Y
1						
2						
3						
Average						

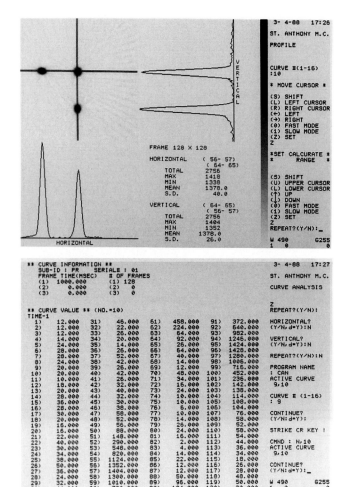

3. Arrange a slice profile through all point sources in both the X and Y directions of each of the three images. (Orienting the phantom such that the line sources fall on the X and Y coordinates allows this to be done in four slice profiles per image rather than six [Fig. 14-26]).
4. Observe the pixel location of each point source (the pixel receiving maximum counts*) in each image in both the X and Y directions (18 observations) by evaluating the count printout of the slice profile.
5. Calibrate the pixels (or the channel of the MCA) by:

$$\text{millimeter/pixel} = \frac{\text{Millimeters between sources}}{\text{Number of channels between peaks}} \text{ or } \frac{75^*}{X}$$

*The NEMA phantom is designed to be 75 mm between sources.

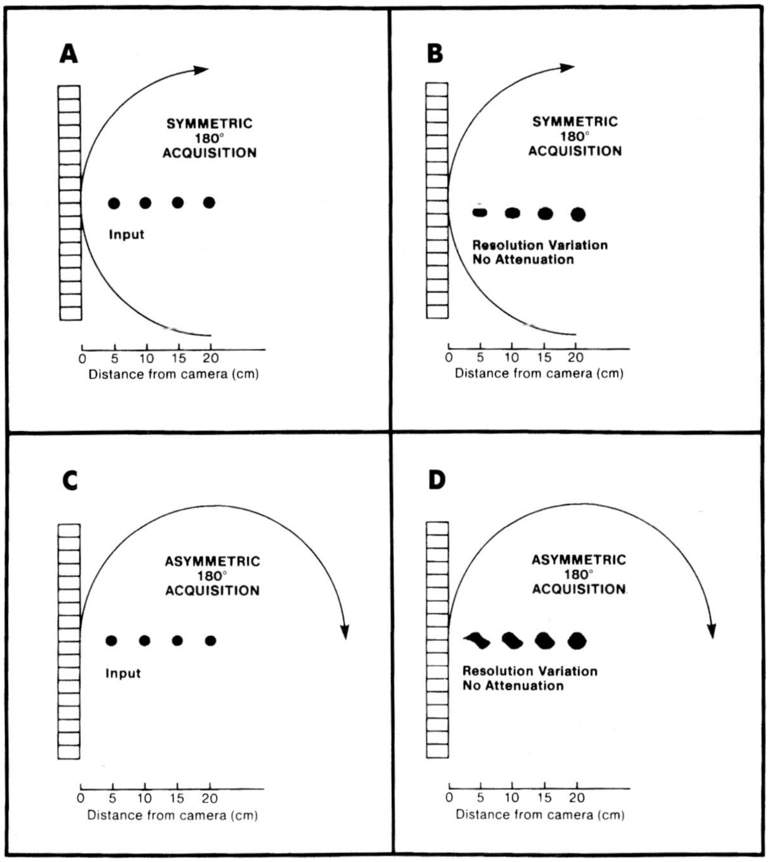

Fig. 14-27. A, Schematic representation of symmetric 180° camera acquisition of four point sources located at 5, 10, 15, and 20 cm from the camera in the anterior view. **B,** Tomographic reconstruction of the symmetric 180° acquisition. **C,** Schematic representation of asymmetric 180° camera acquisition of the four point sources. **D,** Tomographic reconstruction of the asymmetric 180° acquisition. (From Eisner, R.L.: Principles of instrumentation in SPECT, J. Nucl. Med. Technol. 13(3):23-31, March 1985.)

6. Calculate the FWHM for each point source in both the *X* and *Y* directions (18 calculations, 6 calculations per slice) on Table 14-2.
7. The above calculation could also have been figured by using the region of interest (ROI) around each point. In the interest of speed, file all three slices through the ROI before moving to another ROI.
8. Report as follows:
   a. Compute average FWHM values for the tangential slice profiles of the two lateral sources (6 calculations involved, 2 calculations per slice). See Fig. 14-25.
   b. Compute average FWHM values for the radial slice profiles of the two radial sources (6 calculations involved, 2 calculations per slice). See Fig. 14-25.
   c. Compute average FWHM values for both the *X* and *Y* slice profiles of the center source (6 calculations involved, 2 calculations per slice).

Key points

1. Following the resolution study using the NEMA phantom, the activity from the line sources can be removed by withdrawing the plunger on one side. These contents can then be introduced into the water, mixed thoroughly, and used for the SPECT uniformity study.
2. More activity of ^{99m}Tc is required in the center line source than on the periphery because of attenuation at 0.15 cm^{-1}.
3. The persistence scope allows the accurate placement of the radioactivity into the line source.
4. The reconstructed images of the round center source is always round; however, the reconstructed images of the round lateral sources are ovoid. It has been suggested that these distortions are due to inadequate attenuation and resolution correction algorithms. This suggests that distortions also occur in clinical studies and increase as data get farther removed from COR. Figure 14-27 using 180° acquisition shows that the degree of such distortions vary with depth. Distortions worsen if the 180° acquisitions are acquired asymmetrically.

Continued.

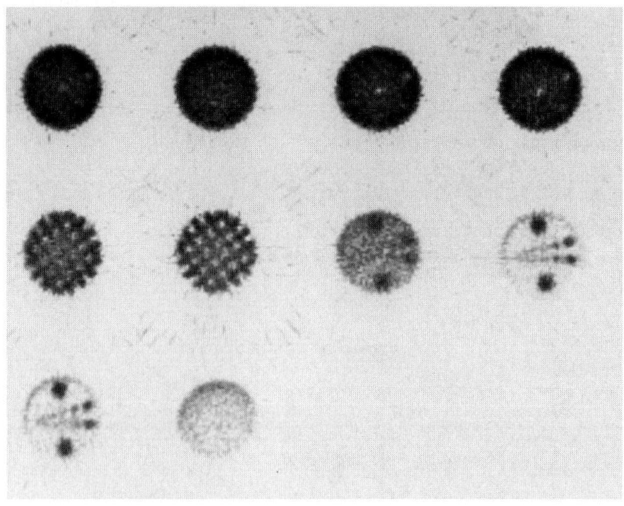

Fig. 14-28. Results of the SPECT phantom generated with count rates more consistent with a clinical study (180k counts/slice × 2 slices).

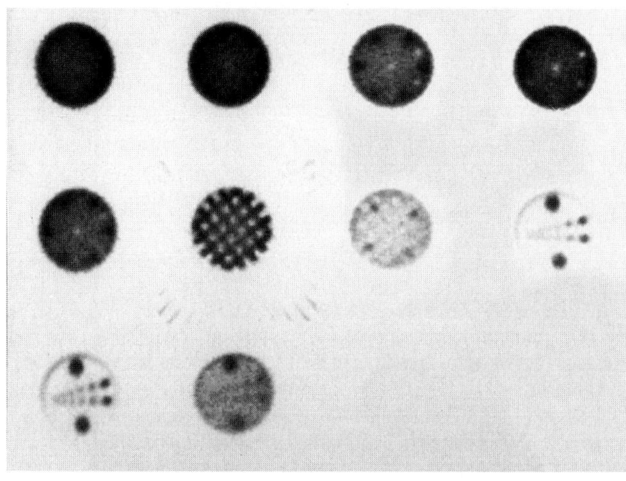

Fig. 14-29. Results of the SPECT phantom generated with high statistical count rates (966k counts/slice × 2 slices).

Procedure 2 (Nuclear Associates or Jasczczak Phantom)

Materials

1. 10 to 20 mCi (370 to 740 MBq) ^{99m}Tc
2. Cylindrical phantom (with hot and cold spots)

Technique

1. Attach an LEHR collimator and confirm an acceptable COR and mechanical alignment.
2. Arrange a 20% window for ^{99m}Tc.
3. Accumulate a 30 million count correction flood at a rate not greater than 30,000 cps on a 64 × 64 matrix (or 120 million count flood on a 128 × 128 matrix).
4. Fill Nuclear Associates (see Fig. 14-19) or Jasczczak phantom with tap water.
5. Introduce approximately 10 mCi (370 MBq) into phantom and mix thoroughly.
6. Arrange the phantom so that the longitudinal axis of the phantom is parallel to the axis of rotation.
7. Set ideal radius of rotation at 150 mm (15 cm) around a 360° circle.
8. Set time per stop so that each slice is approximately 200,000 counts (Fig. 14-28).
9. Repeat the study for high statistical images (i.e., 1,000,000 counts per slice with 128 images) (Fig. 14-29).
10. Repeat the study on a 128 × 128 reconstruction matrix using 128 views.

Data treatment

1. Reconstruct the images with a Ramp filter using appropriate attenuation and uniformity correction factors.
2. Reconstruct slice through the V-shaped block corresponding to hot lesions in a cold field.
3. Reconstruct slice through the grid section, checking for linearity.
4. Reconstruct slice through the plastic rods corresponding to cold lesions in a hot field.
5. Reconstruct slice through the area where no inserts appear, to test for uniformity.
6. Optional: Reconstruct slice through the cold spheres section of the phantom.
7. Repeat for all acquisitions using a Ramp filter.
8. Repeat for all acquisitions using other filters and note which filters work best under some conditions and not under others.
9. Compare results to images on Figs. 14-28, and 14-29. Are there any bull's-eye artifacts (see Fig. 14-17)?

Key points

1. Hot lesions in a cold field simulate brain and bone scans.
2. Cold lesions in a hot field simulate lung and liver scans.
3. The foregoing comparisons should have shown that certain filters prove more effective with high-count-rate studies. Which ones are they?
4. Above comparisons should allow the physician to choose the technique preferred for certain clinical studies.

BIBLIOGRAPHY

Rotating scintillation camera SPECT acceptance testing and quality control, AAPM Report No. 22, New York, 1987, AIP.

Chandra, R.: Introductory physics of nuclear medicine, ed. 4, Philadelphia, 1992, Lea & Febiger.

Croft, B.Y.: Single photon emission computed tomography, Chicago, 1986, Year Book Publishers.

Eisner, R.L.: Principles of instrumentation in SPECT, J. Nucl. Med. Technol. 13(1):23-31, March 1985.

Eisner, R.L., Nowak, D.J., Pettigrew, R., and Fajman, W.: Fundamentals of 180° acquisition and reconstruction in SPECT imaging, J. Nucl. Med. 27:1717-1728, 1986.

English, R.J., and Brown, S.E.: SPECT. single photon emission computed tomography: a primer, ed. 2, New York, 1990, SNM.

Folks, R., Banks, L., Plankey, M., Mattera, J., Greene, R., Brust, K., Graham, M., and Caputo, G.: Cardiovascular SPECT. A continuing education series, J. Nucl. Med. Technol. 13(3):150-162, 1985.

Garcia, E.V.: Digital processing in nuclear medicine imaging, J. Nucl. Med. Technol. 14(1):21-31, 1986.

Go, R.T., MacIntyre, W.J., and Houser, T.S., and others: Clinical evaluation of 360° and 180° data sampling techniques for transaxial SPECT thallium 201 myocardial perfusion imaging, J. Nucl. Med. 26:695-706, 1985.

Greer, K., Jaszczak, R., Harris, C. and Coleman, R.E.: Quality control in SPECT, J. Nucl. Med. Technol. 13(2):76-85, 1985.

Halama, J.R., and Henkin, R.E.: Quality assurance in SPECT imaging, Appl. Radiol., May 1987.

Mueller, S.P., Polak, J.F., Kijewski, M.F., and Holman, B.L.: Collimator selection for SPECT brain imaging: the advantage of high resolution, J. Nucl. Med. 27(11):1729-1738, 1986.

Murphy, P.H.: Acceptance testing and quality control of gamma cameras including SPECT, J. Nucl. Med. 28:1221-1227, 1987.

NEMA standards for performance measurements of scintillation cameras, Pub. No. NU1-1986, National Electrical Manufacturers Association, NEMA, 1986.

Rao, D.V., Early, P.J., Chu, R.Y., Goodwin, P.N., and Graham, L.S.: Radiation control and quality assurance surveys—nuclear medicine a suggested protocol, ACMP Report No. 3, 1986.

Sorenson, J.A., and Phelps, M.E.: Physics in nuclear medicine, New York, 1987, Grune & Stratton, Inc.

Tuscan, M.J., Rogers, W.L., Juni, J.E., and Clinthorne, N.H.: Analysis of gamma camera detector stability and its effect on uniformity correction for SPECT, J. Nucl. Med. Technol. 13(1):1-4, March 1985.

Woronowicz, E.M., Eisner, G.T., Gullberg, G.T., Nowak, D.J., and Mulko, J.A.: Factors affecting single photon emission computed tomography image quality and recommended QC procedures, Milwaukee, Wis., General Electric Medical Systems Operations.

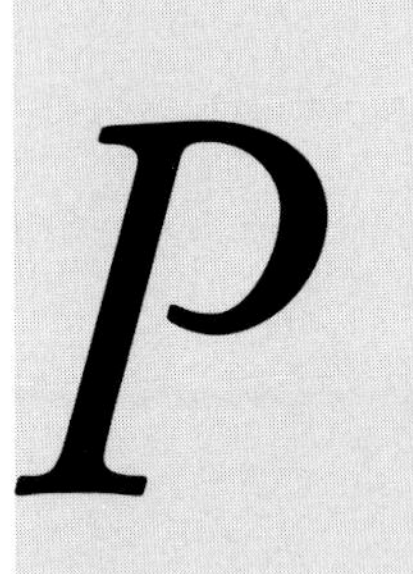

Chapter 15

OSITRON EMISSION TOMOGRAPHY (PET)

PAUL J. EARLY

While positron emission tomography (PET) may seem to be a new modality to the nuclear medicine armamentarium, it is not a newcomer by any means. The value of positron emission and imaging was recognized early by Brownell and Sweet in 1953 with the first positron scanner being developed in 1970 (MGH, Boston). However, it has only recently become clinically useful with the advent of improved instrumentation, development of computer hardware and software, and the birth of "baby" cyclotrons. While all are still quite expensive, the concept of PET centers has moved out of the university research centers and is being viewed by large suburban hospitals and clinics as clinically and financially feasible. Even national radiopharmaceutical companies (e.g., Mallinckrodt Medical, Inc.) have recognized the fiscally rewarding possibility of regional cyclotron centers to provide PET radiopharmaceuticals.

PET is unique in its ability to create "functional" images of blood flow or metabolic processes rather than the more conventional structural or anatomic images produced by x-ray examination, computed tomography (CT), magnetic resonance imaging (MRI), and even single photon emission computerized tomography (SPECT). The functional nature of PET data permits investigation and comparison of events occurring at the cellular level. These data are not attainable by other conventional imaging devices.

With the availability of smaller, effective cyclotrons, it is possible to produce short-lived positron radiotracers of basic organic elements such as carbon (^{11}C), nitrogen (^{13}N), oxygen (^{15}O), and fluorine (^{18}F). These basic elements are "tagged" to common organic molecules found in the body and therefore can be made specifically for a target organ. For example, brain tumors can be imaged using glucose tagged with ^{18}F; the heart can be imaged using ammonia tagged with ^{13}N. Both agents are used to determine function and/or viability of tissue in the brain and heart respectively. While interest in tumor imaging stimulated the early development of PET, recent development of an on-site generator produced positron emitter (^{82}Rb) has stimulated PET studies of the heart and greatly expanded the clinical utility of this new imaging modality. A partial list of routinely used positron-emitting nuclides can be seen on Table 15-1. A partial list of positron-emitting radiopharmaceuticals that could have routine use can be seen on Table 15-2.

■ PRINCIPLES OF PET

The basis of positron emission tomography is the positron—that positively charged beta particle emitted from neutron-poor radionuclides. The end result of that emission is annihilation through interaction with an electron and the total conversion of that combined mass to 1.02 MeV of energy. The unique aspect of this conversion is that the resultant conversion is not one gamma ray of 1.02 MeV but two gamma rays, each equal to exactly one half of that energy—511 keV. Furthermore, these two gamma rays are emitted at 180° to each other. It is these two facts that allow for the external detection of the positron event. Two detectors, placed on each side of the positron-emitting object, can be arranged to absorb both emissions simultaneously and to process their resultant pulses simultaneously. This is performed through the use of a coincidence circuit (the opposite result of the anticoincidence circuit used in routine pulse height analysis). The simultaneous processing of these two events is the key to positron imaging. To be counted, both events must be detected at the same time and be received by the coincidence circuit at the same time. If two events are received in coincidence by this circuit, they will then be "perceived" as being of positron origin, and they will be accepted for further evaluation by the pulse-height analysis and positional analysis circuits. In any counting situation, positron or not, two unrelated events can interact in opposing crystals at the same time, giving false information. These are called *random events*. Keeping them to a minimum is always desirable. This is no different for positron imaging. Once accepted, whether random or true, the electronics will position the event on or

Table 15-1. Positron emitting nuclides common to nuclear medicine

Radionuclide	Half-life (minutes)	Positron yield	Positron energy (MeV)
Cyclotron-produced			
O-15	2.04	99+%	1.72
N-13	9.96	99+%	1.19
C-11	20.4	99+%	0.96
F-18	110.0	96.9%	0.64
Generator-produced			
Rb-82	1.27	96%	3.35
Cu-62	9.8	98%	2.93
Ga-68	68.1	90%	1.90

about a line connecting the centers of the two detectors. If an event is not received in coincidence with another event, it is "perceived" by the system to be not of positron origin and it is rejected. This would occur with background; with scatter photons; or when the annihilation event occurs outside the sensitive volume (the solid angle) of both opposing detectors, in which case only one photon is detected.

This system offers a unique feature to nuclear medicine imaging: no need for collimation. In all other imaging systems, it is necessary to discard a large percentage of events by interposing a lead collimator between the source and the detector to absorb or scatter the unwanted gamma rays and thereby determine the source of the gamma ray. The improvement to sensitivity is between 25- and 100-fold, depending on the size of the positron detectors and system resolution.

■ THE PET CAMERA

A state-of-the-art positron emission tomography (PET) camera (Fig. 15-1) is a device that looks physically like a CT imager but operates differently. A positron camera detects and reconstructs transmitted data. It relies on variations in amounts of radioactivity accumulated in any given area. The CT imager relies on relative attenuation of x-rays between the x-ray tube and the detector. In both cases, however, the data are reconstructed into computer-generated, cross-sectional images using traditional reconstruction algorithms.

The PET camera is a device that uses rings of detectors arranged in a circle around the patient (Fig. 15-2, *A*) or in a hexagonal array (Fig. 15-2, *B*) where the detectors are grouped into "buckets" or "cassettes" (Fig. 15-2, *C*). The contents of each bucket vary with the manufacturer, but there can be as many as 256 discrete crystals being viewed by 16 photomultiplier tubes (four blocks composed of 64 crystals and four PMTs each) (Fig. 15-3, *A, B, C*) with as many as three rings of 16 buckets in a circle (12,288 crystals with 768 PMTs). An alternative design to a bucket is one that uses rings of detectors with 11 crystals in a staggered array being viewed by 6 PMTs (Fig. 15-4, *A* and *B*). To reduce the cost of these cameras, there is some consideration being given to reducing the number of detectors by about 30%, thus necessitating rotating detectors.

In positron imaging, the opposing detectors define the line along which the event occurred, both in the *X-Y* directions and in the *Z* direction (Fig. 15-5). This arrangement precludes the use of collimators and serves to increase the count rate sensitivity. This is often referred to as "electronic

Table 15-2. Positron emitting radionuclides common to nuclear medicine

Radiopharmaceutical	Application
[^{15}O]-O_2	Cerebral oxygen extraction and metabolism
[^{15}O]-CO	Cerebral blood volume Myocardial blood volume
[^{15}O]-H_2O	Cerebral blood flow Myocardial blood flow
[^{13}N]-NH_3	Myocardial blood flow
[^{11}C]-*n*-butanol	Cerebral blood flow
[^{11}C]-palmitate	Myocardial metabolism
[^{11}C]-acetate	Myocardial metabolism
[^{11}C]-glucose	Cerebral glucose metabolism
[^{11}C]-*N*-methylspiperone	Dopamine receptor binding
[^{18}F]-fluorodeoxyglucose	Cerebral glucose metabolism Myocardial glucose metabolism Tumor localization
[^{18}F]-spiperone	Dopamine receptor binding
[^{18}F]-16α-fluoro-17β-estradiol	Estrogen receptor binding
[^{82}Rb]-Rb+	Myocardial blood flow
[^{68}Ga]-citrate/transferrin	Plasma volume

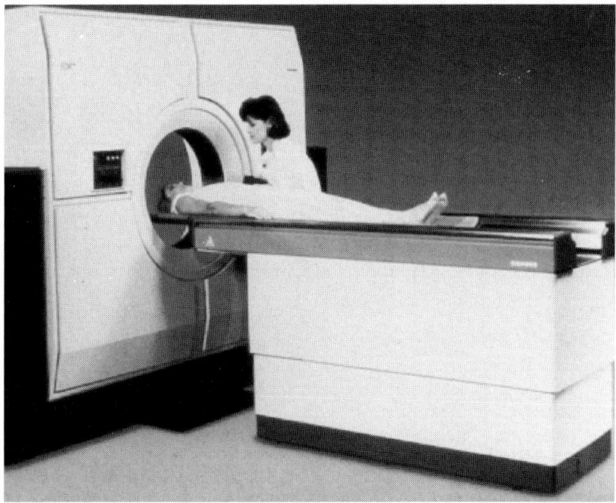

Fig. 15-1. Positron Emission Tomography (PET) camera. (Courtesy, Siemens Medical Systems, Inc.)

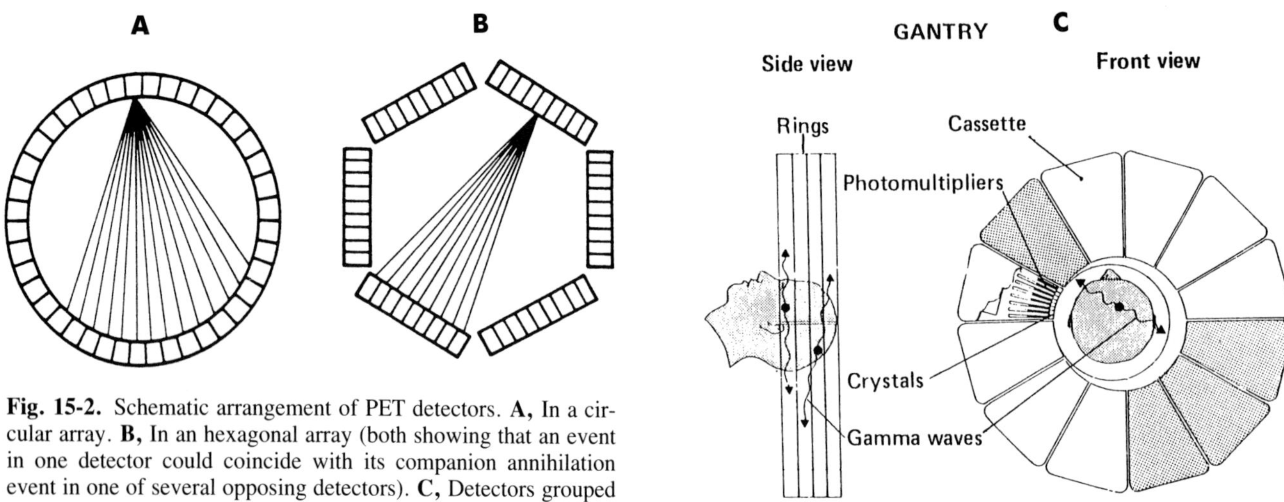

Fig. 15-2. Schematic arrangement of PET detectors. **A,** In a circular array. **B,** In an hexagonal array (both showing that an event in one detector could coincide with its companion annihilation event in one of several opposing detectors). **C,** Detectors grouped into cassettes. (Courtesy Siemens Medical Systems, Inc.)

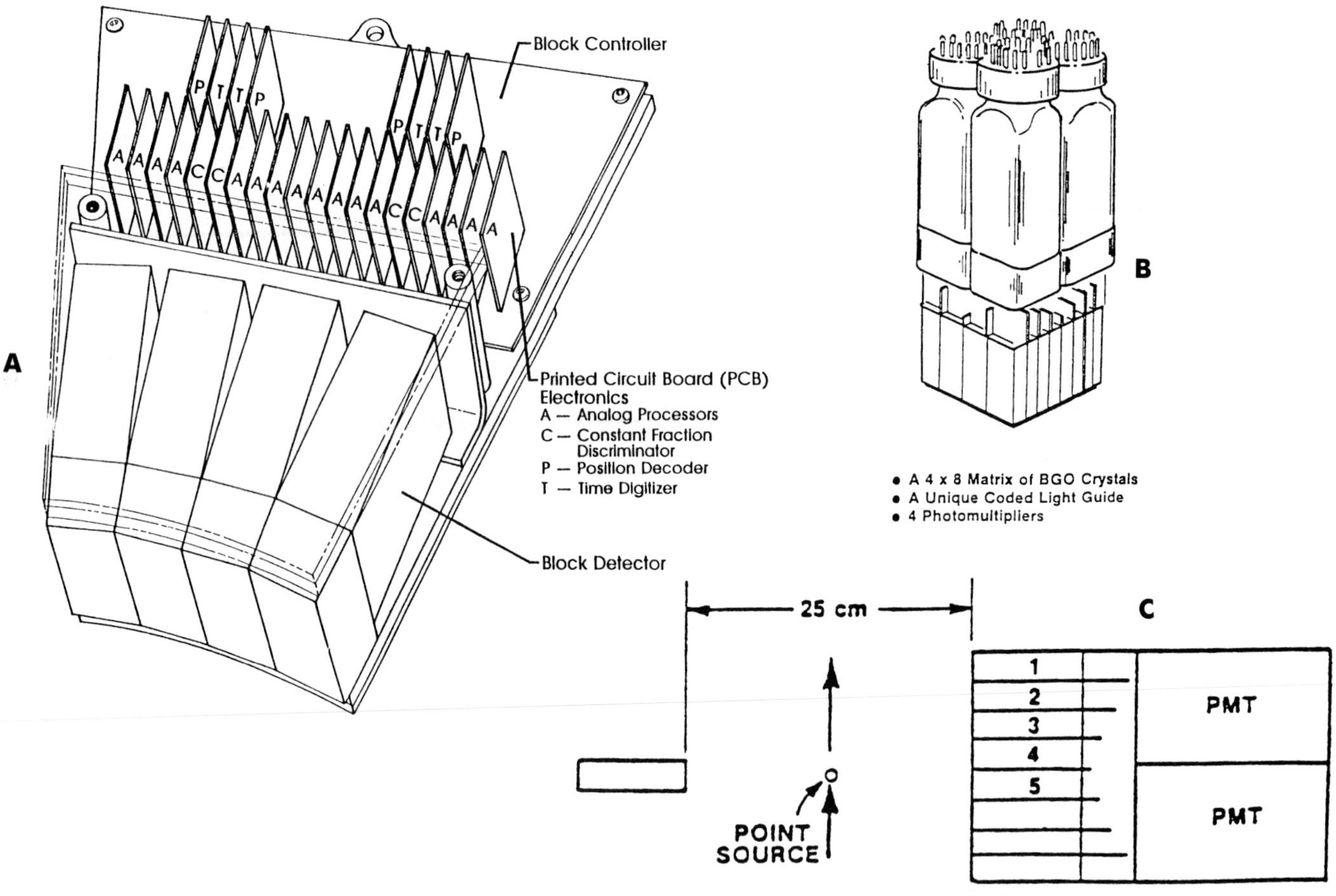

Fig. 15-3. A, Cassette (bucket) containing four block detectors. **B,** Closeup of a multi-crystal block detector. **C,** Schematic showing the relationship of a multiple crystal detector to two photomultiplier tubes (PMTs). (The multiple crystals are formed by making a series of saw-blade cuts into one BGO crystal at varying depths, none of which will extend through the entirety of the crystal.) If the event occurs in crystal #1, approximately 100% of the light produced in the crystal will be received by PMT A while approximately 0% is received by PMT B. If the event occurs in crystal #2, PMT A will receive approximately 93% and B, 7% of the light. If the event occurs in crystal #3, PMT A receives approximately 78% and B, 22%. Light produced in crystal #4 results in PMT A receiving approximately 59% and B, 41%. The remaining crystals have reverse ratios: crystal #5 results in PMT A receiving approximately 41% and B, 59%, etc. In this way, the location of the event can be uniquely identified. (Courtesy Siemens Medical Systems, Inc.)

collimation." Septal rings (Fig. 15-6) made of lead do have some collimation effect, but they are designed primarily for prevention of coincidence crosstalk and to reduce the useless components of count rate (see "Septal Rings" in this chapter).

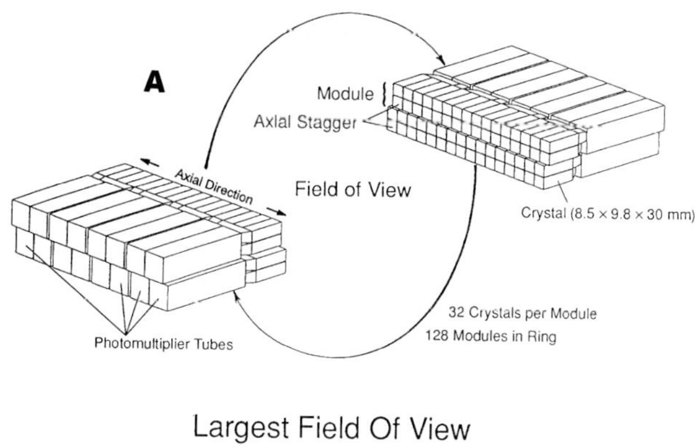

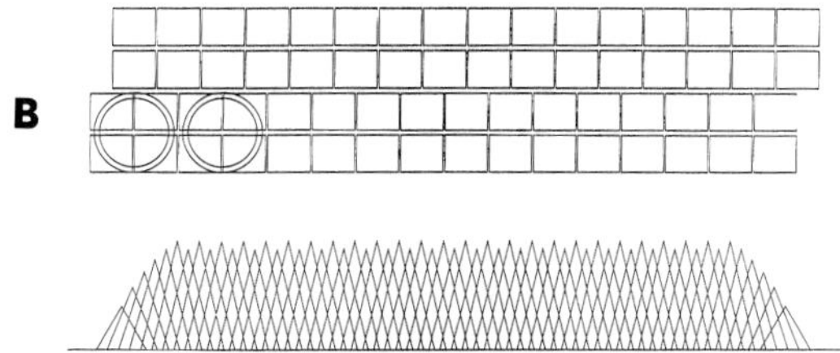

Fig. 15-4. **A,** An innovative PET detector arrangement that provides improved axial sampling. **B,** Schematic showing staggered arrangement of two modular detectors, each containing 32 crystals (rectangles) and 8 PMTs (circles). An event will be seen entirely by one PMT or partially by two PMTs depending upon which detector receives the incident photon, using a one-dimensional light spreading technique. (Courtesy Positron Corp., Houston, Tex.)

■ Time-of-flight versus non–time-of-flight

There have been two major approaches to the determination of positional information (i.e., where the annihilation event occurred). One is the time-of-flight (TOF) method and the other is the non–time-of-flight (NTOF) method.

The TOF method. It is obvious that if two detectors are equidistant from the emission of the pair of gamma rays, the two gamma rays will strike the opposing crystals at exactly the same time and be accepted by the coincidence circuit. However, what happens when an annihilation event occurs that is not equidistant from the two detectors (Fig. 15-7)? In this case, the photon originating closer to the detector will arrive several nanoseconds sooner than the other photon arrives at its detector. (In a 1-m ring, the maximum is 3.3 nsec. For human dimensions, the maximum is 2.2

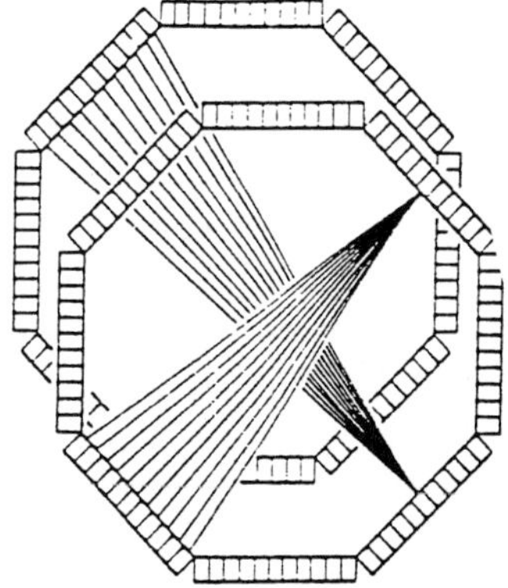

Fig. 15-5. Schematic of two side-by-side rings of detectors showing that an event on one detector could coincide with the detection of its companion annihalation event in one of several opposing detectors in another ring (Z or axial direction).

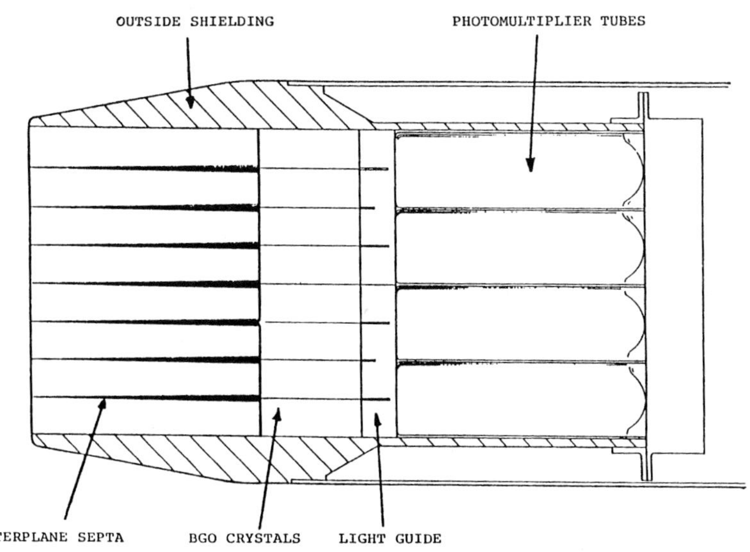

Fig. 15-6. A slice through a detector showing septal rings. (Courtesy Siemens Medical Systems, Inc.)

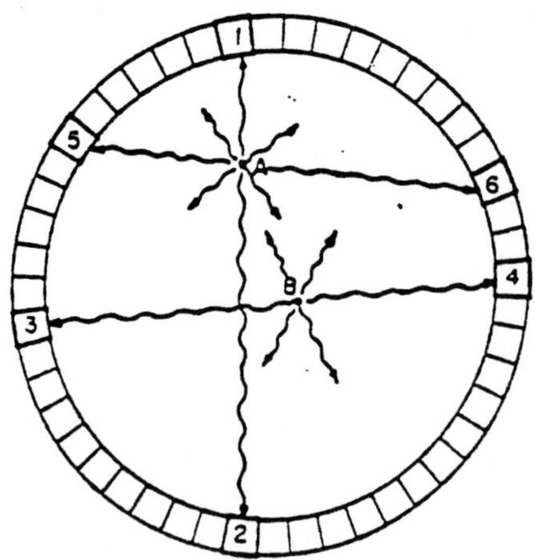

Fig. 15-7. Schematic illustrating "time-of-flight" position analysis.

nsec.) This time "window" is a variable that is defined in the coincidence electronics for the "size" of a human subject. The wider the time window, the less resolution in the final image. Whatever the window size, the time differential can be calculated because photons travel at the speed of light, permitting the event to be used as a valid positioning event. Once the positioning information is complete, the range along the line of response is calculated and positioning signals are sent to the CRT, resulting in the registration of the event. Data can also be sent to the computer matrix as a ray sum that can be subjected to filtering and back projection reconstruction techniques. The range with a 0.5-nsec resolution (best possible result) is uncertain by ± 30 cm/2 $\times$ 0.5 = ± 7.5 cm. This really poor depth resolution is the reason why TOF has failed.

The NTOF method. The method that has become the accepted norm is the non–time-of-flight (NTOF) method. It differs from the TOF method in that the exact X-Y location is not as important as is the line of flight taken by the photons. This is accomplished by identifying the two opposing crystals that shared in the two detection events and "drawing" an electronic vector between the two crystals. Once the line along which the event occurred is identified, all pixels of the computer matrix that represent that line receive the count uniformly. The superimposition of multiple lines from all angles (due to subsequent pairs of 511 keV photons going off at other angles) serves to accentuate the areas of increased or decreased radioactivity (Fig. 12-30). This is further delineated on completion of the image acquisition when the data are subjected to routine filtering and back projection algorithms as seen in SPECT and CT (see Chapter 12). There are arguments for and against both of these techniques. It appears, however, that the differences may be more a result of the crystal that is used in combination with the detection analysis technique than a result of the technique itself. At the very least, it is a combination of crystal and technique.

■ PET DETECTORS

PET detectors are composed of crystals and photomultiplier tubes as previously discussed in Chapter 10. Positron detectors are usually made of much more dense material than that used for lower-energy, single-photon detection. This material includes bismuth germanate or BGO ($Bi_3Ge_4O_{12}$), barium fluoride (BaF_2), and cesium fluoride (CsF). NaI can be used provided it is thick enough (e.g., 1½ inches). There are some characteristics, such as light yield that lend NaI well to PET detection. All of these crystals are about 5 mm wide to provide high-resolution images (Figs. 15-3, *A* and 15-4, *B*). A characteristic of these crystals is their ability to emit light as a result of interaction of the gamma ray similar to NaI. The light is then directed to the photomultiplier tube where it is converted to current as discussed in Chapter 10. Unlike other nuclear medicine equipment with which one crystal is viewed by one or more PMTs, modern PET detectors are composed of multiple crystals being "viewed" by one photomultiplier tube. Variations of this arrangement are used by the manufacturers of the equipment.

■ BGO versus BaF_2

In addition to the consideration of TOF versus NTOF, any discussion of PET detectors must include the type of crystal used. Traditionally, BGO crystals, and recently, NaI crystals, have been used with NTOF technology, and BaF_2 (or CsF) crystals are used with TOF technology. Other combinations, however, are possible. Which crystal is used depends on whether the imaging equipment is to be used in a situation requiring high–count-rate handling capability or highest-quality image (highest signal-to-noise) ratios. These decisions must be based on the four basic parameters of crystal characteristics:

1. Detector sensitivity
2. Random count rate
3. Scatter count rate
4. Light yield
5. Scintillator decay

Detector sensitivity. The purpose of any good PET camera is to keep untrue events as low in number as possible to be able to process more true coincidence events. This is a function of detector sensitivity. Sensitivity varies with detector size and density discriminator threshold level and with multiple coincidence detection capability. Assuming detector size and discriminator threshold levels are the same, the variables become detector material density and multiple coincidence detector capability. BGO has a density of 7.13 g/cm^3, while BaF_2 has a density of 4.89 g/cm^3 (NaI is 3.67 g/cm^3) (Table 15-3). Regardless of where the discriminator threshold is set, the coincidence efficiency of BGO excels that of BaF_2. The coincidence efficiencies (Table 15-4) of BGO and BaF_2 at a threshold setting at the

Table 15-3. Properties of various PET detectors

	Density g/cm³	Decay time (nsec)	Light yield	Hygroscopic
BGO	7.13	300	12	No
BaF_2	4.89	0.8(620)	5	No
CsF	4.64	3	8	Yes
NaI (Tl)	3.67	100	100	Yes

Table 15-4. Coincidence efficiencies of PET detectors

	Threshold of 511 keV	Threshold of 100 keV
BGO	41%	56%
BaF_2	8%	34%

511 photopeak are 41% and 8% respectively. Compare that to a threshold setting of 100 keV in which the values are 56% and 34% respectively, which suggests that BGO has a higher detector sensitivity than BaF_2 regardless of threshold setting. These data also suggest that the threshold setting must be low for BaF_2 to get any coincidence efficiency at all, allowing for the detection of more random and scatter events that cause deterioration of the image.

Random count rate. Random events (termed *randoms*) are photon pairs that reach the detectors at the same time by sheer chance. They may be annihilation gamma rays from two unassociated positron annihilation events or they may be completely unrelated to the pair of annihilation gamma photons and therefore considered undesirable. The more randoms, the worse the image resolution. If the time during which coincidence events are accepted is shortened, fewer randoms interfere with the image and the resolution is improved. Randoms can be eliminated by standard subtraction techniques. Therefore, the higher the threshold discriminator and the narrower the coincidence time window, the fewer randoms are detected. Time resolution is also a function of the detector. BGO has a poorer time resolution than BaF_2 by a factor of about 10, as a result of its scintillation pulse profile. BGO is used with a coincidence time window of 12 nsec while BaF_2 has a window of 3.3 nsec. If two unrelated gamma rays interact with opposing BGO crystals within 12 nsec, a random is recorded.

Scatter count rate. An inspection of the 511 keV energy spectrum with BGO and BaF_2 reveals much more scattered photons because of Comptons in the detector with BaF_2 than with BGO. This suggests that the time spent rejecting all those scatter photons would result in a rejection of the true coincidence counts because of dead-time considerations. With BGO, since there are fewer scatter photons to reject, there is more time to accept true coincidence counts. Therefore, BGO has a lower scatter count rate as well as an increased true coincidence count rate contributing to improved image resolution over the use of BaF_2 crystals. When one or more of the annihilation gamma rays scatter in the object, there exists a possibility that both gamma rays will strike both detectors connected in coincidence. In so doing, data is placed in incorrect locations. This can amount to 15% of the total count rate. However, since these events are spread over a large area (as opposed to true counts concentrated in a small area), the result is a high signal-to-noise ratio (ratio of true-to-scattered). Failure to compensate for these accidental coincidences causes overestimates in measurements of radionuclide concentrations from the image data.

Light yield. Another feature in the consideration of the appropriate crystal for detection of positrons is the amount of light produced per photon interaction. NaI (Tl) has been used for decades because of its high light yield (Table 15-3) holding a relative value of 100. Other PET detectors pale by comparison. This is why there is great interest in using NaI (Tl) crystal for PET detectors even though density, hydroscopicity, and decay times might contraindicate its use. Furthermore, standard pulse-height analysis techniques can be employed to rule out scatter, randoms, etc., and therefore obviate septal rings in the gantry.

Scintillator decay time. All crystals have characteristic scintillation decay times. Scintillator light output is usually seen as a rapid rise in light output followed by a slower light release (decay time), which in some instances reaches exponential rates or even slower. BGO has a scintillation decay time of 300 nanoseconds, whereas BaF_2 has a fast and a slow component measuring 0.8 and 620 nsec respectively (Table 15-3). This fast component has been viewed by many as the primary reason that BaF_2, in combination with the TOF method of detection, is the system of choice for high–count-rate studies. Others have said that although these facts are true, the other parameter favoring BGO and NTOF preclude the use of BaF_2. Currently, as the system producing the highest quality image regardless of the count rate, the BGO-NTOF system is being accepted as the standard of the industry.

■ CHARACTERISTICS OF A PET CAMERA

In addition to the parameters just discussed, there are several other characteristics that affect the quality of an image from PET. These characteristics affect the results after the choice of camera, its detection system, and associated electronics has been made.

■ Spatial resolution

Spatial resolution is a combination of all the features discussed above. In addition, there are two factors that cannot be controlled. They are range of positrons in tissue and annihilation photons that vary from the 180° direction of travel.

Table 15-5. Characteristics of positrons

Nuclide	E_{max} (MeV)	Gammas (singles)	Maximum range in lucite (cm)	Attenuation in H_2O (cm)*	
				50%	95%
^{18}F	0.64	None	0.23	0.038	0.110
^{11}C	0.97	None	0.35	0.074	0.197
^{13}N	1.20	None	0.50	0.097	0.263
^{15}O	1.74	None	0.76	0.160	0.418
^{82}Rb	3.15	11	1.6	. . .	. . .

*From Ellett, W.H., and Humes, R.M.: Absorbed fractions for small volumes containing photon-emitting radioactivity, MIRD Pamphlet No. 8, New York, 1971, Society of Nuclear Medicine.

Range of positrons in tissue. Positrons are emitted with a whole spectrum of energies. Maximum energies of various positron emitters are known, but the actual energy of any positron emitted from the radionuclide varies from that maximum energy all the way to approximately zero energy. Each radionuclide has a different maximum value for its positron. For example, Carbon-11 has a β^+ value of 0.972 MeV as opposed to Fluorine-18, which has a β^+ value of only 0.64 MeV. Table 15-5 lists the significant characteristics of the well-known PET radionuclides. Note that the high energy of ^{82}Rb as well as the presence of 11 "singles" all contribute to a degradation in resolution that is not common to the other four radionuclides. Also, recognize their attenuation characteristics in water (and therefore in tissue). As a result of the energy distribution of positrons (not too unlike the energy distribution of beta particles in Chapter 4), 50% of positrons are attenuated in approximately the first one-third of their maximum path length. As the energy increases, the tissue penetration before annihilation is greater and the resolution decreases.

Variations from 180° emissions. Although classical expressions of the positron annihilation phenomenon suggest that all such photons are emitted at exactly 180° from each other, it is now thought that this is not always the case. Sometimes the positron and the electron will not be completely at rest mass at the time of annihilation, which results in a deviation from the exact 180° emission. At room temperature, this error is about $\pm 0.6°$. The result of this deviation is a reduction in spatial resolution. These two variables (β^+ energy + 180° variations) account for their own contribution to resolution degradation. It has been calculated that the contribution from these two parameters alone can account for resolution inaccuracies of 1.5 to 3.0 mm in PET images. Since some important objects of study are of that size (e.g., myocardium is 8 to 12 mm thick), this represents a serious limitation.

■ Attenuation

The attenuation of annihilation photons is an object of concern in PET imaging, just as it is in SPECT. There is, however, one major exception. Since this is an annihilation event with two photons going in opposite directions, attenuation is independent of source position between the detectors. This is not the case in SPECT. In PET, attenuation is measured for each line of response by using an external source. The loss for each emitted line of response is scaled to compensate and yield attenuation-corrected tomographs directly. The half thickness for annihilation photons in water is about 7 cm. These corrections permit PET tomograms to be used in quantitative assays of radionuclide activity concentrations and in vivo biochemical determinations of function.

■ Stationary versus wobble

As a result of data gaps in early detector systems, both in the *X-Y* (transverse) directions and, more dramatically, in the *Z* (axial) direction, it was perceived early by PET manufacturers that stationary PET imaging devices would be unsatisfactory in certain clinical instances. To overcome this problem, the detectors were designed to oscillate around the center axis in a "wobbling" motion, "filling in" these data gaps. Such systems enhance resolution. Some systems have a staggered crystal arrangement in the axial direction but still require wobbling for the transverse sections. Such studies take longer to perform, but with enhanced resolution as a result. Many users decline to use wobble in newer systems, because clinical resolution differences are difficult to discern. It is argued that stationary acquisitions allow greater freedom in observations of dynamic processes.

■ Dead time

Dead-time losses in PET are more profound than in single-photon systems. They involve not only the coincidence count rates that increase as radioactivity increases, but also random coincidence counts in significant amounts that add to dead time losses well before pileup events paralyze the scanners. The detectors themselves have in the past been a large contributor to dead-time losses. Early models of PET cameras used large detectors in which scatter photons could move within the crystal. With the advent of multicrystal detectors (each detector being only 10 to 20 mm in size) and with the use of lead septa (termed *collimators*), the movement of scatter photons is restricted and light collection is much more efficient. Increases in the number of randoms and scatter also increase dead-time losses. If the circuitry is "tied up" rejecting pileup or scatter, it is not available to accept true coincidence events. Another contribution to dead time may be the choice of radionuclide. ^{11}C is a pure positron emitter and therefore has no single photon, whereas ^{82}Rb has many "singles" in addition to the positron (Table 15-5). The more singles, the greater the coincidence dead time. The largest source of dead-time losses is multiple coincidence (two or more coincidence events that occur at the same time). Because many crystals share the same coincidence circuitry (it is too expensive to have one circuit for each opposing crystal pair), a second coincidence event will be rejected by the system because the circuitry is already occupied with the first coincidence event. Dead-time losses would be reduced if the operator chose to accept only coincidence events that occurred in crystals exactly 180° opposite, but this greatly reduces the count rate and therefore the statistical validity from a clinical study as well. To increase counts, the operator is often able to choose the number of crystals off 180° to include in the imaging process; this is at the expense of dead time, however. The hexagonal-ring PET camera (Fig. 15-4), for instance, has a circuitry configuration in which each bank of detectors is connected in coincidence with all the detectors in the opposing bank; each bank can be expanded to all the detectors in another ring. As the number of crystals used in the detection process increases, the count rate increases. At the same time, dead time losses are increased and resolution decreases. Modern PET systems limit the number of detectors to which the system can be expanded. In so doing, they limit the line of response radii to reduce matrix size and data-transfer time. Dead times can be measured and corrections made on the images. To do anything else would reduce one of the major assets of PET imagery—quantification. The method requires circuitry that measures not only the coincidence counting rates but also the single-channel count rates for each coincidence circuit. If dead-time corrections were not applied, areas of high count rate would appear less in concentration than they really were and would not be a true reflection of count rate differentials between other areas of lesser activity because those areas would have fewer dead-time losses. One approach to directly measuring random event densities is to create a delayed coincidence window and corresponding sinogram frames to be subtracted (after smoothing) from the prompt sinograms. This subtraction is independent of dead-time corrections and yields a true coincidence sinogram that can be properly scaled for dead time and attenuation before filtered back-projection.

■ Septal rings

Septal rings (collimators) are lead disks placed between each ring of detectors (see Fig. 15-6). The outside two disks are usually thicker than the rest to shield the detector from extraneous singles and scatter photons in the room. The inner septal disks are thinner because their purpose is to improve the rates of coincident events to noncoincident events and to reduce the detector solid angle for activity outside the image plane. These septa have been shown to keep the detector-plane-to-detector-plane coincidence crosstalk to somewhere around 2%. These shields are stationary during acquisition and are not easily interchanged. More recent technology suggests that these be removed entirely. In so doing, sensitivity is increased by a factor of 6, but at the expense of an increased scatter fraction. Septa-less PET cameras are also necessary for three-dimensional reconstruction.

■ RADIONUCLIDES USED IN PET

Radionuclides used for PET imaging must of course be positron emitters (Table 15-1). The energy of the positron plays a role in the inherent resolution capability of the system. The higher the energy, the farther it moves away from the point of emission before losing all its energy and causing annihilation. This results in a degradation in resolution. Whether the positron emitter is a pure emitter is also a factor. A pure beta emitter has no companion "singles" to compete in the detection process; therefore, the detector is dedicated to counting the coincident events. Contrast that to the β^+-γ emitter in which the gamma singles are tying up the detector while the coincident events are going undetected. The latter increases dead time and decreases resolution.

It is tempting to regard SPECT and PET as variations in the same imaging modality because they have in common the same image reconstruction process. A distinct advantage of PET over SPECT is the list of positron-emitting radionuclides that are available for labeling biologic and physiologic compounds (Table 15-2). Most compounds of medical significance can be labeled with ^{11}C, ^{13}N, ^{15}O, or ^{18}F—all physiologic radionuclides, all positron emitters, and all readily produced by "baby" cyclotrons. As positron emitters, they are readily detected in vivo to produce high-resolution tomographic images. In addition, no gamma-emitting radionuclides of carbon, nitrogen, or oxygen exist that could be used even to *label* these medically important compounds. SPECT imaging would require the labeling of biologic and physiologic compounds with gamma-emitting radionuclides such as ^{99m}Tc. This usually cannot be accomplished with biologically identical substances and therefore reduces their usefulness. Furthermore, human disease is biochemical in nature; therefore, the most effective treatment is a biochemical solution. It follows then that the most important method of diagnosis addresses the biochemical nature of the disease. For these reasons the future of PET seems secure.

BIBLIOGRAPHY

Budinger, T.: Time-of-flight positron emission tomography: status relative to conventional PET. Teaching editorial, J. Nucl. Med. **24**(1), 1983.

Gould K.L.: Clinical positron imaging of the heart, Houston, Texas, 1987, Univ. of Texas Medical School.

Hawkins, R.A., and Phelps, M.E.: Positron emission tomography for evaluation of cerebral function. Current concepts in diagnostic nuclear medicine, vol. 3, no. 2, New York, 1986, Macmillan Inc.

Hoffman, E.J., Huang, S.C., and Phelps, M.E.: Quantitation in positron emission computed tomography: 1. Effects of object size, J. Comput. Assist. Tomogr. **3**(3):299-308, 1979.

Hoffman, E.J., Huang, S.C., Phelps, M.E., and Kuhl, D.E.: Quantitation in positron emission computed tomography: 4. Effect of accidental coincidences, J. Comput. Assist. Tomogr. **5**(3):391-400, 1981.

Huang, S.C., Hoffman, E.J., Phelps, M.E., and Kuhl, D.E.: Quantitation in positron emission computed tomography: 3. Effect of sampling, J. Comput. Assist. Tomogr. **4**(6):819-826, 1980.

Huang, S.C., Hoffman, E.J., Phelps, M.E., and Kuhl, D.E.: Quantitation in positron emission computed tomography: 2. Effects of inaccurate attenuation correction, J. Comput. Assist. Tomogr. **3**(6):804-814, 1979.

Mazziotta, J.C., Phelps, M.E., Plummer, David, and Kuhl, D.E.: Quantitation in positron emission computed tomography: 5. Physical-anatomic effects, J. Comput. Assist. Tomogr. **5**(5):734-743, 1981.

Mullani, N.A., Gould, K.L., Hartz, R.K., Wong, W.H., and others: Three dimensional volumetric imaging with Posicam™ 6.5 BGO positron camera. Presented as an abstract at the Annual Society of Nuclear Medicine Meeting, San Francisco, 1988.

Phelps, M.E., Mazziotta, J.C., and Schelbert, H.R.: Positron emission tomography and autoradiography, New York, 1986, Raven Press.

Sorenson, J.A., and Phelps, M.E.: Physics in nuclear medicine, ed. 2, New York, 1987, Grune & Stratton, Inc.

Stoub, E.W.: ECAT™ scanner technical introduction, Des Plaines, Ill., 1987, Siemens Gammasonics, Inc.

Ter-Pogossian, M.M.: PET, SPECT and NMRI: competing on complementary disciplines, J. Nucl. Med. **26**:1487-1498, 1985.

Chapter 16

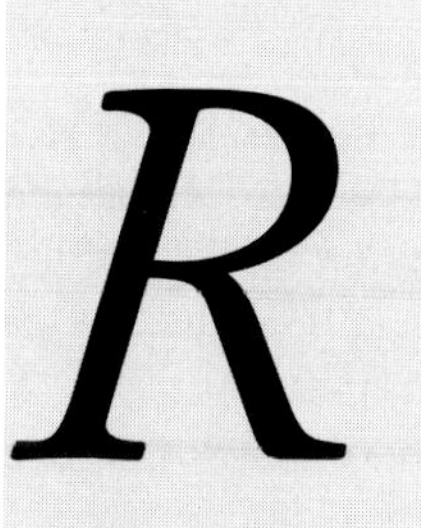

ADIATION SAFETY

PAUL J. EARLY

■ GENERAL CONSIDERATIONS

On April 1, 1987, with the publication in the Federal Register of the new Title 10 of the Code of Federal Regulations, Part 35 (10 CFR 35), many of the regulations dealing with the *medical* use of byproduct material were revised. Some of these regulations had an immediate effect on nuclear medicine departments in states governed by the Nuclear Regulatory Commission (NRC). Other nuclear medicine departments have since felt their effect as their respective states have come into agreement with the attitudes and interpretations of the NRC.

On January 27, 1992, another major change in the thinking of the NRC was instituted with the implementation of the Quality Management Program (QMP). This was an attempt to reduce the number of misadministrations, both diagnostic as well as therapeutic, in the practice of nuclear medicine. In the process, the definition of misadministrations was re-stated.

A more recent development is the revision of Title 10 of the Code of Federal Regulations, Part 20 (10 CFR 20). This revision is an outgrowth of the efforts of the International Commission on Radiological Protection (ICRP) through the publishing of their documents, Pamphlets #26 (1977) and #30 (1979) and affects *all* radiation workers-not just medical radiation workers, as is the case with 10 CFR 35. This document changes the philosophy by which radiation protection is viewed. In the past, radiation protection concerns were simply those of the maximum radiation dose to the critical organ, or to the whole body. The concerns of new Part 20 are to concentrate not just on the limiting of radiation to the reduction of non-stochastic effects. New Part 20 relates these exposures to risks of stochastic effects and attempts to limit their frequency to no greater than these risks incurred in non-occupationally exposed populations. Some of the important aspects of all three of these documents will be discussed in this chapter.

■ TITLE 10, CODE OF FEDERAL REGULATIONS, PART 20 (10 CFR 20)

Effective January 1, 1994, Part 20 (10 CFR 20) was put into effect for all radiation workers, whether they be medical, nuclear reactor, or what. This discussion will reflect on those salient features as they apply to medical applications, but not necessarily at the exclusion of other radiation workers.

■ 2 mrem in any hour to an unrestricted area

This is not a new concept. It existed in old Part 20; however, the application of the concept was changed in new Part 20. Old Part 20 said that any radiation limits were exempt from radiations coming *from* the patient. New Part 20 said that any radiation limits were exempt from radiation *to* the patient. This provision would have been one of the most difficult to meet in the case of nuclear medicine, even diagnostic nuclear medicine, because this regulation would make every diagnostic nuclear medicine patient a "walking restricted area". Since a 20 mCi (740 MBq) dosage yields approximately 10 mrem/hr at the surface of the patient, an in-patient would require a private room, and outpatients would be required to remain in a special radiation-controlled waiting room until their exposures were reduced to this level, or would require hospitalization. The NRC quickly saw this as a conflict with their previously published patient release criteria (10 CFR 35.75) and ruled that since 35.75 is more specific, then 35.75 would take precedence. Therefore, the 2 mrem in any one hour regulation does not apply to radiation from a patient.

■ New exposure limits (see Table 6-3)

The new exposure limits take into consideration the new concepts of stochastic and non-stochastic types of radiation health effects. The exposure limits are identified in 20.1201. These limits are tabulated on Table 6-3. The terminology is explained in Chapter 6 and a flow chart exists in Appendix C, with a supportive internal radiation dose scenario.

■ Records of prior exposure

The licensee is now required under 20.2104 to determine the prior occupational exposure of any new employee prior to beginning work if the past exposure is believed to be > 10%. This may take the form of determining (or estimating) the total occupational radiation dose received during the current year and/or an attempt to obtain the previous exposure records.

■ 100 mrem per year to members of the general public

This limit in new Part 20 is a reduction of these limits in old Part 20 (500 mrem/yr) by a factor of 5. It is an outgrowth of the more recent calculations of the Japanese bomb survivors, where it was determined that the radiobiological effects of the atomic bomb were as a result of radiation exposures that were less than originally believed. This value of 100 mrem per year must now be applied to any *unrestricted* area, which could be areas where members of the general public would be likely to remain for some period of time. Areas such as waiting rooms, lounges, secretarial areas and patient rooms would fall into this area of concern. One important departure from old Part 20 is the fact that one can use *realistic* values such as times of occupancy to calculate anticipated exposures to radiation. In the past, it was necessary to use the most pessimistic (and therefore, usually *unrealistic*) values to determine the need for additional radiation protection measures. This limit does not apply to *restricted* areas. If members of the general public were to enter a restricted area (e.g., a radiopharmaceutical therapy patient's hospital room), they would assume the risk associated with that of a medical radiation worker, and therefore their exposure limit under those conditions would increase to 5000 mrems/yr. At the time of this writing, this interpretation is being challenged with a proposal to limit the exposure of the member of the general public (even in these situations) to the 100 mrem limit. The other concern is that of ^{60}Co teletherapy units. All such units (and they are growing fewer in number each year) were protected with high density concrete and/or lead walls to limit the exposure to the general public to 500 mr/yr. The new requirement applies to these units as well. It is believed by the NRC that, since these teletherapy units were built according to the specification of NCRP Booklet #49, which most agree uses very pessimistic assumptions, and that, with the use of more realistic values, retrofitting of these units will not be necessary. This remains to be seen. If this is not the case, then these units will have to be retrofitted to satisfy these new radiation limits. At the time of this writing, this ruling is also being challenged, in light of the tremendous additional cost that would be incurred by hospitals in this era of hospital cost-containment.

■ Annual exposure reports

It is necessary to provide an annual exposure report to all radiation workers who exceed 10% of the occupational exposure limit (Table 6-3). This regulation takes its direction from 19.13(b) which references 20.2106 which references 20.1502. This annual exposure report must also include exposures that are received by the occupationally exposed person as a result of a second job ("moonlighters").

■ Bioassays

Bioassays will be continued in the same fashion as practiced under old Part 20. The only difference is that there is some relaxation of the bioassay limits using the NRC's Regulatory Guide 8.9, rather than the old Regulatory Guide 8.20. The new ^{131}I limits in Regulatory Guide 8.9 suggest an *Evaluation Level* when any thyroid measurement exceeds 0.133 μCi (2% of ALI limit). An *Investigation Level* is reached when the thyroid measurement exceeds 0.665 μCi (10% ALI). These values are based on an ALI value of 50 μCi (the maximum value), and a thyroid intake retention factor (IRF) for ^{131}I at 24 hours of 0.133 (NUREG 4884). If any single measurement exceeds 0.133 μCi, the RSO will investigate (Level I). Repeat measurements should be made to verify measurements and obtain a better measure of the intake. If any single measurement exceeds 0.665 μCi, the RSO should institute a thorough investigation (Level II). Multiple measurements over several days should be performed. Air sampling and surveys should also be evaluated and compared to the bioassay. Preventative actions should be taken if confirmed. When the total thyroid uptake for an individual reaches 3 μCi in a year, consideration should be made to removing the individual from iodine handling. Certainly, individuals should be removed from iodine handling prior to reaching a total uptake of 6 μCi for the year since this would indicate approaching the limit of one ALI.

■ Pregnancy of a radiation worker

The licensee should develop a pregnancy policy, at least to the extent that these new Part 20 regulations are addressed. This policy should follow the tenets of 20.1208 and 20.2106(e). One of the most significant changes is that the pregnant worker must declare her pregnancy in writing, and include the approximate date of impregnation (20.2106(e)). These records should be maintained in a separate file for reasons of privacy. Without this declaration, the licensee cannot be held responsible for the radiation safety of the fetus. Regulations in 20.1208 state that the licensee must ensure that the dose to the embryo/fetus of a declared pregnant radiation worker must not exceed 500 mrem (5 mSv) during the entire pregnancy. An attempt must be made to avoid substantial variation above a uniform monthly exposure rate to that pregnant worker. If the dose to the embryo/fetus at the time of the declaration is found to exceed 500 mrem (5 mSv) or is within 50 mrem (0.5 mSv) of the limit, the dose for the remainder of the pregnancy period must not exceed 50 mrem. This regulation may infringe on the mother's right to work, which is in violation of her constitutional rights (Ref: U.S. Supreme Court decision re: UAW v. Johnson Controls of Pa.-3/21/93). To avoid any problems along these lines, the NRC has allowed the mother the right to "undeclare" her pregnancy, at which time the institution is absolved of all responsibilities for radiation protection of the embryo/fetus. (This right of "undeclaration" is not found in any section of the CFR; however, it is found in the NRC's set #5 of Questions and Answers regarding Part 20).

■ Receipt of shipments

Part 20 has always addressed the receipt of radioactive shipments regarding the needs to wipe-test and survey the external surfaces of certain shipments. New Part 20 is similar to its predecessor in that it retains the requirement to survey only those radioactive shipments containing > Type A quantities (which are usually > 10 Ci). Be aware that this requirement may be overruled through a license condition (e.g., acceptance of Appendix L of NRC Regulatory Guide 10.8, a licensing guide). New Part 20 departs from old Part 20 in that it requires the wipe-testing of *all* shipments of radioactive materials containing a radioactive label (White I, Yellow II, or Yellow III). The limits of removable contamination have been made more stringent: from 220 dpm/cm^2 × 300 cm^2 (66,000 cpm or 0.03 μCi) to 22 dpm/cm^2 × 300 cm^2 (6600 dpm or 0.003 μCi), a change by one order of magnitude. This new limit is the same as the limits for shipment of radioactive materials in the past.

■ Monitoring of gaseous effluent

The limits for gaseous effluent have been completely changed in accordance with ICRP #26 and #30. This has been accomplished through the introduction of two new terms: Derived Air Concentrations (DAC's) v. the old Maximum Permissible Concentrations (MPC's) and Annual Limit of Intake (ALI). One DAC is defined as that concentration of radionuclide in air which when breathed by reference man for a work year would result in an intake of one (1) ALI. One ALI is defined as the activity of a radionuclide which, if inhaled or ingested by reference man, will result in a dose equal to the ALI value (ALI tables exist in Part 20). These new concepts coupled with the change in philosophy has created DAC values for 767 radionuclides, 65% of which are less restricitve, 26% more restrictive and 9% unchanged. If it can be proven by calculation or actual measurement that a nuclear medicine department can fall within < 20% of the limits for each radionuclide in use, then there is no need to monitor gaseous effluent. This should not be difficult for the routine nuclear medicine department.

■ Disposal into sanitary sewerage systems

In accordance with 20.2003, the method to release radionuclides into the sanitary sewerage system has become much more stringent. Patient excreta continues to be exempt from these limits, however. This method of waste disposal continues to be the most efficient method if the material is soluble or dispersible in water. It is incumbent on the licensee, however, to re-evaluate the disposal limits and ascertain that the institution is still within the limits as described in 20.2003. This will probably be an issue only in large institutions and large RIA laboratories.

■ Placement of film badges

The NRC has finally solved the unsolvable. The question, "Where do I wear my film badge" has been a source of much discussion over the years. Is the proper position under the lead apron? on the collar? The question, "Where do I wear my finger badge?" has been equally disconcerting. Is the proper position on the right hand? left hand? facing the palm? facing away from the palm? New Part 20 has made it clear. It states that the personnel monitor must be placed near the location expected to receive the highest dose (10.1201(c)). It certainly precludes the wearing of the film badge behind the lead apron (except with the use of a second badge in the case of pregnancy) to evaluate the TEDE for the whole body (the DDE for most nuclear medicine technologists). The whole body includes the head and shoulders, which are not covered by the lead apron. It probably precludes the wearing of the finger badge in a position facing away from the palm as well. This regulation would suggest that an evaluation should be made as to where these personnel monitors should be worn.

■ TITLE 10, CODE OF FEDERAL REGULATIONS, PART 35 (10 CFR 35)

This specific portion of the Code of Federal Regulations addresses specifically the medical use of by-product material, and the regulations governing their use. Salient points within these regulations, as they apply to nuclear medicine departments are discussed.

■ Amendment versus Notification versus Ministerial Changes

It is no longer necessary to notify the NRC of all changes relating to the NRC license. "Amendments" are necessary for any significant change in the status of the license *before* the change, but the NRC now allows "notifications" within 30 days *after* some events as well as "ministerial changes" with no notification but adequate documentation. Notifications are required for discontinuation of a licensed user, the Radiation Safety Officer (RSO) or the Teletherapy Physicist, or a name change. Mailing address changes of licensee also apply. Ministerial changes (minor changes in radiation safety procedures that are not potentially important to safety) are allowed without the need for a license amendment, provided a safety review is made, appropriate records are kept, and affected members of the Radiation Safety Committee (RSC) sign off on them. Examples of such instances include a change in film-badge suppliers, a change in the person who calibrates survey meters, a change in waste disposal procedures, or adoption of a model radiation safety procedure as published in a Regulatory Guide.

■ ALARA program

The ALARA program, a program designed to keep exposures to workers and the public *As Low As Reasonably-Achievable*, is now required whereas previously such a program was only suggested by the NRC. This is also an inclusion in the revised Part 20. The program must involve management, the RSO, and all authorized users. The program would be similar to the previous ALARA concepts of radiation safety: summaries of the program, review of personnel exposures, involvement in continuing education of personnel, and changes in radiation safety procedures. The purpose is to ensure that licensees make a reasonable effort to maintain individual and collective personnel exposures ALARA. It is the RSO's responsibility to establish those limits.

■ Radiation Safety Officer (RSO)

Considerable emphasis is placed on the RSO relative to authority and responsibility. Through this individual, licensees shall be able to ensure that radiation safety procedures are being carried out. Therefore the RSO will investigate all overexposures, accidents, losses, misadministrations, or other deviations from good radiation safety. It is the RSO's responsibility to maintain a procedure file on all matters relating to the byproduct material program from receipt to final disposition. This also includes performance checks on survey equipment as well as inservice education. The RSO will review the radiation safety program in its entirety with management once per year. New responsibilities are given to the RSO by way of establishing personnel exposure investigational levels, action levels for area surveys, and action levels for wipe test analyses. If not in a medical institution, the RSO is also responsible for approving minor changes in the radiation safety procedures that are not potentially important to safety. Most important, the licensee will provide the RSO with sufficient freedom and authority to take corrective actions when a radiation safety problem is identified. The RSO is also responsible for the accuracy and completeness of other tasks demonstrated by the requirements for his or her signature on key documents. This does *not* mean the RSO performs the tasks, but rather that the record has been reviewed by a responsible individual with special training and experience. Documents requiring the signature of the RSO are as follows:

1. Sealed-source inventory (10 CFR 35.59[g])
2. Sealed-source leak test (10 CFR 35.59[d])
3. Survey of sealed-source storage area (10 CFR 35.59[i])
4. Dose-calibrator accuracy (10 CFR 35.50[e][2])
5. Dose-calibrator linearity (10 CFR 35.50[e][3])
6. Dose-calibrator geometry (10 CFR 35.50[e][4])
7. Radiation safety program changes (10 CFR 35.31[b])
8. Safety checks for teletherapy facilities (10 CFR 35. 636[c])
9. Radiation surveys for teletherapy facilities (10 CFR 35641[c])

■ Radiation Safety Committee (RSC)

The Radiation Safety Committee (RSC) must maintain a membership that consists of at least three individuals, two of whom must be the Radiation Safety Officer and the management's representative. If either of these latter members are absent, the RSC may not conduct official business. In addition, membership must include an authorized user of each type of use permitted by the licensee and a nursing-service representative. The additional inclusion of the chief nuclear-medicine technologist of the RSC is to be encouraged. In many instances, the chief technologist is the single individual most aware of radiation safety protocols and breaches of same. The technologists are the "front line" radiation workers and therefore may have a practical approach to problems that may not be obvious to other members. A quorum of at least one half the committee's membership must be present, and the minutes must include the names of those members who are both absent and present. The minutes must be provided to each member promptly.

■ Supervision

The term *supervision* has long been a problem in interpretation of the conditions of the NRC license. The biggest problem occurs in the instance of a license listing one single authorized user, who must be absent for some reason. The "visiting authorized user" clause was added to circumvent some of this problem, but the "supervision" clause precluded a physician from using one of his "trainees." It was necessary to use a physician at another institution who was equally licensed but whose level of expertise was perhaps unknown by the vacationing physician. The current interpretation of "supervision" is that the receipt, possession, use (to include prescription, administration, interpretation and follow-up for individual clinical procedures), or transfer of byproduct material by any individual is permitted provided that individual is periodically reviewed by the authorized user, has been instructed in radiation safety practices, and follows the procedure for good radiation safety as established by the RSO. The licensee is the individual who is ultimately responsible for the acts and omissions of the supervised individual.

■ Visiting authorized user

The requirements regarding a visiting authorized user are as follows: A visiting authorized user can be used for 60 days each year provided permission is granted by administration and, if applicable, the RSC; a copy of his or her radioactive material license is on hand; and the clinical procedures are those for which this individual is licensed, as long as the visited institution is also licensed for the procedure.

■ Misadministrations

The NRC has redefined the meaning of misadministrations, effective Jan. 27, 1992. In so doing, they have essentially eliminated misadministrations from anyone's diagnostic regimen, with the exception of dosages greater than 30 μCi ^{131}I and ^{125}I. Since these diagnostic dosages are rare, the possibility of committing a diagnostic misadministration is also rare. Greater concern, of course, is for misadministrations in the dosage range of therapies. The new definitions of misadministrations are as follows:

1. >30 μCi ^{131}I NaI or ^{125}I NaI involving:
   a. Wrong patient
   b. Wrong radiopharmaceutical
   c. Dosage administered is >±20% of the prescribed dosage *and* (for any of the above) the dosage, or the difference in dosage is > 30 μCi.
2. Diagnostic radiopharmaceutical dosage (other than the above) involving:
   a. Wrong patient
   b. Wrong radiopharmaceutical
   c. Wrong route of administration
   d. Wrong dosage
   and (for any of the four possibilities)
   when the dose to the patient's whole body (DDE) is >5 rems *or*
   when the dose to any individual organ (TODE) is >50 rems dose-equivalent.
   By placing these high dose values into consideration, the NRC has essentially ruled out any misadministrations as a result of diagnostic uses.
3. Therapy radiopharmaceutical dosage (other than the above) involving:
   a. Wrong patient
   b. Wrong radiopharmaceutical
   c. Wrong route of administration
   d. Dose administered must be >±20% prescribed.
4. Brachytherapy radiation dose involving:
   a. Wrong patient
   b. Wrong radionuclide
   c. Wrong treatment site (excludes seeds that migrate from site)
   d. Leaking sealed source
   e. One or more sealed sources not removed at completion of treatment
   f. Administered dose >±20% prescribed.

■ Notification of misadministrations

Once a misadministration has occurred, it is an NRC requirement to report the event first within 24 hours, and then within 15 days, as follows:

Within 24 hours, notify by telephone:

1. NRC Operations Center: (201) 951-0550
2. Referring physician
3. Patient or guardian after consulting with the referring physician, or as soon as possible after locating each (in the event of difficulty in locating) unless the referring physician decides to tell patient or it is the opinion of the referring physician that telling the patient or guardian would be harmful to the patient

Within 15 days, submit a written report to:

1. NRC regional Office
2. Patient

■ Recordable event

Also effective Jan. 27, 1992, is definition of a recordable event. This is an event that is usually an error by 50% of that which falls into the misadministration definition. The definition of a recordable event is as follows:

1. >30 μCi of ^{131}I NaI or ^{125}I NaI involving:
   a. Dosage >±10% of that prescribed *and* the difference >15 μCi
   b. No written directive (see QMP below)
   c. No daily dosage record
2. All diagnostic radiopharmaceuticals (including <30 μCi ^{131}I NaI or ^{125}I NaI): None
3. Therapy radiopharmaceuticals (other than the above):
   a. Dosage administered >±10% of that prescribed
   b. No written directive
   c. No daily dosage record
4. Brachytherapy radiation dose:
   a. Dose administered >±10% of that prescribed
   b. No written directive
   c. No daily dose record

The licensee shall evaluate all recordable events within 30 days and prepare an incident report (for in-house use only) addressing:

a. The relevant facts including the cause
b. Identification of the corrective action required to prevent recurrence
c. Inclusion of this information in the annual review for the Quality Management Program (QMP), the details of which will follow

■ QUALITY MANAGEMENT PROGRAM (QMP)

It was the responsibility of every NRC licensee to file a written QMP by Jan. 27, 1992. The purpose of the QMP is to provide high confidence that byproduct material or radiation from byproduct material will be administered as directed by the authorized user. The five objectives of any QMP are:

1. Obtain written directives before the administration of certain radioactive materials
2. Verify patient identification by more than one method
3. Ensure that final plans of treatment and their calculations are in accordance with the written directives
4. Be certain that each administration is in accordance with the written directive
5. Identify and evaluate any unintended deviation from the written directive, and take appropriate action

It is the intent of this program to develop procedures for and conduct a review of the QMP including all misadministration, all recordable events, and a sampling of patient administrations at intervals no greater than 12 months.

■ For all radiopharmaceutical therapies and diagnostic $^{131}I/^{125}I$ >30 μCi

To satisfy the QMP regarding all radiopharmaceutical therapies and diagnostic ^{131}I NaI or ^{125}I NaI greater than 30 μCi, the following conditions must be met:

1. The authorized user must sign and date a written directive before the administration of these radionuclides. The written directive must include the radiopharmaceutical, the dosage, and the route of administration.
2. The authorized user or designee must double-verify the patient to ensure that the correct patient is getting the intended radionuclide. The primary method of identification is to *ask* the patient his or her name. A second method of verification can be through a variety of means such as birth date, address, social security number, signature, ID bracelet, hospital ID card or medical insurance card. Both of these responses are compared with the information on the patient record.
3. The person administering the dose/dosage must verify the details of the administration against the written directive. Details particularly of interest are the radiopharmaceutical, the dose/dosage and the route of administration.
4. Encourage the worker to ask directions if they do not understand the written directive.
5. The user or supervised person must date and sign/initial the written record, which might be the patient chart.
6. Perform an annual review including a random sample (determining the size of the sample based on Acceptance Sampling Tables in 10 CFR 32)

■ For other therapy programs

A similar program is required for brachytherapy, teletherapy, gamma stereotactic radiosurgery, and high dose rate remote afterloaders. The concerns vary with each of these forms of therapy (all having to do with many of the terms above) and in addition, the following:

1. For teletherapy: the total dose, dose per fraction, treatment site, and overall treatment period
2. For high-dose–rate remote afterloaders: the radioisotope, treatment site, and total dose
3. For all other brachytherapy before implantation: the radioisotope, number of sources and source strengths. After implantation but before completion of the procedure: the radioisotope, treatment site, and total source strength and exposure time (or, equivalently, total dose)
4. For gamma stereotactic radiosurgery: target coordinates, collimator size, plug pattern, and total dose

Once the annual review is complete, it is incumbent on the licensee to reevaluate the QMP's policies and procedures to determine whether the program is still effective. If not, its purpose is to identify actions required to make the program more effective, and to implement those changes. These changes should be implemented within a reasonable time after the identification of the problem(s). The intent of the NRC was to make this QMP a program that is performance-based, rather than prescription-based (as are most other NRC programs). As such, the licensee is allowed to make changes in the program without need for license amendment action. Such changes are required to be furnished to the appropriate NRC Regional Office within 30 days after the modification has been made. All other records regarding the QMP annual review and recordable events are required to be kept for 3 years; misadministration records must be kept for 5 years.

■ DIAGNOSTIC USES OF RADIOACTIVE MATERIALS

■ Sources for radioactive materials

The practice of assisting a nearby hospital (not on your NRC license) by sending it an unused patient dosage has been eliminated by regulation. A licensee may use only byproduct material from a licensed manufacturer or distributor of these materials. This has always been a condition of the NRC license, but few hospitals adhered to it. It is now a part of the NRC regulations.

■ Dose calibrator

A dose calibrator is required (even in those instances in which only unit dosages are obtained from a radiopharmacy) to measure the amount of radioactivity administered. Since it is a measuring device, it must be periodically checked for: (1) constancy (daily), (2) accuracy (annually) with at least two long-lived sealed sources, (3) linearity (quarterly) throughout the range of its use between the highest dosage administered and 10 μCi,* and (4) geometry (upon installation). All values cannot exceed 10%. Mathematical corrections are permitted for geometry or linearity errors. Repair or replacement of the dose calibrator is required for accuracy or constancy errors greater than 10%.

■ Survey meters

Survey meters must be calibrated annually through all scales up to 1000 mrem/hr, with two readings on each scale. The regulations further stipulate that an exposure rate from a dedicated check source must be determined at the time of calibration. Furthermore, the licensee will verify calibration by measuring the same check source upon receipt. This requires use of a long-lived radionuclide check source with each instrument. This means that a check source must be purchased for each survey meter and shipped with it after calibration. On receipt, the source is measured to confirm reproducibility and therefore calibration. A point is considered calibrated if the exposure rate differs from the calculated exposure rate by not more than 20%. It is necessary to attach a correction chart or graph to the instrument showing these results.

■ Radiopharmaceutical dosages

The licensee must measure each dosage containing more than 10 μCi of a photon-emitting radionuclide before medical use. This suggests that it is no longer necessary to measure ^{32}P or ^{89}Sr since they are pure beta emitters. Also, the licensee must measure each dosage of 10 μCi or less to verify that the dosage is in fact less than 10 μCi. This makes it necessary to measure blood-volume syringes and Schilling's capsules.

■ Sealed sources

The licensee in possession of sealed sources must leak test the source every 6 months. Leakage is defined as a wipe sample with more than 0.005 μCi of removable radioactivity. This procedure is not required on materials of less than 30 days T_p, gases, less than 100 μCi of beta- or gamma-emitting radionuclides or less than 10 μCi of alpha-emitting radionuclides, sources stored and not being used, and seeds of ^{192}Ir encased in nylon ribbon. Quarterly inventories of all sealed sources, as well as quarterly surveys of storage areas of sealed sources, must be performed.

■ Syringe shields and labels

The licensee must identify the contents of a syringe or the syringe shield by showing at least one of the following:

1. Radiopharmaceutical name
2. Clinical procedure
3. Patient name

*This lower level may be modified to 30 μCi to better fit the Quality Management Program.

Syringe shields are required when preparing a radiopharmaceutical kit or when administering a radiopharmaceutical by injection, unless the use of the shield is contraindicated for that patient. It is not necessary to use a syringe shield for drawing up a dosage. In the case of vials, the vial must be kept in the vial radiation shield and the shield must be labeled to show the radiopharmaceutical name. Color coding alone is no longer adequate.

■ Surveys

Ambient radiation exposure rate. A licensee shall survey with a radiation detection instrument at the end of each day of use all areas where radiopharmaceuticals are routinely prepared for use or administered. This should include the stress lab area. In addition, a survey should be made each week of all areas where radiopharmaceuticals or their waste is stored. The survey instrument must be able to detect exposure rates as low as 0.1 mrem/hr with the licensee (and the assistance of the RSO) establishing appropriate trigger levels for decontamination. The RSO must be notified immediately should a trigger level be exceeded.

Contamination. Once each week, a licensee shall wipe test all areas where radiopharmaceuticals are routinely prepared for use, administered, or stored. A system must be available to detect a wipe sample of 2000 dpm with the licensee (through the assistance of the RSO) establishing appropriate trigger levels. Immediate RSO notification is required when contamination trigger levels are exceeded. NRC Regulatory Guide 8.28 (Table 16-1) could be used in establishing such trigger levels. There is one trigger level that is not left to the option of the licensee or RSO, that of decontamination of the ^{131}I therapy patient room. The maximum permissible level here has been stipulated by the NRC to be 200 dpm/100 cm^2.

■ Storage of volatiles and gases

No fume hood is required if the radiopharmaceuticals and/or radioactive gases are stored in the shipper's shipping container. It is necessary, however, to store a multidose container in a fume hood after drawing the first dosage from it.

■ Decay in storage

A licensee may decay in storage any byproduct material with a physical half-life of less than 65 days before disposal into ordinary trash provided it is held for a minimum of 10 half-lives *and* there is no measurable radiation coming from the waste package. This means that if the decay in storage method is used, the radionuclide must remain in storage for 10 physical half-lives. Although this is not particularly burdensome for some radionuclides, ^{125}I poses a serious problem to the RIA laboratories. Using this method of disposal, the RIA laboratory would necessarily hold the RIA vials and/or liquid for 600 days. In an ordinary RIA laboratory, this may represent an insurmountable storage problem. Should the decay in storage program be adopted,

Table 16-1. Recommended action levels in dpm/100 cm^2 for surface contamination by radiopharmaceuticals

	^{32}P, ^{58}Co, ^{59}Fe, ^{60}Co, ^{75}Se, ^{85}Sr, ^{111}In, ^{123}I, ^{125}I, ^{131}I, ^{169}Yb, ^{198}Au	^{51}Cr, ^{57}Co, ^{67}Ga, ^{99m}Tc, ^{197}Hg, ^{201}Tl
1. Unrestricted areas, personal clothing	200	2000
2. Restricted areas, protective clothing used only in restricted areas, skin	2000	20,000

the labels must be removed or obliterated before final disposal into the ordinary trash. To determine generator background levels, the generators would have to be removed from their protective radiation shielding.

■ Licensure

NRC licensure is ordinarily granted in groups, although individual uses may be granted. This is especially true with therapeutic applications. There are six groups, called *types of use,* which are as follows:

1. 10 CFR 35.100 is comprised of the well-established laboratory techniques (old Group I)
2. 10 CFR 35.200 includes all diagnostic imaging techniques to include Xenon gas plus generators and kits (old Groups II and III)
3. 10 CFR 35.300 includes all radiopharmaceutical therapy, whether hospitalized or not (old Groups IV and V)
4. 10 CFR 35.400 deals with brachytherapy (part of old Group VI)
5. 10 CFR 35.500 includes those sealed sources that are used for diagnosis (the other part of old Group VI)
6. 10 CFR 35.600 includes the use of a sealed source in a teletherapy unit such as ^{60}Co or ^{137}Cs

Given licensure for any radiopharmaceutical types of use, a licensee may use any byproduct material within those groups provided the FDA has accepted a "Notice Of Claimed Investigational Exemption For A New Drug" (IND) or approved a "New Drug Application" (NDA). With the advent of monoclonal antibodies and other biologicals that do not fall into the FDA's definition of drugs, these materials are approved as Product License Applications (PLAs). For this reason, license rhetoric is changing to include the latter.

Types of use

10 CFR 35.100 Use of radiopharmaceuticals for uptake, dilution and excretion studies. This type of use carries with it the requirement that the licensee possess a survey meter capable of detecting dose rates from 0.1 to 100 mR/hr. It is also important to note that the general license for in vivo studies is included under this type of use. The general license for in vitro uses still exists in 10 CFR 31.11.

10 CFR 35.200 Use of radiopharmaceuticals, generators, and reagent kits for imaging and localization studies. This type of use carries with it the need to evaluate the ^{99}Mo concentration such that the licensee may not administer to humans a radiopharmaceutical containing more than 0.15 μCi of ^{99}Mo/mCi of ^{99m}Tc. The licensee who elutes the generator must make this measurement. If prepared radiopharmaceuticals are purchased, there is no need to make this measurement and/or keep records of it. These NRC limits are now in agreement with the molybdenum specifications of the U.S. Pharmacopoeia (U.S.P.). The licensee authorized for this type of use must have in its possession two survey instruments: (1) A portable radiation *detection* survey instrument (e.g., Geiger-Mueller or crystal survey meter) capable of measuring 0.1 to 100 mR/hr and (2) A portable radiation *measurement* survey instrument (e.g., ionization-type survey meter) capable of measuring dose rates from 1.0 to 1000 mR/hr. An energy-compensated G-M survey meter is generally regarded as satisfying both conditions if its maximum capability is 1000 mR/hr or greater.

Aerosols and gases. ^{133}Xe is included in 10 CFR 35.200. It is still necessary to satisfy the conditions and limits for airborne concentrations specified by 10 CFR 20.1203 and 20.1204. Originally, the NRC included both aerosols and gases in this new regulation. Previously, aerosols were not treated as a gas; therefore positive pressure rooms could be used for aerosol studies. By disallowing their use except in negative pressure rooms, it was felt by most that this prevented the use of an important diagnostic modality for the critically ill patient who could not be moved to the nuclear medicine department. In light of this and with the assistance of Mallinckrodt Medical, Inc., a request was made to the NRC to delay application of this regulation to aerosols until such time as a Petition For Rulemaking could be acted on in favor of allowing aerosols to be used in rooms other than those with a negative pressure. The NRC responded to this request on March 23, 1987 (about 1 week before these new regulations were to be in effect) and notified all licensees that the inclusion of aerosols in the conditions of 10 CFR 35.205 be disregarded until further notice. Mallinckrodt Medical, Inc. subsequently filed a Petition for Rulemaking to the NRC, and the NRC responded by removing aerosols from this condition in the regulation.

10 CFR 35.300 Use of radiopharmaceuticals for therapy. In this license group are included the following radionuclides: iodine 131 for hyperthyroidism, cardiac conditions, and thyroid carcinoma; phosphorus 32 (soluble) for polycythemia vera, leukemia, and bone metastases; and phosphorus 32 (colloid) and gold 198 (colloid) for intercavitary uses.

10 CFR 35.400 Use of sources for brachytherapy. In this license group are the various sealed sources for brachytherapy. They are as follows: cesium 137 for topical, interstitial and intercavitary treatment; cobalt 60 for topical, interstitial and intercavitary treatment; gold 198 (seed) for interstitial treatment; iridium 192 (seed) for interstitial treatment; strontium 90 eye applicators; iodine 125 (seed) for interstitial treatment; and palladium 103 (seed) for interstitial treatment.

10 CFR 35.500 Use of sealed sources for diagnosis. This group consists of sealed sources of potentially therapeutic size, used diagnostically. These include bone-mineral analyzers, using iodine 125, americium 241, or gadolinium 153. This group also includes a portable imaging device using iodine 125.

10 CFR 35.600 Use of a sealed source in a teletherapy unit. This group governs the use of cobalt 60 and cesium 137 teletherapy units.

■ RADIOPHARMACEUTICAL THERAPY

In any administration of radioactive materials, it is necessary to always be cognizant of any forbidden radiation health safety practices. This need is magnified when dealing with therapeutic amounts of radioactive materials. Whether the material be in liquid form or solid form, the use of therapeutic amounts of radioactivity carries its own special set of problems and associated solutions. The following is to present a program of good radiation safety that could be used in any modern health-care facility. The requirements contained within conform to the guidelines of the U.S. Nuclear Regulatory Commission. These regulations are also within the guidelines of good common sense and good radiation safety practice and without undue requirements for effective record keeping and handling procedures. Any deviations from a program such as this may well be extended to the more (surely not less) stringent side.

■ Receipt of radioactive shipments

Any receipt of radioactive shipments carries with it the requirements of the Department of Transportation (DOT) to monitor the packages on receipt. These monitoring procedures would include the measurement of the package at surface and at 1 m to determine the levels of external radiation. According to the U.S. DOT regulations, these readings cannot exceed 200 mrem/hr at the surface of the package or 10 mrem/hr at 1 m. In addition, the exterior surface of the inner source container (lead container in which the radioactive material is shipped) must be wipe-tested and determined free of contamination. Contamination is regarded as a wipe test yielding greater than background of removable contamination as measured with a G-M survey meter. If determined to be contaminated, the source and the inner source container must be treated as contaminated throughout the entire use. The radioactive shipment also carries with it an additional wipe-testing requirement—the leak test of the outer surface of the incoming package. This should be no greater than 22 dpm/cm^2 wiped over 300 cm^2 = 6600 dpm or 0.003 μCi of removable contamination. Finally, a measurement should be made of the empty shipment box to determine if there is any residual radioactivity left in the container itself. Once determined free of contamination, this package can have its radioactive materials signs obliterated and thrown into the regular trash. If contaminated, the package must be held for decay until background levels are reached. Once radioactive materials are removed from the shipping box, they should be placed in a shielded area until time of use. If these sources are liquid ^{131}I sources, this storage site should be a fume hood. Before use, and preferably at the time of receipt, the radioactive material should be measured to ensure the proper radioactive dosage to the patient.

■ Administration

In all of the procedures dealing with the use of therapeutic radiopharmaceuticals, it is easiest to think of radioactive iodine 131 because this is the most widely used source of radiopharmeutical therapy and it carries with it most of the problems associated with a therapy application. If the material is in liquid form, it is essential that it be administered to the patient in a closed environment (i.e., a fume hood) because of the volatility of iodine 131. The lid should be removed from the radioactive source in the fume hood to allow the volatilized iodine 131 to escape via the fume hood. Radionuclide administration sets that simulate a closed environment for the use of liquid iodine 131 are available. This may obviate the need for a fume hood. Other choices would be to receive the radioactive material in capsule form. In this form, volatilization and escape of a radionuclide is not considered to be a problem.

■ Following administration

Private room/private bath. If the patient has received an amount of radioactivity that is equal to or greater than 30 mCi (1110 MBq) or that measures 5 mrem/hr at 1 m, it is required that the patient be accommodated in a private room with a private bath. It is obvious that the reason for private bathroom facilities is that the patient will not expose patients in the immediate environs to unnecessary radiation. Further, a private bath is required so that contamination is restricted to the patient and the room in which the patient is accommodated. Once the patient has reached 30 mCi (1110 MBq) or measures less than 5 mR/hr at 1 m, the patient is allowed to go home after being given some basic instructions on keeping safe distances from pregnant women and small children. Should it be necessary for the patient to remain in the hospital for periods longer than the time required to reduce to these radiation levels (for reasons other than the purpose of the radionuclide therapy application), it is no longer necessary to continue this radiation-control program.

Maximum use of disposables. All surfaces within the patient's room and bathroom that possibly could be exposed to patient contamination should be covered with disposable materials having plastic on one side and absorbent material on the opposite. These coverings would include the floor, the area around the toilet, and the area around the sink. In addition, items that would be handled by the patient (since iodine 131 is excreted in the perspiration) would be covered with plastic bags. These would include the telephone, faucet handles, nurse call button, and any other items the patient would be able to touch.

Designated waste container. It is important that a waste container remain within the patient's hospital room to have a ready place to throw contaminated materials. Plastic food trays and plastic glasses would be placed in this container. Bed linens should be disposable and therefore used. Bed linens would also be placed into these designated waste containers. Containers are maintained in the room until such time as the radiation safety officer deems it appropriate to dispose of the contents. Containers should be labeled clearly to prevent anyone from inadvertently throwing away its contents.

Room postings. The hall side of the patient's door should have a "Caution: Radioactive Materials" sign posted, indicating a patient within who contains radioactive materials. Information as to how long the nursing staff and visitors are allowed to remain in the area should also be posted on this door. The door should be kept closed to prevent inadvertent entry into this controlled area. Visits by individuals under age 18 must be authorized on a patient-by-patient basis with the approval of the authorized user after consultation with the radiation safety officer.

Surveys. Once the patient is placed in the bed, the room should be surveyed at the bedside, at 3 feet, at the doorway, and at the nearby patient. 20.1301(a)(1) and (2) states that the TEDE to members of the general public cannot be $>$ 100 mrems (1 mSv) per year, or not $>$ 2 mrems (0.02 mSv) in any one hour. In accordance with ALARA, it is important that the radiation levels outside the room be kept to 2 mrems/hr, with the awareness that the patient next door could not remain in that room at those radiation levels for greater than 50 hours (to prevent exceeding the 100-mrem/yr portion of the NRC regulations). It is best to restrict the radiation levels to the nearby patient to levels as low as possible, but never to exceed 100 mrems for the hospital stay of the patient. Since the radioactive patient is kept in a hospital room which has been declared a restricted area, any persons entering this room assume the same "risks" of the radiation worker; therefore, the above restrictions do not apply.* However, in the interest of ALARA, a suggested approach to visitor control is to establish a 2 mrem/hr line (place yellow radioactive tape on the floor), beyond which the visitor should not go.

The patient should always remain in bed during the times that the visitor(s) is present. Furthermore, the patient must remain in his or her own room the entire time of treatment. Informing the patient of these restrictions will assist the radiation safety control process. Usually these patients are lucid and are willing to assist. Calculations should also be made for the nursing staff. These calculations could take the ALARA approach and determine how long the nurse could remain at bedside and at 3 feet in order to stay within the 2 mrem-in-any-one-hour limit. Usually, however, these staff members are considered radiation workers and wear personnel monitors. As such, their radiation limits could be considered the same as those of all other radiation workers (i.e., 5 rems/yr or 0.05 Sv). Another precaution should be that no pregnant visitors or members of the nursing or housekeeping staff can attend the patient.

Personnel monitors. It is necessary to ensure radiation safety for not only the patient nearby but the nursing and housekeeping staff as well. The Nuclear Regulatory Commission looks most favorably on the use of film badges. While it requires some time to receive a report on data collected from film badges, this does present the radiation safety officer with an unbiased report regarding radiation exposures to the wearer of the film badge. Each person working with the patient must have his or her own film badge. Dosimeters can be used, but these are usually used only as a secondary monitoring device. The reason is that the dosimeters are biased records recorded by the individual exposed. While they do offer an advantage because of the immediacy of their readings, the unbiased aspect of the record is lost. In addition, calibration and leakage of the charge on the dosimeter is always a concern.

Patient excreta. Patient excreta is exempt from any of the NRC regulations regarding disposal of radioactive materials into the sewage system. For this reason, hospitals performing radiopharmaceutical therapy are encouraged to not collect the urine but to allow the patient to use the bathroom facilities as usual. The patient should be instructed to flush the toilet three or four times after use to ensure the removal of the radioactive materials. By allowing the patient to use the toilet, the need to collect urine is obviated and a great potential for contamination and exposure is eliminated.

Release of therapy patient. NRC regulations allow the release of any patient who is given a radiopharmaceutical (diagnostic or therapeutic) from radiation control when the

*This interpretation is being challenged by the NRC at the time of this writing. It is their wishes that, even though the radioactive patient's hospital room is a restricted area, the dose limits for members of the general public should apply. If so, then the ALARA approach to radiation safety would satisfy the usual therapeutic application.

measured dose rate from the patient is less than 5 mrem/hr at a distance of 1 m *or* the radioactivity in the patient is less than 30 mCi. In instances in which greater than 30 mCi of ^{99m}Tc is used in a diagnostic procedure, the first condition of 5 mR/hr at 1 m may be used since it would require about 80 mCi of ^{99m}Tc to receive a meter reading of 5 mR/hr at 1 m. Furthermore, this regulation suggests that at these same levels, radiation safety practices can be discontinued even in the event of a patient being required to remain in the hospital for some reason other than the radiation dose. In the latter instance, the patient would be allowed to be moved from the private room. In the past, patients were released if the radioactivity in the patient was less than 30 mCi. However, if hospitalization of the patient was required after the radioactivity had decayed to the 30-mCi level, it was the recommended practice (NCRP 37) to maintain the radiation safety program until patient dose rates reached 1.8 mR/hr at 1 m.

If <30 mCi (rather than <5 mR/hr at 1 m) becomes the action level used to release therapy patients, the preferred procedure to determine if 30 mCi remains in the patient is as follows: Administer the iodine to the patient and place the patient in the hospital bed, which has been positioned in an area of the room that minimizes radiation levels to nearby patients and other areas housing nonoccupational personnel.

Allow the radionuclide to be absorbed and circulate for 1 to 2 hours. Return to the patient with a G-M survey meter and determine a location in the room where the patient becomes as close to a point source as possible *and* the deflection of the needle is at maximum for that particular meter scale. Mark the spot and return each day for repeat measurements until the deflection is reduced to the equivalent of 30 mCi (e.g., if 100% of the scale represents 100 mCi, then 30% of scale would represent 30 mCi). With this technique, many of the problems of contamination and exposure are eliminated.

Decay disposal. The radioactive materials accumulated during the time of the therapy application should be monitored following the patient's removal from the room. Any bags containing radioactive material that give readings greater than background should be taken to the radioactive decay area, whereas those containers that are decayed to background levels can be thrown into the regular trash. Any radioactive waste going to decay must be labeled as being radioactive with some indication of its origin and the date of sequestration to the decay area. This material should remain for 10 physical half-lives and reaches background levels.

Release of the room. Once the patient has been released from the room and the radioactive trash has been removed, a complete survey should be performed of the patient's room, including the bathroom and sink facilities. Wipe tests should also be performed on all areas surveyed. Acceptable surveys would be those yielding radiation levels equal to or less than background. Acceptable wipe tests are those yielding less than 200 dpm/100 cm^2.

Phosphorus-32 therapies. Because of the beta nature of the radiation from phosphorus 32, radiation safety procedures as already defined should not apply, except when phosphorus 32 is administered in the colloidal form. Since this material is administered with the instillation method, the nurse should be advised to observe the wound and report any drainage to the radiation safety officer. It is presumed that bandages and dressings are contaminated in these situations. It is the responsibility of the radiation safety officer to supervise the changing of the dressings.

Bioassays. The thyroid burden of each individual who helped prepare and/or administer a dosage of iodine 131 (capsule or liquid) of >30 mCi must be measured within 3 days after administering the dosage. Refer to "Bioassays" at the beginning of this chapter. A record must be kept of each test, listing the thyroid burden measurement, its date, the name of the individual whose thyroid burden was measured, and the initials of the individual who made the measurements.

■ SEALED SOURCE THERAPY

The requirements for sealed-source therapies are no less stringent than those of radiopharmaceutical therapies. Many of these requirements are identical. The likelihood of contamination is considerably less because these are sealed sources and therefore not subject to the leakage that occurs with radiopharmaceuticals.

■ Storage

Just as with radiopharmaceutical therapy, safe storage of brachytherapy sources is of paramount interest. For sealed sources, special containers are made to house individual sources so that they do not become lost and so that inventories can be easily performed. To ensure complete accountability, an inventory should be performed listing the number of sources that are on hand at initiation of the therapy procedure, the number of sources that are being used during the therapy procedure (including those sources that are remaining), and the return and inventory of all sources.

■ Administration

The administration of sealed sources does not vary greatly from that of radiopharmaceutical therapy. Differences are pointed out in the following discussion.

Private room/private bath. A private room with a private bath is also a requirement for this form of therapy and for the same reasons as listed above. Contamination is not usually as much of a concern as is radiation exposure to the roommate and the potential loss of a sealed source.

Surveys/postings. The room should be surveyed and posted the same as for radiopharmaceutical therapy. The distinction with this form of therapy is that the change in radiation levels is not as extreme because of the use of long-lived radionuclides. Usually a single measurement on the first day will satisfy the entire treatment period. Release of the room to routine use must be performed by the radiation safety officer in accordance with the aforementioned guidelines.

Personnel monitors. Whole-body badges and ring badges are required to be worn by persons performing the therapeutic application. It is also considered extremely important that all personnel attending the patient wear personnel monitors to determine the amount of radiation exposure. No pregnant persons should be admitted to the therapy room. Persons less than 18 years of age can be admitted on a case-by-case basis.

Transport container. Since the sources are usually transported to the room for insertion, it is important that the container is left in the room of the patient being treated. The reason for this is that, should a source fall on the floor, someone would be able to pick it up with the long-handled forceps (which would also be left in the room) and placed into the storage container for safe harbor. Such an incident should be reported immediately to the radiation safety officer who would take immediate action to remove the source from the immediate environs of the patient's room and return it to the storage area or arrange for reinsertion.

Placarding. The patient's chart should be placarded with signs indicating that the patient is undergoing radioactive therapy treatment. Thus nurses or other attending personnel would know immediately that they were dealing with a patient containing radioactive materials.

Iodine-125 seed therapy. Because of the unique nature of seed therapy and the use of a low-energy gamma-emitter such as iodine 125, a separate radiation safety program is required as follows:

1. General
   Personnel who prepare, insert, or retrieve ^{125}I seeds must wear a finger- or wrist-type monitoring device to monitor radiation exposure to the extremities. To maintain accountability of the seeds, a source inventory should be performed at the following times:
   a. When the seeds are removed from storage
   b. Before and after the seeds are loaded in the applicator
   c. Before and after surgery
   In transporting seeds from storage and/or preparation areas to the place of use, adequate shielding must be employed to ensure good radiation safety practices.
2. Instructions to Nurses (for hospitalized patients)
   a. Nurses should be given a description of the size and appearance of the seeds.
   b. Handle dislodged seeds with a spoon or forcepts, never by hand. Place the dislodged seeds in a shielded container provided by the Radiation Safety Officer.
3. Surgical dressings and bandages used to cover the area of the insertion may be changed only by the attending physician. Dressings should be kept in a basin until checked by the Radiation Safety Officer.
4. All bed linen must be checked with a radiation survey meter before being removed from the patient's room to ensure that no dislodged sources are inadvertently removed.
5. No special precautions are needed for dishes, instruments, or utensils. Collected urine should be monitored for seeds prior to disposal. If found, seeds should be recovered and treated as radioactive waste.
6. The Radiation Safety Officer should be advised immediately of the loss and/or finding of a seed, of the need for emergency surgery, or of the death of the patient.
7. On discharge, the Radiation Safety Officer will perform a survey of the room and contents before housekeeping duties are initiated and before the room is returned to general use.

■ Emergency

In the event that the patient should undergo emergency surgery or die, it is necessary to ensure the safety of others attending the patient. The handling of the patient or body falls into three categories:*

1. Less than 5 mCi (185 MBq): If the patient contains less than 5 mCi in the entire body, no precautions are necessary.
2. Between 5 and 30 mCi (185 to 1110 MBq): If the patient contains 5 to 30 mCi in the entire body, no precautions are necessary in the burial process, the cremating process, or the embalming process. If autopsy is to be considered, however, the Radiation Safety Officer should supervise the proceedings. It is important that the autopsy physician knows he or she is dealing with a person containing radioactivity so that body fluids can be properly treated as contaminated and target organs can be removed during the autopsy process to avoid unnecessary exposure.
3. Greater than 30 mCi (1110 MBq): Should the body contain greater than 30 mCi, burial or cremation is considered possible with no further precautions. If, however, an autopsy or embalming is required, the Radiation Safety Officer should supervise in a manner similar to that in the items listed above.

■ Surveys

All places of sealed-source storage must be surveyed on a quarterly basis. The purpose of the survey is to ensure that ambient radiation levels in the area of storage fall within the bounds of good radiation safety practice.

*NCRP #37.

Table 16-2. Record retention period

Record	Retention	Reference
Receipt	3 years from transfer or disposal	30.51(c)(1)
Transfer	5 years	30.51(c)(3)
Surveys	3 years	20.2103(a)
Personnel monitoring	Indefinitely	20.2106(f)
Radiation Safety Committee minutes	Duration of license	35.22(a)(5)
Patient dosage	3 years	35.53(c)
Area surveys (daily & weekly)	3 years	35.70(h)
Disposal by decay in storage	3 years	35.92(b)
Other disposal	Indefinite	20.2108(b)
^{99}Mo assay	3 years	35.204(c)
Dose calibrator accuracy, linearity & constancy	3 years	35.50(e)
Dose calibrator geometry	Duration of dose calibrator	35.50(b)(4)
Dose/dosage records (written directive)	3 years	35.32(d)(2)
Survey meter calibration	3 years	35.51(d)
Sealed-source leak test	5 years	35.59(d)
Sealed-source inventory	5 years	35.59(g)
Survey of sealed-source storage	3 years	35.59(i)
Recordable event	3 years	35.32(c)(3)
QMP Annual review	3 years	35.32(b)(3)
Dose/dosage records (written directive)	3 years	35.32(d)(2)
Midadministrations	5 years	35.33(d)
Ministerial changes	Until license renewal or termination	35.31(b)
Xenon trap check & ventilation measurements	Undefined	35.205(e)
Instruction for care of patient receiving radiopharmaceutical therapy	3 years	35.310(b)
Room survey of radiopharmaceutical therapy patient (at time of administration)	3 years	35.315(a)(4)
Room survey of radiopharmaceutical therapy patient (on release)	Undefined	35.315(a)(7)
^{131}I bioassay	Indefinitely	35.315(a)(8) (refers to 20.2103(b)(3)
Survey of brachytherapy patient on source removal	3 years	35.404(b)
Survey on implant of implant area and brachytherapy patient for misplaced sources	3 years	35.406(d)
Brachytherapy source use records	3 years	35.406(d)
Instruction for care of brachytherapy patient	3 years	35.410(b)
Survey of brachytherapy patient room and surrounding areas on implant	3 years	35.415(a)(4)

■ Inventory

All sealed sources must be inventoried on a quarterly basis to ensure that their presence can be accounted for at all times. These sealed sources would include not only the therapy sources but any other sealed sources used in other parts of the hospital. A record must be kept of these inventoried sealed sources.

■ Wipe tests

Wipe tests must be performed on all beta and gamma sealed sources containing greater than 100 μCi. Such sealed sources would be the therapy sources, the dose calibrator sealed sources, the strontium 90 eye applicator, cobalt 60 teletherapy, and other items such as cobalt 57 flood discs in the nuclear medicine department. Leak tests are also required on alpha sources contained greater than 10 μCi of activity.

■ Record retention

The NRC has provided complete guidelines for retention of all records generated in a nuclear medicine department. They are as found in Table 16-2.

This chapter has described the Code of Federal Regulations as they pertain to the use of byproduct materials in diagnosis and/or radiopharmaceutical and sealed source therapy. It is imperative that all NRC licensees and users obtain a copy of Parts 20 and 35 and correlate it with statements and conditions of their current NRC license. It would also be helpful to obtain a copy of the NRC Regulatory Guide 10.8 (A guide for the preparation of applications for medical use programs, rev. 2, August 1987). The Guide suggests procedures that will help in maintaining compliance with these regulations. There are situations where the Guide goes beyond the requirements of 10 CFR Part 35. It is important to realize that 10 CFR Part 35 is a regulation;

Regulatory Guide 10.8 is a guide, however, and therefore simply a suggestion. Should the licensee decide to incorporate any or all of the procedures of Regulatory Guide 10.8 into their license application, they now become a procedure that must be implemented by the licensee. That implementation is subject to inspection and enforcement by the Nuclear Regulatory Commission.

REFERENCES

1. Code of federal regulations, Title 10, Parts 20 and 35, Washington, D.C., 1986, The U.S. Nuclear Regulatory Commission.
2. Medical use of byproduct material; final rule, Federal register (10/16/86), vol. 51, no. 200.
3. Precautions in the management of patients who have received therapeutic amounts of radionuclides, 2nd Printing, NCRP Report No. 37, Washington, D.C., 1978, National Council on Radiation Protection and Measurements.
4. Application of bioassy for ^{125}I ^{131}I, Regulatory Guide 8.20 (9/79), revision 1, U.S. Nuclear Regulatory Commission, Washington, D.C.
5. Early, P.J.: Radiation safety and handling of therapeutic radionuclides, Nucl. Med. Biol. 14(3):263-267, 1987. Int. J Radiat. Appl. Instrum. Part B.
6. Guide for the preparation of applications for medical programs, Regulatory Guide 10.8 (10/80), Rev. 1, U.S.Nuclear Regulatory Commission, Washington, D.C.
7. Early, P.J., and Weiss, S.C.: Medical use of byproduct material, Nuclear Regulatory Commission Rep. No. 10 CFR Part 35, revised 1987, J. Nucl. Med. Technol. 16(2):92-97, June 1988.

Part Two

CLINICAL NUCLEAR MEDICINE

Chapter 17

BONE

B. DAVID COLLIER
D. BRUCE SODEE
RALPH G. ROBINSON

B. David Collier and D. Bruce Sodee

Inorganic materials make up 45% of the constituents of bone. These materials include calcium, phosphate, and magnesium. Organic materials make up 30%, and water constitutes 25% of bone weight. Calcium makes up about 15% of the weight of fresh osseous tissue. Bone calcium exists in two forms, calcium carbonate and tricalcium phosphate; the ratio of calcium to phosphate is approximately 2.2:1.

There are two types of ossification—intramembranous and intracartilaginous (endochondral). The cranial vault, maxilla, and mandible are formed through ossification of membranes. The bones of the limbs, trunk, and base of the skull are transformed from cartilage to bone by both forms of ossification. It has been shown that calcium and phosphorus are first laid down in the epiphysis of developing bone and later move to the shaft, or diaphysis. Growth occurs at both ends of the bone. The cells involved in ossification are called *osteoblasts;* cells that deossify bone are called *osteoclasts*. Through the combined action of the osteoblasts and osteoclasts, complete replacement of calcified cartilage results in adult bone.

Hormones control bone formation and bone breakdown. Primarily parathormone, which is elaborated to the parathyroid gland, and thyrocalcitonin, which is produced by the thyroid gland, have roles in bone formation and destruction.

■ ANATOMY

The anatomy of bone has become increasingly important in the technology and practice of nuclear medicine. With the introduction of excellent bone-seeking radionuclides and improvement of instrumentation, a complete knowledge of the gross anatomy and microanatomy of bone is needed by all in this field. Because of the complexity of the 206 bones of the skeleton, the student is referred to basic anatomy textbooks such as *Gray's Anatomy* or to the chapter on the skeleton in *Structure and Function in Man* by Jacob and Francone. Illustrations included in this text introduce the student to the important skeletal structures visualized in bone imaging.

■ PHYSIOLOGY

The skeleton is composed primarily of collagen, cartilage, and osteoid tissues. Collagen is firm and pliable and is made up of reticulum, elastin, and ground substance. This latter compound substance selectively protects and supplies the parenchymal cells it supports. Therefore it becomes an important water-binding agent and plays an *ion-exchange resin* role important in mineral metabolism of bone.

Cartilage is hard, resilient, and made up of collagen fibrils, elastin, and ground substance. Hyalin cartilage is found in relation to bone growth and joint surfaces.

Osteoid is hard and rigid and morphologically identical to collagen. Its differential features are its osteoblasts and the advent of mineralization.

Bone, like every other tissue, is dynamic and is being remodeled throughout life. The histophysiologic resolution of old bone and replacement with new bone is called *internal remodeling of bone*. This requires continuous development of new generations of differentiating cells. Bone morphogenesis is the process of differentiation and organization of progenitor cells into cartilage or woven bone and then reabsorption and replacement of woven bone with a lamellar bone and bone marrow. Bone morphogenesis is the function of the biochemical components of the organic matrix of bone, collectively referred to as *bone morphogenic property*. This property consists of a protein (BMP), support fibrous protein (collagen), and a proteinase (BMPase) that degrades BMP.

The fact that bone is constantly renewed and regenerated in the adult is evidence that embryonic morphogenesis persists throughout life. Morphogenesis in bone is demon-

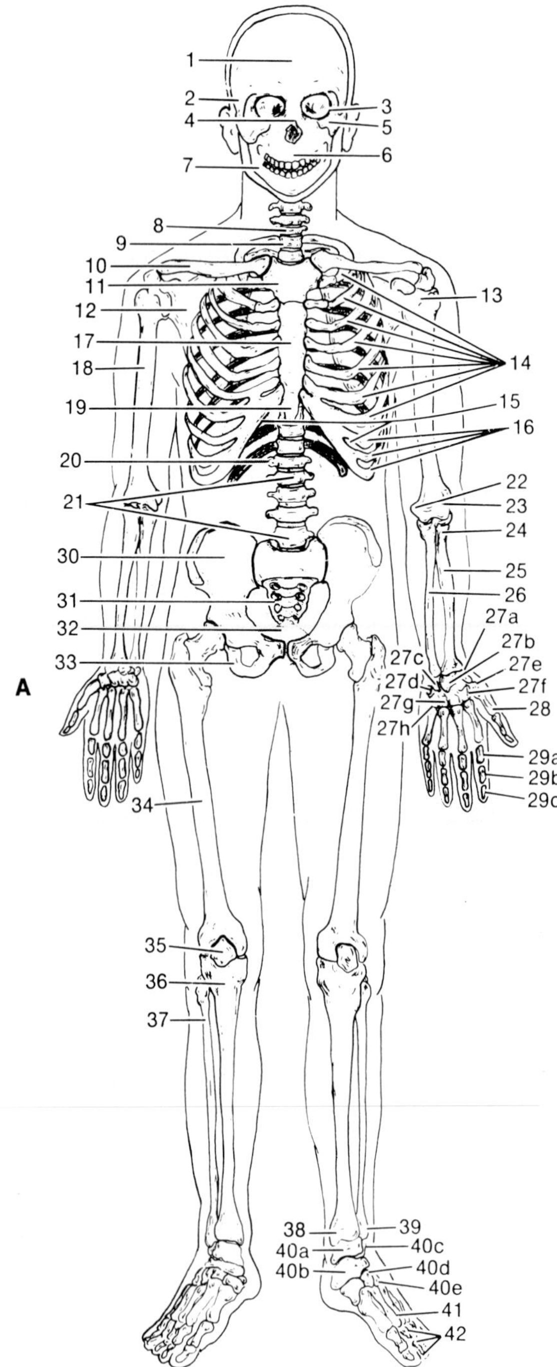

Fig. 17-1. A, Anterior skeleton.

1. Frontal bone
2. Temporal bone
3. Orbit
4. Nasal bone
5. Zygomatic bone
6. Maxilla
7. Mandible
8. Seventh cervical vertebra
9. Thoracic vertebra I
10. Clavicle
11. Manubrium of sternum
12. Shoulder blade
13. Head of humerus
14. True ribs
15. Kidneys
16. False ribs
17. Body of sternum
18. Humerus
19. Xiphoid process
20. Transverse process
21. Lumbar vertebrae
22. Medial condyle of humerus
23. Lateral epicondyle of humerus
24. Capitulum of radius
25. Radius
26. Ulna
27. Carpal bones
    a. Scaphoid bone of hand
    b. Lunate bone
    c. Triangular bone
    d. Pisiform bone
    e. Trapezium
    f. Trapezoid
    g. Capitate bone
    h. Hamate bone
28. Metacarpal bones
29. Finger bones
    a. Proximal phalanx
    b. Middle phalanx
    c. Distal phalanx
30. Iliac bone
31. Sacrum
32. Bladder
33. Ischium
34. Femur
35. Patella
36. Tibia
37. Fibula
38. Medial malleolus
39. Lateral malleolus
40. Tarsal bones
    a. Talus
    b. Navicular bone
    c. Calcaneus
    d. Cuneiform bones I to III
    e. Cuboid bone
41. Metatarsal bones
42. Phalanges of toes

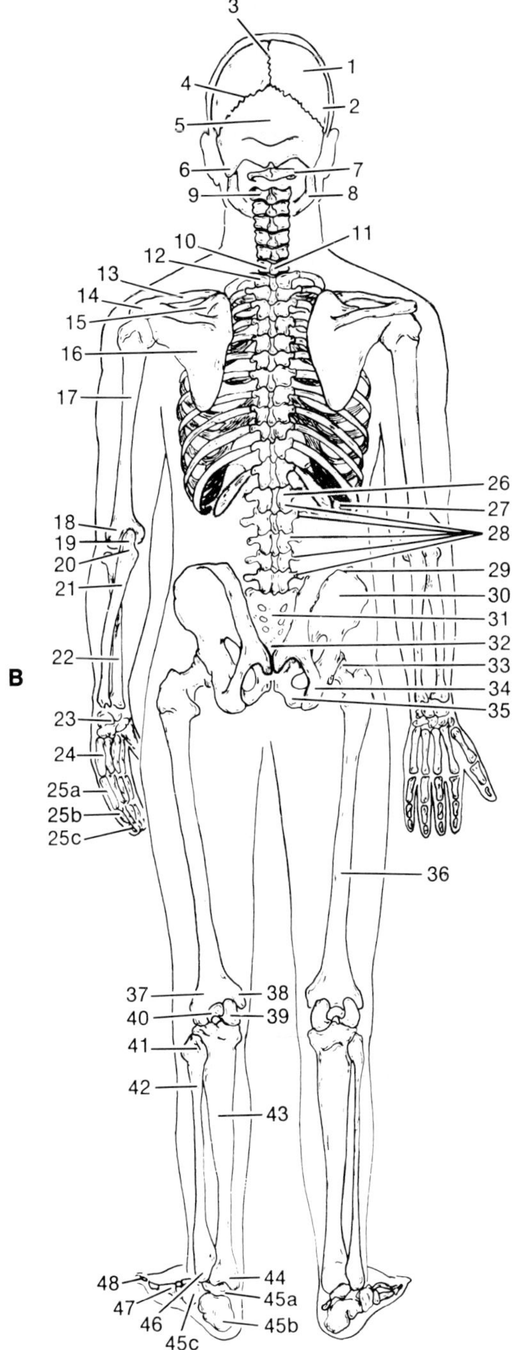

Fig. 17-1, cont'd. B, Posterior skeleton.

1. Parietal bone
2. Temporal bone
3. Sagittal suture
4. Lambdoidal suture
5. Occipital bone
6. Mastoid process
7. Atlas
8. Mandible
9. Axis, or second cervical vertebra
10. Seventh cervical vertebra
11. Spinous process
12. Thoracic vertebra I
13. Clavicle
14. Acromion
15. Spine of scapula
16. Scapula, or shoulder blade
17. Humerus
18. Lateral epicondyle of humerus
19. Olecranon
20. Head of radius
21. Ulna
22. Radius
23. Carpal bones
24. Metacarpal bones
25. Finger bones
    a. Proximal phalanx
    b. Middle phalanx
    c. Distal phalanx
26. Transverse process
27. Kidneys
28. Lumbar vertebrae
29. Iliac crest
30. Upper part of ilium
31. Sacrum
32. Bladder
33. Head of femur
34. Ischium
35. Pubic bone
36. Femur
37. Lateral epicondyle of femur
38. Medial epicondyle of femur
39. Medial condyle of femur
40. Lateral condyle of femur
41. Head of fibula
42. Fibula
43. Tibia
44. Medial malleolus
45. Tarsal bones
    a. Talus
    b. Calcaneus
    c. Cuboid bone
46. Lateral malleolus
47. Metatarsal bones
48. Phalanges of toes (conform of those of hand)

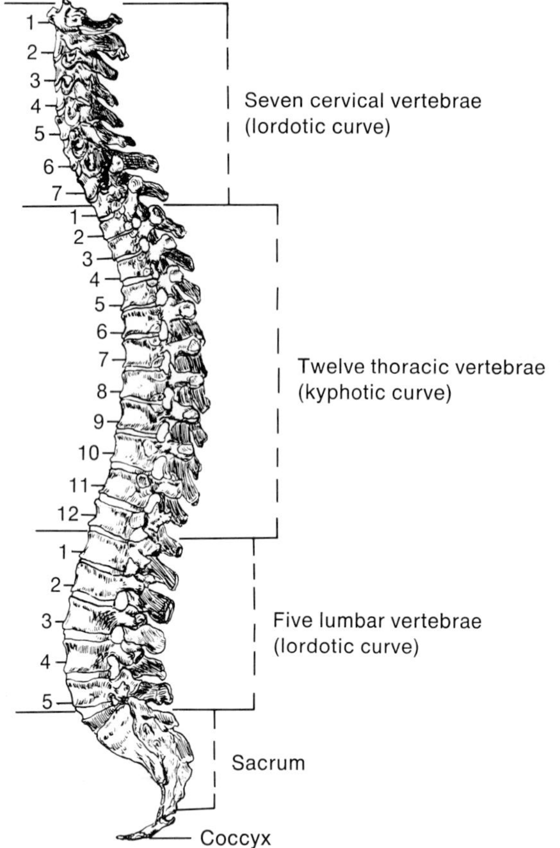

Fig. 17-2. Lateral view of vertebral column.

strated as mesenchymal cells proliferate and differentiate into osteoprogenitor cells, eventually reassembling as osteoblasts and forming new bone and finally interacting with perivascular connective tissue cell populations to develop bone marrow.

■ Formation

Periosteal tissue (the covering of bone) is differentiated into two layers. The cells of the inner layer that lie in contact with bone or cartilage become separated by a homogeneous substance called *osteoid,* which is laid down by cells called *osteoblasts*. The osteoblasts in their elaboration of osteoid become surrounded by osteoid and shrink to compact cells with pyknotic nuclei within their cell spaces, the lacunae, and are known as *osteocytes*. Successive layers of bone are laid down in concentric circles, and each layer is called a *lamina* (Fig. 17-3). Thus compact bone is formed. This manner of bone production is known as *intramembranous ossification*. Almost all the long and flat bones are formed by this method, and worn-out bone is replaced in the same manner. Thus this form of bone accounts for the bulk of the skeletal tissue.

■ Mineralization

Bone mineral exists in an apatite crystal form. Ions are arranged in units, and units are shared by contiguous units in a lattice arrangement much like interior walls of buildings are shared by adjacent rooms. The formula for bone salt is best represented by a hydroxyapatite:

$$3\ Ca_3\ (PO_4)_2 \cdot Ca\ (OH)_2$$

Other ions in trace amounts are Na^+, Mg^{++}, K^+, Cl^-, and F^-.

There is a continuous interchange of ions between the crystal lattice and the fluid that bathes it. Thus bone is a dynamic system in constant flux. Because of the unit structure of the crystalline component of bone, it has an immense surface area, approximating 100 acres in humans.

The factors involved in bone mineralization are still not well understood. The osteoblastic cells elaborate alkaline phosphatase, which plays a role in formation of ground substance but does not enhance mineralization. However, the osteocytes continue to elaborate phosphatase, although buried in a calcified intercellular substance that maintains a high phosphate ion concentration in the tissue fluid in the canaliculi prevents the ionic concentration from falling to a point at which bone salt would go back into solution. The osteocyte may also resorb surrounding bone in a process termed *osteoclytic osteolysis*.

■ Normal lysis

The stress stimulus is the most important factor in the modeling and remodeling of bone. Modeling of bones is completely the result of reorientation of lamellae into haversian systems (Fig. 17-3) laid down in lines of mechanical stress. Stress may be a matter of pressure or tension. The osteoclast is the cell that primarily causes deossification, the disappearance of bone organic matrix and its mineral content. Apparently the osteoclast disintegrates osteoid first, thus releasing the mineral content. Actually alteration of blood supply, mechanical trauma, parathyroid hormone, and vitamin D are also involved in bone destruction.

■ Factors in metabolism

Of the body calcium, 99% is in the skeleton, and less than 1% is in the extracellular fluid, organelles, and membranes. This latter 1% is under the physiologic control of the endocrine systems and transport mechanisms. Most calcium is in the structural calcium in the skeleton. Calcium is ingested in the diet and absorbed from the gut. It is continuously lost from the body through renal excretion, fecal loss, and sweat.

If losses of calcium are smaller than that absorbed, then excess calcium can be deposited in the skeleton. If losses of calcium from the body are greater than that absorbed, then calcium must be mobilized from the skeleton to maintain the homeostatic concentration in the extracellular fluid necessary for life. Vitamin D is the primary governing factor in the gut absorption of calcium and in large doses enhances the exchange of calcium from bone into serum. Mobilization of calcium is influenced by various endocrine glands. Growth hormone controls longitudinal growth of

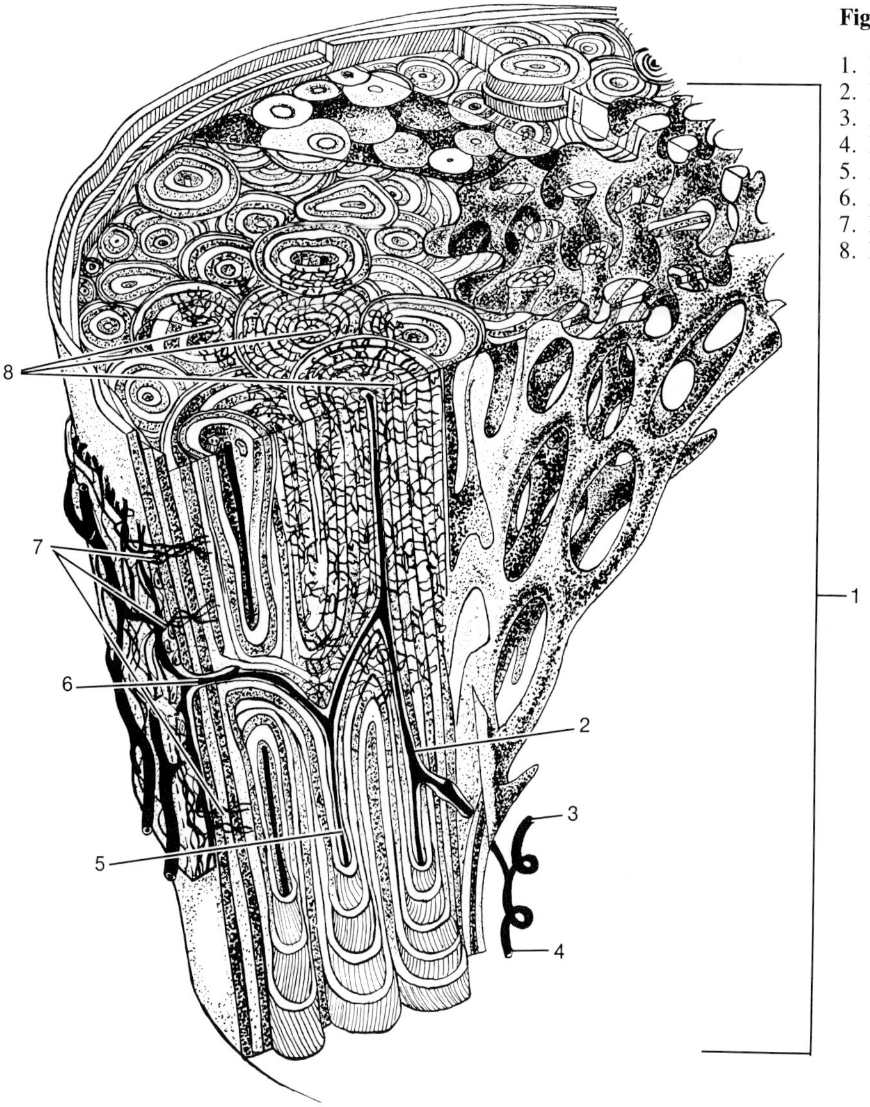

Fig. 17-3. Cross-sectional anatomy of long bone.

1. Medullary cavity
2. Haversian canal
3. Ascending medullary artery
4. Descending medullary artery
5. Arterioles derived from medullary artery
6. Anastomosis
7. Periosteal arteries
8. Haversian system

bone; linear growth is accompanied by remodeling of bone, removal of calcium from formed bone, and redeposition in new epiphyseal areas. Thyroid hormone increases both bone formation and, to a greater degree, bone reabsorption rates. Adrenocortical hormones inhibit bone formation to a greater extent than bone reabsorption. Parathyroid hormones influence bone reabsorption, bone remodeling, and increased bone turnover. Finally, calcitonin, a hormone secreted by cells found in the thyroid, reduces bone turnover, lowering serum calcium. The net effect of all the hormone systems is on the deposition or removal of calcium to and from the skeleton, which provides the homeostatic concentration of calcium in extracellular fluid.

■ Circulation (Fig. 17-3)

The bone-nutrient-arterial system consists of branches of the nutrient artery and the metaphyseal arteries in anastomosis with each other to become the medullary blood supply. The periosteal arterial system is a component of the arterial system that supplies the surrounding muscles. Three fourths or more of the compactum is supplied with blood by the medullary system; therefore the blood flow through bone is normally centrifugal from medulla to periosteum. In animal research it has been shown that if the nutrient system is blocked, the periosteal system is able to reverse the usual flow and convey blood supply to the compactum. Bone is well supplied with nutrients because no bone cell is more than 0.10 mm away from a capillary. Bone is permeated by a system of tiny canals (canaliculi) that extend from one lacuna to another and extend to a bony surface where the capillary is situated. These canals are actually the remnants of the cytoplasmic connecting process of osteoblasts. As osteoid and calcified bone are formed, these processes are retracted, leaving the canals (canaliculi) in their place. Tissue fluid originating from the capillary fills the canaliculi and lacunae. Thus metabolites are brought to the osteocyte, and waste is carried away. This tissue fluid bathes the crystalline component of bone, and ion exchanges are made between this component and the extracellular fluid.

Bone marrow

While bone formation is extending from ossification centers toward each end of the fetal cartilaginous bone model, the periosteum continues to add bone to the sides of the model. As the periphery becomes stronger, the cancellous bone in its central portion is no longer necessary for support, so this bone dissolves and leaves a cavity called the *marrow cavity*. In the fetus the marrow of most bones is red marrow, which derives its color from the vast numbers of red blood cells in various stages of production. During the growth period, the marrow of most bones becomes yellow or filled with large quantities of fat. In the adult, red marrow is found only in the bones of the vault of the skull, flat bones, bodies of the vertebrae, cancellous bone of some of the short bones, and at the ends of long bones. Under conditions in which increased red–blood-cell production is needed, yellow marrow becomes reconverted to red marrow. In red bone marrow, multipotential stem cells called the *primitive reticular cell* and the *endothelial cell* differentiate into the erythrocytic, myelocytic, and megakaryocytic series of cells that generate the adult red blood cell, the granular leukocyte, and the platelet. The vascular supply of bone marrow is derived from the nutrient artery. The arteries divide into capillaries, and the latter run into sinusoids. Sinuses form a system of vessels running from the periphery toward a central longitudinal vein. Hemopoietic tissue lies between the sinuses. Capillaries stemming from marrow arterioles enter the haversian canals to supply endosteal parts of the diaphyseal bone. The blood flow of bone marrow is 0.5 ml/gm/min, as compared to liver blood flow, which is 0.56 ml/gm/min and may be altered by physiologic demand.

BONE IMAGING

LABORATORY APPLICATION

40

ROUTINE IMAGING STUDIES

Purpose

Bone imaging is used to detect skeletal lesions at the earliest possible time, monitor the course of skeletal disease, and evaluate the metabolic activity of skeletal lesions. Bone imaging usually will detect the presence of metastatic disease before radiographs become positive. In addition, early osteomyelitis typically is associated with positive bone images and normal radiographs. As much as 50% of the bone must be decalcified before either tumors or infection can be detected with radiographs. Bone imaging, however, can detect these lesions with as little as 1% decalcification at a much earlier stage. Early stages of avascular necrosis also may be associated with positive bone images and normal radiographs. Stress fractures, an increasingly common sports-related injury, are identified earlier and more frequently with bone imaging than with radiographs. Furthermore, occult fractures of the femoral neck, pelvis, and spine occasionally may be detected by bone imaging even after conventional radiographs have failed to locate the abnormality. Serial bone imaging examinations are an accurate, objective, and convenient way to monitor the activity of skeletal disease that is being treated. For example, the patient who is known to have metastatic bone disease and who is undergoing chemotherapy may benefit from serial–bone-imaging examinations. Other diseases for which serial–bone-imaging examinations may be requested include osteomyelitis and Paget's disease. Bone imaging is used also to evaluate the metabolic activity of skeletal lesions. For example, radiographic findings reported as suspicious but not definite for tumor, infection, or fracture often lead to further investigation with bone imaging. Such lesions if present would produce a positive bone image. Bone imaging provides a functional display of skeletal activity. With rare exceptions, the examination is performed today using ^{99m}Tc-labeled diphosphonates. Diphosphonates are absorbed on the surface of bone in a manner that reflects both local osteoblastic activity and skeletal vascularity. For this reason, metastases, infection, fracture, and other bony lesions that incite an intense osteoblastic response are easily detected by bone imaging. Avascular necrosis, which produces a zone of absent skeletal vascularity and deficient osteoblastic activity, also may be detected with bone imaging.

The kidneys of normal young adults will excrete about half of the injected dose of ^{99m}Tc diphosphonate. However, metabolic bone disease or widespread bone tumors may produce avid skeletal uptake of the nuclide with very little of the injected activity being excreted in the urine. Renal failure also produces low renal clearance of the injected dose. With renal failure the skeleton is imaged with less than the usual clarity because of high background activity in the soft tissues. High-resolution collimation using either pinhole, converging, or straight-bore collimators may at times provide additional important diagnostic information. For pediatric skeletal imaging, pinhole collimators are particularly useful. In addition, image contrast may be slightly increased by using asymmetric camera energy window for ^{99m}Tc. Both ^{67}Ga citrate and ^{111}In-labeled leukocyte imaging have been used to identify sites of osteomyelitis and septic arthritis. In addition, ^{67}Ga citrate may also be used as a tumor-seeking agent in identifying sites of bony malignancy.

Indications

1. Screening of high-risk patients with tumors (e.g., breast, lung, prostate, or kidney cancer) known to metastasize frequently to bone.
2. Detection of early osteomyelitis.
3. Detection of early avascular necrosis.
4. Detection of stress fractures and other occult skeletal trauma.
5. Detection and evaluation of Paget's disease, metabolic bone disease, and other osteopathies.
6. Detection and evaluation of arthritis and internal joint derangements.
7. Evaluation of bone viability when blood supply is in question.
8. Evaluation of bone and joint pain of obscure origin.
9. Evaluation following an elevated alkaline phosphatase level.
10. Evaluation following questionably abnormal skeletal radiographs.
11. Serially following the course of bony response to therapeutic regimens (radiation therapy, antitumor chemotherapy, antibiotic therapy, or other treatments).
12. Differentiation of monostotic from polyostotic primary bone tumors or other skeletal disease.
13. Localization of sites for biopsy.

Procedure

Materials

1. 20 mCi (740 MBq) of ^{99m}Tc
2. Scintillation camera
3. Medium/high-resolution whole-body low energy collimator or single-pass diverging collimator

Patient preparation

1. Inject 20 mCi (740 MBq) of ^{99m}Tc diphosphonate 2 to 3 hours before imaging. Dose-to-imaging time depends on the kit used. A 3-hour waiting period seems to be adequate for most of the kits.
2. Instruct the patient to drink as much water as possible during the waiting period and to void frequently. Hydration seems to reduce the background (labeled phosphate compound not taken up by bone) through renal excretion.
3. Have the patient void immediately before imaging.
4. Explain the entire procedure to the patient.

Technique: flow study and blood-pool imaging

1. Before injecting the ^{99m}Tc diphosphonate, position the patient in front of the camera with the skeletal structures of greatest medical interest in the center of the field-of-view (FOV).
2. Set camera controls for ^{99m}Tc peak energy (140 keV) (20% window).
3. Immediately following the bolus intravenous injection of the ^{99m}Tc diphosphonate, obtain the flow study as 10 or more images for 5 seconds per image. Other imaging sequences such as 15 images for 3 seconds per image are also acceptable.
4. Immediately following the flow study, obtain a 500,000-count blood-pool image.

Technique: whole-body table (single-pass)

1. Make sure the patient has voided before beginning imaging procedure. This diminishes the bladder activity.
2. Center patient in the supine position on table (prone position may be used if patient cannot lie supine). Elevate patient's arms with sheets.
3. Place collimator as close to the patient as possible to increase image quality.
4. Set camera controls for ^{99m}Tc energy (140 keV).

Continued.

5. Set window at 200 (20%).
6. Connect area image table to floor tracks, or center whole-body table to the detector head.
7. Place marker to the left of the patient's head.
8. Make sure the switch is in the single-pass or whole-body position.
9. Check for proper orientation.
10. Determine image speed for desired information density (reasonable time 15 to 30 min/whole-body images).
11. Disengage present counts and time buttons.
12. Reset digital readouts to zero.
13. Set proper intensities.
14. Return collimator to the head of the table. Obtain posterior and anterior whole-body images.
15. Following whole-body images, spot images of the following areas are recommended:
    Accumulate 1 million counts
    - Pelvis, to include femoral heads (anterior and posterior views)
    - Lumbar spine, to include iliac crests and kidneys
    - Dorsal spine, to include superior poles of kidneys
    - Chest, anterior view

    Accumulate 700,000 counts
    - Skull, to include cervical spine (anterior, posterior, and both lateral views)

    Accumulate 500,000 counts
    - Extremities, depending on the clinical symptoms of the patient and/or after carefully examining the whole-body images (additional views may have to be obtained to better delineate the areas of abnormality)

Technique: spot imaging

1. Make sure the patient has voided before beginning the imaging procedure.
2. Place the patient in the prone position on the imaging table.
3. Set the camera controls for ^{99m}Tc peak energy (140 keV) (20%) window.
4. Obtain 1000-K count or 2000 information density images. Set proper intensity and proper orientation.
5. With the patient in the prone position, place the detector head over the upper thoracic vertebrae to include C7 (posterior 1). The collimator surface should be in contact with the patient's back.
6. Take a 1000-K count or a 2000 information density view.
7. Take the following views the same as in step 5. Keep the same intensity throughout the study. The collimator surface should be as close to the patient's body as possible.
   Accumulate 1000-K count views as follows:
   Posterior
   - 2, Lower thoracic vertebrae
   - 3, Lumbar vertebrae
   - 4, Sacrum and coccyx
   - 5, Skull and upper cervical vertebrae
   - 6, Left upper rib cage to include shoulder
   - 7, Left lower rib cage
   - 8, Right upper rib cage to include shoulder
   - 9, Right lower rib cage
   - 10, Pelvic
   - 11, Left hip to include femoral head
   - 12, Right hip to include femoral head
8. With the patient in the supine position, perform the following views with the same intensity as in step 5.
   Accumulate 1000-K count views as follows:
   - 13, Sternum
   - 14, Left upper rib cage to include shoulder
   - 15, Left lower rib cage

16, Right upper rib cage to include shoulder
17, Right lower rib cage
18, Pelvis

9. Anterior 19, with the patient in the supine position: bend the right knee in such a manner as to obtain a lateral view of the knee to include the lower femur and upper tibia and fibula. Take a 500-K count or 800 information density view. Change intensity setting.
10. Take the following views for 500-K counts. Use the same intensity as in step 9.
    Anterior
    20, Right femur
    21, Right tibia and fibula
    22, Left femur
    23, Left lateral knee to include lower femur and upper tibia and fibula
    24, Left tibia and fibula
    25, Right humerus
    26, Right lateral elbow to include lower humerus and upper ulna and radius
    27, Right ulna and radius
    28, Left humerus
    29, Left lateral elbow to include lower humerus, upper ulna, and radius
    30, Left ulna and radius

Technique: routine bone SPECT

1. Perform gamma camera quality control for bone SPECT (Table 17-1).
2. Patient preparation is identical to routine bone imaging, except inject 25 mCi (925 MBq) of ^{99m}Tc diphosphonate.
3. Patient positioning is more critical than for routine bone imaging. For example, if the patient is lying in a rotated or obliqued position on the imaging table, the SPECT study will be more difficult to interpret. Furthermore, patient motion will degrade SPECT image quality. See Table 17-2 for additional details.
4. Low-energy, all-purpose collimator
5. Setup for a circular or elliptical 360-degree rotation that comes as close to the patient as possible.
6. Use 64 × 64 matrix on 400-mm FOV camera or 128 × 128 matrix on 500-mm FOV camera.
7. Data acquisition: 20 sec/projection, 64 projections over 360 degrees.

Table 17-1. Gamma camera quality-control for bone SPECT

Daily
Extrinsic flood for uniformity check.
3.0 million counts 400-mm field-of-view camera
4.5 million counts 500-mm field-of-view camera
Weekly
Update energy correction per manufacturer recommendation
Intrinsic flood for uniformity check:
3.0 million counts 400-mm field-of-view camera
4.5 million counts 500-mm field-of-view camera
Update tomographic center of rotation
Update high count extrinsic flood for uniformity correction:
30 million counts for 64 × 64 matrix
120 million counts for 128 × 128 matrix
Monthly
Image bar phantom for check of planar resolution
Image tomographic phantom (optional)

From Collier, B.D., and others: Bone SPECT, Semin. Nucl. Med. 17(3):248, 1987.

Continued.

Table 17-2. Special patient positioning for bone SPECT

Bony structure	Special positioning	Pitfalls
Knees	2- to 3-in. pad between knees. Secure knees with straps to prevent motion Secure feet in neutral position to prevent rotation	For obese patients both knees may not fit in field of view
Hips and pelvis	Empty bladder before exam Position hips symmetrically and secure knees and/or feet to prevent motion	Bladder filling during exam creates artifacts
Lumbar spine	Keep arms out of field of view A pillow under the knees may relieve back pain	Patients with back pain often move during exam
TMJ	Secure neck in comfortable hyperextension Instruct patient not to talk	Check lateral view to be sure the chin is in field of view

From Collier, B.D., and others: Bone SPECT, Semin. Nucl. Med. 17(3):249, 1987.

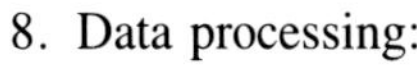

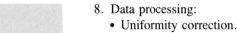

8. Data processing:
   - Uniformity correction.
   - Hanning filter (Frequency cutoff = 0.8 cycle/cm). Do this *before* reconstruction.
   - Reconstruct by filtered backprojection with Ramp filter.
   - No attentuation correction.
   - 6-mm (1 pixel)–thick transaxial, sagittal, and coronal images are produced with the 400-mm FOV camera; 8-mm (2 pixels)-thick, with 500-mm FOV camera.

   NOTE—Some computers may not offer the Hanning filter. If the data are acquired in a 64 × 64 matrix on a 400-mm FOV camera, you may use a standard 9-point smooth for your preprocessing filter.
9. Display:
   - Linear grey scale for most examinations such as lumbar spine, knee, and temporomandibular (TMJ).
   - Log grey scale is useful when searching for femoral head avascular necrosis.

Technique: high-resolution bone SPECT

1. High-resolution collimator
2. Elliptical orbit
3. Data acquisition: 25 sec/projection, 64 projections over 360 degrees
4. Data processing and image display: May be identical to routine bone SPECT technique. If available, distance-weighted reconstruction should be used.

NOTES:

1. High-resolution technique improves the resolution of SPECT examination of the lumbar spine.
2. High-resolution technique provides little or no improvement in TMJ and knee SPECT.
3. High-resolution technique substantially worsens the bladder-filling artifact, which often interferes with hip SPECT.

Interpretation

Normal "hot" areas (Figs. 17-4 and 17-5)

Normally, a high degree of uptake of ^{99m}Tc-labeled diphosphonate compounds occurs in sacroiliac joints, hip joints, the glenoid fossa, the acromioclavicular joints, the sternoclavicular joints, the ends of long bones, growing epiphyses, and over the vertebral column. Fractures and orthopedic surgery produce increased uptake that may persist for 1 or more years. Apparent variations in uptake in the spine are caused by the normal curvatures of the spinal column.

Uptake in soft tissues

^{99m}Tc-diphosphonate bone images show concentration of radioactivity by functioning kidneys with excretion of the agent into the renal collecting systems and bladder. Pronounced renal uptake may

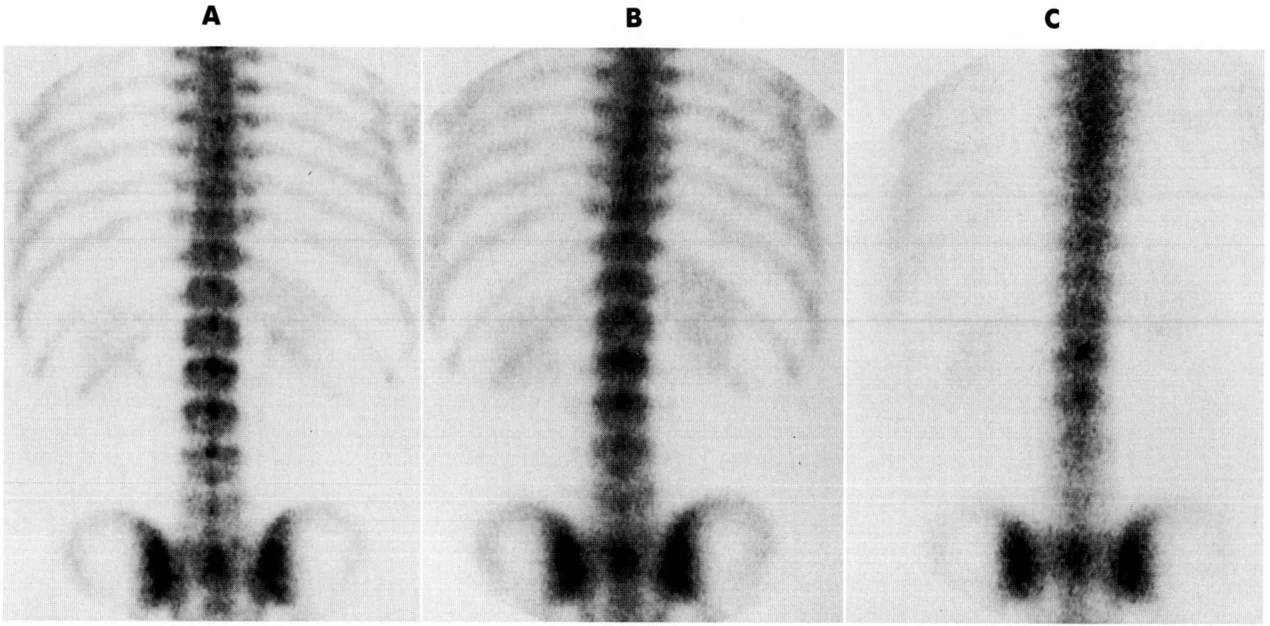

Fig. 17-4. Normal posterior view bone images of the thoracolumnar spine obtained with the collimator **(A)** in close apposition to the patient's back. **B,** 5 inches from the back. **C,** 10 inches from the back. It is apparent that as the collimator is moved away from the patient, spatial resolution decreases and image clarity deteriorates. Both planar and SPECT bone imaging benefit from having the collimator as close to the patient as possible.

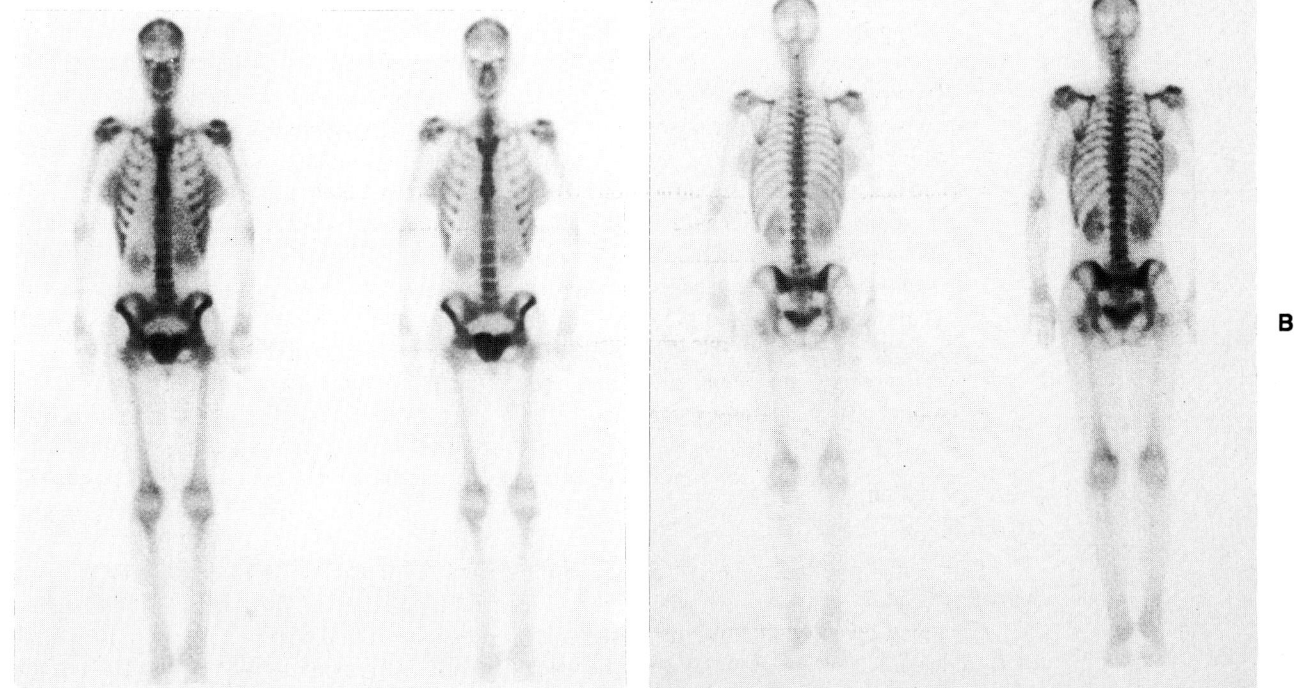

Fig. 17-5. Normal bone study. Bone images performed 2 hours after administration of a 20 mCi (740 MBq) dose of ^{99m}Tc medronate disodium. **A,** Anterior whole-body images. **B,** Posterior whole-body images. Diagnosis—normal study. Breast visualization is normal in young females.

Continued.

indicate poor renal function or obstructive uropathy. Areas of soft tissue necrosis or calcification in addition to tumors may concentrate ^{99m}Tc-diphosphonate compounds.

Abnormal uptake in bones

Neoplastic, traumatic, and inflammatory lesions of bone that incite an osteoblastic response also will produce areas of abnormally increased ^{99m}Tc-diphosphonate concentration. Purely osteolytic lesions (often seen with multiple myeloma and eosinophilic granuloma but only rarely with the common forms of metastatic bone disease) are less likely to be detected as sites of increased scintigraphic activity.

Diagnosis

Increased deposition of bone-imaging agents is not in itself diagnostic of a neoplastic process, nor does a positive bone image differentiate between malignant and benign bone tumors. Nonneoplastic causes of positive bone images include trauma and inflammatory processes. Paget's disease of bone when metabolically active is also associated with positive bone images. In the absence of fractures, the bone image is not positive in osteoporosis; however, it is frequently positive in osteomalacia. The final diagnosis often must be made by correlating the bone image with clinical data and radiographic findings.

Diagnostic pitfalls

Diagnostic "pitfalls" to keep in mind when interpreting bone images include the following:

1. There is increased concentration in areas of normally increased blood flow and osteoblastic activity, such as the metabolically active epiphyses of children.
2. Bone images may be negative in purely osteolytic eosinophilic granuloma, multiple myeloma, and (more rarely) metastatic bone disease.
3. Bone images may be negative when bony healing is completed (e.g., healed fractures, cured osteomyelitis, successfully treated bone metastases). However, it may take 1 or more years for the bone images to return to a normal appearance.
4. When bone images are positive but nonspecific, radiographic correlation is important. Remember, however, that radiographs may remain normal for 6 months or more after a metastatic lesion is detected on the bone image. Serial radiographs or biopsy may be necessary.
5. In breast cancer, the true positive yield with bone imaging in stage I or II disease is usually no more than 3% in the perioperative period. However, 3 to 6 months later the number of metastatic bony sites increases with a steady rise up to 18 months postoperative. It is suggested that all patients with breast cancer undergo a perioperative baseline whole-body ^{99m}Tc-diphosphonate study. A follow-up study at 6 to 12 months can then be compared with the baseline bone images.
6. ^{67}Ga citrate or ^{111}In-labeled leukocyte imaging may be used in conjunction with bone imaging to study osteomyelitis (Fig. 17-6, *A* and *D*). These studies may better define active osteomyelitis and may in addition detect adjacent deep soft tissue infection.
7. ^{99m}Tc-diphosphonate compounds may concentrate at sites of significant soft tissue pathologic conditions such as breast carcinoma (Fig. 17-7), malignant pleural effusion (Fig. 17-8) or ascites, soft-tissue malignancies, myositis ossifications, myocardial infarction, electrical burns, ectopic calcification, intramuscular injections, splenic infarction, and amyloid deposition.

Arthritis

In all of the arthritides there is increased concentration of nuclide in the bone adjacent to the diseased joints. Either synovitis with increased regional blood flow or direct bony involvement may account for this periarticular uptake. Based solely on bone scan findings, it is therefore not possible to distinguish with complete confidence between the various forms of arthritis. However, recognizing certain characteristic patterns of multiple-joint involvement (e.g., carpus and proximal joints of the hand in rheumatoid arthritis as opposed to distal joints of the hand in osteoarthritis) may be of value in confirming the clinical diagnosis and documenting the extent of disease.

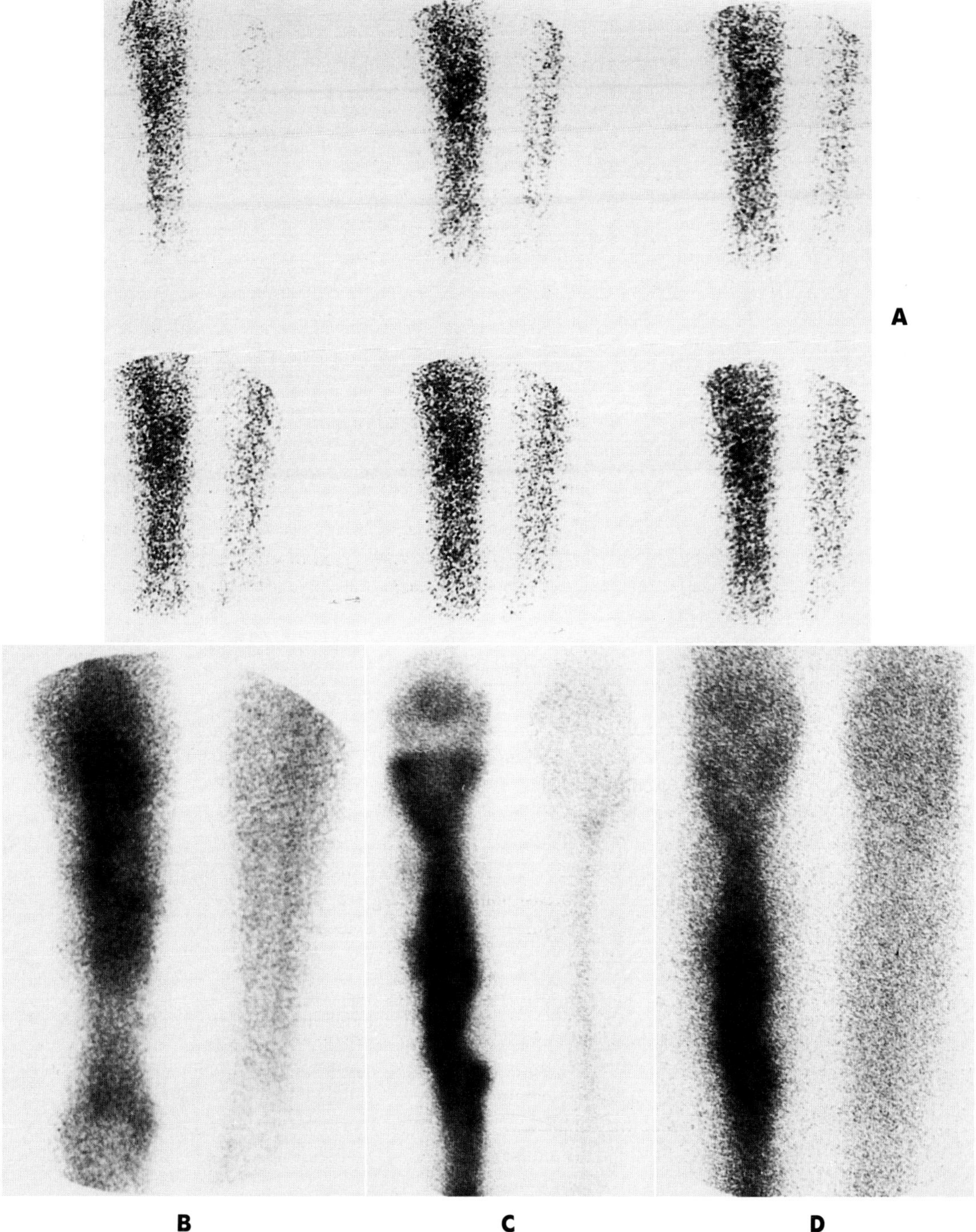

Fig. 17-6. Osteomyelitis of the right tibia. **A,** Anterior flow study (5 seconds/image). **B,** Anterior blood-pool image. Both **A** and **B** show a significant increase in perfusion to both bone and soft tissues of the right calf. **C,** Anterior bone image shows very intense uptake indicating active bony repair. **D,** Anterior gallium-67 image shows significant abnormal uptake in a slightly different distribution than is seen on the bone image. The findings are typical of osteomyelitis.

Continued.

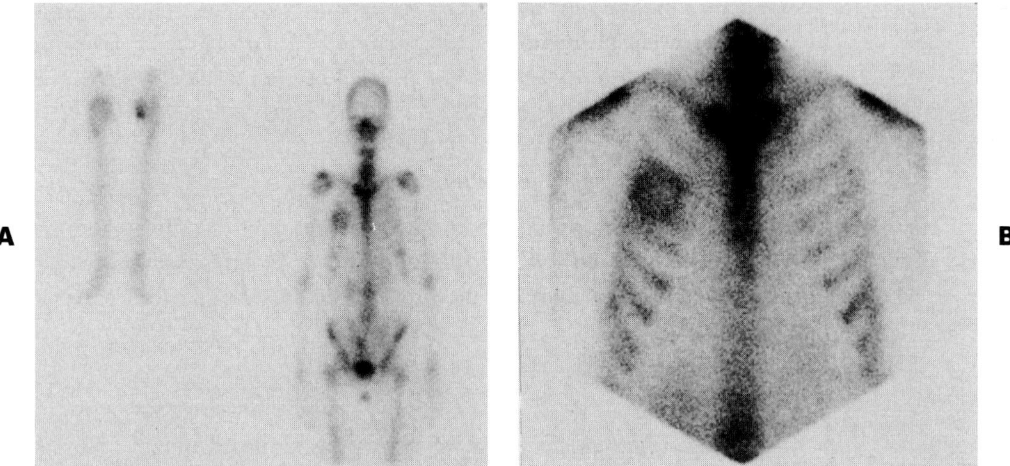

Fig. 17-7. Mastitis or malignancy. Abnormal bone images performed 2 hours after administration of 20 mCi (740 MBq) dose of ^{99m}Tc medronate disodium. There is abnormal soft tissue accumulation of radionuclide in the region of the right breast. **A,** Anterior whole-body. **B,** Spot image of the anterior sternum and rib cage with soft tissue uptake of ^{99m}Tc in the region of the right breast.

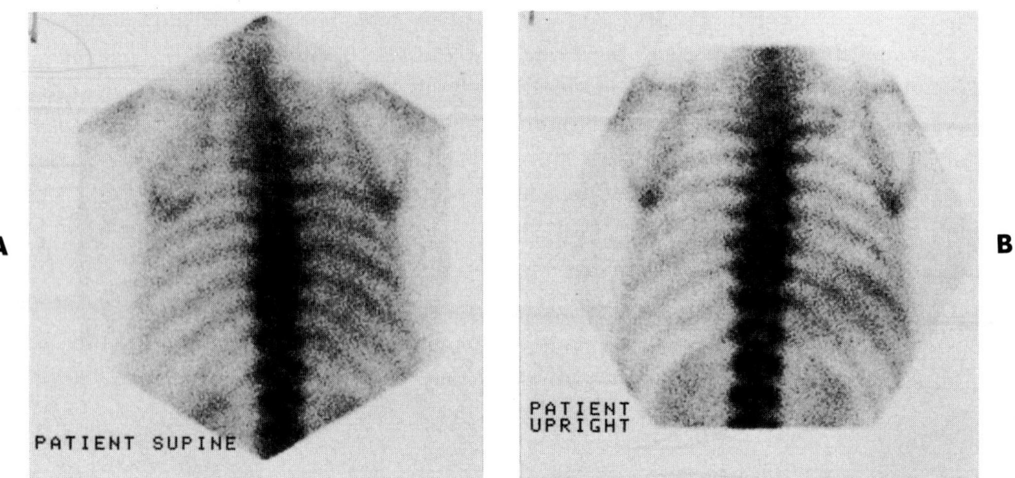

Fig. 17-8. Malignant pleural effusion. Abnormal spot images of the thorax performed 2 hours after the administration of 20 mCi (740 MBq) of ^{99m}Tc medronate disodium. There is a diffuse, increased concentration of radionuclide independently along the right hemidiaphragm. **A,** Spot image of the posterior thorax with the patient recumbent. Note diffuse concentration of ^{99m}Tc medronate disodium throughout right thorax area. **B,** Spot-image posterior thorax with patient in upright position. Diffuse concentration of radionuclide has now settled to right hemidiaphragm area compatible with malignancy associated with pleural fluid.

Avascular necrosis (Fig. 17-9)

Avascularity of the head or metaphysis of long bones may occur spontaneously or may be acquired secondary to fractures, sickle-cell disease, alcoholism, steroid administration, or other less common conditions. Initially there is an absence of accumulation of nuclide in the avascular and infarcted bone. Later there is a healing phase of bony repair with activation of osteoblasts and increased accumulation of nuclide.

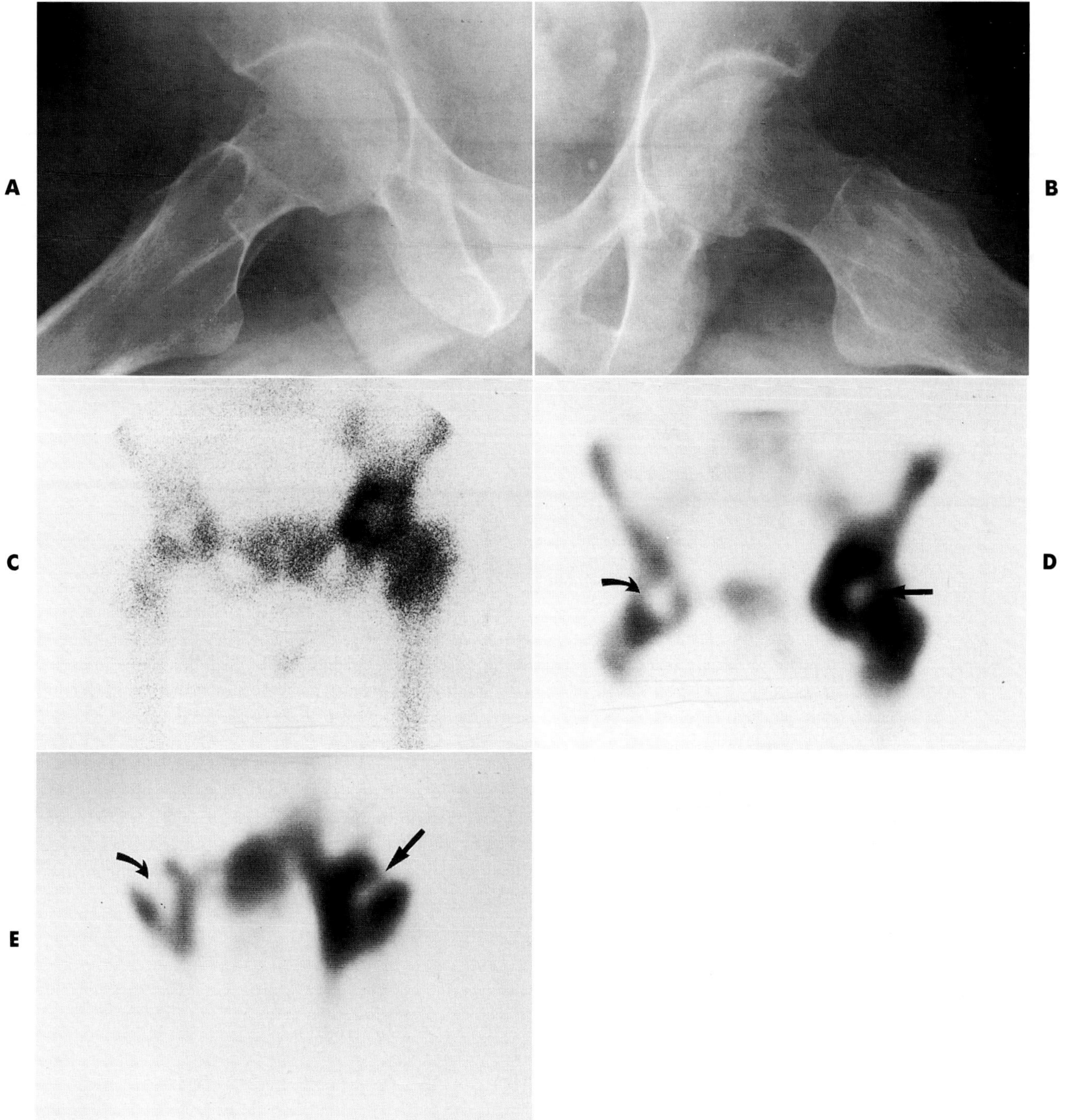

Fig. 17-9. Bilateral femoral head avascular necrosis. **A,** Normal right hip radiograph. **B,** Left hip radiograph shows sclerosis and flattening of the femoral head. **C,** Anterior planar bone image shows increased activity over the acetabulum and proximal left femur without convincing evidence of a photon-deficient defect in the left femoral head. **D,** Coronal SPECT and **E,** Transaxial SPECT bone images through both hips clearly demonstrate a central photon-deficient defect surrounded by increased activity within the left femoral head *(straight arrow)*. In addition, a photon-deficient defect is seen within the asymptomatic right femoral head *(curved arrow)*. (From Collier, B.D., and others: Detection of femoral head avascular necrosis in adults by SPECT, J. Nucl. Med. 26(9):982, 1985.)

Continued.

Avulsions

With sudden overextension there may be avulsions at the bony attachments of major muscle groups. Even though a fracture has not occurred, avulsion of the ligament from the periosteum causes a focal region of increased uptake.

Bone grafts

For several months both donor and graft sites have increased concentration of nuclide. Long segmental bone grafts that are implanted without an arterial anastomosis initially show increased uptake at both ends with absent concentration of nuclide in the center of the graft. During the next several months, osteoblasts usually grow into the graft from both ends. Sequential bone scans will show advancing margins of increased uptake that eventually meet in the middle of the bone graft.

Bone marrow expansion

In patients with bone marrow expansion there is increased concentration of nuclide in the surrounding cortical bone. For example, increased uptake around the knees secondary to the bone marrow expansion in sickle-cell disease is common. Diffuse metastatic replacement of marrow can produce a similar image.

Diabetic gangrene: avascular

In avascular processes such as diabetic gangrene there is an absence of delivery of nuclide to the affected area distal to the occluded vessels. Above the avascular area there usually is a generalized increase in uptake in the affected extremity.

Fibrous dysplasia (Fig. 17-10)

Fibrous dysplasia of bone is a benign overgrowth of fibrous tissue. Sites of skeletal involvement are hypermetabolic and show a significant increase in concentration of nuclide. Bone images show one or more lesions in the face, skull, or long bones having an appearance indistinguishable from metastatic disease. For accurate diagnosis, radiographic correlation is essential.

Fracture

Within 72 hours from the time of injury, most adult and all pediatric patients will have increased concentration of ^{99m}Tc diphosphonate at fracture sites. In geriatric populations, some fracture sites will not show increased uptake until 5 days after the injury. Radiographs will detect most acute fractures. However, femoral neck, pelvis, spine, scaphoid, or other clinically significant fractures

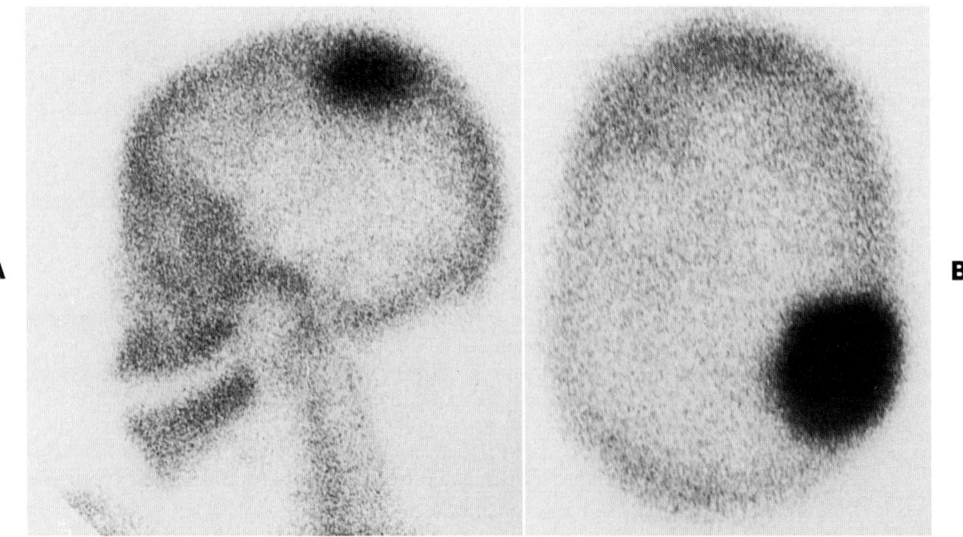

Fig. 17-10. Fibrous dysplasia. **A,** Left lateral of skull. **B,** Vertex of skull. A significant increase in uptake is seen at site of the lesion.

sometimes are not evident on radiographs. In these instances, bone scanning is used to establish the diagnosis. Fractures often occur in characteristic patterns that can be recognized on bone scan. For example, rib fractures usually produce short focal lesions in multiple adjacent ribs (Fig. 17-11), and pelvic fractures usually involve at least two sites in the bony pelvic ring. Bone images also may be used to roughly establish the age of some fractures. For vertebral body compression fractures, 60% return to normal in 1 year, 90% in 2 years, and 95% in 3 years. However, diaphyseal fractures of long bones, particularly when there is an angular deformity, may show increased uptake related to ongoing bony remodeling that persists for many years. Finally, an increasingly important application of bone imaging is the imaging of stress fractures (Fig. 17-12) in athletes and other physically active individuals.

Frostbite

With frostbite there is an increased concentration of nuclide in the involved bones that have retained their blood supply. Avascular zones, however, show no concentration of nuclide.

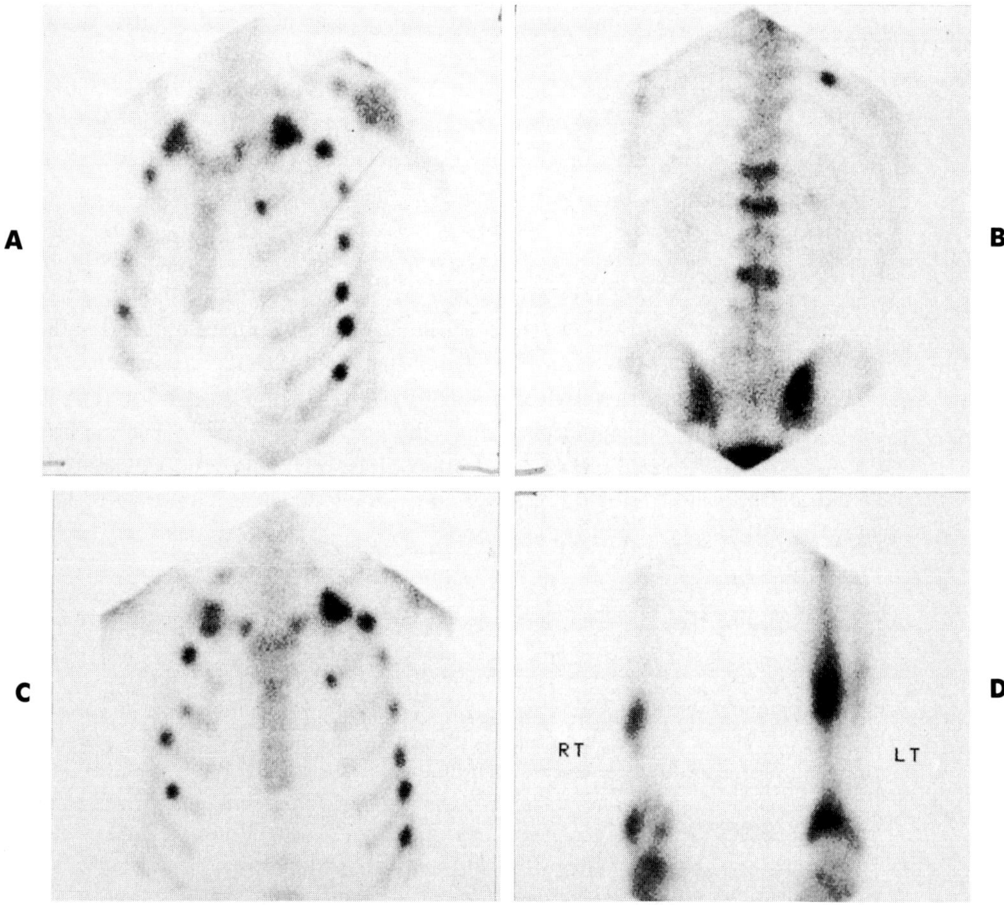

Fig. 17-11. Fracture. Abnormal bone images performed 2 hours after administration of 20 mCi (740 MBq) dose of ^{99m}Tc medronate disodium. There are multiple focal increases of radionuclide in ribs, clavicles, twelfth thoracic vertebra, first and third lumbar vertebra, right sacraliliac joint, left tibia, and right fibula. **A,** Spot image of left anterior oblique rib cage and sternum. **B,** Spot image of thoracic-lumbar-sacral spine. **C,** Spot image of anterior sternum and rib cage. **D,** Spot image of lower third of right and left legs, anteriorly. Images show multiple rib fractures; compression fractures involving T12, L1 and L3, left and right clavicles; fracture involving right sacraliliac joint, lower left tibia, and right fibula. This patient was in an automobile accident.

Continued

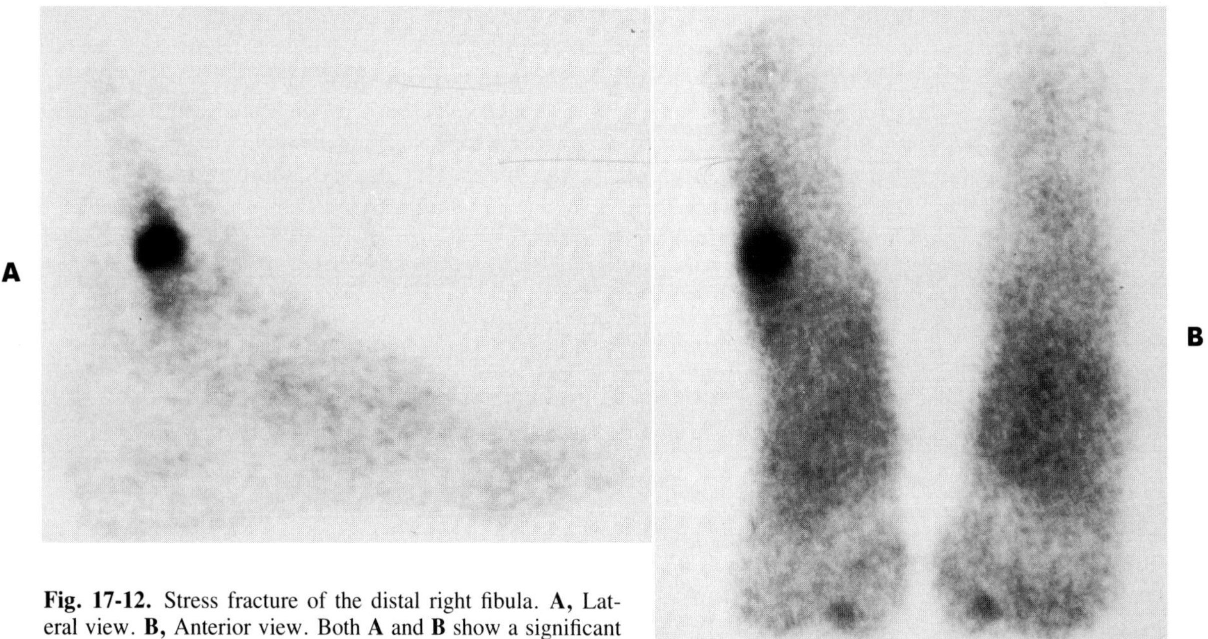

Fig. 17-12. Stress fracture of the distal right fibula. **A,** Lateral view. **B,** Anterior view. Both **A** and **B** show a significant increase in uptake at the site of the stress fracture.

Hyperostosis frontalis interna

Increased concentration of nuclide in the frontal skull, usually symmetric, is present with hyperostosis frontalis interna. This abnormality may be patchy and may extend into the parietal regions.

Hypertrophic pulmonary osteoarthropathy (HPO)

Increased concentration of nuclide along the cortical margins of multiple long bones in association with lung cancer (or rarely with tuberculosis, emphysema, or other chronic lung conditions) should suggest hypertrophic pulmonary osteoarthropathy (HPO). Because HPO may be painful and lung cancer silent, these patients sometimes are sent to the nuclear medicine department for an evaluation of unexplained leg pain. In fact, a bone image showing the typical findings of HPO sometimes is the first indication of lung cancer.

Postpartum sacroiliac and pubic symphysis increased uptake

Following delivery there may be increased concentration of nuclide in the sacroiliac joints and pubic symphysis. This may persist for as long as 18 months after delivery.

Reflex sympathetic dystrophy syndrome (shoulder-hand syndrome)

In the acute phase of RSDS there is a diffuse increase in nuclide concentration within the affected extremity that is most pronounced near the joints. Flow studies at this time also show an increase in perfusion to the affected extremity.

Metabolic abnormalities

Hyperparathyroidism. PTH activates the osteoblasts and produces high bone turnover. Bony uptake of ^{99m}Tc diphosphonate compounds is increased to the point at which the kidneys may not be visualized (i.e., a "super scan"). In a "super scan" all injected activity is in the skeleton and the kidneys are not visualized. Particularly prominent uptake may be seen at sites of skeletal involvement with "brown" tumors of hyperparathyroidism (Fig. 17-13).

Hyperthyroidism. In this process bone turnover rates are significantly increased; therefore there may be an increased accumulation of radionuclide through the skeleton causing a "super scan."

Osteomalacia. There is increased uptake of nuclide that usually is not so marked as to produce a "super scan."

Osteoporosis. In the absence of osteoporotic fractures, the bone scan usually is normal.

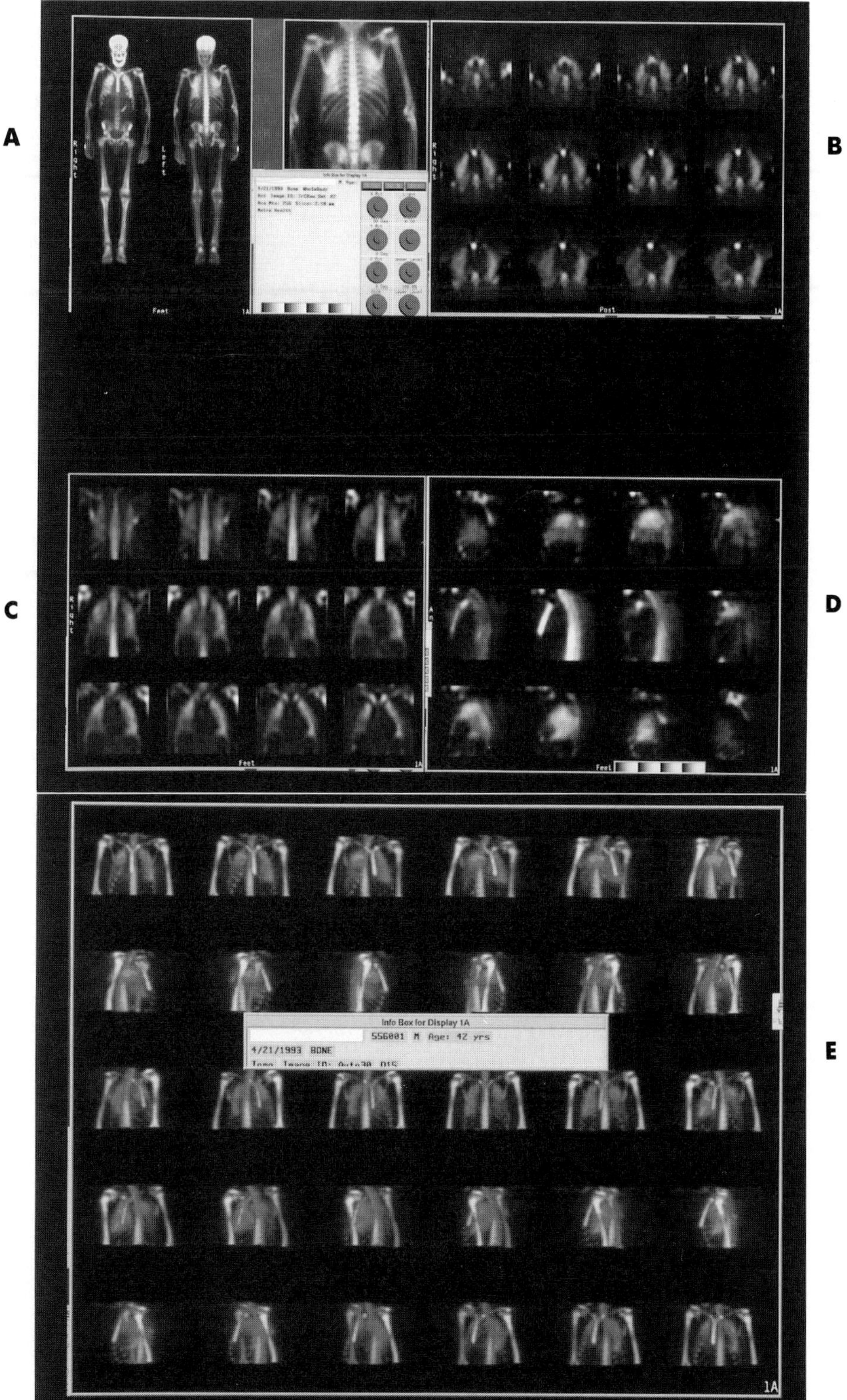

Fig. 17-13. Renal osteodystrophy with secondary hyperparathyroidism. Patients had an elevated serum calcium and renal failure. **A,** Whole-body images and "blow-up" of posterior view. There is significantly increased deposition of nuclide in the skull, mandible, and long bones, and ectopic concentration in the lungs and stomach. Renal visualization is almost absent. SPECT of the thorax. **B,** Transverse slices reveal homogeneous concentration of nuclide throughout the lung fields. **C,** Coronal slices. **D,** Sagittal slices. **E,** Rotational SPECT images.

Continued.

Orthopaedic surgery and prostheses

Repair and remodeling following orthopaedic surgery proceeds at a relatively uniform rate throughout the affected bone. As a rule, the intensity of nuclide concentration that reflects the status of ongoing bony repair is normal or only minimally elevated by 1 year following surgery. Therefore, focal intense uptake at the tip of a femoral prosthesis that has been in place for more than 1 year should raise suspicions regarding loosening. Similarly, a focus of intense uptake within a bony fusion mass that has had more than 1 year to heal raises suspicions regarding possible nonunion or pseudoarthrosis.

Benign bone lesions

Bone cyst. These are usually not visualized on the nuclear study unless the lesion is large enough to cause a photopenic region or there is a fracture through the cyst.

Nonosteogenic fibroma. This is primarily seen in young adults in the lower femur and in the tibia and fibula. Usually there is slight increased concentration of nuclide surrounding the lesion caused by reactive bone formation.

Osteoid osteoma. Osteomas of this type are usually found in young males in the tibia, femur, or vertebral body. Generally there is marked concentration of nuclide caused by reactive new bone formation.

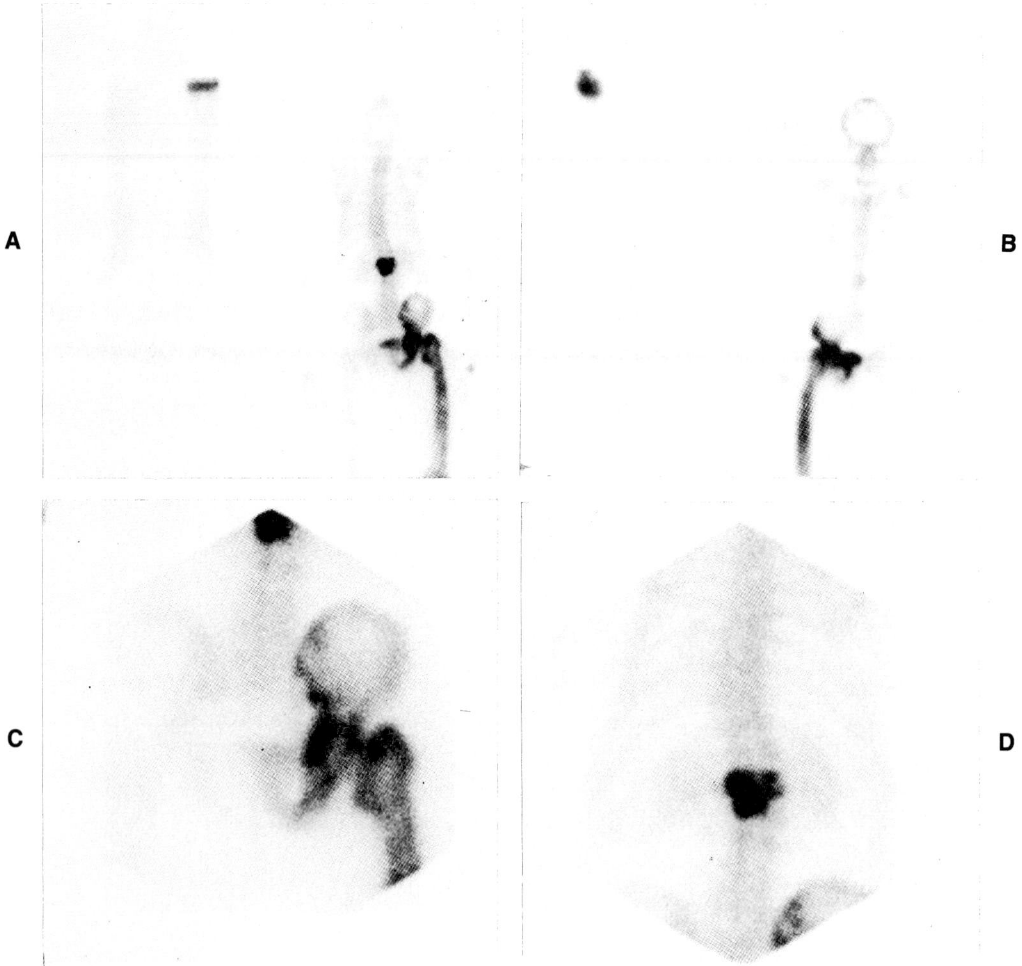

Fig. 17-14. Paget's disease. Abnormal bone images performed 2 hours after administration of 20 mCi (740 MBq) dosage of ^{99m}Tc medronate disodium. There are increased areas of concentration in right hemipelvis and femur, first and second lumbar vertebrae, and skull. **A,** Posterior whole-body image. **B,** Anterior whole-body image. **C,** Spot images of pelvis and femoral heads. **D,** Spot images of thoracic-lumbar spine and ribs.

Osteomyelitis. There is significantly increased concentration of nuclide caused by increased vascularity and reactive new bone formation. Nuclear images usually are positive before there are x-ray abnormalities. There is increased soft tissue vascularity proximal to and surrounding the site of infection. The bone image remains positive during the repair phase, which may last for months or years. As with Paget's disease, there is increased blood flow to bone. A perfusion study may help differentiate this lesion from other entities.

Paget's disease. Paget's disease is a chronic disease causing enlargement and deformity of bones (Fig. 17-14). The pelvis, femur, skull, tibia, vertebrae, or scapula frequently are involved. When long bones are involved, Paget's disease almost always extends to either the proximal or distal end of the bone. There usually is significant concentration of the bone-seeking nuclides at sites of skeletal involvement. In this disease, nuclear images are positive before x-ray changes occur. Paget's disease of bone may, however, enter a late and metabolically inactive phase during which there are dramatic radiographic findings with little or no increased uptake evident on the nuclear images.

Primary malignant bone lesions

Ewing's sarcoma. This is a tumor in children, with the femur being a common site. Bone images are positive early, probably because of periosteal new bone formation. The lesion may be polyostotic and may metastasize to other bones. Bone images are positive early in the disease process.

Osteogenic sarcoma. The region of increased concentration may be larger than the size of the tumor because of adjacent vascularity. The tumor has a predilection for the distal femur and is monostotic.

Reticulum cell sarcoma. The shafts of long bones are primarily involved and the disease is found in patients over the age of 40. Again, early visualization is probably caused by periosteal new bone formation.

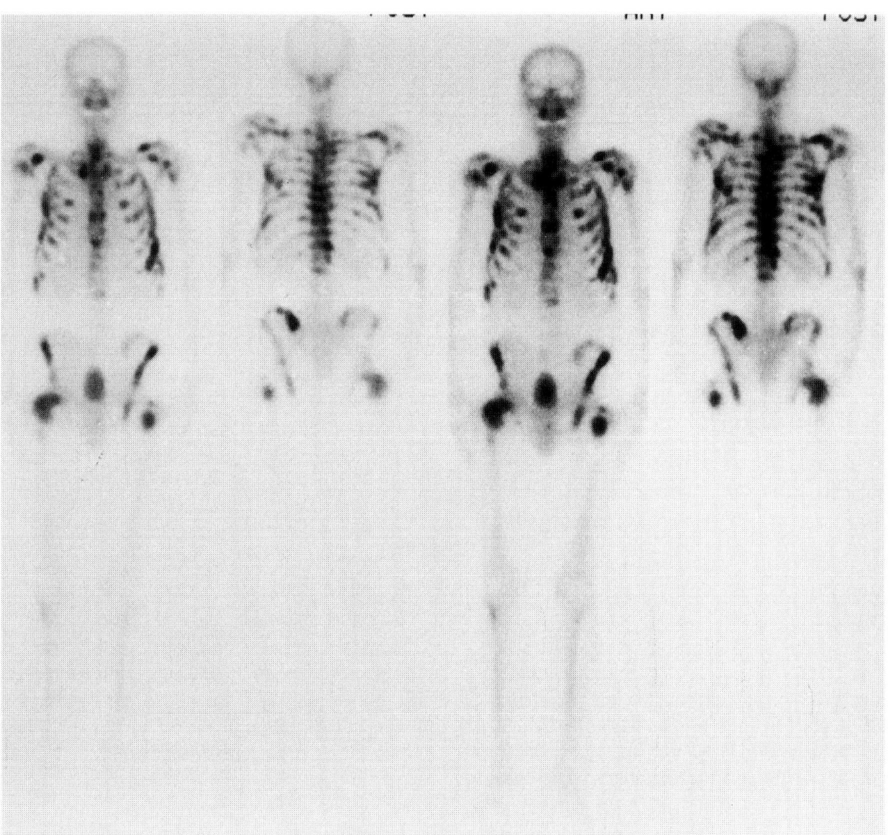

Fig. 17-15. Multiple bony metastases from prostate carcinoma. Decreased activity centrally in the pelvis and in the lower lumbar spine is the site of a radiation therapy portal. Nonvisualization of the kidneys is due to the very avid uptake at the site of bony metastases: the so-called super scan.

Continued.

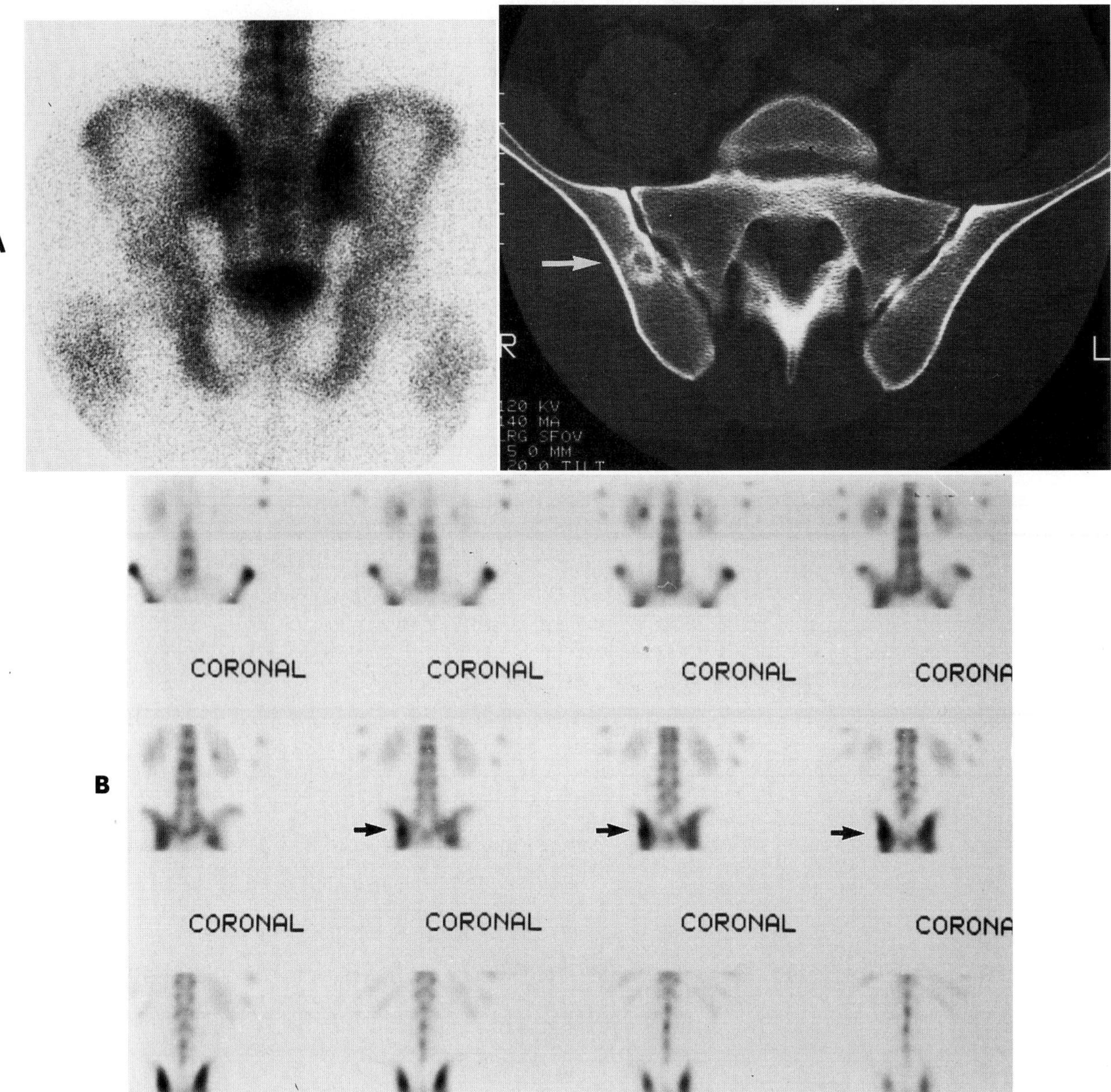

Fig. 17-16. Metastasis to the ilium adjacent to the right sacroiliac joint. **A,** Posterior planar image does not demonstrate the lesion. **B,** Coronal SPECT bone images, displayed consecutively from the level of the anterior vertebral bodies *(upper left image)* to spinous process *(lower right image)*. **C,** Transaxial CT through the sacroiliac joints. The lesion is more easily identified with SPECT *(arrows in* **B**) and is confirmed on CT *(arrow)*.

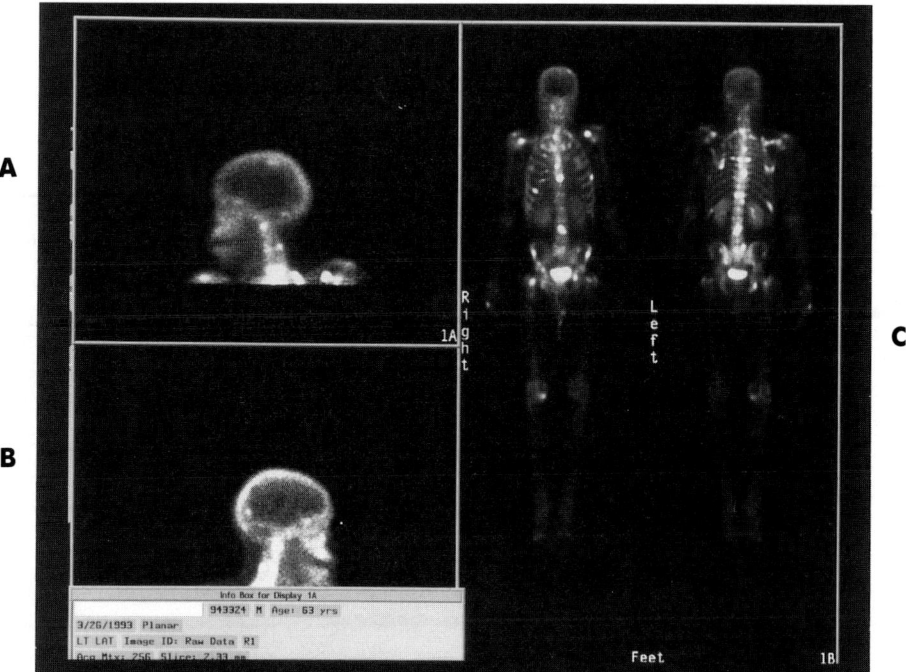

Fig. 17-17. Multiple skeletal metastatic sites from breast carcinoma. Multiple focal sites of increased concentration of nuclide in the vertebral column, ribs, pelvis, skull, right ischium, and neck of right femur. **A,** Left lateral skull and cervical spine. **B,** Right lateral skull and cervical spine. **C,** Anterior and posterior whole-body images.

Metastatic disease to bone. Many soft-tissue malignancies metastasize to bone (Figs. 17-15 to 17-17). ^{99m}Tc-diphosphonate compounds are used primarily to screen patients with primary carcinoma of the breast, lung, prostate, or kidney for metastatic sites in bone. However, bone imaging also may be indicated as part of the evaluation of patients with other malignancies. Most, if not all, oncology patients with unexplained bone pain, elevated bone fraction of alkaline phosphatase, or elevated serum calcium levels should undergo bone imaging. Magnetic resonance imaging and plain radiography are excellent correlative imaging modalities in verifying the presence of metastatic disease.

■ BONE MARROW IMAGING

LABORATORY APPLICATION

41

USING ^{99m}Tc SULFUR COLLOID

Purpose

Bone-marrow imaging with either ^{99m}Tc sulfur colloid, ^{99m}Tc micro-aggregated albumen, or other ^{99m}Tc-labeled tracers that localize in the reticuloendothelial system is sometimes useful. Marrow space disease processes, such as avascular necrosis, infarcts, infection, and tumors may be imaged. Bone marrow imaging has been used to study the functional capacity of the bone marrow in patients with anemia.

Indications

1. Study of the functional capacity of the bone marrow in patients with anemia
2. Study of functional enlargement of the bone marrow space in patients with polycythemia or diseases that would replace normal bone marrow regions and cause ectopic blood-forming activity
3. Search for metastatic sites that may involve bone marrow, primarily or secondarily

Continued.

Procedure

Materials

1. 12 mCi (444 MBq) of ^{99m}Tc sulfur colloid
2. Low-energy, high-resolution collimator and scintillation camera

Patient preparation

1. Explain the entire procedure to the patient.
2. Administer intravenously 12 mCi of ^{99m}Tc sulfur colloid.
3. Wait 1 hour before starting imaging procedure. This time period is necessary for maximum concentration of the colloidal particles in the reticuloendothelial system.
4. Instruct the patient to void before starting images. ^{99m}Tc in the pertechnetate form is also excreted through the kidneys. Hence the bladder should be emptied for better visualization of the pelvic area.

Technique

1. Peak camera for ^{99m}Tc peak energy (primary gamma energy is 140 keV).
2. Adjust intensity setting.
3. Determine proper orientation.
4. With the patient in the prone position, obtain 100,000-count images of the following areas:
   a. Lumbar and upper pelvic area (make sure the liver and spleen are not included on this view)
   b. Left hip to include the femur
   c. Right hip to include the femur
   d. Left shoulder to include the humerus (make sure the liver and spleen are not included on this view)
   e. Right shoulder to include the humerus (make sure the liver and spleen are not included on this view)
5. After completing the above, the images are carefully examined for extension of bone marrow into the long bones. If abnormal concentration is detected, views of the rest of the long bones may be obtained.

Interpretation

Position

Active physiologic bone marrow is usually found in the sternum, vertebral column, and pelvis. When the physiologic bone marrow space is enlarged, bone-marrow activity may be found throughout the rest of the bony skeleton.

Space-occupying lesions: filling defects

Metastatic tumors to bone marrow are difficult to detect unless they are 2 cm in size.

Abscess

These are difficult to detect unless they are 2 cm in size. Areas of atrophy of bone marrow are usually gross, and ectopic areas of bone marrow are visualized.

Femoral head necrosis

In femoral head avascular necrosis there is complete absence of visualization of the bone marrow space normally found in the femoral head.

Diagnosis

The majority of bone-marrow images have been performed at specialized hematology centers with special equipment. These centers are usually close to a reactor site. The radioactive iron bone-marrow studies have correlated with areas of red-cell production and have shown areas of absent production and ectopic bone marrow proliferation. The colloidal-image studies grossly agree with the iron-imaging studies. Technetium sulfur colloid has been used in searching for metastatic disease that involves bone marrow. However, a great amount of the vertebral column is lost to view because of covering liver and spleen images.

Abscess

An *abscess* may or may not reveal abnormal bone-marrow study, depending on the extent of infiltration. Usually infiltration must exceed the usually stated 2 cm.

Bone marrow atrophy

With *bone-marrow atrophy* there is deficient visualization of functioning bone-marrow areas with or without ectopic bone-marrow visualization.

Femoral-head necrosis

With absence of vascularity in *femoral-head necrosis* the normally visualized femoral-head bone-marrow space is not visualized.

Leukemia and lymphoma

There is deficient bone-marrow visualization and probably ectopic bone-marrow visualization with *leukemia and lymphoma.*

Polycythemia

In *polycythemia,* normal bone marrow is visualized with ease and proliferation of bone marrow pattern is noted.

Primary or metastatic disease to bone

Abnormal bone-marrow findings may or may not be revealed, depending on the extent of infiltration. Usually infiltration must exceed the usual stated 2 cm.

Measurement studies

Ralph G. Robinson

Accurate methods to assess bone-mineral content of the skeleton in vivo have been available since 1963. Over the past decade, improved methods to quantitate bone density at several skeletal sites have been developed. These methods have improved to the point at which they are extremely accurate in a clinical setting, with precision of less than 1% in trabecular bone as measured in the lumbar spine. The availability of these safe, rapid, and relatively inexpensive ways to quantitate bone mass has revolutionized the diagnosis and treatment of osteoporosis. Osteoporosis is a descriptive diagnosis for bone that becomes weakened enough for spontaneous fractures to occur. Weakened, osteopenic bones have numerous etiologies. This is not just a disease of postmenopausal females. The consequences of weakened bones—vertebral crush fracture and hip fracture—cost billions of dollars in direct health-care costs annually, not to mention the costs associated with long-term custodial care that is required for a large portion of patients who suffer hip fractures later in life. About 20% of patients who suffer hip fractures over age 45 will die within a year of their fracture and at least half of those who were ambulatory before fracture cannot walk independently following the hip fracture. Only one fourth of those who recover are able to resume normal physical activity after the hip fracture. The lifetime risk of hip fracture in Caucasian women is 15%; for men it is 5%. Vertebral fractures occur, on average, earlier in life than do hip fractures and have significant morbidity in terms of pain, decreased physical activity, and change in physical appearance as a result of reduced height and development of a "dowager's hump" (senile dorsal kyphosis). There are now several effective therapies for osteoporosis. The younger the patient at the time of diagnosis, the more effective the therapy and the milder the condition. It is never too late to make the diagnosis or institute therapy; however, earlier diagnosis and treatment will result in a better outcome. The purpose of this discussion is to acquaint you with several current techniques using both gamma-ray and x-ray absorption to measure bone density at several body sites.

■ NONINVASIVE BONE DENSITOMETRY

Bone-density procedures may be performed in patients of any age. They are not contraindicated in pediatric patients. In pediatric patients through adolescence, single-photon absorptiometry (SPA) is the preferred procedure, because the highest metabolic rate (and therefore the greatest change in bone) is occurring in the long bones. Most other patients should be first studied by a dual-photon technique (DPA or DEXA) with emphasis on the lumbar spine and proximal femur at the hip. The image of the spine study should be carefully evaluated for region of interest placement and proper anatomic numbering of the vertebra. Obvious artifacts, such as overlying metallic objects, will cause falsely elevated results. A usually dense vertebra from severe degenerative disease or previous fracture, injury, or even metastatic cancer should be excluded from the analysis. Degenerative disease with severe facet sclerosis may artificially increase the average density over the vertebra measured, and an unusually heavily calcified overlying aorta may also cause an artificially increased value. Some commercial equipment offers a lateral image to avoid the posterior elements in the field of view, but the accuracy and validity of this technique is not yet established. The usual analysis is to average AP image values of the L2 through L4 vertebrae; other combinations, however, may be used in patients who have focally increased densities in one or more imaged vertebrae. As a last resort, an isolated vertebra may be used for measurement and comparison over time if all other lumbar vertebra are too dense to accurately assess.

LABORATORY APPLICATION

42

BONE-DENSITY DETERMINATION BY SINGLE-PHOTON ABSORPTIOMETRY

Purpose

Single-photon absorptiometry (SPA) utilizes a photon beam from a ^{125}I-sealed source with an energy of approximately 29 keV. Because of the very low energies employed, penetration is adequate for scanning across a patient's limb (such as the forearm) but cannot be used in the larger areas of spine or hip. As the beam of radiation and its detector scan in a rectilinear fashion across the soft tissues and bones (radius) of the distal forearm, some of the photons are absorbed. The greater the density of bone in the scanning path, the greater the number of photons absorbed. The relative absorption can be calibrated to express bone mineral and mass per unit length of bone (gm/cm). Single-photon absorptiometry has also been used to measure bone at the very distal radial site, where there is some trabecular content, and also in the calcaneus. For consistency of measurement, the preferred site for SPA measurement is at the junction of the middle and distal third of the radius. Here the bone is predominantly cortical in nature. The density will change relatively little with minor repositioning of the scanning location.

The SPA procedure is particularly well suited for use in pediatrics. The long bone is where the action is in pediatric patients. In addition to the 10 general indications for bone-density studies listed below, SPA studies of the appendicular skeleton as measured at the radius should be performed in children with chronic renal disease, reduced bone age, delayed growth and development, delayed onset of secondary sexual characteristics, malabsorptive and other gastrointestinal disorders, and who are placed on corticosteroid therapy for inflammatory diseases such as juvenile rheumatoid arthritis.

Indications

1. Premenopausal oophorectomy, premature spontaneous menopause, or estrogen-deficiency conditions including amenorrhea.
2. When the diagnosis of osteopenia is suggested by other means, such as plain x-ray films.
3. Long-term corticosteroid therapy, either planned or already begun.
4. Endocrinopathies known to be associated with osteopenia, such as prolactinoma, hyperparathyroidism, Cushing's syndrome, hyperthyroidism, and male hypogonadism.
5. Unexplained fractures.
6. Postgastrectomy and other malabsorption diseases.
7. Treatment-related osteopenia, such as heparin anticoagulation, long-term administration of antacids for peptic ulcer disease, and anticonvulsant therapy.
8. Long-term immobilization (more than 1 month), either planned or current.
9. Chronic renal disease, particularly in childhood or adolescence.
10. To monitor treatment programs for osteoporosis, including estrogen or estrogen/progesterone, testosterone replacement, calcitonin therapy, exercise, and pharmacologic quantities of vitamin D with calcium.

Regardless of the cause of the osteoporotic condition, the adequacy and effectiveness of the chosen therapy should be evaluated. It should be remembered that absorptiometry is a diagnostic procedure that leads to a therapeutic decision involving costly pharmaceuticals and possible therapy risks, and that the results of these treatments should be monitored.

Procedure

Patient preparation

No special patient preparation is required; however, before beginning the examination, the entire procedure should be explained to the patient.

Technique

The patient's nondominant arm is imaged, unless there is a history of a known fracture at that site. In that case the dominant arm should be studied. If a unilateral neuromuscular problem is present, it may be of interest to scan both forearm sites.

Interpretation

Normal tables for bone-mineral content of the radius by SPA are available for adults and children age 6 and above, both male and female. Published data for radius values under the age of 21 were done with first-generation equipment. Current SPA equipment consistently reads 5% less than first-generation equipment because of an improved ability to detect bone edges. If the older tables are used, the expected normal range should be decreased by 5% to compare with current readings. Values 10% or greater below the mean for the patient's age should be considered mildly osteoporotic no matter what the age of the patient. It is becoming increasingly recognized that to know the degree of osteopenia at several body sites, multiple body sites should be studied. Adults with established osteoporosis in trabecular bone are usually measured at the spine and often in mixed bone at the proximal femur. If osteoporosis is established in an adult, the bone mineral content of cortical bone of the radius should be measured as well. A normal value in cortical bone suggests that the etiology of the reduced trabecular bone content is relatively recent. If the cortical bone is commensurately decreased, this suggests that the cause for skeletal osteoporosis has been present for a long period of time. It is suggested that if the degree of cortical osteopenia significantly exceeds trabecular bone loss, endocrine disorders such as primary or secondary hyperparathyroidism or hyperthyroidism are the etiology for the observed bone loss.

LABORATORY APPLICATION

43

BONE-DENSITY DETERMINATION BY DUAL ENERGY ABSORPTIOMETRY

There are two reliable dual energy absorptiometry techniques available to measure the density of bone in the axial skeleton. The usual site of measurement is the lumbar spine, which is composed primarily of trabecular bone. Because of substantial intervening soft tissue, a dual-energy technique is required to accurately assess bone density at the spine, and also at the proximal femur and hip. The first technique introduced was dual-photon absorptiometry (DPA), which came into general use in 1983. DPA typically uses a radioactive gadolinium-153 source, providing 44 and 100 keV gamma photons. Relative absorption of the two different gamma photons can be calibrated to provide a bone-density value for the lumbar spine that should show a test-retest variation of no greater than 2% in a clinical setting. Precisions as low as 1.5% have been obtained. More recently, dual energy absorptiometry systems using two different x-ray energies have appeared, delivering precisions of less than 1% in the clinic. The dual-energy x-ray absorptiometry systems (DEXA) deliver this improved precision because of increased photon flux and greater stability of the photon source. The flux should remain essentially constant with a DEXA system, whereas with radioactive decay there is a decreasing count rate from the source over time. Dual-energy x-ray absorptiometry (DEXA) is currently superior to DPA. However, further refinements in the amplifiers, circuits, and detector systems of gadolinium-based DPA systems may allow this design to approach or surpass 1% precision as well. Both systems deliver a clinically useful reading in patients. Because most patients show relatively slow changes in bone density over time, the system providing the greatest precision will be the one most accurate in demonstrating small but significant differences in patients on treatment. The DEXA systems have achieved precisions as low as 0.5% in some series. Both DPA and DEXA systems deliver extremely low radiation exposures to the patient, on the order of 1 to 2 mrem of skin entrance dose over the area being scanned. Thus radiation exposure is not a factor in deciding between

Continued.

the two techniques. The availability of radioactive sources and physician preference may dictate which system is chosen. The DEXA systems provide a significantly shortened scanning time (4 minutes for the lumbar spine) and are preferable for patient through-put. Future developments will include multiple detector arrays, which will further decrease patient scan times. Whole-body bone-mineral content determinations in 10 to 20 minutes can also be performed with multiple detector systems. The whole-body capability will become increasingly important in clinical practice. In addition, both DPA and DEXA systems with whole-body capability can perform accurate body composition measurements, including total-body mineral content, percent fat, and lean body mass. This will be an area of significant clinical use for these systems in the future. The purpose of the diagnostic study, as well as the indications, patient preparation, and scanning techniques are similar with both the DPA and DEXA systems. The major differences are the photon source and scan time required. The performance of DPA and DEXA studies are described together.

Purpose

Dual-energy absorptiometry systems determine the bone-mineral content and density of trabecular bone as measured in the lumbar spine and mixed trabecular/cortical bone as found in the proximal femur. Other body sites may also be studied, using a region-of-interest technique.

Indications

1. See indications listed under Laboratory application 42.
2. Onset of menopause. (A better-informed decision as to whether to prescribe estrogen replacement at the time of menopause can be made with the knowledge of the state of the individual's skeleton at that time.)

Procedure

Patient preparation

No special patient preparation is required. The patient should be asked to remove any metallic objects (belt buckles, coins, keys, etc.) that might be in the scanning path. Recent gastrointestinal (GI) studies with barium may also interfere due to the attenuation of the photons by barium.

Technique

1. The patient lies supine on the imaging table (Fig. 17-18). The lower extremities are elevated with a cushion under the lower legs to elevate the knees and flatten the pelvis and lumbar spine against the scanning table.
2. The scan is performed in a rectilinear fashion, generally from L1 through L5, with the dual-energy photon beam beneath the scanning table.

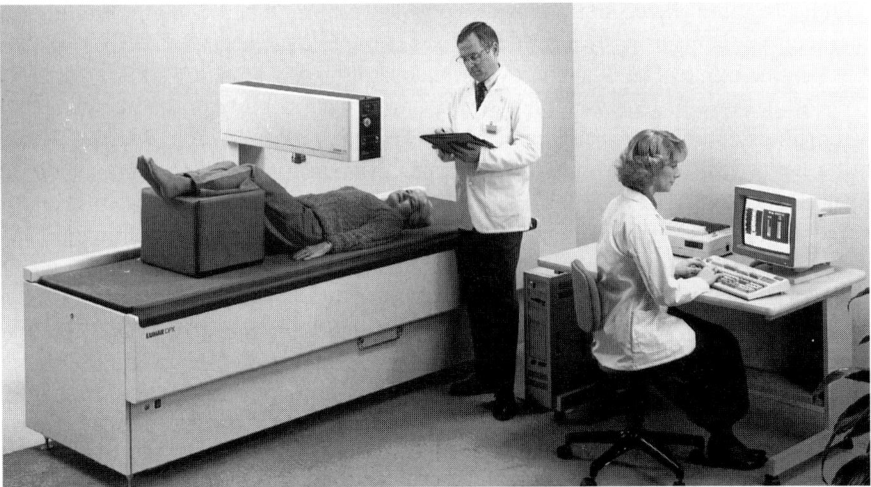

Fig. 17-18. DPX dual-energy x-ray absorptiometry scanner. (Courtesy, Lunar, Madison, Wisc.)

3. The gamma or x-ray beam passes through the soft tissue and bone of the patient and is detected by a scintillation detector on the C-arm above the table.
4. ^{153}Gd is routinely used as the gamma source. Although ^{153}Gd sources may have a useful life of 15 to 18 months, annual replacement is recommended. ^{153}Gd provides two photons at 44 and 100 keV. Dual-energy x-ray tubes give X-ray energies of 35 and 70 keV, or energies approximating ^{153}Gd, depending on the manufacturer.

Interpretation

The internationally recognized definition of osteoporosis is two spontaneously collapsed vertebrae. If the diagnosis of osteoporosis is to be made at an early enough time and age of patient in the course of disease to prevent fracture, a more rigid definition must be adopted. We diagnose osteoporosis in individuals whose vertebral bone density is more than 10% below that expected, considering their age, height, weight, sex and race. The most important comparison is to the patient's own age and sex group. Patients of either sex with values between 0.8 and 0.99 gm/cm^2 (Lunar DPA ranges as examples) have about a 20% predictability for spontaneous fracture while those with an absolute vertebral density below 0.62 gm/cm^2 will be found to already have had at least one spontaneous fracture nearly 100% of the time. Those patients whose values are between 0.62 and 0.80 gm/cm^2 fall between these predictive ranges. A predictive fracture risk estimate can be obtained by interpolation. Results should be reported to two decimal places. Repeat studies done in follow-up should be analyzed over the same area as in the first patient visit. A careful comparison of the two ROI studies should be performed. The latest commercial scanners have the capability of displaying current and prior studies side by side on the analysis display. The improved bone image obtained with x-ray–based systems further improves ROI placement. Densitometry values obtained from the proximal femur show slightly greater variation from visit to visit than do studies of the lumbar spine. There is greater variability in positioning in this region, and precisions of 3% were common with DPA equipment. Dual-energy x-ray studies do not give improved precision in the femur. Standard areas for measurement include a band across the femoral neck, Ward's triangle (an area in the center of the femoral neck), and the trochanteric region. The trochanteric region includes a large section of the greater trochanter. Of the three areas, Ward's triangle is the single most important in describing bone loss in the femur and in predicting hip fracture risk. The values from trabecular bone as measured at the lumbar spine, mixed cortical/trabecular bone in the hip, and primarily cortical bone as measured at the radius provide a constellation of values to more accurately assess the relative degree of bone loss at these several body sites. The important factor in report generation is to call the referring physician's attention to the development of even mild osteopenia. If the physical, psychological, and fiscal costs of osteoporosis are to be prevented, early and patient-specific treatment must be instituted. Early diagnosis is the key. If medically significant osteopenia is found, a search for underlying medical conditions that may be causing or contributing to the bone loss must be made.

Quantitative computed tomography

Quantitative computed tomography (QCT) can also be used to measure vertebral bone density. The CT scanner can be programmed or modified for either a single- or dual-energy technique. A mineral reference standard, usually a K_2HPO_4 solution, is supplied for machine calibration. Bone mineral density values are expressed in milligrams of K_2HPO_4 per cubic centimeter. QCT can provide an accurate assessment of bone-mineral content and has the advantage of limiting its analysis to the vertebral body itself, excluding the posterior elements. However, the radiation exposure (250 to 1000 mrem per study) is much higher than dual-energy absorptiometry methods, and if the more accurate dual-energy QCT systems are used, the x-ray exposure is essentially doubled. Also, much more expensive hardware is required. With the advent of the rapid-scan, dual-energy x-ray systems, it appears that DEXA will become the method of choice for performing bone-density studies. Also, the dual-energy x-ray absorptiometry systems have the added advantage of being able to easily measure the hip. This can be done on QCT examination but is relatively awkward to perform. The DEXA systems may also perform region-of-interest bone-density studies of any bone in the body, opening up their application in a wide variety of orthopedic and metabolic studies that could not be well studied with QCT.

BIBLIOGRAPHY

General

Ashby, D., Di Paola, P., and Hoeffer, P.B.: A comparative study of "small" and "large" field-of-view cameras for bone scanning, Clin. Nucl. Med 6:226, 1981.

Baker, M., and others: Radiographic and scintigraphic skeletal imaging in patients with neuroblastoma: concise communication, J. Nucl. Med. 24:467, 1983.

Bowen, B.M., and Garnett, E.S.: Analysis of the relationship between ^{99m}Tc-Sn polyphosphate and ^{99m}Tc pyrophosphate, J. Nucl. Med. 15:652, 1974.

West, editor: Best & Taylor's physiological basis of medical practice, ed. 12, Baltimore, 1991, The Williams & Wilkins Co.

Bunker, S.R., and others: Pixel overflow artifacts in SPECT evaluation of the skeleton, Radiology 174(1):229-232, 1990.

Citrin, D.L., and others: The use of serial bone scans in assessing response of bone metastases of systemic treatment, Cancer 47:680, 1981.

Coleman, R.E., Ruben, R.D., and Fogelman, I.: Reappraisal of the baseline bone scan in breast cancer, J. Nucl. Med. 19:1045, 1988.

Collier, B.D., Carrera, G.F., Johnson, R.P., and others: Detection of femoral head avascular necrosis in adults by SPECT, J. Nucl. Med. 26:979-987, 1985.

Collier, B.D., Carrera, G.F., Messer, E.J., and others: Internal derangement of the temporomandibular joint: detection by single-photon emission computed tomography, Radiology 149:557-561, 1983.

Collier, B.D., and Fogelman, I.: Bone SPECT case studies, B.C. Decker, Inc., Martin Dunitz Ltd., London, Mosby–Year Book Ltd., St. Louis, 1990.

Collier, B.D., Johnson, R.P., Carrera G.F., and others: Chronic knee pain assessed by SPECT: comparison with other modalities, Radiology 157:795-802, 1985.

Collier, B.D., Johnson, R.P., Carrera, G.F., and others: Painful spondylolysis or spondylolisthesis studied by radiography and single-photon emission computed tomography, Radiology 154:207-211, 1985.

Collier, B.D., Palmer, D.W., Knobel, J., and others: Gamma camera energy windows for ^{99m}Tc bone scintigraphy: effect of asymmetry on contrast resolution, Radiology 151:495-497, 1984.

Collier, B.D., and others: Bone scan: a useful test for evaluating patients with low back pain, J. Skeletal Radiol 19(4):267-270, 1990.

Cuartero-Plaza, A., and others: Abnormal bone scintigraphy and silent radiography in localized reflex sympathetic dystrophy syndrome, Eur. J. Nucl. Med. 19(5):330-333, 1992.

Desi, A., and others: ^{99m}Tc-MDP uptake in nonosseous lesions, Radiology 135:181, 1980.

Disbos, P.E., and Wagner, H.N., Jr.: Normal anatomy normal variant. In Disbos, P.E., and Wagner, H.N., Jr., editors: Atlas of nuclear medicine, vol. 4, Philadelphia, 1978, W.B. Saunders Co., p. 7.

Feiglin, D.H., Levine, M., Stalberg, B., and others: Comparison of planar (PBS) and SPECT scanning in the diagnosis of avascular necrosis (AVN) of the femoral head (FH), J. Nucl. Med. 27:952, 1986 (abstract).

Fogelman, I., and Collier, B.D.: An atlas of planar and SPECT bone scans, Martin Dunitz, London, Mosby–Year Book, St. Louis, 1989.

Fogelman, I., and others: The use of whole-body retention of ^{99m}Tc diphosphonate in the diagnosis of metabolic bone disease, J. Nucl. Med. 19:270, 1978.

Fordham, E.W., and others: Atlas of total body radionuclide imaging, vol. 2, New York, 1982, Harper & Row, Publishers, Inc.

Freeman, L.M., and Blaufax, M.D., editors: Seminars in nuclear medicine, Benign bone disorders, vol. 6, no. 1, New York, 1976, Grune & Stratton, Inc.

Genant, H.K., and others: Bone-seeking radionuclides: an in vivo study of factors affecting skeletal uptake, Radiology 113:373, 1974.

Gold, R. H., and Bassett, L.W.: Radionuclide evaluation of skeletal metastases: practical considerations, J. Skeletal Radiol 15:1, 1986.

Goss, C.M., editor: Gray's anatomy of the human body, ed. 29, (American edition), Philadelphia, 1984, Lea & Febiger.

Guyton, A.C.: Textbook of medical physiology, ed. 6, Philadelphia, 1981, W.B. Saunders Co.

Handmaker, H., and Leonard, R.: The bone scan in inflammatory osseous disease, Semin. Nucl. Med. 6:95, 1976.

Hellman, R.S., Nowak, D., Collier, B.D., and others: Evaluation of distance-weighted SPECT reconstruction for skeletal scintigraphy, Radiology 159:473-475, 1986

Holder, L.E.: Clinical radionuclide bone imaging, Radiology 176(3):607-614, 1990.

Holmes, R.A.: ^{99m}Tc pyrophosphate in demonstrating bone disease of parathyroid dysfunction, J. Nucl. Med. 19:330, 1978.

Howard, J.L., Barron, B.J., and Smith, G.G.: Bone scintigraphy in the evaluation of extraskeletal injuries from child abuse, Radiographics 10(1):67-81, 1990.

Jacob, S.W., Francone, C.A., and Lossow, W.J.: Structure and function in man, ed. 5, 1982, Philadelphia, W.B. Saunders Co.

Jacobson, A.F., and others: Bone scans with one or two new abnormalities in cancer patients with no known metastases: reliability of interpretation of initial correlative radiographs, Radiology 174(2):503-507, 1990.

Jones, A.G., Francis, M.D., and Davis, M.A.: Bone scanning: radionuclidic reaction mechanisms, Semin. Nucl. Med. 6:3, 1976.

Katzberg R.W., O'Mara R.E., Tallents R.H., and others: Radionuclide skeletal imaging, and single photon emission computed tomography in suspected internal derangements of the temporomandibular joint, J. Oral Maxillofac. Surg. 42:782-787, 1984.

Kaye, M., Silverston, S., and Rosenthall, L.: Technetium-99m pyrophosphate: studies in vivo and in vitro, J. Nucl. Med. 16:40, 1975.

Kennan, W.F., Jr., and others: The bone scan in primary care: diagnostic pitfalls, J. Amer. Board of Family Practice 5(1):63-67, 1992.

Khansur, T., and others: Evaluation of bone scan as a screening work-up in primary and local-regional recurrence of breast cancer, Am. J. Clin. Oncol. 10:167, 1987.

Levenson, R.M., and others: Comparative value of bone scintigraphy and radiography in monitoring tumor response in systemically treated prostatic carcinoma, Radiology 146:513, 1983.

Lutwak, L., Singer, F.R., and Urist, M.R.: Current concepts of bone metabolism, Ann. Intern. Med. 80:630, 1974.

Matin, P.: The appearance of bone scans following fractures, including immediate and long-term studies, J. Nucl. Med. 20:1227, 1979.

Mehta, R.C., and Wilson, M.A.: Frostbite injury: prediction of tissue viability with triple-phase bone scanning, Radiology 170(2):511-514, 1989.

Merrick, M.V.: Investigation of joint disease, European J. Nucl. Med. 19(10):894-901, 1992.

Morrison, S.C., and Adler, L.P.: Photopenic areas on bone scanning associated with childhood leukemia, Clin. Nucl. Med. 16:14, 1991.

Piffer, S., Amichetti, M., and Valentini, A.: Skeletal scintigraphy and physical examination in the staging of early breast cancer, Acta. Oncol. 17:21, 1988.

Murray, I.P., and Dixon, J.: The role of single photon emission computed tomography in bone scintigraphy, J. Skeletal Radiol. 18(7):493-505, 1989.

Pollen, J.J., and others: Nuclear bone imaging in metastatic cancer of the prostate, Cancer 47:2585, 1981.

Ram, P.C., and Fordham, E.W.: An historical survey of bone scanning, Semin. Nucl. Med. 9:190, 1979.

Rhinelander, F.W.: Circulation in bone. In Bourne, G., editor: Biochemistry and physiology of bone, ed. 2, vol. 2, New York, 1972, Academic Press, Inc.

Richards, B., Bollack, C., and Bouffioux, C.: The staging of MI disease: the role of bone scan, x-ray and other imaging techniques, Prog. Clin. Biol. Res. 169:233, 1988.

Ritter, M.M.: Granulocytes and three-phase bone scintigraphy for differentiation of diabetic gangrene with and without osteomyelitis, Diabetes Care 15(8):1014-1019, 1992.

Rockett, J.F.: Demonstration of medial meniscus tear by three-phase bone imaging, Clin. Nucl. Med. 16:1, 1991.

Rosenthall, L., and Lisbona, R.: Role of radionuclide imaging in benign bone and joint diseases of orthopedic interest. In Freeman, L.M., and Weissmann, H.S., editors: Nuclear medicine annual, New York, 1980, Raven Press, p. 267.

Rosenthall, L.: Radionuclide bone imaging, Curr. Opin. Radiol. 1(4):440-445, 1989.

Salomon, C.G., Ali, A., and Fordham, E.W.: Bone imaging in patients with unexpected elevation of serum alkaline phosphatase, Clin. Nucl. Med. 14(8):567-570, 1989.

Sham, J.S.T., and others: Nasopharyngeal carcinoma: pattern of skeletal metastases, Br. J. Radiol. 63:202, 1990.

Sham, J.S.T., and others: Role of bone scanning in detection of subclinical bone metastasis in nasopharyngeal carcinoma, Clin. Nucl. Med. 16:14, 1991.

Shapeero, L.G., Henry-Amar, M., and Vanel, D.: Response of osteosarcoma and Ewing sarcoma to preoperative chemotherapy: assessment with dynamic and static MR imaging and skeletal scintigraphy, Invest. Radiol. 17(11):989-991, 1992.

Slizofski, W.J., Collier, B.D., Flatley, T.J., and others: Painful pseudarthrosis following lumbar spinal fusion: Detection by combined SPECT and planar bone scintigraphy, Skeletal Radiol. (in press).

Splittgerber, G.F., Spiegelhoff, D.R., and Buggy, B.P.: Combined leukocyte and bone imaging used to evaluate diabetic osteoarthropathy and osteomyelitis, Clin. Nucl. Med. 14(3):156-160, 1989.

Thibodeau, G.A., and Patton, K.T.: Anthony's textbook of anatomy and physiology, ed. 14, St. Louis, 1994, Mosby–Year Book.

Wardlaw, J.M., Best, J.J., and Hughes, S.P.: Dynamic bone imaging in the investigation of local bone pathology—when is it useful? Clin. Radiol. 43(2):107-112, 1991.

Whaler, J.P., Krook, L., and Nunez, E.A.: Some metabolic considerations in bone disease. In Potchen, E.J., editor: Current concepts in radiology, St. Louis, 1977, Mosby–Year Book.

Williams, P.L., and Warwick, R., editors: Gray's anatomy, ed 37, (British edition), New York, 1989, Churchill Livingstone, Inc.

Williamson, M.R., and others: Osteomyelitis: sensitivity of 0.064 T MRI, three-phase bone scanning and indium scanning with biopsy proof, Magn. Reson. Imaging 9(6):945-948, 1991.

Bone density measurement studies

Cameron, J.R., and Sorenson, G.: Measurements of bone mineral in vivo: an improved method, Science 142:230-232, 1963.

Cameron, J.R., Mazess, R.B., and Sorenson, M.S.: Precision and accuracy of bone mineral determination by direct photon absorptiometry, Invest. Radiol. 3:141-150, 1968.

Cann, C.E., and Genant, H.K.: Precise measurement of vertebral mineral content using computed tomography, J. Comput. Assist. Tomogr. 4:493-500, 1980.

Dalsky, G.P, and others: Weight bearing exercise training and lumbar bone mineral content in postmenopausal women, Ann. Intern. Med. 108:824-828, 1988.

Engesaeter, L.B., and Soreide, O.: Consumption of hospital resources for hip fracture: discharge rates for fracture in Norway, Acta. Orthop. Scand. 56:17-20, 1985.

Eriksen, E.F., Hodgson, S.F., and Riggs, B.L.: Treatment of osteoporosis with sodium fluoride. Chapter 17 in Riggs, B.L, and Melton, L.J., editors: Osteoporosis: etiology, diagnosis and management, New York, 1988, Raven Press.

Ettinger, B., Genant, H.K., and Cann, C.E.: Long-term estrogen therapy prevents bone loss and fracture, Ann. Intern. Med. 102:319-324, 1985.

Ettinger, G., Genant, H.K., and Cann, C.E.: Postmenopausal bone loss is prevented by treatment with low-dosage estrogen with calcium, Ann. Intern. Med. 106:40-45, 1987.

Firooznia, H., and others: Trabecular mineral content of the spine in women with hip fracture, Radiology 159:737-740, 1986.

Genant, H.K., Vogler, J.B., and Block, J.E.: Radiology of osteoporosis. Chapter 7 in Riggs, B.L., and Melton L.J. III, editors: Osteoporosis: etiology, diagnosis and management, New York, 1988, Raven Press.

Heymsfield, S.B., and others: Dual-photon absorptiometry: comparison of bone mineral and soft tissue mass measurements in vivo with established methods, Am. J. Clin. Nutr. 49:1283-1289, 1989.

Hursman, A., James, M., and Francis, R.: The effect of estrogen dose on postmenopausal bone loss, N. Engl. J. Med. 309:1405-1407, 1983.

Johnson, B.E., and others: Contributing diagnoses in osteoporosis, Arch. Intern. Med. 149:1069-1072, 1989.

Johnston, C.C., Jr.: Noninvasive methods for quantitating appendicular bone mass. In Avioli, L.V., editor: The osteoporotic syndrome: detection, prevention and treatment, New York, 1983, Grune & Stratton.

Kiel, D.P., and others: Hip fracture and the use of estrogens in postmenopausal women: the Framingham study, N. Engl. J. Med. 317:1169-1174, 1987.

Lindsay, R., Fey, C., and Haboubi, A.: Dual photon absorptiometric measurements of bone mineral density increase with source life, Calcif. Tissue Int. 41:293-294, 1987.

Martin, P., and others: Partially reversible osteopenia after surgery for primary hyperparathyroidism, Arch. Intern. Med. 146:689-691, 1986.

Melton, L.J., and others: Osteoporosis and the risk for hip fracture, Am. J. Epidemiol. 124:254-261, 1986.

Nilas, L., and others: Usefulness of regional bone measurements in patients with osteoporotic fractures of the spine and distal forearm, J. Nucl. Med. 28:960-965, 1987.

Ott, S.M., Kilcoyne, R.G., and Chestnut, C.H. III: Ability of four different techniques of measuring bone mass to diagnose vertebral fractures in postmenopausal women, J. Bone Min. Res. 2:201-210, 1987.

Pocock, N.A., and others: Recovery from steroid-induced osteoporosis, Ann. Int. Med. 107:319-323, 1987.

Riggs, B.L., and Wahner, H.W.: Bone densitometry and clinical decision-making in osteoporosis, Ann. Int. Med. 108:293-295, 1988.

Ringe, J.D., and Welzel, D.: Salmon Calcitonin in the therapy of corticoid-induced osteoporosis, Eur. J. Clin. Pharmacol. 33:35-39, 1987.

Robinson, R.G.: Dual-photon absorptiometry in clinical practice, J. Nucl. Med. 31:1781, 1990.

Wahner, H., and others: Dual photon (153-Gd) absorptiometry of bone, Radiology 156:203-206, 1985.

Wahner, H.W., and others: Comparison of dual-energy x-ray absorptiometry and dual photon absorptiometry for bone mineral measurements of the lumbar spine, Mayo Clin. Proc. 63:1075-1084, 1988.

Wasnich, R.D., and others: Prediction of postmenopausal fracture risk with use of bone mineral measurements, Am. J. Obstet. Gynecol. 153:745-751, 1985.

Chapter 18

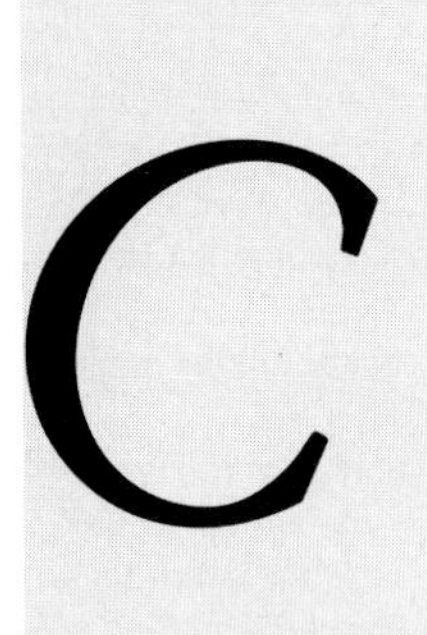

ARDIOVASCULAR SYSTEM

D. BRUCE SODEE
STEVEN C. PORT
JAMES K. O'DONNELL
BAN AN KHAW
JAGAT NARULA
TSUNEHIRO YASUDA
H. WILLIAM STRAUSS

The heart

D. Bruce Sodee

■ ANATOMY (Figs. 18-1 to 18-3)

The heart is a four-chambered (two atria and two ventricles) muscular organ. It is located in the middle mediastinum and is partially overlapped by lung tissue. Anteriorly, the sternum and costal cartilages of the third, fourth, and fifth ribs overlie the heart. Approximately two thirds of the heart is to the left of the midline. The heart is tilted forward and to the left, placing the apex anterior to the rest of the heart. The heart rests on the diaphragm. Posteriorly the heart rests on the bodies of the fifth through the eighth thoracic vertebrae. Its approximate dimensions are: width, 9 cm; length, 12 cm; and depth, 6 cm.

The *right atrium* (a chamber or cavity permitting entrance) is at the right lateral inferior cardiac border; however, most of the inferior border is composed of the *right ventricle*. The *lower left lateral cardiac border* and the *apex* consists of the left ventricle. The *left atrium* is superior and posterior to the *left ventricle* with the left atrial appendage sitting on top of the left ventricle and lateral to the *pulmonary artery*. The atria and ventricles are separated externally by the coronary sulcus or groove. The *right coronary artery,* after leaving the aorta, travels in this sulcus between the right atrium and the right ventricle until it descends on the posterior surface of the heart.

The *left circumflex artery* is found in the coronary sulcus between the left atrium and the left ventricle. The *left anterior descending coronary artery* is in the anterior interventricular sulcus that courses over the interventricular system, which separates the right and left ventricles. It passes around the apex and continues in the posterior interventricular sulcus on the diaphragmatic surface of the heart. The terminal branch of the right coronary artery is found in the posterior interventricular sulcus.

The heart has four major valves: the *aortic valve* at the opening of the aorta in the left ventricle; the *pulmonary valve* at the opening of the pulmonary artery in the right ventricle; the *right atrioventricular valve* (tricuspid) located between the right atrium and the right ventricle; and the *left atrioventricular valve* (mitral or bicuspid) located between the left atrium and left ventricle. The valves are wide and thin and are made up of two layers of the endocardium (lining membrane of the heart) and separated by a small amount of connective tissue. The valves are supported by the chordae tendineae, which attach their free margins to the papillary muscles in the wall of the ventricle. There are semilunar valves that guard the outlet of the left ventricle into the aorta and the right ventricle into the pulmonary artery.

■ Right atrium (Fig. 18-2)

The superior and inferior vena cava deliver venous blood into the right atrium. The blood is delivered into the right ventricle during ventricular diastole through the tricuspid valve. The right atrial wall measures only about 2 mm in thickness.

■ Right ventricle (Figs. 18-2 and 18-3)

The right ventricle propels blood into the pulmonary circulation during ventricular systole. The right ventricle is to

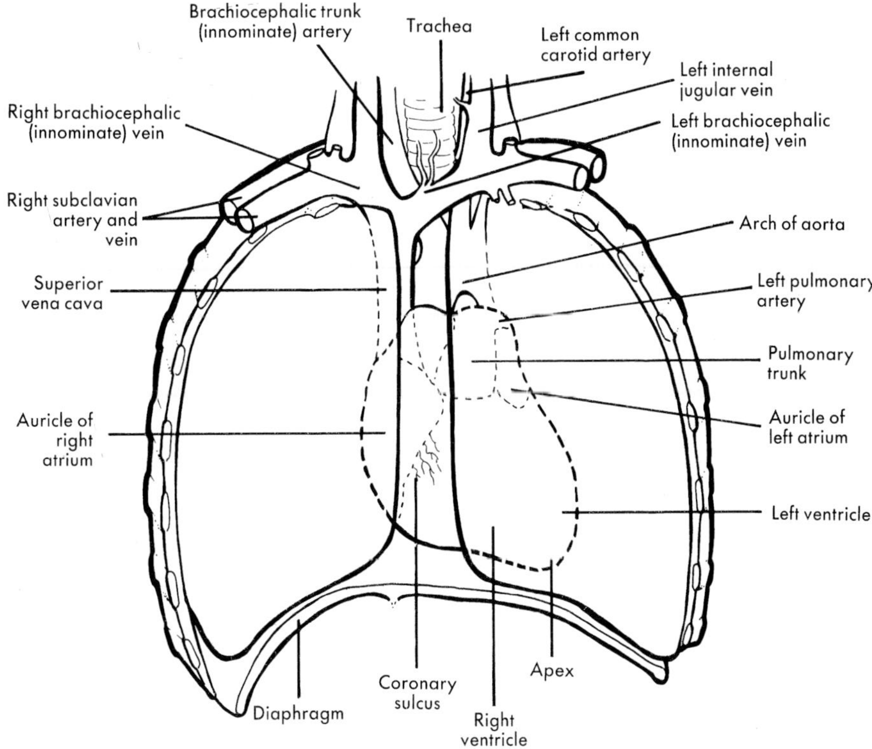

Fig. 18-1. Anterior schematic of the anatomy of the heart and great vessels.

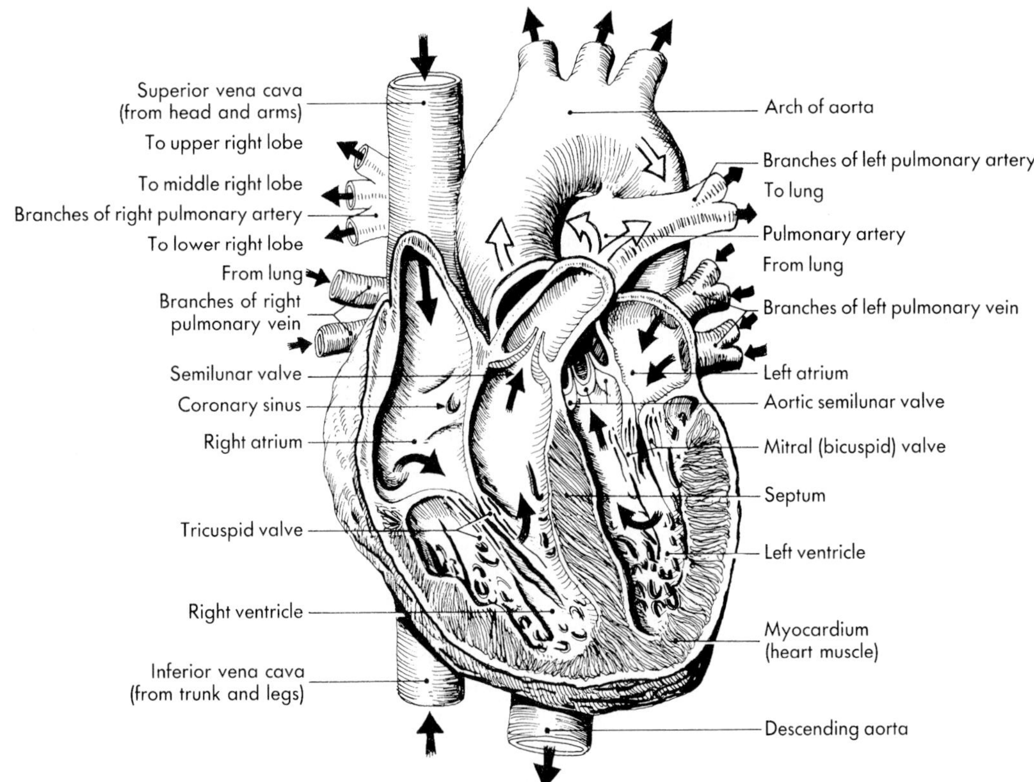

Fig. 18-2. Frontal section of heart showing four chambers, valves, openings, and major vessels. Arrows indicate direction of blood flow. Two branches of right pulmonary vein extend from right lung behind heart to enter left atrium. (From Austrin, M.G., and Austrin, H.R.: Learning medical terminology, a work text, ed. 7, St. Louis, 1991, Mosby–Year Book Inc.)

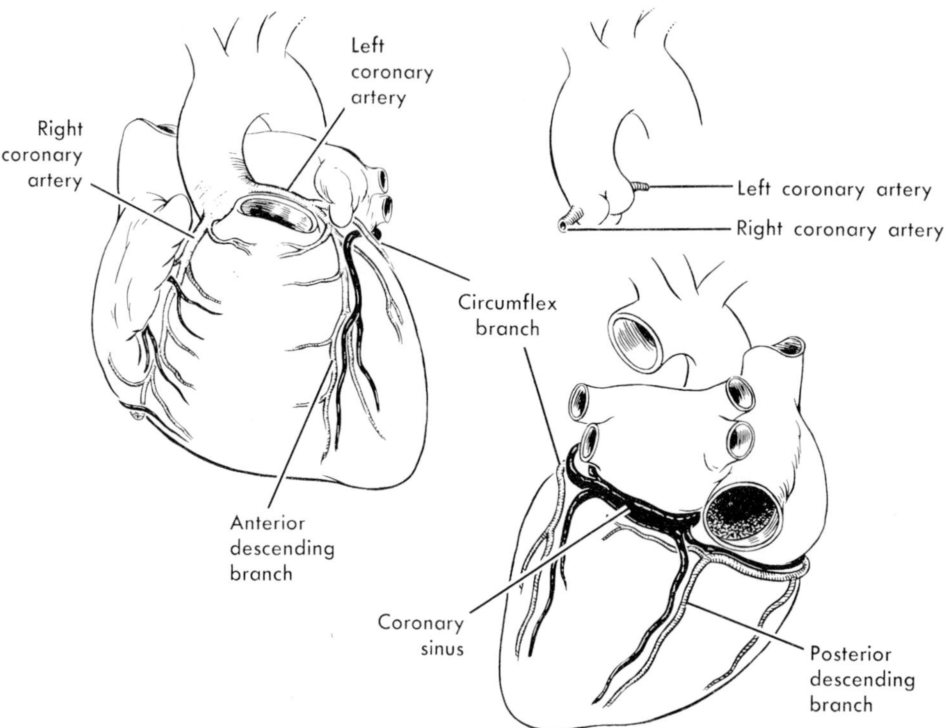

Fig. 18-3. Anterior and posterior view of heart and great vessels. (From King, O.M.: Care of the cardiac surgical patient, St. Louis, 1975, The C.V. Mosby Co.)

the right and anterior to the left ventricle and is just below and medial to the right atrium. The right ventricular wall is thin, measuring 5 mm in thickness. The right ventricular inflow track is made up of the tricuspid valve and the right ventricular muscles of the anterior and inferior walls. The outflow track, called the *infundibulum,* is smooth-walled and forms the superior portion of the right ventricle. During ventricular systole the blood entering the infundibulum is ejected through the pulmonary valve into the pulmonary artery and the pulmonary circulation.

■ Left atrium (Fig. 18-2)

Oxygenated blood is returned to the heart by the pulmonary veins, which enter the left atrium. The left atrial wall is only slightly thicker than the right atrial wall, measuring 3 mm. During atrial systole and ventricular diastole blood is delivered to the ventricle through the mitral valve. A thin septum separates the left from the right atrium.

■ Left ventricle (Fig. 18-2)

The left ventricle fills from the left atrium through the mitral valve during ventricular diastole or the ventricular filling phase. The left ventricle ejects blood into the systemic arterial circulation through the semilunar aortic valve. The wall thickness of the left ventricle is between 8 and 15 mm. Except for the upper third of the septum, the lining of the left ventricle is ridged by interlacing myocardial muscles. Various valve leaflets are attached in both ventricular cavities by chordae tendineae, strong cords of fibrous tissue attached to papillary muscles inserted into the myocardium.

■ Ventricular valves (Fig. 18-2)

The tricuspid and mitral valve leaflets differ in that the mitral leaflets are thinner and harder to separate into well-defined leaflets. The mitral leaflets are of unequal size with the largest leaflet being the anterior leaflet, followed by the septal leaflet, and finally the smallest or posterior leaflet. Their attachments to the papillary muscles and the muscles themselves have a parallel alignment to the ventricular wall, and the leaflets are pulled downward at the onset of isovolemic ventricular systole.

The semilunar aortic and pulmonary valves are similar; however, the aortic cusps (pointed flaps or leaflets) are slightly thicker. They are at the top of their outflow track and are composed of three fibrous cusps. Behind the cusps of the aortic valve the vessel wall bulges outward forming a pouch-like dilation known as the *sinus of Valsalva.* The ostea of the coronary arteries are located in their respective sinuses of Valsalva.

■ Pericardium (Fig. 18-1)

The base of the pericardium is attached to the central tendon of the diaphragm, and the heart is entirely enclosed by the pericardium, a closed membranous sac with two surfaces. The surface in contact with the myocardium is called the *visceral pericardium* or *epicardium*. The external surface of the pericardium is called the *parietal pericardium*. The two pericardial surfaces are lined by serous tissue and are separated by a thin layer of lubricating fluid.

■ Coronary arteries and venous anatomy (Fig. 18-3)

Left coronary artery. The left coronary artery originates from a single ostium found in the upper half of the left coronary sinus of the aorta. The left coronary artery divides into the anterior descending and circumflex rami. The branches of the left main coronary artery are distributed over the free wall of the left ventricle. In rare instances a single major vessel arising from the anterior descending coronary artery crosses diagonally over the anterior wall of the right ventricle. The anterior descending artery generally curves around the apex of the left ventricle into the posterior interventricular sulcus and extends to the posterior surface of the left and right ventricles.

Left circumflex artery. The left circumflex artery usually courses in an opposite direction from the main left coronary artery. It generally provides branches to the posterior surface of the left ventricle, and in 10% of human hearts it continues posteriorly. In such hearts, branches of the left coronary artery supply the entire left ventricle and interventricular septum.

Right coronary artery. The right coronary artery may arise from a single ostium or from two ostia in the right coronary sinus. In 90% of human hearts the right coronary continues past the margin of the right ventricle into the posterior right AV sulcus. It branches posteriorly toward the apex of the heart and with its descending branches along the diaphragmatic surface of the left ventricle. The coronary arteries are small with the largest diameter measurements approximately 3 mm.

Coronary veins. Venous drainage of the left ventricle is usually into the coronary sinus that empties directly into the atrium. A second system, the anterior cardiac veins, forms over the anterior wall of the right ventricle into two or three large trunks draining in the direction of the anterior right AV sulcus. Anastomoses between the cardiac veins and the tributaries are numerous and large.

■ Electrical conduction system of the heart

Sinus node. The pacemaker of the heart is near the junction of the superior vena cava and the right atrium. The sinus node is located only 1 mm beneath the epicardium, and therefore it is extremely vulnerable to damage from diseases that affect the surface of the heart.

AV node. The AV node is between the atria and the ventricles. It triages atrial signals for transmission to the ventricles. The AV node also delays transmission for approximately .04 seconds. Formed by convergents of fibers at the anterior and inferior margins of the AV node is the AV bundle and its proximal and distal branches. Ventricular spread of electric activity is primarily related to specialized cells found in the ventricular myocardium.

■ INNERVATION OF THE HEART

A specialized neuroconducting system involving the sinoatrial (SA) and the atrioventricular (AV) nodes possesses the inherent ability for spontaneous, rhythmic initiation of the cardiac excitation impulse. The autonomic nervous system influences the regulation of the rate of impulse formation and the rate of spread of the excitation impulse, depolarization and repolarization of the myocardium, and the contractility of the atria and the ventricles. The sympathetic nerve fibers supply all the areas of the atria and the ventricle. The vagal nerve fibers are primarily found in the SA and AV nodes; vagal fibers and impulses extend to both ventricles. Normally the parasympathetic influence is the dominant influence on heart rate, whereas the sympathetic nervous system is the dominant influence on ventricular function.

■ Myocardial neuroconduction cells

P cells. P cells microscopically resemble primitive myocardial cells and are the site of pacemaker impulse formation.

Transitional cells. Transitional cells are microscopically between the simple P cells and the more complex working myocardial cells. These cells serve as a link between the P cells and the rest of the heart. The P cells make contact only with one another and with transitional cells. The transitional cells are in contact with one another and all other myocardial cells.

Ameboid cells. Ameboid cells were recently described and their function not as well elucidated as the other cells in the myocardium.

Purkinje cells. Purkinje cells are found principally in the bundle branches as they extend into the myocardium, and they probably relay the electric information to the myocardial cell that is transmitted from the P cell to the transitional cell.

Functional myocardial cells. Working myocardial cells are arranged longitudinally in series with multiple cells forming a fiber-like entity. Cardiac fibers made up of multiple myocardial cells are parallel to one another; however, they have many lateral and end-to-end connections. The working myocardial cells have elongated shapes that are ideal for their main function, mechanical contraction. The myocardial cell contraction is directly related to the dephosphorylation of adenosine triphosphate and calcium reaccumulation by a calcium pump. Since metabolism in the myocardium is so closely linked to oxidative phosphorylation, the myocardium is extremely dependent on appropriate oxygen delivery by the coronary arteries at rest and under stress conditions. The cardiac muscle receives its blood supply primarily by penetrating arteries that extend from the epicardium, although some of the blood supply comes from penetrating vessels from the endocardium.

■ Aorta and the large arterial vessels

The wall of the aorta is considerably thicker than the pulmonary artery. With a microscope many elastic fibers are seen in the aorta. These fibers allow the aorta to function as an expanding reservoir for blood during the rapid ejection from the left ventricle.

Systemic arteries originate from the aorta, and as they branch to become individually smaller, the average velocity of blood flow decreases in the final small arterioles, which are the major source of resistance in the systemic circulation. Arterioles branch into capillary systems that perfuse all tissues.

■ Veins

The veins of the body collect the deoxygenated blood and the perfusate from the tissues and join one another to form progressively larger vessels that return to the heart by way of the superior and inferior vena cava. At rest, about 50% of blood volume is located in the venous portion of the circulation.

■ Lymphatic vessels

Fluid and protein filtered from capillaries do not completely reenter the venous circulation. Lymphatics are specialized vessels that carry unreturned body fluids from the interstitial spaces to the venous circulation. They then return them to circulation through the thoracic duct that joins the left brachial subclavian veins at the junction of the internal jugular and subclavian veins.

■ PHYSIOLOGY

The cardiovascular system consists of the heart and a closed system of arteries, veins and capillaries. Blood is pumped through the body by the heart, carrying with it essential nutrients and substances to all body-system cells and removing metabolic waste products in the process.

■ Cardiac cycle

A complete heartbeat is a two-phase process known as the cardiac cycle. It consists of a contraction (systole) and relaxation (diastole) of both atria and ventricles. The first beat is the systolic contraction that expels blood into the aorta and pulmonary arteries. During diastole, the atria and ventricles relax and dilate to allow the return of oxygenated blood to the heart's chambers. This process is governed by the heart's electrical conduction system.

■ Cardiac performance

Cardiac performance is the result of four determinants: preload, afterload, myocardial contractility, and heart rate.

Preload. The presystolic and end-diastolic volume of the ventricles and the ventricular pressures determine the fiber length of the myocardial cell; these directly influence the strength of the contraction. The force of the ventricular contraction amplifies as the preload increases.

Afterload. Afterload is the arterial resistance against which the ventricle contracts. Forces influencing the performance of afterload include:

a. End-diastolic volume of the ventricle
b. Aortic impedance
c. Arterial resistance
d. Peripheral vascular resistance
e. Amount of blood in the aorta
f. Viscosity of the blood

Afterload indirectly influences diastolic characteristics, filling pressure, and volume or preload of the next beat of the ventricle.

Myocardial contractility. The speed and shortening ability of the myocardium are dependent on loading conditions. The myocardial function is altered by a change in contractility of the muscle independent of change in fiber length.

Heart rate. The rate at which the heart contracts is influenced by many factors, including activity level, blood temperature, disease, and emotions. Cardiac output is the measured response of blood expelled by the ventricles during a contraction.

Myocardial oxygen requirement. The myocardium receives 10% of the cardiac output. Cardiac muscle extracts 70% of the oxygen in every milliliter of blood delivered to it. As mentioned previously, the myocardium functions almost solely on aerobic metabolic pathways, and the deprivation of oxygen for more than 2 minutes results in total cessation of myocardial activity. Myocardial hypoxia produces prompt coronary artery vasodilation.

Electrocardiogram. The electric activity of the heart creates an electric field that is distributed throughout the body. These currents produce potentials on the body surface when electrodes are placed on the body and connected with an appropriate electrocardiograph machine. A graphic recording of the potential differences between the sites can then be obtained. The electrocardiogram form is determined by the sequence of excitation and recovery and the resultant potential differences on the surface of the heart. Excitation of the atrium begins in the region of the sinus node. The electric wave spreads outward over the right atrium and down the interatrial septum. The resultant electrocardiographic wave form is called the *P wave*. Ventricular activation follows the anatomic distribution of the Purkinje system from apex to base, beginning on the left side of the interventricular septum near the apex. This is followed by excitation of the endocardium surface of the right ventricle near the apex. The ventricular QRS complex spreads rapidly over the Purkinje network that circles the cavities of both the right and left ventricles. Midway through the QRS complex the wave form has extended through the epicardium and is completed around the thinner right ventricle. The following T wave is the reverse of excitation, which explains the characteristic feature of the normal electrocardiogram in which the polarity of the QRS and the T wave is the same in most leads.

■ PATHOPHYSIOLOGY

■ Coronary insufficiency

Whenever the demand for energy exceeds the supply, coronary insufficiency results. This may be localized as in coronary atherosclerosis or generalized in the patient with aortic valvular disease or cardiac hypertrophy. In patients with coronary artery disease there is a mixed problem because of the patchy distribution of ischemia and scarring. In coronary artery disease stress evokes a greater than normal increase in coronary flow probably because of an inefficient contractile mechanism in the ischemically damaged myocardium. Areas normally perfused must have an adequate contractile state to compensate for regions of myocardium that have been previously damaged or that do not participate as effectively in contraction.

Slow to normal muscle must increase excessively in relation to its augmented regional activity. This uses up available coronary reserve for lesser degrees of stress than in the normal patient. Since the coronaries penetrate the epicardium and ramify subsequently to the endocardium, the deep layers of the heart are more susceptible to ischemia when the supply and demand balance changes. This depth dependence is manifested by the detection of subendocardial ischemia by ST-segment depression on the electrocardiogram. Regions of myocardium that are ischemic contract less effectively or are not in unison with the remaining normal ventricle. This asynergy underlies the development of congestive failure in many patients with coronary heart disease.

■ Heart failure without myocardial depression

Severe acute hypertension or sudden mitral regurgitation quickly leads to left ventricular pump failure without myocardial depression. This is termed *afterload mismatch with limited preload reserve*. This happens in a normal heart that is fully distended and unable to compensate by increasing its preload.

In chronic mechanical overload such as a large left-to-right shunt, either atrial or ventricular, the patient develops ventricular hypertrophy, and heart failure occurs as a result of longstanding hypertrophy and continued mechanical overload.

■ Impaired cardiac filling

There may be impaired cardiac filling in chronic constrictive pericarditis in an acute cardiac condition. Various restrictive diseases of the ventricular chambers can lead to elevated diastolic ventricular pressures despite normal systolic contractile functions of the myocardium. Mitral and tricuspid valve stenosis, clots, or tumors may also depress cardiac filling.

■ Intrinsic myocardial pathology

Many infiltrative, inflammatory, or tumor stages may influence myocardial contractility, and diseases, such as lymphoma, actually infiltrate into the myocardium. This distorts and interferes with normal myocardial contractility and eventually causes failure of the myocardial pump. Myocardial failure may be the result of a group of diseases called *myocardiopathies* in which there is destruction of the functional myocardial cells. These myocardiopathies are classified as hypertrophic, dilated, and restrictive.

The heart in health or disease has seven mechanisms of cardiac reserve. A change in the *heart rate* is one of the most effective ways of *increasing cardiac output*. However, above certain limits, such as a rate of 170 to 180 beats/min in young people or 140 in older people, cardiac output begins to decline. The decrease is caused by a shortening of the time of diastole, thus foreshortening the time for adequate filling of the ventricles and for coronary blood flow, which occurs primarily during diastole in the left ventricle.

In the normal heart the difference between the left ventricular stroke volume and the end-diastolic volume is termed the *ejection fraction,* which is approximately 50% to 60%. Increased contractility increases the ejection fraction and stroke volume. It may also be increased by a primary increase in venous return. In the early stages of heart failure the end-diastolic volume increases as well as fiber length, which maintains stroke volume, although the ejection fraction is decreased. The decrease in ejection fraction is early evidence of ventricular failure.

As tissue requirements for oxygen increase or supply decreases, the tissue may extract oxygen from each volume of blood passing through the tissue. Since the myocardium already extracts 75% of its arterial oxygen content, this reserve mechanism is of less value to the myocardium.

There is redistribution of cardiac output in the body under conditions of increased demand. This result provides blood flow to the brain and heart as well as to the tissues that acutely require oxygen. The nervous system (sympathetic) under periods of stress increases venous return to the heart and shifts blood from the large venous reservoirs to the heart, arterial system, and active organs.

The majority of the tissues of the body may use anaerobic metabolism as a reserve mechanism, although the value of this mechanism is quite limited in the myocardium. Cardiac dilation and myocardial hypertrophy are forms of compensatory reserve. However, their long-term effects usually lead to cardiac failure.

■ NONINVASIVE NUCLEAR CARDIOLOGY PROCEDURES

Nuclear cardiology procedures currently comprise about 33% to 50% of nuclear procedures performed in a busy clinical nuclear imaging department. These studies are noninvasive and require only the intravenous injection of short-lived radionuclides. They may assess cardiac performance, delineate myocardial perfusion, and measure viability and metabolism, thus having application to the entire field of cardiology. The linking of sophisticated computers to improved scintillation cameras and the availability of sophisticated software have allowed development of quantitative cardiac evaluation unequaled by any other noninvasive or invasive methodology.

Cardiovascular disease is the most common cause of death in this country. The future refinement of nuclear cardiology procedures will have a direct effect on patient management and basic understanding of cardiac pathophysiology.

■ Definitions

Before presenting the various radionuclide cardiac procedures, a few descriptions of the words and phrases used in the performance and interpretation of the studies are presented.

1. *Cardiac cycle*—Complete heartbeat consisting of a contraction (systole) and a relaxation (diastole) of both atria and ventricles.
2. *Cardiac output*—Amount of blood pumped (ejected) per minute by the ventricles. It is determined by the amount of blood ejected from the ventricle with each stroke volume (beat) and the heart rate. The cardiac output (CO) is the stroke volume (SV) multiplied by the heart rate (HR) or:
$$CO = SV \times HR$$
3. *Diastole*—Rhythmic cycle of relaxation and dilation of the heart during which the chambers fill with blood.
4. *Ejection fraction*—Ventricles do not completely empty their blood during contraction. This stroke volume represents a fraction of the total volume reached at end-diastole. The ejection fraction (EF) equals the end-diastolic volume (EDV) minus the end-systolic volume (ESV) divided by end-diastolic volume (EDV) or:
$$EF = \frac{EDV - ESV}{EDV}$$
5. *End-diastolic volume*—Largest volume attained by the ventricle during a cardiac cycle, depicting the capacity of the ventricle following completion of its filling with blood (the end of the diastolic cycle). The end-diastolic volume (EDV) is the stroke volume (SV) divided by the ejection fraction (EF) or:
$$EDV = \frac{SV}{EF}$$
6. *End-systolic volume*—Smallest volume attained by the ventricle during a cardiac cycle. During contraction the ventricle does not completely eject all its blood volume. The end-systolic volume depicts the residual capacity of the ventricle (the end of the systolic cycle). The end-systolic volume (ESV) is the end-diastolic volume (EDV) minus the systolic volume (SV) or:
$$ESV = EDV - SV$$
7. *Pulmonary blood volume*—Mean pulmonary transit time multiplied by cardiac output or:
$$EF = \frac{EDV - ESV}{EDV}$$
8. *Pulmonary transit time*—Time elapsed between visualization of the pulmonary artery and the left atrium and ventricle.
9. *Qualitative*—Represents limited measurement capabilities (positive or negative).
10. *Quantitative*—Capable of being specifically measured (produces a mathematic conclusion).
11. *Redistribution*—Delayed (3 hours) images following myocardial stress images obtained immediately after injection of ^{201}Tl.
12. *Sensitivity*—Number of positive studies divided by patients with proven disease.
13. *Specificity*—Number of true negative studies divided by number of patients without disease.
14. *Systole*—Rhythmic cycle of contraction of the heart during which time blood is expelled from the heart's chambers.

LABORATORY APPLICATION 44

FIRST-PASS RADIONUCLIDE ANGIOGRAPHY

Steven C. Port

Purpose

First-pass radionuclide angiography (RNA) can provide many quantitative, semiquantitative, and qualitative indices of cardiac function as well as important anatomic information. Some of those applications, such as shunt detection and measurement of chamber-to-chamber transit times, are unique to first-pass radionuclide angiography. Some can be performed with a multigated acquisition as well. The specific advantages and disadvantages of first-pass radionuclide angiography will be discussed below, but it is important to recognize that neither first-pass radionuclide angiography nor multigated radionuclide angiography can be applied to all clinical questions. A thorough familiarity with the merits of both modalities allows the operator to use the technique that is most appropriate for a given clinical situation. Not infrequently, it is appropriate to acquire both a first-pass radionuclide angiogram and a gated study at the same time. That approach should be taken routinely when both right ventricular and left ventricular ejection fractions need to be measured at rest.

Advantages of first-pass radionuclide angiography

Since tracer transit through the central circulation is typically less than 20 seconds, first-pass radionuclide angiography acquisition times are short. That offers several distinct advantages. First and foremost, it is less stressful on patients. They don't have to be still for prolonged periods of time, and they don't have to sustain their peak exercise workloads for more than 15 seconds. The latter is particularly advantageous for patients who are experiencing signs or symptoms of severe ischemia or for those limited by pulmonary insufficiency during stress.

Physiologically, the short acquisition time ensures that the data represent one isolated physiologic or pathophysiologic state. During a rapidly changing situation such as progressive, exercise-induced ischemia, a multigated study requiring 2 minutes may result in an averaging of different states of ventricular function. The short acquisition time also lends itself to the use of ultra–short-lived radionuclides. Gold-195m ($t\frac{1}{2}$ = 30.5 seconds) has been used successfully for rapid, sequential first-pass studies. Iridium-191m ($t\frac{1}{2}$ = 4.9 seconds) and tantalum-198 ($t\frac{1}{2}$ = 9.3 minutes) have also been used. With gold-195m and iridium-191m, the patient must be connected directly to the generator and studies require decay correction. Simultaneous injection of gold-195m and thallium-201 allows for acquisition of a first-pass study at peak exercise followed several minutes later by a perfusion scan once the gold-195m has decayed. The recent introduction of technetium-99m myocardial perfusion imaging agents also allow a first-pass study at peak exercise followed by perfusion imaging.

Because of the temporal separation of cardiac chambers, right or left ventricular function can be studied in any view. The shallow right anterior oblique view (a relatively useless view in equilibrium studies) offers excellent atrioventricular separation and a left ventricular radionuclide angiogram that can be directly correlated with contrast left ventriculography.

Another unique aspect of first-pass radionuclide angiography is the ability to study the route taken by a radionuclide bolus through the central circulation. Simple qualitative inspection of tracer transit in either static or dynamic formats may provide important anatomic information especially in cases of congenital heart disease. As will be discussed below, quantitative analysis of first-pass curves can be used to detect and quantify left to right shunts.

Finally, laboratories performing a large volume of rest and exercise radionuclide angiograms will find that, compared to gated exercise studies, patient throughput is significantly greater with first-pass studies.

Disadvantages of first-pass radionuclide angiography

There are several disadvantages of first-pass imaging. First and foremost is the necessity for separate injections of a radionuclide for each view or intervention to be imaged. With technetium-99m, this results in higher radiation doses and limits the number of views or studies to two or at most three on a given day. The long half-life of technetium-99m in relation to the short acquisition time results in high levels of background activity that must be taken into account if more than one injection is made. It is necessary to position patients carefully during radionuclide injection, and the quality of the injection bolus is important. First-pass studies have count-rate and processing requirements that exceed most conventional Anger camera systems. In addition, data processing is more demanding, time consuming, and operator-dependent than is the processing of gated studies. The spatial resolution of first-pass studies in general is not as good as that of high-quality equilibrium studies, although at peak exercise the differences are not as significant because of the limited statistics in the average gated exercise study. In fact, at peak exercise, the first-pass study may be superior to a 1½- to 2-minute gated study.

Continued.

Indications

Coronary artery disease

Rest and exercise first-pass RNA has been extensively applied to both the diagnosis and management of patients with suspected or known coronary artery disease. The diagnosis of chest pain and the prognosis of patients with or without prior myocardial infarction are leading indications for rest and exercise first-pass RNA. A less well documented but widely used practice is the selection of patients with known coronary artery disease for medical or surgical therapy. Technetium-perfusion agents allow assessment of left ventricular function and myocardial perfusion at the same sitting. The roles of first-pass RNA when used adjunctively to perfusion imaging have not been thoroughly explored yet, but there is no doubt that first-pass RNA will add diagnostic and prognostic information to perfusion data and in certain cases will aid in the assessment of myocardial viability.

Resting first-pass radionuclide angiography is particularly useful in the diagnosis of certain complications of acute myocardial infarction, including determination of right ventricular ejection fraction in patients suspected of having right ventricular infarction and detection and quantitation of a left-to-right shunt in patients with suspected interventricular septal rupture.

Valvular heart disease

Resting first-pass radionuclide angiography can be helpful in estimating the severity of aortic or mitral insufficiency and can help in deciding when valve replacement is necessary. Serial resting studies are particularly important for that purpose. Exercise first-pass radionuclide angiography has not been shown to add prognostically significant information in cases of valvular insufficiency. For patients with mitral stenosis, serial measurement of right ventricular size and ejection fraction may be prognostically useful, but little data are available to substantiate such an approach. In aortic stenosis, first-pass RNA can be used to assess left ventricular function, but a gated study is of equal value. First-pass RNA has been used to quantitate tricuspid insufficiency.

Congenital heart disease

Although the overall assessment of patients with congenital heart disease is better served by echocardiography and cardiac catheterization, first-pass radionuclide angiography is ideally suited for the detection and quantitation of left-to-right shunts. As such, it may be reliably used for proving or excluding a significant left-to-right shunt as the cause of an undiagnosed heart murmur. First-pass radionucide angiography is also well suited for following patients who have undergone surgical correction of left-to-right shunts.

Technical and procedural aspects of first-pass radionuclide angiography

Radionuclide

Technetium-99m compounds are traditionally used in first-pass radionuclide angiography. Although the pertechnetate salt can be used for cardiac imaging, ^{99m}Tc DTPA is preferable because of its enhanced excretion rate. It should be emphasized that any radionuclide that can be administered intravenously in a sufficient dose, whether a traditional blood-pool imaging agent or not, could theoretically be used to generate a first-pass study. For example, a first-pass study can be acquired during injection of technetium-99m pyrophosphate and a myocardial infarction scan acquired later. We have used this approach to provide information about the exact location and severity of infarction in patients whose MI scans are subsequently positive. As mentioned above, short-lived radionuclides such as gold-195m, iridium-191m, and tantalum-198 are also suitable although they present other problems related to the generators and collimation.

Electrocardiogram

An electrocardiographic rhythm strip must be acquired before a first-pass study is performed. The cardiac rhythm must be assessed to avoid injecting a patient unnecessarily. Very frequent ventricular or atrial ectopic beats, ventricular bigeminy, or runs of ventricular ectopics may make data processing or clinical interpretation impossible. A multigated study with ectopic beat rejection may be appropriate in such a situation. Otherwise, the study should be postponed. For high–count-rate first-pass studies, an electrocardiogram (ECG) is not necessary. During the acquisition of low–count-rate studies, an ECG is important to generate a so-called gated first-pass acquisition. In that situation the ECG signal is used to help identify end-diastole of individual beats.

Radionuclide administration

The key to successful first-pass imaging of the left ventricle is temporal separation of the cardiac chambers. That places great importance on the site and technique of radionuclide injection. A large peripheral vein, preferably an external jugular or the medial antecubital vein, should be used. If the external jugular vein is used, a 20-gauge, 1-inch teflon cannula is adequate. For the antecubital approach, an 18-gauge, 1- to 1½-inch cannula is desirable. First-pass studies should never be attempted through forearm veins, and use of existing intravenous lines should be discouraged if other suitable veins are available. It is helpful to attach a 6-inch length of intravenous tubing to the IV cannula and place a 3-way stopcock at the other end for ease of administration (Fig. 18-4). The radionuclide should be drawn up in a volume not exceeding 1 to 1½ ml and should be flushed in with 10 to 20 ml of saline. For left ventricular and shunt studies, the bolus should be rapidly and compactly (high specific-activity) injected. For right ventricular studies, a slower injection provides more right ventricular beats for analysis.

The radionuclide dose will vary with body size, collimation, gamma camera dead-time losses, and the type of study to be acquired. A typical first-pass left ventricular study requires 0.3 to 0.4 mCi/kg body weight of ^{99m}Tc. Shunt studies and right ventricular studies can be performed with lower doses.

Instrumentation

The type of imaging device used is crucial to the quality and accuracy of first-pass data. The device must be capable of recording at least 150,000 to 200,000 counts/sec. As such, either a multicrystal gamma camera, a high–count-rate digital single-crystal camera, or a proportional wire chamber are the instruments that are suited for first-pass studies. Conventional gamma cameras can be used, but one should anticipate a high frequency of suboptimal results when the study is acquired to analyze left ventricular function, especially left ventricular wall motion. A high-sensitivity collimator is essential; a collimator whose matrix is matched with the software matrix is preferable. No less than a 1-inch–thick collimator is necessary and for accurate wall motion analysis a 1½-inch–thick collimator is extremely helpful if not mandatory. The computer software must be capable of both a high temporal resolution and a small, 32 × 32 (or smaller) matrix acquisition. The study is most

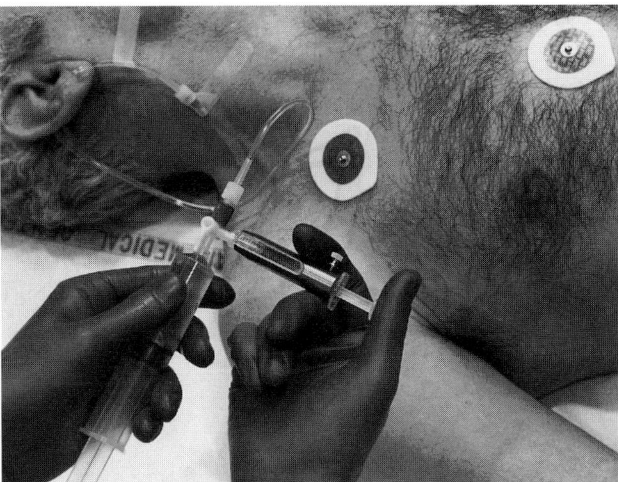

Fig. 18-4. A patient is prepared for a first-pass study by insertion of a 20-gauge, 1½-inch Teflon cannula in the right external jugular vein. Intravenous tubing connects the cannula to the shielded dose syringe and the saline flush syringe via a three-way stopcock.

Continued.

easily acquired in frame mode with 0.02 to 0.05 sec/frame; the higher the heart rate, the shorter the frame time. To avoid confusion in trying to adjust the frame times for each study, a compromise of 0.025 to 0.035 sec/frame can be used successfully for most clinical studies. A list-mode acquisition can also be used. If more than one study is to be acquired within a short period of time, it is important for the software to be able to correct the second acquisition for dead time and for background activity remaining from a previous injection. Some software requires an electrocardiographic signal to be stored with the frame data. However, first-pass data processing can be accurately and reproducibly performed without any electrocardiographic input. Studies should be acquired for a minimum of 30 sec or about 800 to 1200 frames. Once the data are examined, the operator can elect to permanently store fewer frames if appropriate.

Patient orientation and positioning

The patient should be advised about the nature of the study and especially the need for a good injection bolus. Although experienced technologists can usually position the patient to ensure visualization of the entire heart without test doses or transmission images, such aids are extremely important for the less experienced. A 0.5-mCi (18.5 MBq) to 1-mCi (37 MBq) test injection helps identify the position of the ventricular chambers. Alternatively, a large flat flood source can be held behind the chest to easily identify the lungs and mediastinum. For a left ventricular study, the left ventricular apex and some left lung should be included in the field of view.

The most informative and widely used views are the shallow (20° to 30°) right anterior oblique and the anterior views. For left ventricular studies, the right anterior oblique is preferable to the anterior because it provides separation between the descending aorta and the left ventricle. Left anterior oblique or left lateral views can also be acquired and are indicated when there is a specific question about inferobasal or posterolateral left ventricular wall motion. A shunt study should usually be acquired in the anterior view. When a patent ductus is suspected, a shallow left anterior oblique view may allow visualization of the ductus itself. For a shunt study it is important to include as much of the right lung as possible. If inclusion of the right lung excludes the left ventricle, then two injections may be necessary, one to maximize right lung statistics and one to maximize right and left ventricular statistics. Patients should be positioned as close as possible to the collimator and cautioned not to move during acquisition. During bicycle exercise, the patient should be encouraged to move the chest as little as possible. Breathing should not be restricted during exercise because it will lead to great discomfort and a lack of cooperation. In fact, patients should be cautioned against an inadvertent Valsalva maneuver or breath holding since they may compromise the integrity of the radionuclide bolus. To help avoid a delayed injection bolus, a patient injected through an arm vein should be asked to avoid squeezing a bicycle handle or other support device with the arm to be injected.

For treadmill exercise studies, it is necessary to use an external marker applied to the chest wall to track motion. Both americium-241 (window at 50 to 60 keV) or ^{125}I (window at 15 to 55 keV) markers have been used. Dual-energy acquisition of the technetium (140 keV) and the marker is performed, and any detected marker motion is used to correct the technetium data. Without such an approach, first-pass RNA cannot be reliably performed during treadmill exercise.

Post-acquisition procedures

Immediately after acquisition is terminated, one should view the data and make sure that the bolus is acceptable and that the right and left ventricles are within the field of view. Reframing the data at 1-sec intervals helps that assessment. If acceptable, the patient can leave the imaging area or have a subsequent study performed. Once imaging is completed, patients should be encouraged to drink liquids to enhance urinary excretion of the radionuclide.

Data processing

First-pass data processing, in general, is more time-consuming and demanding than processing gated studies. There are three basic routines that are common to processing data for either right or left ventricular analysis (Fig. 18-5). They include generation of a time-activity curve from a region of interest around the ventricle, creating a representative cycle from as many usable beats in the time-activity curve as possible, and correcting that representative cycle for background activity. Once

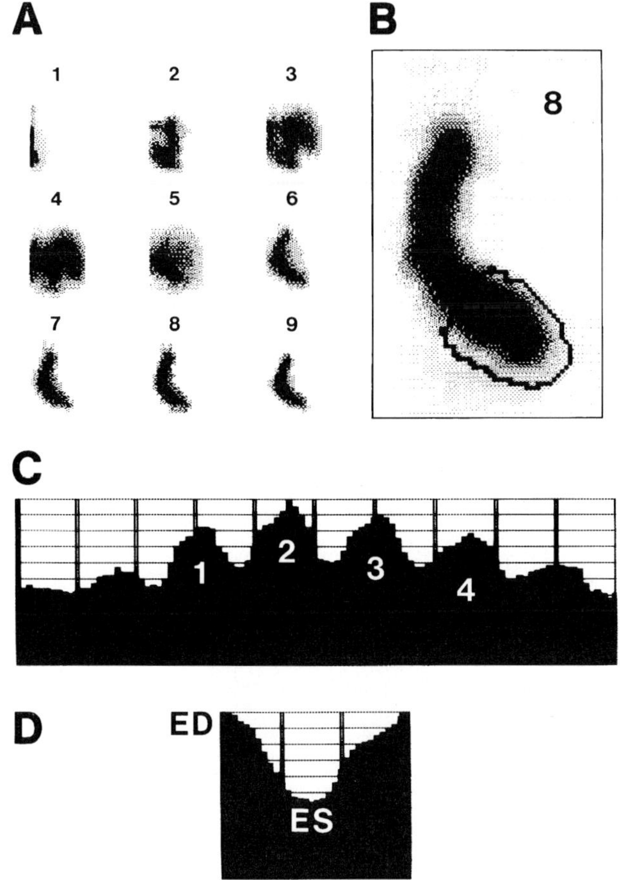

Fig. 18-5. Basic elements of first-pass data processing. A, Data are grouped into 1-second images for identification of the left ventricle. Any typical left ventricular image, in this case image 8, is then displayed in a larger format (B) so that a region-of-interest can be drawn around the left ventricle. That region of interest is used to generate a time-activity curve (C). Individual beats (numbered 1-4) are then selected and cyclically added together to create a representative cardiac cycle from which background is subtracted to give a final representative cycle (D).

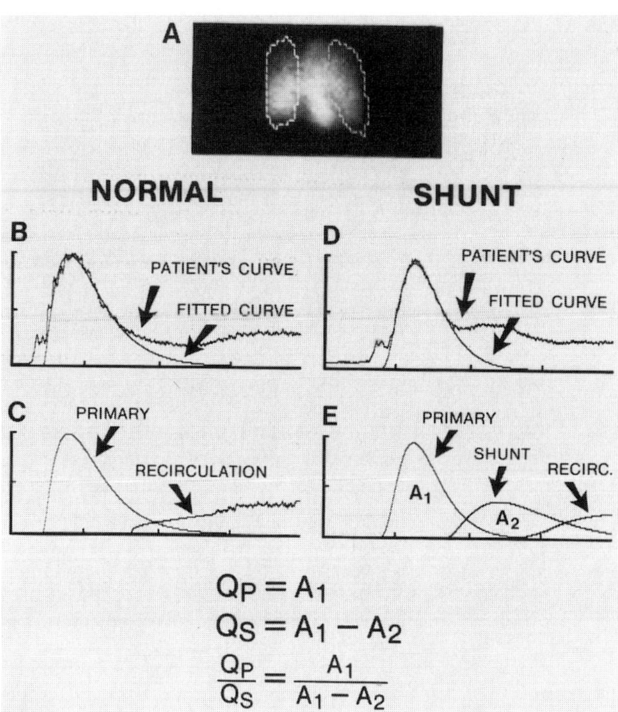

Fig. 18-6. A shows a 1-second image of a first-pass shunt study. The image is selected from the pulmonary phase because of the clear delineation of the lungs. The dotted lines represent manually drawn regions-of-interest around the right and left lungs that are used to generate time-activity curves. B shows such a time-activity curve from a normal subject, while panel D shows a curve from a patient with a left-to-right shunt. In each case a gamma-variate computer fitted curve is also displayed on the primary peak. C shows that after subtraction of the fitted curve from the normal patient's curve, one is left with a primary curve and a recirculation component but no shunt. E shows that after subtraction of the fitted curve from the shunt patient's curve, one has a primary peak, a shunt peak, and a recirculation peak. Note that the shunt peak occurs much earlier than the recirculation peak. The areas of the peaks A1 and A2 are then used to calculate the ratio of pulmonary to systemic blood flow Q_p/Q_s.

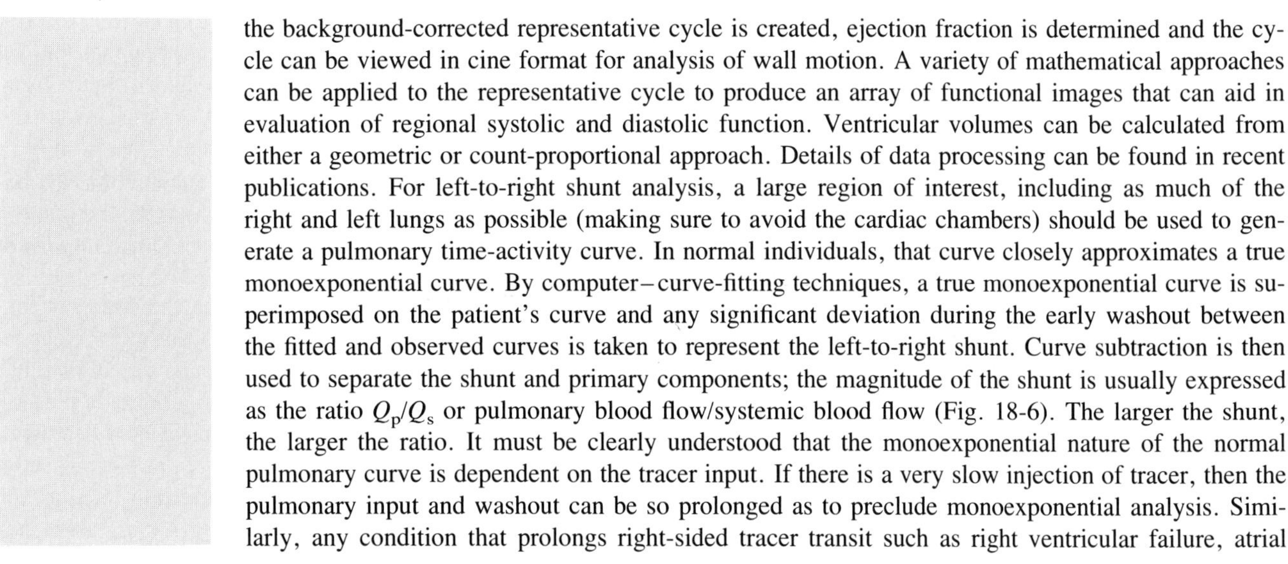

the background-corrected representative cycle is created, ejection fraction is determined and the cycle can be viewed in cine format for analysis of wall motion. A variety of mathematical approaches can be applied to the representative cycle to produce an array of functional images that can aid in evaluation of regional systolic and diastolic function. Ventricular volumes can be calculated from either a geometric or count-proportional approach. Details of data processing can be found in recent publications. For left-to-right shunt analysis, a large region of interest, including as much of the right and left lungs as possible (making sure to avoid the cardiac chambers) should be used to generate a pulmonary time-activity curve. In normal individuals, that curve closely approximates a true monoexponential curve. By computer–curve-fitting techniques, a true monoexponential curve is superimposed on the patient's curve and any significant deviation during the early washout between the fitted and observed curves is taken to represent the left-to-right shunt. Curve subtraction is then used to separate the shunt and primary components; the magnitude of the shunt is usually expressed as the ratio Q_p/Q_s or pulmonary blood flow/systemic blood flow (Fig. 18-6). The larger the shunt, the larger the ratio. It must be clearly understood that the monoexponential nature of the normal pulmonary curve is dependent on the tracer input. If there is a very slow injection of tracer, then the pulmonary input and washout can be so prolonged as to preclude monoexponential analysis. Similarly, any condition that prolongs right-sided tracer transit such as right ventricular failure, atrial

Continued.

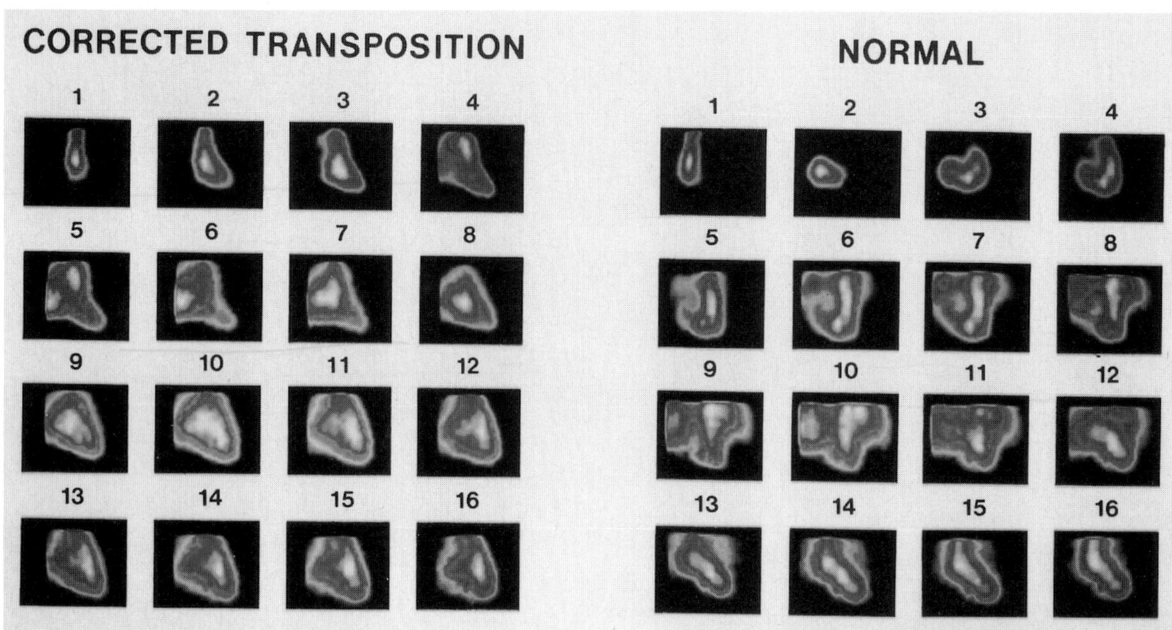

Fig. 18-7. Serial 1-second images from a patient with corrected transposition of the great vessels (CTGV) and from a normal subject. Careful inspection of the images shows that in the patient with CTGV, the tracer appears in the superior vena cava (image 1) but then enters what morphologically looks like a left ventricle (images 3-7). After the pulmonary phase the tracer appears in a chamber that resembles a right ventricle (images 10-16). In addition, one can appreciate the altered position of the pulmonary artery (image 3) and aorta (image 16) by comparison with the normal subject.

fibrillation, or tricuspid or pulmonic insufficiency can also make monoexponential analysis of a pulmonary curve difficult or impossible.

Interpretation

First-pass radionuclide angiography interpretation begins with an inspection of the transit of the radionuclide through the central circulation. That is useful for quality control and may yield important diagnostic information especially in certain forms of congenital heart disease (Fig. 18-7). A significant intracardiac left-to-right shunt can be excluded by a simple inspection of serial static images that shows a clear left ventricle, free of right ventricular activity. Qualitative analysis of left ventricular tracer transit can be helpful in detecting and quantifying left-sided valvular heart disease. Both mitral and aortic insufficiency will prolong left ventricular tracer transit to a degree proportional to the severity of the valvular insufficiency. Factor analysis has recently been applied in this situation to quantify valvular insufficiency. Inspection of the images may distinguish aortic from mitral insufficiency by the appearance of the left atrium or ascending aorta (Fig. 18-8). Serious errors in data interpretation will occur if careful attention is not given to the quality of the bolus, tracer transit through the right heart, and the individual beats of the left ventricular time-activity curve. One should always inspect the left ventricular time-activity curve before background correction for problems such as high background activity, arrhythmias, and patient motion. Examples of such problems are demonstrated in Fig. 18-9.

The most widespread application of first-pass radionuclide angiography is the evaluation of left ventricular function at rest and during upright bicycle exercise. At rest, the left ventricular ejection fraction should range from 0.50 to 0.80 and regional wall motion should be symmetric. With exercise, the ejection fraction usually increases and individual segments contract more forcefully. End-diastolic volume may be unchanged or slightly increased while end-systolic volume should decrease. Exceptions do occur in healthy individuals, especially in elderly subjects. The typical response to exercise in the patient with significant coronary artery disease is a decrease in ejection fraction, an increase in end-systolic volume, and a deterioration in the extent of wall motion in those segments

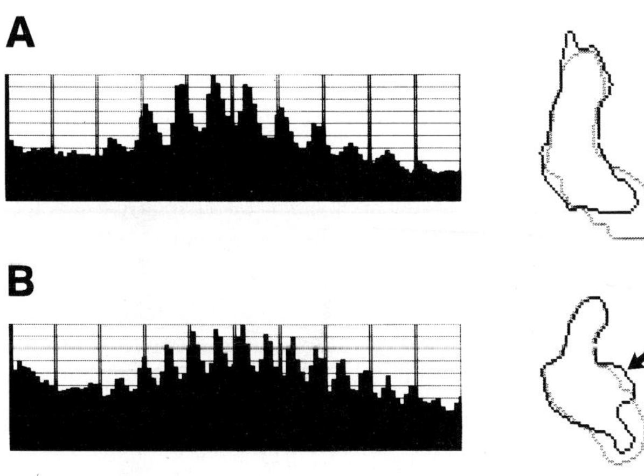

Fig. 18-8. Time-activity curves and end-diastolic and end-systolic perimeter images of the left ventricle are shown from a normal subject in **A** and from a patient with mitral valve disease in **B**. Note the prolonged left ventricular tracer transit in **B** and the markedly dilated left atrium *(arrow)*. The combination is diagnostic of mitral valve disease.

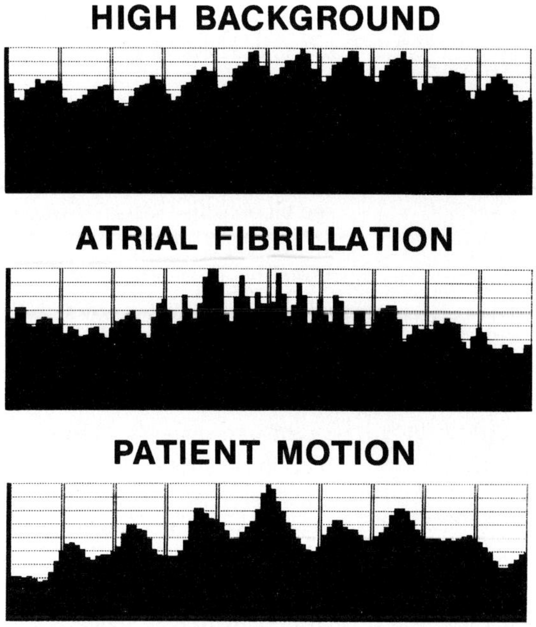

HIGH BACKGROUND

ATRIAL FIBRILLATION

PATIENT MOTION

Fig. 18-9. Representative left ventricular time-activity curves from technically compromised studies. Such data may be difficult or impossible to accurately process.

supplied by stenotic coronary arteries. In general, the more extensive the coronary disease, the lower the exercise ejection fraction. Although decreases in ejection fraction are typical in coronary artery disease, they are not specific. Regional–wall-motion abnormalities are much more specific for coronary disease; for this reason every laboratory should strive for the highest resolution images obtainable. The radionuclide ejection fraction has important prognostic as well as diagnostic applications. Both the resting and the peak exercise left ventricular ejection fractions have been correlated with survival in patients with coronary disease. In one study the first-pass exercise ejection fraction was a more powerful predictor of patient outcome than was data from cardiac catheterization.

As indicated previously, first-pass radionuclide angiography can be useful diagnostically in patients with valvular heart disease, but its overall role is less clear and its application more limited than in patients with coronary artery disease. When valvular disease is suspected, interpretation of first-pass data depends more on chamber volumes, tracer transit, and resting ejection fractions of the right and left ventricles than on exercise data or regional wall motion. For all clinical studies, correct interpretation of first-pass data is highly dependent on a thorough understanding of data acquisition and processing as well as constant attention to statistics and overall study quality.

LABORATORY APPLICATION

45

EQUILIBRIUM GATED RADIONUCLIDE VENTRICULOGRAM

Purpose

The equilibrium-gated–radionuclide ventriculogram is a noninvasive, widely available method to examine the function of the pumping chambers of the heart. Ventricular size (relative or absolute), configuration, and wall-motion information complement measurements of ejection fraction; rates of contraction and relaxation; quantification of the coordination of contraction by parametric imaging such as Fourier phase; and amplitude analysis and timing of specific portions of the time-volume cycle such as isovolumic relaxation period or the rates of fast filling. The fortuitous arrangement of the heart's anatomy makes these measurements much more accurate for the left ventricle than for the right. To obtain good information about the right ventricle's function, the first-pass study has been used as described beginning on page 376. A technique that combines the advantages of both,

Continued.

the *gated* first-pass–equilibrium study with radionuclides that do not pass the pulmonary capillary bed to reach the left ventricle, is discussed at the end of this chapter.

Radiopharmaceutical preparations

An old method of tracing the blood pool employed the intravenous injection (IV) of radiolabeled albumin particles. These tend to degrade and leak from the blood pool much faster than the labeled red blood cells (RBCs). Simple in vivo labeling of the RBCs can be done with an initial injection of 10 to 20 μg of tin (as stannous pyrophosphate) per kilogram of body weight, intravenously, followed by 15 to 30 mCi (555 to 110 MBq) of intravenous ^{99m}Tc-pertechnetate. The labeling will be almost instantaneous, though there will be some pertechnetate uptake in the thyroid gland, stomach, etc. This labeling technique is easy and generally yields a sufficiently good label. There are in vitro labeling techniques that involve the use of stannous chloride in a kit with an anticoagulant. After RBCs are added to the kit, ^{99m}Tc-pertechnetate is added. After incubation the labeled cells are injected intravenously. These methods give the purest label. They are excellent for gastrointestinal bleeding studies in which physiologic excretion of pertechnetate can lead to false positive diagnoses. A compromise involves a modification of these techniques in which the stannous pyrophosphate is injected into the patient and then a sample of RBCs is withdrawn for incubation with ^{99m}Tc-pertechnetate. Precautions should be taken to do all these procedures in a sterile fashion and to ensure that RBCs removed for tagging are returned to the correct patient. Concerns about inadvertent cross transfusions, blood-borne infections, and protection of the technical staff's health are of primary importance. Any of the techniques for labeling will yield a radiopharmaceutical that allows imaging to go on for hours if need be. Doses for resting studies in which time relatively abundant can be held to the 15- to 20-mCi (555 to 740 MBq) range. For studies in which there is a need for rapid acquisition, higher activities can be used. Exercise studies that require acquisitions as short as 2 min can normally be done with adequate statistics with a 30 mCi (1110 MBq) dose.

Acquisition

The equilibrium-gated–radionuclide ventriculogram goes by several names and nicknames in the literature. The names imply several features of the study. A stable radiolabel of the blood pool (as discussed above) is needed. The volume of blood in a given structure is directly proportional to the count intensity in the study. An electrocardiogram gating device triggers frame-by-frame data acquisition with software that averages together hundreds of cardiac cycles into a composite cine style series of images subsequently displayed in a repeating loop. Most gating devices use three leads placed around the anterior chest wall. A frequently successful placement is over the apex of each lung and over the lower left chest. Some systems also use a fourth ground lead placed lower over the upper abdomen. Care should be taken to keep the metal snaps and wires away from the blood pool being imaged. The leads should be adjusted so that a large sharp QRS complex is recognized by the gate. When this is done, multiple technical choices must be intelligently made for the acquisition.

The single most useful image is that obtained in a "best septal" projection, which is most often a left anterior oblique (LAO) view of about 30 to 45 degrees with the patient lying supine. The camera and patient should be maneuvered to show the best separation of the left ventricle (LV) and right ventricle (RV), no matter what the degree of cardiac rotation. This is also known as a "short-axis" view and has a direct correlate in the contrast-angiography short-axis ventriculogram. This is the view from which left ventricular ejection fraction (LVEF) and all other statistical information is measured. A variation on the best septal view that some laboratories find quite satisfactory is the acquisition of the best septal view with a 30-degree slant-hole collimator. With this turned so that the axis of the holes is directed caudad, the average heart will be displayed with the atria projected well clear of the ventricles. Usually this separates the right atrium (RA) from the RV. This view is analogous to the echocardiography "four-chamber" view. Some authors outline the blood pool of the RV for a calculation of right ventricular ejection fraction (RVEF). The problem is that the pulmonary outflow tract is superimposed on the RV blood pool. This introduces errors in the RVEF calculation that cannot be corrected. The left atrium (LA) is partially hidden by the aorta and the pulmonary artery, but the LV is well displayed. The walls seen to best advantage are the septum and the free walls of each ventricle (Fig. 18-10). Simple caudal tilting of the camera may also produce

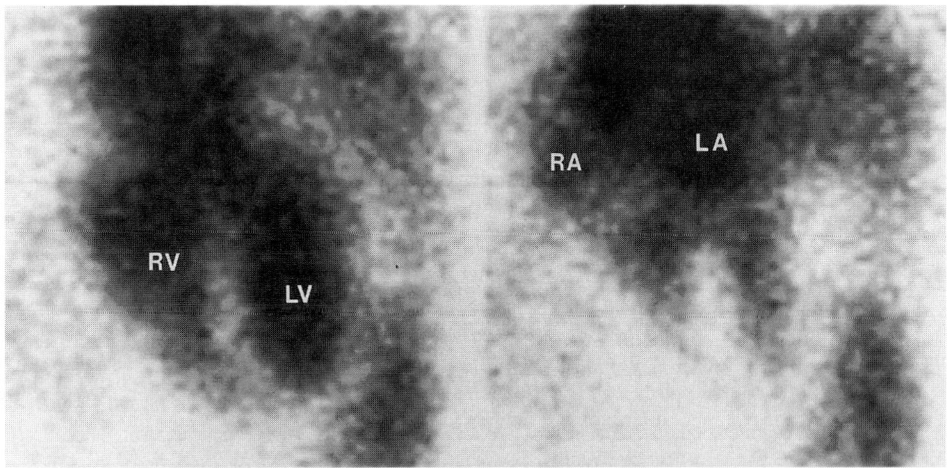

Fig. 18-10. Four-chamber view. End-diastole and end-systole from a standard best septal and a four chamber study of a normal heart. Zoom and low energy all purpose and low energy thirty degree slant collimators were used in this study. The left atrium (LA) and right atrium (RA) are better separated from the right ventricle (RV) and left ventricle (LV) in the four chamber view.

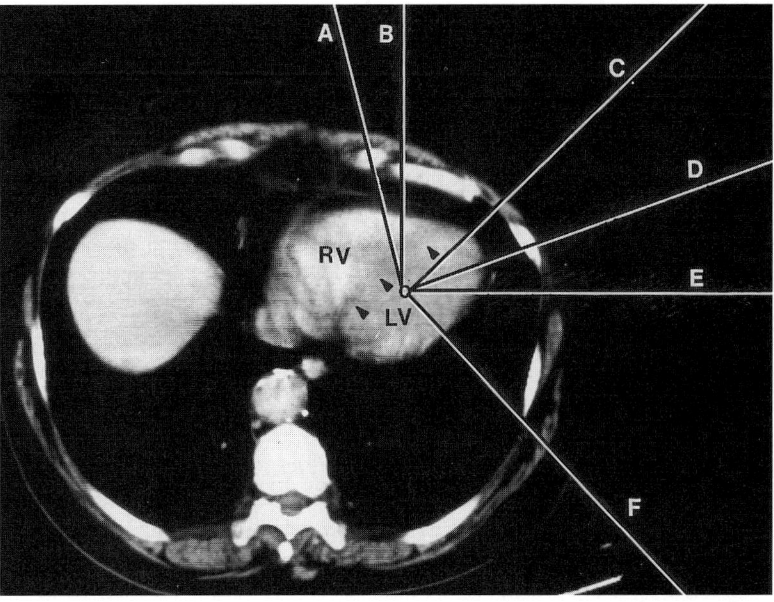

Fig. 18-11. Trans-axial computed tomogram slice through the ventricles displays the axis of acquisition for each lettered view. Note the respective distances (and path through the body) from the center of the LV to the chest where the camera is placed. The septum *(arrowheads)* divides RV and LV. *A* = RAO, *B* = anterior, *C* = best septal, *D* = 70 degrees LAO, *E* = left lateral and *F* = left posterior oblique.

this effect if the camera can be so positioned without backing off the chest wall so far that all resolution is lost. Tall, thin people tend to have a heart that is vertically arranged; a four-chamber view is obtained by simply applying the parallel collimator flush with the chest wall. Those who are more obese or barrel-chested may have ventricles with a long axis perpendicular to the chest wall. Thus the normal best septal LAO view may change in appearance from individual to individual. In many laboratories the standard examination also includes the right anterior oblique (RAO), anterior, steep LAO, left lateral, and/or left anterior oblique (LPO) views (Fig. 18-11). The rationale for these different views is frequently based on the prior experience of the physician and technologist doing the study. The RAO is a natural choice of the cardiologist because the conventional contrast-angiographic long-axis view of the LV is obtained in this projection. Unfortunately the radiation from the LV is partially attenuated in its passage through the RV. What LV radiation is left is added to the radiation arising in the RV. The RAO–long-axis view is a superimposition of both the LV and the RV, which are heavily weighted by the RV. An additional problem is that the RAO is usually done in a fixed degree of rotation, such as 15 or 30 degrees RAO. This makes it a semilong axis that has variable angulation with respect to the best septal LAO–short-axis view.

A more logical long-axis view of the LV is the left posterior oblique (LPO). After a best septal LAO is done with a patient in the supine position, the camera remains in the best septal angulation

Continued.

while the patient is turned to lie on his or her right side. This is to quickly establish a true long-axis view that is orthogonal (perpendicular) to the best septal LAO–short-axis view. If a SPECT camera and table are being used for the study, it is simple to rotate the gantry 90 degrees from the best septal LAO view to gain the LPO view. Occasionally the inferior LV wall in the LPO view will be obscured by the spleen, and a minor degree of caudal tilt will allow the camera to peek over the top of the spleen. Radiation from the RV is superimposed on the image of the LV, but the image will still be dominated by the LV radioactivity. Neither long-axis view is perfect, but the LPO is a better radionuclide demonstration of the left ventricle than is the RAO. The anterior and left lateral views of the ventricles are actually oblique views of the cardiac anatomy. Since the actual cardiac axis is different in each patient, the degree of obliquity with reference to the heart is different in each examination. Perhaps there is some utility to these views if there is a need to compare with the ubiquitous posterior-anterior and left lateral chest radiograph. The steep LAO is usually done at a fixed 70 degrees LAO angulation. Its only imaging correlation is with the customary planar thallium-201 steep LAO.

The collimator and camera to be used for the gated study can vary widely. Large (LFOV) and standard (SFOV) field-of-view instruments can be used. There is a lot of wasted camera if the LFOV is used for a relatively small organ. The accuracy of the study does not rest on high-resolution systems, and it is counterproductive to use a high-resolution/low-sensitivity collimator. The blood pool moves continuously and will never be captured with the precision of a static structure. A low-energy dynamic (low resolution/high sensitivity) or all-purpose collimator is normally sufficient. The only nonrecoverable mistake is to use a nonparallel collimator (i.e., diverging or converging), which variably distorts the image as the ventricles change volume during the cardiac cycle. The intrinsic resolution of the camera used is not as critical as in static detail imaging. Frequently an older, poorer camera with good uniformity will provide a study that is just as accurate as that done with the most expensive new system. The question of the number and size of the frames used for the acquisition of a radionuclide ventriculogram is limited by the hardware and software available and selected by the user within these limits. Acquisition matrices available in nuclear medicine computers vary from 32 × 32 to 64 × 64 or 128 × 128, or even 256 × 256. Most are displayed after video interpolation up to a larger display matrix. Magnification used during the acquisition is very helpful in the subsequent interpretation of the wall motion and calculation of various parameters of function. Nonmagnified images on even an SFOV camera tend to show plenty of structures that are immaterial, including the aortic arch, the lungs, liver, and spleen. The acquisition should be sized so that the majority of what is imaged is pertinent blood pool in the ventricles and atria. There is little reason to use the two larger matrix sizes because the resolution of the camera/computer system is not as good as the minuscule pixel size. The pixel size employed using an SFOV (25-cm diameter) camera with a 1.5× magnification and a 64 × 64 matrix has pixel sizes of about 2.5 × 2.5 mm. This is adequate for the imaging of a beating ventricle. The smallest matrix size (32 × 32) is too coarse for the data display and analysis. The number of frames used per R-to-R interval is variable according to the computer system used. One computer accepts as many as 120 frames/cardiac cycle. Most systems will not allow the acquisition of more than 32. More frames per R-to-R interval provide better temporal resolution but increase acquisition time to obtain a given level of statistical significance. During resting studies there is the luxury of time: the limits placed on the number of frames in a study

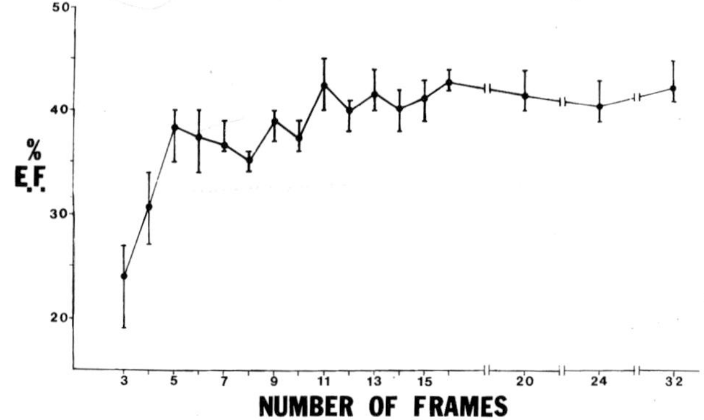

Fig. 18-12. Left ventricular ejection fraction (LVEF) measurement as a function of number of acquired frames. An exceptionally patient patient allowed sequential acquisitions to be performed in increments of one frame from 3 to 16 as well as 20, 24, and 32 frames per R-to-R interval. Then ten different technologists processed the data from each acquisition. Their average LVEF is graphed along with bars that show the maximum range *(not the standard deviation of error)* of the measurements for each study. The studies with few frames per R-to-R interval underestimate this systolic parameter.

may be a factor of the patience of the patient and/or technologist. How many frames should be used? Sampling less than 14 frames in a study with a normal resting heart rate introduces significant errors in the measurement of LVEF. At 16 frames, accurate systolic information (LVEF and rates of contraction) is provided (Fig. 18-12). For exercise studies in which the time at any level of exercise is brief, 16 frames/cycle is a reasonable choice. Smoother cine display of wall motion is better done with smaller temporal increments provided by 24 or more frames/cycle. To accurately measure the complex events of diastole, better temporal resolution from at least 32 frames per R-to-R interval is needed. How long should the acquisition be conducted? The effect of statistical noise in images lessens at higher-count saturations. Too few counts per pixel in the image will result in an image that is highly irregular. It will be difficult to process and interpret. Past some point, increasing the counts in the image produces negligible improvement in image quality. A brief experiment with a typical patient will allow an intelligent choice to be made. Progressive doubling of low-count studies will show the level of counts per image that gives a useable image. Given the 64 × 64 matrix size and an SFOV camera with a 1.5-zoom, a minimum of 100K counts/frame will produce a fair image. 300K in a resting study gives an excellent quality in most systems (Fig 18-13). Simple electrocardiogram R-wave triggering may be done with the computer by simply keeping a running average of the R-to-R interval and predicting the next interval. If the heart rate is 75 beats/min, the R-to-R interval will be 800 ms and each frame of a 16-frame study would be 50 ms long. In forward gating, the first frame of the acquisition sequence begins with the R wave. Data are rapidly transferred to a succession of frames that begin with the new R wave and terminate when the preselected number of frames is finished or when the next R wave has been reached. The average volume curve subsequently generated will show the changing counts (and therefore volume) of the ventricle during systole and diastole. If the interval is highly regular, the end of the last frame will coincide with the next R wave (Fig. 18-14). There is some normal variation in R-to-R intervals that is related to respiration. Breathing produces pressure changes in the chest; these changes cause variations in the rate

Continued.

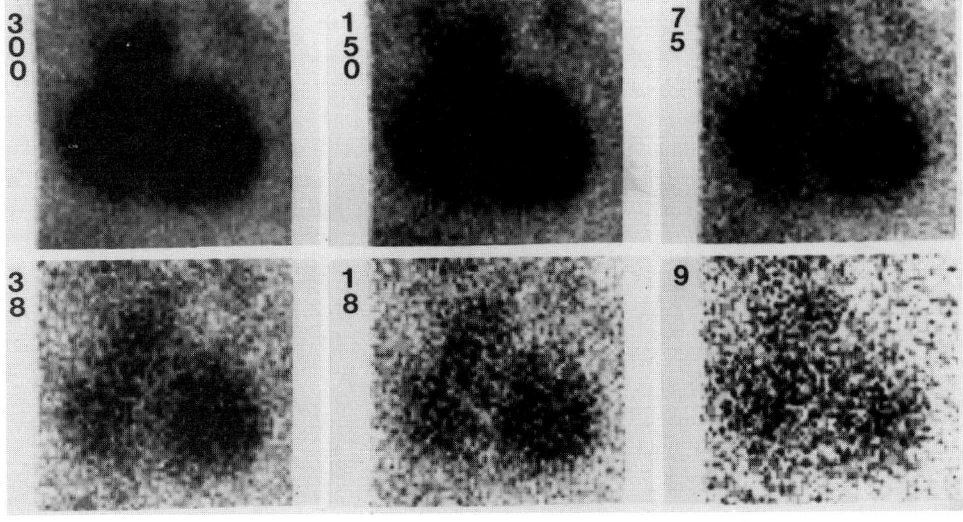

Fig. 18-13. Image quality as a function of pixel count saturation. End diastolic frames from a patient with a dilated LV were acquired with total counts of 300K, 150K, 75K, 38K, 18K, and 9K without altering camera position. Image quality drops progressively as acquisition time is halved.

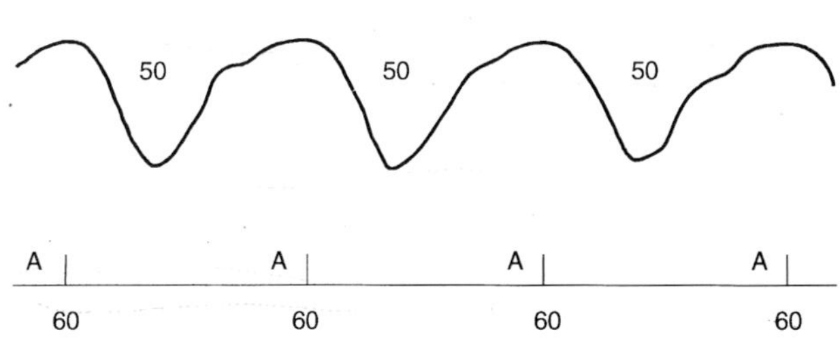

Fig. 18-14. Gating normal sinus rhythm. Successive, regular beats are triggered by R waves *(A)*, which correspond to a heart rate of 60 beats per minute. The LVEF is 50% for each cycle. (The instantaneous heart rate is shown underneath the spike symbolizing each R wave. The LVEF for each cycle is shown over the end systolic points of the curve.)

at which venous blood returns to the heart. The heart changes rate slightly to handle this variable load. As the heart speeds up and slows down slightly, some of the data from the last few frames of the study will be lost. When the cardiac cycle is longer than the average computer-predicted interval, the framing will stop acquisition before diastole is finished. The data in the last few frames will underrepresent the actual volume of the ventricle recorded near end-diastole. When the cycle is shorter than that predicted by the computer, the next R wave will occur (and restart the acquisition at the first frame) before the last frame acquisition is finished. No counts will be recorded in the end-diastole frames cut off by restart of the acquisition. Both effects of cycle variability combine to produce artifactually diminished counts in the last few frames of a resting study. This is seen as "flickering" of the last few frames when the study is replayed in an endless loop cine mode. The LV average-volume curve generated from such data will not show a fully recovered volume at end-diastole. The part of the ventricular cycle representing the "atrial kick" at end-diastole is poorly represented. One way to get around this problem is to use retrospective gating. Data temporarily stored in buffers are assigned to each frame until after the cycle is completed. The slightly different-length cardiac cycles are evenly divided between the given number of frames. This "forward-and-backward" or "rubber-band" gating puts more counts in the frames at the end of the cycle than does the fixed–time-per-frame method. It alters the shape of the average volume curve and changes the ejection fraction and derivative statistics. When the heart has highly regular rhythm, only minimal distortions of the average volume curve result from any gating technique used. It is important to standardize acquisitions and processing.

When the R-to-R interval is highly variable because of arrhythmia, distortions in the average volume curve are marked. To understand the problem it is necessary to understand the beat-to-beat volume changes in a ventricle with an irregular rhythm. Early R waves such as a those in premature ventricular contractions (PVC) and subsequent compensatory pause cycles will mean that the time required for systole is less affected than that for diastole. R waves that come too soon cause the ventricle to begin to contract before it is finished filling. When there is a delay in the R wave, there is prolonged filling. Since the stroke volume of the ventricle is mostly a function of its initial volume, the cycle beginning with a PVC generally has a depressed LVEF while that beginning with a compensatory pause has a very high LVEF. The variation can be striking (Fig. 18-15). Occasional PVCs coupled with compensatory pauses can be excluded from the acquisition by "bad-beat" rejection software that detects R-to-R intervals that are outside a given tolerance (usually by more than 10% different from the predicted R-to-R interval). One, two, or more beats after a PVC can be excluded from the acquisition. This minimizes the impact of an occasional PVC on the average ventricular volume curve. The old technique to deal with irregular heart rates is referred to as "list-mode" acquisition. A disk drive is used as a fast tape recorder and the incoming data from a gated

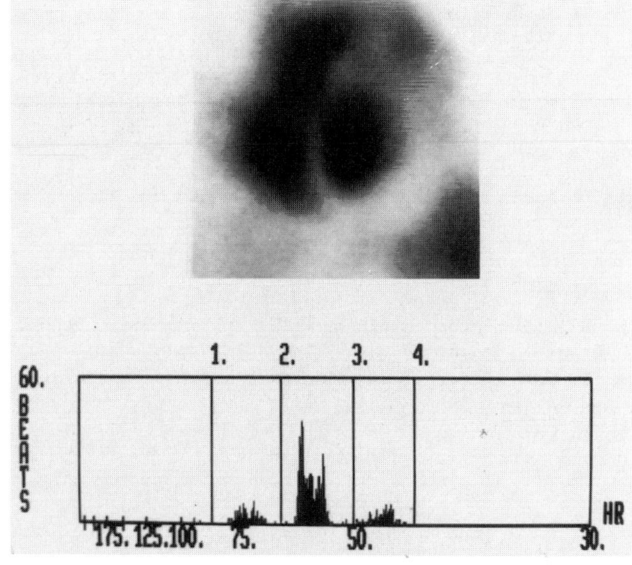

Fig. 18-15. Graphic display from a multi-window acquisition shows the histogram of instantaneous heart rates displayed with normal rhythm between lines 2 and 3. PVCs are collected at heart rates bounded by lines 1 and 2. Compensatory pauses at slow instantaneous rates are shown between lines 3 and 4. The time span of the R-to-R interval is greater from left to right on the horizontal axis so the heart rates marked are tachycardic (fast) on the left and bradycardic (slow) on the right.

study is recorded along with timing information and R-wave trigger signals. These data are acquired at the expense of a tremendous amount of disk space used and requires a long reformatting period. Criteria for accepting or rejecting data to be included in a series of frames are applied according to the tastes of the operator. Gated studies can be tediously dissected out of the most irregular data. This reformatting requires specification of selection criteria, such as the acceptable lengths of R-to-R interval and the number of cycles to be rejected after "bad beats." Acquisition computers with larger memories and faster processing times have replaced the list-mode acquisition. An improvement of the bad-beat–rejection technique calls for temporarily holding the incoming data in buffers and analyzing the length of the cycle to reject cycles that are longer or shorter than a specified range. Those cycles that are inside a specified "window" (ordinarily an average cycle length of ±10%) are added to the frames of a gated study. With large-memory acquisition units, multiple windows may be established to accept data from cycles of given lengths as separate gated studies. This strategy helps when a heart repeatedly changes rates. The variable ejection fractions from different rates are weighted by their respective prevalence to measure the heart's average LVEF. This technique is sometimes called the "on the fly" list mode (Fig. 18-16).

A special case of arrhythmia is bigeminy. Two different heart rates alternate regularly in this condition. Using two separate acquisition windows the LVEF for each half of the beats is calculated. Bearing in mind the principle that long cycles cause increased filling time, note that the higher LVEF occurs during the shorter cycle. The shorter cycle then has less time for filling, so the LVEF is lower during the longer cycle (Fig. 18-17). The worst case for gating a study occurs when the heart beat is irregularly irregular in length, such as in atrial fibrillation. The heart beating in this fashion usually has a depressed LVEF (Fig. 18-18).

A

1. 2. 3. 4. 5. 6.

60. BEATS

175. 125. 100. 75. 50. 30. HR

B

CYCLE LENGTH (HR)	NUMBER of CYCLES	EJECTION FRACTION %
55— 78	563	18
78— 94	785	30
94—117	1099	20
117—134	290	14
134—180	264	18

WEIGHTED E.F. = 21.5%

Fig. 18-16. A, Multiple window "on the fly list mode" acquisition. A dilated LV which switches between five different heart rates at rest is simultaneously acquired as five-gated studies. **B,** The cycle lengths accepted for inclusion in the five simultaneous studies, the number of R-to-R cycles collected, and the LVEF for each study is used to determine a weighted or average LVEF of 21.5 percent.

Continued.

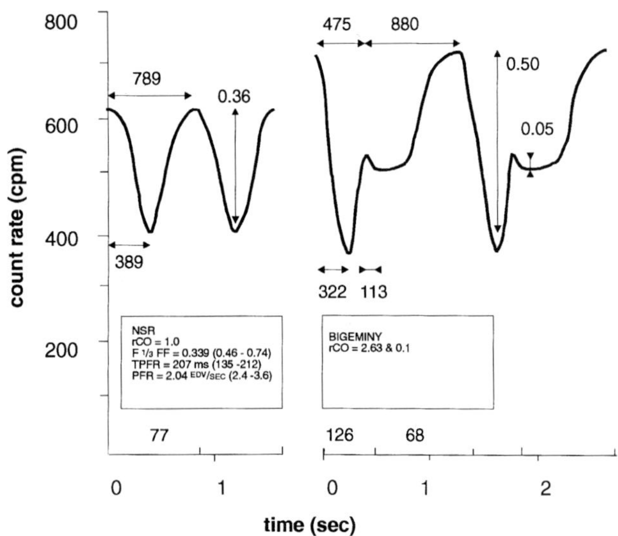

Fig. 18-17. Normal sinus rhythm and bigeminy. On the left is a time/volume curve for a patient with a low LVEF of 0.36 at a steady heart rate of 77 beats per minute. The cycles last 789 milliseconds of which 389 milliseconds are spent in systole. In the box the relative cardiac output is set to one for purposes of comparison with the subsequent study (see text under Exercise Equilibrium Gated Radionuclide Ventriculography for discussion of relative output.) Diastolic parameters are shown along with the normal ranges for the laboratory (see Fig. 18-22). When the patient spontaneously changed to a bigeminy rhythm he alternated between instantaneous heart rates of 128 and 68 beats per minute. The duration of the first cycle was 475 milliseconds with 322 milliseconds devoted to systole. After brief, incomplete diastolic filling another R wave triggers a minimal emptying for a 113 milliseconds systole followed by a very long diastole with a total cycle length of 880 milliseconds. The heart thus alternates between ejection fractions of 0.50 and 0.05 with relative cardiac outputs of 2.63 and 0.1 compared with the normal sinus rhythm study.

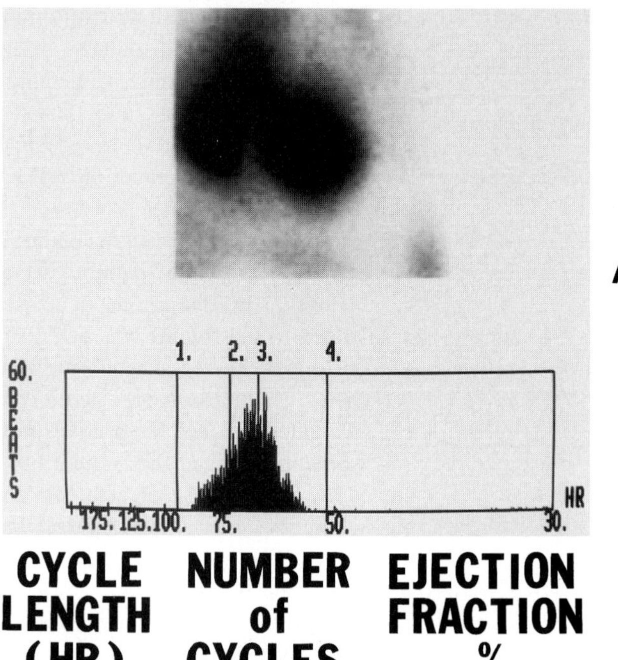

B

CYCLE LENGTH (HR)	NUMBER of CYCLES	EJECTION FRACTION %
50 – 60	852	24
60 – 75	847	20
75 – 90	379	17

WEIGHTED E.F. = 21.1%

Fig. 18-18. A, Atrial fibrillation. A three-window simultaneous acquisition has boundary lines 1 through 4 arbitrarily drawn on the heart rate histogram. **B,** In a manner similar to Fig. 18-16, *B*, a weighted LVEF is calculated. The haphazard rhythm of this heart makes random the amount of LV filling that occurs before each contraction. This is no way to run a ventricle!

Processing

Filtering

Once the study has been acquired, the next step involves the processing of the raw data before interpretation. A simple technique to improve the quality of the images in the acquired frames involves the use of filtered data. Temporal and spatial filtering are done to exclude part of the noise that is superimposed on the study. The intelligent selection of a filter is made easier if one knows the frequencies that are "cut off" the processed study. A filter can be conceived as small strings of coefficients that operate in the neighborhood of each pixel in the raw-data study to generate a filtered study (Fig. 18-19). Rapidly changing count rates in adjacent pixels in space or in the same pixel with time are suppressed while slower cycles are preserved in the output images. The effect is to make broad edges smoother and reduce the shimmering effect of noisy data during cine playback. If filters are used in which all the coefficients in the center pixel and its neighborhood add up to 1, the total counts in the output image will be the same as those in the raw data (nongain filtering). They will be more uniformly distributed, however. The exception to this effect comes when low-count data are filtered with integer arithmetic. Since the answers come out in fractions less than 1,

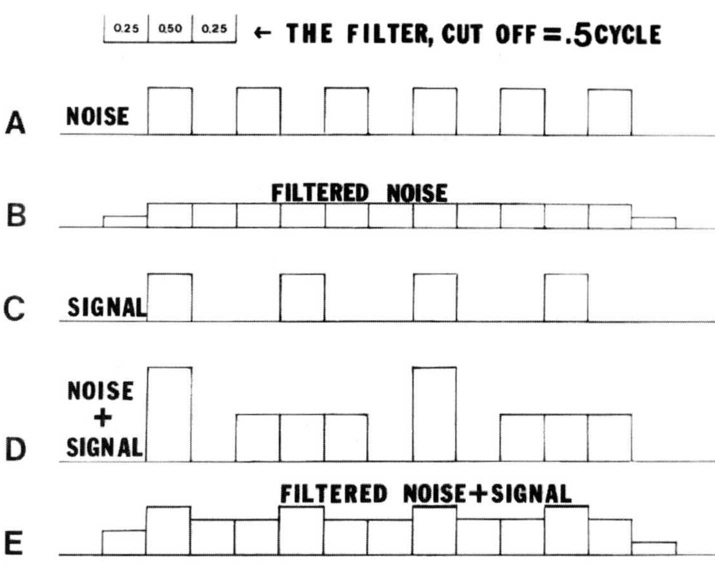

Fig. 18-19. Simple one-dimension filter. A simple filter kernel with coefficients of 0.25, 0.5, and 0.25 is diagrammed at the top of the figure. Noise is diagrammed in row A as a series of pixels that alternate between "on" and "off" or zero and one unit. This noise has a frequency of 0.5 cycles per pixel corresponding to a cycle of one per two pixels. The filter kernel can be conceived as a string of three coefficients that slide along row A one pixel at a time. At each pixel the three coefficients are multiplied by the value of the pixel underneath the coefficient. The sum of these three products is then placed in the pixel under the center of the kernel in an output string diagrammed as row B. Signal is diagrammed in row C as a pixel with the value of one separated by two blank pixels before the next pixel with signal of one. The signal has a frequency of 0.33 cycles per pixel of a cycle of one per three pixels. The signal has an amplitude of $1 - 0 = 1$. When noise from row A is added to the signal from row C the result is row D. The filter kernel is run across row D. The sum of the products of each coefficient and pixel value in row D is graphed in row E. Note that the signal of one "on" and two "off" pixels is preserved. The signal has an amplitude of $1 - 0.75 = 0.25$ units. The noise (0.5 cycle per pixel) has been cut off.

the errors as a result of truncation are relatively large and the output images have significant contour-map–style edges. This problem is best avoided by the acquisition of higher-count studies. Uniform multiplication of sparse raw data before integer filtering tends to prevent truncation losses during filtering but should not be used as a substitute for a good acquisition. Knowing what filter to select requires an understanding of frequency cut-off values. If the smallest object to be included in the image is 5 pixels wide, the limiting frequency desired would correspond to a cycle of 10 pixels (5 pixels with signal and 5 pixels without signal). With a filter that tended to smooth out data that had a cycle length less than 10 pixels, any signal smaller than 5 pixels could be excluded. The cut-off value would be a frequency of 0.1 cycles/pixel. The ultimate "noise" would be a cycle of 2 pixels (one "on" and one "off") with a frequency of 0.5 cycles/pixel. A typical frame from an equilibrium radionuclide ventriculogram is filtered with a spatial filter that has a cut-off frequency of 0.1 cycles/pixel. This is chosen to retain the interventricular septum as the smallest object that needs to be seen in the filtered version of the raw data. Selection of filter cut-off values for temporal filtering of equilibrium-radionuclide ventriculograms depends on the number of frames and the detail to be represented on the average ventricular volume curve. If a 20-frame study is to be processed for measurement of LVEF, the cycle length is 20 frames and a cut-off frequency of 0.05 cycles/pixel is established. To preserve diastolic data in the average volume curve, a higher cut-off frequency is required because the duration of diastolic events (isovolumic relaxation, fast filling, slow filling, atrial kick) may be only a few frames long. For example, in a 32-frame study, the isovolumic relaxation period is about two frames long. An appropriate noise cut-off would correspond to cycle of two frames "on" and two frames "off" at a frequency of 0.25 cycles/pixel. A lower cut-off frequency would tend to smooth out this short event on the average volume curve.

Systolic function parameters

Reliable outlining of the edges of the LV blood pool in each frame is critical to the calculation of the LVEF. This number is the most sought-after piece of information in the entire study and deserves some explanation. One method is to manually draw edges around the largest (end-diastolic) and the smallest (end-systolic) LV images. This method allows for too much observer bias and is not particularly accurate. A more precise method takes a percentage of the maximum counts per pixel in the center of the image and uses that percentage to establish the edges. Radial profiles drawn outward from the center of the blood pool are marked when they reach a preset threshold percentage. About 50% of peak counts might be a reasonable place to declare the LV edge. This or any

Continued.

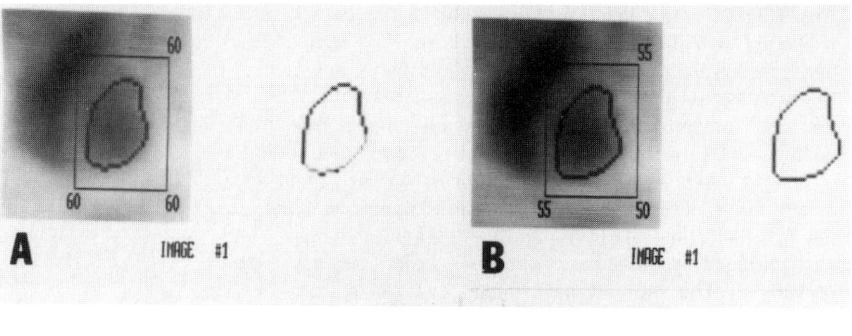

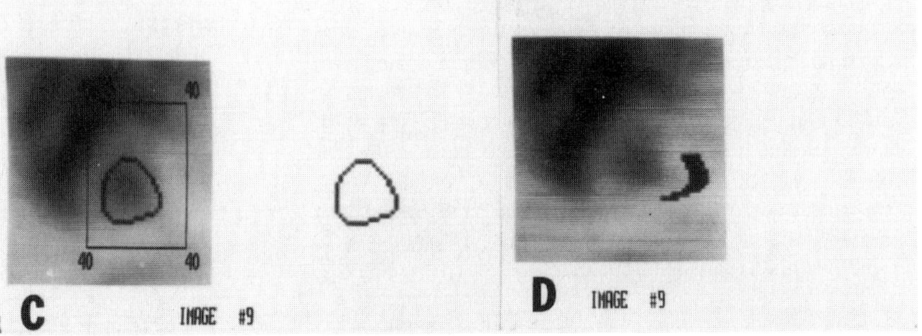

Fig. 18-20. Radial search for second derivative edges. The top two images are end-diastole. The bottom two are end-systole. Starting from a center of the box the computer searches outward along 60 radial lines **(A).** The corners of the box show percentages of the LV center pixel that will halt the search for the edge in each quadrant of the box. Each is started at 60 percent. If a second derivative edge point is found along a radial line before the blood pool drops to 60 percent, a dark point is placed over that pixel. Light colored pixels indicate that the algorithm searching each radial reached the value of 60 percent and stopped searching at that point. The edge in the bottom left and bottom right quadrants is too tight around the blood pool. The search criteria are dropped to 55 percent in the two upper and left lower quadrants and 50 percent in the lower right quadrant **(B).** Second derivative points already found do not change. New second derivative points are found in the bottom two quadrants. The edges in these two quadrants are extended and marked with dark pixels. Similar processing is conducted in every frame of the study including end systole **(C).** That same frame is used to establish a region of interest for background measurement **(D).**

other number is an arbitrary choice. An elegant and reproducible method for edge detection is that done with the second derivative (inflection point) edges placed along the radial profiles drawn out from the center of the blood pool. The beauty of this technique is that it is highly reproducible. Multiple observers will operate such second-derivative–seeking programs and find exactly the same edges. With this method the LVEF measurement gains precision (Fig. 18-20, *A-D*).

Other proprietary software packages use Fourier transform data and other tricks to achieve precision in the calculation of the ejection fraction. Regardless of how the edges are chosen, the best calculations will occur when the basic acquisition of data is done carefully with true "best septal" projections. Significant overlap of chambers because of poor positioning cannot be corrected by any edge-selection technique. Since the number of counts in the LV at end-systole and end-diastole must be corrected for the background activity, a reasonable estimate of that background must be established. This could again be done manually but is subject to individual bias. Using an area displaced slightly to the anatomic left of the end-systolic blood pool to estimate the background is a good first approximation. This area really was behind the blood pool of the end-diastolic frame in most normal studies. Care must be taken to monitor automatic background region-selection routines to see that they do not drape the background region over a tortuous aorta or other large, nonrepresentative blood pool such as the spleen. In these cases a manual selection of a typical background region is more accurate. With the end-diastolic and end-systolic counts corrected by the average background, the difference divided by the end-diastolic counts (again corrected by average background) gives the global ejection fraction. This formula is as follows:

$$\text{LVEF} = \frac{(\text{LVED counts} - \text{Background counts}) - (\text{LVES counts} - \text{Background counts})}{(\text{LVED counts} - \text{Background counts})}$$

In a well-positioned best septal LAO acquisition of a normal heart, most programs will grab the edges of the left ventricle with ease. When there is a slightly rotated ventricle or an unavoidable overlap with another chamber, the study can still be salvaged by intelligent manual correction of obviously errant segments of the edges. If a volume curve is determined region by region for the entire cycle, the first derivative of that curve will yield information about the rates of emptying and filling. Peak rates and average rates are usually measured in units of end-diastolic volumes per second (negative or positive). The systolic average dV/dt is directly proportional to the dP/dt (change in pressure with respect to change in time), which is measured by cardiac catheterization. It is a mea-

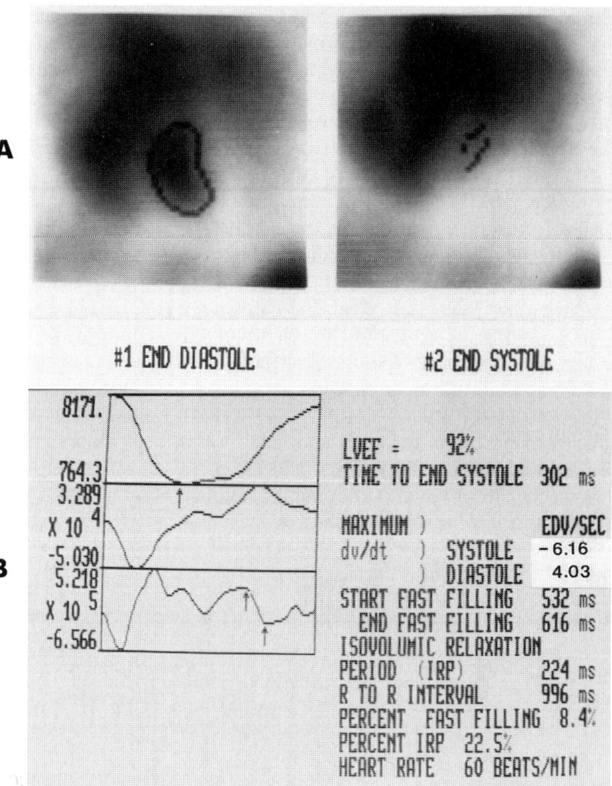

Fig. 18-21. A, Hypertrophic cardiomyopathy. A very high temporal resolution study (70 frames per R-to-R interval) in a patient with concentric hypertrophy of the LV. Regions of interest are superimposed on the images. The blood pool almost disappears in the end-systole frame. **B,** The average volume curve is shown at the top with end systole marked at 302 milliseconds by an arrow. The middle curve is a first derivative curve. The bottom is the second derivative curve that is marked at the beginning and ending of fast filling by a pair of arrows. The time between end systole and the beginning of fast filling is the isovolumic relaxation period (IRP) of 224 milliseconds. This delays myocardial perfusion that occurs in diastole only after fast filling begins and the tension in the LV wall drops below arterial pressure. If this patient exercises, the time for diastole decreases. With too much myocardium to feed and very little diastole, ischemia occurs. Ischemia and arrhythmias in hypertrophic cardiomyopathy may lead to sudden death in a young person with normal coronary arteries.

sure of the velocity and force with which the blood is ejected from the ventricle. The average rate of ejection usually exceeds 1.4 end-diastolic volumes per second (EDV/s) in a normal resting patient. This normal value, as well as all the normal rate values, is best determined in a normal population in each nuclear medicine laboratory with the equipment at hand. Studies done with a minimum number of frames suffer from poor temporal resolution. Measuring rates of emptying and filling requires standardized acquisition, filtering, and processing.

Diastolic function parameters

- ***Isovolumic relaxation period***

Large numbers of frames with time intervals as small as 10 milliseconds are possible with some systems. This allows precise measurement of events such as the isovolumic relaxation period (IRP), which is the interval between end-systole and the beginning of fast filling and normally lasts about 50 ms. In patients with hypertrophic cardiomyopathy, the IRP exceeds 90 ms and may be closer to 200 ms as the heavy wall stays contracted before the beginning of fast filling. The beginning and end of fast filling can be best found by examining the second derivative of the volume curve for points of inflection that mark these points in a reliable manner (Fig. 18-21, *A* and *B*).

- ***Time to peak filling, peak filling rate, and first third filling fraction***

Another measurement that can be done to examine diastolic function is the time between end-systole and peak filling (TPFR), which can be accurately performed on studies with a smaller number of frames (such as 32 per cycle). Normal values of TPFR are about 160 milliseconds and incorporate all of IRP and part of fast filling. TPFR lengthening can be the result of a decrease in compliance of the LV wall. The peak filling rate (PFR) is about 3 EDV/s in a normal patient. Lower PFR is a result of decreased compliance of the LV wall. The amount of ventricular filling during the first third of diastole (the first third filling fraction or F1/3FF) is about 50% to 60% in a normal patient. These are measures of ventricular compliance during filling and can be used to detect early LV dysfunction in dilated cardiomyopathies before systolic parameters such as LVEF change. If there is poor systolic performance these numbers will be abnormal as well (Fig. 18-22).

Continued.

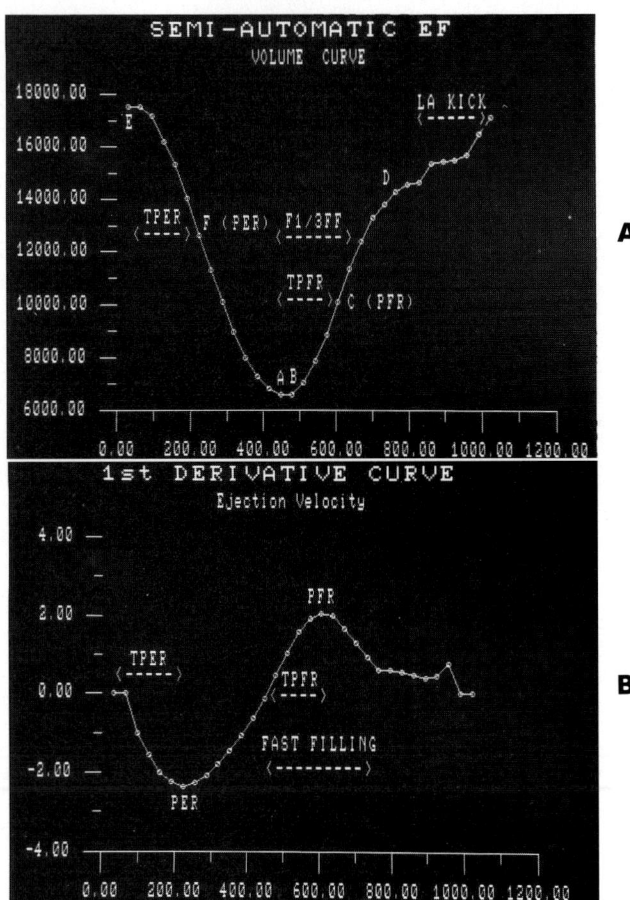

Fig. 18-22. **A**, Diastolic parameters from a 32-frame average volume curve. Points on a volume curve start with end systole (A) and the beginning of fast filling (B). The difference between (A) and (B) is the isovolumic relaxation period. The point (C) is the peak rate of filling (PFR). The distance from (A) to (C) is the time to peak filling (TPFR). Diastole is 600 milliseconds long. The first 200 milliseconds of diastole marks the first third filling fraction (F1/3FF). It returns more than one half of the volume lost during systole. Fast filling ends at (D). The end of the diastolic cycle comes when the LA contracts (LA kick). End diastole (E) commences another cycle of contraction which reaches its peak filling rate (PFR) at F. The time between (E) and (F) is the time to peak filling (TPFR). **B,** The first derivative curve of the average volume curve. Note the first half of the curve is negative as volume is decreasing with respect to time. At end-systole the curve is back to zero and becomes positive during filling. This curve corresponds point for point with that in **A** and shows graphically the PFR, TPFR, TPER, PER and the period of fast filling. The systolic part of the curve is simpler than the diastolic which has a second minor peak during the LA kick.

Regional ejection fractions

Regional–wall-motion analysis can be quantitated with regional–ejection-fraction programs. These programs divide the ventricular blood pool into multiple wedges and then calculate the ejection fraction in each wedge. Presumably the magnitude of the regional ejection fraction reports the vigor of the wall sections in each region. Unfortunately the regions are highly variable in geometry; significantly different ejection fractions can be arranged by moving the center point of the wedges. These programs are also adversely affected by physical translation (side-to-side movement) of the LV during the cycle. An image formed by overlaying the end-systolic and end-diastolic regions around the blood pool performs much the same function as do the multisegment programs. Wall-motion abnormalities in the anterior and posterior/inferior walls can be completely *en face* in the best septal view and can go completely undetected in the regional analysis. Despite the problems, regional assessments of wall motion are widely reported and scored in an attempt to quantify the contractility of the myocardium.

Ejection fraction, stroke volume, and paradox images

A parametric image of the LV in the best septal LAO view that some authors prefer is the ejection-fraction image. Mapping each pixel's ejection fraction is done by applying the LVEF formula (given above) for each pixel instead of for the whole ventricle. In a stroke-volume image, the ventricular end-systolic frame is subtracted from the ventricular end-diastolic frame. Any negative pixels in the resulting image are set to zero so the display only shows pixels that decreased in volume during ventricular systole. The paradox image is calculated by subtracting the ventricular end-diastole frame from the ventricular end-systole frame. Again, any negative pixels in the output image are set to zero. The paradox image could be thought of as an atrial–stroke-volume image. It helps detect areas of ventricular dyskinesia in which counts in a pixel increase while the rest of the ventricle is emptying (Fig. 18-23).

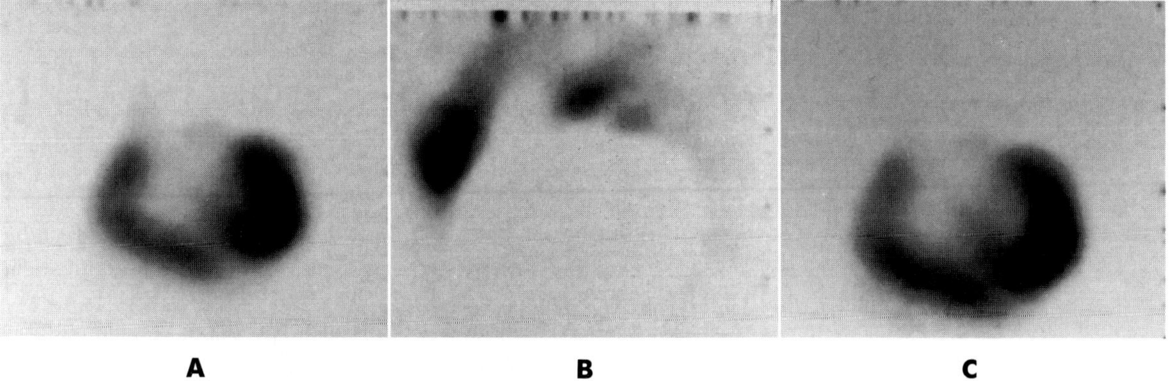

Fig. 18-23. Normal stroke volume, paradox, and ejection fraction images. The stroke volume image (**A**) is end-diastole minus end-systole. Only those pixels with a positive value are displayed. The paradox image (**B**) image is ventricular end-systole minus end-diastole. Only those pixels with a positive value are displayed so that the atria appear in this normal subject. The ejection fraction image (**C**) bears a strong resemblance to the stroke volume image though it is calculated differently. It is really a stroke volume image divided by the end-diastolic image.

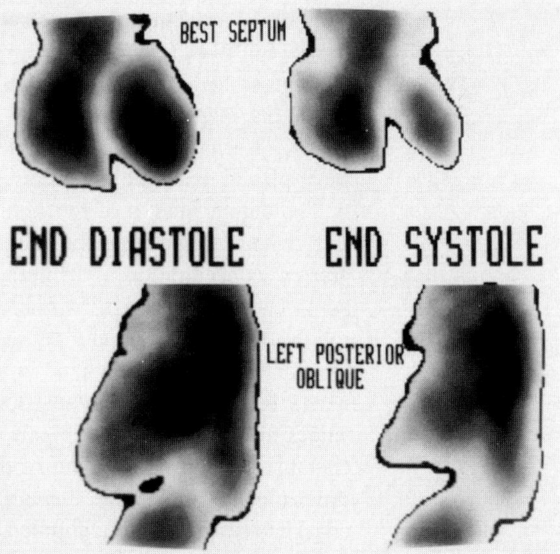

Fig. 18-24. Gray scale representation of the MIKE black/yellow/blue edge enhancement table for end-diastolic and end-systolic frames from a LAO best septal and LPO study. There is no background, a sharp border, and a blood pool with darker shades of gray according to volume.

Specialized display tables for wall motion

A tool for the interpretation of wall motion that is very simple but powerful is the use of a special color-translation table to enhance the edge of the blood pool. For instance, the blood pool can be displayed in a blue scale that is linear from about 30% to 100% of the maximum count per pixel with a bright yellow edge at 30% of the maximum pixel and *no* display color (black) from zero to 30%. This sort of edge table, when used with filtered data, will put a bright-yellow edge at the interface between blood and heart wall. Manipulating the display levels during cine replay is necessary to move the yellow edge to the outer margin of the LV blood pool. The yellow edge contrasts optimally with the black background and the blue blood pool. The linear blue scale preserves the impression of volume within the ventricle as would a grey-scale display. The use of multicolored translation tables can be distracting as the colors shimmer and dance during replay and can be counterproductive. Edge-enhancement grey scales can also be created to emphasize the wall motion (Fig. 18-24). This kind of cine display assists the observer of wall motion who must categorize each area of LV wall movement as normal (converging vigorously on the center of the blood pool during systole), hypokinetic (not moving enough), akinetic (not moving at all), and dyskinetic (moving the wrong way).

Continued.

First harmonic Fourier phase and amplitude analysis

The statistics about the function of the left ventricle can be further developed with the use of Fourier phase and amplitude analysis. The mathematics that create the two characteristic images are not as formidable as one might expect. Each pixel in a frame in the study is followed in time by one in the same location. A time-activity curve could be constructed for each temporal chain of pixels that would show the fluctuation in counts during the cycle for that location. The pixels inside the normal ventricle would have a curve that looked like the average volume curve for the whole chamber. Those pixels covering the atria would show an opposing curve. For a 64 × 64 study, 4096 curves could be generated using a lot of plotting paper but providing little helpful information. In all four pumping chambers, each pixel's time-activity curve looks a bit like a jagged sine or cosine curve. Three numbers specify any given cosine wave. A constant defines its average position in the Y dimension. The amplitude constant of the curve describes the distance between peak and trough. A third constant, the phase shift, defines the displacement of the peak of the curve with respect to $X = 0$, which is conventionally placed at end-diastole. This shift is calculated in angular degrees. The best possible single-cosine wave fit to each of the individual time-activity curves can be established as a function of these three constants. A map of the values for each pixel's amplitude constants represents the degree of count-rate changes during the cycle. A map of the phase angles shows when the peak of the wave occurs with respect to end-diastole. The cycle is not a perfect cosine wave, and more time is spent in diastole than in systole. The fitted first harmonic cosine approximation to the ventricular pixel will frequently have its peak shifted to the left of the end-diastolic frame. For display purposes, the map of phase-shift information may be chosen to run from minus 90 degrees to plus 270 degrees to avoid splitting the information regarding the ventricles. To read the output maps, a color display with many colors is helpful. A "rainbow" map with red, orange, yellow, green, blue, indigo, violet, and black in sequence allows many more subtle time events to be displayed than can be perceived with a gray scale (Fig. 18-25, *A* and *B*).

The output images of the Fourier programs thus encode information about "how much motion" and "when motion occurred" for amplitude and phase images, respectively. In a normal study the greatest concentration of "amplitude" is in the left ventricle with the right ventricle and the atria next. The phase images normally show nearly simultaneous timing information for the ventricles, followed 180 degrees later by a cluster of atrial-timing information. This is a powerful statistical tool for those who understand how to read it. The presence or absence of a wall-motion abnormality would be incorrectly diagnosed without the assistance of Fourier images. Falsely high amplitude values may be assigned to pixels that are changing their count rate only by virtue of the blood-filled chamber sliding into and out of the pixel's view. It is wise not to depend on the Fourier images to the exclusion of the cine display. Quantitation of coordination of left ventricular contraction (synergy) can be done with a simple statistical analysis of the histogram that corresponds to the pixels of the LV-phase image. Phase and amplitude images are calculated within a region of interest around the left ventricle. The histogram of these LV pixels displays the number of pixels with a given phase shift (in degrees) from the R wave. The spread of this curve is measured as a standard deviation. Large values of the standard deviation of the left ventricular phase angle correspond to uncoordinated contractions (Fig. 18-26).

Minimum/maximum images

Other parametric or statistical images can be created with the time-activity curves associated with each pixel from a gated blood-pool study. Minimum/maximum-rate images can be derived to map the relative time at which each pixel reaches its minimum and maximum counts. The relative amplitude of these minimum and maximum counts can also be mapped. Minimum/maximum-rate images can also be created to map the time to maximum-emptying rate and the time to maximum-filling rate. This is done by examining a first-derivative curve for each pixel. An amplitude map is also created for each of the rate maps. These maps include pixel-by-pixel representations of the important diastolic parameters TPFR (time to peak filling) and PFR (peak rate of filling). The most helpful information is contained in the emptying/filling images. These appear to be superficially similar to the Fourier phase/amplitude maps and should also be displayed for interpretation in a color scale with many gradations of color. The information plotted will help detect and confirm areas of wall-motion abnormality that have late times to maximum-emptying rate and low rates of emptying (seen on the corresponding amplitude map). Maximum/minimum-acceleration maps for each pixel

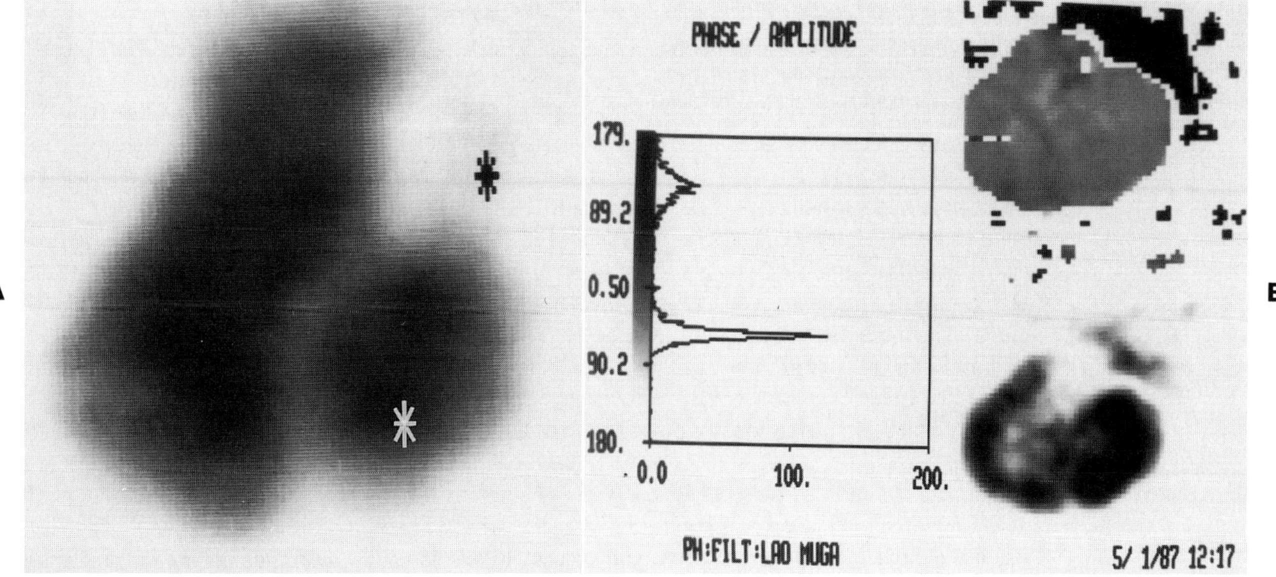

Fig. 18-25. A, Normal Fourier phase and amplitude analysis. A single LV pixel *(white asterisk)* and LA pixel *(black asterisk)* are marked over a best septal LAO study. **B,** The amplitude values plotted for each pixel *(lower right)* show the greatest values in the LV and RV. The display of phase angle values for each pixel *(upper right)* is complimented by a vertical histogram at left that plots the number of pixels with a given value on a gray scale which begins with white at 180 degrees. Note that most of the LV and RV pixels are clustered in the gray area between −90 and below 0. The tight clustering on the histogram and uniform color of the ventricles in the phase image indicate a well coordinated contraction. Later in the cycle there is a cluster of darker atrial pixels graphed between +90 and 180 degrees.

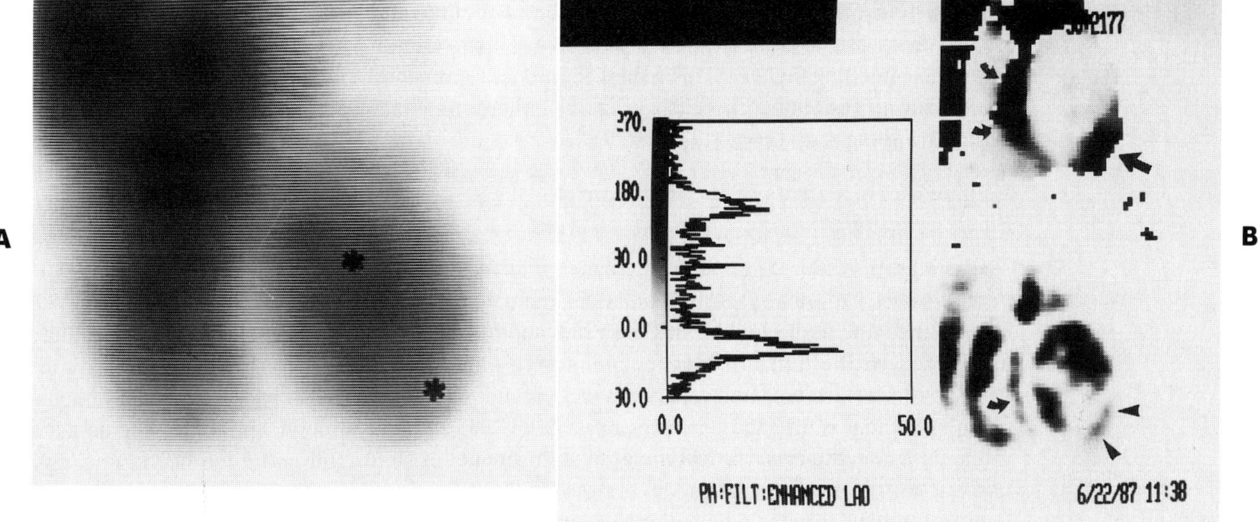

Fig. 18-26. A, Aneurysm of the LV shown by Fourier phase and amplitude analysis. The dilated LV has two individual pixels *(asterisks)*. The apex *(lower asterisk)* is dyskinetic after an extensive myocardial infarction as it moves outward as the rest of the ventricle contracts. **B,** The amplitude image *(lower right)* shows an apical island of amplitude that is separated from the rest of the LV by a diagonal line of pixels *(arrowheads)* with no amplitude. The matching phase image *(upper right)* shows dark pixels at the apex *(arrow)* that have the same phase angle shift as the atrial pixels. (In addition there is an artifactual dark band of pixels along the septum in the amplitude and phase image *[curved arrows]* that corresponds to left-to-right translation or rocking of the ventricles from side to side during contraction.) The histogram curve shows pixels with a wide variety of phase angle values.

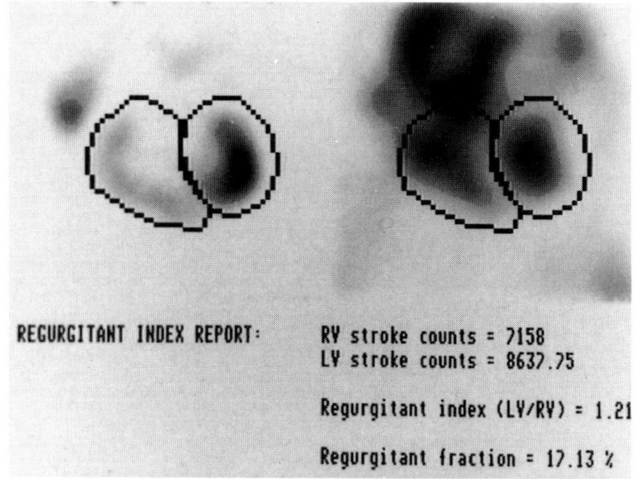

Fig. 18-27. Regurgitant Index. Regions of interest around the ventricles on a Fourier amplitude image *(left)* are used to generate the relative stroke volumes of each ventricle. This is expressed as either a regurgitant index or a regurgitant fraction. The blood pool image *(right)* shows the same regions.

can be calculated from second-derivative curves. These also have amplitude maps. For practical purposes, however, the minimum/maximum rate and acceleration maps have no particular advantage over Fourier amplitude and phase images.

Regurgitation

Quantification of aortic or mitral regurgitation requires estimation of the stroke volume (SV) for both ventricles. Ratio of LVSV to RVSV is theoretically 1 to 1. Except when there is dyskinesia, the Fourier-amplitude images encode numbers for each pixel that are proportional to its SV. By adding up all the values in regions of interest drawn around the LV and RV on an amplitude image made from a best septal LAO acquisition, this ratio can be calculated. The LVSV/RVSV ratio is normally a bit higher than 1. There is usually some overlap of the RA and RV, which causes some RV pixels to have a reduced apparent amplitude because of RA counterpulsations. To prevent this problem, four-chamber acquisitions (discussed above) have been used to help separate RA and RV. Regurgitation can also be expressed as a regurgitant fraction. A LVSV/RVSV = 2 would have a regurgitant fraction = 50%. This means that twice as much blood was ejected from the LV as from the RV during systole but that 50% of it was either going backward into the LA or regurgitating into the LV from the aortic root (Fig. 18-27).

Volume measurements of the left ventricle

Blood sample/attenuation correction methods

There are a variety of ways to calculate the left ventricular end-diastolic volume (LVEDV); however, none is particularly correct or better than the other in terms of accuracy. If the LVEDV is known, it can be multiplied by the heart rate and the ejection fraction to obtain cardiac output (CO), usually reported in terms of liters per minute (L/min). This may be further normalized by dividing output body surface area and reported a cardiac index (L/min/m^2). This absolute measurement of the pump's function is affected by many physiologic and pathophysiologic variables. The demand for a given cardiac output may be answered by adjustments in heart rate, end-diastolic volume, and ejection fraction. It is preferable to know all three. The simplest way to get an estimate of the LVEDV is to use a standard-size acquisition for every study and/or use a ruler in the acquisition. To take advantage of the relationship between LV count rate and volume, the following equation must be solved:

$$\text{LV volume} = \frac{(\text{Blood-sample volume}) \times (\text{LV count rate})}{(\text{Blood-sample count rate})}$$

The tricky part is the calculation of LV count rate. The formula for end-diastolic count rate is:

$$\text{LV count rate} = \frac{(\text{LV counts in the end-diastolic frame}) - (\text{Background})}{(\text{No. of cycles}) \times (\text{Time/frame}) \times [e^{-(\text{mu} \times \text{Dcm})}]}$$

Note that the counts observed in the frame are summed from many cycles. The time per frame is easily calculated from the heart rate and the number of frames per cycle, or it can be found with the acquisition data recorded by most computer systems. The value for "mu" (which has units of cm^{-1}) is discussed below as is the calculation of "D" (depth to the center of the ventricle in centimeters). The volume of an aliquot of the patient's radioactive blood can be accurately determined in cubic centimeters from the syringe in which it is drawn. It is placed in a shallow dish in front of the same camera and collimator used for the acquisition. (A thin layer is used to eliminate self attenuation in the blood.) Count rate per milliliter of blood is measured in the same matrix size as is the gated study. A timed acquisition of 5 to 10 min in a single static frame is sufficient. If the blood is drawn and counted immediately at the end of the gated study, loss of count rate from radioactive decay will be negligible. If there is a significant delay between the gated study and the measurement of aliquot count rate, correction for radioactive decay is necessary. Apparent counts-per-time in the LV end-diastolic frame are derived from the end-diastolic (usually the first) frame in the gated study. Attenuation in the chest wall requires measurement of the distance "D" from the surface of the chest wall to the center of the LV. This can be done directly by measuring in the LPO view (Fig. 18-28, *A* to *D*). An alternative method of measuring the depth to the center of the LV relies on measuring the distance between the apparent center of the blood pool in the best septal LAO projection and in the anterior projection. This distance and the angle of the best septal LAO are two elements of a right triangle. Solving this triangle for "D" is simple (Fig. 18-29). Both techniques rely on accurate location of the center points in the LV and on the chest wall and thus share an opportunity for error. A linear soft-tissue attenuation coefficient, or "mu", of 0.153 is assumed by some investigators. This method is relatively simple. Unfortunately, 0.153 is usually an overestimate of "mu" because there is some air-containing lung between the chest wall and center of the LV. On the average, a value of 0.12 may be more accurate. The correction for attenuation then raises the base of natural logarithm "e" to the negative of the product of "mu" and "D". The error induced by assumptions of "mu" and "D" can be great because of the exponential function. Relatively difficult are techniques that measure the integrated transit of the first-pass bolus of injected activity through the LV to establish the actual value of "mu" for each patient. Another technique uses an LAO image of a radioactive source in a tube in the esophagus to estimate the individual "mu". The distance from esophagus to chest wall is about double that from the LV center to the chest wall. Attenuation of the esophageal source can be measured directly by comparison of an LAO image of the source with a nonattenuated image of the source in air. Complex programs for CT scanners have also approximated this value. These techniques are outside the capabilities of most nuclear medicine clinics.

SPECT methods

An adaptation of single-photon computed tomography (SPECT) has been tomography of the heart blood pool to measure LVEDV. The acquisition can be gated so that only data at end-diastole is accepted. The subsequently reconstructed transaxial slices represent only that stage of the heart cycle. Regions of interest around the LV blood pool are used to generate the area of each slice. The pixel size and slice thickness must be calibrated to determine the volume in each slice. Adding all slice volumes together allows calculation of the LVEDV with no attenuation-correction problems. To make this technique simpler, the study can be done without gating the acquisition. Since the blood pool expands at end-diastole to its maximum dimensions, regions of interest at the outside of the blood pool correspond to the end-diastolic volume (Fig. 18-30).

Count-based ratio method

A more recent method describes a "count-based ratio" technique that depends on the ratio of the maximum pixel activity in the ventricle to the total counts in the ventricle. The mathematics that back this method are intriguing. They assume that LV counts lost to attenuation will be balanced by those added from the background. They also assume that the LV is a sphere with no self-attenuation. The center of the LV should be the pixel with the greatest activity. Accurate calibration of pixel size in the matrix used is necessary. The mathematics of this method are simple. The formula is as follows:

$$\text{LVEDV} = 1.38 \times M^3 \times R^{3/2}$$

where M is the dimensions of a pixel in millimeters and R is the ratio of the total to the maximum pixel counts. This does not require measuring "mu", "D", or the count rate of a blood sample (Fig. 18-31). The standard error of all these methods of LV-volume determination (measured against the

Continued.

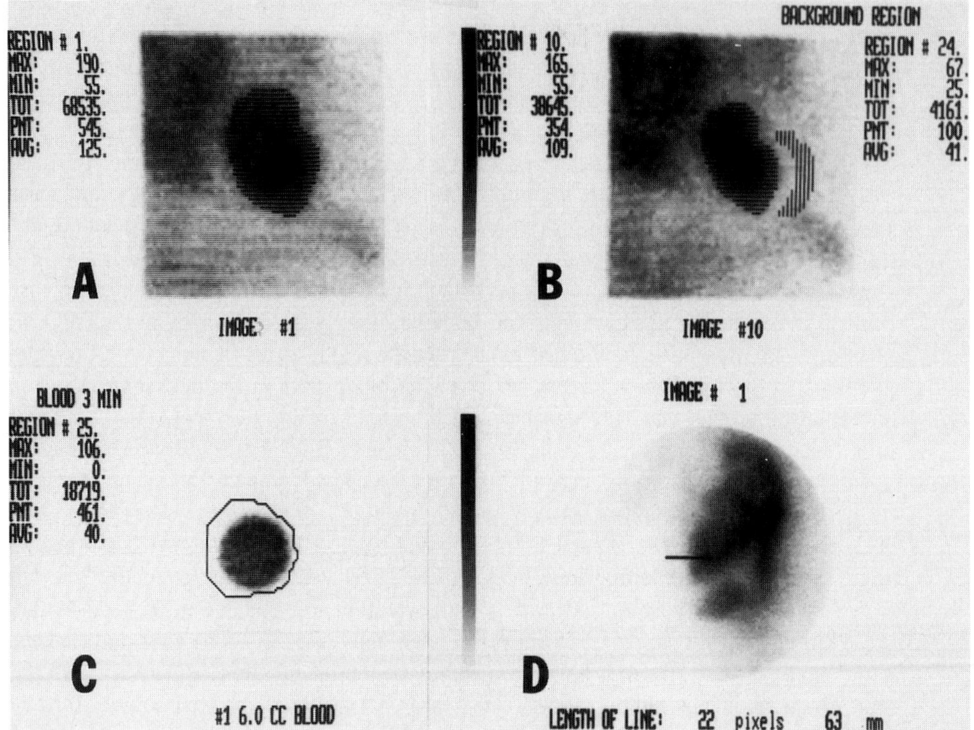

Fig. 18-28. Data collection for cardiac output. The end diastolic raw counts are totaled at 68535 from a region around the LV **(A).** Correction for background is 545 (the number of LV pixels) times 41 (the average background per pixel). The heart rate is 65. The number of frames in the acquisition is 23. The time per frame is 0.040 seconds. The number of cardiac cycles collected in the acquisition is 125. The blood sample of 6 cubic centimeters in a shallow dish **(C)** yields 18719 counts per three minutes or 17.33 counts/sec/cc. In the LPO view the depth from the anterior body wall to the center of the ventricle is 22 pixels or 6.3 cm in this calibrated acquisition **(D).** Correction for attenuation with an assumed "mu" of 0.153 per centimeter raises the base of the natural logarithm to the power $-(0.153 \times 6.3)$. The observed count rate of the LV is:

$$\frac{68535 - (41 \times 545)}{(0.40) \times (125) \times [e^{-(0.153 \times 6.3)}]} = 2422/\text{sec}$$

Multiplying the count rate of an unknown volume by the reciprocal of the known volume's count rate yields the LVEDV:

$$\frac{2422}{\text{sec}} \times \frac{1 \text{ cc}}{17.33/\text{sec}} = 140 \text{ cc LVEDV}$$

The ejection fraction is:

$$\frac{[68535 - (545 \times 41)] - [38645 - (354 \times 41)]}{[68535 - (545 \times 41)]} = 0.48$$

The cardiac output is:

$$1\text{L}/1000\text{cc} \times 140 \text{ cc/beat} \times 65 \text{ beats/min} \times 0.48 = 4.37 \text{ L/min}$$

The patient's body surface area is 1.5 m^2 so the cardiac index is:

$$(4.37 \text{ L/min})/1.5\text{m}^2 = 2.9 \text{ L/min/m}^2$$

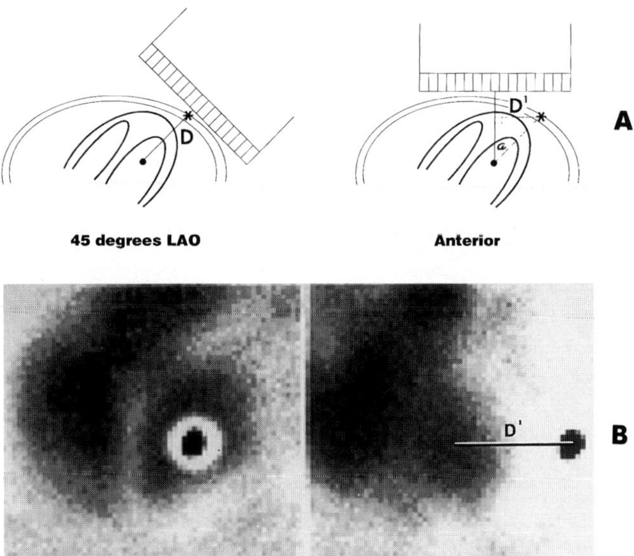

Fig. 18-29. Right triangle solution for measuring the depth to the center of the LV. Camera placement is diagrammed **(A)** and corresponding images shown **(B).** A right triangle is created by placing a radioactive marker on the chest wall over the center of the LV in the best septal LAO projection *(left)*. The camera is rotated camera back to the straight anterior projection *(right)*. An image taken in the anterior projection is used to measure the distance from the marker to the center of the LV. This distance ("D′") and the angle *(a)* of the best septal view is used to calculate the depth to the center of the LV "D" for attenuation correction:

$$D = D'/\sin(a)$$

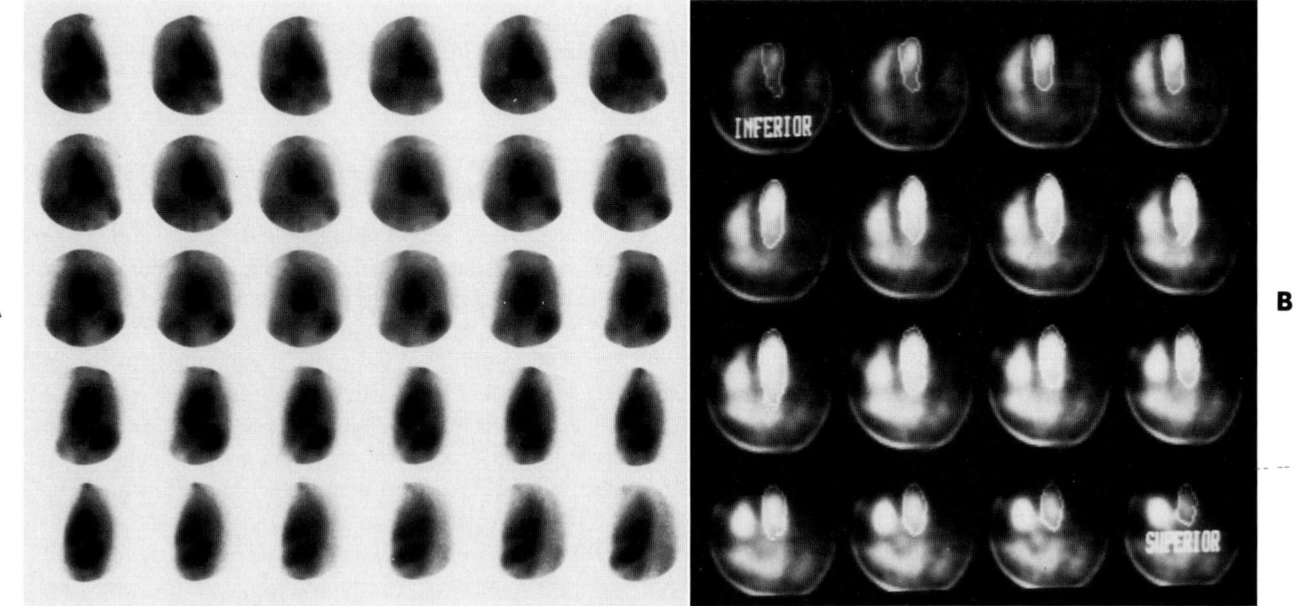

Fig. 18-30. LVEDV measurement by SPECT. An ungated SPECT acquisition of thirty frames spaced six degrees apart over 180 degrees from RAO to LPO **(A)** is used to create trans-axial slices **(B)** of the LV blood pool. The pixels (which are really three dimensional volume elements known as "voxels") in each region of interest around the LV in each slice are added up to measure the volume.

Continued.

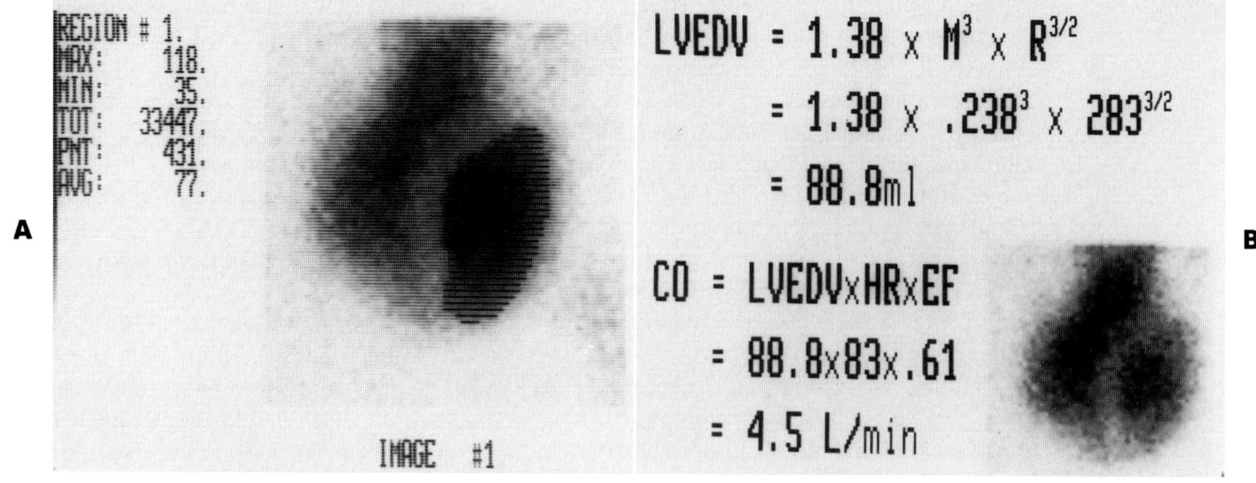

Fig. 18-31. A, Count based ratio method of LV volume measurement. The region of interest from an end-diastolic frame has a total of 33447 counts with a maximum pixel of 118. **B,** The total/maximum count ratio (R) is 283. The calibration of pixel size (M) is 0.238 millimeters per pixel. The value 1.38 is a constant. The LVEDV measured at 88.8 ml is multiplied by the heart rate of 83 and the LVEF of 0.61 to obtain a cardiac output (CO) of 4.5 L/min.

questionable standard of contrast angiography) is about the same. If there are a dozen methods to estimate a value in nuclear medicine, not one of them is clearly the best. If one were best, only one method would exist! Nevertheless, there is value in calculating LVEDV as part of the resting gated ventriculogram. With LVEDV the calculation of cardiac output is easy:

$$\text{Cardiac Output (L/min)} = \text{LVEDV(L)} \times \text{Heart Rate (min}^{-1}) \times \text{LVEF}$$

The perceptive reader has realized by now that all the LVEDV methods above could be adapted to calculate LV end-systolic volume (LVESV). The more perceptive reader realizes that the complement of the LVEF allows calculation of LVESV as follows:

$$\text{LVSV} = \text{LVEDV} \times (1 - \text{LVEF})$$

The LV stroke volume (LVSV) is simply as follows:

$$\text{LVSV} = \text{LVEDV} \times \text{LVEF}$$

Exercise equilibrium-gated–radionuclide ventriculography

An adaptation of the radionuclide ventriculogram to study the function of the LV during exercise can be accomplished with the addition of a bicycle ergometer in either supine or a semi-erect, seated posture. The two biggest technical problems with exercise studies are limited exercise tolerance and patient motion relative to the camera face. Dosages of 30 mCi (1110 MBq) of ^{99m}Tc-labeled red cells; a high-sensitivity collimator; and 16-frame, 3-minute acquisitions combine to get a useful data at each level of exercise. Starting with rest, successive levels of exercise are begun every 3½ minutes. After a 30-second equilibration period, a 3-minute gated study is acquired. Carefully graded levels in exercise (adding 25 watts of resistance per level), with an attending physician monitoring patient symptoms, electrocardiogram, pulse, and pressure, are required to do the procedure safely. In some laboratories a final study is done during the immediate postexercise period as the patient "cools off." Imaging filtering and processing for LVEF is accomplished at each stage.

There are lots of variations in techniques using the exercise equilibrium-gated–radionuclide ventriculography. In some laboratories the study is limited to a rest–and–peak-exercise acquisition. Peak-exercise effort may produce excessive body motion as the patient strains against restraining straps and the bicycle pedals. Electrical artifact from muscle contraction may hamper the ECG gating at the same time. The criteria for a normal rest/maximum-exercise study include a minimum increase in ejection fraction of 5 percentage points with normal wall motion. The LVEDV should not appear to increase significantly during exercise because the normal response is to decrease end-systolic volume to gain a higher stroke volume. (The heart rate should also rise.) As should be obvious, the exercise study cannot really be normal if it is not normal to begin with at rest. Exercise-gated studies were tried for years as the method for detecting ischemic myocardium in the face of atherosclerotic coronary artery disease (CAD). Although the study is fairly sensitive for CAD, the exercise myocardial-perfusion scans with thallium-201 or the newer ^{99m}Tc-myocardial agents are more specific for this diagnosis. The exercise radionuclide ventriculogram is still a fine way to demonstrate the functional reserve of the left ventricular pump. It has application in diagnosis of valvular lesions, restrictive heart disease, cardiomyopathy, a variety of medications, and other conditions that alter the functional response of the LV to exercise. The pattern of LV exercise response shows many patients actually reach their best LV function before their "maximum" level of exercise. This is especially true of poorly conditioned but well-motivated patients who last for only a few levels of exercise. It is also seen in athletes who exert super-maximal effort. With an analysis of each level of exercise, an elegant physiologic study can be obtained with both systolic and diastolic parameters. A modification of the mathematics discussed under the section on cardiac output is used. The individual variations in "mu" and "D" were discussed as the largest source of error in the blood-sample method of LV-volume determination. These values can be safely assumed to remain constant during exercise. Relative changes in LV volume may be made without knowledge of either value and without drawing a blood sample. The formula for relative LV end-diastolic volume (rLVEDV) is as follows:

$$\text{rLVEDV} = \frac{(\text{LV counts in the end diastolic frame}) - (\text{Background})}{(\text{No. of cycles}) \times (\text{Time/frame})}$$

An extension of this calculation allows calculation of the relative LV end systolic volume (rLVESV) simply as follows:

$$\text{rLVESV} = \text{rLVEDV} \times (1 - \text{LVEF})$$

The relative LV stroke volume (rLVSV) is calculated as follows:

$$\text{rLVSV} = \text{rLVEDV} - \text{rLVESV}$$

These three relative LV volumes can be tabulated along with the relative cardiac output (rCO):

$$\text{rCO} = \text{rLVEDV} \times \text{LVEF} \times \text{Heart rate}$$

Recording these data along with each exercise level's heart rate, blood pressure, and double product (heart rate × systolic blood pressure = double product, which is proportional to heart work) is advisable (Table 18-1).

Table 18-1. Exercise equilibrium-gated–radionuclide ventriculogram data*

	Absolute measurements				Relative measurements			
Work level	**Heart rate**	**Blood pressure**	**Double product**	**LVEF**	**rLVEDV**	**rLVESV**	**rLVSV**	**rCO**
Rest	80	110/70	8.6K	0.52	1.00	1.00	1.00	1.00
I	94	112/76	10.5K	0.59	1.13	0.96	1.29	1.50
II	100	124/88	12.4K	0.63	1.00	0.98	1.21	1.50
III	119	140/90	17.1K	0.71	0.95	0.58	1.30	1.94
IV	139	156/94	21.7K	0.72	0.81	0.47	1.11	1.95
V	167	170/96	28.4K	0.78	0.79	0.36	1.19	2.48
VI	161	180/100	32.6K	0.82	0.75	0.28	1.18	2.67
Post	149	149/94	25.3K	0.74	0.82	0.44	1.17	2.17

*Diastolic dysfunction during exercise equilibrium-gated–radionuclide ventriculography. The patient is a young male athlete who is having progressively more difficulty with endurance running. Exercise levels are in increments of 25 kW on a bicycle ergometer. Note that the patient has normal systolic function as described by a progressively increasing heart rate, double product (measured in thousands), and LVEF. The volume and cardiac outputs are relative to resting measurements. Each level is indexed to a value of 1.0 at rest. (Remember that the actual volume is not measured with this technique.) During exercise, relative left ventricular end-diastolic volume (rLVEDV) rises slightly at work level I, which is normal. Then rLVEDV falls progressively with further exercise, indicating that the ventricle is not filling well during diastole. The relative left ventricular end-systolic volume (rLVESV) drops progressively in a normal fashion. The combination of both rLVEDV and rLEVSV falling dictates a meager rise in relative left-ventricular stroke volume (rLVSV) of about 20%. The relative cardiac output (rCO) goes up only 2.5× baseline. This study demonstrates the abnormal left ventricular diastolic performance of a hypertrophic cardiomyopathy. Failure to quickly fill the ventricle during diastole limits exercise in an otherwise healthy patient.

Continued.

Gated "equilibrium" first-pass right ventriculogram

It is not the purpose of this section to present fast dynamic first-pass and gated first-pass ventriculography. A fascinating adaptation of the gated technique allows the isolated examination of the RV with a hybrid of the equilibrium-gated and first-pass techniques. The gated-equilibrium first-pass technique extends the advantages of multicycle, gated-equilibrium ventriculogram accuracy to the RV.

A slow intravenous infusion of krypton-81m or xenon-133 dissolved in saline will establish an equilibrium level of radioactive blood in the RV. These dissolved noble gases have a partition coefficient that strongly favors the gaseous phase. On arrival at an alveolus, they change phase and are almost completely eliminated by the lungs. Xenon-133 dosages of 20 to 30 mCi (740 to 1110 MBq) diluted in 20 ml of normal saline are infused slowly from the antecubital vein over 60 sec and then followed with an additional slow bolus of normal saline. As the Xenon-133 mixes with venous blood returning to the heart, an equilibrium acquisition of up to 2 minutes can be done. The RAO projection is optimal since this allows separation of the right atrium and the pulmonary outflow tract from the RV. Precise aiming of the camera is assisted by injection of a small preacquisition radiotracer bolus, which is observed on the camera's persistence scope. A slight degree of caudal tilt will keep the RV projected below the activity in the base of the left lung. The LV will not enter the picture unless there is a right-to-left shunt. Sixteen frames are used because the acquisition is relatively short and the counts collected will be sparse by comparison with equilibrium-gated LV studies. The acquisition is manually terminated when the bolus clears from the subclavian vein. Processing after temporal and spatial filtering includes outlining of the RV blood pool in the same fashion used for LV-gated equilibrium–blood-pool studies. The normal RV ejection fraction (RVEF) can be determined and is considerably lower than the LVEF. The normal RV wall motion is different from the LV because the pulmonary outflow tract does not have the same mobility as the other walls. RV Fourier phase and amplitude images can also be calculated (Figs. 18-32, 33).

Interpretation

Faced with the numerous parameters that can be calculated, one should still begin an interpretation of the study with a visual evaluation of the cine display of the gated study. The LV wall's

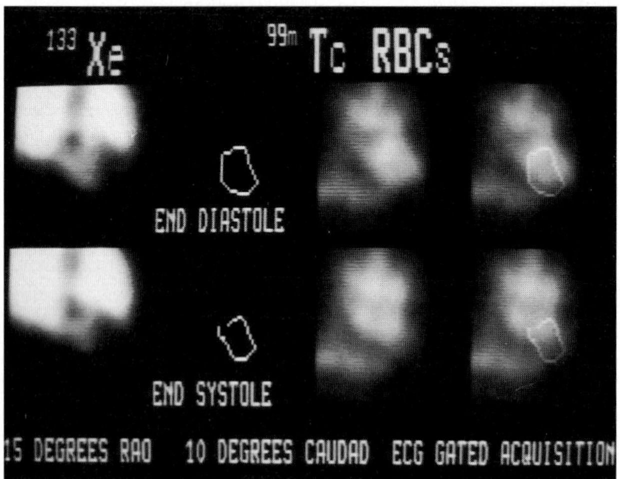

Fig. 18-32. ^{133}Xe in saline gated equilibrium radionuclide ventriculogram of the RV. A sixteen-frame gated acquisition of the RV shows the ventricle projecting below the bases of the lungs. The upper row shows an end-diastole ^{133}Xe image, its end-diastolic region of interest and end-diastole frames from a subsequent ^{99m}Tc RBC blood pool with and without the same region derived from the ^{133}Xe study. The bottom row shows matching systolic images.

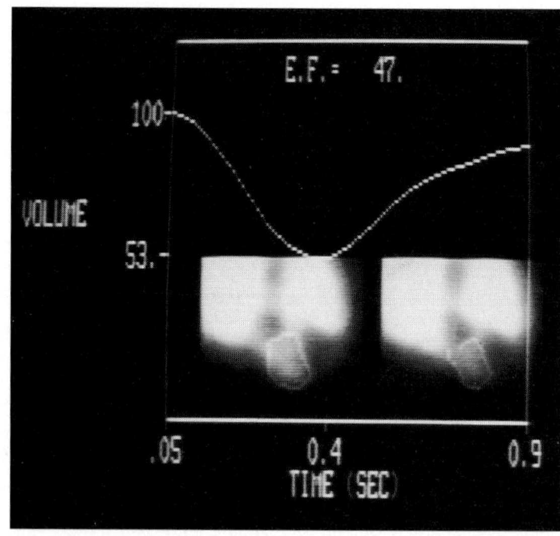

Fig. 18-33. A normal ^{133}Xe in saline equilibrium gated study with its average volume curve and regions of interest around the RV in end-diastolic *(left)* and end-systolic *(right)* images. The RVEF is 47 percent.

efforts are indirectly displayed as the blood pool moves. Either the raw or filtered data can be displayed, and simultaneous display of the different projections can be very helpful in triangulating abnormal wall motion. The training of the human eye to read wall motion is easy. In motion, the radionuclide ventriculogram is much easier to understand than when viewed as a series of static images. The most difficult aspect of illustrating this section is the inability to display motion images on the printed page. This is also a problem when archiving of data is limited to what can be photographed or printed on static media.

Chamber size and configuration can be reported by visual estimate and assisted by one of the volumetric estimates quoted above. The heart rate is also one of the three important parts of the equation that leads to calculation of the cardiac output. The last factor (and the one most frequently sought) is the LVEF, which is either reported as a percentage or as a decimal. Some nuclear medicine clinics report cardiac output with each study. The normal LVEF range is a bit different in each laboratory, but an average of 65% with 5% for a standard deviation (range = 55% to 75%) is representative. Those with LVEFs above this value at rest may be afflicted with hypertrophic cardiomyopathy, valvular insufficiency, and (less commonly) high output states. Hypertrophic cardiomyopathy has a normal or decreased LVEDV. Valvular insufficiency (aortic insufficiency or mitral regurgitation) commonly has an abnormally high LVEDV. The high output states are usually seen with high heart rates, not with high ejection fractions. The LVEFs that are too low are generally the result of prior infarctions or cardiomyopathies that damage the contractility of the heart wall. When the LVEF is low, compensation is usually by increased LVEDV. Increased heart rate can also help sustain cardiac output.

Inspection of the average volume curve's diastolic shape and parameters assists in detection of hypertrophic and early dilated cardiomyopathy. As with other measurements, each nuclear medicine clinic should establish standard acquisitions, standard processing, and normal ranges before these numbers are used in evaluation of LV function. The observer's impression of the quality of wall motion is confirmed by functional and parametric images. There are too many of these discussed above to make it practical to routinely do them all. When the observer becomes familiar with several of them in normal and abnormal ventricles, they become an objective "second observer" to help keep him or her honest. When the statistics and images have been discussed in the report, it is preferable to place the information in the context of the clinical problem. Which coronary artery distribution is abnormal, whether there is improvement or degradation in the function of the ventricle, and prognostic implications of the findings should be reported. Clarification of these issues with the referring physician leads to as much intelligent interpretation of the gated radionuclide ventriculogram as afforded by any nuclear medicine examination.

LABORATORY APPLICATION

46

MYOCARDIAL IMAGING

James K. O'Donnell

Anatomy (Figs. 18-34 to 18-36)

The development of cross-sectional tomographic imaging techniques including transmission-computed tomography (CT), magnetic resonance imaging (MRI), single-photon emission-computed tomography (SPECT), and positron emission tomography (PET) has revealed the need for familiarity with sectional anatomy of the heart.

The normal anatomic position of the heart is mostly to the left of midline in the mediastinum, with the apex angled forward and to the left. This position is somewhat variable, depending on the position of the diaphragm, the volume of the lungs, and the relative sizes of the cardiac chambers themselves in health or disease. Position can change in the individual (for example, as a result of simple exercise with increased diaphragmatic excursion and cardiac-chamber contractility).

Image sections oriented to the transverse (or axial), coronal, or sagittal planes of the body will thus "slice" the heart in an oblique fashion depending on its axis relative to the body at the time of imaging. For reproducibility and for accurate comparison of cardiac anatomy in serial studies (such as stress and redistribution ^{201}Tl images), it is necessary to realign the image planes along the short or long axes of the heart itself. Computer software can accomplish this for most imaging modalities.

Continued.

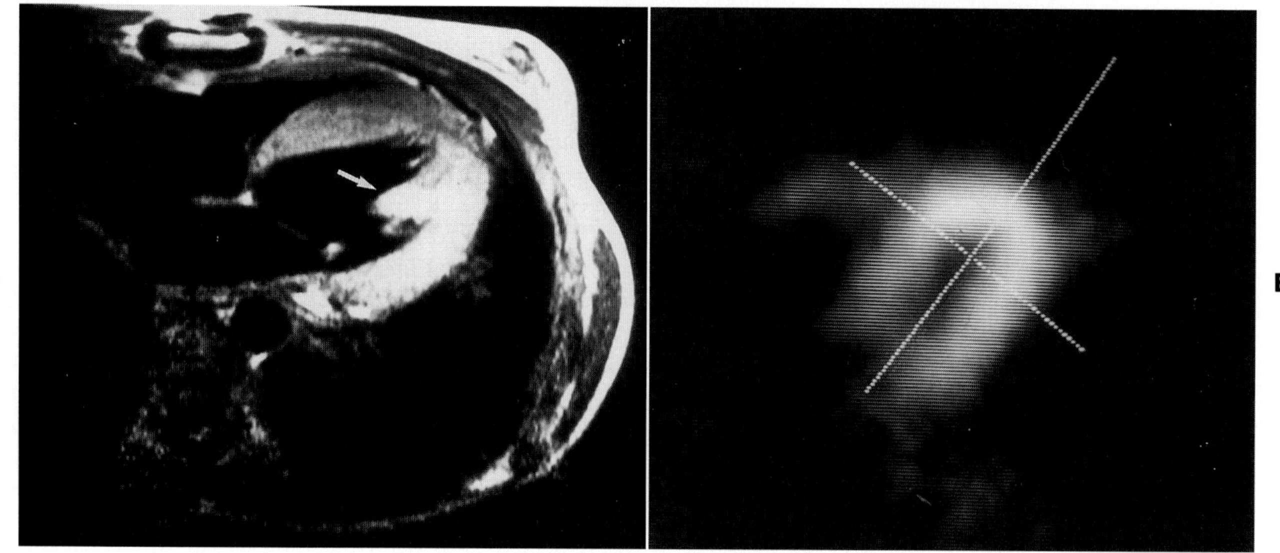

Fig. 18-34. **A,** Cardiac MRI transverse image demonstrating a somewhat thickened left ventricle in the normal body axis position. Note the hypertrophied papillary muscle *(arrow)*. **B,** Thallium-201 transverse SPECT image demonstrating the obliquely angulated left ventricle in body axis position but with short and long cardiac axes identified.

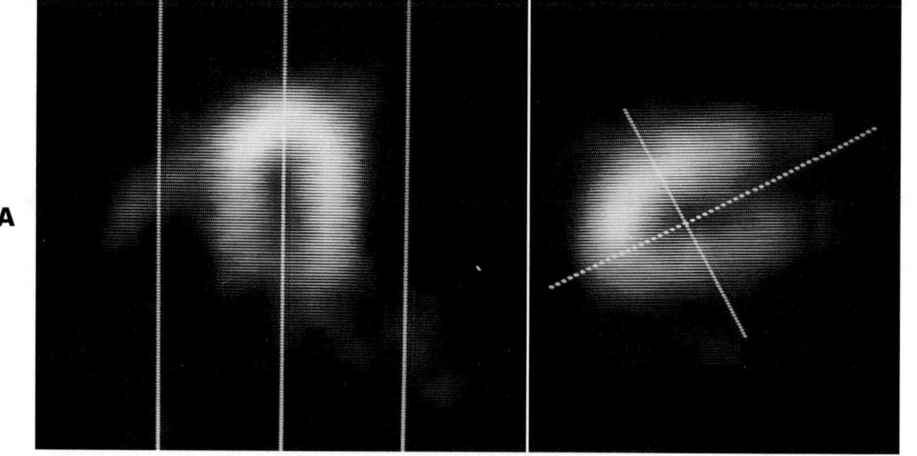

Fig. 18-35. **A,** Initial rotation of Fig. 18-34, *B*, preparing it for short axis reconstruction. **B,** Thallium-201 vertical long axis SPECT image in body axis position with short and long cardiac axes identified.

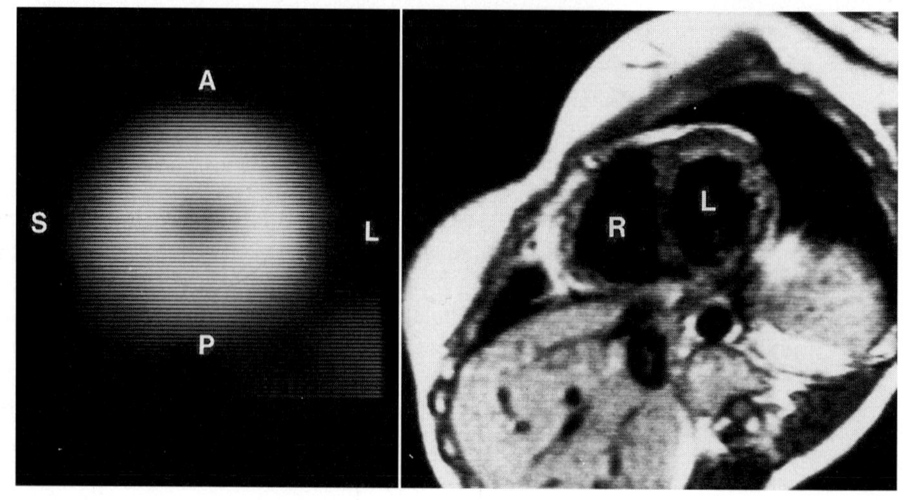

Fig. 18-36. **A,** Final reconstruction of ^{201}Tl SPECT image along the cardiac short axis. This is a single section or "slice" through the left ventricle with easily identified anterior (A), posterior (P), septal (S), and lateral (L) segments. **B,** Similar electronically angulated MRI cardiac short axis image showing relationship between left and right ventricles.

Image interpretation is then much easier and more accurate. To standardize image analysis and displays, efforts are being made to promote a universal system of nomenclature for cardiac-axis tomography. These terms are as follows:

New standard	Previous variations
Short axis	Transverse or coronal
Vertical long axis	Sagittal
Horizontal long axis	Coronal or transverse

Cardiac short-axis images of the left ventricle are the most clinically relevant for the majority of diagnostic imaging purposes. These images can best be understood by considering them as "slices of bread," with the top of the "loaf" as the anterior ventricular wall and the bottom as the posterior/inferior wall. The most common orientation for images is then with the septum on the left and lateral wall on the right of the viewer. Sequential images move from the base of the ventricle at the valvular plane progressively toward the apex. Additional vertical long-axis and horizontal long-axis image series demonstrate anatomic slices by cutting the ventricular "loaf" lengthwise from top to bottom or from side to side, respectively.

Tomographic studies allow much more detailed estimation of the size of abnormalities (area or volume) as well as the detection of more subtle findings such as papillary muscle involvement, aneurysmal dilatation, and dysynchronous contraction of ventricular segments during wall-motion analysis.

Purpose

Accurate imaging of regional and global myocardial perfusion can be an invaluable aid for the diagnosis and management of coronary artery disease. Functional imaging with thallium-201 and other radiopharmaceuticals directly reflects the delivery of blood to myocardial tissue and provides physiologic information to compare with the anatomic estimation of coronary artery stenoses obtained from coronary artery angiography. Multiple studies have confirmed the improved sensitivity and specificity of thallium-201 myocardial perfusion imaging over other diagnostic tests such as stress electrocardiography alone.

Thallium-201 is a cyclotron-produced analog of potassium (Kallium) with a physical half-life of 73 hours. Following intravenous injection of ^{201}Tl chloride, there is rapid clearance of the nuclide from the blood. Normal myocardial tissue extracts about 85% of the amount present in the coronary artery blood in the first pass through the heart. Distribution within the heart is according to regional myocardial blood flow and myocardial cell viability. Like potassium, ^{201}Tl relies on cell-membrane integrity and active metabolic transport for its uptake into cells of the myocardium. About 3% to 5% of the total injected dose localizes in myocardial tissue when ^{201}Tl is administered during exercise. After initial localization, there is rapid redistribution of ^{201}Tl in the heart and throughout the body as the intracellular and extracellular concentrations move toward an equilibrium that parallels that of potassium.

The kinetics of ^{201}Tl allow its use in stress myocardial perfusion studies wherein the nuclide is administered to a patient at peak exercise on a treadmill or bicycle ergometer. Initial images are then acquired immediately after exercise to obtain regional myocardial perfusion information. Repeated images in the redistribution phase 2 to 4 hours later demonstrate any changes in the ^{201}Tl distribution. Early stress-induced defects, which later normalize in redistribution images, imply myocardial ischemia. Persistent defects indicate scarring.

The combination of ^{201}Tl-stress–myocardial imaging with standard stress electrocardiography has improved the sensitivity and specificity for detecting coronary artery disease from 65% to about 85%. Various methods have been developed to quantify further the relative uptake of ^{201}Tl in distinct myocardial segments. These generally involve a graphic representation of maximum counts in myocardial segments or in a circumferential profile within a region of interest around the left ventricular myocardium. Such techniques have further improved accuracy as well as reproducibility over visual estimation alone.

An additional technical advance has been the development of single-photon emission computed tomography (SPECT). Using a gamma camera mounted on a rotating gantry and interfaced to a computer, multiple images of the heart are acquired as the camera head travels in a transaxial rota-

Continued.

tion around the thorax. Typical protocols call for a 64-frame acquisition over 360 degrees or a 32-frame acquisition over 180 degrees. New multihead gamma camera designs (for example, triple-head SPECT systems) acquire data from more than one angle simultaneously and can shorten acquisition times considerably. These frames of raw data are then reconstructed by computer algorithms to provide multiple 5- to 6-mm–thick image "slices" parallel to the short and long axes of the heart. SPECT has increased sensitivity for ^{201}Tl perfusion abnormalities to about 90% by lessening the common problems of overlying soft-tissue or breast artifact and of superimposed uptake by normal myocardium on areas of decreased activity (both inherent problems in planar imaging with ^{201}Tl).

Pharmacologic stress has also begun to play a role in myocardial-perfusion imaging, allowing accurate diagnostic studies to be performed in patients unable to achieve adequate treadmill exercise levels. Dipyridamole and adenosine are potent coronary vasodilators that increase normal coronary blood flow by a factor of 2 to 3 during intravenous infusion. There is less or no change in blood flow through significantly stenotic arteries. Therefore, a differential between normal and stenotic coronary vessels can be demonstrated when ^{201}Tl injection follows an intravenous infusion of either of these vasodilators. The diagnostic accuracy is similar to images acquired after treadmill stress. Some symptoms of chest pain or headache may occur in 20% to 30% of patients, but significant clinical complications from the use of vasodilators as a pharmacologic stress are minimal. Intravenous aminophylline promptly reverses the vasodilator effect and any clinical symptoms such as angina. When using the shorter-acting adenosine, simply discontinuing the infusion is usually enough to alleviate symptoms.

Two new classes of ^{99m}Tc-labeled pharmaceuticals for myocardial perfusion imaging have recently been approved for clinical use (Table 18-2). Sestamibi (Cardiolite, DuPont Co., Billerica, Mass.) is an isonitrile compound extracted from the coronary artery circulation in proportion to blood flow and is bound to intracellular proteins. There is no significant redistribution as there is with ^{201}Tl. Thus for several hours after the injection of this compound, imaging will reflect areas of decreased perfusion because of ischemia or infarction present at the time of injection. Various published protocols have used Sestamibi in combination with treadmill or pharmacologic stress to detect ischemia as opposed to scar. By appropriate adjustment of doses at rest and during stress, same-day procedures can be completed in about the same time frame as for ^{201}Tl. Because of its retention in the myocardium, ECG-gated wall-motion evaluation can be performed by either planar or SPECT techniques.

Teboroxime (CardioTec, Squibb Diagnostics, Princeton, N.J.) is a boronic-acid (BATO) derivative whose uptake within myocardial cells is also determined by coronary artery blood flow. This is a neutral lipophilic compound that passively diffuses across the cell membrane but then washes out rapidly. Because of this rapid washout, imaging must begin within 2 to 3 minutes after intravenous injection and be completed within 8 to 10 minutes. A potential advantage is faster patient throughput, especially with less time required between stress and rest imaging phases.

Clinical evaluation of myocardial perfusion using positron-emission tomography (PET) and short

Table 18-2. Single-photon myocardial perfusion radiopharmaceuticals

	Thallium-201	**^{99m}Tc-Sestamibi**	**^{99m}Tc-teboroxime**
Compound	Potassium analog	Isonitrile	BATO
Physical half-life	73 hours	6 hours	6 hours
Dose (total)	2-4 mCi (74-148 MBq)	30-60 mCi (1110-2220 MBq)	35-50 mCi (1295-1850 MBq)
Imaging time after injection	Immediately to 5 min	45-90 min*	Immediately
Imaging energy	68-80 keV	140 keV	140 keV
Myocardial washout	Some	Minimal	Rapid
Redistribution	Yes	No	No
Myocardial extraction efficiency	85%	65%	90%
Absorbed dose (Avg. study) Whole body (70-kg subject)	0.68 rad	0.50 rad	0.83 rad

*Same-day protocol:
8-10 mCi (296-370 MBq) ^{99m}Tc-Sestamibi resting
25-30 mCi (925-1110 MBq) ^{99m}Tc-Sestamibi stress

half-life positron-emitting radiopharmaceuticals has begun to show great promise. PET studies employing another potassium analog, rubidium-82 from a strontium-rubidium generator, have proved equivalent to or slightly better than ^{201}Tl in assessing myocardial perfusion. This and other agents, including fluorine-18 deoxyglocose (FDG), have further demonstrated myocardial metabolism and allowed differentiation between salvageable and irreversibly damaged myocardium in cases of severe coronary artery stenosis or infarction. Ongoing and further studies are expected to evaluate and accurately quantify absolute myocardial blood flow and metabolism.

Indications

Resting ^{201}Tl imaging

1. To detect the presence and extent of myocardial damage in the initial 6-hour (almost 100% sensitive) to 24-hour (about 75% sensitive) period after suspected acute myocardial infarction.
2. To evaluate patency of coronary artery bypass grafts in the early postoperative period.

Exercise or pharmacologic stress ^{201}Tl- or ^{99m}Tc-myocardial imaging

1. To screen patients at high risk for coronary artery disease.
2. To evaluate the functional significance of anatomic stenoses found during coronary angiography.
3. To estimate the degree of myocardial damage and possible residual ischemia after recovery from myocardial infarction.
4. To determine a prognosis and to help plan rehabilitative therapy after acute myocardial infarction.
5. To evaluate and follow patients who have undergone coronary artery bypass grafting (CABG), percutaneous transluminal coronary angioplasty (PTCA) dilatation, or thrombolytic therapy.
6. To differentiate ischemic from other causes of cardiomyopathy.
7. To provide adjunctive information in the evaluation of left ventricular hypertrophy; idiopathic hypertrophic subaortic stenosis (IHSS) or asymmetric septal hypertrophy (ASH); right ventricular hypertrophy; or congenital heart disease.

Procedure

Materials

1. Scintillation camera with low-energy, medium- or high-resolution, parallel-hole collimator
2. 2 to 4 mCi (74 to 148 MBq) ^{201}Tl chloride (or ^{99m}Tc myocardial radiopharmaceuticals [Table 18-2])
3. Imaging device for hard copy and computer for digital data acquisition
4. Treadmill for exercise stress or intravenous dipyridamole for pharmacologic stress
5. Cardiopulmonary resuscitation equipment in case of emergency

Patient preparation

1. Explain the entire procedure to the patient.
2. The patient is given nothing by mouth except for water for at least 3 to 4 hours before the procedure.
3. If possible, patients should discontinue any beta-blocker medication 48 to 72 hours before the procedure.
4. Insulin-dependent diabetic patients should have their insulin doses and food intake adjusted appropriately by their primary physician.
5. If pharmacologic stress with vasodilator infusion is to be employed, the patient should discontinue any Xanthine medications such as aminophylline, theophylline, or caffeine, at least 48 hours before the procedure.

Technique

1. Establish a secure intravenous line in a peripheral arm vein.
2. Set the imaging device for static images.
3. Prepare the computer for data acquisition using appropriate software for planar or SPECT images.

Continued.

4. When the patient has achieved the desired level of treadmill stress or when significant symptoms or signs intervene (e.g., chest pain or hypotension) as determined by the attending physician, inject the dosage of ^{201}Tl chloride intravenously followed by a saline flush.
5. If pharmacologic stress with dipyridamole or adenosine is employed instead of treadmill stress, inject the dosage of ^{201}Tl chloride or ^{99m}Tc myocardial radiopharmaceuticals intravenously at the appropriate point in the protocol.
6. Have the patient continue treadmill exercise for at least 60 seconds following ^{201}Tl or ^{99m}Tc myocardial radiopharmaceutical administration.
7. Begin imaging as soon as possible after exercise. Imaging should begin no more than 5 minutes after termination of exercise with ^{201}Tl if at all possible. With Teboroxine, imaging is immediate; with Sestamibi, wait 30 to 90 minutes.
8. Acquire images for a preset time of 600 sec/view for a planar study.
9. Acquire images in the 45-degree left anterior oblique, anterior, and 70-degree left anterior oblique (and/or lateral) positions.
10. Acquiring the 45-degree left anterior oblique image first will give the best early stress representation of the separate territories supplied by the three major coronary arteries.
11. For SPECT acquisition, follow the procedure recommended by the manufacturers of the individual gamma camera/computer combination.
12. Repeat a redistribution phase image series at 2 to 4 hours after the initial injection of ^{201}Tl. Use the identical acquisition protocol and the exact patient position in which the stress images were acquired. Some institutions now routinely employ a second ("re-injection") dosage of ^{201}Tl before acquisition of the second image series. This may improve the sensitivity in detecting ischemia over redistribution imaging alone.
13. The patient should consume only small amounts of clear liquids between stress and redistribution imaging. A heavy meal will direct more of the cardiac output toward the gut and possibly prevent ^{201}Tl redistribution to an ischemic myocardial segment.
14. Process the computer-acquired data using available ^{201}Tl quantification software for planar images or SPECT reconstruction and display programs for a tomographic study.
15. If ^{99m}Tc Sestamibi is used, the protocol will usually be either a same day rest-stress series with a resting dose of 8-10 mCi (296-370 MBq) followed by a stress dose of 25-30 mCi (925-1110 MBq) or a two-day protocol stress-rest series using 25-30 mCi (925-1110 MBq) each on separate days.
16. For a resting study without exercise or pharmacologic stress, simply inject the ^{201}Tl-chloride dose intravenously and begin image acquisition immediately. It may be more appropriate to repeat the image series at a shorter interval than the usual stress-redistribution study, typically at 30 to 60 minutes after injection.

Interpretation (Figs. 18-37 to 18-50)

Thallium-201 uptake in a normal heart after stress will result in images with a fairly uniform distribution of activity to all myocardial segments. There may be a slightly uneven pattern as a result of variability of up to 20% in differential uptake within individual segments. Moderate uptake by the right ventricle is normally seen in stress images. Redistribution phase images are more likely to be uneven because of varying rates of ^{201}Tl washout in normal myocardial segments.

Correlation of the ^{201}Tl uptake in left ventricular myocardial segments with actual coronary artery anatomy is difficult and imprecise. Only about two thirds of patients have the standard right coronary artery dominant circulation. Others have either left dominant or balanced coronary circulations. Thus, the classical correlation is anterior and septal segments: left anterior descending artery; posterior and inferior segments: right coronary artery; posterolateral and lateral segments: left circumflex artery. However, these correlations should be considered only approximations; especially for the ventricular apex, they are quite variable.

Interpretation of abnormal ^{201}Tl myocardial perfusion images is based on a comparison of the stress and redistribution or reinjection phases. Segmental or global decreases in ^{201}Tl uptake after stress indicate the presence of either myocardial scarring or ischemia. Later redistribution images demonstrate persistent defects if myocardial scarring from infarction is present. If there is viable but ischemic myocardium present, the redistribution images will demonstrate partial or complete nor-

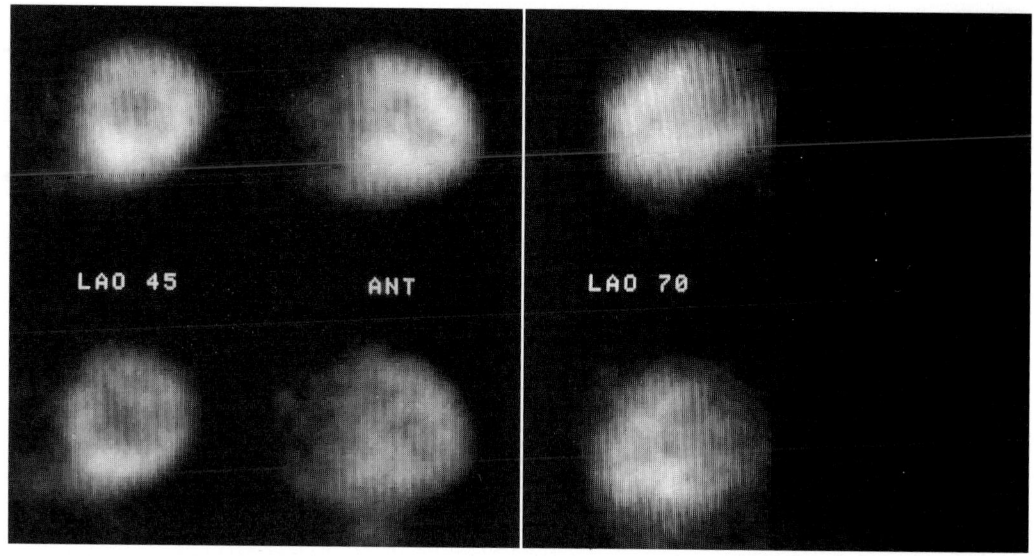

Fig. 18-37. Normal planer ^{210}Tl myocardial images in both stesss (upper) and redistribution (lower) phases after injection of 2.0 mCi (74m Bq) of ^{201}Tl chloride at peak treadmill exercise.

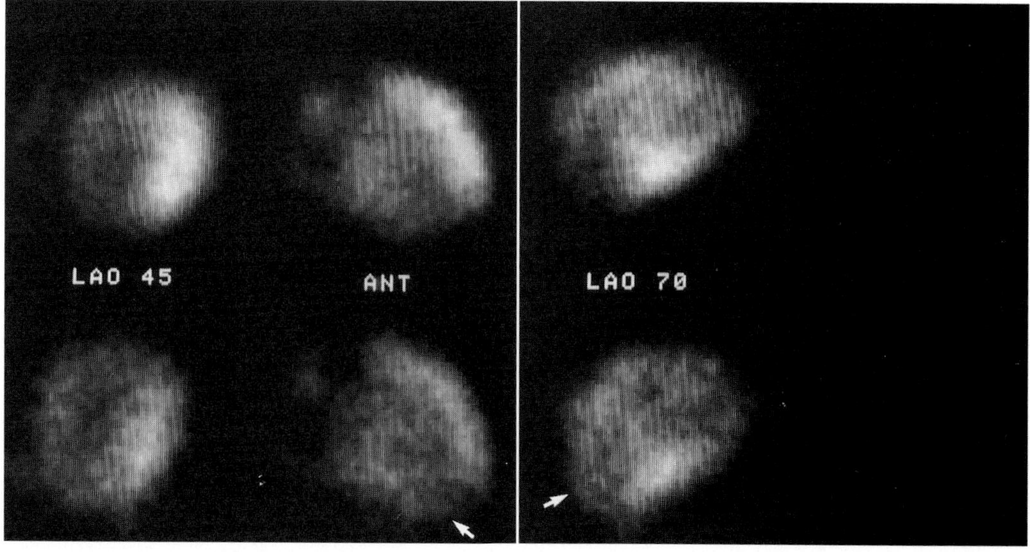

Fig. 18-38. Combination of scar and ischemia in a patient with recurrent angina after myocardial infarction. ^{210}Tl images demonstrate persistent septal and inferior defects with partial interoapical and apical redistribution *(arrows)*.

Continued.

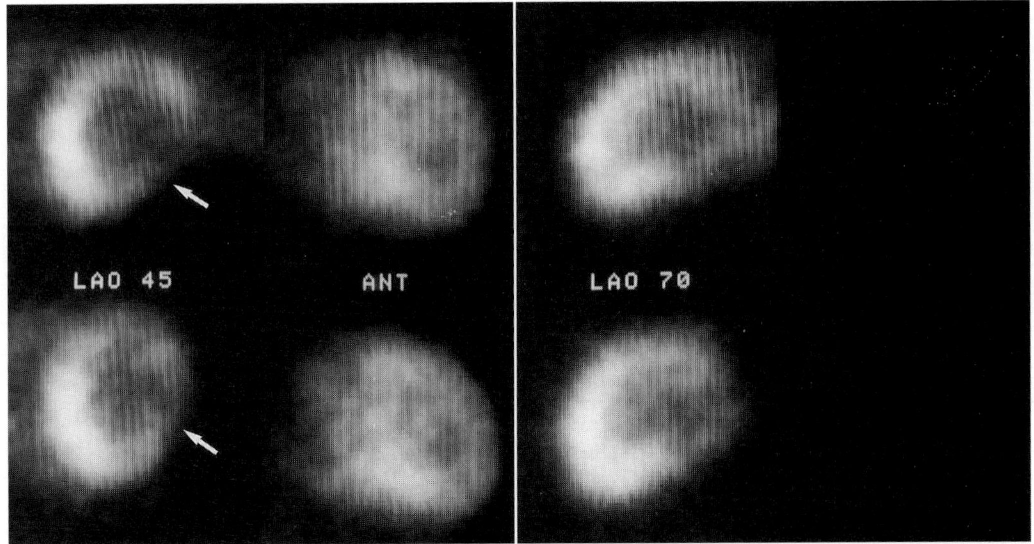

Fig. 18-39. Myocardial scarring in a patient with previous infarction. There are persistent ^{201}Tl defects in the lateral and inferolateral segments *(arrows)*.

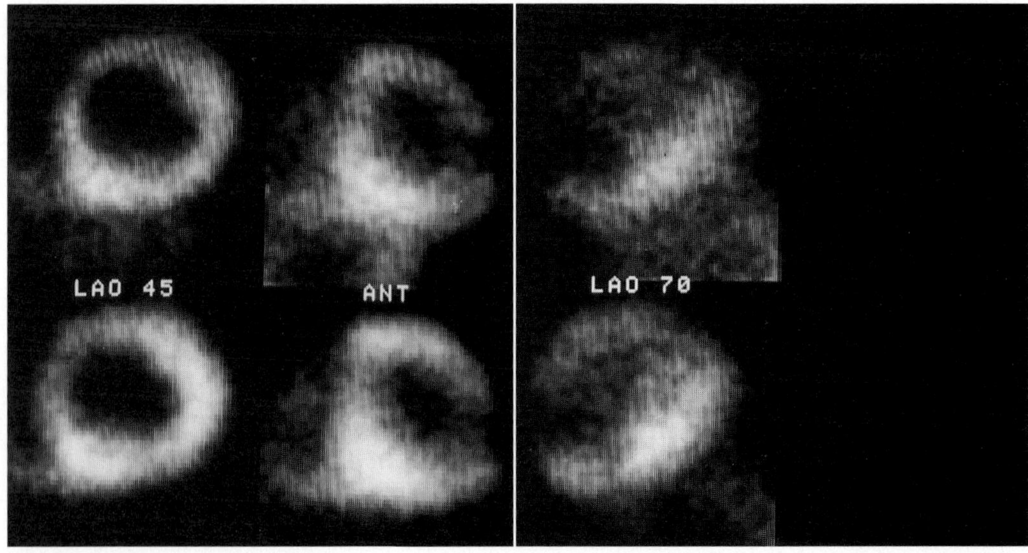

Fig. 18-40. Extensive myocardial scarring with stress-induced ventricular dysfunction. ^{201}Tl images show persistent defects in the septal, anterior, and apical segments with moderate chamber dilatation.

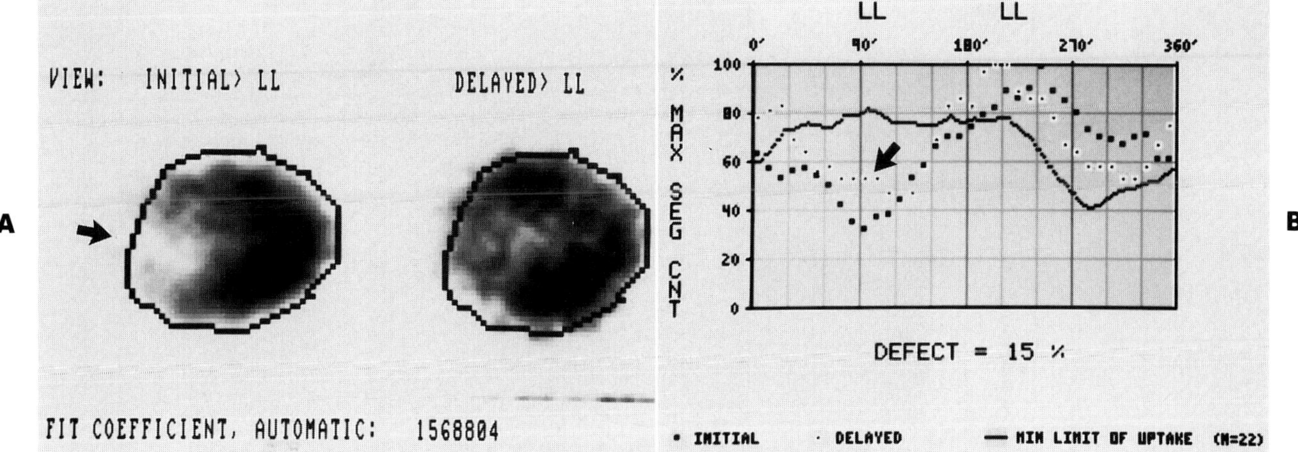

Fig. 18-41. Quantitative ^{201}Tl myocardial image analysis. **A,** Left lateral view demonstrating a large anteroapical and apical perfusion defect *(arrow)* with partial redistribution in a patient with recurring angina after infarction. **B,** Circumferential ^{201} Tl profile confirming an ischemic redistribution pattern *(arrow)* superimposed on a persistent scar pattern.

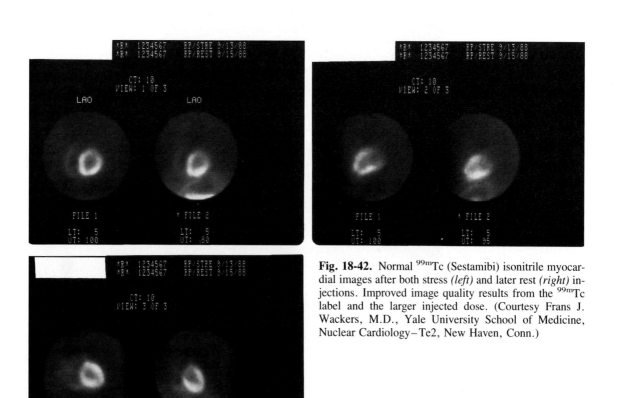

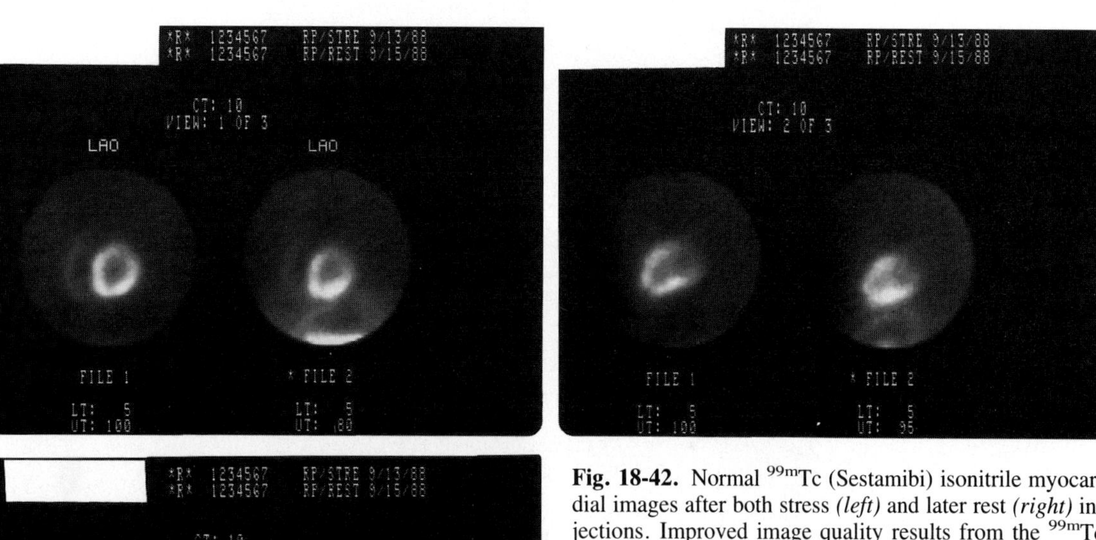

Fig. 18-42. Normal ^{99m}Tc (Sestamibi) isonitrile myocardial images after both stress *(left)* and later rest *(right)* injections. Improved image quality results from the ^{99m}Tc label and the larger injected dose. (Courtesy Frans J. Wackers, M.D., Yale University School of Medicine, Nuclear Cardiology–Te2, New Haven, Conn.)

Continued.

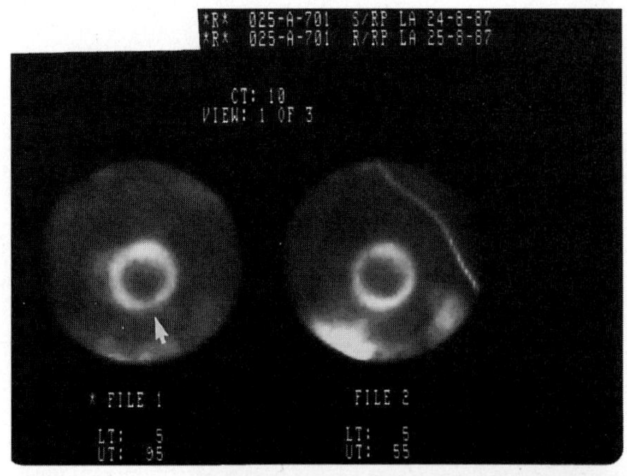

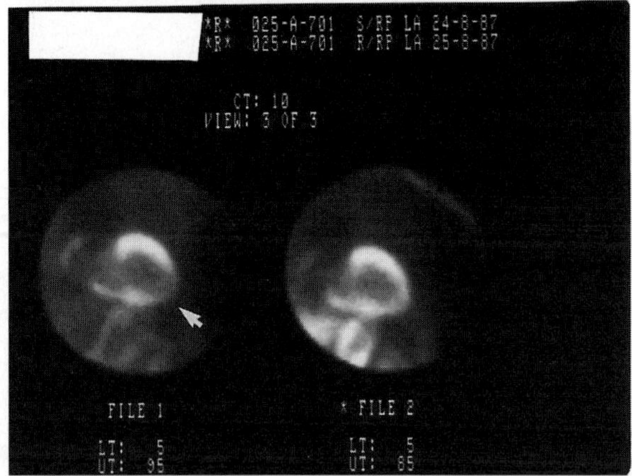

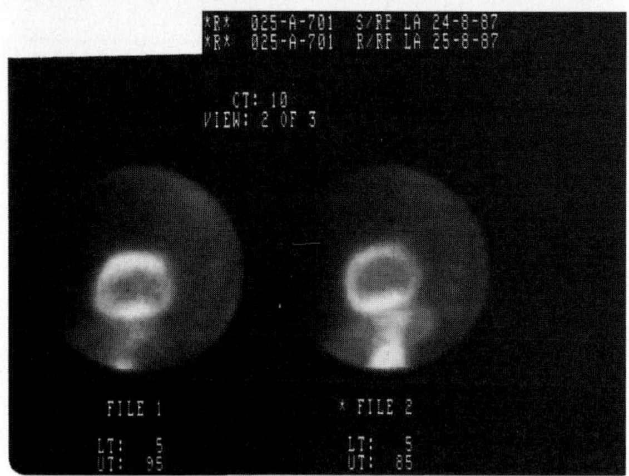

Fig. 18-43. Abnormal planar ^{99m}Tc (Sestamibi) isonitrile images showing stress-induced ventricular chamber dilatation as well as inferior and apical defects *(arrows)*. Later images after reinjection at rest demonstrate improved perfusion and document ischemia. (Courtesy Frans J. Wackers, M.D., Yale University School of Medicine, Nuclear Cardiology–Te2, New Haven, Conn.)

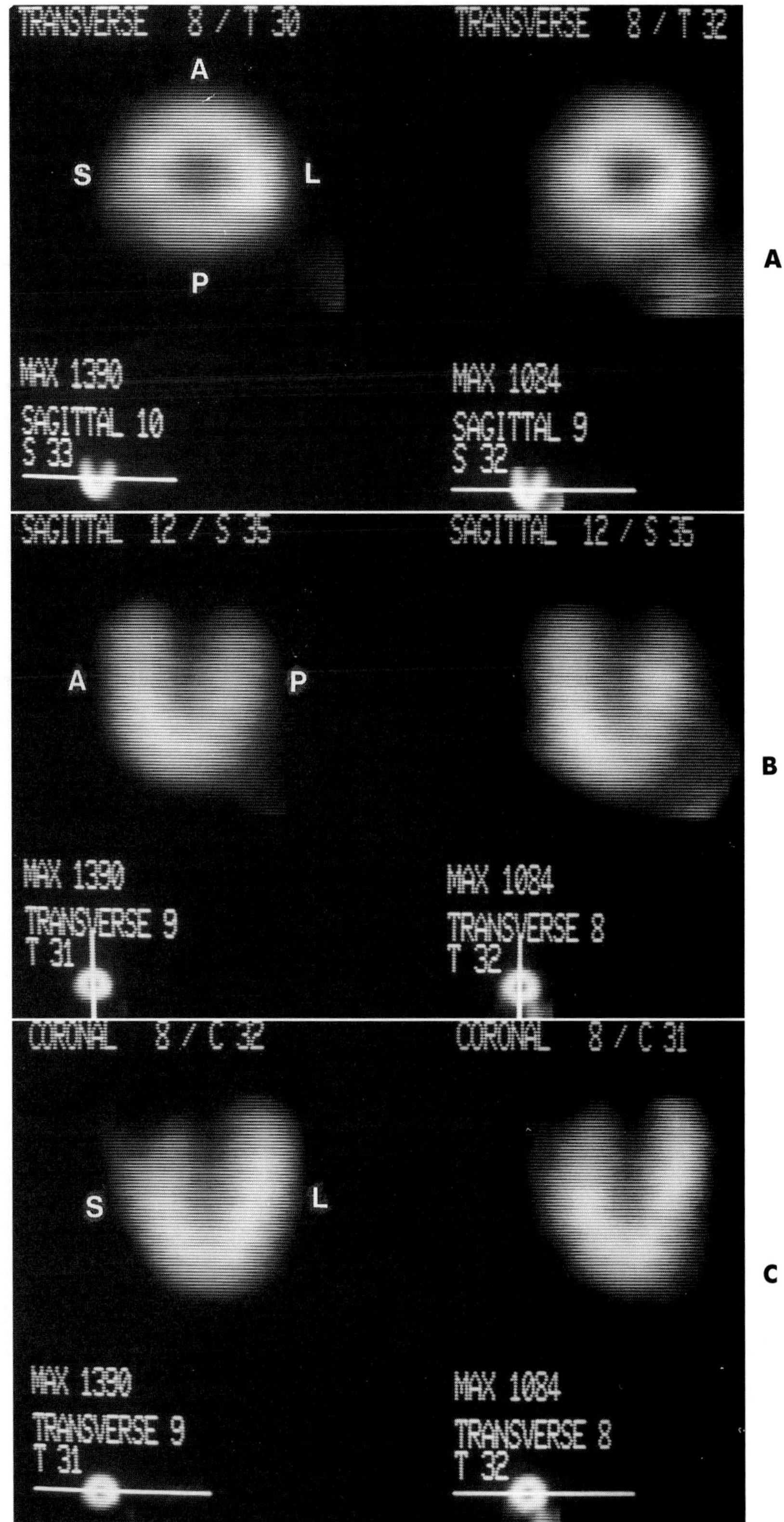

Fig. 18-44. Normal SPECT ^{201}Tl myocardial images in both stress *(left)* and redistribution *(right)* phases. **A,** Short axis section selected from mid-left ventricle demonstrating anterior (A), posterior (P), septal (S), and lateral (L) segments. **B,** Vertical long axis section through the mid portion of the anterior (A) and posterior (P) segments. **C,** Horizontal long axis section through the mid portion of the septal (S) and lateral (L) segments. (The printed transverse, sagittal, and coronal legends on the illustration are standard computer legends and do not apply to the myocardial anatomic position as described in the text.)

Continued.

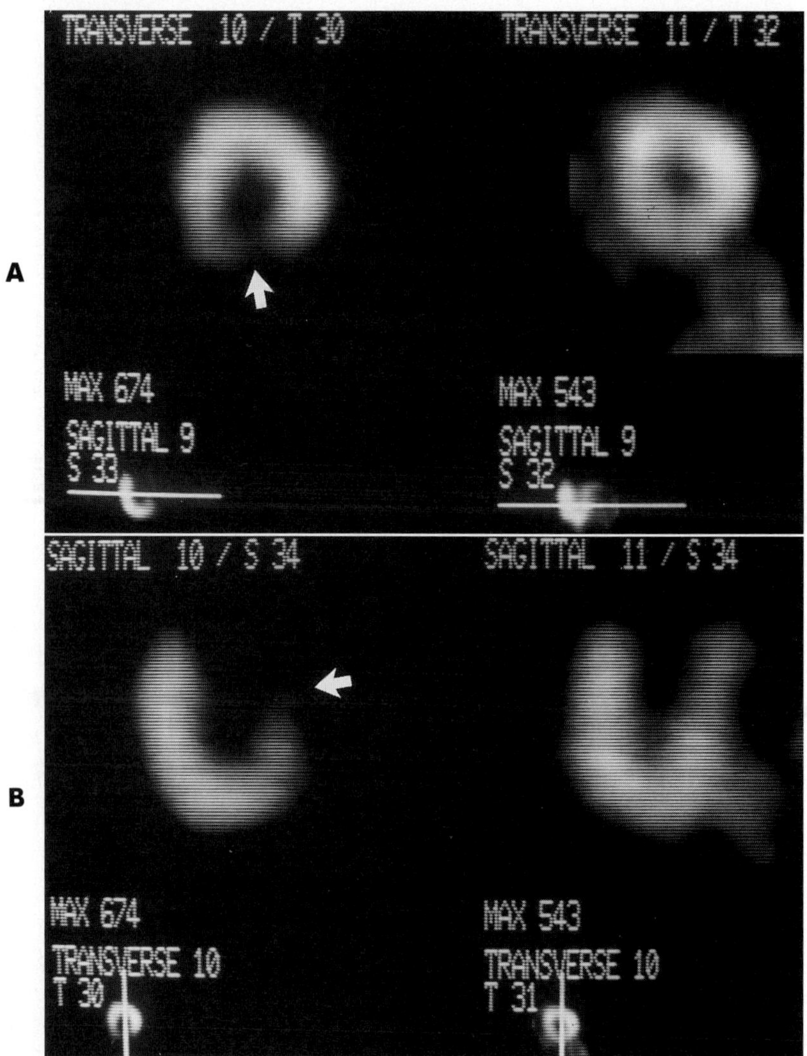

Fig. 18-45. Posterior myocardial ischemia. **A,** Short axis ^{201}Tl SPECT section shows inferior stress defect (arrow) with improvement in redistribution. **B,** Vertical long axis section best demonstrates the extent of the defect from base to mid-ventricle *(arrow)*. (The printed transverse, sagittal, and coronal legends on the illustration are standard computer legends and do not apply to the myocardial anatomic position as described in the text.)

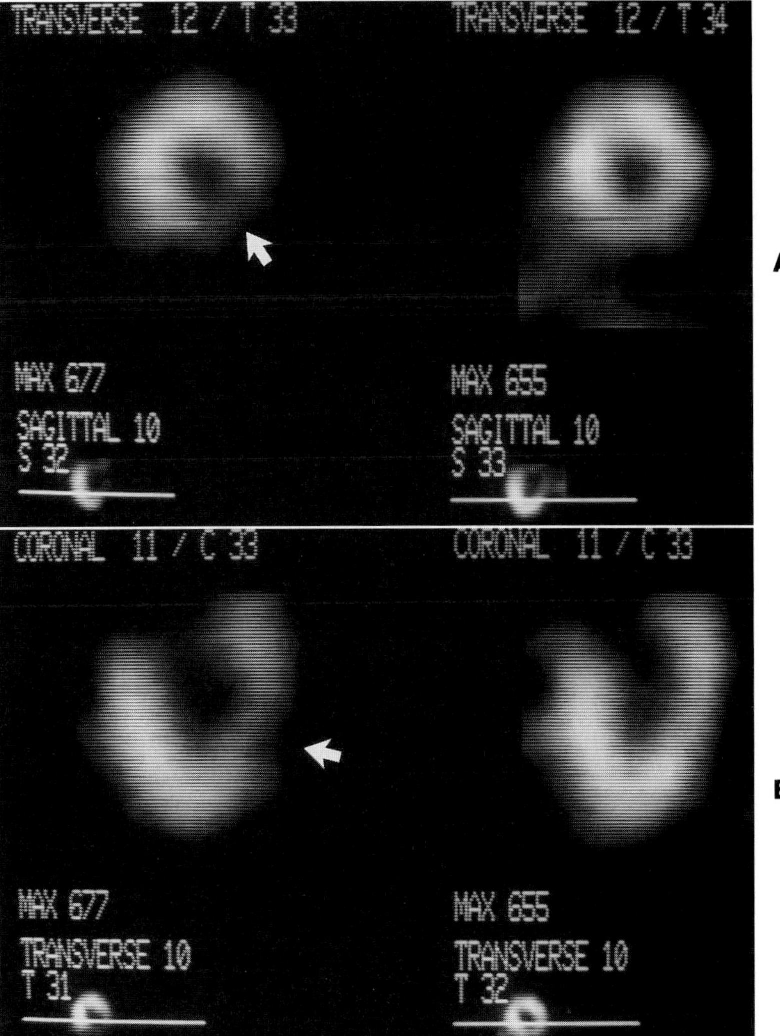

Fig. 18-46. Inferolateral myocardial ischemia. **A,** Short axis ^{201}Tl SPECT section shows inferolateral stress defect (arrow) with improvement in redistribution. **B,** Horizontal long axis section here best demonstrates the extent of the defect in mid-portion of ventricle *(arrow)*. (The printed transverse, sagittal, and coronal legends on the illustration are standard computer legends and do not apply to the myocardial anatomic position as described in the text.)

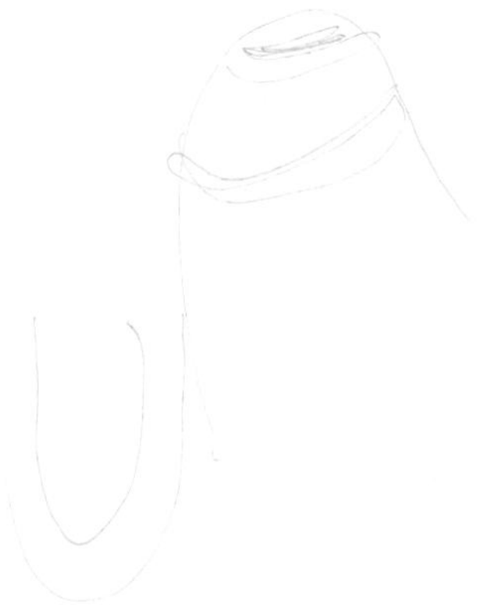

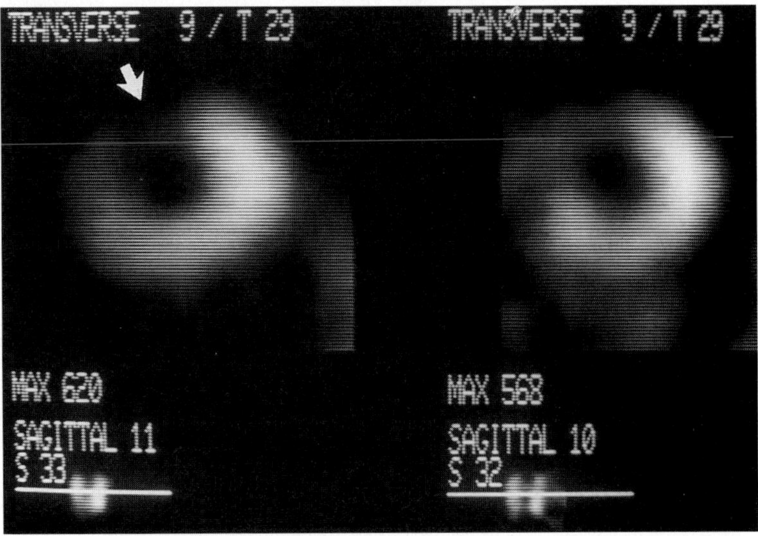

Fig. 18-47. Anteroseptal myocardial scar. Representative ^{201}Tl short axis SPECT section through the mid-portion of the left ventricle demonstrates persistent defects *(arrows)*. (The printed transverse, sagittal, and coronal legends on the illustration are standard computer legends and do not apply to the myocardial anatomic position as described in the text.)

Continued.

Fig. 18-48. Posterior myocardial scar and inferior ischemia. **A,** Short axis ^{201}Tl SPECT section shows a persistent posterior defect *(arrows)*. **B,** Vertical short axis section best demonstrates the extent of the persistent defect and also shows slight inferoapical ischemia in redistribution *(arrow)*. (The printed transverse, sagittal, and coronal legends on the illustration are standard computer legends and do not apply to the myocardial anatomic position as described in the text.)

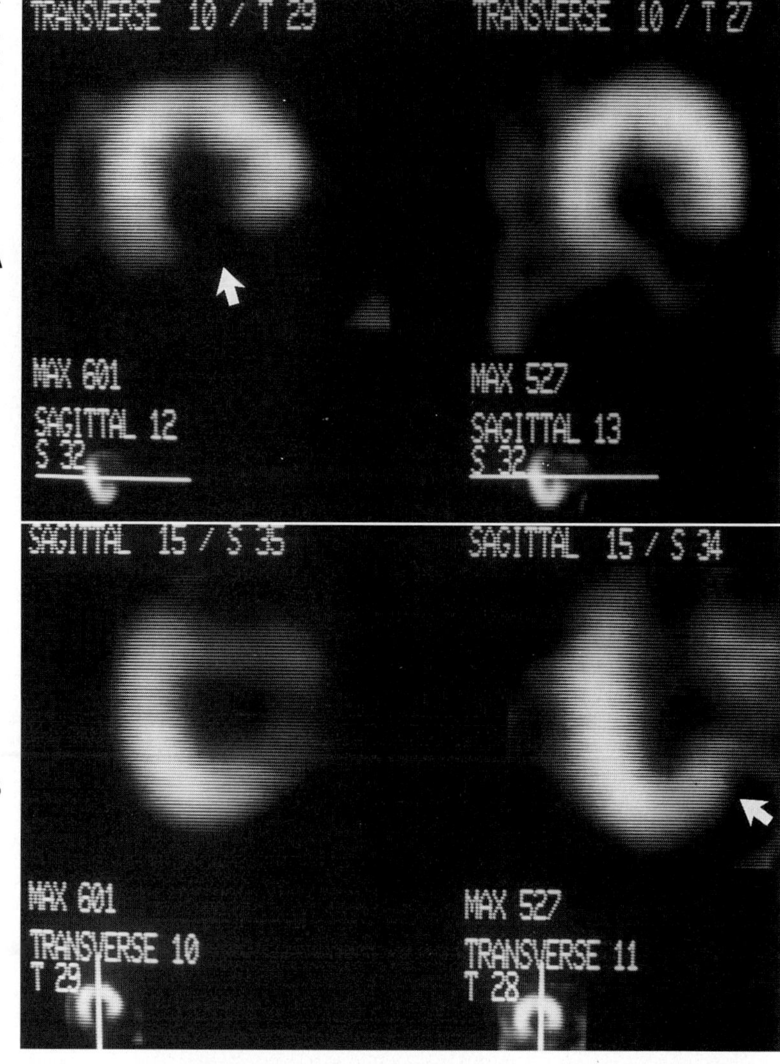

Fig. 18-49. Three-dimensional reconstruction of normal ^{99m}Tc (Sestamibi) isonitrile SPECT myocardial perfusion images. The SPECT image slice data are used to construct a surface rendering of the entire heart which can be rotated or "tumbled" through multiple projections. (Courtesy Picker-Ohio Imaging Corporation, Cleveland, Ohio.)

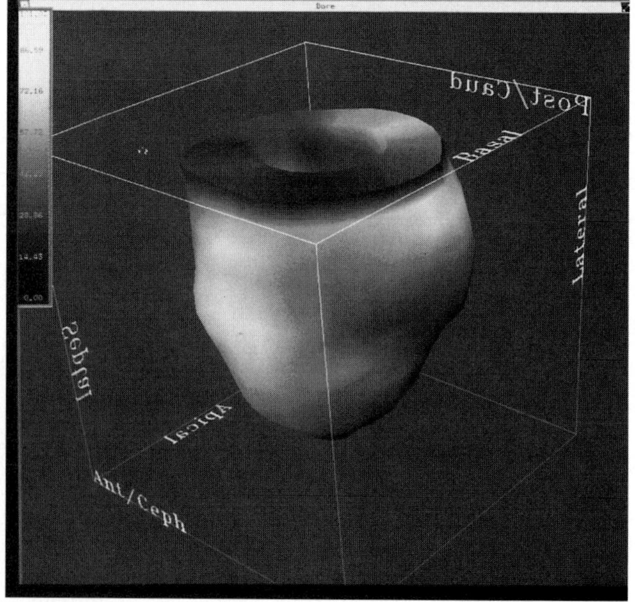

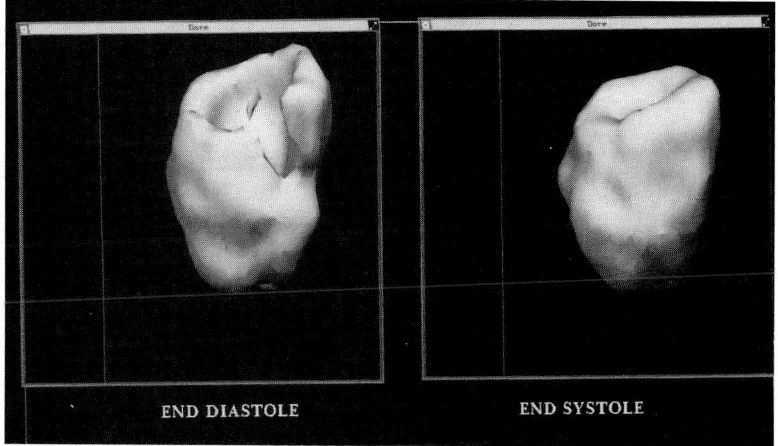

Fig. 18-50. Three-dimensional reconstruction of ECG-gated ^{99m}Tc (Sestamibi) isonitrile SPECT images at both end-diastole and end-systole. The end-diastolic image demonstrates a prominent posterior perfusion decrease. (Courtesy Picker-Ohio Imaging Corporation, Cleveland, Ohio.)

malization of ^{201}Tl activity in the ischemic areas as relative coronary artery perfusion improves in the 2 to 4 hours subsequent to treadmill stress. In some cases in which coronary artery stenosis is severe, a ^{201}Tl defect may also persist for longer than this 2- to 4-hour period after stress. Thus if ischemia alone or superimposed on prior infarction is strongly suspected clinically, further delayed images, sometimes as long as 24 hours after stress, may document the expected late improvement in ^{201}Tl uptake.

Several recent reports have demonstrated that a significant improvement in sensitivity for myocardial ischemia can be achieved by dividing the ^{201}Tl dosage and giving a second injection of ^{201}Tl just before the redistribution phase of imaging. This split-dose technique will detect a reversible ischemic pattern in many cases where even late redistribution images would have shown a persistent defect (i.e., a false negative for ischemia).

Severe triple-vessel coronary artery disease can potentially result in a false-negative ^{201}Tl pattern as a result of a universal decrease in uptake with no apparent segmental abnormalities. However, secondary findings are usually present, including ventricular chamber dilatation from stress-induced dysfunction and incipient congestive failure, excessive right ventricular ^{201}Tl uptake, and a poor myocardium: lung uptake ratio. Symptomatic and ECG changes during stress also usually cause the diagnosis of triple-vessel disease to be considered.

Other causes of false-negative stress myocardial perfusion studies include inadequate stress or the use of beta-blocker medications. False-positive studies sometimes result from mitral valve prolapse, left ventricular hypertrophy, or nonischemic cardiomyopathies. Typical patterns of ^{201}Tl uptake may help to differentiate these causes. For example, idiopathic hypertrophic subaortic stenosis (IHSS) shows asymmetric bulbous enlargement of the septal area, infiltrative cardiomyopathies such as amyloidosis often show concentric biventricular enlargement, and hypertensive hypertrophy shows left ventricular enlargement alone.

Artifactual changes in ^{201}Tl-perfusion images are common. Decreased activity in the posterior and inferior segments can be a result of diaphragmatic attenuation of the low-energy ^{201}Tl photons. Likewise, a linear anterior decrease often results from overlying breast attenuation artifact in female patients. SPECT imaging techniques lessen these difficulties but do not eliminate them entirely. Some centers adopt procedures such as compressing breast tissue away from the precordium or positioning patients in the right lateral decubitus for the lateral views to decrease diaphragmatic interference.

Additional attempts to analyze ^{201}Tl uptake and washout patterns by computer manipulation and quantification techniques are helpful. Background subtraction, image smoothing, contrast enhancement, the use of color displays, and quantification by segments or by circumferential profile analysis are all refinements available in various forms in commercially distributed software packages. Their use can significantly improve diagnostic accuracy over simple visual estimations of stress and redistribution activity.

The growing use of SPECT ^{201}Tl studies reflects their value both in improved detection of abnor-

Continued.

malities and in the estimation of the area and/or volume of the perfusion abnormality made possible by the inspection of multiple-image slices.

Three-dimensional reconstructions of radiopharmaceutical distribution within the myocardium are among the newest computer software developments. These whole-ventricle representations from the SPECT data may prove useful in area and volume determinations.

Another (less common) use of myocardial perfusion imaging is in patients with suspected acute myocardial infarction. Resting ^{201}Tl perfusion imaging has been shown to be nearly 100% sensitive in detecting acute transmural infarcts within the first 6 hours of onset. Sensitivity decreases slightly in the 6- to 24-hour period postinfarction and is considerably less for nontransmural infarction. The finding of a defect is nonspecific, however. A perfusion defect may result from severe resting ischemia or an old myocardial infarction. The concomitant finding of significant right ventricular uptake on a resting study is ominous and usually indicates ventricular failure. In some cases, additional delayed imaging after the initial resting image series may show an ischemic component with evidence of redistribution. Resting ^{201}Tl studies may also benefit in the acute clinical setting by aiding in the differentiation of left versus right ventricular infarction, by helping to establish a prognosis after infarction and in planning rehabilitative therapy, or by providing noninvasive follow-up of patients after PTCA or thrombolytic interventions.

Although the documentation of an image pattern is the mainstay of interpretation for myocardial perfusion imaging, the ultimate estimation of the presence and extent of coronary artery disease depends on the integration of this data with all the clinical information available. Thus the finding of a persistent anterior segment defect on stress ^{201}Tl imaging could be interpreted as myocardial scarring in an elderly patient with known previous infarction and normal stress ECG; as severe ischemia with poor redistribution in a middle-aged male with a negative prior history but classical angina and stress ECG changes; or as normal with breast attenuation artifact in a young female with atypical pain and a normal stress ECG.

The ongoing development of ^{99m}Tc radiopharmaceuticals and the further applications of emission tomography, both SPECT and PET, are expected to refine and enhance the clinical applications of myocardial perfusion imaging.

LABORATORY APPLICATION

47

MYOCARDIAL INFARCT IMAGING

D. Bruce Sodee

Purpose

^{99m}Tc stannous pyrophosphate is a bone-imaging agent; however, it was found in 1975 that this radiopharmaceutical localized in areas of acute myocardial infarction. In the peripheral zones of myocardial infarction there is calcium accumulation within the mitrochondria as well as within the cytoplasm of necrotic cells, and this accumulation correlates well with sites of maximum pyrophosphate deposition. It has also been noted that pyrophosphate binds to macromolecules (denatured protein), which are also part of the necrotic process. Accumulation is also related to myocardial blood flow. Maximum concentration is found when myocardial blood flow drops to 30% to 40% of normal. In areas completely avascular pyrophosphate accumulation is not found. The time of maximum deposition of pyrophosphate is usually 48 to 72 hours after infarction.

Indications

1. For defining areas of myocardial infarction several days after the acute event
2. For patients whose electrocardiographic or laboratory results are equivocal
3. For patients with bundle branch blocks in whom electrocardiographic changes of infarction are difficult to interpret
4. For defining right ventricular infarction
5. For visualizing infarctions following coronary artery surgery

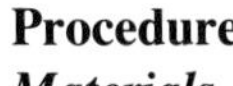

Procedure

Materials

1. Scintillation gamma camera with high-resolution, low-energy parallel-hole collimator (140 keV)
2. 15 to 20 mCi (555-740 MBq) of ^{99m}Tc stannous pyrophosphate
3. Imaging device and computer for data acquisition

Patient preparation

1. Explain the entire procedure to the patient.

Technique

1. Three hours before imaging, inject 15 to 20 mCi (555-740 MBq) of ^{99m}Tc stannous pyrophosphate intravenously.
2. With camera set for ^{99m}Tc (140 keV), place the patient in an anterior position, centering the entire left chest to the field of view.
3. Set the photographic unit for static image. Prepare the computer for data acquisition.
4. Collect 1 million counts.
5. Repeat in the left anterior oblique and left lateral views.

Interpretation (Figs. 18-51 and 18-52)

The following interpretative criteria are used in reporting pyrophosphate myocardial studies:

0 = No cardiac uptake
1+ = Diffuse cardiac region concentration less than rib concentration
2+ = Focal diffuse myocardial uptake equal to rib concentration
3+ = Myocardial uptake equal to sternal concentration
4+ = Myocardial concentration greater than sternal concentration

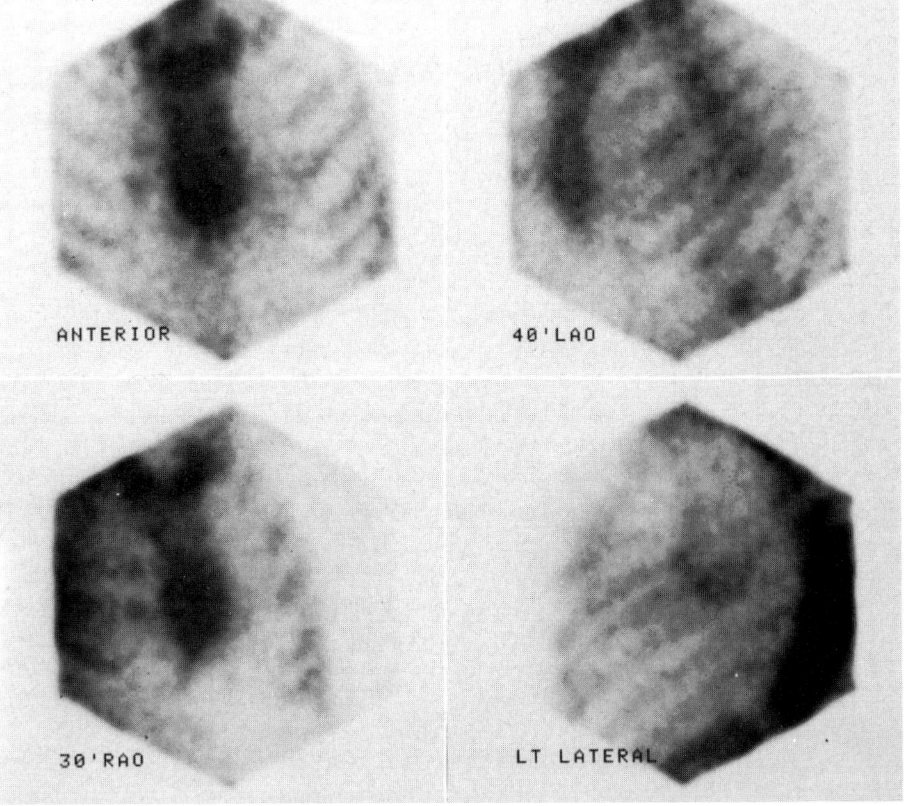

Fig. 18-51. Following intravenous administration of 15 mCi ^{99m}Tc stannous pyrophosphate, images of thorax are negative. There is no concentration of nuclide in region of myocardium.

Continued.

Fig. 18-52. Markedly abnormal PYP ^{99m}Tc images of thorax in patient with clinical and laboratory evidence of anterior wall infarction. There is 4+ increased concentration of PYP ^{99m}Tc in antero-lateral left ventricular myocardium with central region of absent activity. This halo type of concentration is compatible with a poor prognosis.

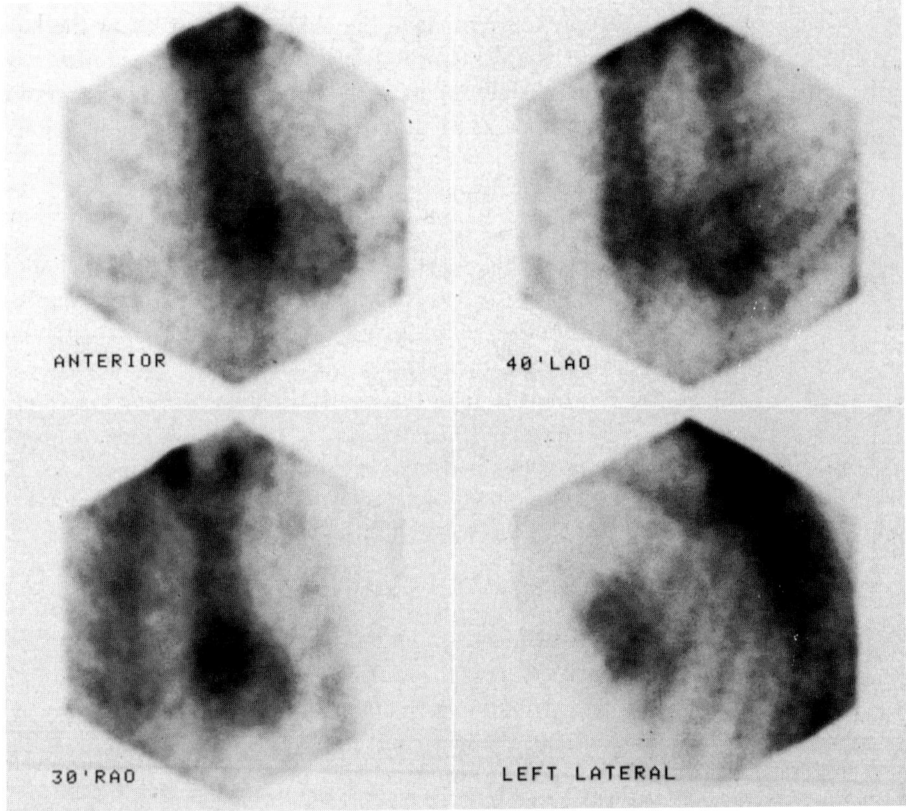

Using the classifications just given, 3 to 4+ concentrations are associated with acute transmural myocardial damage. Subendocardial infarction or chronic angina has a 2+ diffuse concentration. A 2+ relatively focal concentration is usually visualized in patients with subendocardial infarction. The 2+ diffuse pattern seen in patients with unstable angina becomes a real problem in separating subendocardial infarction from unstable angina. It has been shown pathologically that patients with unstable angina have focal areas of myocardial necrosis, although they have no laboratory evidence of myocardial damage.

In skeletal muscle damage, contusion of the myocardium, and cardiomyopathy there may be pyrophosphate accumulation. Continued concentration of pyrophosphate for prolonged periods after myocardial infarction and the doughnut sign (a ring of pyrophosphate concentration surrounding large anterior wall infarcts) are grave prognostic signs.

In the coronary care unit, selected patients may benefit from thallium imaging and 48- to 72-hour pyrophosphate imaging after admission.

LABORATORY APPLICATION

48

MONOCLONAL ANTIBODIES FOR IMAGING MYOCARDIAL NECROSIS

Ban An Khaw, Jagat Narula, Tsunehiro Yasuda, and H. William Strauss

Purpose

To date there are several myocardial infarct avid-imaging agents. The most established of these is technetium-99m-labeled pyrophosphate. However, none of these agents is optimal or totally specific for the delineation of necrotic myocardium. Although there is extensive literature describing the sensitivity and specificity of ^{99m}Tc-labeled pyrophosphate for the diagnosis of acute myocardial infarction, anomalous localization of pyrophosphate in nonnecrotic but highly ischemic myocardium has also been seen by various investigators. Localization of pyrophosphate has been reported in patients

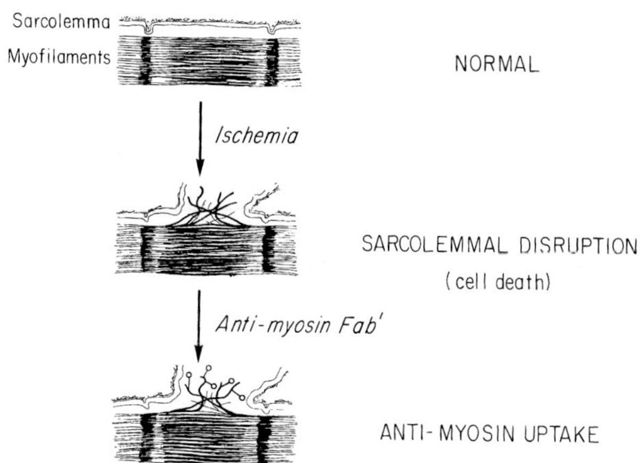

Fig. 18-53. Diagramatic representation of the concept of the binding of antimyosin to the necrotic myocytes through regions of membrane disruption. (From Khaw, B.A., et. al, Irreversible Ischemic Injury in Anoxic Cultured Myocytes. In: E.I. Chazov, et. al, Cardiology, 1984: 1135-1147, Plenum Publishing, New York.)

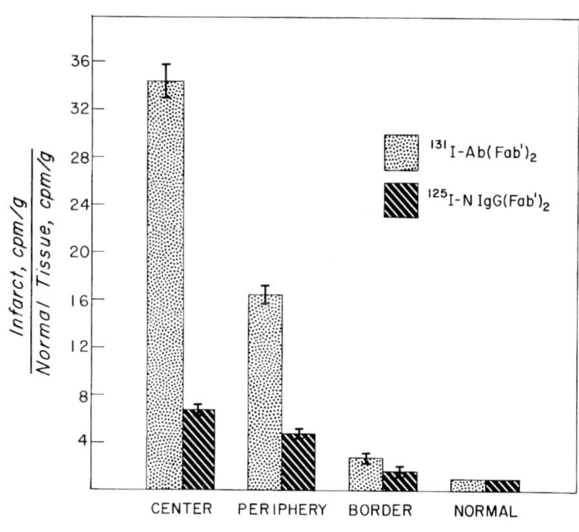

Fig. 18-54. Ratios of radioactivity (cmp/g) in test region to that in normal myocardium for I-131-Antimyosin (Fab')2 and I-125-Normal IgG (Fab')2 injected simultaneously into animals with acute experimental myocardial infarcts. The test region of the myocardium was divided into center, periphery and border zones by visual inspection of the triphenyl tetrazolium chloride stained heart slices. The differences in the ratios of radioactivity between I-131-antimyosin (Fab')2 and I-125-normal IgG (Fab')2 are highly significant ($p < 0.001$). (From Khaw B.A. et al, Early imaging of experimental myocardial infarction by intracoronary administration of 131-I-labeled anticardiac myocin (Fab')2 fragments. Circulation 58:1137, 1978. By permission of the American Heart Association, Inc.)

with stable angina without infarction and in regions of old myocardial infarcts several months after the acute episode. These observations led to the suspicion that, although pyrophosphate accumulated in necrotic myocardium, severely comprised but viable myocytes may also accumulate this agent. To develop a highly specific and sensitive method for detection of myocardial necrosis, an immunologic approach was chosen because of the exquisite specificity and high affinity of antibodies for selected target antigens. An intracellular cardiac protein, myosin, was chosen because of its abundance and immunologic specificity and because, in normal myocytes, the myosin molecules exist as myofilaments segregated from the extracellular environment by the intact cell membrane. Following myocyte necrosis, the intracellular myosin molecules are exposed to the extracellular milieu. If antibodies specific for myosin are then introduced in the extracellular fluid, the antibodies will bind to the exposed myosin in the necrotic myocardium. Once again, if these antibodies are appropriately radiolabeled, the areas of myocyte necrosis can be located by determining the areas of radioactivity (Fig. 18-53). This hypothesis is not exclusive for the detection of acute myocardial infarction. It is also applicable whenever myocyte necrosis occurs, such as in myocarditis, acute heart transplant rejection, anthracycline cardiotoxicity, Lyme carditis, rheumatic carditis, Churg-Strauss disease, and pheochromocytoma.

***Background** (Experimental)*

It has been demonstrated that localization of antimyosin is highly specific for the necrotic myocardium by various in vivo and in vitro methods. Fig. 18-54 shows that the average ratio of specific localization (determined as radioactivity in the test tissue) to radioactivity in normal posterior left ventricular myocardium was approximately 32:1. Nonspecific sequestration was only about 5:1 at 24 hr after simultaneous administration of the mixture of specific and nonspecific antibodies. The

Continued.

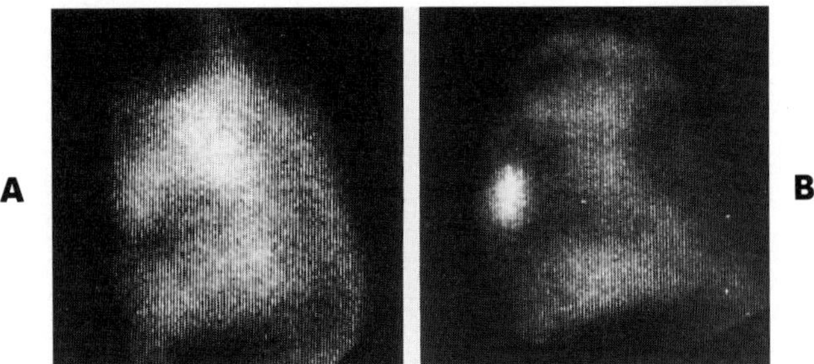

Fig. 18-55. Left lateral gamma images taken of two dogs with acute experimental myocardial infarction. **A,** Dog injected with ^{111}In labeled monoclonal antibody Fab not specific for myosin. **B,** Dog injected with ^{111}In labeled monoclonal antimyosin Fab. The images were obtained five hours after IV administration of the radiolabeled antibodies. The infarct can be clearly visualized with antimyosin Fab, whereas only blood pool can be seen with antibody Fab not specific for myosin. (From Khaw, B.A., et al, Myocardial imaging with radiolabeled monoclonal antibodies In: CJF Spry (ed.), Immunology and Molecular Biology of Cardiovascular diseases, MTP Press, Lancaster, United Kingdom, 1987.)

requirement of specificity of the antibody for successful imaging can also be demonstrated. Figure 18-55 shows that only the dog injected with monoclonal antimyosin Fab radiolabeled with ^{111}In showed unequivocal infarct localization, whereas the animal injected with a similarly radiolabeled monoclonal antibody Fab that wasn't specific for myosin showed no localization in the region of the infarct. Only blood-pool images were obtained.

Indications

1. Diagnosis and localization of acute myocardial infarction is from time of onset of chest pain to about 30 days. Although antimyosin positivity has been reported to last up to 9 months after the acute event, the intensity of uptake decreases significantly after the first 2 or 3 weeks.
2. Confirmation of acute myocardial infarction in patients with equivocal laboratory and/or electrocardiographic evidence.
3. Determination of myocardial salvage or conversely the extent of myocardial necrosis acutely after thrombolytic therapy.
4. Noninvasive diagnosis of acute myocarditis.
5. Noninvasive diagnosis of acute heart transplant rejection.
6. Diagnosis of drug-induced cardiotoxicity.
7. Diagnosis of myocyte necrosis associated with various other noncoronary artery-related cardiomyopathies such as Lyme carditis, rheumatic carditis, etc.

Procedure

Materials

1. Scintillation gamma camera with a medium-energy collimator. A gamma camera with single-photon emission computed-tomographic (SPECT) capabilities may facilitate interpretation of equivocal cases.
2. ^{111}In (indium) chloride.
3. DTPA-antimyosin Fab kits (Myoscint, Centocor, Malvern, Pa.) currently approved in Western European countries.

Patient preparation

Acquaint the patient with the procedure of a single intravenous injection on ^{111}In-labeled antimyosin Fab. At about 12 to 24 hours following intravenous injection of the ^{111}In-labeled antimyosin

Fab, the patient will be imaged for diagnosis of acute myocardial infarction. For diagnosis of myocarditis, heart transplant rejection and other noncoronary, artery-related cardiac disorders, the patient will be imaged with a gamma camera at about 44 to 52 hours after intravenous injection of the radiolabeled antibody.

Technique

1. 1.8 mCi (66.6 MBq) is prepared for intravenous administration, by addition of approximately 2 mCi (74 MBq) in 0.1 m citrate (pH 5.0) to 500 μg DTPA-antimyosin Fab in 0.2 ml of phosphate-buffered saline as supplied in the kit from Centocor. Efficiency of radiolabeling as determined by ascending thin-layer chromatography should be greater than 90% at 30 min of incubation at room temperature. At this efficiency of radiolabeling, 1.8 mCi may be withdrawn directly from the kit and administered intravenously. It has been our practice to perform skin tests before administration of the full radiolabeled antimyosin dosage. An aliquot containing 6 to 10 μg (50 to 100 μl) of the radiolabeled antibody preparation is injected subcutaneously in the forearm. If no wheal and flare reaction is observed after 15 to 30 min, the full dosage is administered. Recent studies have elected to forego skin testing because no adverse reaction to antimyosin administration has been seen in 1000 or more patients and because the practice of intradermal injection for skin testing may also function as immunization to produce human antimurine response.
2. At 12 to 24 hours for acute myocardial infarct imaging and at 44 to 54 hours for either myocarditis, acute heart transplant rejection, or other noncoronary artery related cardiomyopathy imaging, the patient is imaged using a gamma camera, preferably one with SPECT capabilities.
3. *Planar imaging*—The camera may be set for either or both at 173 and 247 keV photopeaks of ^{111}In. The camera detector head is then placed over the heart in the anterior position, and the acquisition time is set for 4 min. The data acquired may be stored digitally.
4. Repeat data acquisition in the 45-degree left anterior oblique position for the same time of acquisition (left lateral acquisition may at times expedite interpretation).
5. *SPECT*—Single-photon emission-computed tomography is completed using the smallest circle that can be circumscribed by the detector of a rotating gamma camera. A series of 60 or 120 images at 6- or 3-degree increments respectively were recorded for 30 sec each into a 128 × 128 matrix. The images are reconstructed with a filtered backprojection algorithm to transverse, sagittal, and coronal projections with a thickness of about 1 cm (3 pixels).
6. Semiquantitation of antimyosin uptake for objective diagnosis can be obtained by comparison of the ratios of the count density in the heart to that in the lungs. Count density is obtained by assigning a region of interest over the cardiac silhouette, as well as one over the right lung base or left upper-lung region by computer planimetry. Avoidance of sternal, hepatic, and on occasion rib activity regions would allow accurate assessment of the H/L ratios.

Diagnosis

Acute myocardial infarction

Localization of the radiolabeled antimyosin Fab can be easily assigned to the anterior, inferior, or posterior wall in most transmural infarcts (Fig. 18-56). However, in certain patients who underwent successful thrombolytic therapy in which the damage may be minimally patchy or subendocardial, visualization of the region of damage may be feasible at 24 hours after intravenous administration but unequivocal diagnosis is best performed from the 48-hour postantimyosin antibody administration images (Fig. 18-57). Antimyosin imaging may also be used to rule out myocardial infarction in patients who had precordial chest pain of 30 min or longer, who had a small but significant total creatine kinase enzyme elevation but who had an electrocardiogram not indicative of acute myocardial infarction (such a case is shown in Fig. 18-58). The patient shown in Fig. 18-58 was diagnosed (from the antimyosin scan) with a posterior myocardial infarction. The extent of myocyte necrosis has also been reported to be the best predictor of the prognostic outcome. Recently simultaneous dual-isotope imaging (with thallium-201– and indium-111–labeled antimyosin antibody) has been performed before discharge to differentiate ischemic from necrotic myocardium in patients with myocardial infarction. Johnson and co-workers proposed that early identification of myocardium at jeop-

Continued.

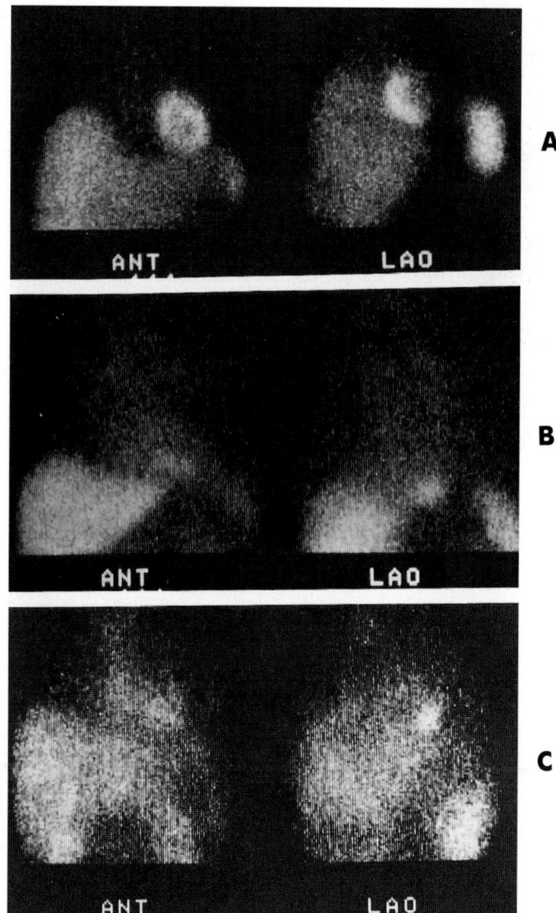

Fig. 18-56. Planar anterior and 45 degrees left anterior oblique gamma scintigraphic images of three patients with **(A)** anterior, **(B)** inferior, and **(C)** posterior acute myocardial infarction. The images were obtained approximately 24 hours after IV administration of the radiolabeled monoclonal antimyosin Fab.

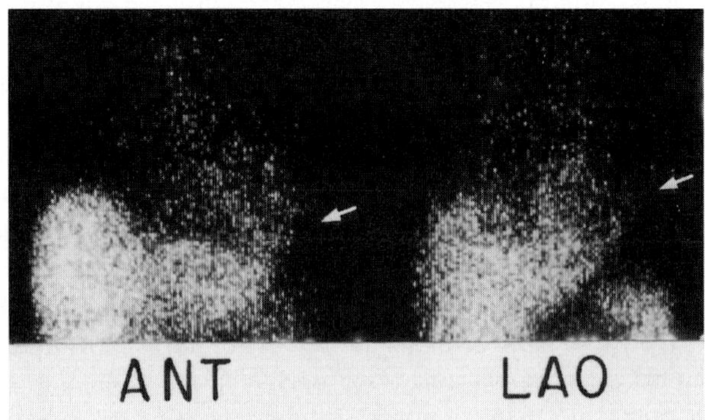

Fig. 18-57. Anterior and 45 degree LAO gamma scintigrams of a patient with an anterior myocardial infarction obtained 48 hours after antibody administration. The images show minimal, diffuse and patchy uptake of In-111 activity in the anterior myocardium *(arrows)* of the patient who underwent spontaneous reperfusion. The patient's total peak CK was 990 IU with 9% CK-MB. (From Khaw, B.A., et al, Acute myocardial infarct imaging with Indium-111-labeled monoclonal antimyosin Fab. J Nucl Med 28:1671, 1987.)

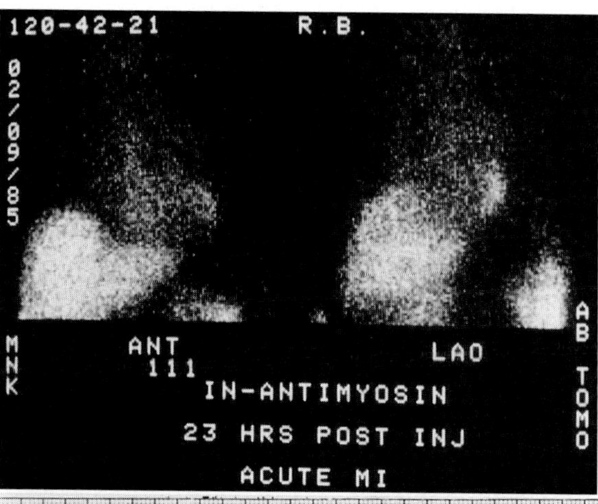

A

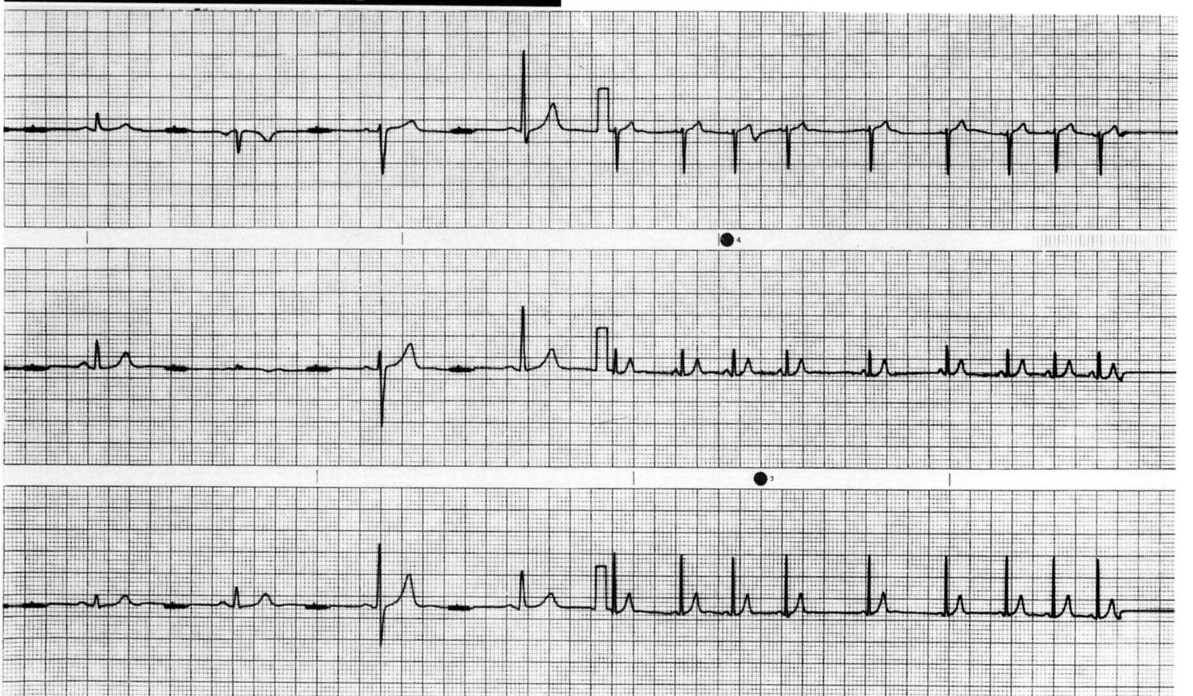

B

Fig. 18-58. A, Anterior *(left)* and 45 degree LAO *(right)* gamma scintigrams of a patient with an inferoposterior infarction. **B,** The patient's acute electrocardiogram was not diagnostic of acute myocardial infarction. (From Khaw, B.A., et al, Acute myocardial infarct imaging with Indium-111-labeled monoclonal antimyosin Fab. J Nucl Med 28:1671, 1987.)

ardy would facilitate early intervention in these patients. Antimyosin uptake corresponding exactly to thallium-deficient zone indicates necrotic zone. On the other hand, the area of mismatch between the two radio tracer delineation represents the ischemic myocardium. An overlap is indicative of an admixture of viable and necrotic myocardial tissues, which may be subject to further ischemic insult. Patients who were not reperfused demonstrated either a match or a mismatch pattern, while patients who underwent successful thrombolysis showed an overlap or a match pattern. Patients with a match pattern followed an event-free course. Since simultaneous SPECT imaging with thallium and antimyosin can provide landmarks for reference of the LV territory, identification of antimyosin uptake in the right ventricle also became feasible.

Acute myocarditis

The definition of acute myocarditis requires myocyte necrosis as well as white-cell infiltration. The current gold standard for diagnosis of acute myocarditis is ventricular endomyocardial biopsy with subsequent histopathologic examination by an experienced pathologist. The method is invasive and lacks sensitivity. Therefore, a method that is noninvasive and more sensitive would be highly desirable. Since myocyte necrosis is a prerequisite for diagnosis of acute myocarditis, antimyosin

Continued.

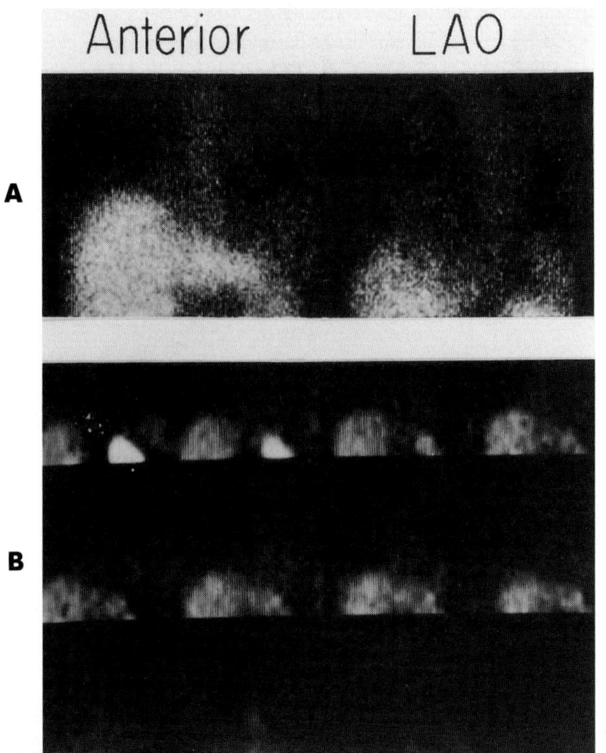

Fig. 18-59. A negative ^{111}In antimyosin image. No tracer accumulation is seen in the region of the myocardium in either **(A)** the planer images or **(B)** the coronal tomographic reconstruction. (From T. Yasuda, et al, Indium-111 monoclonal antimyosin antibody imaging in the diagnosis of acute myocarditis. Circulation 76:306, 1987. (By permission of the American Heart Association, Inc.)

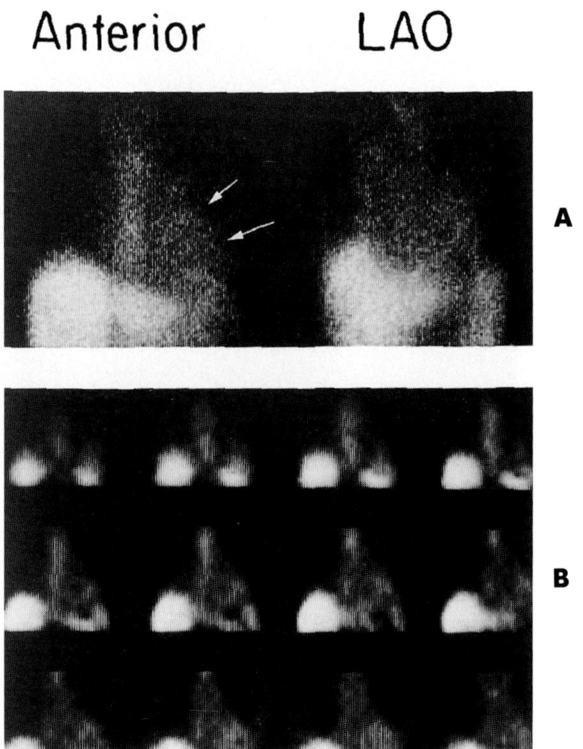

Fig. 18-60. A positive antimyosin image. Diffuse uptake in the cardiac region is seen in **(A)** the planar images and **(B)** the coronal tomographic reconstructions. (From T. Yasuda, et al, Indium-111 monoclonal antimyosin antibody imaging in the diagnosis of acute myocarditis. Circulation 76:306, 1987. (By permission of the American Heart Association.)

Fab should also localize in the myocarditic hearts. Thus a noninvasive method may be available for diagnosis of myocarditis. Figure 18-59 shows negative images where no radio tracer concentration is seen in the region of the myocardium 48 hours after intravenous administration of ^{111}In-labeled antimyosin Fab. This patient also showed negative results for myocarditis from the biopsy data. However, Fig. 18-60 shows significant tracer concentration in the region of the myocardium of a patient with a positive biopsy for myocarditis. Although unequivocal positive scans are easy to read, borderline positive cases may require SPECT tomographic analyses to differentiate minimal residual blood-pool activity from myocardial activity. Studies by Carrio and colleagues indicated that the use of heart-to-lung count-density ratios obtained by computer planimetry can provide a semiquantitative diagnostic alternative to subjective interpretation of either the planar or SPECT images. A cutoff point of 1.55 was used by these investigators. Multiple administration of the monoclonal antimyosin Fab for diagnostic purposes appears to be safe. To date, patients have been injected several times without any adverse reactions or antimurine Fab antibody activity. Myocarditis frequently presents as acute onset of dilated cardiomyopathy. In a recent report of the diagnostic accuracy of antimyosin scintigraphy in such a subset of patients, a negative scan was almost always associated with a biopsy-negative result for myocarditis. On the other hand, all patients with biopsy-verified myocarditis had positive antimyosin scans. However, there were many patients with positive antimyosin scans who had negative biopsies. This discordance may be the result of the insensitivity of the biopsy procedure or the occurrence of myocyte necrosis without inflammation in dilated cardiomyopathy resulting from subendocardial ischemia in dilated hearts. Whatever the explanation, it has been demonstrated that patients with positive scans have more likelihood of improvement in their left ventricular systolic function over time regardless of the biopsy results as compared with those patients with negative antimyosin scans. Furthermore, occasionally myocarditis can present with chest pain mimicking acute myocardial infarction. Recurrent or intractable episodes of chest pain in spite of optimal therapy continue to occur in these patients. Coronary angiography is required for possible intervention or for the exclusion of coronary artery disease. Normal coronary artery anatomy usually leads to the discharge of the patient from the hospital without a definitive diagnosis. Antimyosin scintigraphy in this clinical context can offer a discriminatory test. Typical diffuse, faint, and global uptake in the myocardium would denote myocarditis, whereas localized antimyosin uptake in a coronary vascular territory would denote an acute myocardial infarction.

In rare instances, life-threatening ventricular tachyarrhythmias or sudden cardiac death can be the first and only manifestation of myocarditis. In such cases, myocarditis has been reported only at necropsy. Antimyosin scintigraphy may identify such patients even when the left ventricular function is still preserved.

Heart transplant rejection

Similar to the noninvasive diagnosis of acute myocarditis, the diagnosis of acute heart transplant rejection required biopsy evidence of white-cell infiltration and myocyte necrosis. Therefore, the application of radiolabeled antimyosin Fab for the diagnosis of acute rejection of heart transplants should be feasible. Adonizzio and co-workers have reported imaging of rejecting heterotopically transplanted hearts in dogs with ^{111}In-labeled antimyosin Fab. First et al reported the first clinical application of ^{111}In-labeled monoclonal antimyosin Fab for noninvasive diagnosis of acute heart transplant rejection. A surprising observation was the basal level of antibody activity in all transplanted hearts. This activity was greater than the possible residual blood-pool activity that might remain. However, concurrent with the episode of acute rejection, the intensity of ^{111}In antimyosin Fab localization increased. Recently Ballester and colleagues demonstrated that antimyosin studies ($n = 97$) performed on acute heart transplant patients were positive when the scans were performed between 1 and 3 months after transplantation (H/L = 1.95 ± 0.7). The H/L ratios decreased with time and by 24 months showed near normalization (1.58 ± 0.2). There were different patterns of antimyosin positivity in the transplant patients. The decreasing pattern of antimyosin uptake was associated with clinical course free of complications related to rejection. However, the persistent or increasing pattern of antimyosin uptake (H/L) were consistent with the potential of rejection-related complications. Furthermore, these investigators noted that there appear to be no sudden bouts of rejection episodes by antimyosin uptake criteria, but rejection appears to be a steady-state activity that usually decreased with time. This phenomenon of gradual unresponsiveness to the graft has been referred to as *tolerance*. Although dependence on H/L ratios has standardized the semiquantitative diagnosis of myocardial necrosis associated with transplant rejection and other noncoronary artery-related cardiac disorders, blind acceptance of the heart-to-lung ratio may lead to erroneous diagnosis especially in immunocompromised patients with accompanying pulmonary infections. Thus it appears that antimyosin imaging may be of assistance in noninvasive assessment of the degree of allograft rejection as well as for the identification of patients who are likely to develop tolerance.

Doxorubicin cardiotoxicity

Doxorubicin is an effective chemotherapeutic agent used alone or in combination for treatment of breast cancer, lymphomas, and various solid tumors. The efficacy of doxorubicin depends on the cumulative dose but is limited by the appearance of cardiac toxicity. Doxorubicin cardiotoxicity is currently evaluated by serial measurements of the left ventricular ejection fraction or by performance of sequential endomyocardial biopsies. The role of antimyosin scintigraphy has recently been reported for early recognition of cardiomyocyte damage inflicted by doxorubicin. Antimyosin uptake has been demonstrated to precede systolic dysfunction. Significant antimyosin uptake was observed at intermediate cumulative doxorubicin doses when left ventricular systolic function was still maintained. There was a direct correlation between the dose of doxorubicin and the magnitude of myocyte damage as reflected by antimyosin uptake. Furthermore, patients with greater myocardial antimyosin antibody uptake had higher likelihood of developing congestive failure at maximal doxorubicin dosage. Also, patients treated with continuous doxorubicin infusion had less antimyosin uptake than those treated with bolus administration at all levels of comparison. Currently we cannot recommend antimyosin scintigraphy for the detection of doxorubicin toxicity because almost all pa-

Continued.

tients at intermediate cumulative dosage have a positive scan and they cannot be withdrawn from the therapy based on antimyosin positivity. However, greater antimyosin uptake at the intermediate dose may predict possible systolic dysfunction at the maximal dose. Such patients may benefit from continuous infusion of the drug.

Cardiac involvement in systemic disorders

Structural and functional cardiac abnormalities are integral components of various systemic disorders. Systemic manifestations usually dominate clinical presentation, and myocardial lesions are often identified as incidental abnormalities at necropsy. Occasionally, cardiac involvement presents as electrocardiographic abnormalities, arrhythmias, or congestive heart failure. In these clinical situations, early recognition of cardiac involvement before the onset of overt heart disease may have significant therapeutic and prognostic implications. Since myocyte necrosis or degeneration with or without inflammatory cellular infiltration may be the underlying cardiac pathologic condition in these disorders, antimyosin antibody imaging may be useful in the recognition of the cardiac involvement. Positive antimyosin scans have been reported in various systemic disorders such as Lyme disease, rheumatic fever, Churg-Strauss disease, and pheochromocytoma. These reports have been studied in patients with systemic disorders who had overt cardiac involvement. Additional studies are required in patients without clinically obvious cardiac involvement, to establish the diagnostic value of this test for detection of similar injury before the development of symptoms or signs of cardiac disease.

LABORATORY APPLICATION

49

VENOGRAPHY: DORSAL VEIN PROCEDURE

D. Bruce Sodee

Purpose

The purpose of this study is to visualize the deep venous system of the lower extremity as well as the internal iliacs. By using ^{99m}Tc-labeled MAA or ^{99m}Tc HAM, the lung may also be imaged to help establish or rule out pulmonary embolization.

Procedure

Materials

1. Scintillation gamma camera with 140 keV parallel-hole collimator
2. Area scan
3. ^{99m}Tc MAA, 2 to 3 mCi
4. Two- or three-way stopcocks
5. Four tourniquets applied above the ankles and knees so that the dose seeks a deep venous system
6. Butterflies, 20- to 21-gauge
7. Normal saline solution dose (2 to 3 ml) for flushing intravenous tubing

Patient preparation

1. No special preparation is required.
2. Explain the entire procedure to the patient.

Technique

1. Insert a 21-gauge butterfly into the dorsal vein of each foot. Flush with a small amount of saline solution.
2. Connect the stopcocks, MAA syringes, and saline solution syringes to the tubing.
3. Place the patient with his feet at the lower edge of the table and centered to the camera.
4. Set the area scan controls and recording devices. The distance should be enough to travel from the feet to the midabdomen (approximately 130 cm).
5. Set the area scan speed to 64 cm/min.
6. Apply tourniquets at the ankles and just below the knees.
7. Start the camera and inject MAA in approximately 5 to 10 seconds. Immediately follow with

saline solution injection and close stopcocks. There is a short delay after starting the camera before it begins imaging.

8. When the camera reaches the level of the knees, reduce the speed to 48 cm/min.
9. Reduce the speed to 16 cm/min for the pelvis and abdomen.
10. When the image is complete, remove the tourniquets.
11. Perform a 1000K anterior view of the lungs with the patient in the supine position.
12. During the lung image, instruct the patient to exercise the lower extremities.
13. Repeat the area scan of the legs at 120 cm/min.
14. Photograph all images.
15. Remove the butterflies from the patient.

Interpretation

The nuclear image of the deep venous system of the leg lacks the resolution or the anatomic surety that normal channels have been filled. However, thrombosis of any part of the deep venous system is usually portrayed by radionuclide venography, and abnormal collateral circulation is displayed. Partially occlusive thrombi are usually not visualized on the first-pass study. The delayed image of the extremities has the ability to visualize as hot spots the adherence of particulate matter or microspheres to the clot or damaged endothelium.

With inadequate tourniquet application the superficial venous system may be enhanced, thus clouding the interpretation of the deep venous system. The radiopharmaceutical may be delayed at the valves of the deep venous system, causing a false positive result.

LABORATORY APPLICATION

50

VENOGRAPHY: EQUILIBRIUM ^{99m}Tc RED CELL PROCEDURE

D. Bruce Sodee

Purpose

The majority of blood volume in the lower extremities is found in the deep venous system of the leg. Using the same equilibrium technique as that employed in gated cardiac studies, ^{99m}Tc-tagged red-cell images of the lower extremities give an excellent depiction of the deep as well as the superficial venous system. The large deep venous system (iliacs, femorals, popliteals, and saphenous veins) is visualized without difficulty, and the smaller deep venous system of the calf may be also visualized employing the high-resolution cameras available today. This noninvasive technique requires injection of ^{99m}Tc in the upper extremity, eliminating the discomfort and difficulty associated with the injection of the dorsal veins of the feet. Blockade, partial blockade, and collateral flow in the venous system may be established. A valuable part of the study is viewing arterial perfusion to the area of interest (thigh or calf) following the injection of ^{99m}Tc, and this aids in the diagnosis of acute thrombophlebitis.

Procedure

Materials

1. Scintillation gamma camera with high-resolution, low-energy parallel-hole collimator (140 keV), and area scan
2. Imaging device and computer for data acquisition
3. 20 mCi of ^{99m}Tc pertechnetate, 1.0 ml of stannous pyrophosphate for in vivo labeling of patient's red cells

Patient preparation

1. No special preparation is required.
2. Explain the entire procedure to the patient.

Technique

1. Twenty to thirty minutes after the intravenous administration of stannous pyrophosphate, position the patient's lower extremity in preparation for the flow study (should be performed in the area of pain, inflammation, or redness).

Continued.

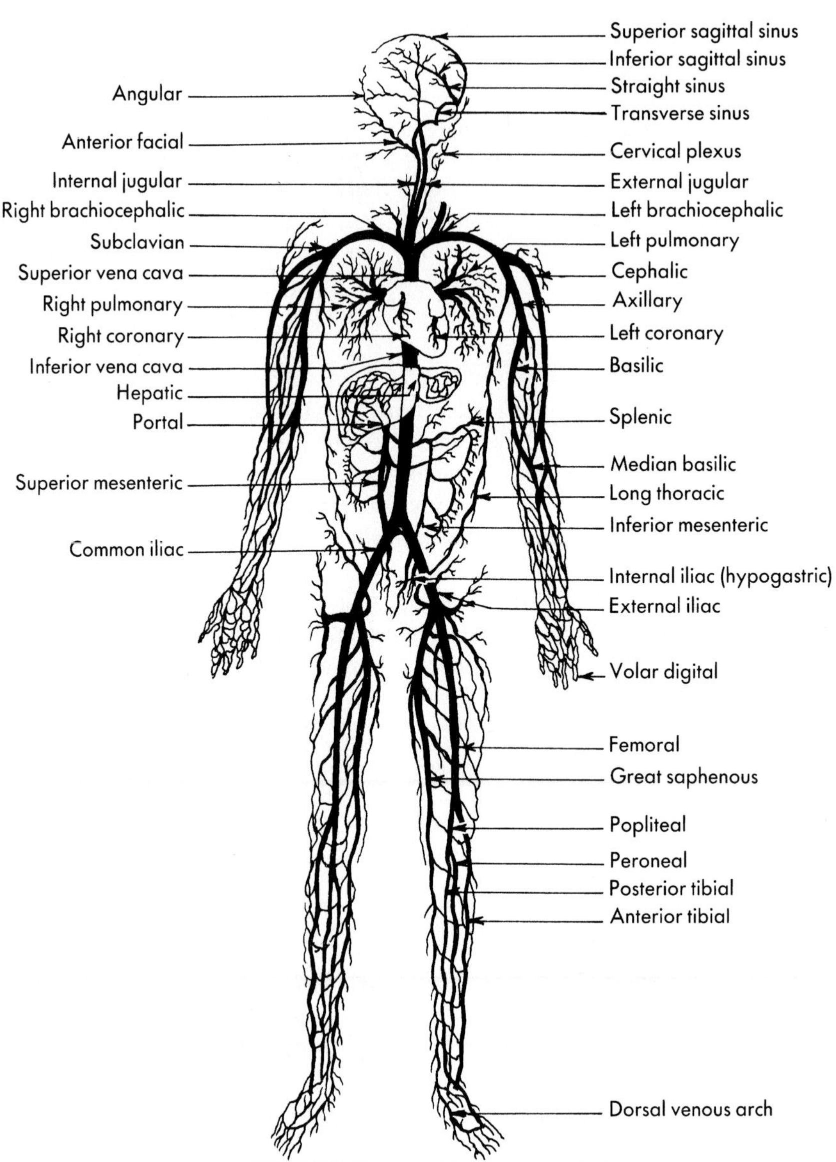

Fig. 18-61. Normal whole-body venous anatomy, anteriorly. (From Austrin, M.G., and Austrin, H.R.: Learning Medical Terminology, A worktext, ed.7, St. Louis, 1991, Mosby-Year Book, Inc.)

2. Set the camera for the proper window (140 keV).
3. Prepare the computer and photographic device for 60 1-second sequential images. Set the proper orientation. Press reset count and time.
4. Inject 20 mCi of ^{99m}Tc pertechnetate intravenously.
5. Begin imaging 8 to 10 seconds after administering the dose.
6. Immediately following the flow study, begin whole-body images, anteriorly and posteriorly of femorals, popliteals, calves, and feet (set the area scan speed to 15 to 20 cm counts/min).
7. If static images are acquired, accumulate 1000K for each static image both anteriorly and posteriorly of femoral, popliteals, calves, and feet.

Interpretation (Figs. 18-61 to 18-63)

Using a partial whole-body or static imaging technique of the venous system of the lower extremities gives excellent resolution of the deep venous system and collateral circulation. Combined with the initial perfusion images of the region of interest (either the thigh or calf region), information as to the amount of inflammation in the region can be obtained and is extremely helpful in establishing diagnosis of acute thrombophlebitis.

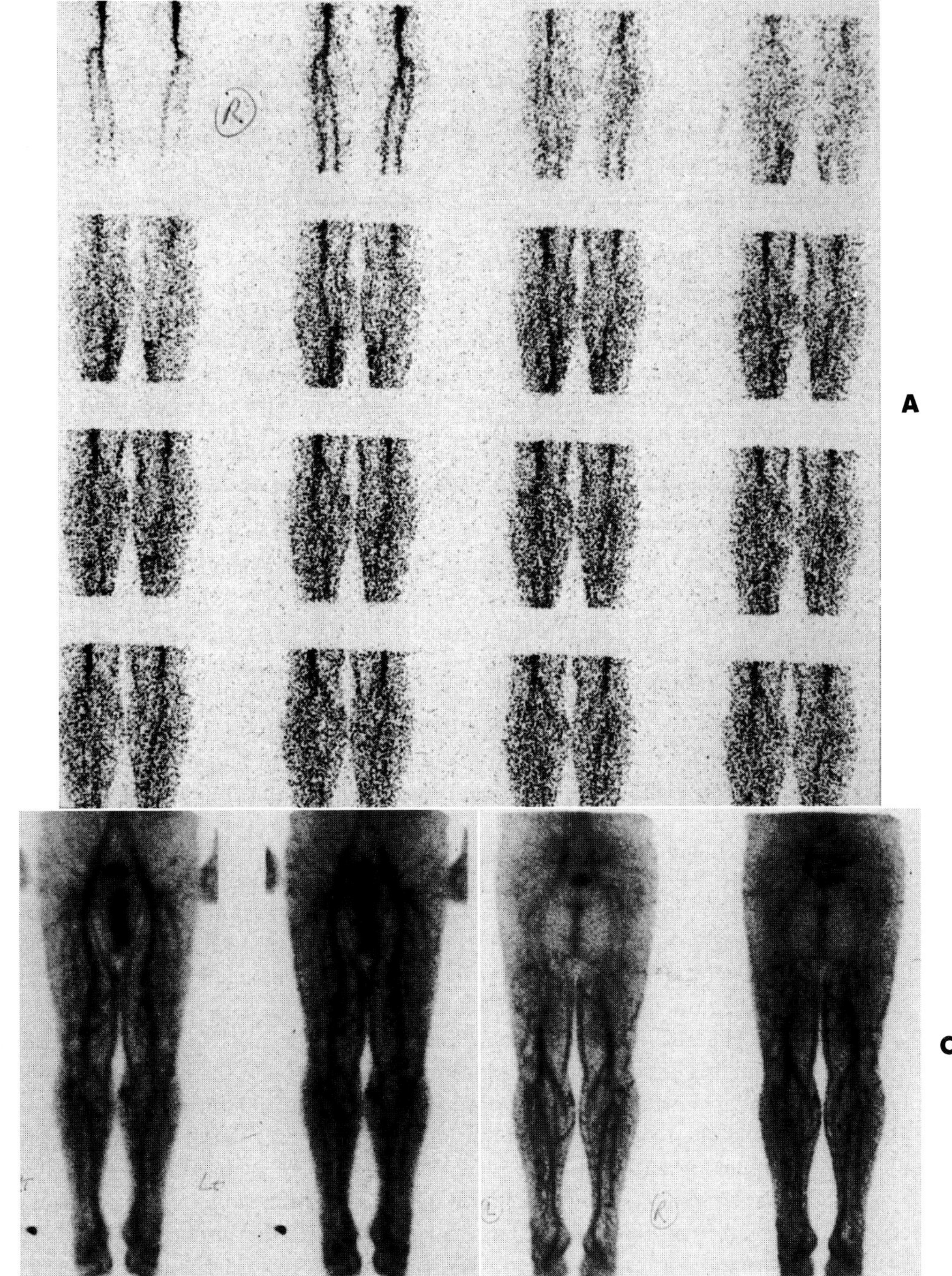

Fig. 18-62. Normal visualization of venous system in lower extremities following injection of 200 mCi of sodium pertechnetate. Thirty minutes before, patient is given 1.0 ml stannous pyrophosphate, which tagged red blood cells. In vivo tag then takes place with ^{99m}Tc and PYP-tagged red blood cells, giving ^{99m}Tc-labeled red blood cells. **A,** Four-second posterior sequential image perfusion study of lower extremities is normal. **B,** Lower half of body venous anatomy, anterior view. **C,** Posterior venous anatomy.

Continued.

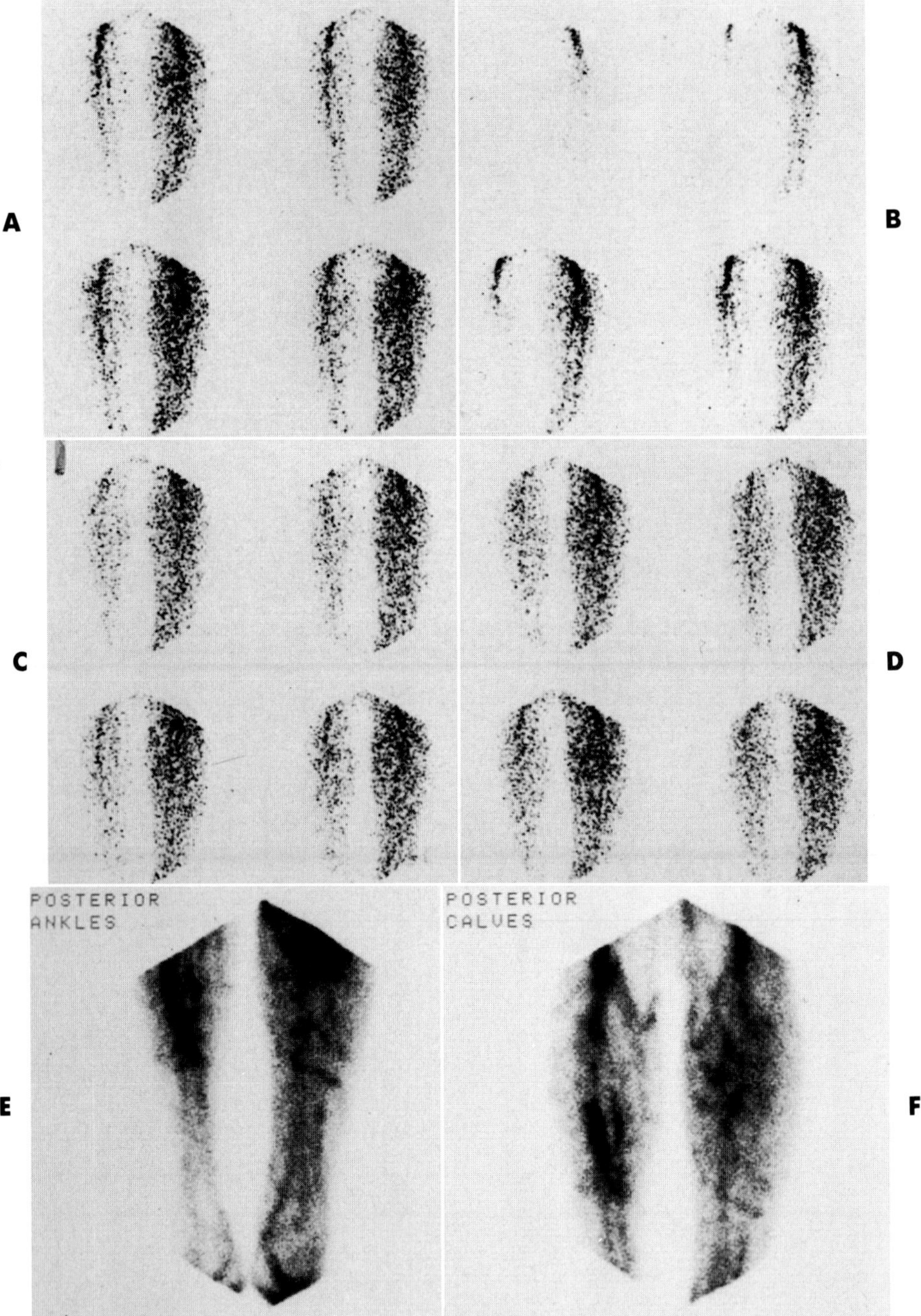

Fig. 18-63. Abnormal visualization of venous system in lower extremities following injection of 20 mCi of sodium pertechnetate. Thirty minutes before, patient is given 1.0 ml stannous pyrophosphate intravenously. Diagnosis is thrombophlebitis of right lower extremity. **A** to **D,** Four-second sequential images perfusion study of lower extremities is abnormal. Increase in flow down right lower extremity as compared to left. **E** and **F,** Posterior static images of ankle and calf regions reveal normal vascular structure in the left leg. Right leg reveals absence in flow in anterior tibial vein laterally with corresponding collateral flow throughout right calf. Edema is noted in right calf when comparing its size to left calf.

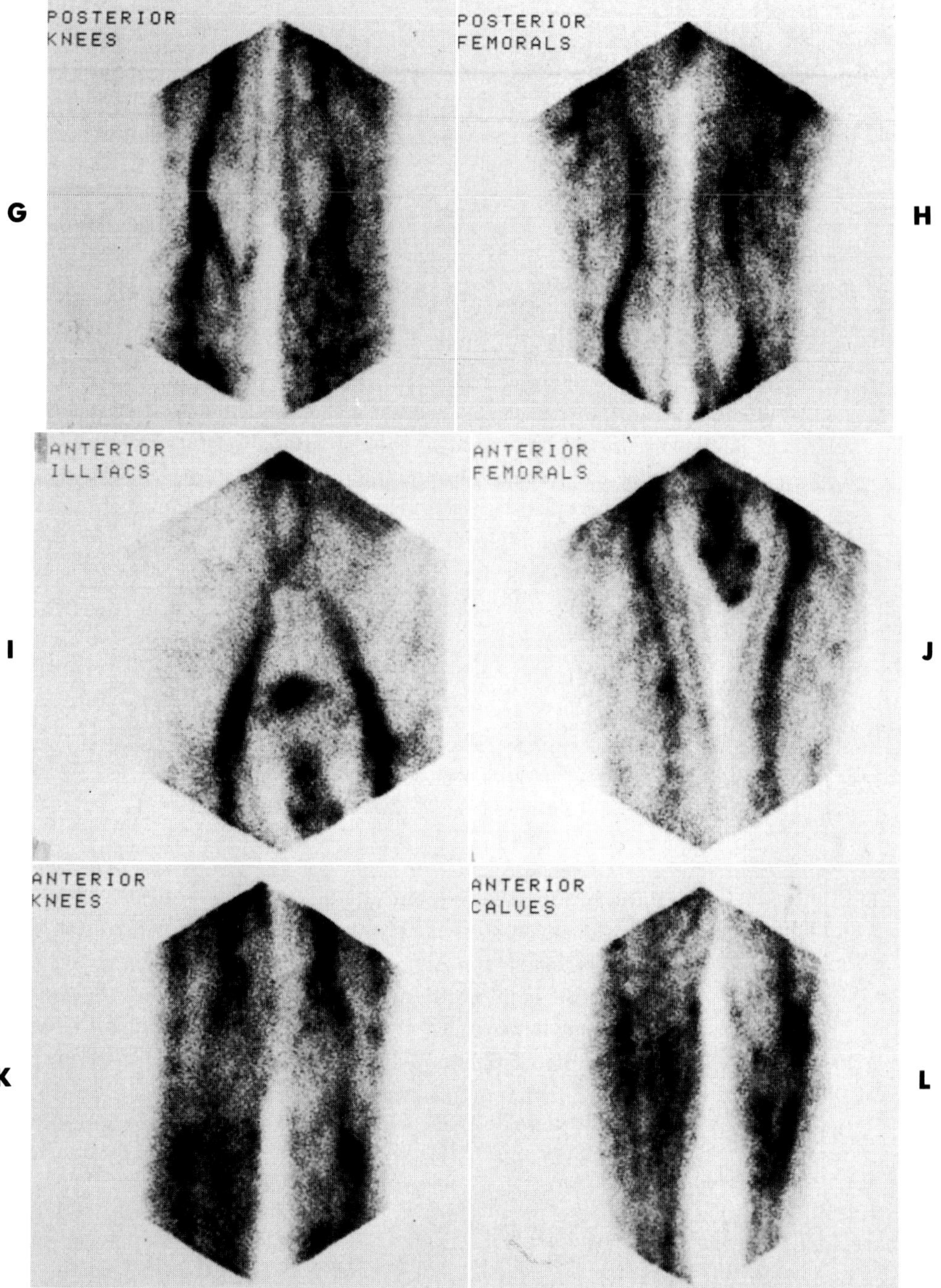

Fig. 18-63, cont'd. G, Posterior static image in region of knees shows decrease in flow of right popliteal vein when compared to left. **H,** Posterior static images of femoral vein laterally with greater saphenous vein along medical border of thighs. **I,** Anterior static image of iliac veins as they pass through pelvis. Bladder uptake and vascular flow to penis can be seen. **J,** Anterior static image of femoral veins with corresponding branches. **K,** Anterior static images of knees. **L,** Anterior static image of calves showing extensive collateral perfusion throughout right calf.

Continued.

The quality of information obtained on the venous image of the lower extremity is initially confusing, since the superficial and the deep venous systems are demonstrated. It is therefore important that the interpreter keep an image of the deep venous system (particularly of the calf) sharply in mind. Thrombi are not visualized; however, the decrease in flow in the venous system or the obstruction to the deep venous system is readily apparent and is comparable to radiographic venography information. Increased perfusion can be visualized during the arterial injection phase and thus provides significant information for the diagnosis of acute thrombophlebitis. This information cannot be obtained from the radiographic venography. On either partial whole-body or spot-images, the adequacy of flow in the inferior vena cava may also be ascertained.

LABORATORY APPLICATION

51

THROMBUS LOCALIZATION: ^{125}I FIBRINOGEN

D. Bruce Sodee

Purpose

This study is performed to localize fresh thrombus formation in the extremities. As fibrinogen takes part in clot formation, the labeled fibrinogen will be incorporated into freshly formed clots. This makes possible the early detection of thrombi in the extremities.

Procedure

Materials

1. 100 μCi of ^{125}I fibrinogen in approximately 1 mg of fibrinogen
2. Hand-held scintillation detector
3. Linear graph paper

Patient preparation

1. Block the thyroid with 8 to 10 drops of Lugol's solution. This may be administered just before beginning the study.
2. Explain the entire procedure to the patient.

Technique

1. Give the patient 100 μCi of ^{125}I fibrinogen intravenously.
2. Take the counts once on the day of injection and every day thereafter for 7 days. This may be extended to 2 weeks for high-risk patients, but a second injection may be required after 7 days because of in vivo survival of fibrinogen.
3. The patient should be recumbent with the leg to be scanned elevated 15 degrees for 5 minutes before monitoring. This decreases venous pooling and gives better access to the calf of the leg.
4. Each leg should be marked in 2-inch segments extending from the middle of the inguinal ligament down the thigh, following the femoral vein to the posterior portion of the knee and then following the widest portion of the calf and ending at a point just posterior to the internal malleolus of the ankle. Use an indelible marker on the patient's legs to reproduce counts daily. Each site can be given a number, starting with number 1 in the inguinal region.
5. Record the counts over the heart daily, and use this as a reference count.
6. Divide each leg count by the heart count and record the percent uptake. A rate meter calibrated to read 100% when placed over the heart may also be used. The detector is then held over the leg sites and gives a reading expressed in percent.
7. On a daily basis plot the percent uptake versus the site of uptake on linear graph paper.

Key points

1. If a thrombus is indicated, daily counting can be continued to determine whether the thrombus is increasing in size or dissolving or to assess the effect of therapy.
2. The condition of the patient's legs should be noted. Surgical procedures, ulcers, hematomas, arthritis, and fracture can give false positive results because of fibrinous deposits. Radiopaque venography may also cause inflammation of the vein, leading to false positive results.

3. A major difficulty is detecting thrombi forming in the upper thighs because of attenuation of ^{125}I fibrinogen by overlying tissue and of scatter from ^{125}I in the bladder.
4. This test is only positive in an actively forming thrombus. Well-established thrombi may be missed.

Interpretation

Normal studies demonstrate a gradual decrease in percent from the inguinal ligament down to the ankle. A slight increase may be seen over the knee. These readings do not increase on subsequent days.

Abnormal studies are indicated by an increase of 15% to 20% over a site from the previous day and a persistence of these counts during the next 24 hours. Thrombophlebitis may be indicated when there is a difference in uptake in comparison with the same site on the opposite leg, adjacent sites, or earlier uptake over the same site. Thrombi in the proximal femoral-pelvic region will not be identified because of the high background in this region.

This procedure is of questionable cost-effectiveness because of the time devoted to the study and the large group of patients in the hospital who are prone to venous thrombosis. In those diseases or in surgical procedures known to be a factor in venous thrombosis, many physicians by treating their patients with low-dose heparin therapy are apparently decreasing the incidence of this complication with minimum adverse effects.

BIBLIOGRAPHY

General references

Guyton, A.G.: Textbook of medical physiology, ed. 8, Philadelphia, 1990, W.B. Saunders Co.

Hurst, J.W., editor: The heart—arteries and veins, ed. 8, New York, 1993, McGraw-Hill, Inc.

Thibodeau, G.A. and Patton, K.T.: Anthony's textbook of anatomy and physiology, ed. 14, St. Louis, 1994, Mosby–Year Book.

First-pass radionuclide angiography

Bonow, R.O., Picone, A.L., McIntosh, C.L., Jones, M., and others: Survival and functional results after valve replacement for aortic regurgitation from 1976 to 1983: impact of preoperative left ventricular function, Circulation 72:1244, 1985.

Corbett, J.R., Dehmer, G.J., Lewis, S.E., Woodward, W., and others: The prognostic value of submaximal exercise testing with radionuclide ventriculography before hospital discharge in patients with recent myocardial infarction, Circulation 64:535, 1981.

DePace, N.L., Iskandrian, A.S., Hakki, A., Kane, S.A., Segal, B.L., and others: Value of left ventricular ejection fraction during exercise in predicting the extent of coronary artery disease, JACC 1(4):1002, 1983.

Dymond, D.S., Elliot, A.T., Platman, P.W., and others: The clinical validation of gold-195m: a new short half-life radiopharmaceutical for rapid sequential, first-pass angiography in patients, JACC 2:85, 1983.

Gal, R., Grenier, R., Carpenter, J., Schmidt, D.H., and Port, S.C.: High count rate first-pass radionuclide angiography using a digital gamma camera, J. Nucl. Med. 27:198, 1986.

Gal, R., Grenier, R., Schmidt, D.H., and Port, S.: Count-based left ventricular volume measurement without blood sampling or attenuation correction from first-pass radionuclide angiography, J. Nucl. Med. 27(6):912, 1986b (abstract).

Gal, R., Grenier, R.P., Schmidt, D.H., and Port, S.C.: Background correction in first-pass radionuclide angiography: a comparison of several approaches, J. Nucl. Med. 27:1480, 1986c.

Holman, B.L., Neirinckx, R.D., Treves, S., and Tow, D.E.: Cardiac imaging with tantalum-178, Radiology 131:525, 1979.

Johnson, L.L., Rodney, R.A., Vaccarino, R.A., Egbe, P., Wasserman, L., Esser, P.D., Posniakoff, T.A., and Seldin, D.W.: Left ventricular perfusion and performance from a single radiopharmaceutical and one camera, J. Nucl. Med. 33(7):1411-1416, 1992.

Jones, R.H., McEwan, P., Newman, G.E., Port, S., and others: Accuracy of diagnosis of coronary artery disease by radionuclide measurement of left ventricular function during rest and exercise, Circulation 64:586, 1981.

Jones, R.H., Floyd, R.D., Austin, E.H., and Sabiston, D.C.: The role of radionuclide angiocardiography in the preoperative prediction of pain relief and prolonged survival following coronary artery bypass grafting, Ann. Surg. 197(6):743, 1983.

Konishi, Y., Tatsuta, N., Hikasa, Y., Tamoki, N., Ishii, Y., and Torizuka, K.: Assessment of severity of tricuspid regurgitation by analog computer analysis of dilution curves recorded by scintillation camera, Jap. Circ. J. 4(11):1147-1153, 1982.

Lacy, J.L., Verani, M., Ball, M., Boyce, T., Gibson, R., and Roberts, R.: First-pass radionuclide angiography using a multiwire gamma camera and tantalum-178, J. Nucl. Med. 29(3):293, 1988.

Marshall, R.C., Berger, H.J., Costin, J.C., Freedman, G.S., and others: Assessment of cardiac performance with quantitative radionuclide angiography, Circulation 56:820, 1977.

Narahara, K.A., Mena, I., Maublant, J.C., Brizendine, M., and Criley, J.M.: Simultaneous maximum exercise radionuclide angiography and thallium stress perfusion imaging, Am. J. Cardiol. 53:812, 1984.

Philippe, L., Mena, I., Darcourt, J., and French, W.J.: Evaluation of valvular regurgitation by factor analysis of first-pass angiography, J. Nucl. Med. 29:159-167, 1988.

Port, S., Cobb, F.R., Coleman, R.E., and Jones, R.H.: Effect of age on the response of the left ventricular ejection fraction to exercise, N. Engl. J. Med. 303:1133, 1980.

Port, S.C., Oshima, M., Ray, G., McNamee, P., and Schmidt, D.H.: Assessment of single vessel coronary artery disease: results of exercise electrocardiography, thallium-201 myocardial perfusion imaging and radionuclide angiography, JACC 6:75, 1985.

Pryor, D.B., Harrell, F.E., Lee, K.L., Rosati, R.A., Coleman, R.E., Cobb, F.R., Califf, R.M., and Jones, R.H.: Prognostic indicators from radionuclide angiography in medically treated patients with coronary artery disease, Am. J Cardiol. 53:18, 1984.

Schad, N.: Nontraumatic assessment of left ventricular wall motion and regional stroke volume after myocardial infarction, J. Nucl. Med. 18:333, 1977.

Schad, N., Andrews, E.J., and Fleming, J.W.: Colour Atlas of First Pass Functional Imaging of the Heart, Hingham, 1985, MTP Press Ltd.

Strauss, H.W., Zaret, B.E., Hurley, P.J., Natarajan, T.K., and Pitt, B.: A scintiphotographic method for measuring left ventricular ejection fraction in man without cardiac catheterization, Am. J. Cardiol. 28:575, 1971.

Treves, S., Cheng, C., Samuel, A., Lambrecht, R., and others: Iridium-191 angiocardiography for the detection and quantitation of left-to-right shunting, J. Nucl. Med. 21:1151, 1980.

Equilibrium gated radionuclide ventriculogram

Abdulmassih, S.I., Jaekyeong, H., Segal, B.L., and Askenase, A.: Left ventricular diastolic function: evaluation by radionuclide angiography, Am. Heart J. 115:924-929, 1988.

Arrington, E.R., Hartshorne, M.F., Eisenberg, B., and others: The two-view radionuclide ventriculogram: advantages of the LPO view, Clin. Nucl. Med. 17:371-374, 1992.

Ahnve, S., Gilpin, E., Henning, H., and others: Limitations and advantages of the ejection fraction for defining high risk after acute myocardial infarction, Am. J. Cardiol. 58:872-878, 1986.

Bacharach, S.L., Green, M.V., Vitale, D., and others: Optimum Fourier filtering of cardiac data: a minimum error method, J. Nucl. Med. 24:1176-1184, 1983.

Baker, J.B., Shubao, C., Clarke, S.E., and others: Radionuclide measurement of right ventricular function in atrial septal defect, ventricular septal defect and complete transposition of the great arteries, Am. J. Cardiol. 57:1142-1146, 1986.

Betocchi, S., Bonow, R.O., Bacharach, S.L., and others: Isovolumic relaxation period in hypertrophic cardiomyopathy: assessment by radionuclide angiography, JACC 7:74-81, 1986.

Bhargava, V., Slutsky, R., Costello, D., and others: Peak rate of left ventricular ejection by a gated radionuclide technique: correlation with contrast angiography, J. Nucl. Med. 22:506-509, 1981.

Bonow, R.O., Frederick, T.M., Bacharach, S.L., and others: Atrial systole and left ventricular filling in hypertrophic cardiomyopathy: effect of verapamil, Am. J. Cardiol. 51:1386-1391, 1983.

Bonow, R.O., Rosing, D.R., Bacharach, S.L., and others: Effects of verapamil on left ventricular systolic function and diastolic filling in patients with hypertrophic cardiomyopathy, Circulation 64:787-796, 1981.

Borer, J.S., Miller, D., Schreiber, T., and others: Radionuclide cineangiography in acute myocardial infarction: role in prognostication, Semin. Nucl. Med. 17(2):89-94, 1987.

Boykin, M., Hartshorne, M.F., Baum..n, J.M., and Byrd, B.F.: The last surviving wall, Clin. Nucl. Med. 12:751-754, 1987.

Brown, J.M., White, C.J., Sobol, S.M., and others: Increased left ventricular ejection fraction after a meal: potential source of error in performance of radionuclide angiography, AJC 51:1709-1711, 1983.

Bunker, S.R., Hartshorne, M.F., Schmidt, W.P., and others: Left ventricular volume determination from single photon emission computed tomography, AJR 144:295-298, 1985.

Caputo, G.R., Graham, M.M., Brust, K.D., and others: Measurement of left ventricular volume using single-photon emission computed tomography, Am. J. Cardiol. 56:781-786, 1985.

Choi, B.W., Berger, H.J., Schwartz, P.E., and others: Serial radionuclide assessment of doxorubicin cardiotoxicity in cancer patients with abnormal baseline resting left ventricular performance, Am. Heart J. 106(part 1):638-643, 1983.

Clements, I.P., Sinak, L.J., Gibbons, R.J., Brown, M.L., and O'Connor, M.K.: Determination of diastolic function by radionuclide ventriculography, Mayo Clin. Proc. 65:1007-1019, 1990.

Cokkinos, D.V., DePuey, E.G., Rivas, A.H., and others: Correlations of systolic time intervals and radionuclide angiography at rest and during exercise, Am. Heart J. 109:104-111, 1985.

Dilsizian, V., Rocco, T.P., Bonow, R.O., Fischman, A.J., Boucher, C.A., and Strauss, H.W.: Cardiac blood-pool imaging II: applications in noncoronary heart disease, J. Nucl. Med. 30:10-22, 1990.

Druck, M.N., Gulenchyn, K.Y., Evans, W.K., and others: Radionuclide angiography and endomyocardial biopsy in assessment of doxorubicin cardiotoxicity, Cancer 53:1667-1674, 1984.

Fearnow, E.C., Stanfield, J.A., Jaszczak, R.J., and others: Factors affecting ventricular volumes determined by a count-based equilibrium method, J. Nucl. Med. 26:1042-1047, 1985.

Foster, R.: Min/max functional images: their derivation and application, Softwhere 2:13-19, 1983.

Frais, M., Botvinick, E., Shosa, D., and others: Phase image characterization of localized and generalized left ventricular contraction abnormalities, J. Am. Cardiol. 4:978-998, 1984.

Freeman, A.P., Giles, R.W., Walsh, W.F., and others: Regional left ventricular wall motion assessment: comparison of two-dimensional echocardiography and radionuclide angiography with contrast angiography in healed myocardial infarction, Am. J. Cardiol. 56:8-12, 1985.

Gibbons, R.J., Morris, K.G., Lee, K., and others: Assessment of regional left ventricular function using gated radionuclide angiography, Am. J. Cardiol. 54:294-300, 1984.

Greenberg, J.M., Murphy, J.H., Okada, R.D., and others: Value and limitations of radionuclide angiography in determining the cause of reduced left ventricular ejection fraction: comparison of idiopathic dilated cardiomyopathy and coronary artery disease, Am. J. Cardiol. 55:541-544, 1985.

Ham, H.R., Franken, P.R., Georges, B., and others: Evaluation of the accuracy of steady-state krypton-81m method for calculating right ventricular ejection fraction, J. Nucl. Med. 27:593-601, 1986.

Holman, B.L., Wynne, J., Idoine, J.D., and others: The paradox image: a noninvasive index of regional left-ventricular dyskinesia, J. Nucl. Med. 20:1237-1242, 1979.

Holman, B.L., Wynne, J., Zielonka, J.S., and Idoine, J.D.: A simplified technique for measuring right ventricular ejection fraction using the equilibrium radionuclide angiocardiogram and the slant-hole collimator, Radiology 138:429-435, 1981.

Lavine, S.J., Follansbee, W.P., and Shreiner, D.P., and others: Pattern of left ventricular diastolic filling in chronic aortic regurgitation: a gated blood-pool assessment, Am. J. Cardiol. 55:127-132, 1985.

Marzullo, P.O., Parodi, O., Schelbert, H.R., and others: Regional myocardial dysfunction in patients with angina at rest and response to isosorbide dinitrate assessed by phase analysis of radionuclide ventriculograms, JACC 3:1357-1366, 1984.

Massardo, T., Gal, R.A., Greiner, R.P., and others: Left ventricular volume calculation using a count-based ratio method applied to multigated radionuclide angiography, J. Nucl. Med. 31:450-456, 1990.

Meizlish, J.L., Berger, H.J., Plankey, M., and others: Functional left ventricular aneurysm formation after acute anterior transmural myocardial infarction: incidence, natural history, and prognostic implications, N. Engl. J. Med. 311:1001-1006, 1986.

Miller, T.R., Goldman, K.J., Sampathkumaran, K.S., and others: Analysis of cardiac diastolic function: application in coronary artery disease, J. Nucl. Med. 24:2-7, 1983.

Morris, K.G., Palmeri, S.T., Califf, R.M., and others: Value of radionuclide angiography for predicting specific cardiac events after acute myocardial infarction, Am. J. Cardiol. 55:318-324, 1985.

Morris, K.G., Rozanski, A., Berman, D.S., and others: Noninvasive prediction of the angiographic extent of coronary artery disease after myocardial infarction: comparison of clinical, bicycle exercise electrocardiographic, and ventriculographic parameters, Circulation 70:192-201, 1984.

Moss, A.J., and others (The Multicenter Postinfarction Research Group): Risk stratification and survival after myocardial infarction, N. Engl. J. Med. 309:331-336, 1983.

Nicod, P., Corbett, J.R., Firth, B.G., and others: Radionuclide techniques for valvular regurgitant index: comparison in patients with normal and depressed ventricular function, J. Nucl. Med. 23:763-769, 1982.

Nickoloff, E.L., Perman, W.H., Esser, P.D., and others: Left ventricular volume: physical basis for attenuation corrections in radionuclide determinations, Radiology 152:511-515, 1984.

Okada, R.D., Kirshenbaum, H.D., Kushner, F.G., and others: Observer variance in the qualitative evaluation of left ventricular wall motion and the quantitation of left ventricular ejection fraction using rest and exercise multigated blood pool imaging, Circulation 60:128-136, 1980.

Plotnick, G.D., Becker, L.C., and Fisher, M.L.: Value and limitations of exercise radionuclide angiography for detecting myocardial ischemia in healed myocardial infarction, Am. J. Cardiol. 56:1-7, 1985.

Qureshi, S., Wagner, H.N., Alderson, P.O., and others: Evaluation of left ventricular function in normal persons and patients with heart disease, J. Nucl. Med. 19:135-141, 1978.

Rigo, P., Alderson, P.O., Robertson, R.M., and others: Measurement of aortic and mitral regurgitation by gated cardiac blood pool scans, Circulation 60:306-312, 1979.

Robeson, W., Alcan, K.E., Graham, M.C., and others: Clinical evaluation of the RNCA study using Fourier filtering as a preprocessing method, Clin. Nucl. Med. 9:324-331, 1984.

Rocco, T.P., Dilsizian, V., Fischman, A.J., and Strauss, H.W.: Evaluation of ventricular functions in patients with coronary artery disease, J. Nucl. Med. 30:1149-1165, 1989.

Rozanski, A., Diamond, G.A., Berman, D., and others: Declining specificity of exercise radionuclide ventriculography, N. Engl. J. Med. 309:518-522, 1983.

Rozanski, A., Diamond, G.A., Jones, R., and others: A format for integrating the interpretation of exercise ejection fraction and wall motion and its application in identifying equivocal responses, J. Am. Coll. Cardiol. 5:238-248, 1985.

Schneider, R.M., Jaszczak, R.J., Coleman, R.E., and others: Disproportionate effects of regional hypokinesia on radionuclide ejection fraction: compensation using attenuation-corrected ventricular volumes, J. Nucl. Med. 25:747-754, 1984.

Schneider, R.M., Weintraub, W.S., Klein, L.W., and others: Multistage analysis of exercise radionuclide angiography in coronary artery disease, Am. J. Cardiol. 58:36-41, 1986.

Schneider, R.M., Weintraub, W.S., Klein, L.W., and others: Rate of left ventricular functional recovery by radionuclide angiography after exercise in coronary artery disease, Am. J. Cardiol. 57:927-932, 1986.

Schocken, D.D., Blumenthal, J.A., Port, S., and others: Physical conditioning and left ventricular performance in the elderly: assessment by radionuclide angiocardiography, AJC 8:359-364, 1984.

Shen, W.F., Fletcher, P.J., Roubin, G.S., and others: Relation between left ventricular functional reserve during exercise and resting systolic loading conditions in chronic aortic regurgitation, Am. J Cardiol. 58:757-761, 1985.

Slutsky, R., Karliner, J., and Battler, A.: Reproducibility of ejection fraction and ventricular volume by gated radionuclide angiography after myocardial infarction, Radiology 132:155-159, 1979.

Srivastava, S.C., and Chervu, L.R.: Radionuclide-labeled red blood cells: current status and future prospects, Semin. Nucl. Med. 14(2):68-82, 1984.

Stadius, M.L., Williams, D.L., Harp, G., and others: Left ventricular volume determination using single-photon emission computed tomography, Am. J. Cardiol. 55:1185-1191, 1985.

Starling, M.R., Dell'Italia, L.J., Walsh, R.A., and others: Accurate estimates of absolute left ventricular volumes from equilibrium radionuclide angiographic count data using a simple geometric attenuation correction, J. Am. Cardiol. 3:789-798, 1984.

Starling, M.R., Crawford, M.H., Henry, R.L., and others: Prognostic value of electrocardiographic exercise testing and noninvasive assessment of left ventricular ejection fraction soon after acute myocardial infarction, Am. J. Cardiol. 57:532-537, 1986.

Sutherland, G.R., Driedger, A.A., Holiday, R.L., and others: Frequency of myocardial injury after blunt chest trauma as evaluated by radionuclide angiography, Am. J. Cardiol. 52:1099-1103, 1983.

Taylor, A., Bedont, R.A., Verba, J., and others: Application of Fourier analysis to nuclear cardiology, Appl. Radiol. 3:49-57, 1986.

Turner, D.A., Shima, M.A., Ruggie, N., and others: Coronary artery disease: detection by phase analysis of rest/exercise radionuclide angiocardiograms, Radiology 148:539-545, 1983.

Vitale, D.F., Green, M.V., Bacharach, S.L., and others: Assessment of regional left ventricular function by sector analysis: method for objective evaluation of radionuclide blood pool studies, Am. J. Cardiol. 52:1112-1119, 1983.

Wieshammer, S., Delgardelle, C., and Sigel, H.A.: Limitations of radionuclide ventriculography in the non-invasive diagnosis of coronary artery disease: correlation with right heart haemodynamic values during exercise, Br. Heart J. 53:603-610, 1985.

Wong, D.F., Natarajan, T.K., Summer, W., and others: Right ventricular ejection fraction measured by first-pass intravenous krypton-81m: reproducibility and comparison with technetium-99m, Am. J. Cardiol. 56:776-780, 1985.

Yianniakas, J., MacIntyre, W.J., Underwood, D.A., and others: Prediction of improvement in left ventricular function after ventricular aneurysmectomy using Fourier phase and amplitude analysis of radionuclide cardiac blood pool scans, Am. J. Cardiol. 55:1308-1312, 1985.

Zatta, G., Tarolo, G.L., Palagi, B., and others: Computerized analysis of equilibrium radionuclide ventriculography time-activity curve in the assessment of left ventricular performance: comparison of two methods, Eur. J. Nucl. Med. 10:198-202, 1985.

Myocardial imaging

Beller, G.A.: Pharmacologic stress imaging, JAMA 25:633, 1991.

Botvinick, E.H., and others: Dipyridamole perfusion scintigraphy, Semin. Nucl. Med. 21:242, 1991.

Brown, K.A., and others: Extent of jeopardized viable myocardium determined by myocardial perfusion imaging best predicts perioperative cardiac events in patients undergoing noncardiac surgery, J. Am. Coll. Cardiol. 21:325, 1993.

DePasquale, E.E., and others: Quantitative rotational thallium-201 tomography for identifying and localizing coronary artery disease, Circulation 77:316, 1988.

Dilsizian, V., and Bonow, R.O.: Current diagnostic techniques in assessing myocardial viability in patients with hibernating and stunned myocardium, Circulation 87:1, 1993.

Dilsizian, V., and others: Enhanced detection of ischemic but viable myocardium by the reinjection of thallium after stress-redistribution imaging, N. Engl. J. Med. 323:141, 1990.

Gerson, M.C., editor: Cardiac nuclear medicine, ed. 2, New York, 1991, McGraw-Hill, Inc.

Gould, K.L.: Identifying and measuring severity of coronary artery stenosis: quantitative coronary arteriography and positron emission tomography, Circulation 78:237, 1988.

Haronian, H.L., and others: Myocardial risk area defined by technetium-99m Sestamibi imaging during percutaneous transluminal angioplasty: comparison with coronary angiography, J. Am. Coll. Cardiol. 22:1033, 1993.

Heo, J., and others: Comparison of same-day protocols using technetium-99m Sestamibi myocardial imaging, J. Nucl. Med. 33:186, 1992.

Iskandrian, A.S., and others: Independent and incremental prognostic value of exercise single-photon emission computed tomographic (SPECT) thallium imaging in coronary artery disease, J. Am. Coll. Cardiol. 22:665, 1993.

Kaul, S., and others: Prognostic utility of the exercise thallium-201 test in ambulatory patients with chest pain: comparison with cardiac catheterization, Circulation 77:745, 1988.

Leppo, J., and others: Dipyridamole-thallium-201 scintigraphy in the prediction of future cardiac events after myocardial infarction, N. Engl. J. Med. 310:1014, 1984.

Maddahi, J., and others: Myocardial perfusion imaging with technetium-99m Sestamibi SPECT in the evaluation of coronary disease, Am. J. Cardiol. 66:55E, 1990.

Nohara, R., and others: Stress scintigraphy using single-photon emission computed tomography in the evaluation of coronary artery disease, Am. J. Cardiol. 53:1250, 1984.

O'Donnell, J.K., and others: Clinical evaluation of thallium-201 SPECT with cardiac short axis display, J. Nucl. Med. 25:P61, 1984.

Rockett, J.F., and others: Intravenous dipyridamole thallium-201 SPECT imaging methodology, applications, and interpretations, Clin. Nucl. Med. 15:712, 1990.

Rozanski, A., and Berman, D.S.: The efficacy of cardiovascular nuclear medicine exercise studies, Semin. Nucl. Med. 17:104, 1987.

Saha, G.B.: Fundamentals of nuclear pharmacy, ed. 3, New York, 1992, Springer-Verlag.

Schelbert, H.R., and Buxton, D.: Insights into coronary artery disease gained from metabolic imaging, Circulation 78:496, 1988.

Seldin, D.W., and others: Myocardial perfusion imaging with technetium-99m SQ30217: comparison with thallium-201 and coronary anatomy, J. Nucl. Med. 30:312, 1989.

Special Report: Standardization of cardiac tomographic imaging, Circulation 86:388, 1992.

Sporn, V., and others: Simultaneous measurement of ventricular function and myocardial perfusion using the technetium-99m isonitriles, Clin. Nucl. Med. 13:77, 1988.

Steingart, R.M., and others: Nuclear exercise testing and the management of coronary artery disease, J. Nucl. Med. 32:753, 1991.

Strattman, H.G., and others: Exercise technetium-99m Sestamibi Tomography for cardiac risk stratification of patients with stable chest pain, circulation 89:615, 1994.

Varetto, T., and others: Emergency room technetium-99m Sestamibi imaging to rule out acute myocardial ischemic events in patients with nondiagnostic electrocardiograms, J. Am. Coll. Cardiol. 22:1804, 1993.

Verani, M.S.: Pharmacological stress with adenosine for myocardial perfusion imaging, Semin. Nucl. Med. 21:266, 1991.

Myocardial infarct imaging

Al-Sultan, S., and others: The value of SPECT in identifying false-positive PYP myocardial imaging due to DC burn: a case report, Clin. Nucl. Med.12(9):755, 1987.

Bell, D., and others: Radiopharmaceuticals for myocardial infarct imaging: a clinical comparison of ^{99m}Tc-pyrophosphate and ^{99m}Tc-dimethylaminomethylene diphosphonate, Br. J. Radiol. 61(727):646, 1988.

Fujiwara, Y., and others: Quantitative analysis of acute myocardial infarction using single photon emission computed tomography using technetium-99m pyrophosphate, J. Cardiogr. 16(3):555, 1986.

Gerger, H.H., and Higgins, C.B.: Quantitation of size of myocardial infarctions by computerized transmission tomography: comparison with hot-spot and cold-spot radionuclide scans, Invest. Radiol. 18:238, 1983.

Hashimoto, T., and others: Early estimation of acute myocardial infarct size soon after coronary reperfusion using emission computed tomography with technetium-99m pyrophosphate, Am. J. Cardiol. 60(13): 952, 1987.

Intenzo, C.M., and others: Septal infarction demonstrated on technetium-99m, PYP SPECT, Clin. Nucl. Med. 11(2):82, 1986.

Jansen, D.E., and others: Quantification of myocardial injury produced by temporary coronary artery occlusion and reflow with technetium-99m-pyrophosphate, Circulation 75(3):611, 1987.

Karp, K., and others: Technetium-99m pyrophosphate single-photon emission computed tomography of the heart in familial amyloid polyneuropathy, Int. J. Cardiol. 14(3):365, 1987.

Kondo, M., and others: Clinical significance of early myocardial ^{99m}Tc-pyrophosphate uptake in patients with acute myocardial infarction, Am. Heart J. 113(2, Part 1):250, 1987.

Lyons, K.P., and others: Pyrophosphate myocardial imaging, Semin. Nucl. Med. 10:168, 1980.

Lyons K.P., and others: Myocardial infarct imaging in patients with technetium-99m 2,3-dimercaptosuccinic acid: superiority of technetium-99m pyrophosphate, Clin. Nucl. Med. 12(7):514, 1987.

Minamiji, K., and others: Prognostic value and limitation of doughnut pattern of technetium-99m pyrophosphate myocardial uptake in acute anterior infarction, Jpn. Circ. J. 51(4):363, 1987.

Nishimura, T., and others: Incidence, severity and clinical course of right ventricular involvement after acute inferior myocardial infarction; assessment by sequential ^{99m}Tc-pyrophosphate scan and gated blood pool scan, Nucl. Med. Commun. 7(12):887, 1986.

Radhakrishnan, S., and others: Technetium stannous pyrophosphate imaging in acute ischaemic syndromes, J. Assoc. Physicians India 35(5):345, 1987.

Schofer, J., and others: Thallium-201/technetium-99m pyrophosphate overlap in patients with acute myocardial infarction after thrombolysis: prediction of depressed wall motion despite thallium uptake, Am. Heart J. 112(2):291, 1986.

Silva, R., and others: Recognition of reversible and irreversible myocardial injury by technetium pyrophosphate extraction kinetics, J. Thorac. Cardiovasc. Surg. 94(1):104, 1987.

Volpini, M., and others: Diagnosis of acute myocardial infarction by indium-111 antimyosin antibodies and correlation with the traditional techniques for the evaluation of extent and localization, Am. J. Cardiol. 63(1):7, 1989.

Monoclonal antibodies for imaging myocardial necrosis

Abelman, W.H., and Roberts, W.C.: Cardiomyopathy and specific heart muscle disease. *In* Hurst, J.W.: The heart, New York, 1989, McGraw-Hill, Inc., p. 1313.

Addonizio, L.J., Michler, R.E., Marboe, C., Esser, P.E., Johnson, L.L., Seldin, D.W., Gersony, W.M., Alderson, P.O., Rose, E.A., and Cannon, P.J.: Imaging of cardiac allograft rejection in dogs using indium-111 monoclonal antimyosin Fab, J. Am. Coll. Cardiol. 9:555, 1987.

Aretz, H.T., Billingham, M.E., Edwards, W.D., Factor, S.M., Fallon, J.T., Fenoglio, J.J., Olson, E.G.J., Schoen, F.J.: Myocarditis: a histopathologic definition and classification, J. Cardiovasc. Pathol. 1:3-14, 1986.

Ballester, M., Obrador, D., Carrió, I., Moya, C., Augé, J.M., Bordes, R., Martí, V., Bosch, I., Berná-Roqueta, Estorch, M., Pons-Lladó, Camara, M.L., Padró, J.M., Arís, A., Caralps-Riera, J.M.: Early postoperative reduction of monoclonal antimyosin antibody uptake is associated with absent rejection-related complications after heart transplantation, Circulation 85:61-68, 1992.

Berger, H.J., and Antimyosin Multicenter Trial Group 1988b: Prognostic significance of the extent of antimyosin uptake in unstable ischemic heart disease: early risk stratification, Circulation 78:II-131 (Abstract).

Bhattacharya, S., Liu, X.J., Senior, R., Jain, D., Leppo, J.A., and Lahiri, A.: 111-indium antimyosin antibody uptake is related to the age of myocardial infarction, Am. Heart J. 122:1583-1587, 1991.

Bianco, J.A., Kemper, A.J., Taylor, A., Lazewatsky, J., Tow, D.E., Khuri, S.F.: Technetium-99m (Sn^{2+}) pyrophosphate in ischemic and infarcted dog myocardium in early stages of acute coronary occlusion: histochemical and tissue-counting comparisons, J. Nucl. Med. 24:485, 1983.

Bristow, M.R., Mason, J.W., Billingham, M.E., Daniels, J.R.: Dose-effect and structure-function relationship in doxorubicin cardiomyopathy, Am. Heart J. 102:709-718, 1981.

Buja, L.M., Parkey, R.W., Dees, J.H., Stokely, E.M., Harris, R.A., Bonte, F.J., and Willerson, J.T.: Morphologic correlates of technetium-99m stannous pyrophosphate imaging of acute myocardial infarctions in dogs, Circulation 52:596, 1975.

Carrió, I., Berná, L., Ballester, M., Estorch, M., Obrador, D., Cladellas, M., Abadal, L., and Ginjaume, M.: TI: Indium-111 antimyosin scintigraphy to assess myocardial damage in patients with suspected myocarditis and cardiac rejection, J. Nucl. Med. 29(12):1893-1900, Dec. 1988.

Carrio, I., Pousa, A.L., Estorch, M., and others: Detection of doxorubicin cardiotoxicity in patients with sarcomas by 111-indium-antimyosin monoclonal antibody studies, J. Nucl. Med. 1993 (in press).

Casans, I., Villar, A., Almenar, V., and Blanes, A.: Lyme myocarditis diagnosed by indium-111 antimyosin antibody scintigraphy, Eur. J. Nucl. Med. 15:330-331, 1989.

Codini, M.A., Turner, D.A., Battle, W.E., Hassan, P., Ali, A., and Messer, J.V.: Value and limitations of technetium-99m stannous pyrophosphate in the detection of acute myocardial infarction, Am. Heart J. 98:752, 1979.

Coleman, R.E., Klein, M.S., Roberts, R., and Sobel, B.E.: Improved detection of myocardial infarction with technetium-99m stannous pyrophosphate and serum MB creatine phosphokinase, Am. J. Cardiol. 37:732, 1976.

Cowley, M.J., Mantle, J.A., Rogers, W.J., Russel, R.O., Rackley, C.E., Logic, J.R.: Technetium-99m stannous pyrophosphate myocardial scintigraphy: reliability and limitations in assessment of acute myocardial infarction, Circulation 56:192, 1977.

Dec, G.W., Palacios, I.F., Yasuda, T., and others: Antimyosin antibody cardiac imaging; its role in the diagnosis of myocarditis, J. Am. Cardiol. 16:97-104, 1990.

Finck, H.: Immunochemical studies on myosin. III: Immunochemical comparison of myosins from chicken skeletal, heart and smooth muscles, Biochem. Biophys. Acta 111:231, 1965.

Frist, W., Yasuda, T., Segall, G., Khaw, B.A., Strauss, H.W., Gold, H., Stinson, E., Oyer, P., Baldwin, J., Billingham, M., McDougal, I.R., and Haber, E.: Noninvasive detection of human cardiac transplant rejection with indium-111 antimyosin (Fab) imaging. Circulation 76 (suppl V):V81, 1987.

Gerber, K.H., and Higgins, C.B.: Quantitation of size of myocardial infarcts by computerized transmission tomography: comparison with hot-spot and cold-spot radionuclide scans, Invest Radiol. 18:238, 1983.

Hesse, B., Folke, M., and Mortensen, S.A.: Antimyosin uptake in the lungs in heart-transplanted patients with pulmonary infections, First International Congress of Nuclear Cardiology, 4226, 1993.

Holman, B.L., Chisholm, R.J., and Braunwald, E.: The prognostic implications of acute myocardial infarct scintigraphy with ^{99m}Tc-pyrophosphate, Circulation 57:320, 1978.

Jaffe, A.S., Klein, M.S., Patel, B.R., Siegel, B.A., and Roberts, R.: Abnormal technetium-99m pyrophosphate images in unstable angina: ischemic versus infarction? Am. J. Cardiol. 44:1035, 1979.

Jansen, D.E., Corbett, J.R., Buja, L.M., Hansen, C., Ugolini, V., Parkey, R.W., and Willerson, J.T.: Quantification of myocardial injury produced by temporary coronary artery occlusion and reflow with technetium-99m pyrophosphate, Circulation 75:611, 1987.

Jain, D., Lahiri, A., and Raftery, E.: 1990b: Immunoscintigraphy for detecting acute myocardial infarction without electrocardiographic changes, BMJ 300:151-153.

Johnson, L.L., Seldin, D.W., Keller, A.M., Wall, R.M., Bhatia, K., Bingham, C.O. III, and Tresgallo, M.E.: Dual isotope thallium and indium antimyosin SPECT imaging to identify acute infarct patients at further ischemic risk, Circulation 81:37-45, 1990.

Johnson, L.L., Seldin, D.W., Tresgallo, M.E., and others: Right ventricular infarction and function from dual isotope indium-111 antimyosin/thallium-201 SPECT and gated blood pool scintigraphy, J. Nucl. Med. 32:1018, 1991 (abstract).

Khaw, B.A., Gold, H.K., Leinbach, R.C., Fallon, J.T., Strauss, H.W., Pohost, G.M., and Haber, E.: Early imaging of experimental myocardial infarction by intracoronary administration of 131-I–labeled anticardiac myosin $(Fab')_2$ fragments, Circulation 58:1137, 1978.

Khaw, B.A., Gold, H.K., Yasuda, T., Fallon, T.J., Leinbach, R.C., Barlai-Kovach, M., Strauss, H.W., and Haber, E.: Imaging with antibodies. In Fozzard, H.A., Haber, E., Jennings, R.B., Katz, A.M., and Morgan, H.E., editors: The heart and cardiovascular system, vol. 1, New York, 1986, Raven Press, pp. 453-468.

Khaw, B.A., Strauss, H.W., Moore, R., Fallon, J.T., Yasuda, T., Gold, H.K., and Haber, E.: Myocardial damage delineated by indium-111 antimyosin in Fab and technetium-99m pyrophosphate, J. Nucl. Med. 28:76, 1987.

Khaw, B.A., Yasuda, T., Gold, H.K., Leinbach, R.C., Johns, J.A., Kanke, M., Barlai-Kovach, M., Strauss, H.W., and Haber, E.: Acute myocardial infarct imaging with Indium-111–labeled monoclonal antimyosin Fab, J. Nucl. Med. 18:1671, 1987.

Krause, T., Schumichen, C., Beck, A., Lang, B., Hohnloser, S., and Moser, E.: Scintigraphy using ^{111}In-labeled antimyosin in Churg-Strauss vasculitis with myocardial involvement, Nuklearmedizin 29:177-179, 1990.

Malhotra, A., Narula, J, Yasuda, T., and others: Indium-111 monoclonal antimyosin antibody imaging for diagnosis of rheumatic myocarditis, J. Nucl. Med. 31:84, 1990 (abstract).

Mukherjee, A., Buja, L.M., Kulkarni, P., Nicar, M., Chien, K.R., and Willerson, J.T.: Relationship of mitochondrial alterations and Tc-99m pyrophosphate uptake during myocardial ischemia, Am. J. Physiol. 243:H268, 1982.

Narula, J., Khaw, B.A., Dec, G.W., and others: Acute myocarditis masquerading as acute myocardial infarction, N. Engl. J. Med. 328:100, 1993.

Narula, J., Yasuda, T., Khaw, B.A., and others: Role of antimyosin scintigraphy in recognition of myocardial abnormalities in life threatening ventricular tachyarrhythmias, Circulation 82:736, 1990 (abstract).

Olson, H.G., Lyons, K.P., Aronow, W.S., Brown, W.T., and Greenfield, R.S.: Follow-up technetium-99m stannous pyrophosphate myocardial scintigrams after acute myocardial infarction, Circulation 56:181, 1977.

Parkey, R.W., Bonte, F.J., Meyer, S.L., Atkins, J.M., Curry, G.L., Stokely, E.M., and Willerson, J.T.: A new method for radionuclide imaging of acute myocardial infarction in humans, Circulation 50:540, 1974.

Parrillo, J.E., Aretz, H.T., Palacios, I.F., Fallon, J.T., and Block, P.C.: The results of transvenous endomyocardial biopsy can frequently be used to diagnose myocardial disease in patients with idiopathic heart failure: endomyocardial biopsies in 100 consecutive patients revealed a substantial incidence of myocarditis, Circulation 69:93, 1984.

Samuels, M.A., and Southern, J.F.: 1988. Case records of the Massachusetts General Hospital, case 15, N. Engl. J. Med. 318:970-981, 1988.

Schelbert, H.R., Ingwall, J.S., Sybers, H.D., and Ashburn, W.L.: Uptake of infarct-imaging agents in reversibly and irreversibly injured myocardium in cultured fetal mouse heart, Circulation 39:860, 1976.

Schwartz, R.G., McKenzie, B., Alexander, J., and others: Congestive heart failure and left ventricular dysfunction complicating doxorubicin therapy: seven year experience using serial radionuclide angiocardiography, Am. J. Med. 82:1109-1118, 1987.

Stokely, E.M., Buja, M., Lewis, S.E., Parkey, R.W., Bonte, F.J., Harris, R.A., and Willerson, J.T.: Measurement of acute myocardial infarcts in dogs with Tc-99m-stannous pyrophosphate scintigrams, J. Nucl. Med. 17:1, 1976.

Tamaki, N., Yamada, T., Matsumori, A., and others: Indium-111 labeled antimyosin antibody imaging for detecting different stages of myocardial infarction: comparison with Tc-pyrophosphate imaging, J. Nucl. Med. 31:136-142, 1990.

Wheelan, K., Wolfe, C., Corbett, J., Rude, R.E., Winniford, M., Parkey, R.W., Buja, L.M., and Willerson, J.T.: Early positive technetium-99m stannous pyrophosphate images as a marker of reperfusion after thrombolytic therapy for acute myocardial infarction, Am. J. Cardiol. 56:252, 1985.

Yasuda, T., Palacios, I.F., Dec, G.W., Fallon, J.T., Gold, H.K., Leinbach, R.C., Strauss, H.W., Khaw, B.A., and Haber, E.: Indium-111 monoclonal antimyosin antibody imaging in the diagnosis of acute myocarditis, Circulation 76:306, 1987.

Zaret, B.L., Dicola, V.C., Donabendian, R.K., Puri, S., Wolfson, S., Freedman, G.S., and Cohen, L.S.: Dual radionuclide study of myocardial infarction: relationships between myocardial uptake of potassium-43, technetium-99m stannous pyrophosphate, regional myocardial blood flow and creatine phosphokinase depletion, Circulation 53:422, 1976.

Venography

Dhekne, R.D., and others: Radionuclide venography in pregnancy, J. Nucl. Med. 28:1290, 1987.

Gomes, A.S., Webber, M.M., and Buffkin, D.: Contrast venography vs radionuclide venography: a study of discrepancies and their possible significance, Radiology 142:719, 1982.

Hirsh, J., and Russell, D.H.: Comparative value of tests for the diagnosis of venous thrombosis. In Bernstein, E.F., editor: Non invasive diagnostic techniques in vascular disease, ed. 2, St. Louis, 1981, Mosby–Year Book.

Kakkar, U.V.: Fibrinogen uptake test for detection of deep vein thrombosis: a review of current practice, Semin. Nucl. Med. 7:229, 1977.

Lisbona, R., Stern, J., and Derbekyan, V.: ^{99m}Tc red blood cell venography in deep vein thrombosis of the leg, Radiology 143:771, 1982.

Rao, M.G.: Tc-99m red blood cell venography in deep vein thrombosis of the leg (Letter to the editor), Radiology 148:577, 1983.

Ramchandani, P., and others: Deep vein thrombosis: significant limitations of noninvasive tests, Radiology 156:47, 1985.

Uphold, R.E., and others: Radionuclide venography as an outpatient screening test for deep venous thrombosis, Ann. Emerg. Med. 9:613, 1980.

Chapter 19

LUNG

ANTONIO PALLA
SABAH S. TUMEH
CARLO GIUNTINI

■ ANATOMY

The outer surfaces of the lung are completely covered by a visceral layer of pleura (Fig. 19-1). External to the visceral pleura is the parietal pleura, which lines the entire thoracic cavity. There is a minimal amount of pleural fluid in the pleural space, which prevents friction as the lungs expand. The lungs are cone-shaped and extend from a point just above the rib margins to the diaphragm. Their medial surface is concave to allow for mediastinal structures and for the heart. The bronchi and pulmonary blood vessels enter each lung medially at the lung hilum. The left lung is divided by a fissure into an upper and a lower lobe, while the right lung is divided by two fissures into the upper, middle, and lower lobes. The trachea terminates and divides into the right and the left main-stem bronchi, which in turn divide and branch into the lobes of the lung and, finally, into lung segments. The terminal division elements are called bronchioles, which end in microscopic branches that divide into alveolar ducts; these in turn terminate in a group of alveoli. The alveoli are composed of a single layer of endothelial cells enmeshed in a capillary network well suited for gaseous transport. Approximately 250 to 300 million alveoli are present in the two lungs. The pulmonary artery, which supplies blood to the capillary network in the alveoli, divides in a manner similar to that of the trachea. The branches of the pulmonary artery and those of the bronchial tree follow each other closely; hence, each lung segment receives also a segmental artery. For practical purposes (e.g., the interpretation of pulmonary scintigraphy), each lung may be considered to have nine segments (Fig. 19-2).

■ PHYSIOLOGY

■ Ventilation

Air moves into the gas exchange units of the lungs (i.e., the alveoli) as contraction of the inspiratory muscles generates enough force to expand the chest wall and the lungs to overcome the resistance and the inertia of the respiratory system. The volume of gas that reaches the alveoli is determined by the mechanical properties of the lung parenchyma, the airways, and the chest wall, as well as the force provided by the respiratory muscles. The amount of air that enters the lung with each breath is called the *tidal volume*. The volume of gas contained in the lungs when they are fully expanded is called the *total lung capacity*. The maximal volume of gas a normal person can exhale is called *vital capacity*, and the amount of gas remaining in the lungs is called *residual volume*. The amount of gas in the lungs at the end of a normal breath is called the *functional residual capacity*.

Resistance to airflow is affected by the caliber of the airways. Airway narrowing can result from bronchospasm, edema of the bronchial lining, or retained secretions within the lumen of the bronchi. The first mechanism is seen in asthma; the last two prevail in bronchitis. It is known that reduction can occur in the caliber of the small peripheral airways without having much effect on total airway resistance. The normal elastic recoil of the lung tissue following a deep inspiration is decreased in patients with emphysema as a result of alveolar destruction. Alveolar destruction, in addition to causing loss of recoil, also destroys the capillary network in the alveolar walls. This reduces the perfusion in emphysematous spaces so that the ventilation-perfusion ratio may be better preserved than in peripheral airway obstruction. For this reason, gas exchange is less impaired in emphysema than in bronchitis.

■ Distribution of ventilation

When breathing is normal, more inspired air is distributed to the dependent regions of the lungs than to the superior regions. When inspiration continues to the total lung

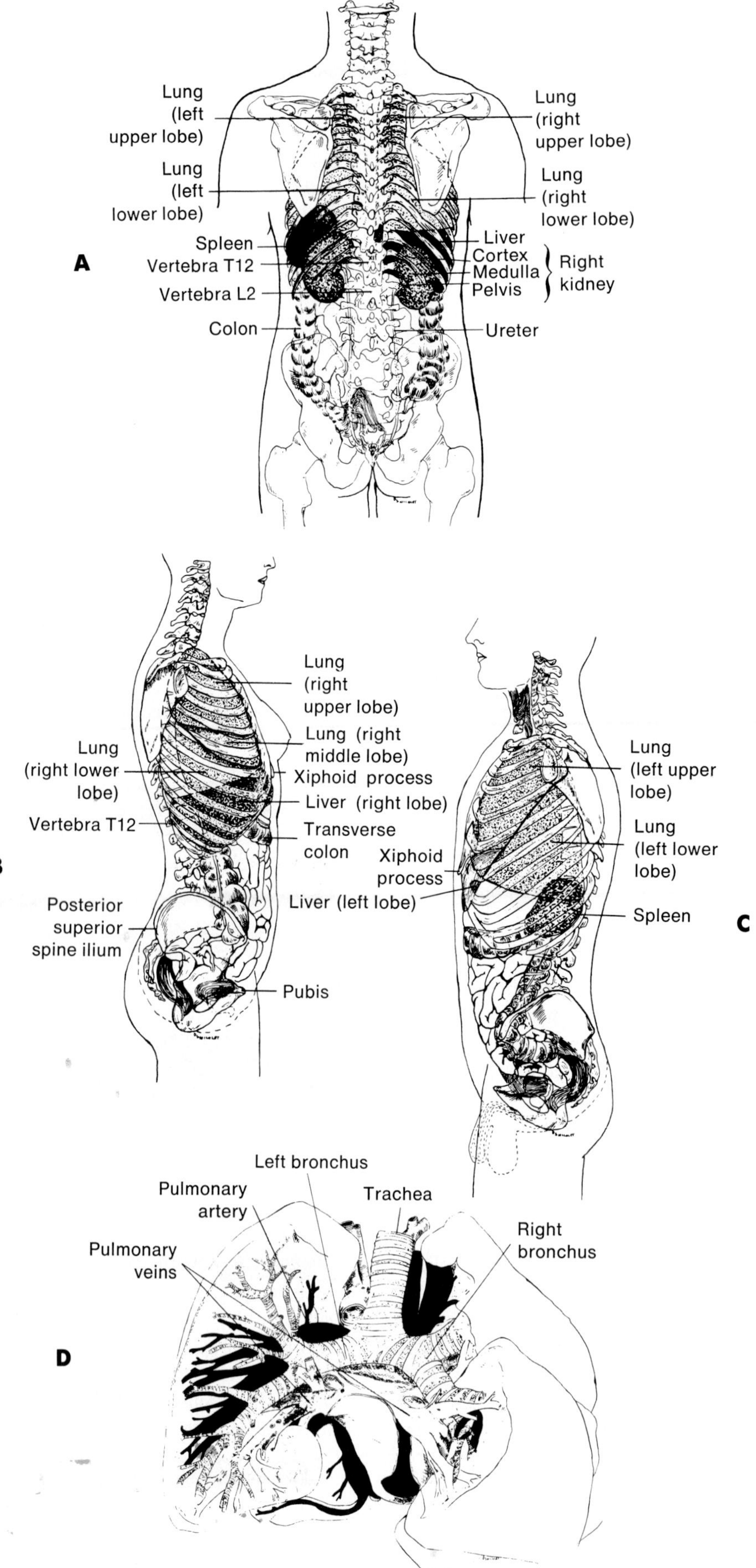

Fig. 19-1. **A**, Posterior anatomic relationships of large organs. **B,** Right lateral relationships. **C,** Left lateral relationships. **D,** Posterior view of tracheobronchial tree.

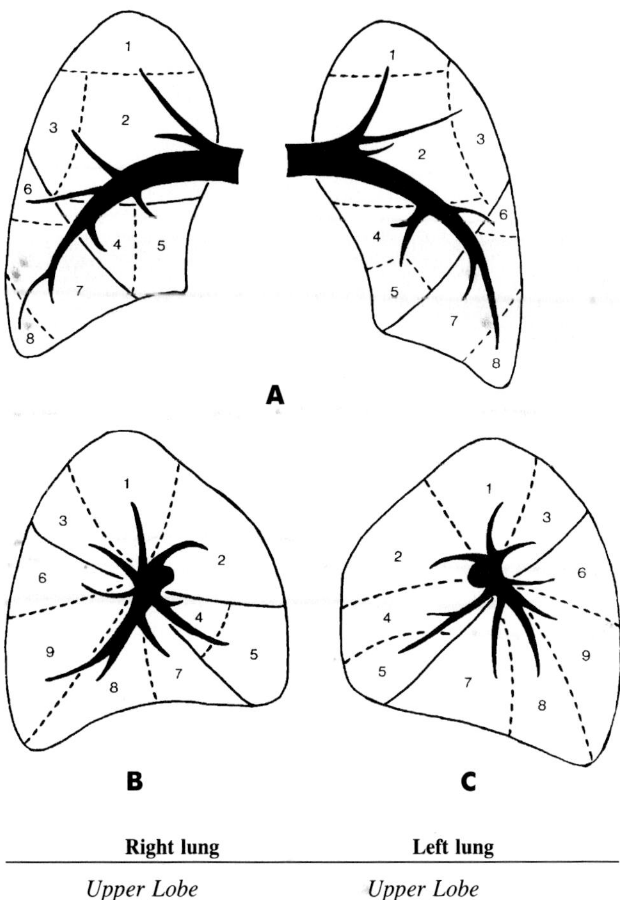

Right lung	Left lung
Upper Lobe	*Upper Lobe*
Apical (1)	Apical (1)
Anterior (2)	Anterior (2)
Posterior (3)	Posterior (3)
Middle Lobe	*Lingula*
Lateral (4)	Superior (4)
Medial (5)	Inferior (5)
Lower Lobe	*Lower Lobe*
Superior (6)	Superior (6)
Anterior basal (7)	Anterior basal (7)
Lateral basal (8)	Lateral basal (8)
Posterior basal (9)	Posterior basal (9)

Fig. 19-2. Schematic representation of pulmonary segments and arterial branches of both lungs. **A,** Anterior view. **B,** Right lateral view. **C,** Left lateral view.

capacity, the alveoli in the upper lobes and in the lower lobes inflate to nearly the same size. During expiration, the pressure surrounding the small airways in the dependent regions of the lung overcomes the internal pressure, causing airways in those regions to close down first. In patients with decreased caliber of peripheral airways and/or loss of elastic lung recoil, there is an increase in closing volume in the affected regions.

■ Perfusion

Blood is pumped into the pulmonary artery by the right ventricle. The finest branches of the pulmonary artery supply the alveolar capillaries. These drain through the pulmonary veins into the left atrium. Obstruction of the pulmonary circulation at the level of the arterial tree (e.g., emboli) or of the lung parenchyma (e.g., bronchitis, emphysema, fibrosis) causes arterial hypertension. Obstruction at the level of the veins or of the left atrium or ventricle causes venous and arterial hypertension. In both types of obstruction, vascular resistance to blood flow increases.

■ Distribution of perfusion

In the sitting and standing positions, pulmonary specific perfusion (blood flow per unit lung volume) physiologically prevails in the lower lung lobes. The ratio between specific perfusion in the upper and lower thirds of the lung (U/L ratio) averages 0.54 ± 0.10. In patients with left heart disease (valvular, ischemic, or myocardial), perfusion is redistributed toward the upper lung regions, with the U/L ratio becoming greater than 1:0 and following the regional redistribution of pulmonary vascular resistance.

■ Diffusion

Diffusion is defined as the movement of molecules from a region of higher concentration to one of lower concentration. In the lung, oxygen moves by diffusion from alveolar gas into pulmonary capillary blood. Oxygen diffusion is impaired to various degrees in patients with emphysema and with interstitial lung disease.

■ PATHOPHYSIOLOGY

■ Chronic obstructive pulmonary disease

Chronic obstructive pulmonary disease (COPD) usually results from some combination of chronic obstructive bronchitis and pulmonary emphysema. COPD is a disorder characterized by abnormal tests of expiratory flow that do not change significantly over periods of several months of observation; this qualification distinguishes COPD from asthma. The airflow may be structural or functional. The following disorders are incorporated in COPD: chronic bronchitis, peripheral airway obstruction, and emphysema. Patients with the latter condition also cough and have various degrees of dyspnea on exertion and irreversible airflow abnormalities as measured by FEV_1 (forced expiratory volume in the first second). In addition, these patients also demonstrate abnormalities at the air/blood interface as determined by carbon monoxide uptake tests (diffusion tests) and hyperinflation, judged clinically by physical examination and by measurements of total lung capacity. With severe emphysema there are bullae or air spaces made up of coalesced, broken-down alveoli.

Smoking is usually the main risk factor in the development of COPD. Other risk factors are familial, acute respiratory infections in childhood, air pollution, occupational exposures and low socioeconomic status. A rare hereditary form of COPD is found in families that have alpha$_1$-antitrypsin deficiencies that demonstrate significant defects on ventilation and perfusion in the lower lobes.

■ Asthma

Asthma, as defined by the American Thoracic Society, is a clinical syndrome characterized by increased responsiveness of the tracheobronchial tree to a variety of stimuli. The major symptoms of asthma are paroxysms of dyspnea, wheezing, and cough, which may vary from very mild and almost undetectable to severe and unremitting (status asthmaticus).

■ Localized airway obstruction

Localized obstruction of airflow may result from compression of airways or from intraluminal obstruction (mucous plug, foreign bodies). These partial or complete obstructions cause partial or complete atelectasis of the involved lung region, with reduction or absence of ventilation. Pulmonary perfusion is also grossly impaired.

■ Interstitial lung disease

A broad group of inflammatory pulmonary disorders of known or unknown etiology are characterized by an initial alveolitis, followed by a progressive substitution of the delicate alveolar structures with fibrous tissue. Collectively, these are known as interstitial lung disease. As they progress, gross abnormalities of lung function may affect ventilation, perfusion, and diffusion. Among interstitial lung diseases of known etiology, asbestosis, silicosis, talcosis, and farmer's lung are a few. In the case of asbestosis, pleural reaction may also ensue, and a pleural cancer called mesothelioma may develop. Among interstitial lung diseases of unknown etiology is idiopathic pulmonary hemosiderosis, a disorder characterized by chronic, recurrent loss of blood in the pulmonary tissues. Another disease in this group is sarcoidosis. Although this is a systemic disease, characterized by noncaseating granulomas in many body tissues, it is commonly recognized as a pulmonary disorder first.

■ Pulmonary bacterial, viral, or fungal infection

The infectious pneumonias can cause severe pulmonary dysfunction, depending on the size of the area involved when exudates fill the alveoli or the interstitial spaces. In bacterial pneumonia ventilation is usually more impaired than is perfusion, with development of low ventilation-perfusion ratio in the affected alveoli as well as arterial hypoxemia. Pneumonias of different kinds, including tuberculosis, are often observed in patients with acquired immunodeficiency syndrome (AIDS).

■ Adult respiratory distress syndrome

Adult respiratory distress syndrome (ARDS) is an acute and progressive clinical disorder characterized by non–cardiogenic-pulmonary edema (increased permeability pulmonary edema), severe dyspnea, arterial hypoxemia rather resistant to high concentration oxygen inhalation, arterial hypocapnia (low CO_2 tension), reduced lung compliance (lung tissue is less distensible), and radiographic evidence of diffuse bilateral lung infiltrates. Sepsis, trauma, burns, and inhalation of fumes are the most common risk factors. Obstruction of the peripheral branches of the pulmonary arterial tree is a feature of ARDS.

■ Pulmonary embolization

Pulmonary embolism is a common medical emergency because the lung arterial tree is often a site of embolization. Thrombi usually form in the deep veins of the lower extremities, break loose and travel via the inferior vena cava through the right heart and then fragment under pressure. The fragmented emboli lodge in the pulmonary arterial tree or capillary bed, depending on their size. Large emboli may lodge in the large branches (trunk, right and left pulmonary arteries, lobar and segmental arteries) in the initial phase of embolization. These thrombi may break down and move into smaller and more peripheral vessels later. Patients with pulmonary embolism develop arterial hypoxemia and hypocapnia. Pulmonary infarction is uncommon because of the dual blood supply (bronchial and pulmonary); only 10% of patients with pulmonary embolism develop infarction.

■ Left heart failure

Pulmonary circulation is unique in that it is exposed to alveolar air, with which it exchanges O_2 and CO_2, accepts the entire cardiac output, and empties directly into the left atrium of the heart via the pulmonary veins. Any left-sided cardiac disease that raises left atrial pressure causes a rise in pressure within the pulmonary venous, capillary, and arterial sections. When there is increased pressure in the left heart and pulmonary veins, the primary consequence is cardiogenic or hydrostatic pulmonary edema (i.e., accumulation of excess extravascular water first in the interstitium and then in the alveoli). Excess extravascular water cannot be removed efficiently from the interstitial space of the lungs by the lymphatics alone because of the very limited fluid output of the lymphatic system. The main function of the lymphatic system is to turn over the proteins of the interstitial space. When the protective mechanisms of the interstitium are overcome—i.e., there is increase in hydrostatic pressure and a decrease in protein osmotic pressure—fluid accumulates in the alveolar spaces, resulting in significant reduction in lung compliance, lung volume, and arterial O_2 tension. These changes are much less severe at the stage of interstitial edema. Thus, as the patient develops left ventricular failure or as the left arterial pressure rises above normal, he or she becomes dyspneic, or short of breath, because of the restricted lung movement and resultant drop in O_2 tension. The increased fluid in the peripheral airways leads to arterial CO_2 retention.

The secondary consequence of raised pressure in the left heart and pulmonary veins is the development of increased pulmonary vascular resistance, especially in the dependent lung regions. This is due to functional and pathologic changes in the lung vessels and interstitium of these regions. It leads to redistribution of lung perfusion from base to apex (elevation of U/L ratio) with some alteration of the ventilation perfusion ratio.

■ Lung tumors

The most common lung tumor is bronchogenic carcinoma, which primarily involves the large bronchi. As the tumor increases in size it partially or completely occludes the involved bronchus or bronchi and the neighboring branch or branches of the pulmonary artery. As a consequence, a dysventilatory syndrome with atelectasis and/or infection develops. This leads to shunting of blood from that segment; a perfusion defect distal to the obstruction may appear. With further tumor extension, reduction or abolition of ventilation and perfusion to the whole lung may ensue.

■ Metastatic neoplasms of the lung

Carcinomas and sarcomas from distant organs frequently metastasize to the lung. Usually such metastases have considerably smaller effects on ventilation and perfusion than do primary lung tumors.

LABORATORY APPLICATION

52

PERFUSION-LUNG IMAGING

Purpose

Perfusion-lung imaging is a noninvasive method for evaluating pulmonary arterial blood flow. The radiopharmaceutical macroaggregated albumin ^{99m}Tc is used for lung-perfusion imaging. The particle size range for ^{99m}Tc macroaggregated albumin is 10 to 90 U; injected intravenously, it lodges in the pulmonary arterioles giving a map of the pulmonary circulation. The recommended number of particles per injection is 200,000 to 700,000 which occludes transiently 1 in 1500 arterioles in the lung.

Thrombi—usually from the deep venous system of the lower extremities, globules of fat, and particulate amniotic fluid—can embolize the pulmonary arteries and produce acute pulmonary hypertension. Pulmonary embolism is a difficult clinical diagnosis. The normal lung-perfusion–imaging study virtually eliminates the diagnosis of pulmonary embolization. Conversely, an abnormal perfusion lung image is found in almost all diseases mentioned under lung pathophysiology. Over the last decade, physicians have set parameters as visualized on the lung images to improve the specificity of lung imaging in the diagnosis of pulmonary embolism. The ventilation study performed with ^{133}Xe, ^{127}Xe, ^{87m}Kr, or particulate aerosols, if performed in conjunction with the lung-perfusion images, improves the sensitivity of the lung perfusion image up to 90%. As a general rule, normal ventilation is usually found in regions of pulmonary embolization.

Lung-perfusion imaging in conjunction with ventilation imaging has added a noninvasive component to the proper evaluation of patients with bronchitis or obstructive forms of chronic pulmonary disease.

Bronchogenic carcinoma, the most common form of lung carcinoma, causes a decrease or absence of pulmonary blood flow to the affected bronchial segment. Lung-perfusion images, therefore, can provide a direct quantitative estimate of how much perfusion remains in the total lung field to enable a prediction as to whether the patient will become a respiratory cripple if the portion of the lung involved in the malignant process is surgically removed. Left ventricular failure or acquired mitral stenosis propagates an increased pressure gradient via pulmonary veins, producing an abnormal lung-perfusion image. Pulmonary arteries to lower lobes are more richly endowed with smooth muscle in their walls than are the pulmonary artery tributaries in the upper lobes. Left heart disease causes functional-anatomic alterations more prominent in the vessels of the lower regions; on lung-perfusion images there is a shift of perfusion pattern from the lower lobes to the upper lobes.

From the above discussion it is apparent that lung-perfusion images cannot be used as the sole diagnostic modality. Knowledge of the patient's clinical status, chest radiographic findings, and the results of a scintigraphic ventilation study must be known by the technologist and the interpreting physician.

Continued.

Indications

1. For evaluation of patients for possible pulmonary embolism
2. For evaluation of pulmonary-flow recovery after therapy, in patients with embolism
3. For evaluation of perfusion changes secondary to lung malignancies
4. For evaluation of perfusion changes found in other lung-disease states, such as emphysema, chronic bronchitis, asthma, and inflammatory disease
5. For evaluation of perfusion changes secondary to acquired cardiac disease
6. For preoperative pulmonary evaluation

Procedure for Large–field-of-view anger scintillation camera imaging

Materials

1. Large field-of-view Anger scintillation camera
2. Parallel-hole collimator (low-energy)
3. ^{99m}Tc-macroaggregated albumin (MAA); 2 to 4 mCi (74 to 148 MBq) ^{99m}Tc-labeled products are better for imaging purposes for the following reasons:
   a. a smaller radiation dose is administered to patient, and
   b. a larger quantity of activity can be administered and the views can be obtained with higher ID in a shorter length of time

If ^{99m}Tc-labeled products are used, the manufacturer's directions for labeling and administering must be followed precisely.

Patient preparation

1. No special patient preparation is required; however, the entire procedure should be explained to the patient before beginning the examination.

Special note

It has been found that certain patients suffer severe respiratory distress after receiving an injection of ^{99m}Tc MAA. These patients are generally women whose ages range from about 30 to 50 and who are suffering from acute, severe chest pain. If the patient meets these criteria, check tactile temperature of the patient's hands and look for signs of cyanosis. Question the patient about cold, tingling hands. If in doubt, reduce the dose of ^{99m}Tc MAA to 1 mCi (37 MBq).

Technique

1. Set camera controls for correct energy level (^{99m}Tc-energy is 140 keV).
2. Preset count for 500K.
3. Set orientation according to patient position and set proper intensity. If the patient has large and/or abnormal lungs, the intensity should be increased to compensate.
4. Administer the correct dose intravenously, with patient lying supine and breathing deeply. Care is needed to be certain that blood is not drawn into the syringe and mixed with the radiopharmaceutical agent; this may cause the radiopharmaceutical to clump and the blood to clot.
5. Imaging may be performed with the patient sitting up or lying down. For best results, perform views with the patient in the upright position to reduce compression of the lungs by the abdominal structures. If the patient is unable to tolerate this position, perform the study with the patient lying on a cart and note the position on the patient history sheet. The procedure may be performed with the patient in an upright position, either standing, sitting on a chair or stool, or sitting on a cart. It is important to immobilize the patient as much as possible. If the patient is unable to sit up for imaging, it is important that he or she be in a true lateral position for the lateral images of the lungs.
6. Position the patient using a variable persistence scope. In positioning for all views, it is important to have the patient's shoulders in a downward position to maintain a proper distance (collimator should be as close to patient as possible).
7. Obtain all images accumulating 500K or a 1000 to 2000 ID. If an ID slice is used, the slice should run through the widest area of the lungs.

8. Eight views should be obtained, with a completion of the same sequence in each study performed. If the sequence is changed, the views should each be labeled as to the position.
   a. *Anterior view:* The patient should be without a pillow to keep the head and face away from the collimator.
   b. *Right lateral view:* The patient must be in a true lateral position with the arm closest to the camera out of the field of view. In this position, if the shoulders are too high for the proper distance, the collimator can be rotated to maintain the proper distance.
   c. *Left lateral view:* Same as for right lateral view.
   d. *Posterior view:* The patient is in the prone position and without a pillow, to keep the head and face from the collimator. This view is very important because the majority of lung tissue is posterior.
   e. *Right posterior oblique:* 45 degrees.
   f. *Left posterior oblique:* 45 degrees.
   g. *Right anterior oblique:* 45 degrees.
   h. *Left anterior oblique:* 45 degrees.

Procedure for SPECT imaging

SPECT scintigraphy of the lungs is a relatively new technique that offers advantages over planar imaging along with some disadvantage. It gives better contrast, edge definition, and separation of target from background, thereby providing information on size, shape, and distribution of perfusion and, possibly, ventilation defects in patients suffering from pulmonary embolism or other respiratory diseases. Furthermore, SPECT permits quantitative measurement of radionuclide uptake in a defined volume of the lung. However, acquiring SPECT images takes longer (about 20 to 25 minutes) than does planar scintigraphy and therefore requires the patient to stay still for the same period of time.

Materials

1. Large–field-of-view camera with rotating head
2. Dedicated computer and software
3. Low-energy all-purpose collimator
4. 2 to 4 mCi (74 to 148 MBq) of ^{99m}Tc macroaggregated albumin

Patient preparation

1. No special preparation is required; however, because of its length the procedure should be explained fully to the patient.

Technique

- ***Acquisition***

1. Check the table-detector alignment.
2. Administer dose to the patient as for the traditional planar scintigraphy.
3. Raise the patient's arms above the head and ask him or her to stay still in the supine position.
4. Check the patient alignment or positioning.
5. Check the patient orientation.
6. Set a 360° circular orbit to acquire 64 projections on a 64 × 64 matrix (20 sec/projection).
7. Make the source-to-detector distance as short as possible along the rotation.
8. Start acquisition.

- ***Reconstruction***

1. Prefilter with a Hanning filter, using a 0.5-cutoff frequency.
2. Reconstruct into transaxial slices 6.3 mm thick.
3. Filter by a Ramp filter and employ the technique of convoluted back-projection.
4. Reorient images into coronal and sagittal planes 6.3 mm thick.

Continued.

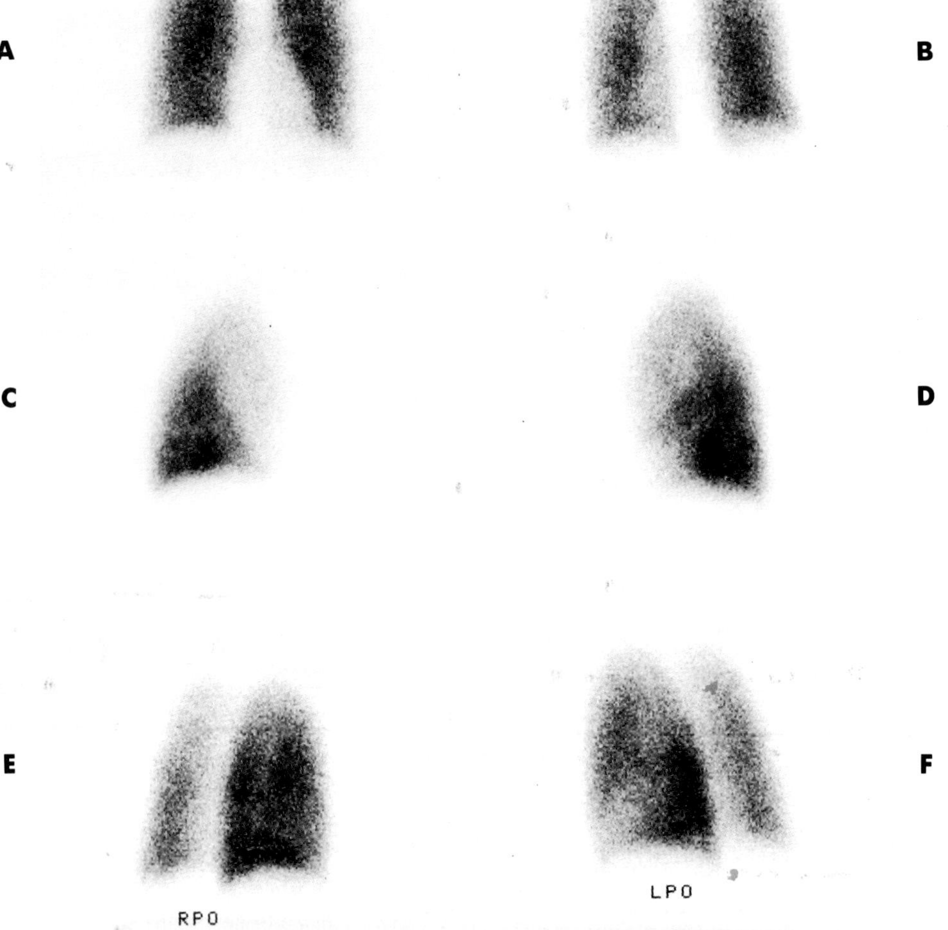

Fig. 19-3. Lung-perfusion images using ^{99m}Tc MAA demonstrates normal distribution of radionuclide over both lung fields. **A,** Anterior view. **B,** Posterior view. **C,** Right lateral view. **D,** Left lateral view. **E,** Right posterior oblique view. **F,** Left posterior oblique view.

Interpretation (Fig. 19-3)

In normal subjects, the patterns of perfusion lung scan are influenced by age, changes in gravity, and depth of respiratory effort. Even a small, ill-defined perfusion defect may be clinically significant in a young patient while it would be considered insignificant in a middle-aged patient.

Regional blood flow is higher in the most dependent regions of the lungs—that is, in the lower lobes if the patient was injected in the sitting position and in the posterior zones if the patient was injected in the supine position. During shallow respiration, pulmonary blood flow is greater in the central area; as the depth of respiration increases, this flow is likely to increase peripherally. The effect of gravity and respiration on the distribution of regional blood flow is more accurately appreciable by SPECT.

Planar imaging

Anterior view

The lungs are normally cone-shaped with a horizontal cutoff at the level of the diaphragm, since the bases are not seen on the anterior view. Aortic and cardiac silhouette are visualized as a photopenic area centrally.

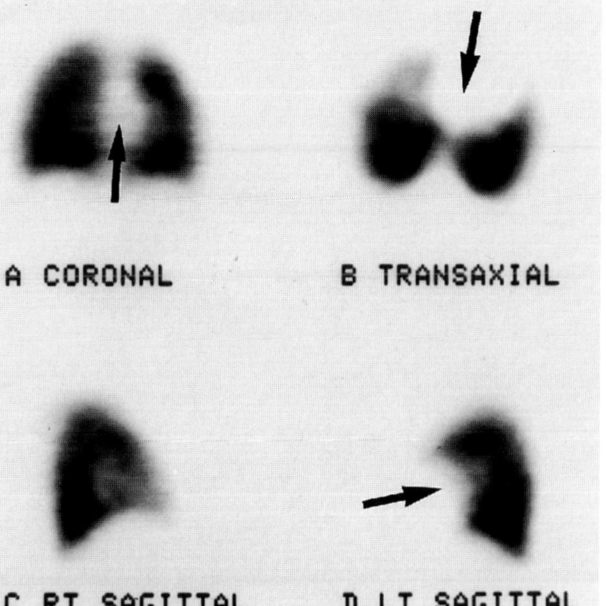

Fig. 19-4. Normal SPECT perfusion scintigraphy showing the four views routinely obtained. The arrows point to the photopenic area caused by the heart silhouette.

Posterior view

Most lung tissue is located posteriorly. The bases of the lung are seen in the posterior view. The vertebral column appears as an area of decreased or absent perfusion. On both the anterior and the posterior projections, different segments in the same lung are superimposed and thus difficult to separate from each other.

Lateral view

On the lateral view, the lung usually follows the contour of the thorax and the diaphragm. If these are normal in position, any absence of perfusion is abnormal. Although the lateral view is excellent for the demonstration of defects in some lobes such as the right middle lobe, "shine-through" from the other lung may obscure small defects.

Oblique view

Peripheral segmental lesions are better visualized on oblique views. On these projections, one lung projects away from the other and perfusion defects in the near lung field can be easily demonstrated.

SPECT imaging (Fig. 19-4)

Tomographic reconstruction allows good visualization of all segments because it eliminates the overlapping of normal tissue and photopenic area representing the defect. The three different planes shown by SPECT (coronal, sagittal right, sagittal left, and transaxial) provide complementary information about the size and location of the segments.

Diagnosis

Emboli, severe emphysema, pneumonia, bronchogenic carcinoma, or cardiac disease may all cause similar perfusion defects discernible on lung-perfusion images. Differential diagnosis may be made by careful clinical and radiographic examination as well as by radionuclide ventilation studies or pulmonary arteriography. The interpreter should know the patient's position at the time the images were obtained. If the anterior or the posterior view is taken with the patient on his side, the dependent lung is compressed, and rib and diaphragmatic motion is limited. Accurate positioning on the lateral views is necessary; otherwise, the contralateral base is seen with falsely abnormal results on the image. When there is a gross decrease in perfusion in one lung, the lateral image on the

Continued.

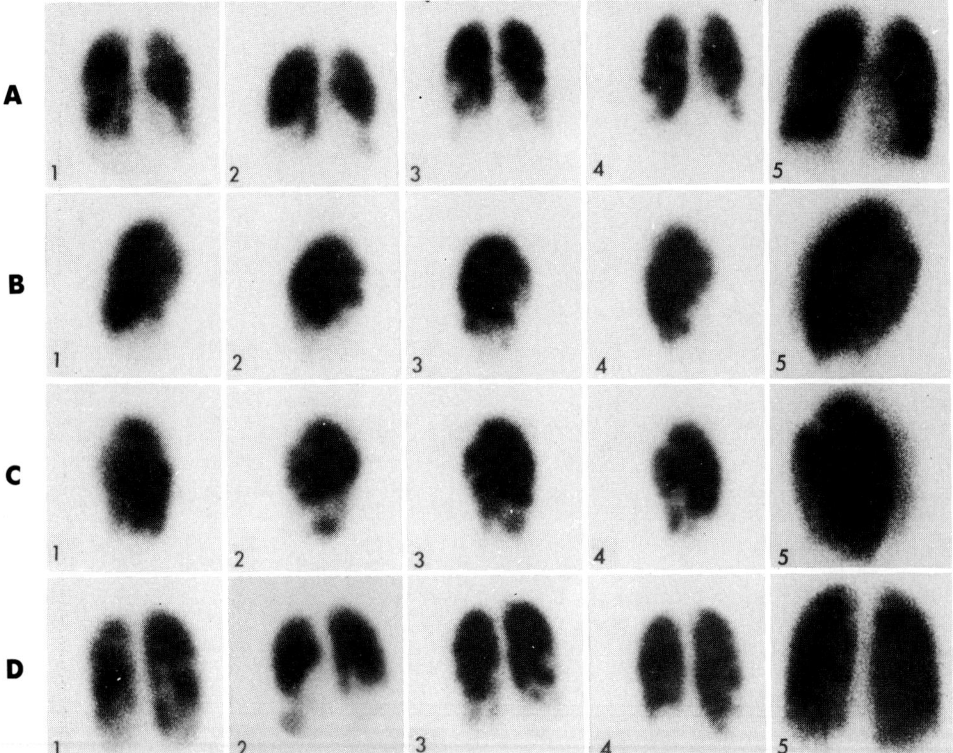

Fig. 19-5. Lung images. **A,** Anterior view. **B,** Right lateral view. **C,** Left lateral view. **D,** Posterior view. *1,* Multiple segmental defects in perfusion in all lobes. Patient placed on heparin therapy. *2,* (7 days later) Gross loss of perfusion to lower lobes with partial reperfusion of upper lobe defects. *3,* (14 days after initial study.) Improvement in perfusion. Views on *(4)* and *(5)* performed still later reveal further improvement. Comment: Second perfusion study illustrates reperfusion "steal" phenomenon. With massive embolization in this patient, upper lobe arterial segments were completely occluded and lower lobe segments partially occluded. With recanalization of upper lobe segments, lower lobe segments partially occluded were "uncovered" as perfusion shifted to now more normally perfused upper lobes.

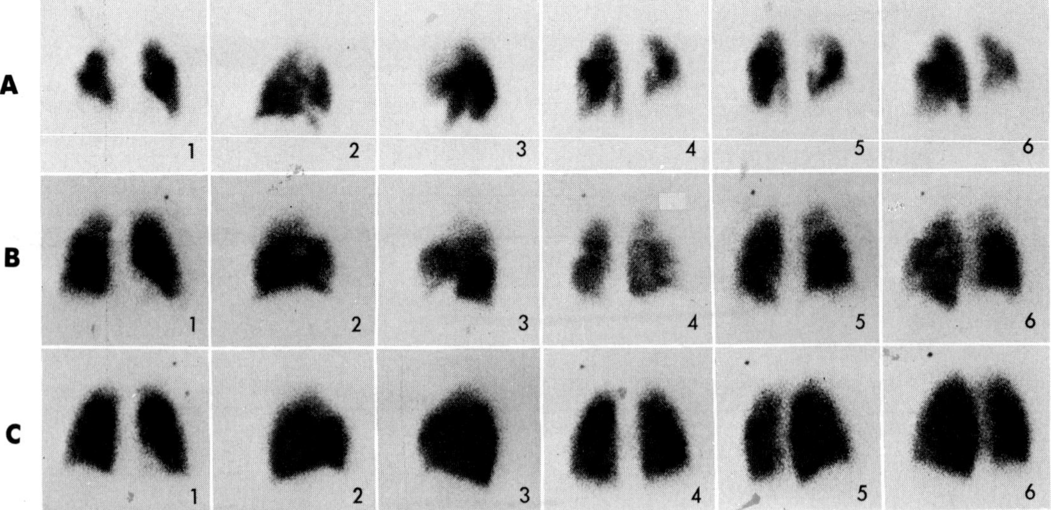

Fig. 19-6. Multiple pulmonary emboli. Study *was* performed with 3 mCi of ^{99m}Tc MAA. *1,* Anterior view; *2,* right lateral view; *3,* left lateral view; *4,* posterior view; *5,* right posterior oblique view; *6,* left posterior oblique view. **A,** (initial study) Multiple segmental defects in all lobes. **B,** Rapid early reperfusion of all embolized regions. **C,** (10 days later) Complete reperfusion of all embolized regions. Images are within normal limits.

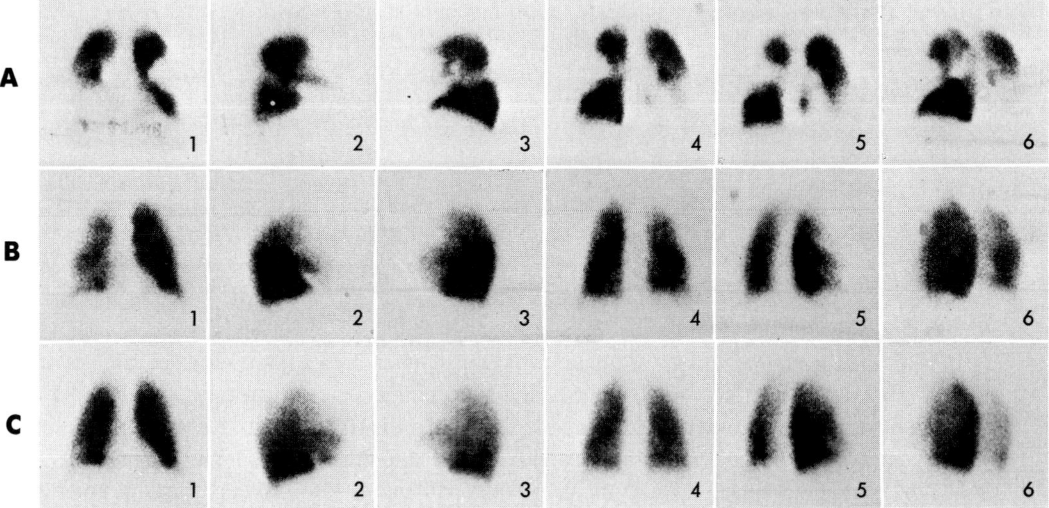

Fig. 19-7. Multiple pulmonary emboli. The study was performed with 3 mCi of ^{99m}Tc MAA. *1,* Anterior view; *2,* right lateral view; *3,* left lateral view; *4,* posterior view; *5,* right posterior oblique view; *6,* left posterior oblique view. **A,** (initial study) Multiple segmental defects and absent perfusion of right middle lobe and right lower lobe. **B,** (9 days later) Early reperfusion of all embolized regions. **C,** (26 days later) Almost complete reperfusion of all embolized regions.

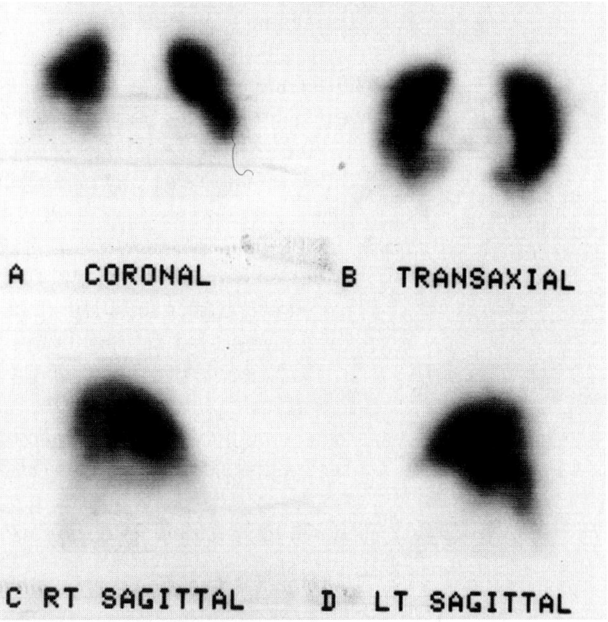

Fig. 19-8. SPECT perfusion scintigraphy in a 64-year-old male with right-sided chest pain and dyspnea. A scan performed after the I.V. injection of 3 mCi of ^{99m}Tc MAA shows multiple segmental defects in the lower lobes bilaterally. Chest x-ray was normal and planar perfusion scintiscans showed nonsegmental defects in both lower lobes. Pulmonary angiography confirmed the presence of emboli in branches to lower and middle lobes and the anterior segment of the upper lobe on the right.

affected side may appear falsely normal as we visualize the opposite normal lung. Injections must be clean. If blood is drawn back into the syringe and clots form, the radiopharmaceutical will adhere to the clots which, on injection, will form "hot spots" on the image. Injection into either plastic tubing or special catheters should be avoided for the same reason.

Pulmonary embolism (Figs. 19-5 to 19-8)

Depending on their size, pulmonary emboli may cause subsegmental, segmental, or lobar perfusion defects. Emboli are usually multiple and most often bilateral. Peripheral defects may be seen when emboli are small. Central, large emboli may completely block perfusion of several segments, lobes, or even a whole lung. Central emboli may break up and on lateral images appear as multiple peripheral emboli. Serial perfusion scintiscans are therefore useful primarily in patients receiving

Continued.

Table 19-1. Probability of pulmonary embolism associated with different scan patterns

High	Moderate	Low	Indeterminate
(1) Multiple large subsegments, or (2) Multiple segments, or (3) Lobar *V/Q* mismatches	One or two subsegments, or Single segment of V/Q mismatches	Nonsegmental perfusion defects	Matching radiographic abnormalities, or Severe COPD

heparin or fibrinolytic therapy. Perfusion impairment as a result of pulmonary embolization may be quantified from the number of unperfused lung segments; in a large series of patients it corresponded to an average obstruction of about 50% of the pulmonary arterial tree. The number of unperfused lung segments in patients with embolism shows a distribution that resembles the normal error frequency function, the so-called Gauss' bell, suggesting that embolism has a continuous spectrum from one or two unperfused lung segments on the one hand to 15 or 16 unperfused segments on the other. Although chest radiographs are normal in most cases of pulmonary embolism, they may show abnormalities highly suggestive of pulmonary embolism, such as significant enlargement of a descending pulmonary artery, elevation of the hemi-diaphragm, atelectatic lines, or focal hyperlucencies. In some cases, pulmonary infarction takes place and appears as a lung density, the shape and size of which is variable and is not diagnostic of embolization. Furthermore, it may be confused with inflammatory lung disease. A normal perfusion scintiscan virtually excludes the diagnosis of pulmonary embolism. Conversely, any lung pathologic condition may cause a decrease in perfusion. With correlating radiographs and radionuclide ventilation studies, the diagnostic value of lung imaging is greatly enhanced. Table 19-1 summarizes the probability of pulmonary embolism associated with different ventilation-perfusion scintiscan patterns. If the clinical suspicion of acute embolism is high and scintigraphy is inconclusive, pulmonary arteriography should be done. Despite its high sensitivity and specifity, angiography is expensive and potentially dangerous for the patient. Investigation of lower limb veins may be a useful adjunct, because it has been shown that patients with diagnosed lower limb thrombi have high probability of positive arteriography for pulmonary embolism.

SPECT may be able to improve the scintigraphic diagnosis of pulmonary embolism because of its ability to separate overlying radioactivity that would obscure defects. However, although SPECT has shown greater sensitivity than planar scintigraphy in identifying segmental perfusion defects, it has not improved the specificity.

Perfusion defects associated with pulmonary embolism may change with time. Reperfusion may take place rapidly or slowly, being promoted by adequate treatment or delayed by underlying pathologic conditions and recurrence of emboli. Reperfusion may be quantified by considering the number and the extension of unperfused lung segments in the eight routine views. Pulmonary blood flow begins to recover early after embolization in most patients, reaching a maximum within the first month and continuing to improve slowly for another 6 months.

Pulmonary hypertension secondary to cardiac disease (Fig. 19-9)

Left heart disease and chronic left ventricle failure cause functional-anatomic alterations more prominent in the lower regions of the lungs. The degree of these alterations as expressed by the increase in pulmonary vascular resistance is reflected on the perfusion lung scintiscans by a reversal of blood perfusion from the basal to the upper regions. This reversal of normal perfusion pattern is an important indicator of lung involvement due to acquired heart disease. Pulmonary edema, a factor commonly associated with the reversal of blood flow, is not as important as medial hypertrophy and intimal fibrosis of the resistance vessels in causing flow redistribution.

Congenital heart disease

Congenital heart disease usually does not affect a clear shunt of perfusion to the upper regions of the lung, but an even gradient from the apex to the base may be seen. If a defect between the right and the left cardiac cavities is suspected, the technologist should check for activity in the renal and brain areas because the macroaggregates may escape from the pulmonary filter through the defect

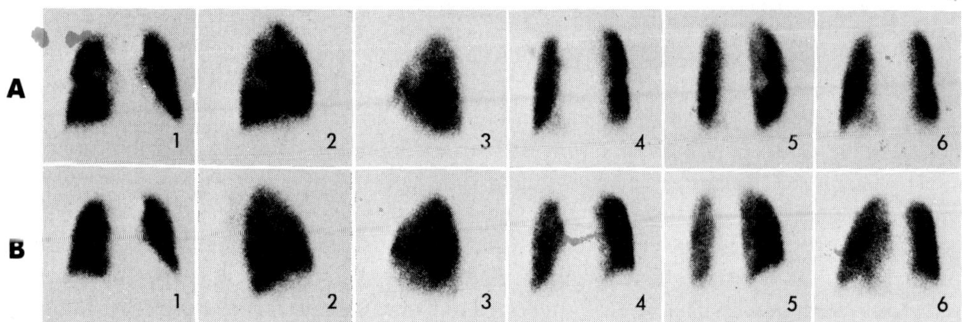

Fig. 19-9. Congestive heart failure. Study performed with 3 mCi of ^{99m}Tc MAA. *1,* Anterior view; *2,* right lateral view; *3,* left lateral view; *4,* posterior view; *5,* right posterior oblique view; *6,* left posterior oblique view. **A,** Marked cardiomegaly. There is decreased perfusion surrounding hilar regions; patchy, nonsegmental decreased perfusion in all lobes; and visualization of interlobar fissures. Study is most compatible with congestive heart failure with pulmonary edema. **B,** (5 days later) Size of heart is reduced. Previous regions of decreased perfusion have now reperfused. Study is compatible with resolving congestive heart failure.

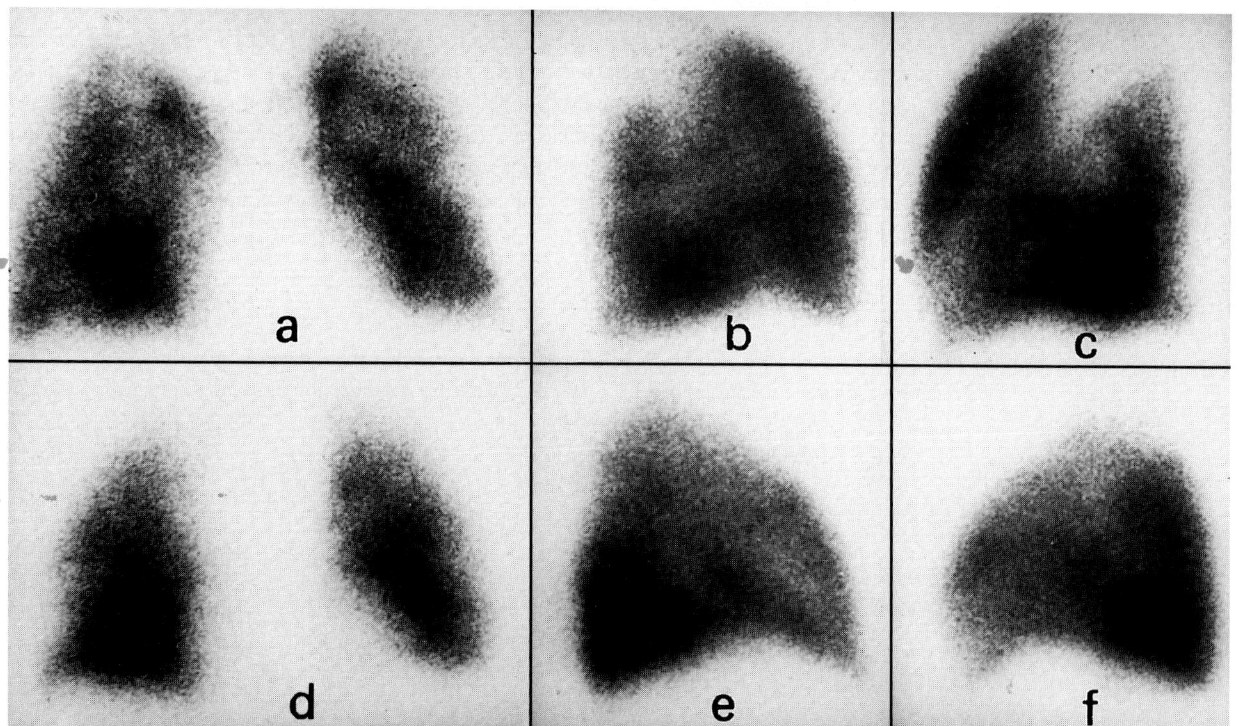

Fig. 19-10. Planar perfusion scintigraphy of a 21-year-old male who developed ARDS in the course of viral pneumonia. On the first examination **(a, b, c),** large bilateral, nonsegmental perfusion defects are visualized in the apical, central, and dorsal regions of the lungs. Regional lung perfusion is redistributed toward the anterosuperior zones. The repeated lung scan **(d, e, f)** shows the persistence of residual perfusion defects. Pulmonary blood flow distribution has not yet completely regained the physiologic configuration. (Courtesy of Drs. M. Pistolesi and M. Miniati, CNR Institute of Clinical Physiology, Pisa, Italy.)

Continued.

and lodge in systemic capillary beds. Primary pulmonary hypertension also causes an even gradient from the apex to the base.

Adult respiratory distress syndrome (ARDS) (Fig. 19-10)

Pulmonary vascular obstruction is a common angiographic and pathologic finding in patients with adult respiratory distress syndrome. It has been found that the presence of filling defects at angiography correlates with the increase of pulmonary artery pressure and resistance, and with respiratory failure, diffuse intravascular coagulation, and mortality. While pulmonary angiography can visualize only a portion of the entire vascular bed, perfusion scintigraphy offers an overall visualization of pulmonary blood flow and gives detailed information about regional distribution patterns. The presence of nonsegmental perfusion defects, mostly in peripheral and dependent areas with redistribution of blood flow to nondependent regions, may be considered a typical pattern of ARDS. Perfusion scintigraphy may be easily repeated to evaluate the effect of treatment and follow the course of the disease.

Bronchial asthma

Bronchial asthma causes a decrease in perfusion of the area(s) aeriated by affected bronchial segment(s). Scans should be performed before and after asthmatic symptoms have been relieved by proper therapy. If the segmental perfusion defects depicted on the initial lung scintiscan improve following appropriate therapy, it would be reasonable to assume that those defects were secondary to bronchial spasm.

Chronic obstructive pulmonary disease (Fig. 19-11)

Chronic bronchitis causes a patchy nonsegmental decrease of perfusion in the lung. Defects may be located everywhere in the lungs but they appear more frequently in the lower regions. Most often abnormalities due to chronic bronchitis are visible on chest radiograph and ventilation studies. Repeated studies after prolonged hospital treatment are useful to show the reversibility of vascular lesions. Pulmonary emphysema causes significant inhomogeneity of distribution of pulmonary blood flow and increase of lung size. In massive bullous emphysema, there is absence of perfusion in the area(s) of bullous formation.

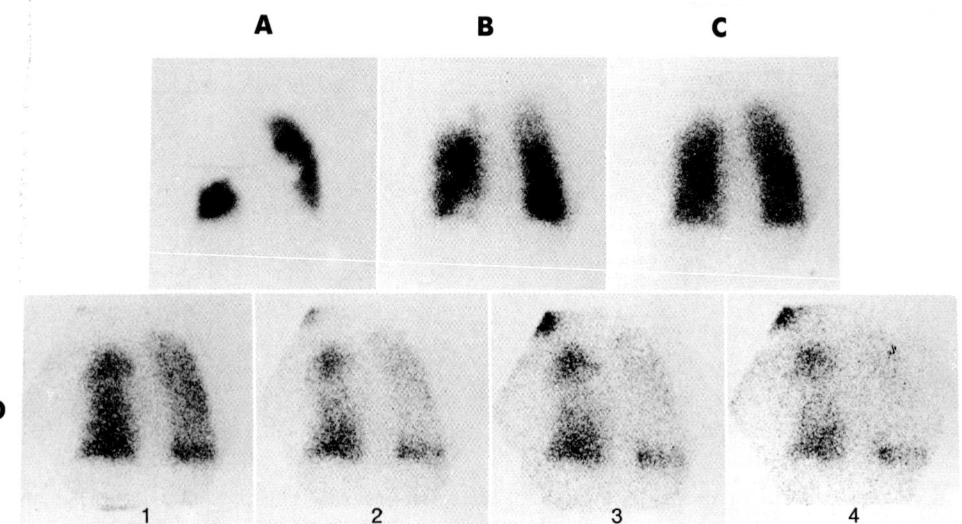

Fig. 19-11. Patient, 74 years of age, with moderately severe COPD (emphysema), history of acute chest pain, and increasing shortness of breath. **A,** Posterior perfusion (^{99m}Tc MAA) lung image reveals absent perfusion in left upper lobe and superior left lower lobe as well as in mediastinal region of right lung. **B,** ^{133}Xe ventilation study (posterior position). Inhalation phase—note ventilation of left lung and mediastinal portion of right lung. **C,** ^{133}Xe equilibrium phase. Even distribution of ^{133}Xe throughout both lung fields. **D,** Washout phase. Note delayed washout of ^{133}Xe from areas of increased dead air space (emphysema). Combined studies imply that patient has pulmonary embolization superimposed on COPD.

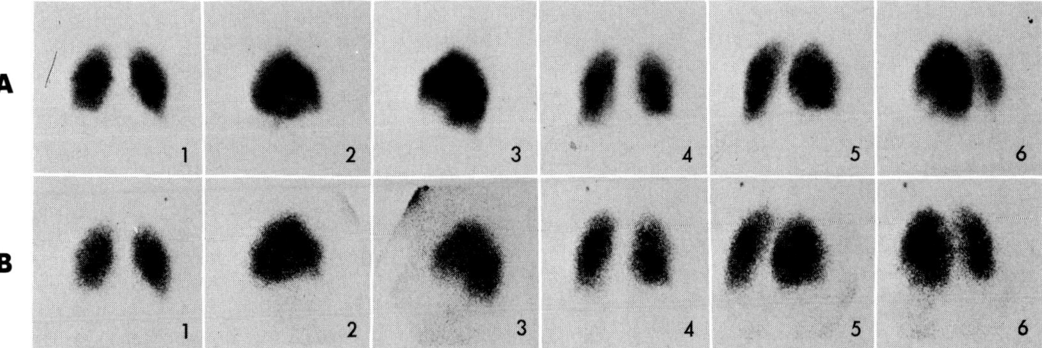

Fig. 19-12. Right pleural effusion study performed with 3 mCi of ^{99m}Tc MAA. *1,* Anterior view; *2,* right lateral view; *3,* left lateral view; *4,* posterior view; *5,* right posterior oblique view; *6,* left posterior oblique view. **A,** (Initial study) Note on right lateral and right posterior oblique views there is absent perfusion at base of right lobe. On x-ray study pleural effusion was visualized. **B,** (Following day) Following thoracentesis, perfusion images show significantly improved visualization of right base, thus ruling out hidden lesion or pulmonary embolus.

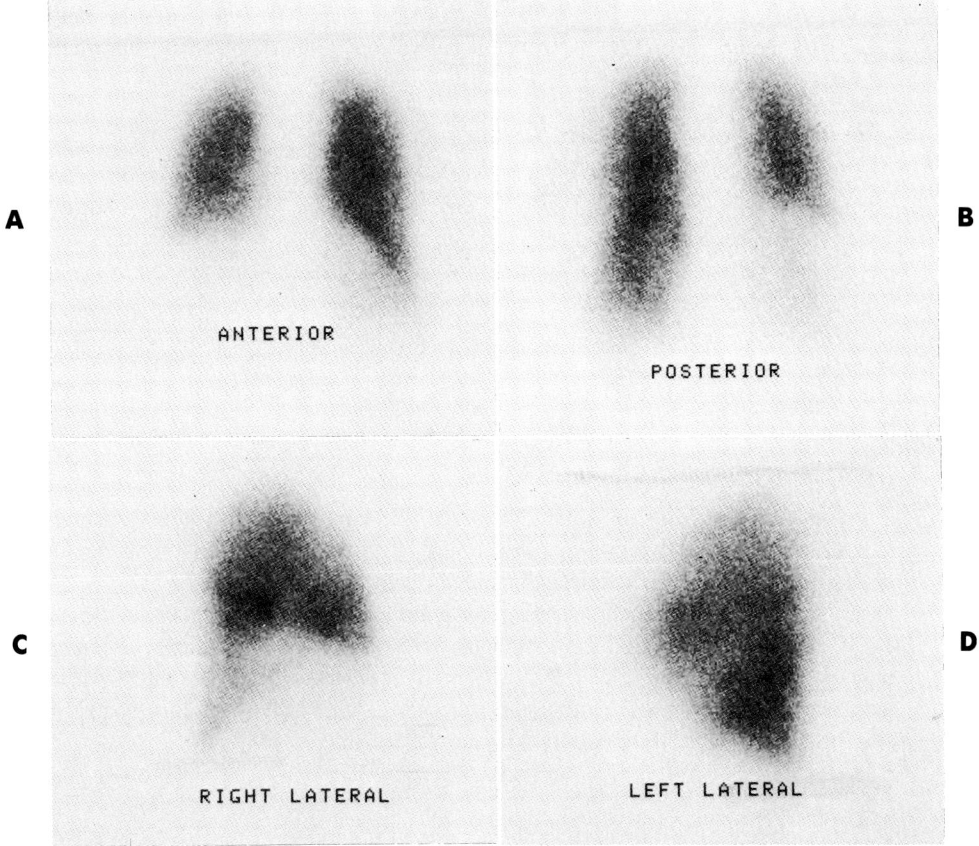

Fig. 19-13. Patient 71 years old with history of bronchogenic carcinoma involving middle and lower lobes of right lung. Perfusion images using MAA ^{99m}Tc are abnormal. There is decreased perfusion in right middle lobe and in anterior basilar segment of right lower lobe. Left lung shows normal distribution of nuclide. **A,** Anterior. **B,** Posterior. **C,** Right lateral. **D,** Left lateral. **E,** Right posterior oblique. **F,** Left posterior oblique.

Quantitative analysis of pulmonary perfusion demonstrates approximately 64% perfusion to left lung and approximately 36% perfusion to right lung. Typically, left lung receives 45% of total perfusion and right lung receives 55%.

G, Computer-assisted quantitative analysis of posterior lung fields using regions of interest drawn manually over both lungs. Total counts in region A (left lung), is 204,653 and total counts in region B (right lung), is 130,208. Therefore 38% of perfusion is to left lung, 62% to right lung.

Continued.

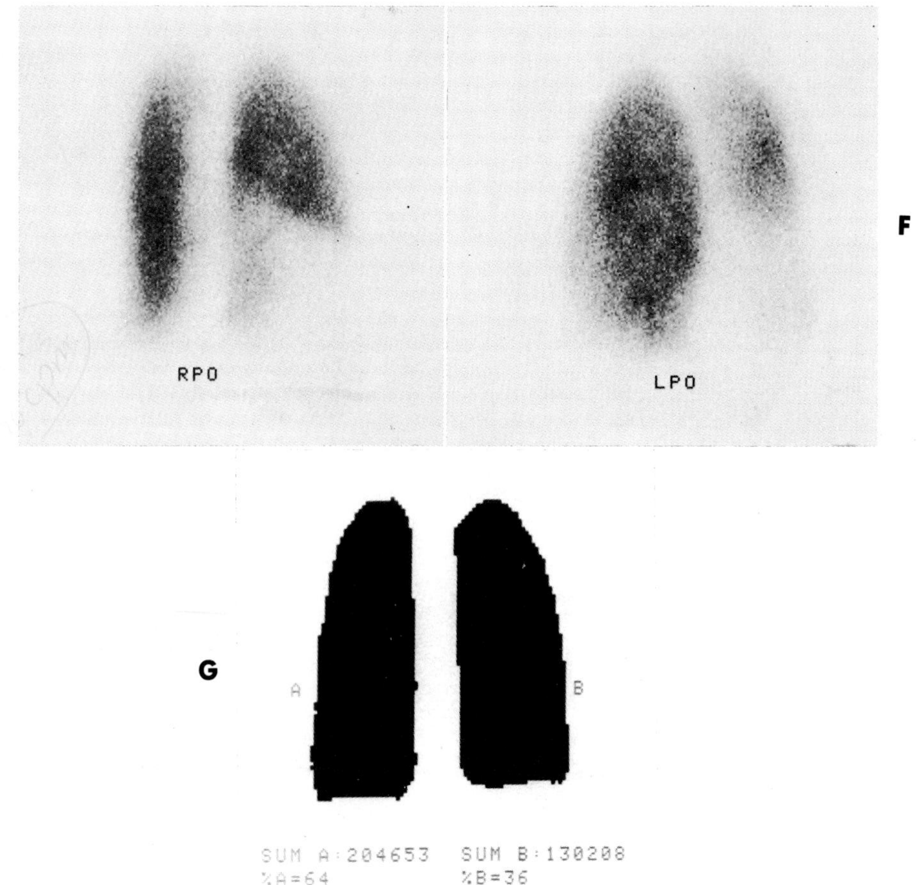

Fig. 19-13, cont'd. For legend see page 457.

Inflammatory disease of the lung

Acute or chronic inflammatory diseases of the lung may cause nonsegmental decrease of perfusion in areas of inflammation that are usually seen on a chest radiograph. Pneumonia causes a reduction of perfusion characteristically smaller than the density seen on chest radiograph; this appearance should distinguish the diagnosis from pulmonary infarct. However, in some cases detected very early, pneumonia may produce ventilation-perfusion defects that mimic pulmonary embolism. Pulmonary fibrosis produces either inhomogeneity of distribution or absence of perfusion, depending on the severity of the disease. Pulmonary sarcoidosis causes a large cone-shaped reduction of perfusion, usually located in the superior regions of the lung.

Pleural effusion (Fig. 19-12)

Large pleural effusions cause mild peripheral reduction of perfusion only, while loculated effusions displace lung tissue in a small area and may produce a picture of a perfusion defect on lung scintiscans.

Primary lung carcinoma (Figs. 19-13 and 19-14)

Centrally located lung carcinoma causes complete absence of perfusion in the segment, lobe, or lung involved that is unusual for other disease processes except possibly massive bullous emphysema. Peripheral lung carcinoma causes focal reduction of perfusion unless mediastinal lymph nodes are involved; in this case, complete absence of perfusion of the whole lung is often visible. Superimposed pulmonary emboli may be found with primary lung carcinoma. Pulmonary scintigraphy

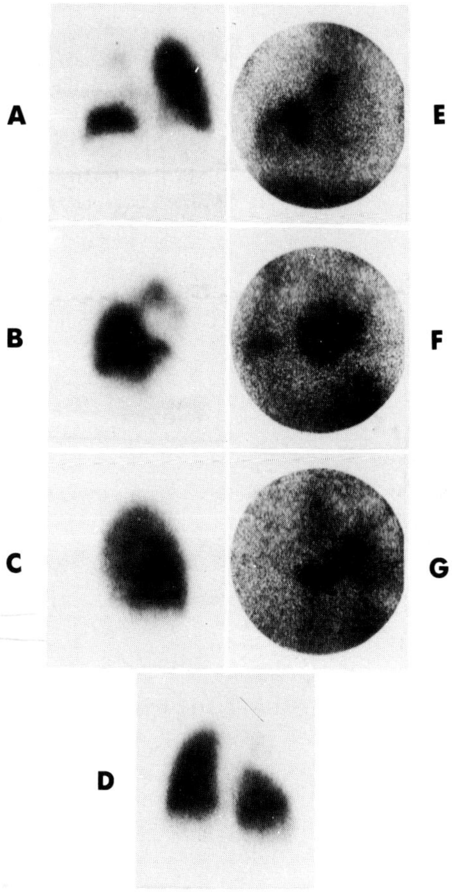

A E

B F

C G

D

Fig. 19-14. ^{99m}Tc HAM lung images. **A,** Anterior view. **B,** Right lateral view. **C,** Left lateral view. **D,** Posterior view. Comment: Almost total absence of perfusion in right upper lobe. ^{67}Ga citrate images 24 hours after administration of dose. **E,** Anterior view. **F,** Right lateral view. **G,** Posterior view. Comment: (Anterior view) 6-cm concentration of gallium in right upper lobe and superior mediastinal concentration. Lateral and posterior views also reveal increased concentration in seventh dorsal vertebra. Diagnosis: Bronchogenic carcinoma of right upper lobe with metastases.

may be useful in the preoperative evaluation of patients with lung carcinoma and compromised pulmonary function.

Metastatic carcinoma of the lung

Metastatic carcinoma of the lung may cause areas of mildly decreased perfusion on lung scintiscans; usually the chest radiograph is abnormal in this group of patients.

LABORATORY APPLICATION

53

VENTILATION/INHALATION IMAGING

Purpose

Ventilation/inhalation studies using radioactive gases are a quantitative and qualitative external method of studying lung physiology. The inert gases ^{133}Xe, ^{127}Xe, or ^{81m}Kr are used in many nuclear medicine departments. Nebulized aerosols are currently being used in most large institutions because of the cost of the test and NRC regulations. Various radiopharmaceuticals, particulate and nonparticulate, have been administered by aerosol using positive pressure. ^{99m}Tc-labeled DTPA (diethylenetriaminepentaacetate) and sulfur colloid are probably the most extensively used; however, larger-size particles such as red blood cells labeled with ^{99m}Tc or with ^{113m}In may be employed to evaluate patients affected by COPD and to study the function of tracheobronchial epithelium. With proper aerosol administration, particle size may be made small enough to reach the alveoli. In normal subjects, the smallest particles reach the alveoli and the larger particles adhere to the larger segments of the tracheobronchial tree. Valuable information related to COPD as well as the possibility to distinguish COPD-related perfusion defects from those secondary to pulmonary embolization can be obtained from these results.

Continued.

Indications

1. Gases and small-size particles may be used to add specificity to the lung-perfusion images for assessing the probability of pulmonary embolism in patients who may have underlying bronchial or pulmonary abnormalities.
2. Larger particles are more useful to stage and follow patients with COPD, lung carcinoma, and other forms of bronchial obstruction and/or lung pathology.
3. Submicron aerosols of DPTA have also been recently used to evaluate pulmonary permeability in restrictive lung disease or pulmonary edema by monitoring their clearance from the lungs.

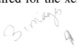

Procedure for ^{133}Xe and ^{127}Xe ventilation

Materials

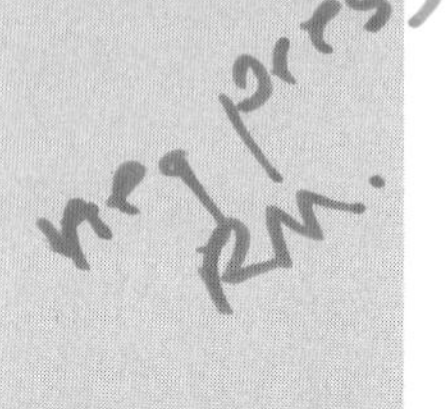

1. ^{133}Xe or ^{127}Xe gas, 10 to 15 mCi (370 to 555 MBq); enclosed ventilation system with appropriate mouthpiece or face mask (this can be a spirometer or a closed system from a commercial supplier)
2. Exhaust system for removing xenon from the room in case of accidental release of exhaled gas
3. Oxygen tank necessary to add oxygen to some systems before performance of the study
4. Scintillation camera with appropriate collimator. For cameras with a large field of view, use a low-energy parallel-hole collimator for ^{133}Xe and medium energy collimator for ^{127}Xe
5. Photographic recording device and/or data storage system

Patient preparation

1. No special preparation is required; however, the entire procedure should be explained to the patient before beginning the examination.

Technique

1. Turn exhaust system on. This is done in case of accidental release of xenon in the room. In case of accidental release of xenon, the room must be closed off in accordance with the exhaust system used and the Nuclear Regulatory Commission (NRC) license.
2. Set camera and photographic controls.
3. Peak camera for radionuclide energy level. ^{133}Xe has a 80-keV gamma, ^{127}Xe has a 202-keV gamma
4. Position patient for posterior view in upright position. The Xe dose may be used to perform a transmission image to check the patient position. The routine view for performance of this study is the posterior view. If the patient has recently undergone perfusion-lung imaging, the patient should be ventilated in the position that depicts the perfusion defects best. Because of the higher energy of ^{127}Xe, a combined perfusion and ventilation study can be performed. Complete the perfusion image first; then, without moving the patient, complete a ventilation study for comparison.
5. Place face mask on patient and hold firmly in place, covering nose and mouth. A mouthpiece may also be used with a clamp on the patient's nose.
6. Attach xenon delivery system for injection of xenon and collection of exhaled xenon.
7. Instruct patient to take a deep breath. At the same time inject the xenon. Have patient hold the breath for 15 seconds and record the image. This is a 15-second inspiration image.
8. Instruct patient to exhale and stop breathing for 15 seconds. Record the image. This is a 15-second expiration image.
9. Instruct patient to breath normally and obtain a 60-second image. This is a 60-second equilibrium image.
10. Change controls on the system so the patient may inhale room air through the mask or mouthpiece and exhale into the closed system.
11. Record three to six 60-second images until the bulk of the xenon has left the lungs. These are 60-second washout images.
12. Close off xenon delivery system and remove mask from the patient's face.
13. Dispose of xenon according to system used and the NRC license. When using ^{127}Xe, additional shielding may be required for the xenon traps.

Procedure for ^{81m}Kr inhalation

Materials

1. Krypton ^{81m}Kr gas generator
2. Oxygen tubing with appropriate mouthpiece or face mask
3. Humidified oxygen supply; as oxygen passes through rubidium generator, krypton flows directly to the patient (flow rate of 3 L/min)
4. Scintillation camera with appropriate collimator; for cameras with a wide field of view, use a low-energy, parallel-hole collimator or a medium-energy, parallel-hole collimator
5. Photographic recording device and/or data storage system

Patient preparation

1. No special preparation of the patient is required; however, the entire procedure should be explained to the patient before beginning the examination.

Technique

1. Set camera and photographic controls.
2. Peak camera at energy level (^{81m}Kr has a 191-keV gamma).
3. Before administering ^{81m}Kr, give the patient 3 mCi (111 MBq) of ^{99m}Tc macroaggregated albumin (see perfusion-lung–imaging procedure).
4. With the patient in an upright position and face mask or nasal cannula in place, a perfusion and an inhalation study can be alternated.
5. Perform the anterior perfusion; then, without moving the patient, adjust the gamma camera energy setting for ^{81m}Kr. Administer the ^{81m}Kr and image for 300K to 500K. This technique should continue for the remainder of views (right lateral, left lateral, posterior, right posterior oblique, and left posterior oblique).
6. The recommended dose for ^{81m}Kr is 1 to 10 mCi (37 to 370 MBq) administered by continuous inhalation. (Refer to manufacturer's guidelines for maximum millicuries per minute.)
7. Turn humidified oxygen supply off and remove mask from patient's face.
8. Place ^{81m}Kr generator in appropriate storage area.

Procedure for ventilation with aerosols

Materials

1. Scintillation gamma camera with low-energy, parallel-hole, medium- or high-resolution collimator
2. Imaging device and computer for data acquisition
3. Positive pressure nebulizer (driven by compressed air or oxygen at a flow rate of 10 to 15 L/min)
4. Disposable tubing
5. Y connectors
6. Baffle within nebulizer
7. One-way breathing valves
8. Mouthpiece or face mask
9. Bacteria filter
10. ^{99m}Tc-labeled DTPA, 25 to 35 mCi (925 to 1295 MBq), in a volume of 3 to 4 ml

Patient preparation

1. Explain the entire procedure to the patient.
2. Instruct the patient to breathe normally and relax.

Technique

1. Support nebulizer in upright position in an appropriate shield.
2. Connect nebulizer to oxygen or air supply through standard tubing.

Continued.

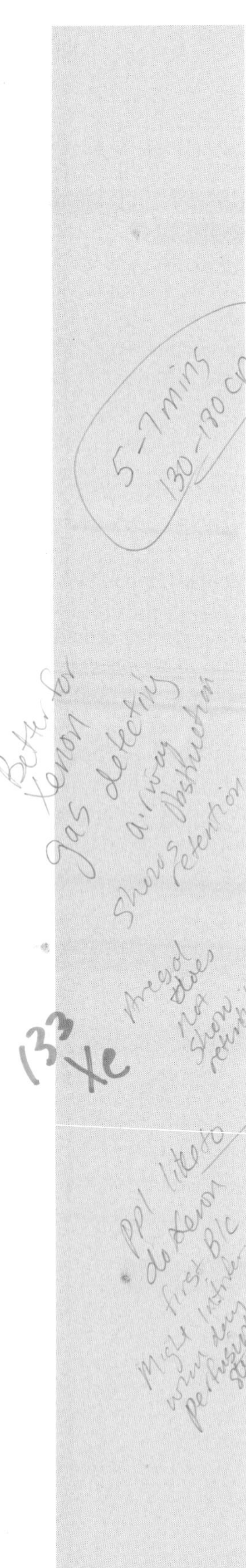

3. Introduce 25 to 35 mCi (925 to 1295 MBq) of ^{99m}Tc DTPA in 2 to 3 ml through the opened end of the Y valve (at the top of the shield) leading into the nebulizer. With the needle, press aside the rubber valve diaphragm and slowly inject the aerosol. Do not use a needle longer than 1½ inches.
4. The patient can be in the supine or sitting position. Instruct him or her to breathe by mouth; the valve diaphragm should be opening and closing.
5. If the mouthpiece is used, the nose must be clamped shut. A tight-fitting mask may be used in place of the mouthpiece; for an uncooperative patient a face mask is preferable.
6. Turn on oxygen or air flow at rate of 10 to 12 L/min. (The pressure must be greater than 30 psi.)
7. The ventilation procedure can be done either before or after the perfusion study.
   a. For preperfusion study, the patient should breathe tidally for 5 to 7 minutes. This is sufficient to deposit 0.70 to 1 mCi (25.9 to 37 MBq) of ^{99m}Tc in the lungs (130,000 to 180,000 cpm)
   b. For postperfusion study, the patient should breathe tidally for 5 to 7 minutes. This is sufficient to deposit 2 to 3 mCi (74 to 111 MBq) of ^{99m}Tc in the lungs (300,000 to 500,000 cpm).
8. Turn off the gas flow to nebulizer.
9. If face mask is being used, wipe patient's face with damp washcloth. Have the patient expel any saliva into a disposable washcloth to reduce gastric accumulation of the drug.
10. Dispose of unit (nebulizer, mouthpiece) into a plastic bag and place in low-level waste disposal.
11. Obtain the same anatomic views as done in perfusion study.
12. When using larger size aerosols (HAMM), obtain an additional set of views 4 hours later.

Diagnosis (Figs. 19-15 to 19-18)

Anatomy is not as clear-cut on ventilation images as on perfusion studies because chronic lung disease, like pulmonary emphysema, crosses segmental lung boundaries, which may distort the images. Xenon ventilation images are limited to one view, usually chosen from the perfusion study to demonstrate the defect(s) to best advantage. One of the main advantages of gas over aerosol is that it detects regions of airway obstruction by showing retention of the gas during the clearance phase, while aerosols and krypton do not show such retention. Because of the short half-life of ^{81m}Kr, inhalation studies using this gas may be repeated to match the six-view lung-perfusion study. The use of the aerosols allows a direct comparison of perfusion and ventilation in multiple views. Compared to ^{81m}Kr, aerosols are less expensive and more readily available. Some people advocate doing a ^{133}Xe-ventilation study before the perfusion because of the possibility of interference between the two energies if this order is reversed. We do not find this to be a real problem, and we prefer to do the perfusion study first for two reasons. First, if the perfusion study is normal it obviates the need for a ventilation study. Second, we perform the ventilation study with the patient in the position that shows the defect(s) to best advantage. Ventilation studies done with technetium-labeled aerosol should be obtained before the perfusion because both are done with the same radionuclide. However, accurate computer techniques of subtraction may prevent the overlap of activity from the perfusion and ventilation studies. With the advent of ^{127}Xe, the xenon ventilation may follow the ^{99m}Tc-macroaggregated lung-perfusion images because of the different energies of the two nuclides. However, ^{127}Xe is expensive and not readily available.

Pulmonary embolism (Fig. 19-19)

The ventilation study is classically normal in patients with pulmonary embolization. Accordingly, patients with two or more segmental perfusion defects and normal ventilation have high probability (more than 85%) of embolism. In patients with severe COPD or with radiographic abnormalities matching the perfusion defects, the probability of embolism is indeterminate. When the ventilation study is also indeterminate, and if the clinical suspicion of embolism is still present, pulmonary arteriography or digital subtraction angiography should be performed. In everyday practice most nuclear medicine departments utilize modifications of prospective investigation of pulmonary embolism diagnosis (PIOPED) criteria to state the probability of pulmonary embolization. Based on its

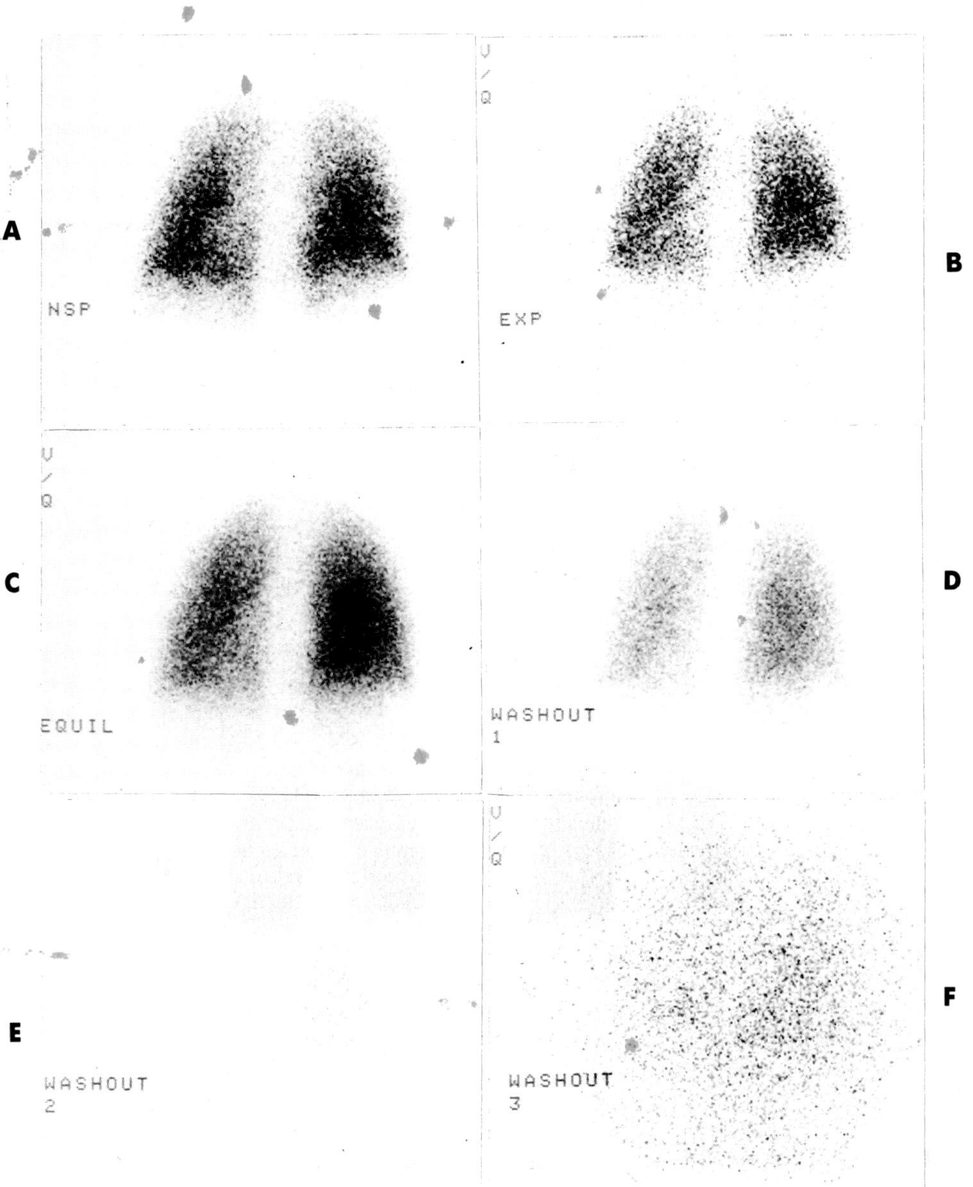

Fig. 19-15. ^{127}Xe ventilation images demonstrate initial minimal decrease in apices; however, equilibrium reveals more uniform distribution. No significant trapping in washout views. This is essentially negative ventilation study. **A,** Inspiration view. **B,** Expiration view. **C,** Equilibrium view. **D,** Washout 1. **E,** Washout 2. **F,** Washout 3.

Continued.

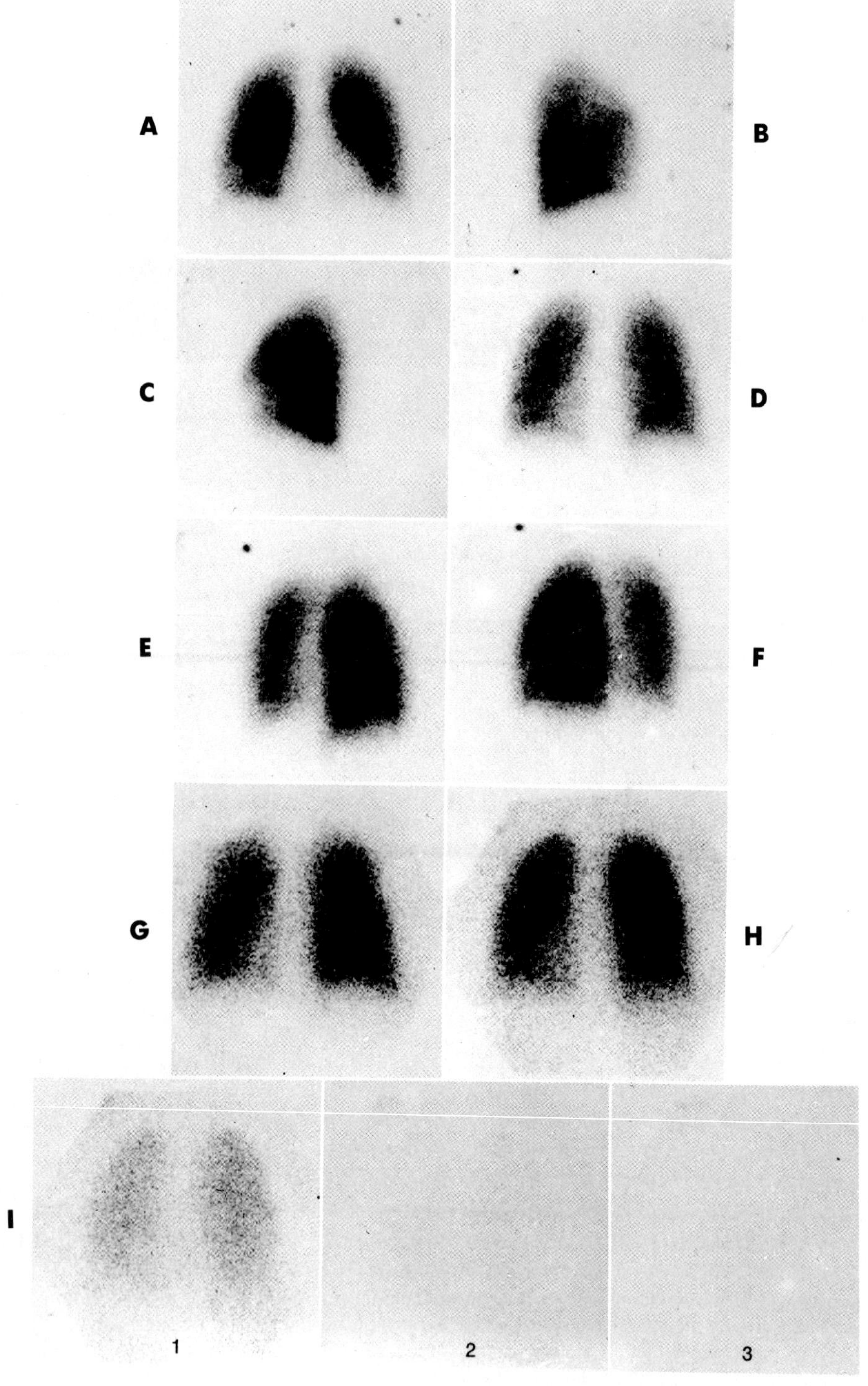

Fig. 19-16. Moderately obese young patient with short history of left chest pain. Perfusion lung images (^{99m}TC MAA) are within normal limits. **A,** Anterior view (slight decrease at right lateral base because of fold of fat). **B,** Right lateral view. **C,** Left lateral view. **D,** Posterior view. **E,** Right posterior oblique view. **F,** Left posterior oblique view. ^{133}Xe ventilation study is normal. Studies were performed in posterior position. **G,** Inhalation. **H,** Equilibrium. **I,** Washout phase.

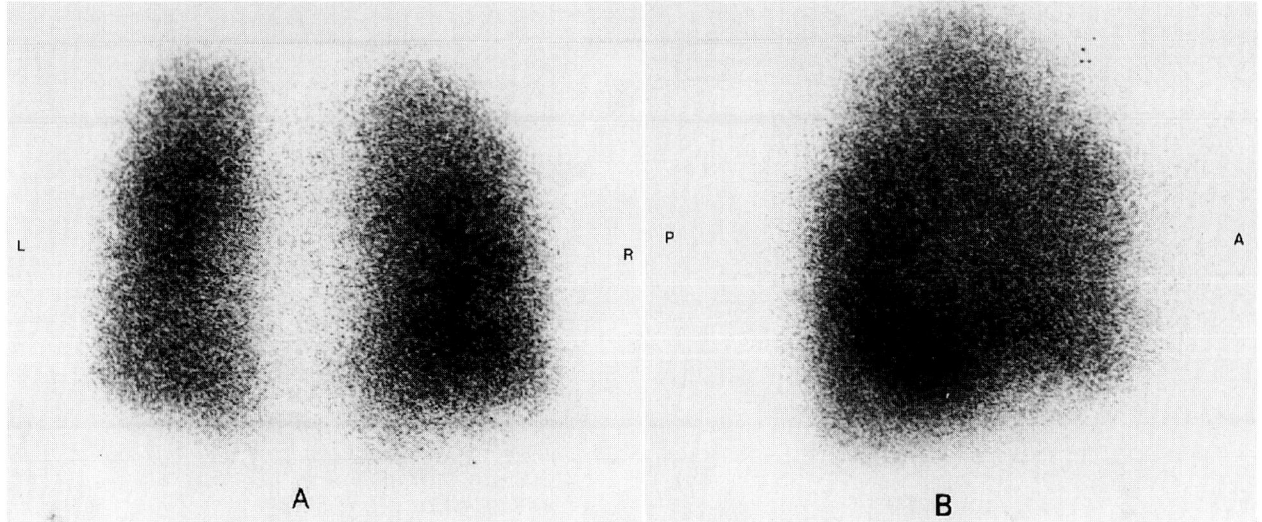

Fig. 19-17. ^{81m}Kr ventilation images of a normal subject demonstrate uniform distribution of gas to both lungs. Multiple views may be obtained; only two are shown here for the sake of brevity. **A,** Posterior view. **B,** Right lateral view.

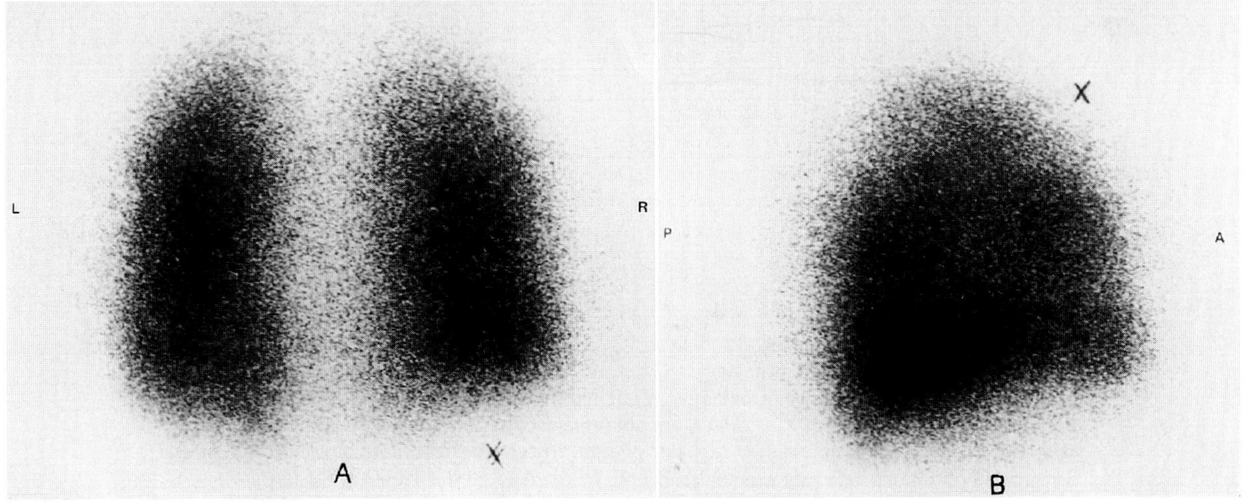

Fig. 19-18. ^{99m}Tc HAMM ventilation images of a normal subject showing uniform distribution of minimicrospheres to both lungs. Multiple views may be obtained; only two are reported here for the sake of brevity. **A,** Posterior view. **B,** Right lateral view.

Continued.

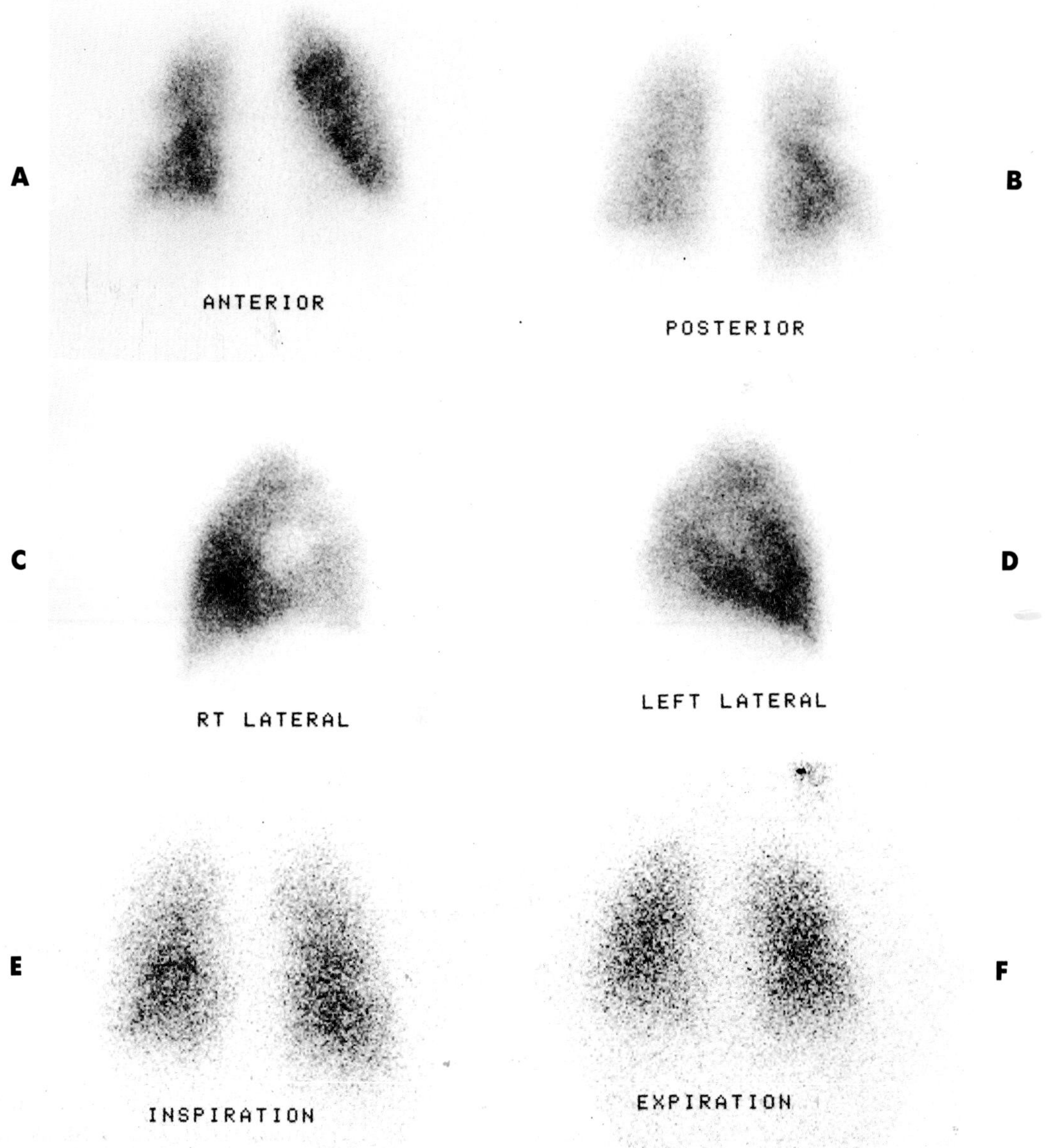

Fig. 19-19. Patient has history of phlebitis in left lower leg and recent onset of right chest pain. Perfusion lung images using ^{99m}Tc MAA are abnormal. There is sharply defined absence of perfusion in general region of superior segment of right lower lobe with normal concentration and distribution of radionuclide over remainder of lung fields. **A,** Anterior view. **B,** Posterior view. **C,** Right lateral view. **D,** Left lateral view.

On deep inspiration, ^{133}Xe ventilation images reveal a minimal area of decreased ventilation in region of superior segment of right lower lobe. Expiration and equilibrium images are normal. Washout images are also normal. Studies were performed in posterior position. **E,** Inspiration. **F,** Expiration. **G,** Equilibrium. **H,** Washout 1. **I,** Washout 2. Combined with sharply defined defect on pulmonary perfusion imaging, the Xe study suggests strong possibility of solitary pulmonary embolus in right lung.

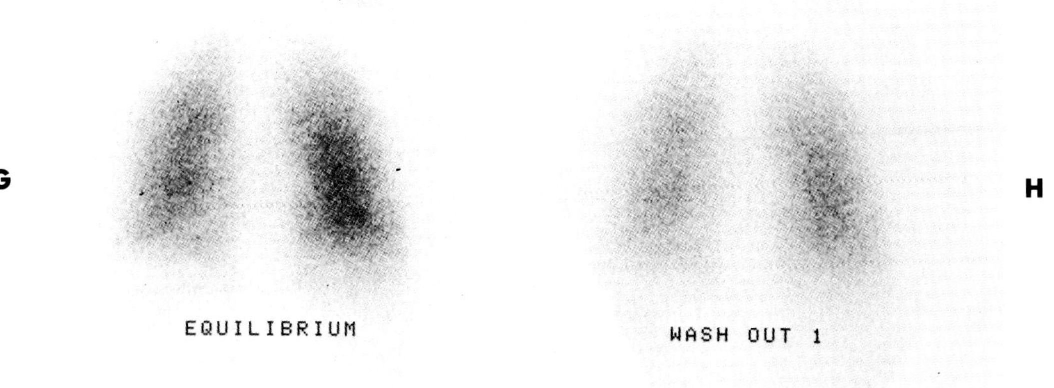

Fig. 19-19, cont'd. For legend see opposite page.

ability to separate target organ from background activity, SPECT also has been employed in conjunction with radiolabeled aerosols (DTPA or sulfur colloid) or ^{81m}Kr to obtain pulmonary ventilation and ventilation/perfusion ratio. Available results suggest that SPECT finds regions of abnormal deposition not seen on conventional imaging; these data, however, need to be confirmed in larger clinical studies.

Chronic obstructive pulmonary disease (Figs. 19-20 to 19-23)

In mild airway obstruction, ^{133}Xe-ventilation studies show uneven and delayed entry of the gas; the equilibrium phase is approached only after several minutes. During the washout phase, ^{133}Xe is cleared slowly and unevenly and that underlines the presence of an obstructive state. In severe bullous disease, xenon may still be in the regions of bullous formation for up to 15 minutes. ^{81m}Kr does not show the delay of activity clearance, but it is useful for dynamic studies after administration of bronchodilators. Regardless of which agent is used, ventilation and perfusion are typically matched in patients with obstructive airway disease.

Bronchogenic carcinoma

The main role of ventilation/perfusion imaging in lung carcinoma is quantification of differential pulmonary function, useful in determining whether a patient should have a pneumonectomy. Since there is partial occlusion of the bronchus, there is decreased delivery of xenon to the region of the lung distal to the carcinoma during inhalation and retention during the washout phase of the study. With either small (DTPA) or larger (HAMM) particles, significant reduction of ventilation distal to the carcinoma may be visualized. The use of SPECT may help detect defects of ventilation in regions that are otherwise difficult to explore, such as apices or areas near the mediastinum.

Continued.

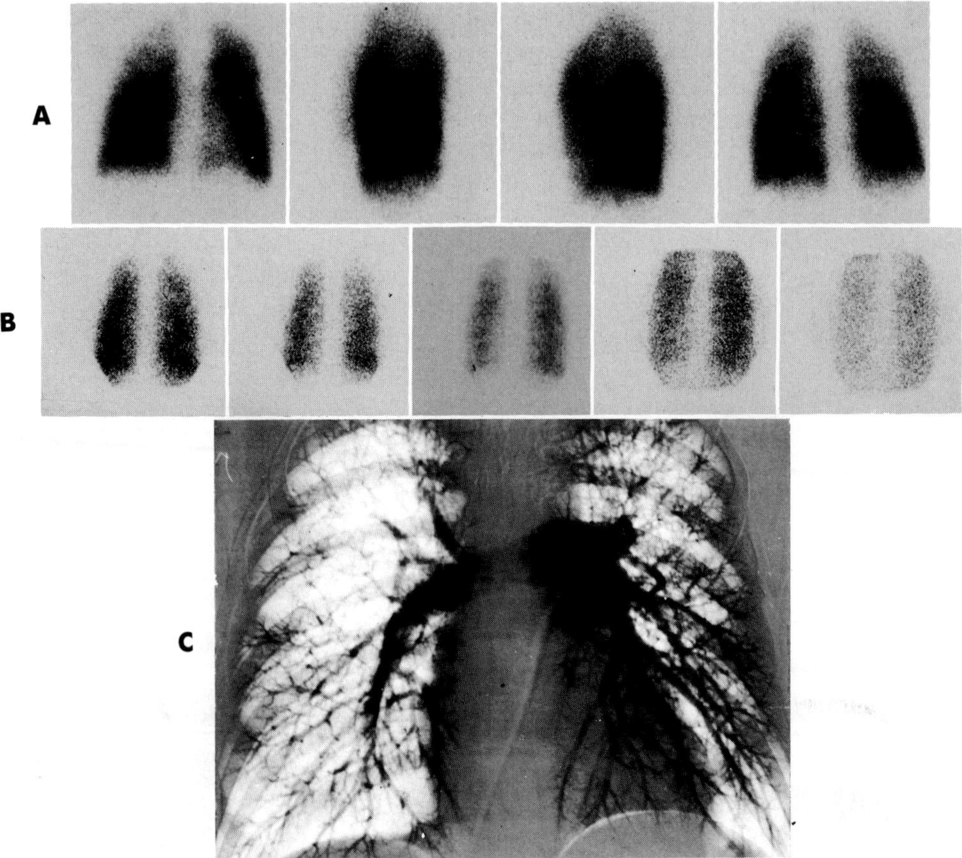

Fig. 19-20. COPD. **A,** Lung-perfusion images reveal nonsegmental decreased perfusion of both upper lobes. **B,** Xe ventilation study. *From left to right:* Inspirational view reveals expanded lung volume and uneven distribution in upper lobes and superior right lower lobe; expiration view reveals decreased compliance; equilibrium view reveals uneven distribution; and two washout views reveal prolonged washout of left upper lobe, right upper lobe, and superior right lower lobe. Chest x-ray study was negative. **C,** Pulmonary angiogram reveals slight decrease of perfusion of left and right upper lobes, but greater decrease of perfusion is noted in right upper lobe. No segmental perfusion defects suggestive of pulmonary embolization are seen.

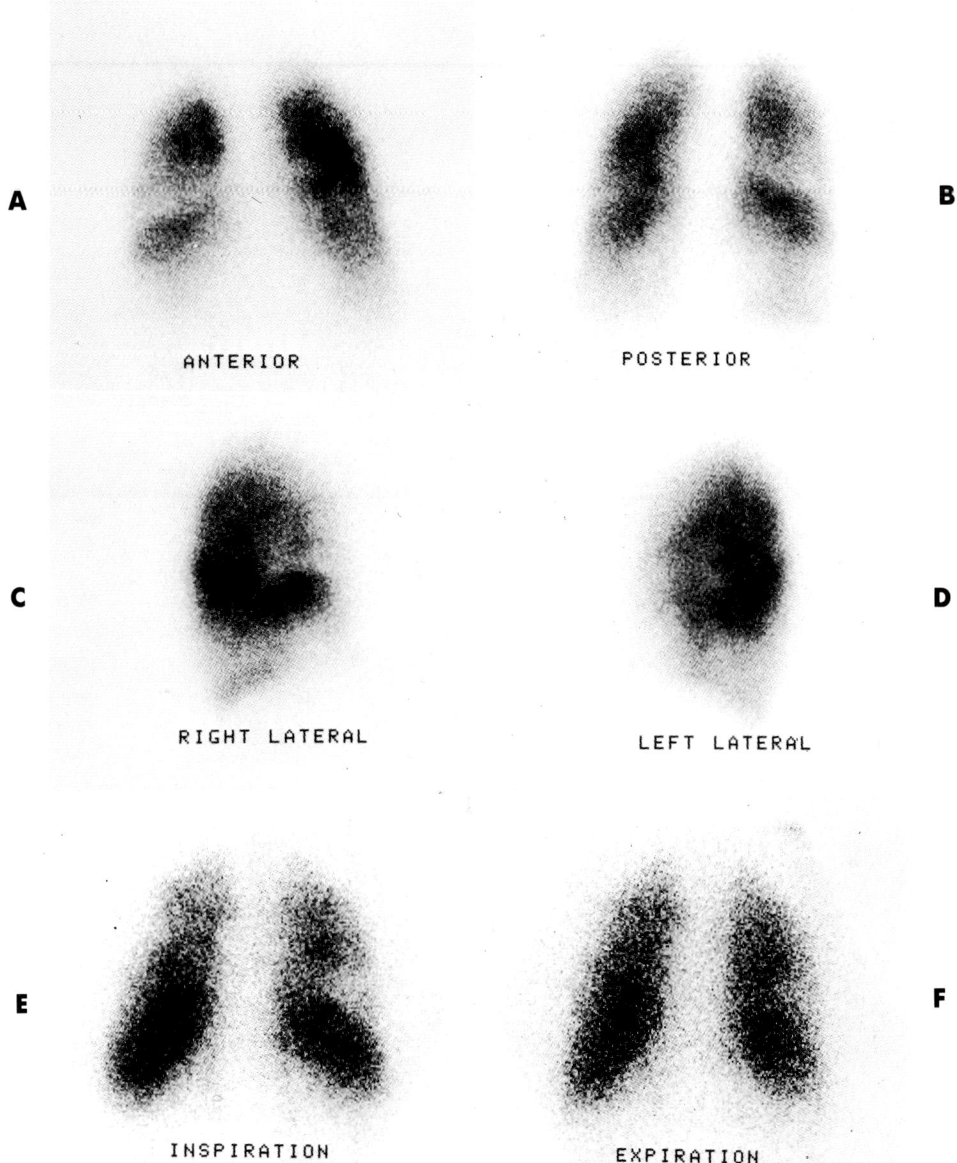

Fig. 19-21. Patient is 74-year-old male with moderately severe COPD (emphysema), history of acute chest pain, and increasing shortness of breath. Lung-perfusion images are abnormal. There are multiple nonsegmental regions of decreased perfusion visualized bilaterally. This is almost absent perfusion in region of basilar lower lobe. **A,** Anterior view. **B,** Posterior view. **C,** Right lateral view. **D,** Left lateral view.

^{133}Xe ventilation images are abnormal. On deep inspiration there is significant bilateral decrease in inspiratory volume in upper lobes. Equilibrium phase is normal. Sequential washout images are abnormal with prolonged washout of xenon from areas of increased dead air space (emphysema) in basilar portions of both lower lobes and in midlung fields, primarily on right. Studies were performed in posterior position. **E,** Inspiration. **F,** Expiration. **G,** Equilibrium. **H,** Washout 1. **I,** Washout 2. **J,** Washout 3. **K,** Washout 4. **L,** Washout 4, intensity increased. Combined studies demonstrate matched defects of perfusion and ventilation of COPD.

Continued.

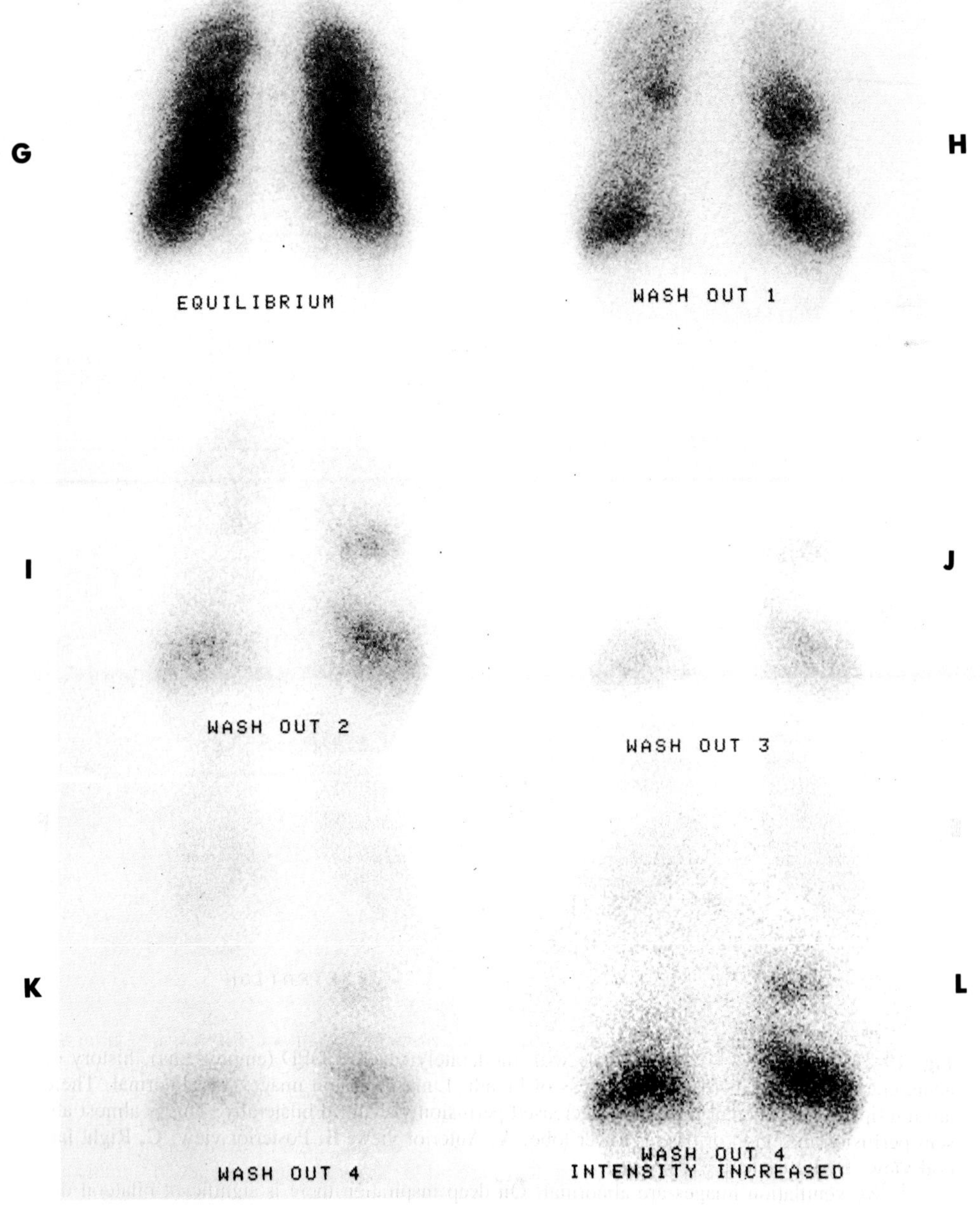

Fig. 19-21, cont'd. For legend see page 469.

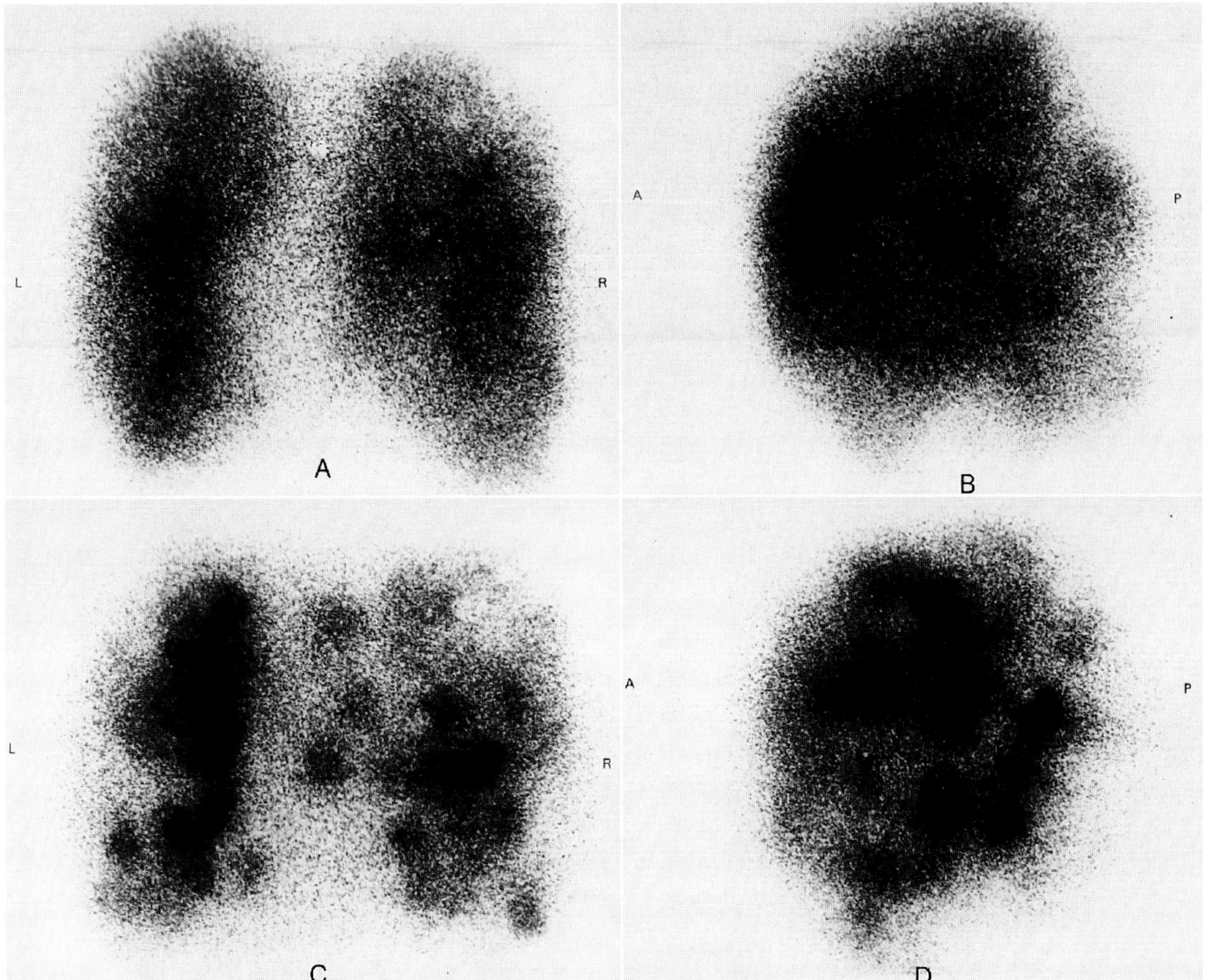

Fig. 19-22. ^{81m}Kr ventilation study in a patient affected by severe chronic bronchitis. The distribution of gas shows inhomogeneity and absence of ventilation in most regions of left lower lobe. **A,** Posterior view. **B,** Left lateral view. ^{99m}Tc ventilation study in the same patient shows a typical "spotty" deposition as a result of the significant inhomogeneity of ventilation. Minimicrospheres (HAMM) have a mean diameter of 0.75 μm and, unlike gases, their intrapulmonary deposition is affected by gravitational settling in respiratory units. Pathologic changes in the airways may influence their pattern of deposition. **C,** Posterior view. **D,** Left lateral view.

Continued.

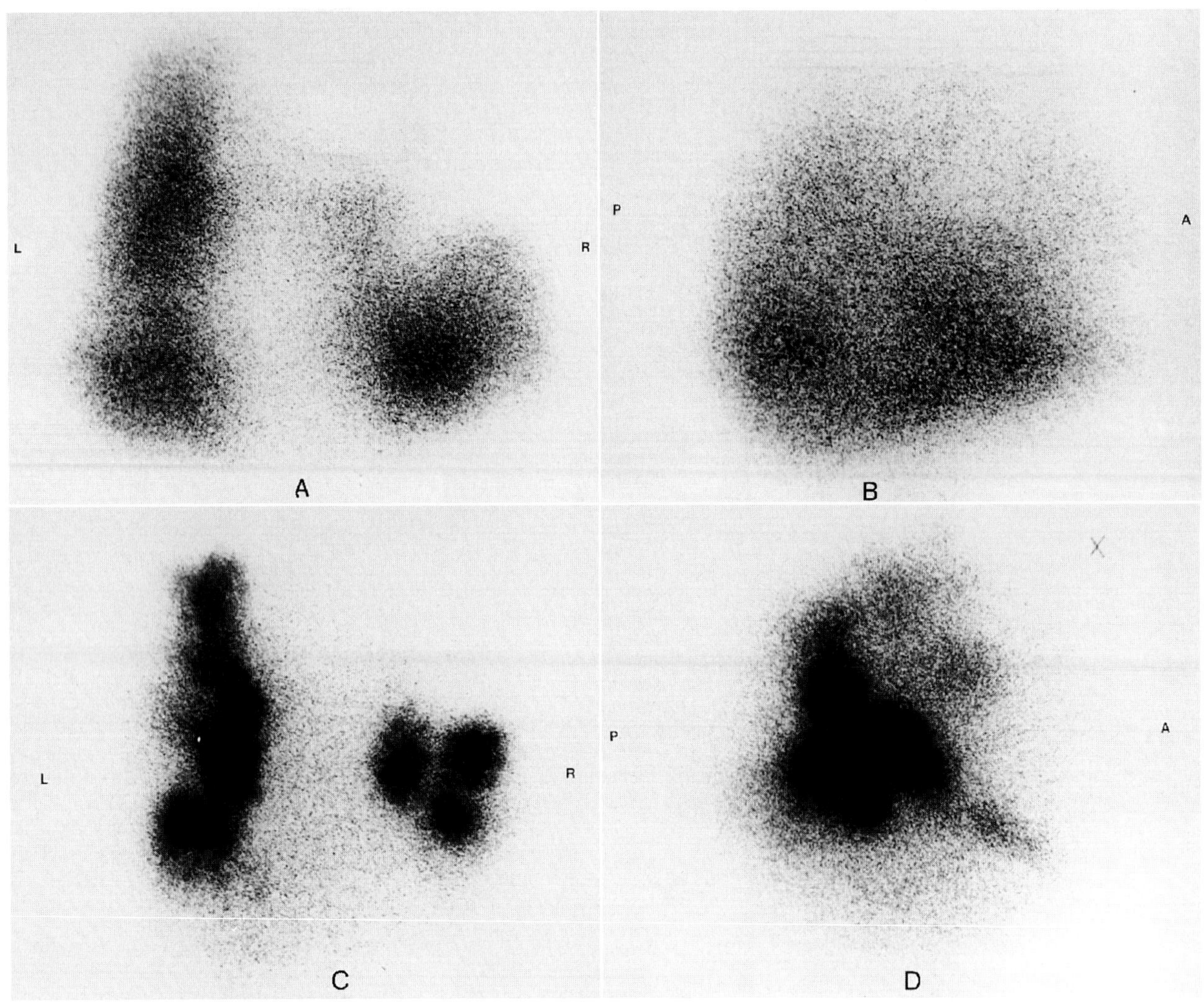

Fig. 19-23. ^{81m}Kr ventilation study in a patient with bronchial asthma. Beside the inhomogeneity of gas distribution, notice the absence of ventilation in the upper regions of the right lung. **A,** Posterior view. **B,** Right lateral view. ^{99m}Tc HAMM ventilation study in the same patient shows a typical "central" deposition of particles in large bronchi while the peripheral lung regions are not visualized because of airway obstruction. **C,** Posterior view. **D,** Right lateral view.

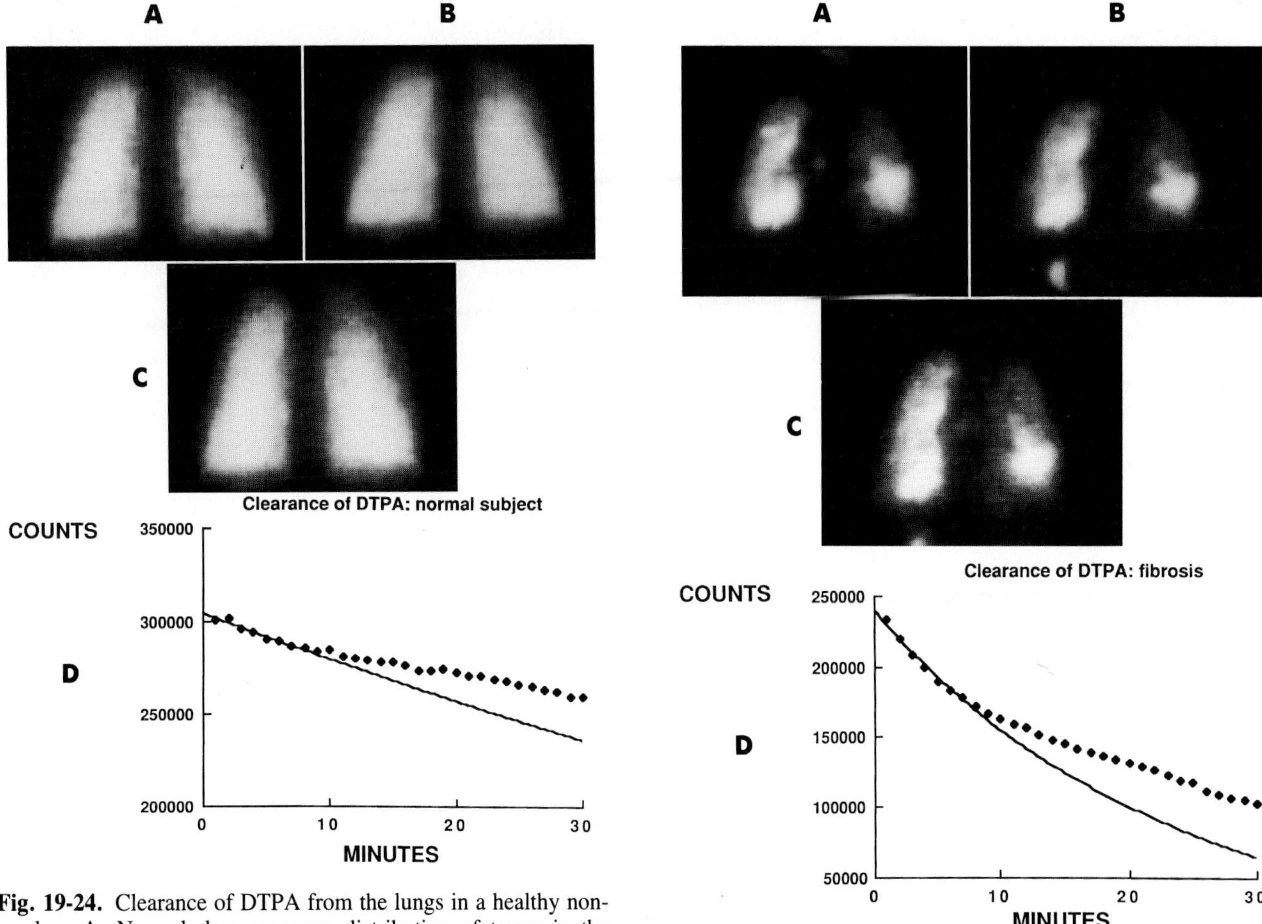

Fig. 19-24. Clearance of DTPA from the lungs in a healthy nonsmoker. **A,** Normal, homogeneous distribution of tracer in the lungs (anterior view) obtained at **(A)** Time 0; **(B)** 15 min; and **(C)** 30 min after inhalation. **D,** Time/activity curve in the same subject. The fitting was calculated over the first 8 min to avoid the problem of recirculating DTPA. (Courtesy of Drs. A.M. Santolicandro and S. Ruschi, CNR Institute of Clinical Physiology and 2nd Medical Clinic, University of Pisa, Italy.)

Fig. 19-25. Clearance of DTPA from the lungs in a patient with pulmonary fibrosis. Markedly inhomogeneous distribution of tracer in both lungs and hypoventilation of upper regions. Images (anterior view) were obtained at (**A**), Time 0′; (**B**), 15 min; and (**C**), 30 min after inhalation. **D**, Time/activity curve in the same patient. The fitting was calculated over the first 8 min only. The steeper slope of the curve is due to the accelerated DTPA clearance. (Courtesy of Drs. A.M. Santolicandro and S. Ruschi, CNR Institute of Clinical Physiology and 2nd Medical Clinic, University of Pisa, Italy.)

Pneumonia, pulmonary fibrosis, and space-occupying lesions

In pneumonia, pulmonary fibrosis, or in regions of lung parenchymal space-occupying lesions, there is an absence of xenon as well as krypton or aerosols in the abnormal regions involved in all phases of the study.

OTHER USES OF AEROSOLS

Changes in alveolar-capillary permeability (Figs. 19-24 and 19-25)

Available data on the use of ^{99m}Tc-labeled aerosols suggest that the clearance rate of DTPA from the lungs varies with changes in alveolar-capillary permeability. In normal subjects, this permeability may be reversibly increased by cigarette smoking. Accelerated clearance of DTPA particles may be found in patients with chronic interstitial lung disease or with inflammation of the lung such as ARDS and pneumocystis pneumonia.

Continued.

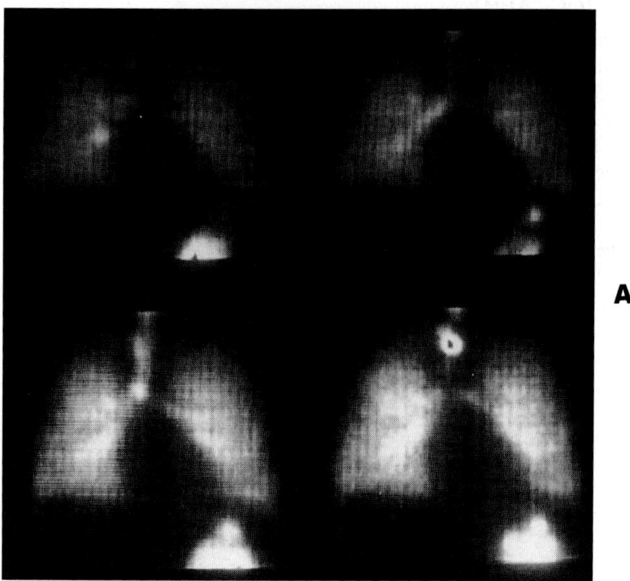

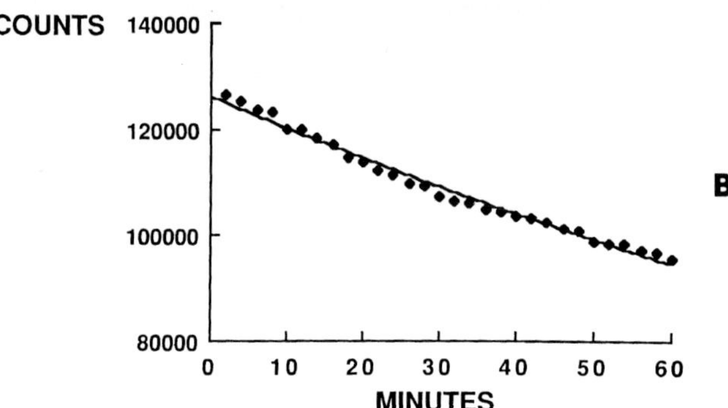

Fig. 19-26. Tracheobronchial clearance of HAMM in a healthy nonsmoker. **A,** Images (anterior view) of tracheobronchial clearance over a 60-min period.

- Soon after inhalation (upper left): lungs are homogeneously ventilated; early phase of tracheobronchial clearance of HAMM is shown in the main right bronchus as a rounded hot spot due to particle accumulation.
- 20 min later (upper right): the particle accumulation has moved up toward the carina
- 40 min later (lower left): the particle accumulation has reached the carina
- 60 min later (lower right): the particle accumulation has been eliminated from the bronchi

B, Time/activity curve in the same subject. After 60 min, about 25% of the intrapulmonary deposition has been cleared away by the tracheobronchial clearance. (Courtesy of Drs. A.M. Santolicandro and S. Ruschi, CNR Institute of Clinical Physiology and 2nd Medical Clinic, University of Pisa, Italy.)

Tracheobronchial clearance (Fig. 19-26)

Particulate aerosols have been used in pulmonary medicine to study tracheobronchial clearance as an index of bronchial epithelium function. Large-size particles deposit along the bronchi and are cleared away by the endothelial cells. Although the rate of removal of particulate material is largely dependent on deposition site, it is also dependent on the presence of airway disease.

Metabolic activity of the lung

In addition to the function of external gas exchange, the lung also has a metabolic function. It activates, deactivates, or synthesizes many metabolites, such as vasoactive amines, peptides, and cyclic nucleotides within the endothelial cells. Recent data have demonstrated that radiolabeled amines are accumulated in the lung by saturable, receptor-specific mechanisms. By following the accumulation of radiolabeled amines in the lung, it is possible to study the regional pulmonary metabolism and the regional lung function in both health and disease. Most recently, a synthetic basic compound with high affinity for lung tissue, the *N,N,N′*-trimethyl-*N′*-(2-hydroxy-3 methyl-5-iodobenzyl)-1,3-proranendiamine (HIPDM) labeled with ^{123}I has demonstrated different behavior in healthy nonsmokers, in asymptomatic smokers, and in patients with other pulmonary disorders. The differences may reflect an increased number of cellular binding sites or may be the expression of hindered HIPDM biotransformation. The investigation of these mechanisms offers the basis for future promising studies. For that purpose, SPECT may represent a useful ancillary technique because it allows one to quantify the pulmonary metabolism with possible intriguing clinical implications.

BIBLIOGRAPHY

Alderson, P.O., and others: Tc-99m-DTPA aerosol and radioactive gases compared as adjuncts to perfusion scintigraphy in patients with suspected pulmonary embolism, Radiology 153:515, 1984.

Coates, G., and Nahmias, C.: Xenon-127, a comparison with Xe-133 for ventilation studies, J. Nucl. Med. 18:221, 1977.

Effros, R.M., and others: Tc-99m-DTPA aerosol deposition and clearance in COPD, interstitial disease, and smokers, J. Thorac. Imag. 1(2):54, 1986.

English, R.J., and Brown, S.E.: Single photon emission computed tomography: a primer, New York, 1986, The Society of Nuclear Medicine, Inc.

Ellis, D.A., and others: Role of lung scanning in assessing the resectability of bronchial carcinoma, Thorax 38:261, 1983.

Fazio, F., and Jones, T.: Assessment of regional ventilation by continuous inhalation of radioactive krypton-81m, BMJ 3:673, 1975.

Giuntini, C., and others: Factors affecting regional pulmonary blood flow in left heart vascular disease, Am. J. Med. 57:421, 1974.

Gottschalk, A., and others: Ventilation-perfusion scintigraphy in the PIOPED study—Part II: Evaluation of the scintigraphic criteria and interpretations, J. Nucl. Med. 34:1119, 1993.

Guyton, A.G.: Textbook of medical physiology, ed. 6, Philadelphia, 1981, W.B. Saunders Co.

Mandell, C.H.: Scintillation camera lung imaging: an anatomic atlas and guide, New York, 1976, Grune & Stratton, Inc.

McNeil, B.J.: A diagnostic strategy using ventilation-perfusion studies in patients suspect for pulmonary embolism, J. Nucl. Med. 17:613, 1976.

Mellins, R.B.: Metabolic functions of the lung and their clinical relevance, Am. J. Roentgenol. 138:999, 1982.

Osborne, D.R.S., and others: Single photon emission computed tomography and its application in the lung, Radiol. Clin. North Am. 21:789, 1983.

Palla, A., and others: Follow-up of pulmonary perfusion recovery after embolism, J. Nucl. Med. Allied Sci. 30:23, 1986.

Parker, J.A., and others: Pulmonary perfusion after rt-PA therapy for acute embolism: early improvement assessed with segmental perfusion scanning, Radiology 166(2):441-445, 1988.

Pistolesi, M., and others: Perfusion lung imaging in the adult respiratory distress syndrome, J. Thorac. Imag. 1(3):11, 1986.

Santolicandro, A., and others: Imaging of ventilation in chronic obstructive pulmonary disease, J. Thorac. Imag. 1(2):36, 1986.

Sasahara, A.A., and others: New developments in the detection and prevention of venous thromboembolism, Am. J. Cardiol. 43:1214, 1979.

Thibodeau, G.A., and Patton, K.T.: Anthony's textbook of anatomy and physiology, ed. 14, St. Louis, 1994, Mosby–Year Book.

Worsley, D.F., Alavi, A., and Palersky, H.: Role of radionuclide imaging in patients with suspected pulmonary embolism, Radiol. Clin. North Am. 31:849, 1993.

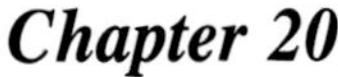

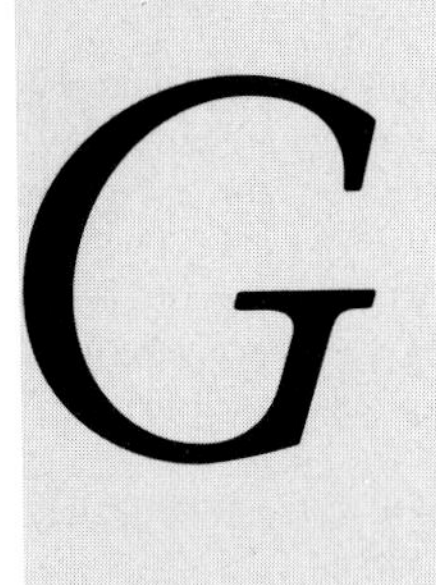

Chapter 20

GASTROINTESTINAL SYSTEM

D. BRUCE SODEE
MICHAEL G. VELCHIK
RICHARD B. NOTO
JOHN REILLEY
ABASS ALAVI

The Liver

D. Bruce Sodee

■ ANATOMY (Figs. 20-1 and 20-2)

The liver is the largest organ in the body, weighing between 1500 and 1800 gm. It is located in the right hypochrondium and epigastrium and may extend into the left hypochondriac region. Its upper surface fits with the under surface of the diaphragm, and the posterior concave surface of the liver fits over the right kidney, the upper portion of the ascending colon, and the pylorus.

The liver connects to the caudal surface of the diaphragm and the anterior walls of the abdomen by five ligaments. The liver is divided into four lobes: the right lobe, the smaller left lobe, the quadrate lobe, and the caudate lobe.

The liver is composed of many units called lobules. Each lobule is composed of cords of hepatic cells loosely held together by alveolar connective tissue that carries capillaries from the portal vein and the hepatic artery and also carries nerves and hepatic ducts. The cords of hepatic cells radiate toward a central or an interlobular vein with branches of hepatic artery and branches of the portal vein being at the periphery of the lobule. Thus small capillaries are in close connection with the hepatic secretory cell, and the cells capable of forming a secretion are in close contact with ducts that empty the secretion from the lobule.

The portal venous system brings blood derived from the stomach to the liver, spleen, pancreas and intestine. In the liver the portal vein divides into a vast number of branches that form the interlobular plexus in the spaces between the hepatic lobules. The portal blood then enters the lobule and converges toward the center. These channels are termed *sinusoids*. The sinusoids empty into the central veins, which continue to empty into the hepatic vein, which enters the inferior vena cava.

Arterial blood is brought to the liver via the hepatic artery. It subdivides in the same manner as the portal vein, mixing in the sinusoids and emptying into the intralobular veins. The liver has a lymphatic system that begins in spaces in the lobules, forms a network around the lobule, and runs centrifugally from the center of the lobule outward. The bile ducts are formed by grooves in the hepatic cells. The grooves on two adjacent hepatic cells fit together and form a passage into which bile is emptied as soon as it is formed by the hepatic cells. The intercellular biliary passages radiate to the circumference of the lobule where they empty into interlobular bile ducts that unite and finally form the right and left main hepatic ducts. The right and left hepatic ducts join just above the point where the cystic duct—the connection with the gallbladder—and the common hepatic duct join. Past this point the duct is called the *common bile duct;* this enters the duodenum after passing behind the head of the pancreas. At its entrance into the duodenum the common bile duct has a muscular sphincter called the *sphincter of Oddi*.

The liver is covered by an outer layer of fibrous tissue called *Glisson's capsule* and is almost entirely enclosed by tissue derived from the peritoneum. Pain fibers are only found in Glisson's capsule; thus pain of hepatic origin is caused by massive enlargement of the liver.

The vascular sinusoids in the hepatic lobule are lined by reticuloendothelial cells called *Kupffer cells*. The hepatic artery, the portal vein, and the common bile duct can all be found in relation to the porta hepatis, which is at the division point of the right and left lobes of the liver.

■ PHYSIOLOGY

This single largest organ of the body has multiple and varied functions, which may be summarized as follows:

1. Secretory and excretory
2. Circulatory
3. Storage
4. Metabolic

■ Secretory and excretory function

The hepatic cells form and secrete approximately 1 liter of bile per day. This bile is made up of bile salts, choles-

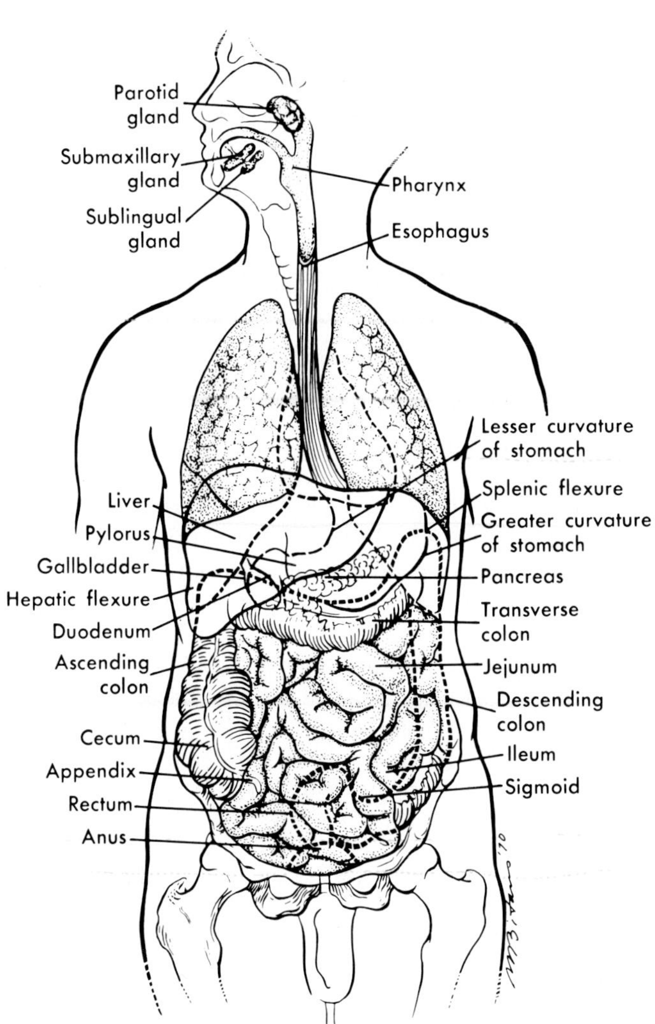

Fig. 20-1. Digestive tract and adjacent organs. (From Austrin, M.G. and Austrin, H.R.: Learning medical terminology, ed. 7, St. Louis, 1991, Mosby–Year Book.)

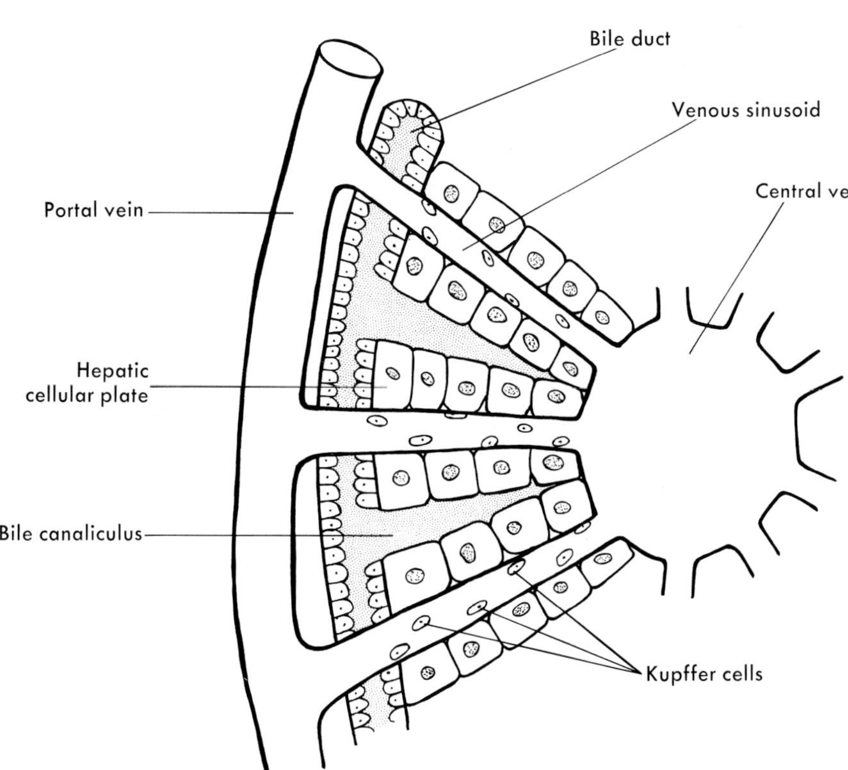

Fig. 20-2. Liver lobule and the relationship of the hepatocyte to the canaliculi and the Kupffer cells to the venous sinusoids. (From Phipps, W., Long, B., and Woods, N.F.: Medical-surgical nursing, concepts and clinical practice, ed. 2, St. Louis, 1983, Mosby–Year Book.)

terol, bile pigments, and water. The bile salts perform a function in the intestinal phases of digestion. Bile pigments are formed from the hemoglobin of degenerating red blood cells.

■ Hemopoietic (circulatory function)

The liver aids in regulation of blood volume by controlling the volume of blood leaving the liver through the hepatic vein. The liver also stores erythrocyte-maturing factor needed in the development of red blood cells, and in the embryo this factor forms red blood cells. The liver produces important coagulation factors such as prothrombin and fibrinogen.

■ Hepatic storage function

Vitamins A, D, and B_{12} are stored in the liver as well as trace elements such as iron, copper, and magnesium.

■ Hepatic metabolic function

The liver synthesizes glycogen, converts glycogen to glucose, and stores glycogen, which is synthesized primarily from glucose, fructose, and lactose. The liver is a primary organ for fat metabolism, since it oxidizes fatty acids; synthesizes cholesterol, phospholipids, and ketones; and synthesizes fats from glucose. The liver synthesizes proteins, converts amino acids into glucose, and deaminizes amino acids, thus synthesizing urea.

■ Detoxification

The liver detoxifies products of digestion using chemical reactions such as oxidation reduction and conjugation. The liver also eliminates drugs in the bile and reduces the toxicity of morphine and strychnine by storing and freeing them slowly. Kupffer's cells found in the sinusoid have phagocytic action; thus the liver plays a significant role in the defense mechanism of the body.

■ PATHOPHYSIOLOGY

A sign of severe liver damage is jaundice, a yellowing of the skin and sclera of the eyeballs. This is caused by an elevation of serum bilirubin. Hepatocytes conjugate bilirubin into a soluble glucuronide that is excreted into the bile; however, bilirubin is also produced by the reticuloendothelial cells. Following degradation of the red cells, hemoglobin polypeptides are split by the reticuloendothelial system producing biliverdin, which is reduced by the reticuloendothelial system to bilirubin, which binds to albumin or alpha-1 globulin in the plasma for transport to the liver. Bilirubin glucuronide is detectable by its reaction with Ehrlich's diazo reagent. This is the so-called *direct van den Bergh reaction*. Unconjugated protein-bound bilirubin reacts only after being solubilized with alcohol, and this is termed the *indirect van den Bergh reaction*. Thus elevated serum concentrations of indirect reacting bilirubin are characteristic of accelerated hemolysis, whereas elevated levels of conjugated bilirubin are seen in hepatocellular liver disease or in obstructions of the draining biliary tract. This is an example of how one sign, jaundice, which the layperson commonly attributes to liver damage, may have a multiplicity of causes.

The liver is one of the few human tissues that has regenerative powers. In most types of liver disease, hepatic tissue continuously regenerates in an attempt to maintain a functional volume. Most regenerative powers take place in the left lobe of the liver in disease states such as alcoholic damage or in chronic hepatitis. The nodularity of the liver of alcoholic cirrhosis is due to the macroscopic elevations of regenerative liver tissue. Liver diseases associated with jaundice may be divided into hepatocellular disease and cholestatic (bile stasis) disease. Hepatocellular jaundice is associated with significantly elevated serum transaminases with only a minimum increase in serum alkaline phosphatase. These patients have a history of exposure to a hepatotoxin or drug or have positive viral hepatitis serologic findings. Cholestatic jaundice may be evident without general failure of hepatic function, and it resembles obstructive jaundice. In these patients the serum alkaline phosphatase is noticeably elevated, and the serum transaminase is minimally increased.

■ Drug induced liver disease

The liver is predisposed to toxicity from drugs because it is a site of biotransformation of drugs. This biotransformation may lead to intracellular hepatocyte damage, to hepatocyte necrosis, or to the formation of a hepatocellular carcinoma. Carbon tetrachloride, acetaminophen, and methyldopa cause hepatocellular necrosis. Estrogens, anabolic steroids, erythromycin, or chlorpromazine may cause cholestasis with little or no flow of bile in the canaliculi, the smallest of the biliary ducts. Phenytoin, quinidine, and the sulfonamides may cause diffuse lymphoid hyperplasia in the liver with focal necrosis of hepatocytes.

■ Alcoholic liver disease

The principal organ for the metabolism of ethanol is the liver. The by-products of ethanol metabolism have important effects on intermediary metabolism in the hepatocyte. The morphologic hepatic changes in chronic alcoholism show up as a diffuse fatty liver in the majority of patients and as alcoholic hepatitis and cirrhosis in the minority of chronic alcoholic patients. Alcoholic hepatitis, a prerunner of cirrhosis, microscopically is seen in the liver as necrosis and inflammatory cells in the central lobular region with fibrosis around the terminal venules and sinusoids. As fatty infiltration and the damage just described continue, the patient develops the well-known features of the chronic alcoholic: portal hypertension, enlargement of the spleen, and dilation of esophageal varices.

■ Acute viral hepatitis

Hepatitis A. There is a short incubation in this disease process, which is spread by the fecal or oral route and in endemic fashion. The virus is found in stools during the incubation period, rapidly disappears with clinical symptoms, and is gone by the time jaundice develops. Viremia is transient, and no chronic disease or carrier state occurs.

Hepatitis B. There is a long incubation phase, usually 1 month to 6 weeks, is spread by parenteral, venereal routes or by close contact. Fifty percent of the hepatitis cases are caused by this agent. In the liver the virus replicates and is found in the blood as the whole virus or Dane particle and associated antigens to the intact virus. Hepatitis B surface antigen is the excess surface coat of the virus. The hepatitis B core antigen does not freely circulate; however, antibodies to the core antigen appear early in the infectious period and persist for the duration of the infection. Hepatitis B surface antigen antibodies appear after an interval following the disappearance of infection, and they persist. Patients who are immunosuppressed, newborns, patients having renal dialysis, and male homosexuals are likely to develop chronic infection. Approximately 10% to 12% of the patients with acute hepatitis B become chronic carriers.

Non-A, Non-B hepatitis. Twenty-five percent of cases of hepatitis and 90% of cases of posttransfusion hepatitis are associated with a negative serology for hepatitis A and B. Chronic hepatitis develops in up to 20% of sporadic cases and up to 60% of posttransfusional cases of this disease. Half of these patients develop chronic active hepatitis.

Chronic active hepatitis. Patients with chronic active hepatitis develop sporadic necrosis of hepatocytes and progressive fibrosis leading to cirrhosis. Another form of chronic hepatitis is called *chronic persistent hepatitis,* but this disease is self-limited and does not progress to cirrhosis. These diseases may be drug induced, have an autoimmune basis, or be related to previous infection with hepatitis B or non-A, non-B hepatitis.

■ Genetic liver diseases

Rare hereditary diseases, such as primary hemochromatosis, which causes an inappropriately high iron absorption, result in increased iron deposition in the hepatocyte, causing progressive hepatic fibrosis. In Wilson's disease there is a massive copper overload of the liver that causes progressive hepatic damage.

■ Metastatic carcinoma

Since one of the primary functions of the liver is to filter particles from the bloodstream, the liver filters out hematogenous tumor cells. If the cancer cell is not destroyed, it begins to grow locally and thus becomes a liver metastasis. Approximately 50% of all patients with cancer develop metastatic disease to the liver. The most common primary tumors to metastasize to the liver are the gastrointestinal tumors, lung tumors, and breast tumors.

Tumor cells usually have a diameter between 10 and 30 μmm. The doubling time of tumor cells is between 20 and 120 days with periods of rapid growth and periods of quiescence. When a metastatic lesion in the liver reaches a 1-cm diameter, it has been in the liver for approximately 9 years. To reach a 2-cm size would take 1 more year. The liver may also be infiltrated with Hodgkin's lymphoma or non-Hodgkin's lymphoma. This type of infiltration is usually throughout the liver with secondary liver enlargement.

■ Primary hepatic carcinomas

Hepatomas or primary carcinomas of the liver usually follow long-standing cirrhosis of the liver caused by postnecrotic cirrhosis, hemochromatosis, or Laënnec's cirrhosis. These primary tumors are usually slow-growing. They have also been associated with chronic viral hepatitis infection. Hepatomas typically have an increase in blood flow.

■ Benign lesions of the liver

Hemangiomas or vascular malformations are commonly found in the liver and are usually of no significance. Adenomas of the liver, which are benign, are associated with the long-term use of oral contraceptive agents.

LABORATORY APPLICATION

54

LIVER IMAGING

Purpose

Radionuclide liver imaging is primarily performed using the radiopharmaceutical ^{99m}Tc sulfur colloid or ^{99m}Tc human albumin microspheres. Technetium sulfur colloid is found in the liver in close proximity to Kupffer's cells, which line the sinusoids of the liver and are part of the reticuloendothelial system. Technetium sulfur colloid therefore is found normally in the spleen and bone-marrow space. In the disease states outlined in the section on pathophysiology, profound changes occur in the delivery of blood supply to the liver as hepatocytes are destroyed, infiltrates are formed, and resultant inflammatory scarring takes place. Thus in something like profound cirrhosis, the perfusion of the liver is grossly distorted, and the technetium sulfur colloid deposition is extremely irregular because it cannot be delivered to the sinusoidal Kupffer's cells. Therefore the alternate reticuloendothelial system of the spleen and bone marrow space receives an increased quantity of the radionuclide for deposition. Disease processes in the liver are in no way uniform. Areas of destruction may alternate with other relatively normal areas, and in chronic diseases such as alcoholic cirrhosis, there are whole regions of collapse with intervening areas of hepatic tissue undergoing regeneration.

Continued.

Common systemic diseases, such as diabetes and sarcoidosis, cause hepatomegaly or enlargement of the liver. The pathologic condition that causes the enlargement is microscopic and far beyond the resolution of nuclear medicine systems.

Currently, nuclear physicians have two completely different ways of imaging the liver. Up until the last 4 or 5 years, planar imaging has been the routine way of imaging hepatic anatomy. This method images the entire volume of the liver, historically from different directions (anteriorly, obliquely, posteriorly, or laterally). Since the entire volume of the liver is being imaged, it is obvious that small lesions cannot be seen because of the superimposition of normal hepatic uptake of Tc sulfur colloid; therefore, if the lesion was situated on the surface or deep in the hepatic parenchyma, it was not unusual to miss these lesions. Theoretically, 2- to 3-cm lesions, if in the proper plane, could be imaged. With the advent of single-photon emission computed tomography, in theory and in practice 1- to 2-cm lesions may be imaged without difficulty, whether they be superficial or deep in the hepatic parenchyma. With computer technology, the volume of the liver is sliced into 8-mm to 1-cm slices, in transverse, sagittal, and coronal slices. Therefore, lesions that could not be imaged by standard planar technology are now easily imaged with SPECT technology. As well as visualizing the lesions, one can accurately depict the volume of the lesion numerically. It is thus much easier to follow the progress of chemotherapy on metastatic lesions. SPECT images also give the nuclear physician a sensitive index of uneven, nonhomogeneous distribution of radionuclide in diseases that affect the entire liver (including cirrhosis, hepatitis, and fatty infiltration of the liver). The smallest focal lesion that can be visualized on a nuclear medicine image today is approximately 1 cm in diameter. Even with single-photon emission computed tomography, a smaller lesion is difficult to localize.

With agents such as technetium sulfur colloid, which are evenly distributed throughout the liver, any visualized abnormality is just an absence or decrease in concentration in the confines of the three-dimensional liver. Primary carcinoma, metastatic carcinoma, cystic disease of the liver, hemangiomas, and other space-occupying lesions can only be described as space-occupying lesions and must be further interpreted only with knowledge of the patient's clinical condition, history, and results of clinical laboratory studies (such as the level of the alkaline phosphatase, which is usually elevated in metastatic disease). Blood-pool scintigraphy may also be used to help in the interpretation of the imaged liver. Following the injection of ^{99m}Tc-tagged red cells, images are obtained every 2 to 4 seconds. Malignant lesions get their blood supply primarily from the hepatic artery; therefore, blood flow in primary or metastatic tumors will be seen earlier than in normal hepatic tissue. Hemangiomas will have an increased blood-pool activity very early following injection; adult hemangiomas are visualized best two hours following injection of tagged red cells.

Ultrasound and/or radiologic computed tomography done in correlation with the nuclear liver image enhances correct diagnosis. In today's practice computed tomography is used as the primary screening study, with ultrasound and nuclear imaging further evaluating the regions of abnormality. The nuclear image may also be used to localize an appropriate abnormal area for biopsy.

Indications

1. Differential diagnosis of hepatomegaly and abdominal masses
2. Preoperative evaluation for liver metastases in patients with known malignancies
3. Workup of patients with diffuse liver diseases such as cirrhosis or hepatitis
4. Evaluation of liver position and shape in patients with an elevated and/or abnormally shaped right diaphragm on chest x-ray film
5. Examination of patients with ascites of unknown origin
6. Diagnosis of patients with jaundice
7. Diagnosis of patients with suspected hepatic abscesses
8. Localization of hepatic lesions for needle biopsy or abscesses for drainage
9. Follow-up of patients with liver malignancies who are undergoing chemotherapy, radiotherapy, or partial resection and follow-up of the course of antibiotic or drainage therapy for hepatic abscesses
10. Examination of trauma patients with suspected liver rupture or hematoma

Procedure for planar imaging

Materials

1. Scintillation camera and low-energy collimator
2. ^{99m}Tc sulfur colloid or ^{99m}Tc human albumin microspheres, 2 to 6 mCi (74 to 222 MBq) with images begun 15 min after the dose is administered
3. Two 10 × ¼-inch lead strips, or ^{57}Co rulers used to localize costal margins

Patient preparation

1. No actual preparation is necessary; however, when using ^{99m}Tc sulfur colloid, it has been found that if the patient has had any type of barium studies, the barium in the colon could interfere with the liver image and lead to a false positive study.
2. Explain the entire procedure to the patient.

Technique

1. Calibrate for radionuclide.
2. Adjust intensity and determine proper orientation.
3. When using ^{99m}Tc sulfur colloid, set preset counts for 1 million.
4. Perform ^{99m}Tc sulfur colloid liver and spleen study, and use variable persistence scope for positioning.
5. Place lead markers on right and left costal margins. These markers are used to check for liver and/or spleen indentation by the rib cage and mobility of the liver on inspiration and expiration images.
6. Perform 11 views of the liver with a standard field-of-view camera or 4 to 6 views with a large–field-of-view camera.
   a. Anterior liver with marker
   b. Anterior spleen with marker
   c. Anterior liver (without markers)
   d. Anterior spleen
   e. Left anterior oblique view of the spleen
   f. Right lateral liver
   g. Posterior liver; record time
   h. Posterior spleen; record time
   i. Combined liver-spleen image using a camera with a wide field of view, which enables the views to be performed on the same image
7. Determine liver-spleen ratio from posterior images. Increased splenic concentration greater than 1:1 indicates expanded bone-marrow space.
8. If the spleen has increased concentration either visually or according to the ratio, take 40,000- to 100,000-count images of the shoulder and pelvis.
9. On completion of the study, process and label all views.

Procedure for SPECT imaging

Materials

1. Scintillation camera and SPECT table (single-head)
2. Nuclear computer with SPECT capabilities and array processor
3. ^{99m}Tc sulfur colloid, 8 to 12 mCi (296 to 444 MBq)

Preparation

1. Explain entire procedure to the patient.

Technique

A. Camera and patient set-up
   1. Calibrate camera for radionuclide peak. Predefined calibration and flood information should be stored before the initiation of the SPECT acquisition. Most software packages require predefined center of rotation calibration. With the wide variance of SPECT equipment now avail-

Continued.

able, extrinsic (collimator) uniformity may not be required if the system allows for high-count intrinsic flood-field uniformity storage that can be applied to the SPECT acquisition data.

2. Set proper orientation for SPECT acquisition.
3. Remove preset count or time.
4. 15% to 20% window (depending on camera).
5. 1.4 to 1.5 magnification in the center of the field of view.
6. Position SPECT table in the same position as it was when the center of rotation was acquired.
7. Adjust closest possible camera radius to patient abdomen to circumvent patient and SPECT table—a complete 360-degree circular arc for cameras without body-contouring capabilities.
8. For body contouring (noncircular, elliptical), a 1-, 2-, or 3-point setup is usually required through the software manufacturer. An elliptical orbit to match the patient's body contour is much preferred because resolution is improved by having the radioactive source closer to the collimator face; this also reduces scatter.
9. When patient is properly positioned, set camera position to 0° and level the detector.

B. Computer Setup

1. Most software packages allow acquisition and reconstruction "on the fly." This option should be selected to save processing time.
2. Enter patient data.
3. Acquisition matrix can either be 64 × 64 or 128 × 128, depending on user/physician preference.
4. Angular range should be 360° with the number azimuths (angles) being 64, 120, or 128, depending on the matrix selected and the software used.
5. Acquisition time can vary from 10 to 20 sec/angle depending on dosage given and count density (statistics) preferred.
6. Whether the software allows prefiltering or postfiltering of the data, a third-order Butterworth filter with a 0.3 cut-off value has given the best image resolution (signal information) with the least amount of noise (unwanted signal or frequency). The Butterworth filter offers the best trade-off between smoothness and sharpness of edge.
7. Choose the thickness of the transverse or transaxial slices. Thicker slices contain more counts and are less noisy. Thinner slices contain less counts but have the greatest resolution. Since thicker slices will be more uniform, three pixel slices are preferred (with Technicare 560 version 4.0 software in a 128 × 128 matrix, this calculates to about 8.1 mm or 2.7 mm/pixel). Accepted practice in most nuclear medicine facilities is 6- to 12-mm–slice thicknesses.

C. Computer Processing

1. Once the transaxial or transverse images have been acquired, an attenuation or scattering correction should be applied. The more tissue the gamma photons have to penetrate from the center of the source (liver) to the detector, the more those photons will be attenuated or scattered. Correction has to be made, otherwise the center of the patient organ will appear less radioactive than the patient organ actually is.
2. For 140-keV–gamma photons emitted from the liver, an attenuation correction of 0.11 or 0.12 reciprocal cms is preferred.
3. Sagittal and coronal projections can then be created from the stored transaxial data. Use the same slice thickness as the transaxial slices; in this case, 3 pixels (8.1 mm).
4. Photographic techniques should allow for the greatest amount of information to be transferred to hard copy (film). The films, to include transverse, sagittal, and coronal images, should include the largest range of gray scale to allow for the subtlest of changes. Overexposures or underexposures will result in the loss of detail.
5. Intensity settings should remain consistent through each set of images (transverse, sagittal, and coronal). Two sets of images may be required when either the liver or spleen has much more activity per pixel than the other.

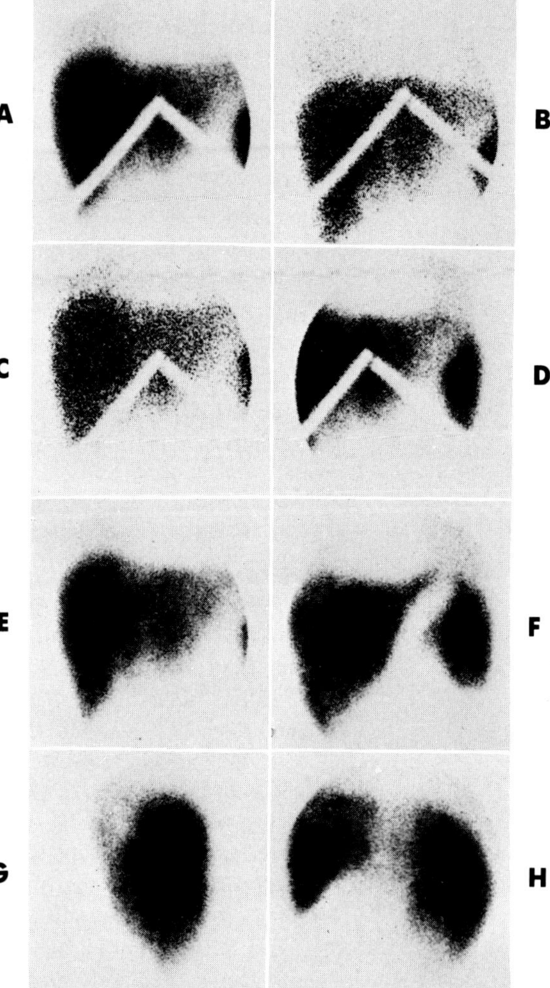

Fig. 20-3. Normal liver and spleen images. Study was performed with 6 mCi (222 MBq) of ^{99m}Tc sulfur colloid administered intravenously. **A,** Anterior view with costal margin marker. **B** and **C,** Inspiration/expiration views. **D,** Anterior view of spleen with costal margin marker. **E,** Anterior view of liver without marker. **F,** Left anterior oblique view of the spleen. **G,** Right lateral view. **H,** Posterior view of liver and spleen.

Interpretation: planar position, shape, and size (Fig. 20-3)

Anterior view

On the anterior liver image the normal-size liver is usually found above the right costal margin if the right hemidiaphragm is in a normal position. The enlarged liver extends below the right costal margin. The normal-size spleen is visualized in the left quadrant above the left costal margin.

The liver is a pliable organ and its shape can be distorted by external pressure; that is, an enlarged right kidney, gallbladder, or head of the pancreas, or any other mass in the porta.

In many patients a normal gallbladder bed or an exaggerated division between the right and left lobes may be visualized. In the region between the right and left lobes (that is, the porta), the portal vein and the inferior vena cava may have an imprint. The anterior view is the best view to judge the size of the liver.

In a minority of patients a Riedel's lobe, an elongation of the right lobe, may be visualized extending down into the pelvis. The normal left lobe is only approximately 15% of the volume of the right lobe of the liver, and since it is anterior, it is usually best visualized on the anterior view.

Right lateral view

The right lateral view of the liver usually reveals the left lobe superimposed on the anterior portion of the right lobe; this may obscure anterior right lobe lesions.

The normal costal margin imprint on the inferior right lobe may give the appearance of a false space-occupying lesion.

Continued.

Oblique lateral view

A shallow anterior oblique position may demonstrate lesions in the anterior right and left lobes. The lateral oblique position with the camera rotated or the patient rolled slightly anteriorly is the best position to demonstrate the true lateral surface of the right lobe. In this position the spleen is visualized posteriorly to the dorsal surface of the liver.

Posterior view

In the posterior view the diaphragmatic surface of the liver, the region of the right renal bed, and the medial right lobe are demonstrated well. Left-lobe visualization is obscured by vertebral bodies.

The spleen is well visualized on this view, since it is a posterior organ and the quantitation of the amount of the radionuclide in the liver and spleen is best done in this position.

Left lateral view

In the left lateral view the spleen is seen well posteriorly, and the anterior surface of the left lobe can be demonstrated.

SPECT position, shape, and size (Fig. 20-4)

Transverse section views

The SPECT transverse views are comparable to the standard radiographic CT slice images. Standard transverse slice images are 8-mm cuts, beginning at the lower portion of the right lobe and progressing to the diaphragm. In the normal liver (Fig. 20-4), the initial fifth to sixth 8-mm slices are images of the inferior right lobe of the liver. Slices 7 to 9 depict the posterior right renal fossa impression. The next four images (slices 10 to 13) depict anteriorly the beginning of the inferior left lobe and the gallbladder bed; they then serially depict the superior right lobe and the majority of the left lobe. In the central posterior region progressively, the main portal vein and the right and left tributaries of the portal vein are seen sectionally moving through the hepatic parenchyma. The biliary tree per se is not visualized unless dilated. The biliary tree is in close association with the portal venous system. The spleen is visualized usually at the level of the beginning visualization of the left lobe. Depending on the orientation of the liver, serial cuts at times show the portal-vein system in cross section and may be mistaken for a small space-occupying lesion unless the observer tracks the various sections above and below the pseudo space-occupying lesion section to follow the course of the portal venous system. Note the smooth border of the lateral and posterior diaphragmatic surface of the right lobe of the liver.

If there is excessive shunting of ^{99m}Tc sulfur colloid to the spleen, the acquired images may have to be photographed twice, in varying intensities, to allow visualization of the hepatic structure. It is important when completing repeat studies on the same patient to maintain the same camera settings as obtained on the first study.

Sagittal images

Sagittal reconstruction images begin on the right of the liver and progress to the left at 8-mm increments. The initial slices 3 and 4 of the normal liver reveal the lateral and central right lobe. Note the smooth superior and posterior border of the diaphragmatic surface of the liver. The gallbladder bed is visualized on about the fifth to sixth slice as an anterior structure compressing the inferior medial right lobe. At the same time, the right portal vein is visualized centrally and anteriorly. It can be followed through the following slices as the right branch of the portal vein is visualized (as a rounded 6- to 7-mm area of decreased to absent concentration of radionuclide) through the junction of the portal venous system and finally into the left portal vein as it progresses from the inferomedial left lobe through the superior left lobe. On about the sixth to seventh slices, the left lobe becomes visible anteriorly and superiorly, with progressive slices revealing more and more of the left lobe structure. The sagittal slices superbly allow visualization of small diaphragmatic surface space-occupying lesions. The spleen in the normal case is small; it is visualized posterior to the left lobe, at times progressing past and laterally to the visualized left lobe of the liver. The sagittal slices will also reveal superficial lesions on the anterior surface of the right and left lobes of the liver. On slice 17, the bone marrow is visualized by increasing the photographic intensity.

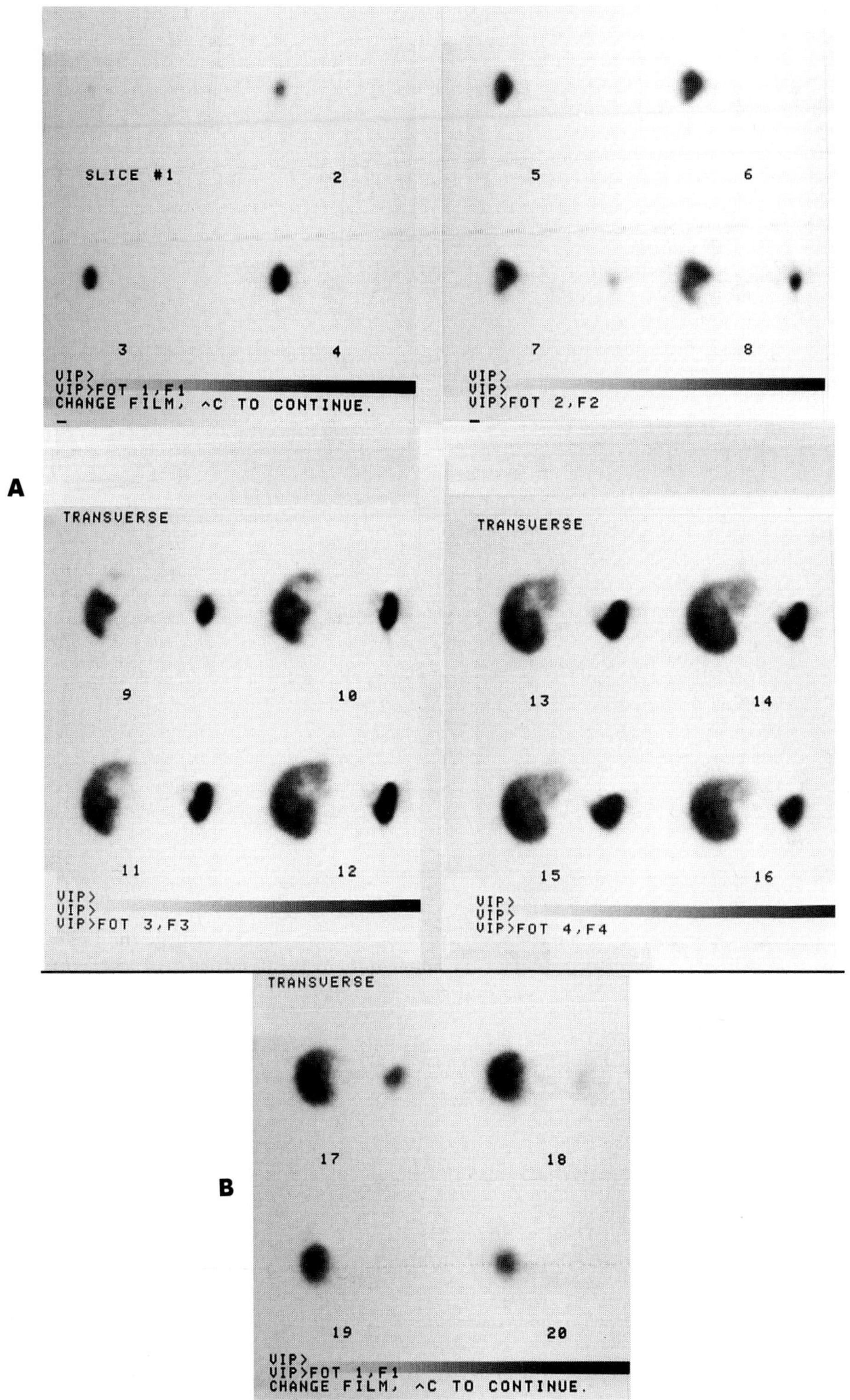

Fig. 20-4. Normal liver and spleen images performed by SPECT following the administration of ^{99m}Tc sulfur colloid. Each 8-mm section is viewed separately; however, with computer techniques sections can be added together into a composite three-dimensional surface image. **A** and **B,** Transverse 8-mm sections 1 to 18.

Continued.

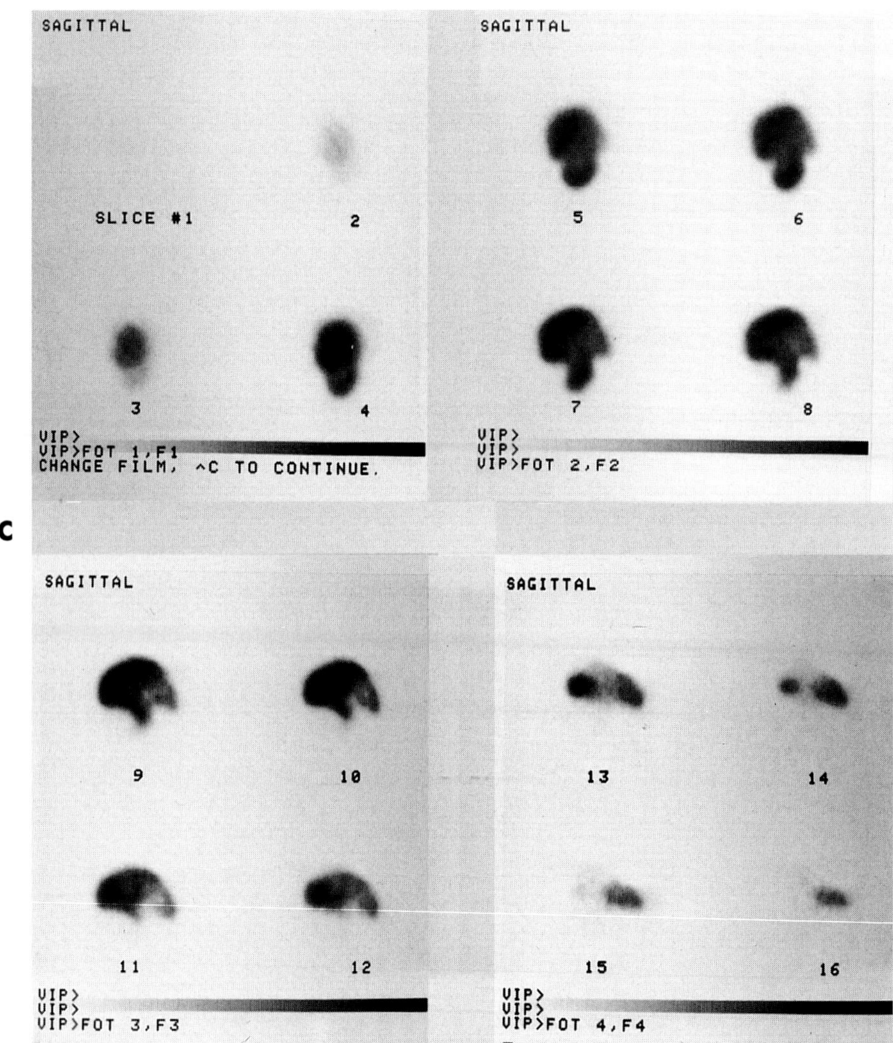

Fig. 20-4, cont'd. C and **D,** Sagittal 8-mm sections 1 to 32.

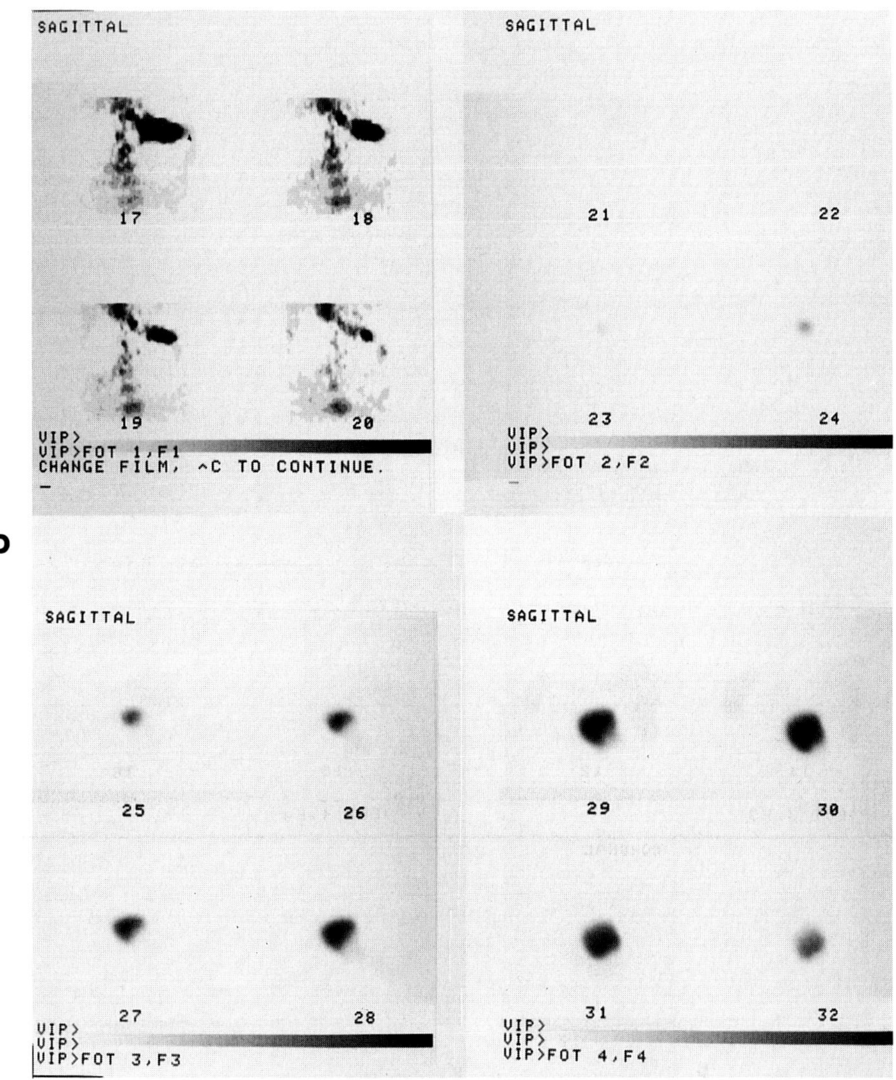

Fig. 20-4, cont'd. For legend see opposite page.

Continued.

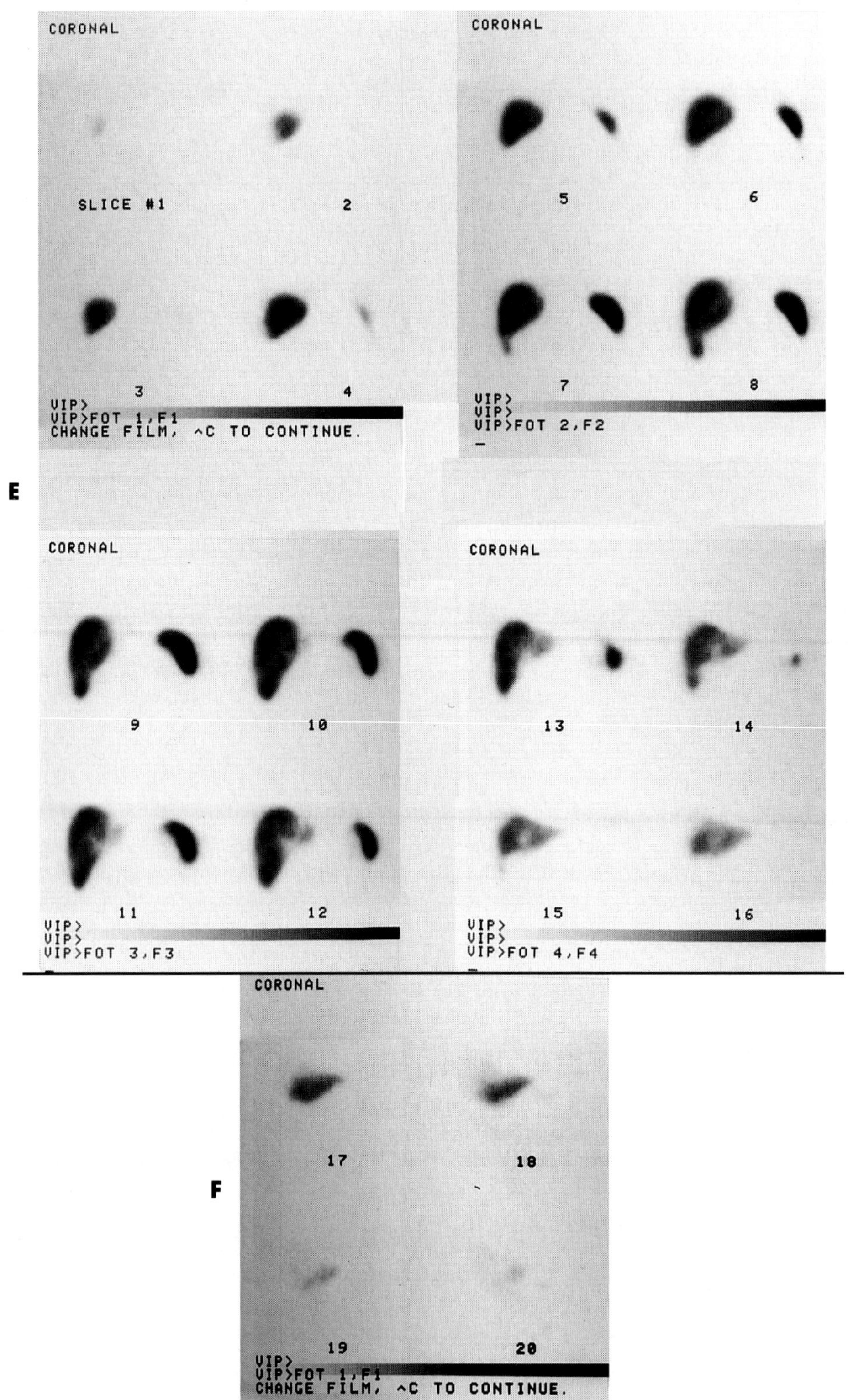

Fig. 20-4, cont'd. E and **F,** Coronal 8-mm sections 1 to 20.

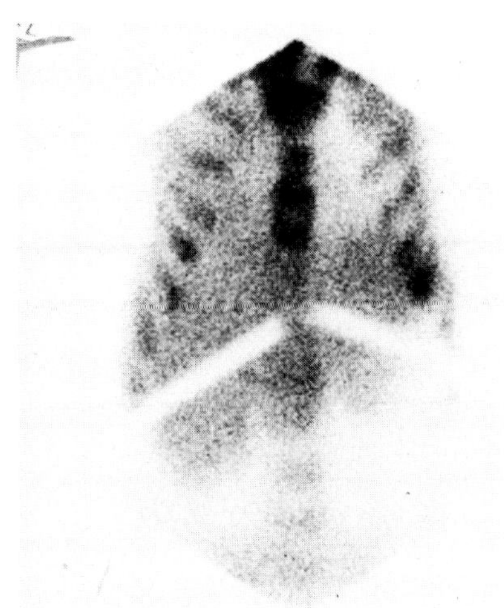

Fig. 20-5. Acute alcoholic (toxic) hepatitis. Anterior liver image following the intravenous administration of 6 mCi (222 MBq) ^{99m}Tc sulfur colloid reveals significant hepatomegaly with diffuse decreased concentration of radioactivity throughout enlarged liver. Spleen is normal size with significant increased concentration of radioactivity. Entire skeleton is visualized because of the marked expansion of bone-marrow space. This study is compatible with significant hepatocellular injury with shunting of technetium sulfur colloid to the spleen and entire bone-marrow space of the skeleton, which has been expanded.

Coronal images

Coronal SPECT images give the best overall visual impression of hepatic and splenic sizes. Systems software systematically picks slices, beginning at the posterior surface of the liver and progressing anteriorly in 8-mm increments. The most posterior slices will depict the right renal fossa impression on the inferior right lobe medially, with the spleen being visualized as a posterior organ. On about slice 10, the main portal vein begins visualization in the region of the medial porta hepatis, and progressively on the next two slices the right portal vein is visualized. The gallbladder is a relatively anterior organ and is visualized on slice number 12 as the left lobe begins visualization. The left portal vein is then seen progressing from the porta hepatis and on slice number 15 is visualized in cross-section in the medial mid left lobe. Note the smoothness of the hepatic diaphragmatic surface superiorly and laterally.

Diagnosis

Acute hepatitis (Fig. 20-5)

Acute hepatitis may be viral-induced or toxic. The condition acutely causes both lobes of the liver to enlarge, and particularly with viral hepatitis there is increased visualization of the spleen as a result of enhanced reticuloendothelial activity of the spleen.

Chronic hepatitis

Chronic hepatitis, which may be viral-induced or nutrition/alcohol-based has many common denominators on the ^{99m}Tc sulfur colloid liver image. A common early finding in these livers is fatty infiltration that causes global hepatomegaly. As the disease progresses, there is primarily enlargement of the left lobe over enlargement of the right lobe, and enlargement of the caudate and quadrate lobes is visualized. As the disease process further progresses, there is shunting of technetium sulfur colloid, since the normal circulation to the reticuloendothelial system is impaired in the liver and technetium sulfur colloid is deposited in the spleen. The quantitative or qualitative concentration of the spleen in contrast to the concentration in the liver reflects the activity of the disease. SPECT imaging has increased both the sensitivity and specificity of the ^{99m}Tc sulfur colloid images, particularly in patients with fatty infiltration of the liver. On planar images, the deposition of ^{99m}Tc sulfur colloid in the liver appears to be homogeneous while on SPECT images the nonhomogeneous distribution of radiopharmaceutical is appreciated. There is usually a shift of ^{99m}Tc sulfur colloid to the spleen; therefore, with the combination of nonhomogeneous concentration within the liver and increase in ^{99m}Tc sulfur colloid visualized in the spleen, the fatty infiltrative process may be suspected in drug-induced or early hepatitis. There is also localization of the lesions to the periportal portions of the liver, and this may also be recognized on the SPECT images.

Continued.

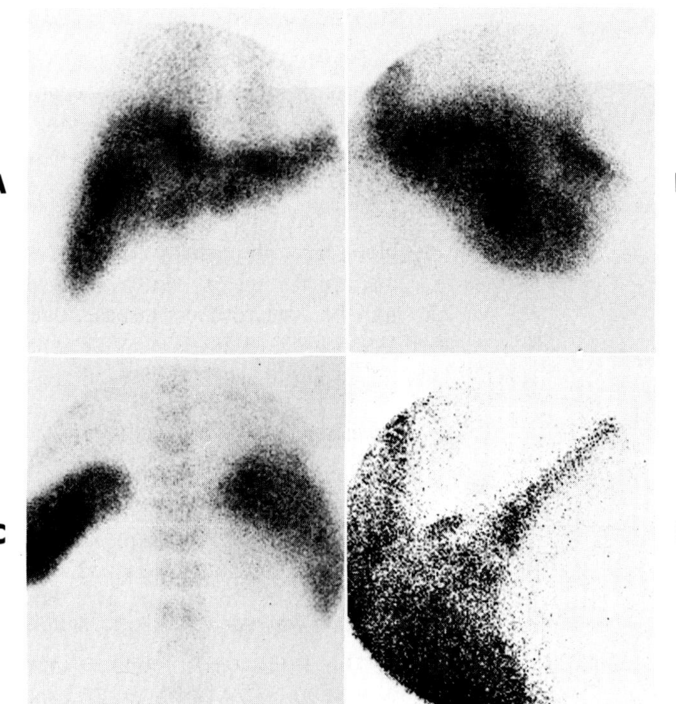

Fig. 20-6. Cirrhosis. **A** to **C,** Small scarred liver with significantly uneven distribution of nuclide in the liver; areas of increased activity alternate with areas of almost absent activity. Splenomegaly is present with increased concentration of radioactivity caused by portal hypertension. There is increased visualization of bone marrow into long bones. **D,** View reveals marrow space extending into shaft of humerus. There is also radioactivity in the lung, which suggests an active form of hepatitis.

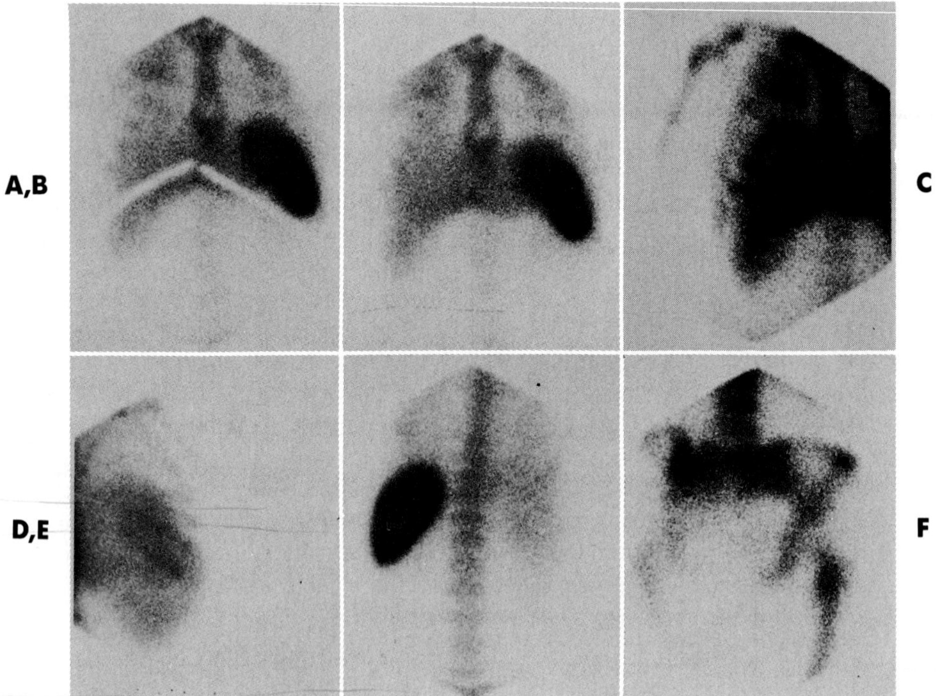

Fig. 20-7. Cirrhosis. Severe Laënnec's cirrhosis with portal hypertension. No expansion of bone marrow space. **A,** Anterior view with costal market. **B,** Anterior view without costal marker. **C,** Anterior liver area. **D,** Right lateral view. **E,** Posterior view. **F,** Bone marrow—pelvis and femur.

Hepatic cirrhosis (Figs. 20-6 and 20-7)

Hepatic cirrhosis or necrosis of portions of the liver with fibrotic replacement again can have multiple etiologies. Chronic hepatitis B, non-A and non-B hepatitis, nutritional (alcoholic), chronic biliary obstruction, toxic hepatitis, hemochromatosis, or Wilson's disease can all lead to hepatic cirrhosis. The cirrhotic liver usually has bands of fibrosis alternating with areas of regenerated nodules of liver tissue. The patient in the end stage of cirrhosis usually has a small right lobe with an enlarged left lobe with hypertrophy of the accessory lobes. Because of the interference with portal blood flow, the patient in the end stage of cirrhosis has portal hypertension with secondary enlargement of the spleen, which is visualized on the technetium sulfur colloid image. Although cirrhosis may be a microscopic disease, over half of the patients with cirrhosis have pseudospace-occupying lesions on a technetium sulfur colloid liver image. Secondary to the severity of the disease, there is increasing visualization of the bone-marrow space.

Abscesses

Hematogenous or blood-borne abscesses may form in the liver because of bacteria or infective agents such as *Entamoeba histolytica*. Abscesses may be single or multiple and can be described as cold space-occupying lesions. The etiology of the space-occupying lesion usually is known because of other findings in the patient and the clinical history.

Primary hepatocellular, gallbladder, and biliary carcinoma (Figs. 20-8 to 20-10)

The primary carcinomas of the liver and associated biliary tree may appear as a solitary space-occupying lesion; however, metastatic disease from the primary carcinoma may also be present. There is an increased incidence of primary hepatic carcinoma in patients with cirrhosis. Since the image findings (such as patchy or large cold areas throughout the liver) may be similar, the diagnosis of primary carcinoma in a patient with cirrhosis is difficult to make on a technetium-99m sulfur colloid liver image.

Hepatic adenoma and focal nodular hyperplasia

Hepatic adenoma and focal nodular hyperplasia are two relatively rare disease entities that show up on liver imaging as space-occupying lesions (that is, cold lesions) in over half of the cases reported.

Benign tumor (Fig. 20-11)

Cysts and hemangiomas, both of which are relatively frequent conditions, appear as single or multiple space-occupying lesions on the liver image. The cavernous hemangioma can be well diagnosed by following the technetium sulfur colloid study with a technetium tagged red blood cell imaging series, since the abnormal vessels are seen either on the flow or on the later static images.

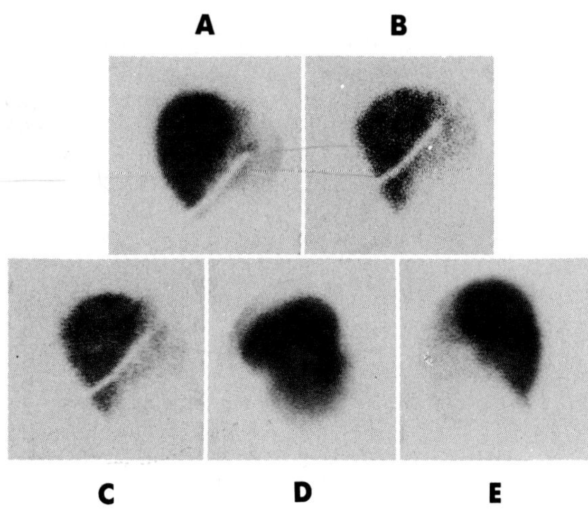

Fig. 20-8. Hemangiosarcoma of liver. Study was performed with ^{99m}Tc sulfur colloid. Liver images reveal destructive lesion of left lobe with extension into right lobe. Perfusion and gallium studies would be indicated with this type of presentation. **A,** Anterior view with costal marker. **B** and **C,** Inspiration and expiration views show absence of right lobe pliability and significant infiltration of right lobe. **D,** Right lateral view. **E,** Posterior view.

Continued.

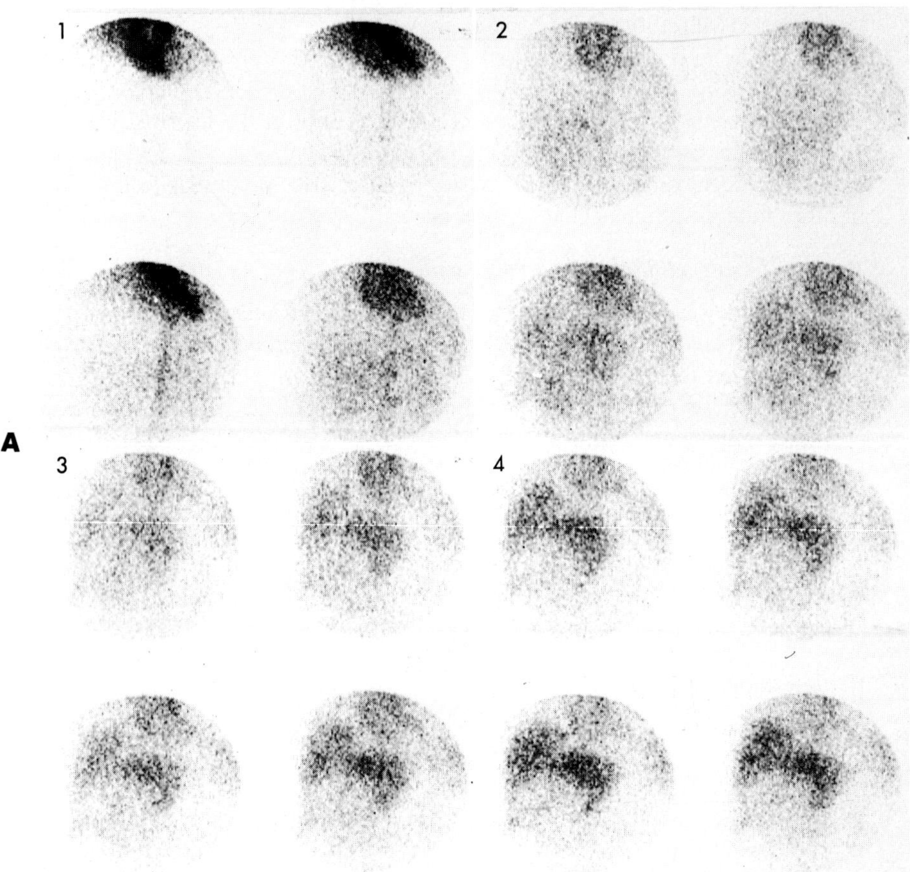

Fig. 20-9. Hepatoma. **A (1-4),** Liver perfusion images and **B (5-10),** static images performed following intravenous administration of 6 mCi ^{99m}Tc sulfur colloid reveal 12-cm anterior and inferior right lobe space-occupying lesions. Static images reveal lesion to be semilobular with low-level concentration of nuclide as compared with normal liver tissue. Right lobe laterally is compressed and left lobe is compressed superiorly by the mass, which extends over inferior left lobe and below level of hepatic contour.

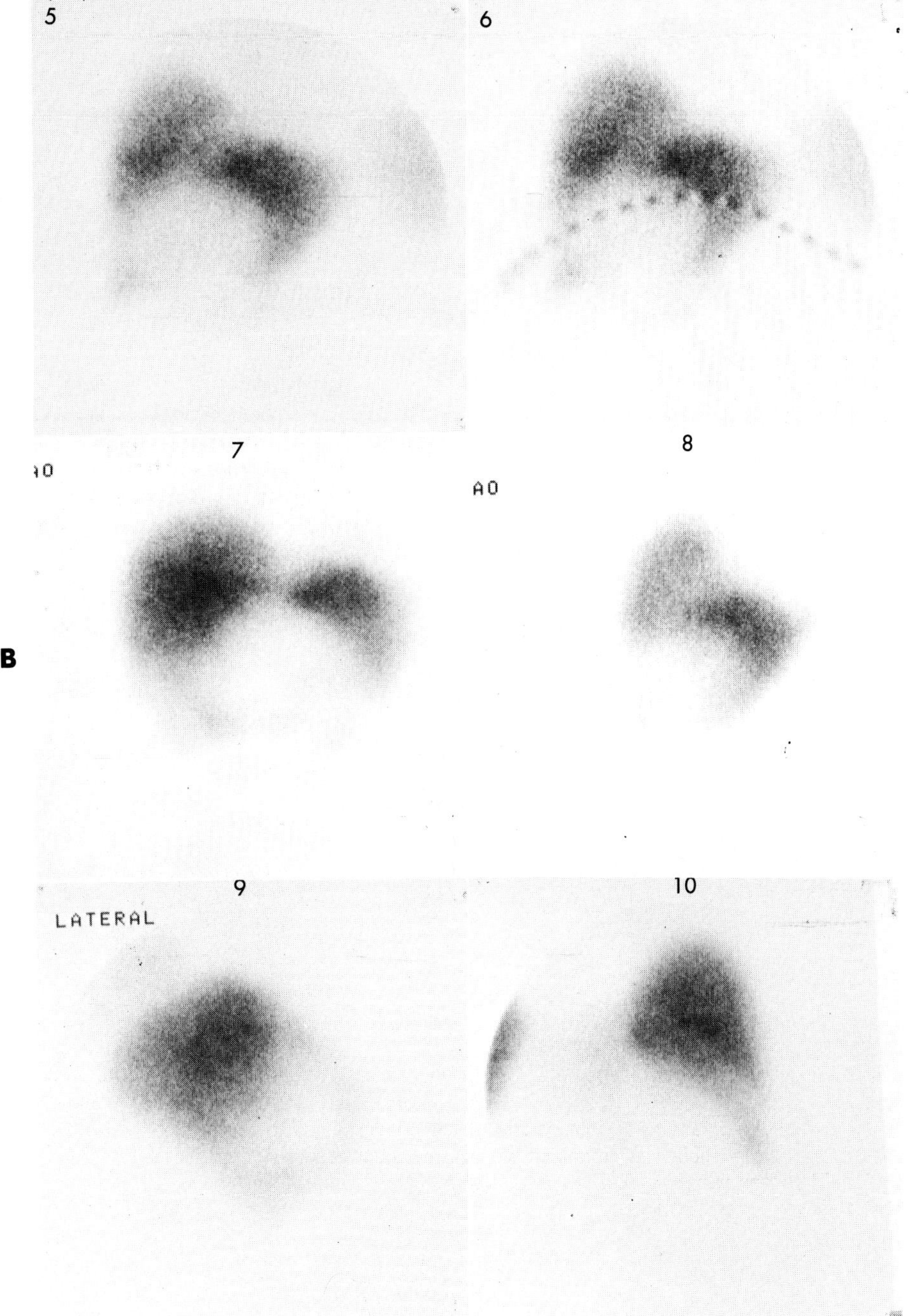

Fig. 20-9, cont'd. For legend see opposite page.

Continued.

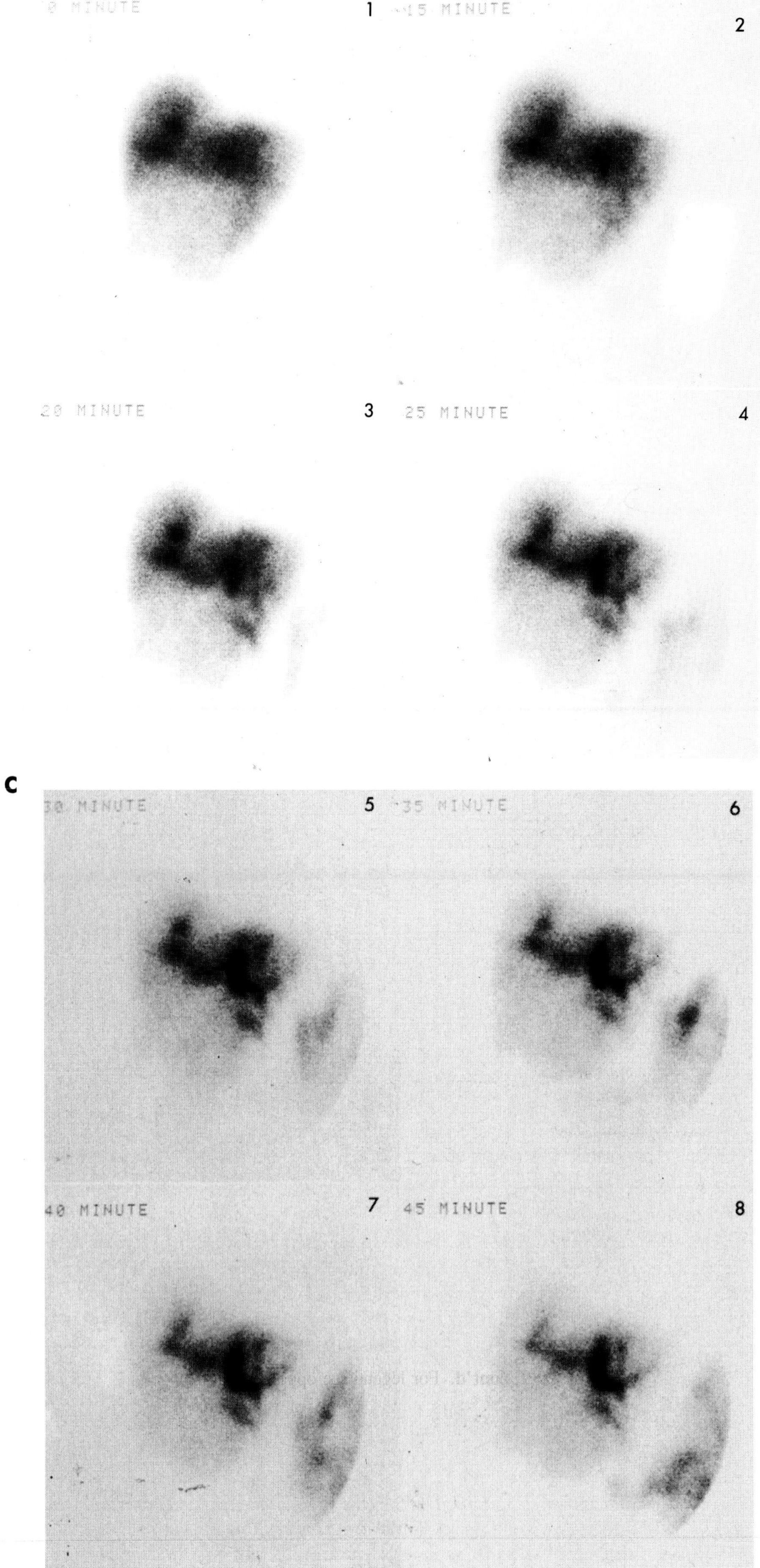

Fig. 20-9, cont'd. For legend see opposite page.

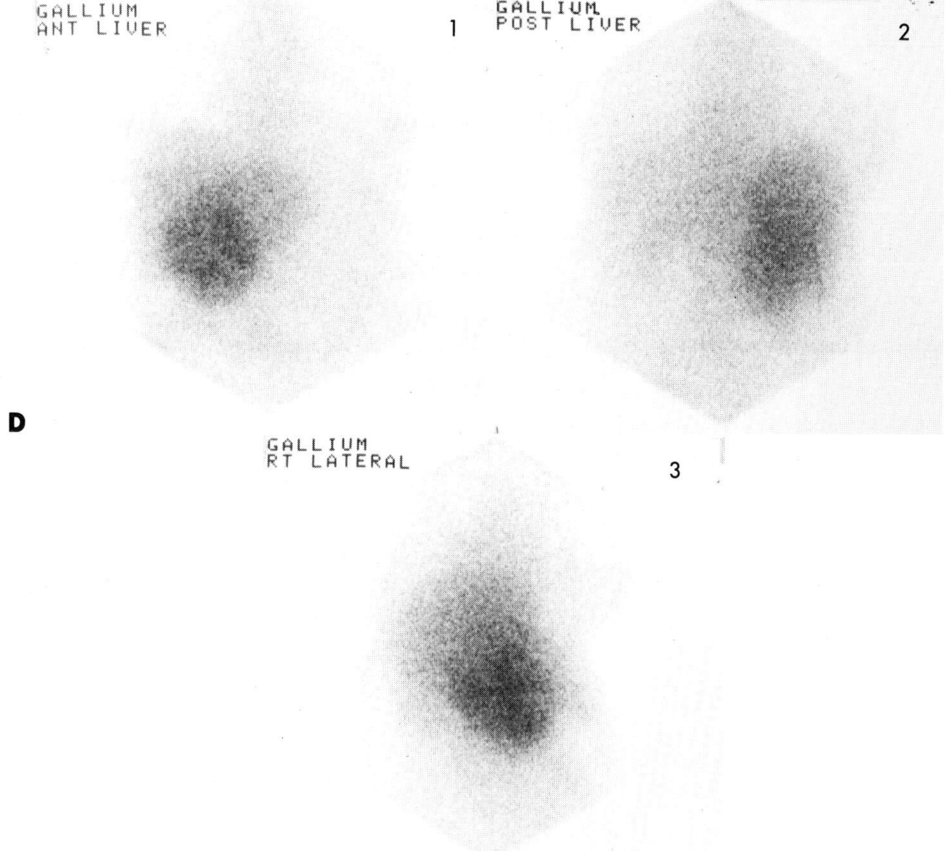

Fig. 20-9, cont'd. C (1-8), Biliary images performed following intravenous administration of 6 mCi (222 MBq) ^{99m}Tc disofenin reveal hypoperfusion of large lesion. Immediate parenchymal view reveals normal concentration in superior right and left lobes with some retention of parenchymal activity in the lesion. At 15 minutes intrahepatic biliary tree is visualized and is pushed medially and superiorly by the lesion. Common hepatic and bile ducts are pushed past the porta. Apparent gallbladder is visualized in low porta position, completely pushed out of position. Common hepatic duct is mildly dilated; common bile duct is not. There was prompt loss of biliary activity into gastrointestinal (GI) tract. The functional activity noted in lesion slowly dissipates through 1-hour study but is still present, whereas normal hepatic tissue has cleared disofenin. **D (1-3),** Gallium images performed 48 hours following intravenous administration of 5 mCi (185 MBq) ^{67}Ga citrate reveal evenly 6+ increase in concentration of nuclide in large right lobe lesion. Diagnosis: hepatoma.

Continued.

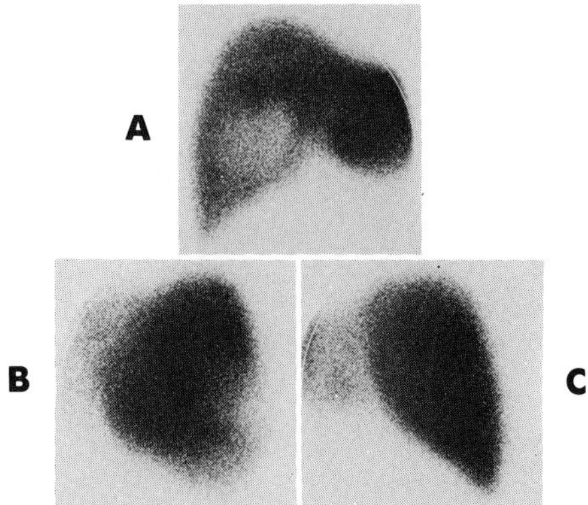

Fig. 20-10. Gallbladder carcinoma. **A,** Anterior view reveals right lobe with large space-occupying lesion extending from porta hepatis and gallbladder bed. Lesion is larger than dilated gallbladder. **B,** Lateral view shows anterior indentation of lesion. **C,** Lesion is not seen well on posterior view.

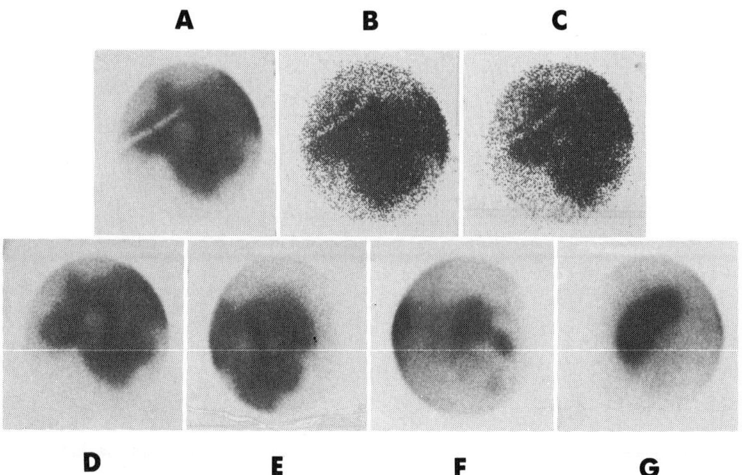

Fig. 20-11. Polycystic disease of liver. Study was performed with technetium sulfur colloid. **A,** Anterior view with costal margin marker. **B,** Inspiration view. **C,** Expiration view—pliability retained. **D,** Anterior view with costal margin marker removed. **E,** Right lateral view. **F,** Posterior view (466 seconds). **G,** Posterior spleen view (223 seconds). Comment: Here are multiple round space-occupying lesions. Pliability of liver is normal. There is no evidence of intrahepatic arteriovenous shunting. If this had been metastatic disease with this degree of destruction, arteriovenous shunting would have been expected.

The Tc-tagged red blood cell SPECT images have made the confirmation of hemangiomas relatively simple (Fig. 20-12). Benign hemangiomas are picked up relatively often on screening ultrasonic images of the gallbladder and liver. By ultrasound criteria, abnormalities can take many forms and at times are quite difficult to distinguish from metastatic sites. In children, the hemangioma is almost always visualized as an increased area of flow on the hepatic perfusion series; again, in almost all cases this can be recognized as a hypervascular region on SPECT imaging. On SPECT imaging, lesions 1 cm in size may be localized while on planar imaging the lesions must be 3 to 4 cm in size. In about 50% of adult cases the lesions will not be localized on either the flow or the immediate SPECT images; however, the majority of the lesions may be recognized on delayed images (i.e., 2 to 3 hours postinjection). It is therefore recommended that in adults the SPECT imaging series be started 2 to 3 hours postinjection. Lesions such as hepatomas do have an increased hepatic artery flow and may blush on the initial perfusion images. On SPECT imaging, however, the vast majority of the hepatomas will have a decrease in vascular flow as compared with normal hepatic tissue.

Fatty infiltration of the liver

Diffuse-and-patchy fatty infiltration of the liver will always produce a normal nuclear liver image, while patchy fatty infiltration will cause abnormalities on CT and ultasound images.

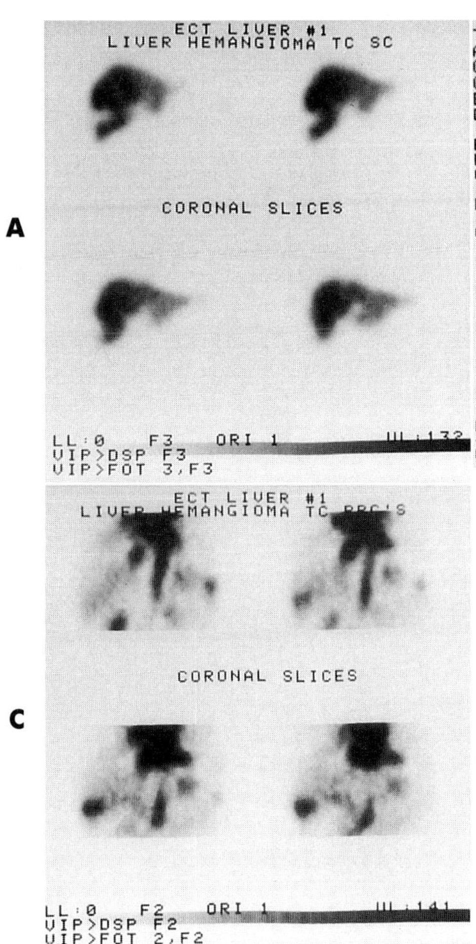

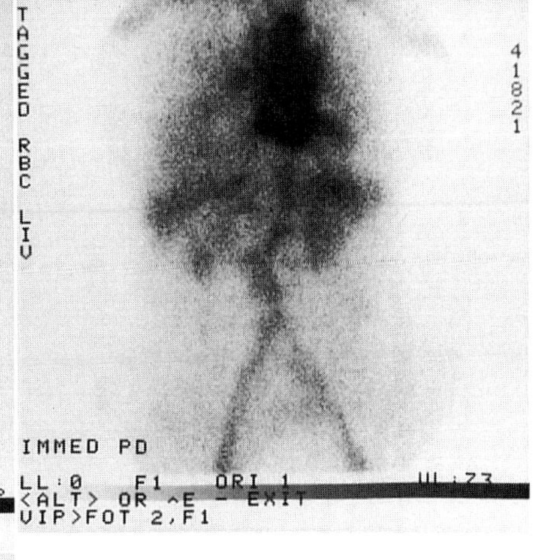

Fig. 20-12. Intrahepatic hemangioma. Ultrasound of the liver revealed a 2 × 21/2 cm echogenic lesion in the lateral inferior right lobe of the liver. **A,** ^{99m}Tc sulphur colloid SPECT coronal liver image reveals a photopenic region in the lateral inferior right lobe of the liver. **B,** Immediate planar anterior image following the administration of ^{99m}Tc tagged RBCs reveals a concentration of tagged red blood cells in the inferior right lobe of the liver. Normal activity is visualized in the heart, large vessels, spleen, and kidneys. **C,** One-hour post ^{99m}Tc RBC injection a SPECT coronal image reveals the hemangioma in the inferior lateral right lobe of the liver.

Metastatic carcinoma (Figs. 20-13 to 20-17)

Searching for metastatic carcinoma in the liver is a primary reason for the use of planar and SPECT technetium-sulfur-colloid images of the liver. About 50% of patients who die from malignancy will have hepatic metastatic disease. The most common liver metastases are the result of malignancies of the primary colon, lung, genitourinary tract, pancreas, and breast. In using planar imaging, the detection rate for metastatic disease of the liver ranges between 80% and 90%.

Routine SPECT hepatic imaging has been taking place since 1983. In a comparison of routine planar images and routine SPECT images, it has been found that SPECT images do increase the accuracy of definition of space-occupying lesions in the liver by about 10% in our metastatic patients. Ultrasound or CT examination will have slightly less sensitivity than will the SPECT hepatic image in the detection of small metastatic sites; however, the specificity improves with directed CT or ultrasound evaluation.

The reason for the improved sensitivity of SPECT imaging over planar imaging is obvious (Figs. 20-16 and 20-17). There is inherent contrast enhancement in SPECT imaging as well as and the approved ability to detect small superficial lesions and the small lesion that is deep in the hepatic parenchyma. The true volume of liver involvement is much better visualized on SPECT images; on SPECT imaging lesions may be measured in volume to better estimate the effects of chemotherapy. The literature states that a 1- to 1.5-cm lesion may be visualized on planar images. In any large series this type of lesion is difficult if not impossible to visualize on planar images. On SPECT imaging, 1-cm lesions may theoretically be visualized. The smallest single space-occupying lesion visualized by SPECT images measured 2 cm × 4 mm; it was a superficial lesion. When multiple lesions are present, the 1-cm lesion may be visualized without difficulty. The majority of imaging

Continued.

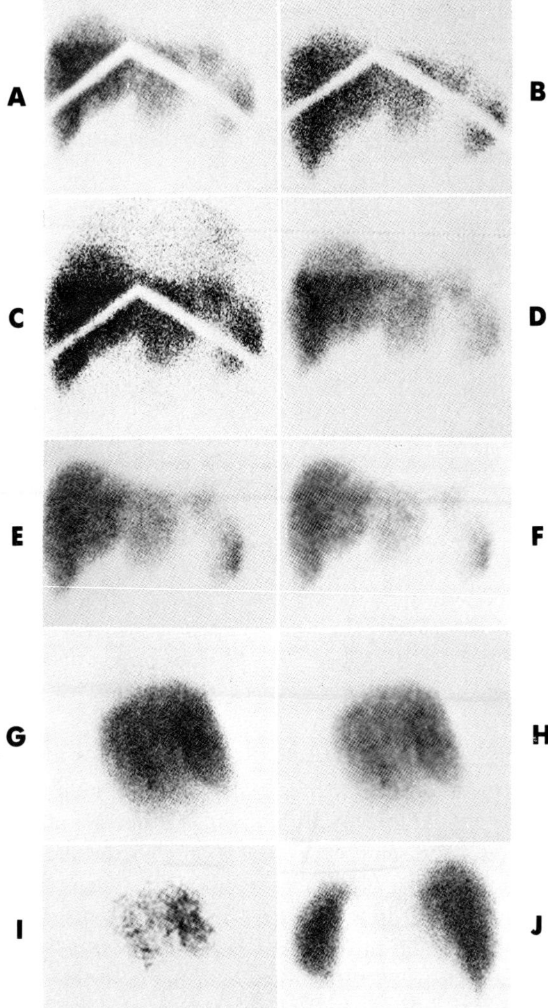

Fig. 20-13. Focal metastatic disease. **A,** Anterior view with costal marker. **B** and **C,** Inspiration/expiration view. Comment: There is decreased pliability of superior right lobe. **D,** Anterior view, breast shadow on superior right lobe. **E,** Anterior view, breast elevated. **F,** Nine-point computer smoothing accentuating small focal areas of decreased concentration. **G,** Right lateral view. **H,** Nine-point computer-smoothed image. **I,** Post-image enhancement. Comment: Computer enhancement reveals multifocal space-occupying lesions. **J,** Posterior liver/spleen view.

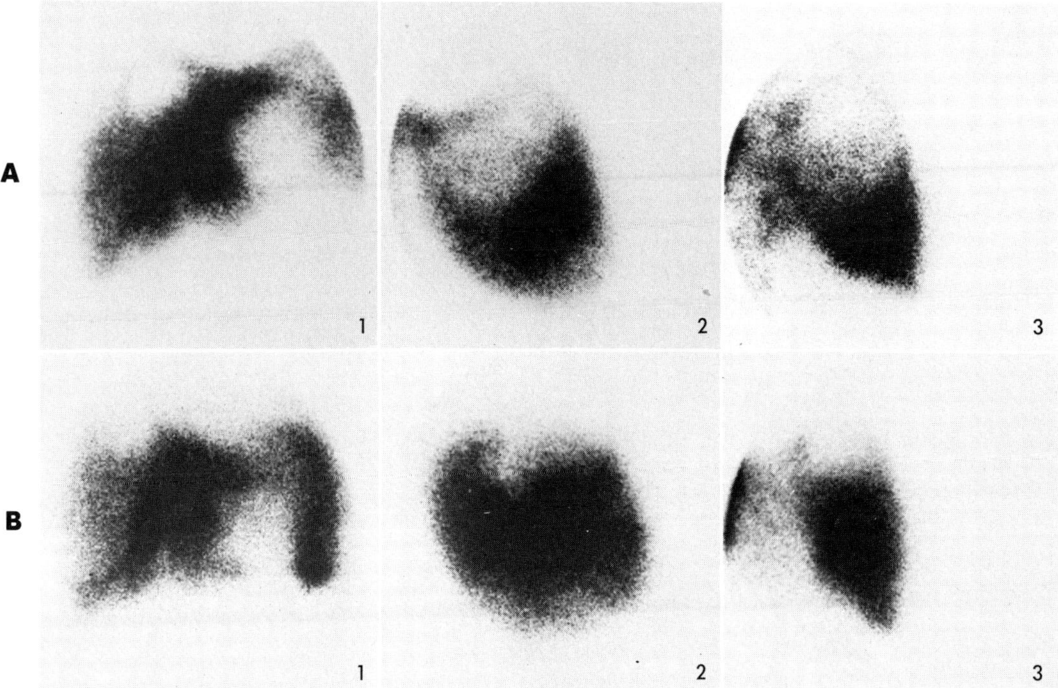

Fig. 20-14. Metastatic disease. *1,* Anterior view. *2,* Right lateral view. *3,* Posterior view. **A,** February 1979 images. Comment—there are multiple conglomerate metastatic lesions in superior right and left lobes. **B,** August 1979, follow-up images (following intensive course of chemotherapy). Comment—using a computer, volume of metastatic disease in the liver can be quantitated. There was a 45% decrease in size in metastatic deposits in left lobe and a 61% decrease in size in metastatic deposits in right lobe.

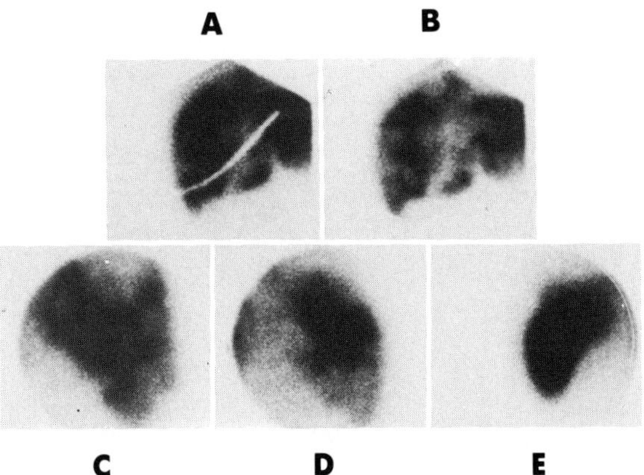

Fig. 20-15. Metastatic disease. **A** and **B,** Anterior views of the liver using ^{99m}Tc sulfur colloid. **A,** With lead costal marker. **B,** Without costal marker. **C,** Right lateral view. **D,** Posterior view of liver. **E,** Posterior view of spleen. There is infiltrative metastatic disease with multifocal space-occupying lesions. Note in this case increased count rate in spleen (posterior liver 300,000/96 seconds, posterior spleen 300,000/76 seconds). When liver has been almost totally replaced by metastatic disease, there is increased intrahepatic arteriovenous shunting.

Continued.

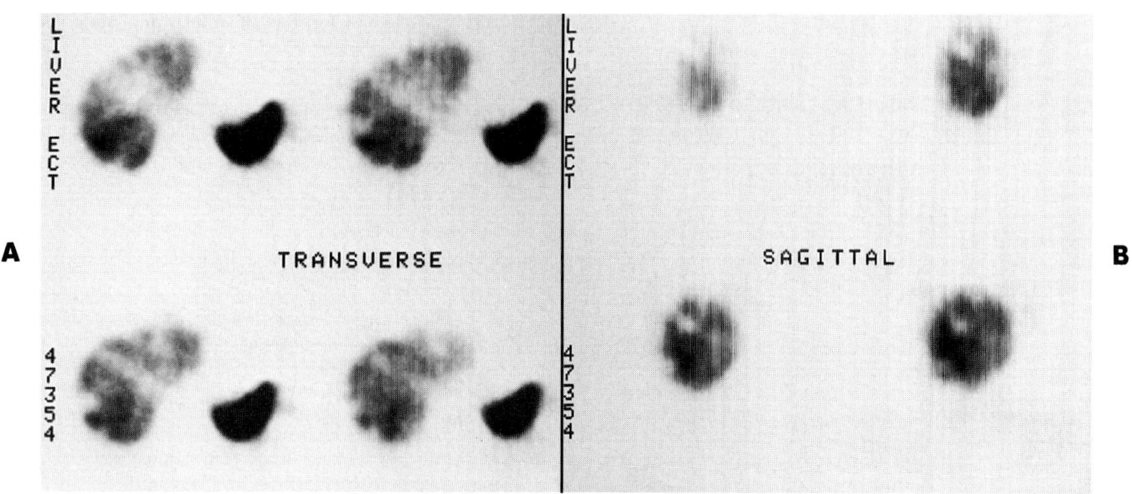

Fig. 20-16. Following the administration of ^{99m}Tc sulfur colloid. **A,** SPECT transverse and **B,** Sagittal 8-mm slices depicting tiny multiple metastatic sites in the liver, the largest measuring 2 cm × 2.5 cm in diameter. The peripheral metastatic sites could not and cannot be visualized on planar images. This patient was referred for SPECT imaging with a known pancreatic carcinoma.

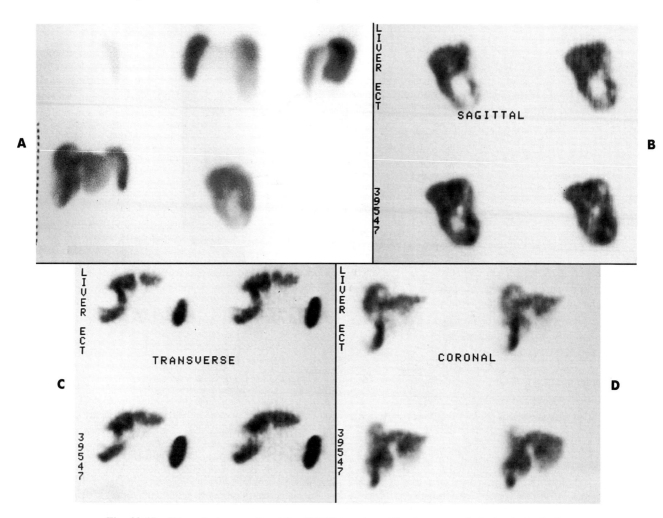

Fig. 20-17. This patient was referred for SPECT imaging with a known cystic lesion in the body of the pancreas. **A,** The planar liver/spleen images revealed splenomegaly with an increased concentration of ^{99m}Tc sulfur colloid. Anterior and posterior images reveal no specific evidence of a space-occupying lesion. The lateral image does reveal a lesion that appears to be on the anterior surface of the right lobe. **B,** SPECT images reveal a large conglomerate metastatic lesion on the anterior surface of the right lobe, which is well demonstrated on the sagittal slices. Multiple other metastatic sites are visualized on the surface of the right lobe and deep in the left lobe on transverse **(C)** and coronal slices **(D).**

specialists at this time recommend the use of the radionuclide imaging as the initial diagnostic procedure in the search for metastatic disease of the liver. This recommendation should also state that SPECT imaging should be used routinely in the search for hepatic metastatic sites.

Hepatic trauma

Because of the proximity of the liver to the rib cage, the liver is frequently traumatized in a crushing injury. In an emergency setting the liver image visualizes areas of hematoma formation.

Superior vena cava obstruction and other related disease processes

In superior–vena-cava obstruction, the intravenously injected nuclide is routed through collateral thoracic veins to subdiaphragmatic collaterals that include the umbilical vein. If the umbilical vein has remained open, it empties into the liver above the porta where it does not branch throughout the liver but ends abruptly in the region of the liver in the porta, primarily the caudate lobe. In the case of superior vena cava obstruction, the liver image shows a "hot" or increased concentration of nuclide in this focal area of the liver. In the Budd-Chiari syndrome (that is, hepatic vein thrombosis), a similar small region of increased concentration of nuclide is visualized because it is the only remaining functional liver surrounded by the liver with decreased function. A similar porta-hepatitis increased concentration is seen in inferior–vena-cava obstruction.

Extrahepatic disease

Right pleural effusion or depression of the hemidiaphragm by an emphysematous lung may cause displacement of the liver inferiorly with flattening of the dome of the liver and disappearance of the normal cardiac impression. Rarely seen is upward displacement of the right lobe with the liver shaped like a police hat (chapeau de gendarme) because of eventration of the right diaphragm. A large tumor of the right kidney may compress the liver and cause a large pseudomass in the right lobe of the liver.

The Biliary Tree

Michael G. Velchik

■ ANATOMY AND PHYSIOLOGY (Fig. 20-18)

The smallest of the bile ducts are formed as grooves as two adjacent hepatic cells fit together. Bile is emptied into this grooved space, and the continuum of the bile space, called *bile canaliculi,* radiate to the circumference of the lobule where they empty into interlobular bile ducts that unite and form the right and left main hepatic ducts. The right and left hepatic ducts join centrally to form the common hepatic duct. The cystic duct that leads from the gallbladder joins the common duct at this point; the duct continues distally as the common bile duct, which enters the duodenum after passing behind the head of the pancreas. The terminal end of the common bile duct is guarded by the muscular sphincter of Oddi.

The gallbladder is an approximately 2.5 cm × 7 cm sac that holds about 50 ml of bile. The gallbladder is lined by a mucous membrane and has sparse muscular fibers between the mucous membrane, which is serous and derived from the peritoneum. The majority of bile secreted by the liver enters the gallbladder where it is concentrated and stored. The gallbladder has rhythmic contractions that occur at a rate of 2 to 6/min; when stimulated it has tonic contractions that last from 5 to 30 minutes. Water and inorganic salts are actively absorbed through the gallbladder wall. The bile pigments, bile salts, and cholesterol of bile are not absorbed. Bile in the gallbladder has 10 times more solids than the bile found in the hepatic duct. The gallbladder also increases the viscosity of bile by the secretion of a thick mucous material. Gallbladder contraction is under neural and hormonal control. The primary hormone that causes gallbladder contraction is elaborated by the duodenum and is called *cholecystokinin.*

■ PATHOPHYSIOLOGY

■ Gallstone formation

The bile secreted by the liver is responsible for the formation of cholesterol gallstones. Cholesterol stone formers secrete a bile saturated or supersaturated with cholesterol. Bile salts and lecithin normally maintain cholesterol in solution in bile, and in stone-formers the cholesterol content exceeds the concentration of bile salts and lecithin. There is nucleation and precipitation of cholesterol crystals with growth of these crystals in the gallbladder lumen. Small gallstones may pass through the cystic duct into the common hepatic duct; if small enough they will pass through the sphincter of Oddi. If they lodge at the level of the sphincter, biliary spasm and signs of partial or complete obstruction of the biliary tree will be present. If the stones

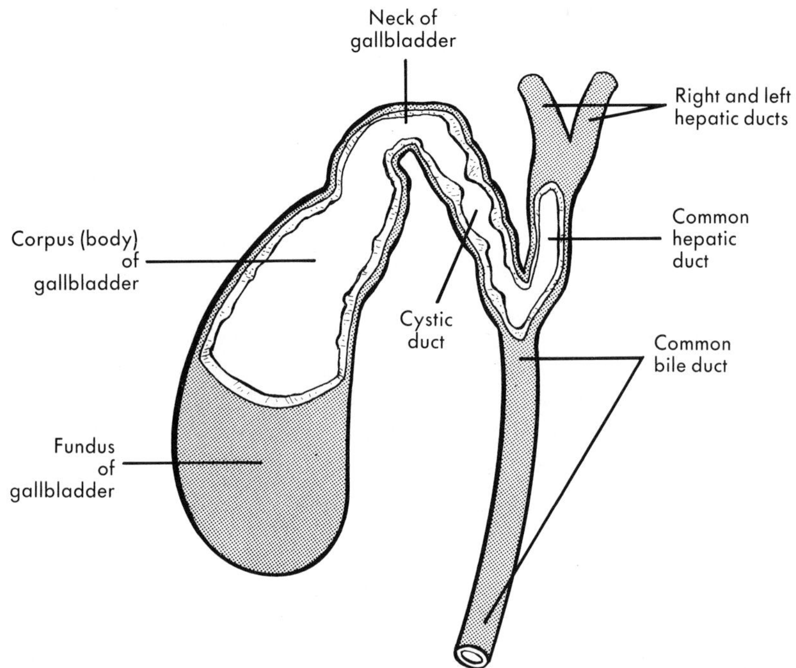

Fig. 20-18. Relationship of gallbladder's cystic duct as it joins common hepatic duct.

lodge in the cystic duct, they will produce the signs and symptoms of acute cholecystitis.

■ Cholelithiasis

Cholelithiasis, the formation of stones in the biliary tree, is a relatively common disease. The majority of gallstones are composed primarily of cholesterol, which usually is in solution in bile. However, if the bile becomes supersaturated, stones will form and usually will reside in the gallbladder. If the stones pass into the biliary tree, they cause biliary colic, which is a sudden epigastric or right upper quadrant pain that lasts several hours. Impaction of a stone in the cystic duct can cause acute cholecystitis.

■ Acute cholecystitis

A patient with acute cholecystitis usually has acute right subcostal pain and tenderness. Ninety-five percent of the patients have gallstones with obstruction of the cystic duct. Bacteria are usually present in the gallbladders of patients with chronic stones, and the infection of an obstructed gallbladder may lead to overwhelming infection and perforation. In less than 5% of patients with acute cholecystitis, gallstones are not found. The cystic duct obstruction may cause hydrops of the gallbladder, and the gallbladder is distended with uninfected mucus; this is not a common occurrence, however.

■ Acute or chronic obstruction of the extrahepatic biliary tree

Ampullary carcinoma, pancreatic carcinoma, biliary duct carcinoma, metastatic or primary carcinoma of the liver, as well as biliary stones can cause complete, partial, or intermittent obstruction of the biliary tree. With acute obstruction there is usually biliary-type pain emanating from the hypogastrium as a result of biliary spasm. However, in intermittent or chronic obstruction, there is little in the way of symptomatology except that the patient has a progressive elevation of serum bilirubin with jaundice. As the intrabiliary tree pressure increases, the hepatocyte is unable to secrete bilirubin. With the buildup of bilirubin and bile salts in the hepatocyte, a toxic chemical hepatitis ensues. Ascending cholangitis caused by bacteria in the biliary system may complicate biliary obstruction.

LABORATORY APPLICATION

55

HEPATOBILIARY IMAGING

Purpose

This section discusses hepatobiliary imaging (cholecystography) and its role in the workup of patients with suspected acute cholecystitis, chronic cholecystitis, cholestasis, and trauma, and of the postoperative patient. Its relative advantages and limitations are described compared with other radiologic studies such as oral cholecystogram (OCG), ultrasound (US), and computed tomography (CT). A suggested algorithm is presented whenever possible for the diagnostic evaluation of such conditions.

The reader is expected to derive an understanding of the optimal instrumentation and method for the performance of cholescintigraphy, the mechanism that results in a normal or abnormal image, the findings expected for various disease entities (including expected sensitivity, specificity, and accuracy), the patient radiation exposure, and the advantages and disadvantages of cholescintigraphy compared with other radiologic examinations.

Radiopharmaceuticals for cholecystography

Mebrofenin (Fig. 20-19), disofenin, and idofenin, all labeled with technetium-99m, are the radiopharmaceuticals used for cholecystography. The main advantage of the iminodiacetic acid (IDA) agents over previous hepatobiliary agents is their ability to be labeled with technetium-99m. In addition, they are easy to prepare and are relatively stable. The IDA agents are rapidly cleared from the bloodstream (T ½ = 3 min) by the hepatocytes (polygonal cells) of the liver by an anion active transport mechanism similar to bilirubin; they are excreted unconjugated into the bile. The primary route of excretion is through the hepatobiliary system (80% to 90%) with the secondary route being the urinary tract (10% to 20%). The relative percent excreted through the primary route as compared with the secondary route depends on the alkyl or "R" group of the IDA derivative, and the bilirubin level. There is a shift from the primary hepatobiliary route to the secondary renal route, with rising bilirubin level as a result of competitive inhibition.

Radiation dosimetry

The estimated absorbed radiation dose for an average (70 kg) patient after an intravenous injection of 5 mCi (185 MBq) of Tc-mebrofenin is shown in Table 20-1. Thus, in a normal subject (bilirubin <1.5 mg/dl), the critical or target organ is the colon, followed by the small intestine and gallbladder. This is directly attributable to the amount of radioactivity present and its residence time.

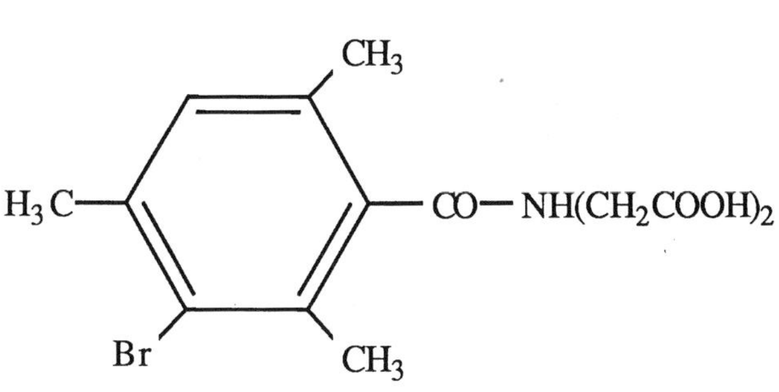

Fig. 20-19. Choletec (Mebrofenin) trimethylbromoiminodiacetic acid.

Table 20-1. ^{99m}Tc-Mebrofenin dosimetry*

	Normal subjects	Jaundiced patients
Tissue	**RAD/5 mCi (185 MBq)**	**RAD/5 mCi (185 MBq)**
Total body	0.10	0.08
Liver	2.35	0.45
Gallbladder wall	0.69	0.63
Small intestine	1.50	0.80
Upper colon	2.37	1.24
Lower colon	1.82	0.99
Bladder wall	0.15	1.21
Ovaries	0.50	0.32
Testes	0.25	0.05
Bone marrow	0.17	0.13

Modified from Loberg, M.D. and Buddemeyer, E.V.: Application of pharmacokenetic modeling to the radiation desimetry of hepatobiliary agents. In Third International Radiopharmaceutical Dosimetry Symposium, FDA No. 81-8166, U.S. Dept. of Health and Human Services, Public Health Service, FDA Bureau of Radiological Health, Rockville, Md., 1981, pp. 318-332.

Continued.

In severely jaundiced patients (bilirubin >10 mg/dl), there is a shift from the primary hepatobiliary route to the secondary renal route of excretion. Consequently, in these patients the radiation dose to the bladder approaches that of the colon. Therefore, the radiation exposure of various tissues and organs varies in health and disease and also with the different IDA derivatives, but the overall dosimetry is well within the diagnostic range and compares favorably with that of other radiologic examinations of the hepatobiliary tree (with the exception of ultrasound [US], which obviously has no associated radiation exposure).

Indications

1. To aid in the diagnosis of acute cholecystitis
2. To establish the function of the gallbladder in patients with chronic cholecystitis
3. To aid in the differential diagnosis of acute hepatitis versus acute biliary obstruction
4. In the follow-up of patients who have had biliary diversionary procedures or stints placed through obstructions in the biliary system
5. To visualize abnormal biliary leakage
6. To establish the presence of biliary reflux into the proximal duodenum and stomach following gastric surgical procedures
7. To visualize choledochal cysts
8. To aid in the diagnosis of biliary atresia

Contraindications

1. There are no absolute contraindications to cholescintigraphy, only the relative contraindication of pregnancy. Allergic reactions are extremely rare, unlike the high incidence of reactions to IV/oral-contrast material employed for intravenous cholangiography (IVC), computed tomography (CT), or oral cholecystography (OCG).

Procedure

Materials

1. Large–field-of-view (LFOV) gamma camera (SPECT optional) and low-energy, all-purpose (LEAP) collimator interfaced to a computer (optional)
2. ^{99m}Tc mebrofenin (or radiopharmaceutical of choice) 5 mCi (185 MBq) administered intravenously. Recommended dosage is 5 mCi (185 MBq) for average (70 kg) patient, which may be increased to 10 mCi (370 MBq) in severely jaundiced or obese patients

Patient preparation

1. Patient must be NPO for at least 2 hours before the examination. (Recent food ingestion may result in gallbladder contraction and consequently a potential false positive diagnosis. However, most patients with RUQ pain and suspected acute cholecystitis have not eaten recently or are receiving IV fluids.)
2. Explain the entire procedure to the patient.

NOTE—Bowel preparation is unnecessary because the intestinal gas and fecal material that may interfere with US, IVC, OCG, or CT does not interfere with cholescintigraphy. Similarly, skin wounds and surgical incisions that may interfere with US or metallic clips that may interfere with CT or magnetic resonance imaging (MRI) do not adversely affect hepatobiliary scintigraphy.

Technique

1. Calibrate for radionuclide being used (^{99m}Tc energy 140 keV).
2. Adjust intensity and determine proper orientation.
3. Position patient under the camera in the supine position with the right upper quadrant of the abdomen centered. A camera with a large field of view is best for this study. A diverging collimator may be necessary on a camera with a small field of view.
4. Images begin immediately after intravenous injection; however, an optional flow study or radionuclide angiogram that may detect vascular lesions is performed by obtaining a series of frequent images (1 image/2 to 5 seconds) for a total duration of 1 min after an IV bolus of 5 mCi (185 MBq) of the radiopharmaceutical.

5. The imaging sequence is not crucial as long as a series of images are obtained during the course of an hour.
6. Usually images may be obtained for 500,000 counts each at 15-min intervals in the anterior projection including a right lateral at 1 hour postinjection. The latter is often helpful in differentiating radioactivity in the gallbladder (which is anteriorly located) from activity in the second portion of the duodenum (which is located in the midline) or activity in the collecting system of the right kidney (which is posterior in location). In the anterior projection, radioactivity in the duodenum or right kidney may simulate gallbladder activity, resulting in a false negative diagnosis in a patient with acute cholecystitis and non-visualization of the gallbladder. Oblique views or giving water by mouth (which flushes out duodenal activity but doesn't alter gallbladder activity) may be helpful in this regard.
7. Alternatively, one may obtain sequential images of 1-minute duration each, which provides a visual impression of the clearance of activity from the bloodstream initially and subsequently the hepatic parenchyma (since the images are obtained for the same time rather than counts). Obtaining images at frequent intervals (e.g., 1 every minute rather than 1 every 15 minutes) is especially helpful in evaluating the progression of radioactivity from the bloodstream to the liver, bile ducts, and intestine, as well as in identifying bile leaks, fistulas, bilomas, obstruction and patency of surgical anastomoses. It may also help to distinguish between activity within the gallbladder (which tends to progressively increase over time or remain relatively static) from activity in the second portion of the duodenum (which tends to fluctuate or vacillate up and down during the course of the examination). If a computer is used, the images may be played back sequentially in the form of a cine loop, which enhances one's perception of tracer progression. If one desired to perform the minimum number of images, for example in a very sick patient, the most crucial images are the anterior and right lateral images obtained at 60 minutes postinjection.
8. The administration of a fatty meal or a slow dose of cholecystokinin (CCK, 0.02 μgm/kg) (Sincalide™) administered intravenously 30 minutes following administration of the radiopharmaceutical may be helpful in (1) the diagnosis of acalculous cholecystitis, (2) the differentiation of radioactivity in the gallbladder from duodenal activity (the former decreases and the latter is unaltered), (3) the distinguishment between acute and chronic cholecystitis, and (4) the evaluation of hepatobiliary kinetics.
9. The opioid drug morphine induces contraction of the sphincter of Oddi; this will accelerate visualization of the gallbladder. Morphine administered slowly intravenously (0.04 mgm/kg) 30 to 40 minutes postadministration of the radiopharmaceutical may enhance gallbladder visualization, shorten the procedure, and rule out the diagnosis of cystic duct obstruction.
10. Delayed images beyond 1 hour postinjection are an alternative to CCK in helping to separate chronic from acute cholecystitis and may be useful in postoperative patients, jaundiced patients, and patients with a suspected bile leak, choledochal cyst, common bile duct obstruction, or a cystic duct remnant.
11. Computer acquisition and analysis is advantageous for: (1) quantification (gallbladder ejection fraction, hepatobiliary kinetics), (2) image processing (color scale, background subtraction, smoothing, image addition and subtraction, filtering, generation of regions of interest, time/activity curve construction, etc.), and (3) dynamic cine loop replay.

Diagnosis

The normal nuclear cholecystogram

After IV administration in normal subjects, hepatobiliary radiopharmaceuticals are rapidly cleared from the bloodstream (17% residual in blood at 10 minutes postinjection) by the hepatocytes (polygonal cells) of the liver. The majority (90% to 95%) is excreted unconjugated into the bile with the remainder excreted in the urine (average = 1% injected dosage during the first 3 hours). If an image or radionuclide angiogram is performed immediately after injection, blood-pool activity is seen in the heart, liver, spleen, kidneys, and major vessels. The liver is clearly visualized by 5 minutes postinjection with the optimal hepatocyte phase occurring at 11 minutes postinjection. The extrahepatic bile ducts and gallbladder are normally visualized at 10 to 15 minutes with small intestine activity at 30 to 60 minutes. For a study to be considered normal, the gallbladder and small bowel must be visualized within an hour. The mechanism of gallbladder visualization in a normal

Continued.

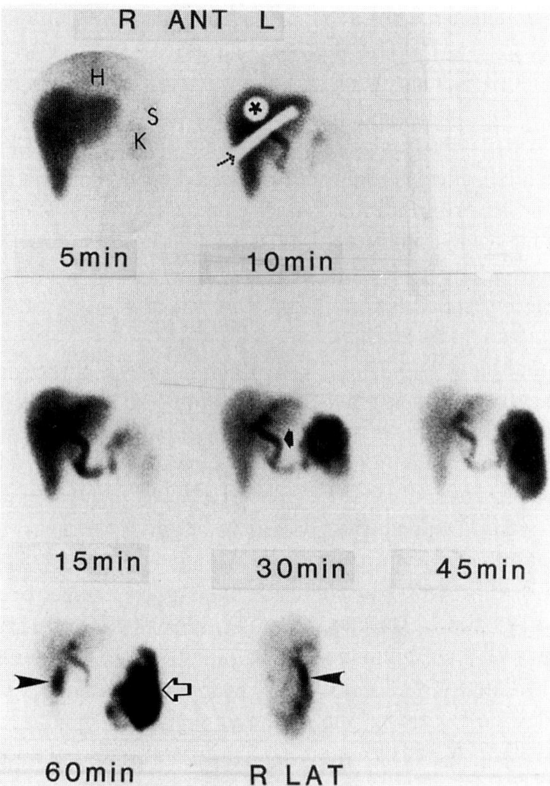

Fig. 20-20. Normal cholescintigram. Following the intravenous administration of 5 mCi (185 MBq) of ^{99m}Tc Mebrofenin, multiple images of the abdomen, taken over the course of 1 hour, reveal normal uptake, distribution, and clearance of radioactivity in the liver, common bile duct *(closed arrow),* gallbladder *(arrowhead),* and small bowel *(open arrow).* The 10-minute image contains a 5-cm lead size marker(*) and lead-strip, costal-margin marker *(dotted arrow).* Note the blood-pool activity in the heart (H), spleen (S), and left kidney (K) in the 5-minute image.

Indications for cholescintigraphy

I. Cholecystitis
  A. Acute
  B. Chronic
II. Jaundice
  A. Obstructive vs. nonobstructive
  B. Neonatal hepatitis vs. biliary atresia
  C. Acute common bile duct obstruction
  D. Choledochal cyst
III. The postoperative patient
  A. Postcholecystectomy syndrome
    1. Cystic duct remnant
  B. Biliary-enteric bypass (portoenterostomy)
    1. Hepatic perfusion
    2. Hepatocyte function
    3. Patency/obstruction
    4. Bile leak
    5. Preferential route of bile flow
  C. Gastroenterostomy
    1. Gastric reflux
    2. Afferent loop syndrome
  D. Liver transplantation
    1. Hepatic perfusion
    2. Hepatocyte function
    3. Patency/obstruction
    4. Bile leak
    5. Preferential route of bile flow
IV. Trauma
V. Biliary dyskinesia

image may be entirely explained on the basis of simple "plumbing" and is completely independent of gallbladder function. Since the gallbladder is connected via the cystic duct to the common bile duct, radioactivity simply diffuses into the gallbladder. It does not involve active secretion by the gallbladder mucosa. A normal cholescintigram is illustrated in Fig. 20-20.

Acute cholecystitis

A list of the possible indications for cholecystography is included in the box above. The most important indications for which it is the initial diagnostic study of choice is right upper quadrant pain and suspected acute cholecystitis. Cholecystitis is the most common indication for abdominal surgery and the fourth most common cause for hospitalization in adults. Twenty million Americans (10%) have gallstones, and about 0.5 million cholecystectomies are performed each year. Early diagnosis and prompt cholecystectomy reduces morbidity; nonoperative therapy is associated with significant morbidity and mortality especially in elderly patients.

Traditionally, the oral cholecystogram (OCG) was the radiologic study of choice for the evaluation of gallbladder disease. However, more recently this has been replaced by ultrasound because of certain inherent limitations: (1) Nonspecificity for acute cholecystitis, (2) Dependency on intestinal absorption and hepatic function (conjugation), both of which may lead to false positive diagnoses, (3) Dependency on serum bilirubin level (>4 mg% precludes a satisfactory examination), (4) False negative rate of 6% to 8%, (5) 25% of patients require a second dosage resulting in a delay of 24

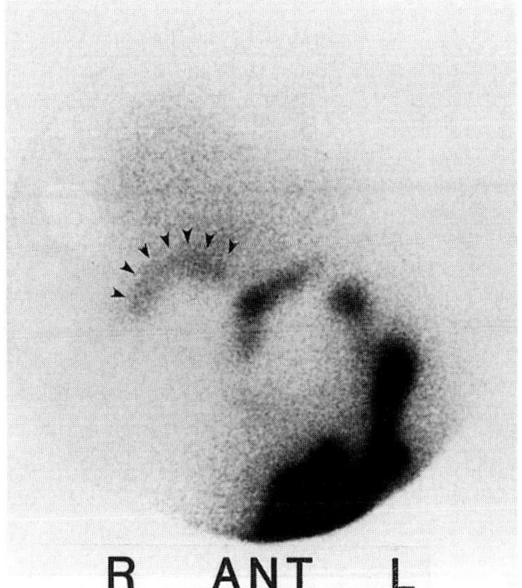

Fig. 20-21. Acute cholecystitis. An anterior view of the abdomen obtained about 60 minutes after the intravenous injection of 5 mCi (185 MBq) of ^{99m}Tc Mebrofenin shows a "rim" *(arrowheads)* of increased radioactivity in the gallbladder fossa with nonvisualization of the gallbladder.

hours, and (6) Associated side effects (nausea, vomiting, diarrhea, allergic reactions). Ultrasound is the best examination for the evaluation of gallstones and chronic cholecystitis, but it has limitations with respect to the diagnosis of acute cholecystitis. It provides purely anatomic information. Although it is excellent in detecting gallstones, it must be remembered that in the 10% of Americans who have gallstones, most are asymptomatic. Therefore, merely demonstrating gallstones does not necessarily imply the presence of acute cholecystitis. Furthermore, ultrasound cannot answer the key functional question concerning whether or not the cystic duct is obstructed. Gallstones in the region of the gallbladder neck and cystic duct are the most difficult to detect because of anatomic considerations (proximity of gas in the duodenum), but they are most important with respect to the diagnosis of acute cholecystitis. The examination is highly operator-dependent and may be compromised by excessive bowel gas (ileus is common in patients with RUQ pain), rib artifacts, and obesity. The false negative rate for the detection of gallstones is 1% to 5% and varies with the equipment and expertise of both the technologist and physician performing the examination. Many secondary signs of cholecystitis have been described in the ultrasound literature, but none is pathognomonic of cystic duct obstruction and acute cholecystitis. Samuels and others compared ultrasound to cholescintigraphy for the diagnosis of acute cholecystitis and found no significant difference in sensitivity (97% for both); however, cholescintigraphy had better specificity (93% vs. 64%) and predictive value (77% vs 40%). They concluded that cholescintigraphy is the procedure of choice for suspected acute cholecystitis.

The advantages of ultrasound include: (1) lack of exposure to ionizing radiation, (2) independence from bilirubin level, (3) superior spatial resolution and depiction of regional anatomy (the majority of patients with RUQ pain have an etiology other than acute cholecystitis, e.g., pancreatitis, renal calculous, liver metastases, etc.), and (4) short examination time (10 to 15 minutes). Its cost is similar to that of cholescintigraphy for the evaluation of the gallbladder in most institutions, but cost is significantly greater if the entire abdomen is evaluated.

Acute cholecystitis is caused by an obstructed cystic duct in 98% of cases. Cholescintigraphy is the only noninvasive diagnostic examination that can accurately determine functional patency of the cystic duct. Weissmann and others reported a sensitivity of 95.2%, specificity of 99.2%, and overall accuracy of 97.6% for the diagnosis of acute cholecystitis by cholescintigraphy in a study of 296 patients. It has therefore become the initial diagnostic study of choice in patients with right upper quadrant pain and suspected acute cholecystitis. Cholescintigraphy is noninvasive, safe, readily available, easy to perform, and free of adverse effects or contraindications; in addition, it may accurately rule out acute cholecystitis within 30 to 60 minutes.

The most common cholescintigraphic appearance of acute cholecystitis is nonvisualization of the gallbladder (Fig. 20-21). For nonvisualization to be diagnostic of acute cholecystitis, there must be

Continued.

evidence of radioactivity in the small intestine. Nonvisualization of the gallbladder at 1 hour postinjection implies cholecystitis but does not distinguish between acute or chronic cholecystitis at that point. Although the vast majority (97%) will have cystic duct obstruction and acute cholecystitis, a small percentage (3%) will prove to have partial or intermittent obstruction and chronic cholecystitis. However, these two groups (acute vs. chronic) may be separated by obtaining delayed images at 4 hours post injection (thereby avoiding a potential false positive diagnosis of acute cholecystitis in a patient with chronic cholecystitis. Delayed visualization of the gallbladder beyond 1 hour postinjection occurs most commonly in patients with chronic cholecystitis, whereas persistent nonvisualization at 4 hours postinjection suggests complete cystic duct obstruction and acute cholecystitis with a high degree of accuracy. Rarely, a patient with chronic cholecystitis will have gallbladder visualization beyond 4 hours postinjection. Therefore, Drane and others have taken this one step further by suggesting that one routinely obtain delayed images up to 24 hours postinjection. Most nuclear physicians stop at 4 hours postinjection, accepting the fact that 1 out of 100 to 200 patients with nonvisualization of the gallbladder at 4 hours postinjection will have chronic cholecystitis.

Another alternative to obtaining delayed images when there is nonvisualization at 1 hour involves the stimulation of gallbladder contraction with either a fatty meal or administration of cholecystokinin (CCK) followed by a repeat injection of the radiopharmaceutical. The premise is that in patients with acute cholecystitis, the gallbladder will remain nonvisualized because of complete cystic duct obstruction, whereas patients with chronic cholecystitis and partial or intermittent cystic duct obstruction (with viscous bile and sludge filling the gallbladder) will empty and subsequently visualize. There is some controversy concerning which stimulus is best. Initial reports suggested that an injection of CCK is more reliable, predictable, and reproducible than the oral ingestion of a fatty meal that is dependent on intestinal absorption, which may be variable. However, subsequent reports have suggested that the fatty meal may be as reliable as the injection of CCK and may be preferable because it is more physiologic. Of interest is that the use of a stimulus for gallbladder contraction in a patient with a potentially obstructed cystic duct is controversial. However, physicians who have employed CCK or a fatty meal routinely in this situation have not reported any significant adverse effects, complications, or exacerbation of symptoms.

The opioid drugs meperidine and morphine, commonly administered to patients with right upper quadrant pain and suspected acute cholecystitis, induce contraction of the sphincter of Oddi, resulting in increased biliary pressure and delayed clearance of radioactivity from the common bile duct and delayed visualization of the small bowel (Fig. 20-22). This pattern may be mistaken for partial obstruction of the common bile duct. However, gallbladder visualization is enhanced and accelerated. Therefore, some investigators have suggested routinely employing narcotic premedication to decrease imaging time and reduce the number of false positive results due to chronic cholecystitis.

Several investigators have described a "rim sign" thought to be highly suggestive of acute cholecystitis, especially severe gangrenous cholecystitis (Fig. 20-21). Bushnell and others found that the sign was associated with a positive predictive value of 94% for acute cholecystitis and suggested that if it is seen in association with a nonvisualized gallbladder at 1 hour postinjection, the patient may be assumed to have acute cholecystitis and delayed images are unnecessary. Smith and Brachman both found a high association of the sign with severe gangrenous cholecystitis and perforation.

Nonvisualization of the gallbladder that is associated with a prominent photon-deficient gallbladder fossa and mass-effect–producing medial displacement of the second portion of the duodenum and/or common bile duct, has been reported in hydrops, empyema, and carcinoma of the gallbladder.

Cholecystography has a false-negative rate of about 1% to 5%. A list of potential causes of false-negative cholecystograms is presented in a box on page 509. Rarely, patients with acute cholecystitis will have gallbladder visualization and a false-negative cholescintigram presumably because of incomplete cystic duct obstruction. Acalculous cholecystitis, which comprises about 5% of all cases of acute cholecystitis (95% calculous), has been reported as a potential cause of false-negative cholecystograms. However, the majority (93%) of patients with acute acalculous cholecystitis will have a functionally obstructed cystic duct and therefore a nonvisualized gallbladder on cholescintigraphy, resulting in a true positive diagnosis. In the minority of patients with acute acalculous cholecystitis who have a gallbladder visualized by cholecystography, a potential false-negative diagnosis may be avoided by the use of CCK or a fatty meal. An abnormal response (absence of gallbladder contrac-

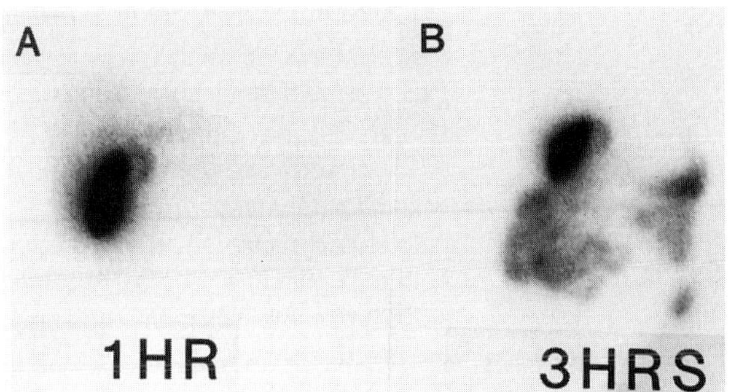

Fig. 20-22. Partial (functional) common bile duct obstruction. **A,** An anterior view of the abdomen obtained 1 hour after the IV administration of 5 mCi (185 MBq) of ^{99m}Tc Mebrofenin in a patient treated with Demerol for right upper quadrant pain shows preferential filling of the gallbladder with delayed small bowel visualization at 3 hours postinjection **(B).**

False-negative cholecystograms (false-negative rate = 1% to 5%)

1. Acute calculous cholecystitis
2. Acute acalculous cholecystitis
3. Right hydronephrosis
4. Duodenal diverticulum
5. Accessory hepatic duct
6. Dual gallbladder
7. Biliary duplication cyst

False-positive cholecystograms (false-positive rate < 1%)

1. Recent food ingestion
2. Prolonged fasting >24 hrs (hyperalimentation)
3. Alcoholism
4. Pancreatitis
5. Chronic cholecystitis
6. Low-fat diet
7. Hyperbilirubinemia
8. Gallbladder agenesis/atresia
9. Ectopic gallbladder
10. Obstructing neoplasm
11. Nicotinic acid ingestion

tion; ejection fraction <35%; nonvisualization after repeat radiopharmaceutical injection) is highly suggestive of acalculous cholecystitis. Occasionally, radioactivity in the second portion of the duodenum or right kidney may mimic gallbladder radioactivity in the anterior projection. This potential pitfall (false-negative diagnosis due to misinterpretation) may be avoided by obtaining right lateral or oblique projections, having the patient drink a glass of water (duodenal activity will change but not gallbladder activity), administering CCK or a fatty meal, or obtaining delayed images.

The reported false-positive rate for the detection of acute cholecystitis by cholecystography is <1%. Causes of potential false-positive cholescintigrams are listed in the box above, right. Recent food ingestion (<2 to 4 hours before injection) may result in gallbladder contraction and consequently a false positive examination. In contrast, prolonged fasting (>24 to 48 hours before injection) and hyperalimentation may result in gallbladder nonvisualization due to an atonic gallbladder filled with viscous bile that impedes the diffusion of radiopharmaceutical into the gallbladder. This pitfall may be avoided by the prior administration of CCK. Patients with chronic cholecystitis may have delayed gallbladder visualization. If the study is terminated prematurely (before 4 hours postinjection), the condition may be misdiagnosed as acute cholecystitis. Alternatively, an IV injection of CCK (or fatty meal) followed by reimaging may be performed. Some investigators have recommended routine pretreatment with CCK; however, this decreases one's sensitivity for the detection of chronic cholecystitis and is unnecessary in normal patients.

Chronic cholecystitis

Patients with suspected chronic cholecystitis and/or gallstones are best evaluated by ultrasound, which has replaced the traditional screening examination, the oral cholecystogram, in this circumstance. As previously mentioned, cholecystography is normal in the majority of patients with chronic cholecystitis and it therefore has poor sensitivity for its detection. All except the very largest gallstones escape detection by cholescintigraphy. Therefore, a normal cholecystogram does not exclude chronic cholecystitis or gallstones. The second most common cholecystographic finding in patients with chronic cholecystitis is delayed gallbladder visualization (>1 hour).

Continued.

Jaundice

In jaundiced patients, it is of paramount importance to distinguish between intrahepatic (nonobstructive) and extrahepatic (obstructive) cholestasis, which are treated medically and surgically, respectively. Ultrasound is the initial diagnostic procedure of choice. It is highly accurate (85% to 95%) in detecting obstruction and can identify the site and cause in the majority of cases. Ultrasound does not expose the patient to ionizing radiation and is independent of bilirubin level. Computed tomography is best used when ultrasound cannot define the site or nature of the obstruction. If both ultrasound and computed tomography fail to clearly delineate the site and cause of obstruction, percutaneous transhepatic cholangiography (PTC), although more invasive, may directly visualize the bile ducts and diagnose the etiology of obstruction in addition to possibly treating it. Endoscopic retrograde cholangiopancreatography (ERCP) is reserved for when a contraindication to PTC exists (bleeding diathesis/sepsis) especially if obstruction of the distal common bile duct or pancreatic duct is suspected.

The main advantage of cholecystography in the evaluation of the jaundiced patient is the functional, physiologic nature of the information it provides. It provides information about hepatic perfusion, hepatocyte function, bile kinetics, preferential route of bile flow, obstruction, bile leaks or collections (bilomas), etc. Unlike ERCP, PTC, or T-tube cholangiograms, it is physiologic and does not require pressure contrast injections or retrograde flow. It is indicated in conjunction with ultrasound to differentiate obstructive from nonobstructive jaundice (including biliary atresia versus hepatitis in neonates), acute common bile duct obstruction, and choledochal cysts.

Cholecystography

Cholescintigraphy has an overall accuracy of 85% to 90% in distinguishing obstructive from nonobstructive jaundice. This has important therapeutic implications. Rosenthall and others found that cholecystography has a predictive accuracy of 77% to 90% for nonobstructive jaundice, 74% to 78% for partial obstruction, and 98% to 100% for complete common bile duct obstruction. The typical cholescintigraphic patterns seen in hepatocellular disease, partial obstruction, and complete obstruction are illustrated in Figs. 20-22, 23, and 24, respectively. Hepatocellular disease is characterized by increased background radioactivity, decreased hepatic uptake, increased renal excretion, and reduced or delayed small-bowel visualization (Fig. 20-25). Both partial (Fig. 20-22) and acute complete common bile duct obstruction (Fig. 20-23) have a high target-to-background ratio (low background activity, high hepatic activity) with delayed (beyond 1 hour) and absent small bowel activity, respectively. In the former, there may be prolonged bile duct visualization (beyond 1 hour), whereas in complete obstruction, the bile ducts are usually not visualized. The gallbladder is usually visualized in partial obstruction but not in complete obstruction. Complete obstruction therefore appears like a liver image (Fig. 20-23). The key differential point in distinguishing between hepatocellular disease and obstruction is the visualization of small-bowel activity in the former and absence in the latter. However, long-standing severe hepatocellular disease may be impossible to differentiate from chronic obstruction since bowel radioactivity may be significantly reduced in the former and the target-to-background ratio will be poor in both.

Acute common bile duct obstruction is readily detected by cholecystography but may be missed by ultrasound because the former reflects functional obstruction whereas the latter depicts anatomy and morphologic dilatation of the common bile duct (the sonographic sign of obstruction) may lag behind the actual functional obstruction. Weissmann and others found that 70% of patients with proven acute common bile duct obstruction by cholecystography had normal-caliber bile ducts by ultrasound. In contrast, dilatation of the common bile duct may be present in the absence of functional obstruction (postoperative, prior obstruction) resulting in a potential false positive diagnosis by ultrasound.

The differential diagnosis of jaundice in neonates includes biliary atresia (obstructive) and hepatitis (nonobstructive). The former is a surgical emergency whereas the latter is treated medically. The prognosis in biliary atresia is directly related to prompt diagnosis and surgical intervention. Nonsurgical therapy of biliary atresia eventually leads to irreversible liver damage (cirrhosis) and death. Fine-needle biopsy is frequently unable to distinguish between the two entities, while cholecystography does distinguish between them.

Fig. 20-23. Complete acute common bile duct obstruction. An anterior image of the abdomen obtained 24 hours after the IV administration of 5 mCi (185 MBq) of ^{99m}Tc Mebrofenin shows nonvisualization of the bile ducts, gallbladder, and small intestine. Note the good uptake of tracer in the liver with high target-to-background ratio and prominent bladder **(B)** activity. Acute obstruction was caused by a distal common bile duct stone.

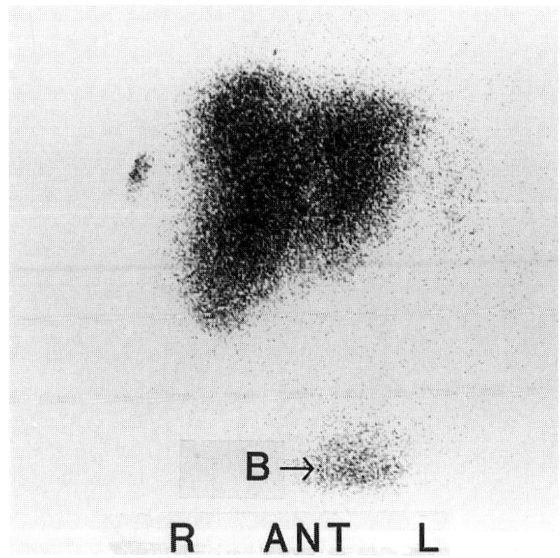

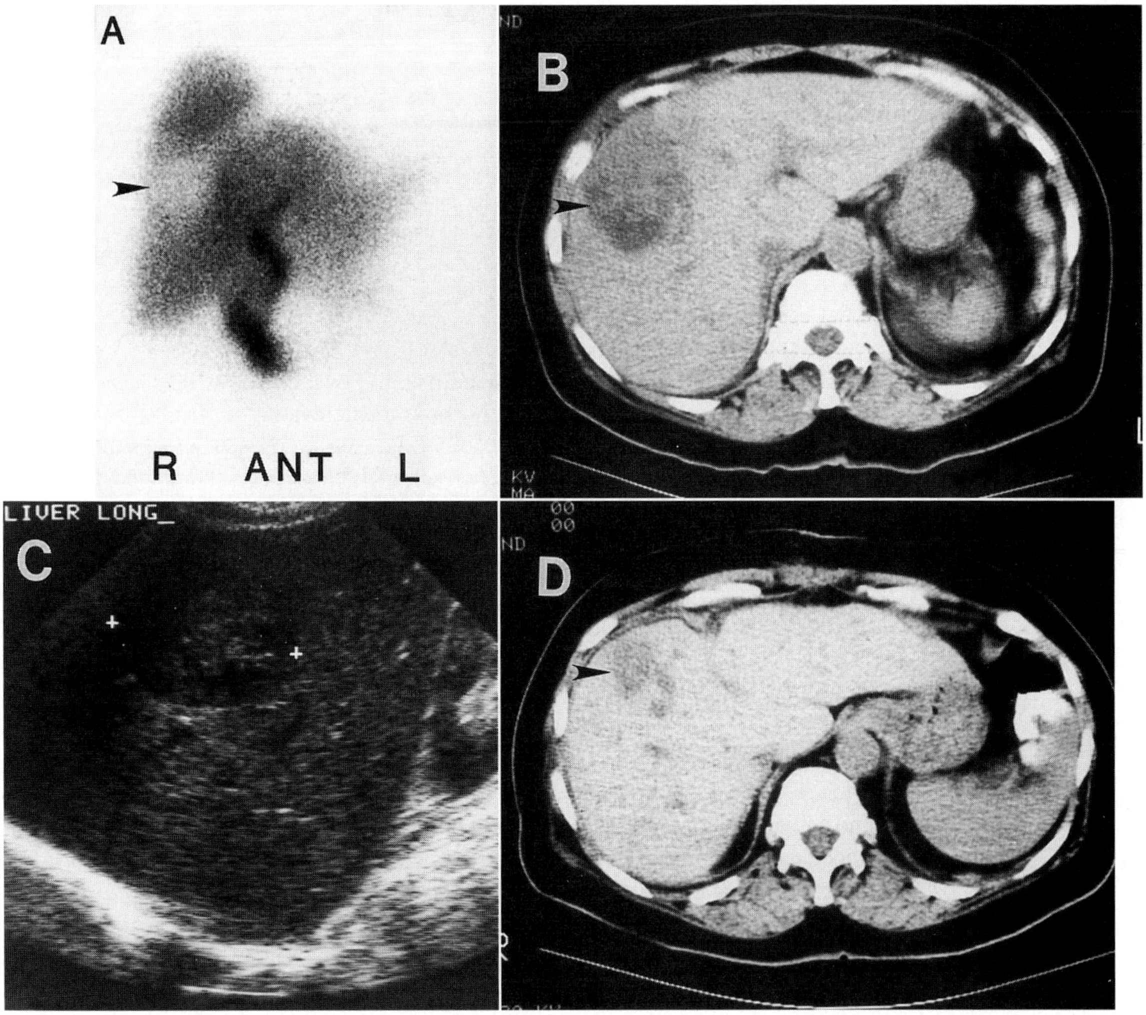

Fig. 20-24. Abscess. **A,** Cholescintigram. An anterior image of the abdomen obtained 15 minutes after the IV administration of 5 mCi (185 MBq) of ^{99m}Tc Mebrofenin in a patient with right upper quadrant pain and suspected acute cholecystitis shows a focal defect (nonfunctioning "cold" space occupying mass) *(arrowhead)* measuring approximately 5 cm in the right lobe. **B,** Computed tomography. A CT scan shows a low-density lesion *(arrowhead)* in the anterior segment of the right lobe corresponding to the abnormality seen by cholescintigraphy. **C,** Ultrasound. A sagittal sonogram of the liver shows a complex mass in the right lobe (crosshairs) corresponding to the other exams. **D,** Computed tomography. Followup CT examination after treatment with antibiotics and percutaneous drainage shows partial resolution.

Continued.

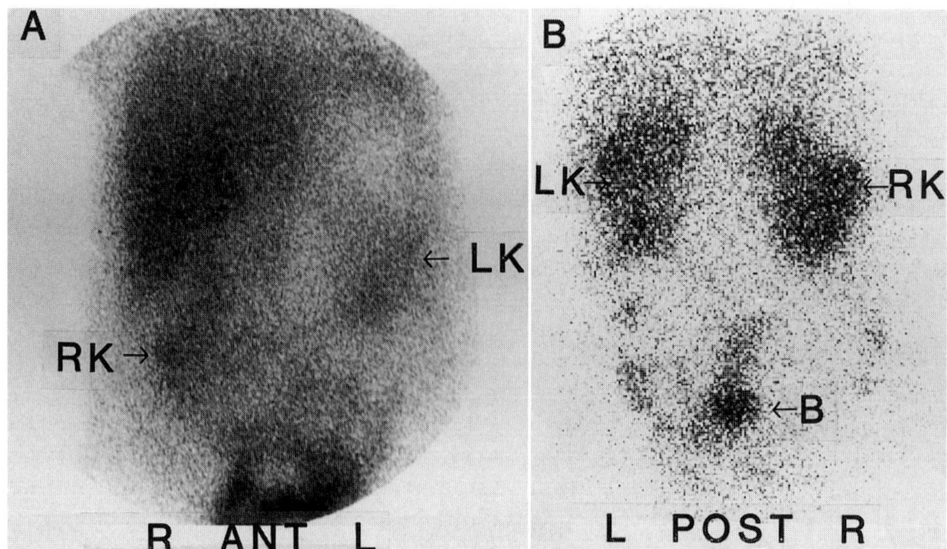

Fig. 20-25. Hepatocellular disease. **A,** An anterior image of the abdomen obtained 60 minutes after the IV injection of 5 mCi (185 MBq) of ^{99m}Tc Mebrofenin in a patient with hepatocellular disease and elevated bilirubin level (12.5 mg%) shows increased background activity and a shift to the secondary renal route of excretion (RK = right kidney, LK = left kidney). **B,** The posterior image shows the renal radioactivity to better advantage. The study is nondiagnostic with respect to the gallbladder, which is not visualized because of the reduced hepatobiliary excretion (B = bladder).

In addition, hepatobiliary scintigraphy is helpful in the evaluation of the success of the surgical procedure (closed portoenterostomy = Kasai; open portoenterostomy = Suruga) by providing information about hepatic perfusion, function, patency of the anastomosis, bile leaks, etc. Ductal dilatation or absence of the gallbladder by ultrasound examination suggests the diagnosis of biliary atresia; however, the gallbladder may be present in up to 20% of patients with biliary atresia and ductal dilatation is usually absent. Ultrasound provides information that is complementary to that of cholecystography and is especially helpful in cases of hepatitis with severe hepatocellular decompensation that might potentially result in a false positive cholecystographic diagnosis of biliary atresia. Some investigators have recommended the use of a fatty meal or CCK in this circumstance to promote gallbladder emptying and subsequently small-bowel visualization in patients with hepatitis. Premedication with phenobarbital (5 mg/day PO × 3 days) has also been advocated to enhance hepatobiliary excretion of the radiopharmaceutical in patients with hepatitis. The key cholecystographic finding is the presence (hepatitis) or absence (biliary atresia) of small bowel radioactivity. Patients with neonatal hepatitis also tend to have more background radioactivity and a poorer target-to-background ratio because of hepatocellular dysfunction than do patients with early biliary atresia. However, this difference becomes obscured in patients with chronic untreated biliary atresia.

Choledochal cysts are rare congenital anomalies that occur more frequently in girls than in boys. Although jaundice is present in the majority of patients, the typical clinical triad of pain, abdominal mass, and jaundice is uncommon. They are caused by anomalous development of the sphincter of Oddi and the junction of the pancreatic and common bile ducts, which permit the reflux of pancreatic juice into the common bile duct to result in inflammation, fibrosis, obstruction, and consequent dilatation. The two best noninvasive procedures for making the diagnosis include cholescintigraphy and ultrasound. The typical cholecystographic appearance is a photon-deficient mass in the region of the porta hepatis that fills in on delayed images (2 to 4 hours postinjection). Ultrasound shows a fluid collection that communicates with the common bile duct or fusiform dilatation of the common bile duct. The treatment is surgical excision and Roux-en-Y anastomosis to establish separate drainage for the liver and pancreas. The gallbladder is usually removed at the time of surgery because of the increased incidence of adenocarcinoma in these patients.

Postoperative patient

Cholecystography provides useful information about hepatic perfusion, function, biliary integrity, and bile flow kinetics after a variety of gastrointestinal surgical procedures (cholecystectomy, biliary-enteric bypass, gastroenterostomy, portoenterostomy (Kasai/Suruga), hepatic resection, and liver transplantation.

Postcholecystectomy syndrome has been reported to affect up to 50% of patients who have had their gallbladders removed. Cholecystography can identify postoperative complications such as common bile duct obstruction, cystic duct remnant, bile leaks and fistulas. Cholescintigraphy is physiologic and demonstrates the true preferential route of bile flow, unlike T-tube cholangiograms, PTC, or ERCP which require artificial retrograde pressure injections of contrast material. Cholecystography does not have any associated adverse side effects commonly associated with radiologic studies requiring iodinated contrast material. In addition, it is more sensitive than the corresponding radiologic contrast study in detecting bile leaks and fistulas. This is because of inherent differences in the techniques.

In patients post–biliary-enteric anastomosis, cholecystography can provide information about hepatic perfusion, hepatic function, anastomotic patency or obstruction, and the identification of bile leaks. As previously mentioned, this applies to patients with biliary atresia who have had open (Suruga) or closed (Kasai) portoenterostomies. In patients postgastroenterostomy, cholecystography can help to elucidate enterogastric bile reflux as a possible cause of postoperative gastritis in addition to afferent and/or efferent loop obstruction, and bile leaks. Bile reflux, commonly seen in patients with Billroth II anastomoses, is rare in patients with Roux-en-Y anastomoses. Stasis of radioactivity in the afferent loop beyond 2 hours postinjection is abnormal and suggests the possibility of afferent loop obstruction.

In liver-transplant recipients, cholecystography has been reported to be useful in evaluating hepatic blood flow, hepatic function, biliary-enteric patency, bile leaks or fistulas, and in the differentiation of rejection and obstruction.

Trauma

Cholescintigraphy can evaluate the integrity of the hepatobiliary system and detect space-occupying lesions such as hematomas or bilomas. It can also determine whether or not the latter communicate with the biliary system. This has important prognostic and therapeutic implications and is not possible with CT or ultrasound. No patient preparation is required. Lacerations and wounds do not interfere with the study, as they do in ultrasound. The "physiologic" route of bile flow is demonstrated, including the presence or absence of bile leaks, fistulas, obstruction, etc. This is especially helpful in patients with blunt trauma and no access for a contrast injection. Zeman and others detected bile leaks in 7 of 21 patients (33%) who had sustained abdominal trauma. Perforation of the gallbladder and/or bile ducts may also be detected.

Unexpected findings

Although the main indication for cholecystography is the diagnosis of acute cholecystitis in patients with right upper quadrant pain, a great deal of additional information may be derived from the image. In one study, nonbiliary pathologic findings were incidentally detected in 42 of 294 patients (14.3%) with suspected acute cholecystitis.

The hepatobiliary image may be subdivided into four phases: (1) The vascular or blood-pool phase, (2) The parenchymal phase, (3) The renal phase, and (4) The intestinal phase. During the vascular phase (0 to 5 minutes), unsuspected vascular abnormalities such as aneurysms, arteriovenous malformations, and hypervascular tumors may be seen. Abnormal fluid collections including ascites and pleural and pericardial effusions appear as photon-deficient regions or halos surrounded by background blood-pool activity. The size and shape of abdominal organs (liver, spleen, kidneys) may be evaluated as a result of resident blood-pool activity even though the spleen and kidneys do not contain hepatocytes and do not actively concentrate the tracer. The size, shape, and position of the liver is best evaluated during the hepatocyte or parenchymal phase (5 to 20 minutes). In addition, space-occupying lesions (hepatoma, abscess [Fig. 20-24], metastasis, hematoma, hemangioma, focal nodular hyperplasia, etc.), which may be responsible for the patient's right upper quadrant pain, may be detected. The majority of these lesions will appear as photon-deficient areas because they do not

Continued.

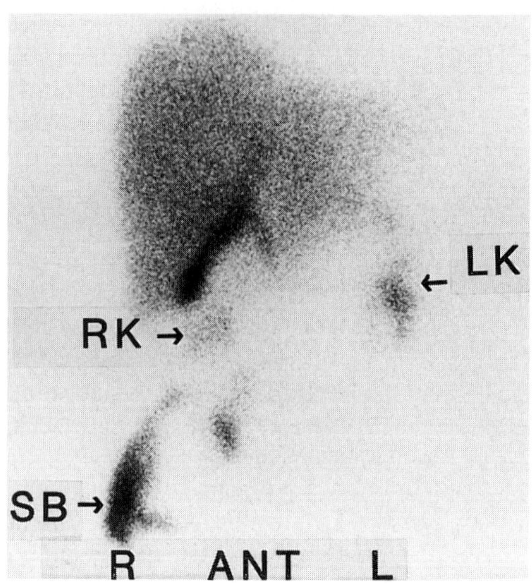

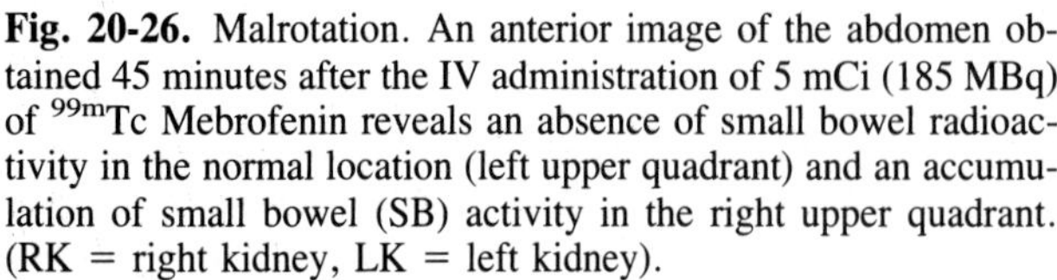
Fig. 20-26. Malrotation. An anterior image of the abdomen obtained 45 minutes after the IV administration of 5 mCi (185 MBq) of ^{99m}Tc Mebrofenin reveals an absence of small bowel radioactivity in the normal location (left upper quadrant) and an accumulation of small bowel (SB) activity in the right upper quadrant. (RK = right kidney, LK = left kidney).

contain functioning hepatocytes. However, the majority of hepatic adenomas are predominantly composed of hepatocytes and will therefore accumulate IDA agents and appear as warm or even hot areas. However, adenomas will appear as focal defects on liver/spleen images because of a relative deficiency of Kupffer cells. A minority of hepatomas may contain functioning hepatocytes and may accumulate IDA agents, but the majority are composed of abnormal hepatocytes and therefore will appear as photon-deficient lesions. Focal nodular hyperplasia will usually appear as a focal defect by cholescintigraphy because of a relative deficiency in hepatocytes but will appear warm or hot by liver/spleen imaging because of a predominance of Kupffer cells. Extrahepatic lesions may occasionally be identified indirectly by contour impressions. Situs inversus is readily identified. If a renal pathologic condition is suspected, an image in the posterior projection should be obtained during the renal phase (5 to 15 minutes) of the study. Renal number, size, shape, position, and function may be evaluated. Unsuspected renal masses or obstruction may occasionally be detected because about 10% of the IDA agents is excreted through the kidneys. During the intestinal phase (30 to 60 minutes), malrotation (Fig. 20-26), intraabdominal masses, and gastric reflux may be detected.

LABORATORY APPLICATION

56

MECKEL'S DIVERTICULUM IMAGING

Richard B. Noto, John Reilley, and Abass Alavi

In the embryo the fetal intestine joins the yolk sac by the primitive yolk duct. If the duct does not close completely, a Meckel's diverticulum may form. This abnormality is found in 2% of the population and is more common in males than in females.

Meckel's diverticulum may vary in length from 0.5 to 13 cm and lies proximal to the ileocecal valve. The diverticulum usually contains ileal mucosa but may contain gastric, duodenal, colonic, or pancreatic tissue. Approximately 50% of the Meckel's diverticula contain gastric mucosa. The most common symptom found in these patients is bleeding, as peptic ulceration may develop in the ileal mucosa adjacent to the Meckel's diverticulum because of the unbuffered secretion from the ectopic mucosa.

Purpose

The majority of Meckel's diverticula that become symptomatic are apparent at an early age, most by age 2. Gastrointestinal (GI) bleeding is the most common presentation, and the condition is difficult to diagnose radiographically with either barium studies or angiography.

The localization of ^{99m}Tc pertechnetate takes place only in those diverticula that contain ectopic gastric mucosa, but most symptomatic Meckel's diverticula, especially those that present with bleeding, do contain gastric mucosa.

Certain drugs may be useful in best demonstrating the ectopic gastric mucosa; these include pentagastrin (stimulates gastric uptake of pertechnetate), glucagon (decreases peristalsis and thereby increases persistence of activity in the ectopic mucosa) and cimetidine (may decrease release of pertechnetate from the ectopic mucosa into the bowel lumen).

Indications

1. Gastrointestinal (GI) bleeding in children and young adults.

Procedure

Materials

1. Large–field-of-view gamma camera with low-energy all-purpose parallel-hole collimator
2. Digital computer system for data storage and analysis
3. Technetium-99m pertechnetate, 15 mCi (555 MBq) for adults; 200 uCi (7.4 MBq)/kg with a minimum dosage of 2 mCi (74 MBq) for pediatric patients
4. Pentagastrin (6 μg/kg) and potassium perchlorate (6 mg/kg)

Patient preparation

1. Patient must be NPO for 4 hours before the study (infants should miss one feeding before the study).
2. Explain the entire procedure to the patient.

Technique

1. Administer pentagastrin (6 ug/kg) subcutaneously 20 minutes before radiopharmaceutical administration.
2. Have patient empty his or her bladder.
3. Set gamma camera for 2-second images for 60 seconds with energy setting of 140 keV with a 20% window for flow phase.
4. Set computer for 1-second acquisition per image for 60 seconds using a 64 × 64 matrix (byte mode) for flow phase.
5. Administer technetium-99m pertechnetate intravenously as a bolus and acquire flow images.
6. After flow phase, acquire dynamic images on computer at 15 seconds per frame for 29 minutes.
7. Simultaneously, acquire 500,000-count static anterior images of the abdomen (including xiphoid to pubis) every 5 minutes for 30 minutes.
8. After 30 minutes, a posterior view and right lateral view are obtained.
9. A repeat anterior view may be obtained after voiding, if necessary. Additional lateral or oblique views may also be necessary, depending on the findings.
10. Potassium perchlorate (6 mg/kg) should be given orally at the conclusion of the study to minimize thyroid uptake of pertechnetate.

Interpretation (Fig. 20-27)

Focal persistent uptake in the abdomen in a structure outside of the normally visualized organs is characteristic of a Meckel's diverticulum. Normal blood-pool activity is visualized on early images in the vessels, liver, spleen, and kidneys and persistent activity may be seen in the kidneys (especially if obstruction is present) and bladder. On images obtained after the blood-pool phase, there is progressively increasing normal gastric activity that becomes very prominent; if a Meckel's diverticulum is present, it should be visualized at the same time as the stomach activity. Abnormal uptake in a Meckel's diverticulum is most commonly seen in the right lower quadrant of the abdomen and is anterior to the retroperitoneal structures on the lateral view.

On the flow phase of the study, vascular abnormalities such as large arteriovenous malformations, vascular tumors, or hemangiomata may be noted; however, if an abnormality is noted on the flow images with rapidly decreasing activity thereafter, the diagnosis of a Meckel's diverticulum is highly unlikely.

Many different findings can lead to false positive results, but the frequency of false positive diagnoses is actually quite low (95% specificity in a review of 226 surgically proved cases by Sfaki-

Continued.

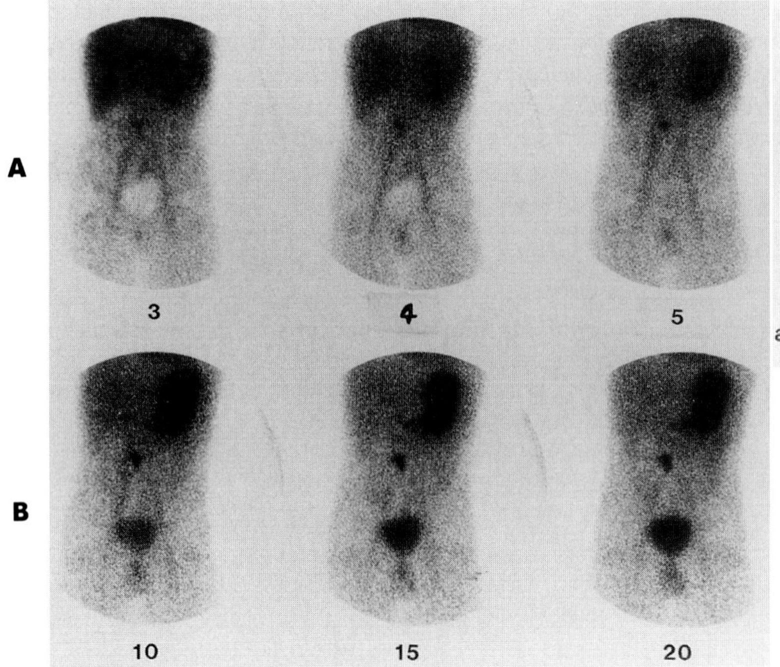

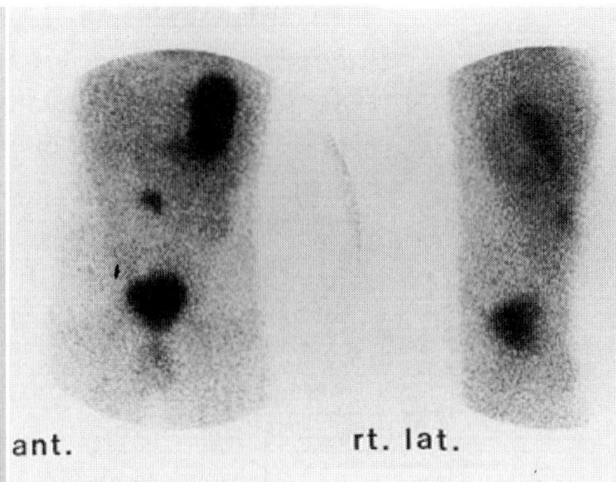

Fig. 20-27. Positive Meckel's diverticulum image. **A,** Images obtained during the first 20 minutes after injection reveal a small focus of increased activity in the midabdomen just to the right of the midline appearing between 3 and 5 minutes after ^{99m}Tc pertechnetate injection. The findings are consistent with a Meckel's diverticulum. Activity in the Meckel's diverticulum is first noted at about the same time that gastric activity appears. **B,** Anterior and right lateral images obtained at 30 minutes after injection reveal persistence of uptake in the Meckel's diverticulum. On the lateral view, the Meckel's diverticulum is seen to be located anteriorly. (Courtesy Dr. S. Heyman, Children's Hospital of Philadelphia.)

anakis and Conway). Causes of false positive results include intussusception, appendicitis, small-bowel obstruction, Crohn's disease, ulcers, vascular tumors, and AVMs.

In addition, various urinary tract abnormalities such as hydronephrosis, extrarenal pelvis, ectopic kidney, and bladder diverticula may cause false positive results, but the lateral view may be helpful in identifying the more posteriorly located urinary structures. Other abnormalities apart from Meckel's diverticula may occasionally contain ectopic gastric mucosa (including various cysts and duplications), and pertechnetate will also localize in these structures.

False negative images may be caused by pretreatment with oral perchlorate, since perchlorate will suppress uptake of pertechnetate by gastric mucosa; for this reason, perchlorate should be withheld until the completion of the study. Other false negative results may occur if gastric mucosa is not present in the Meckel's diverticulum; these cases will not be detected with pertechnetate, but bleeding from Meckel's diverticula that does not contain gastric mucosa is rare. Rapid bleeding may also cause a false negative result by washing away activity from the Meckel's diverticulum. Fortunately, these situations are unusual and the overall sensitivity is about 85%.

LABORATORY APPLICATION

57

GI TRACT BLEEDING IMAGING

Richard B. Noto, John Reilley, and Abass Alavi

Anatomy and physiology

The GI tract is lined with sensitive mucosa. GI secretions used to break down nutrients are caustic to the mucosa if for some reason there is not proper buffering of the secretions. Drugs, such as aspirin, may in some patients cause focal erosion of the gastric mucosa and secondary bleeding. Twenty-five percent of the patients with duodenal ulcers develop GI bleeding. Colonic diverticula, common in the older age groups, also may occur with GI bleeding. In the older age groups, angiodysplasias occur in the colon (primarily in the right colon), which also may cause profound GI bleeding. A problem that may interfere with proper localization of the bleeding site is that bleeding may be intermittent in nature regardless of the cause.

Purpose

Successful management of patients with acute gastrointestinal bleeding often depends on accurate localization of the bleeding site. In the upper GI tract, flexible endoscopy and selective arteriography provide accurate diagnoses in most cases. However, in suspected lower GI bleeding (jejunum, ileum, and colon), imaging techniques are the screening methods of choice because they are highly sensitive. Radionuclide studies may detect bleeding rates as low as 0.05 to 0.1 ml/min, while angiography will only demonstrate active bleeding at a rate of greater than 0.5 ml/min.

If the nuclear image is positive, angiography may be helpful subsequently to further characterize the bleeding site and occasionally for therapeutic reasons, such as intraarterial pitressin.

Technetium-99m sulfur colloid and technetium-99m-labeled red blood cells are each effective in demonstrating GI bleeding sites. ^{99m}Tc sulfur colloid is used primarily in "active" bleeds, while ^{99m}Tc-labeled red blood cells are best for suspected "intermittent" bleeds.

Indications

1. Suspected lower GI bleeding.

Procedure ^{99m}Tc-labeled red blood cells

Materials

1. Large–field-of-view gamma camera with low-energy, all-purpose parallel-hole collimator
2. Digital computer system for data collection and analysis
3. 20 mCi (740 MBq) ^{99m}Tc pertechnetate
4. Kit available for in vitro labeling of red cells

Patient preparation

1. No preparation is required.
2. Explain the entire procedure to the patient.

Procedure for RBC labeling

1. Draw 3 ml of whole blood into a heparinized syringe and add to 10-ml reaction vial containing stannous chloride provided with kit. Mix and allow to react for 5 minutes.
2. Add contents of the other two syringes provided with the kit to the reaction vial, mixing contents after adding each syringe.
3. Add 20 mCi (740 MBq) of ^{99m}Tc sodium pertechnetate and incubate for 20 minutes.
4. Set gamma camera setting to 140 keV with a 20% window.
5. Set computer for 1-minute acquisition per image for 60 minutes, using a 64 × 64 matrix.
6. Place patient in the supine position with the gamma camera above the patient for anterior imaging.
7. Position patient so that the lower border of the liver and spleen are at the top of the field of view.
8. Inject radiopharmaceutical and begin computer acquisition.
9. Obtain a 500,000-count image in the anterior projection and repeat every 5 minutes for 60 minutes.
10. If a focus of bleeding is located, the study is continued with images every 2 minutes until the direction of movement of the extravasated activity is localized.
11. Reposition the patient in either the left anterior oblique or the right anterior oblique position, depending on the area of localization of the bleed, and obtain a 1,000,000-count image.
12. If no focus of bleeding is located after steps 11 and 13, then obtain a 500,000-count anterior image at frequent intervals thereafter to include at least images at 2 and 24 hours after injection.
13. Repeat 500,000-count anterior images are obtained if the patient's clinical findings indicate active bleeding.

Procedure for ^{99m}Tc sulfur colloid

Materials

1. Large–field-of-view gamma camera with a low-energy, all-purpose parallel-hole collimator
2. Digital computer system for data storage and analysis (optional)

Continued.

3. 10 to 15 mCi (370 to 555 MBq) ^{99m}Tc sulfur colloid for adults; 200 uCi (7.4 MBq)/kg with a minimum dosage of 2 mCi (74 MBq) for pediatric patients.

Patient preparation

1. No preparation is required.
2. Explain the entire procedure to the patient.

Technique

1. Set gamma camera energy setting to 140 keV with a 20% window.
2. Set computer for 1-minute acquisition per image for 30 minutes using a 64 × 64 matrix.
3. Place patient in the supine position with the gamma camera above the patient for anterior imaging.
4. Position patient so that the lower abdomen is within the field of view.
5. Inject the radiopharmaceutical intravenously and begin the computer acquisition.
6. Obtain a 500,000-count image. Repeat every 2 minutes for a total of 5 to 10 images.
7. Reposition patient so that the field of view encompasses the lower border of the liver and spleen.
8. Obtain a 1,000,000-count image. Repeat every 2 minutes for a total of three images.
9. Reposition patient once more for a left anterior oblique projection to minimize hepatic activity in the field of view.
10. Obtain a 1,000,000-count image.
11. If a focus of bleeding is localized, continue the study with images every 2 minutes with the patient in the position in which the focus was identified to determine movement of activity. The study is completed at 30 minutes after injection or when the direction of the radiopharmaceutical movement is determined.
12. If no focus of bleeding is located after step 10, perform an anterior abdominal image and a left anterior oblique image for 500,000 counts at 30 minutes and for 1,000,000 counts at 45 minutes.
13. Repeat the above procedure if bleeding recurs any time later. Note: In all images acquired, bone-marrow activity should be clearly visualized for optimal results.

Interpretation (Figs. 20-28 to 20-30)

If the patient is actively bleeding at the time of the study, the bleeding site will be visualized as a focal area of abnormal accumulation of the radiopharmaceutical with either technetium sulfur colloid or technetium-labeled red blood cells. For the diagnosis of GI bleeding to be made, the extravasated activity should be seen to move in an antegrade or retrograde fashion in the bowel lumen. Potential false positive findings include accessory spleen (with technetium sulfur colloid), kidney and bladder activity (secondary to free pertechnetate with technetium-labeled red blood cells), and blood-pool activity in varices or other vascular abnormalities; however, all of these will not show movement in the bowel lumen on sequential images. Visualization of intraluminal transit of extravasated activity is also helpful in determining the exact location of the bleeding site by defining which segments of bowel are adjacent to the site of extravasation. Cinematic replay of the computer acquisition may be especially helpful in evaluating the intraluminal transit of activity and in identifying subtle bleeds.

Technetium-99m sulfur colloid is an ideal agent for demonstrating sites of active bleeding because of the rapid clearance of radioactivity from the background by the liver, spleen, and bone marrow; when there is extravasation secondary to bleeding, activity at the bleeding site increases exponentially while background activity decreases exponentially. Bleeding is best demonstrated in the first 12 to 15 minutes after injection with technetium-99m sulfur colloid; after that time most of the dosage has been cleared from the circulation.

Technetium-99m–labeled intravascular tracers, especially technetium-99m–labeled red blood cells, are also useful in detecting lower GI bleeding. The labeled red blood cell technique has the advantage of a longer potential imaging period during which bleeding may be visualized if intermittent. However, delayed images obtained several hours after technetium-99m labeled–red blood cell

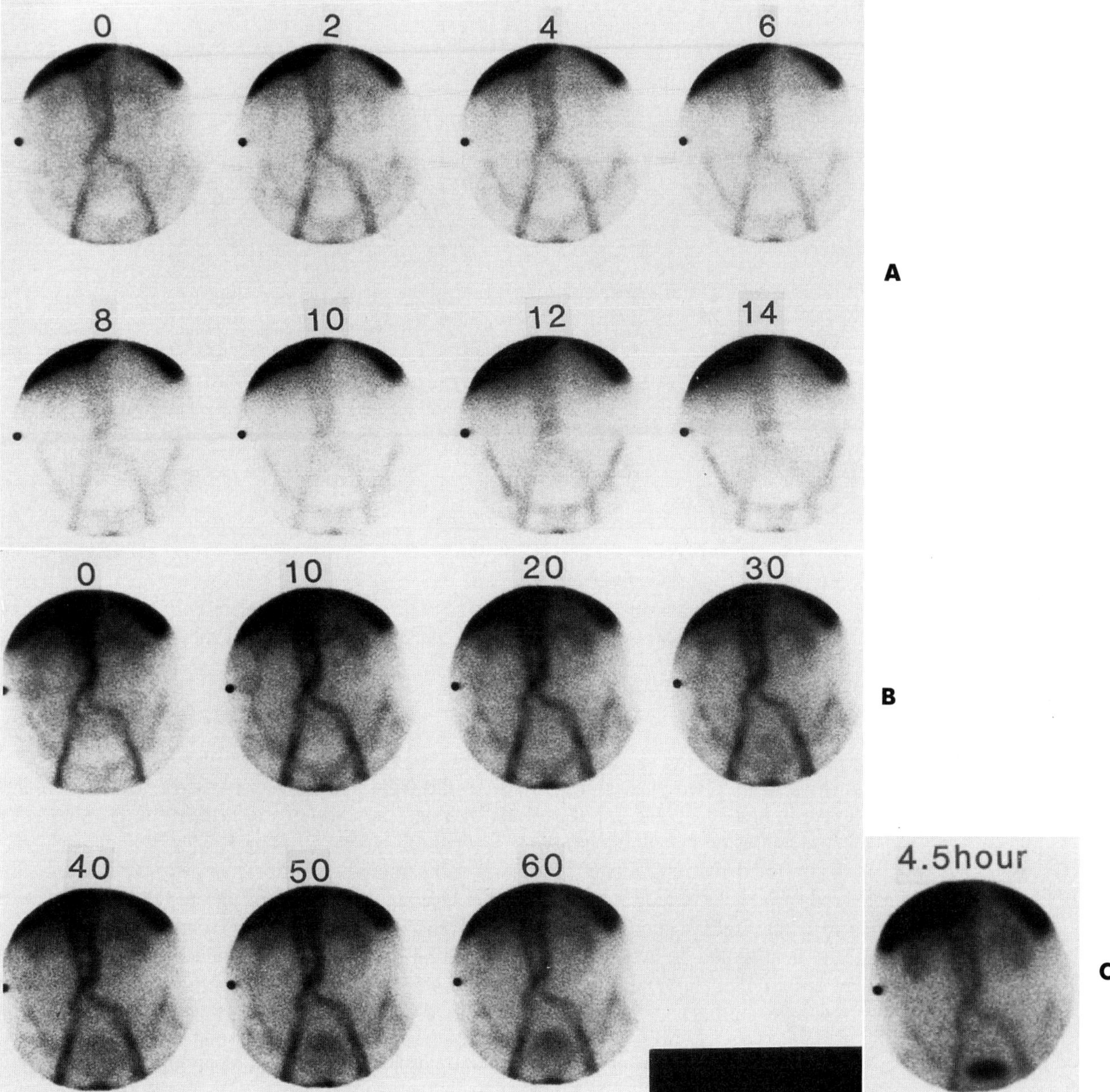

Fig. 20-28. Negative GI-bleeding images. ^{99m}Tc sulfur colloid performed first **(A),** followed immediately thereafter by ^{99m}Tc in vitro labeled red blood cells **(B** and **C). A,** Sequential images obtained every 2 minutes after ^{99m}Tc sulfur colloid injection show normal activity in the liver and spleen, as well as normal activity in the blood vessels on early images and in the bone marrow on later images. **B,** Sequential images obtained every 10 minutes after ^{99m}Tc-labeled red blood cell injection in the same patient show normal activity in the blood vessels. **C,** An image obtained 4½ hours after ^{99m}Tc-labeled RBC injection shows a normal distribution of activity. No focal collections of activity are noted outside of normal locations on either the ^{99m}Tc sulfur colloid or the ^{99m}Tc-labeled red blood cell study to suggest active GI bleeding.

Continued.

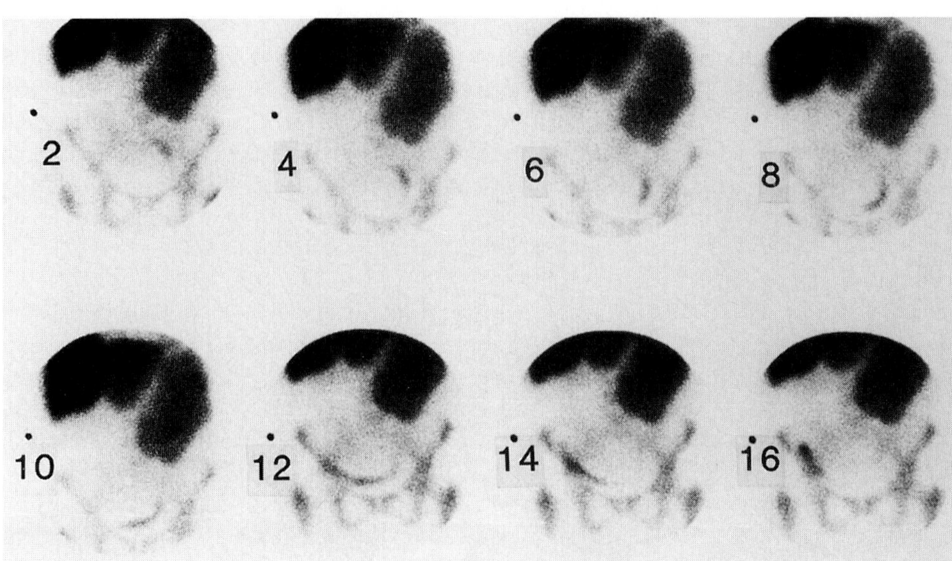

Fig. 20-29. Positive ^{99m}Tc sulfur colloid GI-bleeding image. A focal collection of increased activity is present, first appearing in the left lower quadrant of the abdomen almost immediately after injection. This collection is noted to move intraluminally into the right lower quadrant on sequential 2-minute images; the findings are consistent with a bleeding site in the small bowel. The spleen is massively enlarged in this patient with lymphoma.

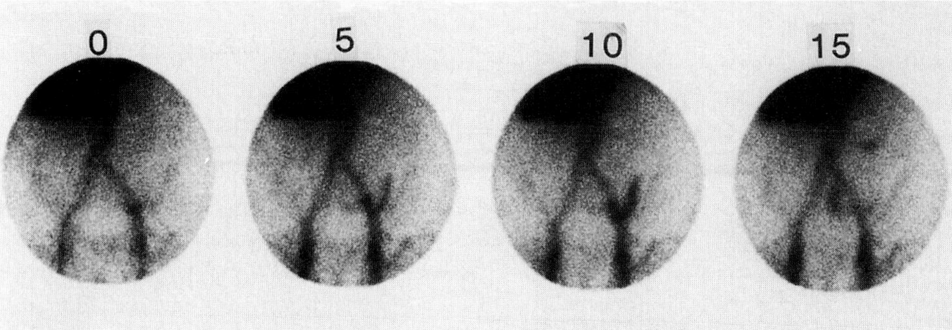

Fig. 20-30. Positive ^{99m}Tc-labeled red blood cell GI-bleeding image. A focal collection of increased activity is noted in the left lower quadrant (overlying the left iliac vessels) on the initial image, with subsequent intraluminal transit. The findings are consistent with an active bleeding site in the sigmoid colon.

administration are often misleading because of the rapid transit of extravasated blood in the intestinal lumen in both antegrade and retrograde fashions. In addition, free activity in the stomach may also cause confusion on technetium-99m–labeled red blood cell images.

A negative GI bleeding image with either technetium-99m sulfur colloid or technetium-99m labeled red blood cells is indicative of no active bleeding at the time of the study in the vast majority of cases. Other studies, such as angiography, are usually not useful if the radionuclide study is normal, and thus should be avoided until the bleeding has been scintigraphically detected (unless the patient is unstable). Preferably, the nuclear medicine study would be repeated at the first sign of recurrent bleeding if technetium-99m sulfur colloid is used. If the technetium-99m labeled red blood cell technique was performed, it is not possible to repeat the image in the first 36 to 48 hours. In addition, delayed images frequently do not help to localize the bleeding site because of the presence of activity diffusely in the bowel lumen.

LABORATORY APPLICATION

58

ESOPHAGEAL TRANSIT IMAGING

Richard B. Noto, John Reilley, and Abass Alavi

The esophagus is a muscular structure extending approximately 25 to 30 cm in length from the pharynx to the stomach with striated muscle present in the upper one third and smooth muscle in the lower two thirds. The process of swallowing is a complex series of responses that begins with the voluntary propulsion of a bolus of food into the pharynx by the tongue muscles. This is followed by a series of reflex-muscle contractions that propel the food from the pharynx into the esophagus. It is then carried by peristaltic waves through the extent of the esophagus. A ring of musculature called the lower esophageal sphincter is normally contracted; this relaxes in the process of swallowing to allow the bolus to pass into the stomach. Various abnormalities can affect esophageal motor function, including primary muscle disorders (e.g., myasthenia gravis), primary neurologic disorders (e.g., brainstem strokes), achalasia, collagen vascular diseases (e.g., scleroderma), and diffuse esophageal spasm. There may also be changes in esophageal motor function secondary to chronic gastroesophageal reflux. In addition, any cause of mechanical esophageal obstruction such as primary or secondary tumors or stricture will cause alteration in esophageal transit.

Purpose

Radionuclide esophageal transit studies attempt to noninvasively quantitate the motor function of the esophagus. Barium examinations of the esophagus are excellent for detecting mechanical obstruction, but they are often not adequate to detect and categorize motor abnormalities. Manometry can evaluate esophageal motor function, but it is relatively invasive and expensive and may be most appropriate for further evaluating disorders that have been detected scintigraphically.

It is possible to reliably identify abnormalities secondary to disorders such as achalasia, scleroderma, diffuse esophageal spasm, and some cases of reflux esophagitis with radionuclide studies. Nuclear images may also allow a quantitative assessment of response to therapy for esophageal motor dysfunction.

Indications

1. Dysphagia or suspected esophageal motor abnormality.

Procedure

Materials

1. Large–field-of-view gamma camera with low-energy, all-purpose collimator or standard field-of-view gamma camera with low-energy diverging collimator
2. Digital computer system for data storage and analysis
3. 300 uCi (11.1 MBq) ^{99m}Tc sulfur colloid in 25 ml of tap water

Patient preparation

1. Patient must be NPO from midnight prior to the study.
2. Explain entire procedure to the patient.

Technique

1. Set gamma camera at 140 keV with a 20% window.
2. Set up computer system to acquire images every second for the first 15 seconds, and every 15 seconds for the following 10 minutes with 64 × 64 matrix.
3. Place the patient in the supine position under the gamma camera, which is placed over the thorax.
4. Instruct the patient to turn his or her head to the side to receive the straw from the cup containing the radioactive mixture. Direct the patient to receive and hold the liquid in his or her mouth.
5. Instruct the patient to swallow the liquid as a bolus and start the computer acquisition at the same time.
6. Explain to the patient the need to dry swallow every 15 seconds on command.

NOTE:

1. Since 15 ml of fluid within the esophagus is required to generate secondary peristalic waves, it is necessary to start with a 25-ml volume in the cup because about 10 ml will remain in the cup after the patient drinks through the straw.
2. Explain the instructions and rehearse the study with the patient before starting procedure.
3. Use an audible timer to indicate when the patient is to swallow.

Continued.

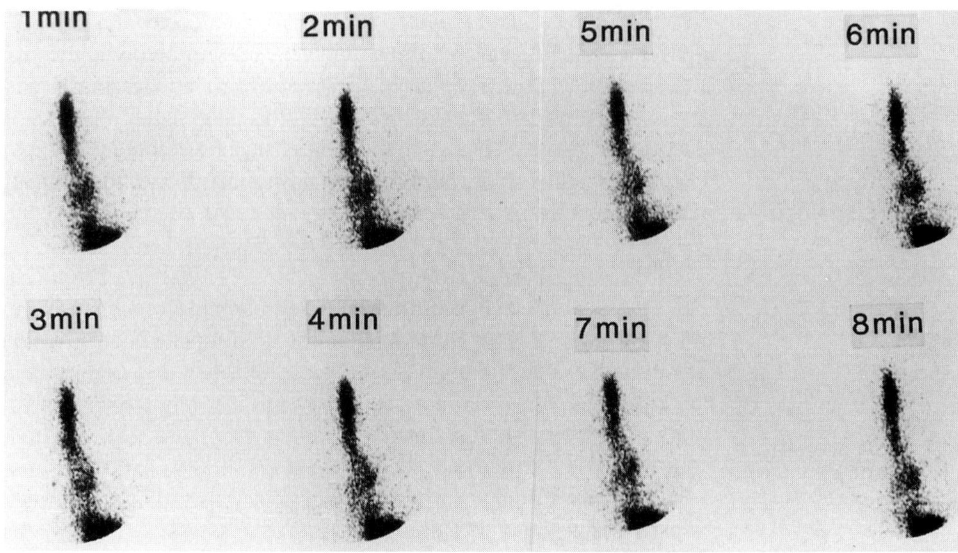

Fig. 20-31. Abnormal esophageal-transit study. Sequential 1-minute images obtained in a patient with scleroderma show significant retention of activity throughout the esophagus through 8 minutes after ingestion of ^{99m}Tc-sulfur-colloid–labeled water. There was 24% transit at 2 minutes, which is significantly decreased.

Interpretation (Fig. 20-31)

The percent esophageal transit at any time t can be measured by the following equation:

$$\% \text{ Esophageal transit} = \frac{(\text{Maximum esophageal activity} - \text{Esophageal activity at time t}) \times 100}{\text{Maximum esophageal activity}}$$

The esophageal activity is measured by drawing a region of interest around the esophagus on the digital computerized image.

In normal individuals, esophageal activity should no longer be visualized by 15 seconds after the first swallow. Calculations of percent transit should be greater than 90% by eight swallows (2 minutes) after ingestion.

Patients with achalasia or scleroderma have an adynamic pattern on the image with significantly decreased percent transit both on single swallow and after multiple swallows; these patients may occasionally be separated diagnostically by reevaluation in an erect position, where scleroderma patients may show some improvement in transit. Diffuse esophageal spasm and esophagitis that has resulted in manometrically demonstrable esophageal motor dysfunction will also result in decreased transit, although this is usually not as severe as in cases of achalasia or scleroderma. It is also possible to divide the esophagus into three regions of interest (proximal, middle, and distal thirds) and plot time/activity curves for each to trace the progress of activity through the esophagus. This may be helpful in further characterizing various abnormalities that have delayed transit or in localizing an abnormality to a particular area of the esophagus.

LABORATORY APPLICATION 59

GASTRIC EMPTYING IMAGING

Richard B. Noto, John Reilley, and Abass Alavi

Anatomy and physiology

The stomach is fixed just below the diaphragm and at the pylorus where it joins the duodenum. The lesser curvature of the stomach is adjacent to the liver.

The stomach's upper portion as it joins the esophagus, called the *cardia,* which dilates into the fundus of the stomach, merges with the body of the stomach, extends into the antrum, and terminates at the pylorus, which joins the duodenum.

The surface epithelium of the gastric mucosa is made up entirely of columnar epithelial cells and is pierced by numerous glands that secrete into the lumen of the stomach. The gastric glands are numerous from the fundus to the antrum of the stomach and are composed of mucous neck cells, parietal cells, and chief cells.

The stomach has four basic functions: secretion, reservoir, motility, and antibacterial barrier.

Gastric secretion

The gastric secretions are mucous fractions, proteolytic enzymes (pepsin and cathepsin), acid, intrinsic factor, water and electrolytes, and gastrin (a hormone).

Reservoir function

The normal stomach's capacity is between 1000 and 1500 ml. The stomach progressively dilutes a meal by secretion as it acidifies.

Gastric motility

The stomach's motor function is involved in grinding and kneading the food to prepare it for entrance into the small intestine. Gastric motility is affected by conditions in the duodenum. If the duodenum has an increased acid content in its lumen, it affects the stomach and slows down gastric emptying.

Antibacterial barrier

Although not well understood, after partial or total gastrectomy the small bowel, normally sterile, is filled with a variety of bacteria.

Gastric secretion and motility are depressed in patients with diabetes, and in advanced diabetes there may be paresis of the stomach. These patients may also have diminished gastric secretion with atrophic gastritis.

In some patients who have undergone vagotomy and partial gastrectomy with a subsequent gastrojejunostomy, there may be profound interference with gastric motility and a delay in gastric emptying times.

Other conditions that may lead to altered gastric emptying include peptic ulcer disease, anorexia nervosa, gastric tumors or inflammation, and a variety of medications.

Purpose

The radionuclide gastric emptying study provides a simple noninvasive means of quantitating gastric emptying. Various other techniques do exist for measuring gastric emptying, including barium studies and various intubation techniques, but radionuclide studies are currently the method of choice.

Multiple different meals, radionuclides, and imaging protocols have been used to scintigraphically quantitate gastric emptying. Solid gastric emptying studies have been determined to be superior to liquid alone in adults; however, dual radionuclide solid-liquid studies are also satisfactory. In infants, technetium-99m-sulfur-colloid–labeled milk is the agent of choice for determining both gastric emptying and gastroesophageal reflux during the same study.

The best possible solid meal in terms of binding stability remains chicken liver labeled with technetium-99m sulfur colloid in vivo. However, this procedure is logistically difficult. Technetium-99m-sulfur-colloid–labeled egg albumin is almost as stable and is the commonly used meal at this time. Meal size will cause significant variations in gastric emptying rate and should not be varied once a protocol has been established.

The technique of acquiring images in both the anterior and posterior projections and determining the geometric mean is considered the most accurate because it corrects for soft tissue attenuation and depth variation.

Indications

1. Determination of possible delayed gastric emptying and quantitation of gastric emptying rate in patients with suspected gastroparesis or other motility problems.
2. Evaluation of response to therapy in those patients who have proven delayed gastric emptying.

Materials

1. Large–field-of-view gamma camera with low-energy, all-purpose parallel-hole collimator.
2. Digital computer system for data storage and analysis.
3. 200 to 500 uCi (7.4 to 18.5 MBq) of ^{99m}Tc sulfur colloid bound to egg albumin, or radio-

Continued.

labeled, solid 300-calorie meal as follows:

Egg whites: 2	248 gm	128 calories
White bread	40 gm	110 calories
Butter (salted)	6 gm	60 calories
		Total: 298 calories
Deionized water	180 cc	

Patient preparation

1. The patient must be NPO from midnight prior to the study.
2. Explain the entire procedure to the patient.

Technique

1. Set gamma camera for 1-minute images with energy setting of 140 keV with a 20% window.
2. Set computer for 1-minute acquisition per image, using a 64 × 64 matrix.
3. Following the (overnight) fast, the patient ingests the radiolabeled meal.
4. With the patient in the erect position, obtain images of the stomach in both the anterior and posterior projections, each for 1 minute. Begin the first image as soon as the patient completes the meal. This is time 0.
5. Take anterior and posterior images for 2 hours, every 15 minutes from the time of meal completion.

Interpretation (Fig. 20-32)

The interpretation of gastric emptying studies is quite variable from institution to institution, depending on the technique used. Each institution should determine its own range of normal values because of variations secondary to meal type, meal size, imaging protocol, and department environment. In addition, a solid-liquid dual radionuclide protocol will yield different results from either solid or liquid alone, with the liquid component emptying before the solid.

With a 300-calorie solid meal of technetium-99m sulfur colloid egg albumin and bread and butter, the average value for solid gastric emptying in normal volunteers is 63% at 1 hour with a standard deviation of 11%. When it is necessary to use a liquid meal of technetium-99m-sulfur-colloid–labeled orange juice, the normal value is approximately 80% at 1 hour.

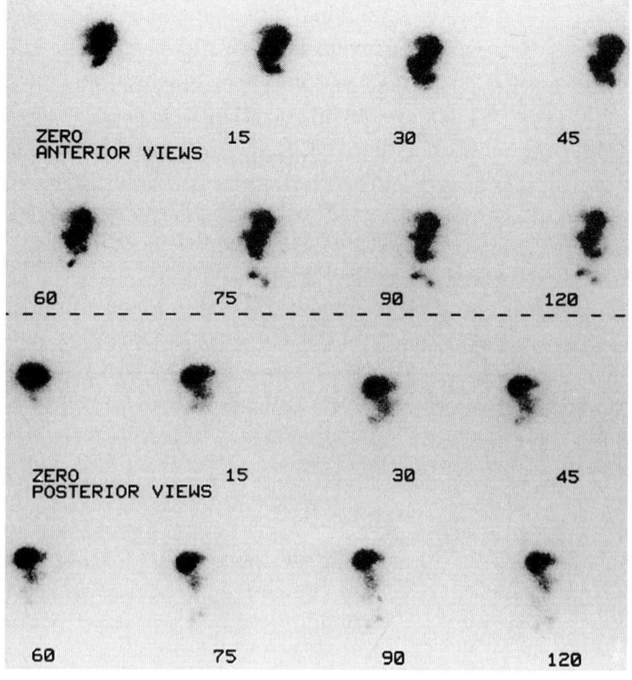

Fig. 20-32. Abnormal gastric-emptying study. Sequential 15-minute anterior and posterior images through 2 hours after ingestion of a ^{99m}Tc-sulfur-colloid–labeled solid meal show significantly delayed gastric emptying in this patient who is status-post–Billiroth II surgery. The 1-hour gastric emptying is 8% and the 2-hour gastric emptying is 14%; these are both significantly decreased.

The calculation of gastric emptying is performed with digital computer display of each image followed by region-of-interest calculation of the activity that remains in the stomach. The percent of gastric emptying at any time t is calculated by determining the geometric mean of the anterior and posterior views as follows:

$$\text{Geometric mean} = \sqrt{\text{Anterior view counts} \times \text{Posterior view counts}}$$

$$\%\ \text{Gastric emptying at time t} = \frac{(\text{Geometric mean at time 0} - \text{Geometric mean at time t}) \times 100}{\text{Decay correction factor} \times \text{Geometric mean at time 0}}$$

While calculating the percent of gastric emptying, make note of any unusual characteristics of the sequential images obtained; such incidental findings may include esophageal retention of activity or reflux, filling defects in the stomach, or anatomic variations secondary to previous surgery that may alter the interpretation.

Significant findings may be noted in the temporal pattern of gastric emptying. There is normally a slight delay or "lag period" before solids begin to empty rapidly from the stomach; no such "lag period" exists in normal patients with liquids. Certain patients may have an extended "lag period" but normal emptying thereafter; other patients will have delays in all phases of gastric emptying.

Delayed gastric emptying has various etiologies that include both mechanical obstruction and functional disorders. Partial mechanical obstruction may allow normal liquid emptying but will significantly delay solid gastric emptying. Common causes of delayed gastric emptying include neuropathic diseases, such as diabetes mellitus, and systemic illnesses, such as scleroderma.

Gastric emptying studies are useful in quantitating the effect of medical and surgical therapeutic interventions. The potential benefit that may be derived from a medication in a specific patient can be evaluated by obtaining radionuclide gastric emptying studies both before and after the start of therapy.

LABORATORY APPLICATION

60

GASTROESOPHAGEAL REFLUX IMAGING

Richard B. Noto, John Reilley, and Abass Alavi

Anatomy and physiology

The entire esophagus is lined with squamous epithelium, and its function is to transmit food from the mouth to the stomach. The lower end of the esophagus has a function of preventing reflux of acid from the stomach into the esophagus. In the normal patient the oblique angle of entry of the esophagus into the stomach, called the *angle of His,* is important because any increase in internal volume in the stomach inflates the stomach upward and to the right, thus compressing and closing the end of the esophagus and preventing reflux. The esophagus also has a sphincter muscle that straddles the diaphragm; this tends to prevent reflux.

Pathophysiology

Normal infants and young children may have reflux into the esophagus after a meal, since the gastroesophageal barrier is not fully established in a child. Hiatal hernias or herniation of the stomach above the diaphragm again is not unusual in children and is common after the age of 50. The reflux of gastric acid into the esophagus causes erosion of the squamous lining of the esophagus and subsequent inflammatory esophagitis.

Respiratory problems in children related to aspiration may also be caused by gastroesophageal reflux.

Purpose

Many different techniques are available to evaluate possible reflux esophagitis; these include barium studies, endoscopy with or without biopsy, and various tests involving infusion of acid through a nasogastric tube, including the acid perfusion test and the acid reflux test. The radionuclide technique for evaluating gastroesophageal reflux has the advantage of being simple, noninvasive, and accurate; it can also be easily quantitated. The quantitation of scintigraphic studies is especially helpful in evaluating the severity of reflux and the response to therapy.

Continued.

Pediatric reflux studies are often performed in combination with evaluation of esophageal transit and gastric emptying; all of these can be quantitated using a single dose. The most common reason to perform reflux studies in pediatric patients is to evaluate chronic respiratory problems such as recurrent pneumonias or asthma; aspiration of gastric contents has been implicated in these cases. Therefore, it is also helpful to image over the lungs intermittently for up to 24 hours to look for evidence of aspirated activity in the lung fields.

Indications

1. Symptoms of reflux esophagitis such as chest pain and regurgitation
2. Evidence of possible aspiration in children
3. Evaluation of response to medical or surgical therapy for reflux

Procedure for adults

Materials

1. Large–field-of-view gamma camera with low-energy, all-purpose collimator or standard field-of-view gamma camera with low-energy diverging collimator
2. Digital computer system for data storage and analysis
3. 300 uCi (11.1 MBq) of technetium-99m sulfur colloid
4. 150 ml of orange juice
5. 150 ml of 0.1 N hydrochloric acid
6. Abdominal binder and sphygmomanometer (available from Baum Co., Copiague, N.Y.; bladder cuff and bulb).

Patient preparation

1. The patient must be NPO from midnight before the study.
2. Explain the entire procedure to the patient.

Technique

1. Set up gamma camera at 140 keV with a 20% window.
2. Set up computer to acquire six 30-second static images, using a 64 × 64 matrix.
3. After an overnight fast, instruct the patient to drink 300 ml of acidified orange juice containing 150 ml of orange juice and 150 ml of 0.1 N hydrochloric acid, mixed with 300 uCi (11.1 MBq) of technetium-99m sulfur colloid.
4. Place abdominal binder on patient.
5. Obtain a 30-second gamma camera exposure with the patient in the upright position so that gastric activity is seen in the lower third of the gamma camera image.
6. Inflate the abdominal binder to 20 mm/Hg pressure and obtain another 30-second exposure.
7. Without deflating the binder, the process is continued at 20/mm Hg increments of the abdominal binder until 100 mm/Hg, at which time the sixth 30-second exposure is obtained and the binder is rapidly deflated.
8. The procedure is then repeated in the supine position.

NOTE—The abdominal binder should be placed below the rib margin to prevent rib fracture.

Procedure for pediatric patients

Materials

1. Large–field-of-view gamma camera with low-energy, high-sensitivity or all-purpose collimator
2. Digital computer system for data storage and analysis
3. Minimum of 150 uCi (5.55 MBq) and maximum of 1 mCi (37 MBq) technetium-99m sulfur colloid. The dosage should be added to the volume of milk or formula that the patient normally receives with a concentration of approximately 5 μCi (0.185 MBq)/ml.

Patient preparation

1. The procedure should be performed at the time of a usual feeding; the patient should not eat immediately before the study.
2. Explain the entire procedure to the parent or guardian.

Technique

1. Place the patient in a semirecumbent position with his or her back to the collimator at an angle of 45 degrees, with the mouth and stomach both in the field of view.
2. Place the radiolabeled milk in a lead-shielded bottle and allow the patient to begin drinking.
3. Set gamma camera for 2-second images for 120 seconds with energy setting at 140 keV with a 20% window (optional).
4. Set computer for 0.5-second acquisitions per image for 120 seconds using a 64 × 64 matrix in byte mode (optional).
5. Allow the patient to complete the feeding (with optional computer acquisition of swallowing phase as above), and then administer unlabeled milk or formula to wash activity from the mouth and esophagus.
6. Place the patient supine and position camera to obtain an anterior view with the mouth and stomach in the field of view.
7. Set gamma camera for 1-minute acquisitions for 60 minutes using a high-intensity setting.
8. Set computer for 3-second acquisition per image for 60 minutes using a 64 × 64 matrix, word mode.
9. After 1 hour, obtain 5-minute anterior and posterior images of the lungs to look for evidence of aspiration. If any abnormal foci are identified, these must be carefully checked to make sure they are in the lungs and not caused by contamination.
10. Obtain repeat static anterior and posterior images of the lungs at 2 hours (for 5 minutes each) and 24 hours (for 10 minutes each) to look for evidence of aspiration.

Interpretation

In adults, the gastroesophageal reflux index is calculated for various levels of increasing abdominal binder pressure. This index is calculated by drawing regions of interest around the esophagus,

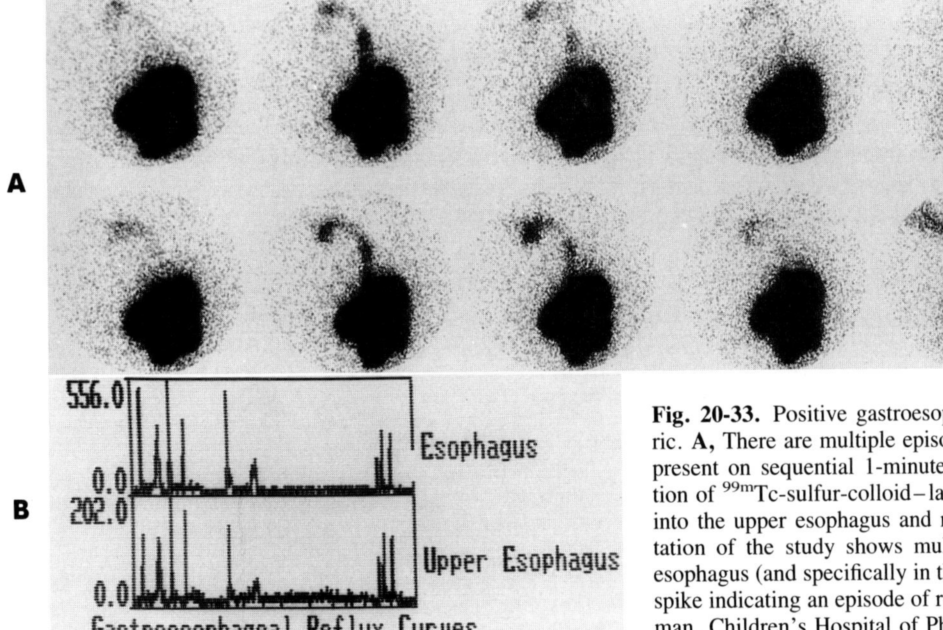

Fig. 20-33. Positive gastroesophageal reflux image—pediatric. **A,** There are multiple episodes of gastroesophageal reflux present on sequential 1-minute images following administration of ^{99m}Tc-sulfur-colloid–labeled milk. The reflux extends into the upper esophagus and mouth. **B,** A graphic representation of the study shows multiple spikes of activity in the esophagus (and specifically in the upper esophagus), with each spike indicating an episode of reflux. (Courtesy of Dr. S. Heyman, Children's Hospital of Philadelphia)

Continued.

esophageal background, and stomach on the digital computerized image and using the following formula:

$$\text{Reflux index at time t} = \frac{(\text{Esophageal counts at time t} - \text{Esophageal background counts}) \times 100}{\text{Maximal gastric counts}}$$

With external abdominal pressures of up to 100 mm Hg, the normal reflux index should be less than 4%. In one series of patients with documented gastroesophageal (GE) reflux, the average reflux index at 100 mm Hg was 11.8%, while normal controls had an average reflux index of 2.2% at the same pressure. If reflux is evident visually, this usually corresponds to a reflux index of 4% or more and the study is considered abnormal. The abdominal pressure generated by the binder is helpful in bringing out subtle cases of reflux; it is believed to generate a pressure gradient at the GE junction that is comparable to that developed when bending over or performing a Valsalva maneuver. Under certain circumstances, such as with young children or after recent abdominal surgery, one may wish to avoid using the abdominal binder; multiple sequential images obtained in the supine position may be analyzed for visual evidence of gastroesophageal reflux.

In pediatric patients (Fig. 20-33) the milk scan is probably the most satisfactory technique because it is a simple and physiologic means of evaluating gastroesophageal reflux. In young children a small amount of reflux may be normal; however, repeated episodes of reflux during the study, especially if the reflux extends into the upper esophagus, should be considered abnormal. Any evidence of activity in the lungs is highly specific for aspiration; however, the absence of detectable activity in the lungs does not rule out the possibility of aspiration.

LABORATORY APPLICATION 61

LEVEEN SHUNT PATENCY IMAGING

Richard B. Noto, John Reilley, and Abass Alavi

Anatomy and physiology

In patients with intractable ascites (often secondary to hepatic cirrhosis), surgical placement of a permanent peritoneovenous shunt, such as the LeVeen shunt, is often helpful in relieving excess ascites. The LeVeen shunt, introduced in 1974, consists of a collecting tube placed into the peritoneal cavity. It drains through a one-way valve into a venous tube placed through the jugular vein into the superior vena cava. The one-way valve opens when the intraperitoneal pressure exceeds the pressure in the superior vena cava, causing intermittent pumping of fluid through the shunt, especially with appropriate breathing exercises.

Pathophysiology

Reaccumulation of excess ascitic fluid after the placement of a LeVeen shunt may be caused by mechanical obstruction, either secondary to valve malfunction or to thrombosis of the venous tubing, or it can be secondary to other factors such as increased sodium consumption, inadequate diuretics, or worsening liver or heart failure.

Purpose

Radionuclide imaging of LeVeen shunt patency attempts to separate mechanical shunt failure (obstruction) from nonmechanical reasons for increasing ascitic fluid.

Indications

1. Increasing ascites, possible obstruction of LeVeen shunt

Procedure

Materials

1. Large–field-of-view gamma camera with a low-energy, all-purpose parallel-hole collimator; camera set at 140 keV with a 20% window
2. Digital computer system for data storage and analysis (optional)
3. 3 mCi (111 MBq) ^{99m}Tc MAA

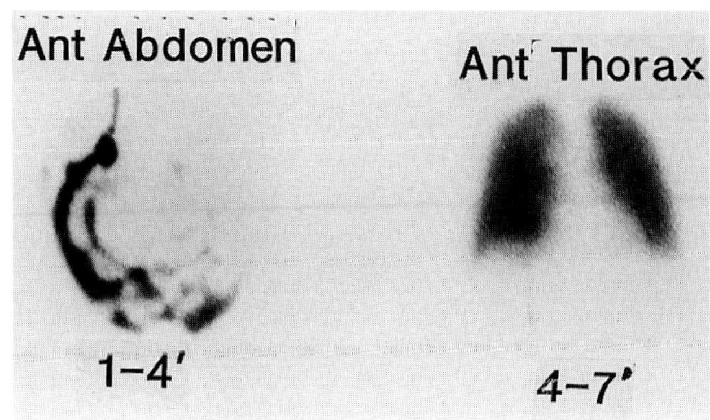

Fig. 20-34. Normal LeVeen shunt study. The 1- to 4-minute image reveals intraperitoneal activity with bowel loops outlined by the injected ^{99m}Tc MAA. The 4- to 7-minute image has the appearance of a normal lung image, indicating normal return of the ^{99m}Tc MAA from the LeVeen shunt into the venous system. The shunt tube can be seen in the right upper abdomen on both images.

Patient preparation

1. Explain the entire procedure to the patient.

Technique

1. Cleanse the patient's abdomen, using Betadine in a sterile manner.
2. The physician performs an intraperitoneal injection of the radiopharmaceutical with the patient in a supine position.
3. Obtain a 500,000-count image of the anterior abdomen immediately following the injection.
4. At 15 minutes, 30 minutes, 1 hour, and if needed, 2 and 4 hours postinjection, obtain images of the abdomen and anterior chest.
5. The procedure is complete when activity is visualized in the lungs.

Interpretation (Fig. 20-34)

If the technetium-99m MAA that is placed intraperitoneally is draining through the shunt into the venous system, activity will rapidly be visualized in the lungs (as with any other IV injection of technetium-99m MAA). Therefore, rapid visualization of lung activity indicates shunt patency, and absence of lung visualization indicates mechanical shunt obstruction. Occasionally, one may visualize the shunt tubing, but this is an unreliable sign dependent on shunt-flow rates. In some institutions, the procedure is performed with technetium-99m sulfur colloid instead of technetium-99m MAA using the liver as the target organ, but this may cause confusion in interpretation because of difficulty separating the liver from the ascites.

LABORATORY APPLICATION

62

BARRETT'S ESOPHAGUS IMAGING

Richard B. Noto, John Reilley, and Abass Alavi

Anatomy, physiology, and pathophysiology

Normally, the mucosa of the esophagus consists of stratified squamous epithelium; in cases of chronic reflux of gastric contents into the esophagus, the esophageal mucosa undergoes conversion to columnar epithelium, identical to that found in the stomach. This abnormality is termed *Barrett's esophagus*. The columnar epithelium is prone to peptic ulceration and stricture. In addition, patients with Barrett's esophagus have about a 2% to 10% risk of adenocarcinoma of the esophagus, which is extremely rare otherwise.

Purpose

Apart from radionuclide methods, the only reliable means of diagnosing Barrett's esophagus is endoscopic biopsy. Barium studies may show ulcers or strictures that suggest the diagnosis, but imaging of the thorax with pertechnetate is more specific and may make biopsy unnecessary in some cases. Technetium-99m pertechnetate is accumulated by the gastric mucosa in the diseased section of the esophagus. While parietal cells are present in only about half of patients with Barrett's esophagus, mucous-secreting cells are almost always present and these are felt to be the primary cell type that localizes pertechnetate.

Continued.

Indications

1. Findings on barium esophagram suggestive of Barrett's esophagus.
2. Chronic reflux esophagitis.

Procedure

Materials

1. Large–field-of-view gamma camera with low-energy, all-purpose parallel-hole collimator.
2. Digital computer system for data storage and analysis (optional).
3. 15 mCi (555 MBq) technetium-99m pertechnetate.
4. Potassium perchlorate (approximately 500 mg).

Patient preparation

1. Patient must be NPO for 4 hours before the study.
2. Explain the entire procedure to the patient.

Technique

1. Administer technetium-99m pertechnetate intravenously.
2. Position patient in erect position to minimize gastric reflux into the distal esophagus.
3. Acquire 500,000-count static anterior images of the chest, including the entire esophagus and the superior aspect of the stomach every 5 minutes for 60 minutes.
4. Administer potassium perchlorate (approximately 500 mg) at the conclusion of the study to minimize thyroid uptake of pertechnetate.

Interpretation

Accumulation of pertechnetate superior to the level of the gastroesophageal junction should create high suspicion of Barrett's esophagus. The uptake in the Barrett's esophagus should occur at about the same time that normal gastric activity is seen. False positive results can be caused by swallowed saliva or by reflux from the stomach; therefore, the patient is asked to minimize swallowing (oral suction may be used) and the examination is performed with the patient erect to minimize reflux.

LABORATORY APPLICATION

63

RETAINED ANTRUM IMAGING

Richard B. Noto, John Reilley, and Abass Alavi

Anatomy, physiology, and pathophysiology

In patients who have had Billroth II surgery for peptic ulcer disease, the gastric remnant is connected to the jejunum (the efferent loop) with an afferent loop of duodenum also extending from the anastomotic site.

In about 5% of cases, recurrent ulcers will develop near the anastomosis, almost always on the jejunal side. Some cases of recurrent ulceration are associated with a high circulating level of gastrin, which then causes increased acid secretion. The increased gastrin may be secondary to a gastrin-secreting tumor, as in Zollinger-Ellison syndrome, or may be secondary to retained gastric antrum at the end of the duodenal stump. If a cuff of gastric antrum is still present in the afferent loop, the retained antrum will constantly secrete gastrin because it will no longer be in contact with acidic gastric juices that normally serve as a feedback mechanism for stopping gastrin secretion. For this reason, retained gastric antrum will very frequently cause anastomotic ulcers.

Purpose

Retained antrum may be diagnosed by endoscopic biopsy of the duodenal stump, but this is an invasive and difficult procedure. Radionuclide studies with technetium pertechnetate are technically simple; they were shown in one large series to have a 73% sensitivity and 100% specificity for detecting retained antrum. When retained antrum is identified, it alerts the surgeon to the cause for the recurrent ulceration and the retained antrum can be surgically removed.

Indications

1. Recurrent ulceration after Billroth II surgery, especially if an increased serum gastrin level is demonstrated

Procedure

The procedure is identical to the procedure for Barrett's esophagus detection, except that static images of the mid-abdomen (instead of images of the chest) are obtained.

Interpretation

An area of focal increased uptake in the right upper quadrant adjacent to, but separate from, the stomach should be considered positive for retained antrum. Retained antrum should visualize at the same time as normal gastric mucosa. Antral cuffs as small as 1 cm may be demonstrated using this technique.

BIBLIOGRAPHY

General

Best & Taylor's physiologic basis of medical practice, ed. 12, Baltimore, 1991, The Williams & Wilkins Co.

Guyton, A.G.: Textbook of medical physiology, ed. 7, Philadelphia, 1986, W.B. Saunders Co.

Sleisenger, M.H., and Fordtranm, J.S.: Gastrointestinal disease. In Pathophysiology–diagnosis–management, ed. 2, Philadelphia, 1978, W.B. Saunders Co.

Spior, H.M.: Clinical gastroenterology, New York, 1970, Macmillan Publishing Co., Inc.

Thibodeau G.A., and Patton, K.T.: Anthony's textbook of anatomy and physiology, ed. 14, St. Louis, 1994, Mosby–Year Book.

Liver imaging

Alstead, E.M., and others: Is SPECT of the spleen worthwhile in the evaluation of liver disease severity?, Nucl. Med. Commun. 8(1):33, 1987.

Brendel, A.J., and others: Single photon emission computed tomography (SPECT), planar scintigraphy, and transmission computed tomography: a comparison of accuracy in diagnosing focal hepatic disease, Radiology 153(2):527, 1984.

Buell, U., and others: Single-photon emission computed tomography (SPECT) for assessment of hepatic lesions: its role in the diagnostic work-up, J. Nucl. Med. 24(8):746, 1983.

Brodsky, R.I., and others: Hepatic cavernous hemangioma: diagnosis with ^{99m}Tc-labeled red cells and single-photon emission CT, Am. J. Roentgenol 148(1)125, 1987.

Carrasquillo, J.A., and others: Single-photon emission computed tomography of the normal liver, Am. J. Radiol. 141(5):937, 1983.

Chhabria, P.B., and Chandnani, P.C.: "Hot" spot on radiocolloid scan of the liver, Clin. Nucl. Med. 1(7):258, 1976.

Clouse, M.E.: Roentgenographic techniques for the diagnosis and management of liver tumors, Semin. Oncol. 10(2):159, 1983.

Dhawan, V.M., and others: Pseudo-Budd-Chiari syndrome, Clin. Nucl. Med. 3(1):30, 1978.

Dendy, P.P., and Gemmell, H.G.: An evaluation of the contribution of single photon emission computed tomography (SPECT) to radionuclide imaging of the liver, Ann. Radiol. (Paris) 26(1):72, 1983.

Dodo, Y., and others: (Comparative study of scintigraphy, single photon emission CT, and computed tomography in the evaluation of space occupying lesions of the liver), Nippon Igaku Hoshasen Gakkai Zasshi 44(1):61, 1984.

Freeman, L.M., and Blaufox, M.D., editors: Gastrointestinal disease uptake. 1. Liver and biliary tract, Semin. Nucl. Med. 12(1):(entire issue), 1982.

Henke, C.E., and others: Vascular dynamics in liver scan "hot spot", Clin. Nucl. Med. 3(7):267, 1978.

Jacobsson, H., and others: Specific considerations in the interpretation of single-photon-emission computed tomography of the normal liver, Eur. J. Nucl. Med. 11(8):309, 1985.

Kavanagh, G.J., and others: Automated volume determination of the liver and spleen with Tc-99m colloid SPECT imaging. Quantification of the liver functional and nonfunctional tissue in disease, Clin. Nucl. Med. 15(7):495-500, 1990.

Kudo, M., and others: Small hepatocellular carcinomas in chronic liver disease: detection with SPECT, Radiology 159(3):697, 1986.

Lutzker, L.G.: Radionuclide imaging of the injured spleen and liver, Semin. Nucl. Med. 13(3):184, 1983.

MacCarty, R.L., and others: Hepatic imaging by computed tomography. A comparison with ^{99m}Tc-sulfur colloid, ultrasonography and angiography, Radiol. Clin. North Am. 17:137, 1979.

Manabe, T. and others: A comparative study of planar, SPECT, x-ray CT and angiographic imaging in detecting space-occupying lesions (SOL) of the liver, Rinsho Hoshasen 31(7):773, 1986.

Marmolya, G.A., and others: Focal fatty infiltration of the liver appearing as a defect on a liver-spleen scintigram. Case report, Clin. Nucl. Med. 17(4):300-302, 1992.

Matumoto, T., and others: SOL-detectability of liver SPECT—analysis of the structure of ROC-curve, Radioisotopes 34(9)486, 1985.

Matumoto, T., and others: SOL-detectability of liver SPECT—analysis by SOL detection model, Radioisotopes 34(8):414, 1985.

Oratz, M., Rothschild, M.A., and Schreiber, S.S.: Hepatic radionuclide planar imaging, Semin Liver Dis 9(1):7-15, 1989.

Parker, L.A., and Banning, B.: Focal nodular hyperplasia of the liver. Scintigraphic demonstration with technetium-99m sulfur colloid emission computed tomography, Clin. Nucl. Med. 10(8):601, 1985.

Patton, D.D.: Current status of liver scintigraphy for space-occupying disease. In Freeman, L.M., and Weissman, H.S., editors: Nuclear Medicine annual 1982, New York, 1982, Raven Press.

Pettigrew, R.I., and others: Single photon emission computed tomograms of the liver: normal vascular intrahepatic structures, Radiology 150(1): 219, 1984.

Shih, W.J., and Riley, C.: Examples of complementary roles of abdominal CT and radiocolloid liver imaging, Clin. Nucl. Med. 14(7):532-536, 1989.

Snow, J.H., and others: Comparison of scintigraphy, sonography and computed tomography in the evaluation of hepatic neoplasms, Am. J. Roentgenol. 132(6):915, 1979.

Sodee, D.B., and Ballistrea, M.: Diagnostic accuracy of nuclear medicine SPECT imaging, Nucl. Med. Biol. 14(3):191, 1987, Int. J. Radiation Appl. Instrum., Part B.

Strauss, L., and others: Single-photon emission computed tomography (SPECT) for assessment of hepatic lesions, J. Nucl. Med. 23(12):1059, 1982.

Triger, D.R., and others: Hepatic reticulo-endothelial function: a correlation of radioisotopic and immunohistochemical assessment, Liver 9(2):86-92, 1989.

Tumeh, S.S., and others: Cavernous hemangioma of the liver: detection with single-photon emission computed tomography, Radiology 164(2): 353, 1987.

Van Heertum, R.L., and others: Hepatic SPECT imaging in the detection and clinical assessment of hepatocellular disease, Clin. Nucl. Med. 17(12):948-953, 1992.

Weisgrau, R.A., and Guiberteau, M.J.: The diagnosis of acute complicated cholecystitis by Tc-99m sulfur colloid liver imaging, Clin. Nucl. Med. 15(4):240-242, 1990.

Ziessman, H.A., and others: Improved detection of small cavernous hemangiomas of the liver with high-resolution three-headed SPECT, J. Nucl. Med. 32(11):2086-2091, 1991.

Hepatobiliary

Aburano, T., and others: The role of Tc-99m IDA hepatobiliary and Tc-99m colloid hepatic imaging in primary biliary cirrhosis, Clin. Nucl. Med. 16(1):4-9, 1991.

Andersson, A., Bergdahl, L., and Boquist, L.: Acalculous cholecystitis, Am. J. Surg. 122:3-7, 1971.

Bennet, R.J., Stadalnik, R.C., and Mcgahan, J.P.: Perihepatic abscess detection on cholescintigraphy, Clin. Nucl. Med. 6:393-394, 1981.

Berk, R.N., Loeb, P.M., and Goldberger, L.E.: Oral cholecystography with iopanoic acid, N. Engl. J. Med. 290:204-210, 1974.

Bolt, R.J.: Cholecystitis and cholelithiasis, Curr. Ther. 26:321-324, 1974.

Brachman, M.B., Tanasescu, D.E., Ramanna, L., and Waxman, A.D.: Acute gangrenous cholecystitis: radionuclide diagnosis, Radiology 151:209-211, 1984.

Brown, P.H., Krishnamurthy, G.T., Bobba, V.V.R., and others: Radiation dose calculation for five Tc-99m-IDA hepatobiliary agents, J. Nucl. Med. 23:1025-1030, 1982.

Brown, P.H., Krishnamurthy, G.T., Bobba, V.V.R., and Kingston, E.: Radiation dose calculation for Tc-99m-HIDA in Health & Disease, J. Nucl. Med. 22:177-183, 1981.

Bushnell, D.L., Perlman, S.B., Wilson, M.A., and Polcyn, R.E.: The rim sign: association with acute cholecystitis, J. Nucl. Med. 27:353-356, 1986.

CHOLETEC product information (package insert). Squibb Diagnostics and Medi+physics.

Cramp, C.: The incidence of gallstones and gallbladder disease, Surg. Gynecol. Obstet. 53:447-452, 1931.

D'Alonzo, W.A., and Velchik, M.G.: Post cholecystectomy syndrome due to a cystic duct remnant diagnosed by hepatobiliary scintigraphy, Clin. Nucl. Med. 9:719, 1984.

Doo, E., and others: Quantification of hepatobiliary function as an integral part of imaging with technetium-99m-mebrofenin in health and disease, J. Nucl. Med. 32(1):48-57, 1991.

Drane, W.E., Nelp, W.B., and Rudd, T.G.: The need for routine delayed radionuclide hepatobiliary imaging in patients with intercurrent disease, Radiology 151:763-769, 1984.

Ferrucci, J.T., Jr., Adson, M.A., and Mueller, P.T.: Advances in the radiology of jaundice: a symposium and review, Am. J. Roentgenol. 141:1-20, 1983.

Fonseca, C., Rosenthall, L., and Greenberg, D.: Differential diagnosis of jaundice by Tc-99m-IDA hepatobiliary imaging, Clin. Nucl. Med. 4:135-142, 1979.

Fig, L.M., and others: Morphine-augmented hepatobiliary scintigraphy in the severely ill: caution is in order, Radiology 175(2):467-473, 1990.

Freeman, L.M., Sugarman, L.A., and Weissmann, H.S.: Role of cholecystokinetic agents in Tc-99m-IDA cholescintigraphy, Semin. Nucl. Med. 11:186-193, 1991.

Glenn, F.: Acute acalculous cholecystitis, Ann. Surg. 189:458-465, 1979.

Gliedman, M.L., and Wilk, P.J.: A surgeon's view of hepatobiliary scintigraphy, Semin. Nucl. Med. 12:2-4, 1982.

Harvey, E., Loberg, M., and Cooper, M.: Tc-HIDA: a new radiopharmaceutical for hepatobiliary imaging, J. Nucl. Med. 16:533, 1975.

Hawkins, R.A.: Radionuclide studies of the liver and hepatobiliary system, Curr. Opin. Radiol. 1(4):499-507, 1989.

Henderson, R.W., Telfer, N., and Halls, J.M.: Gastrobiliary fistula: pre and post operative assessment with Tc-99m-PIPIDA, Am. J. Roentgenol. 137:163-165, 1981.

Herry, J.Y., Brissot, P., and LeJeune, J.J.: Evaluation of a liver transplant by Tc-99m-Dimethyl-IDA Scintigraphy, J. Nucl. Med. 21:657-659, 1980.

Itoh, H., and others: Assessment of hepatic excretory function in chronic liver disease by hepatobiliary scintigraphy, Ann. Nucl. Med. 3(3):139-142, 1989.

Jarvinen, H.J., and Hastbacka, J.: Early cholecystectomy for acute cholecystitis: a prospective randomized study, Ann. Surg. 191:501-505, 1980.

Klingensmith, W.C., and Ashdown, B.C.: Cholescintigraphy in the diagnosis of intrahepatic cholestasis: how specific is it? Clin. Nucl. Med. 16(9):621-626, 1991.

Klingensmith, W.C., Fritzberg, A.R., Spitzer, V.M., Kuni, C.C., Williamson, M.R., and Gerhold, P.: Work in progress: clinical evaluation of Tc-99m-trimethylbromo-IDA and Tc-99m-disopropyl-IDA for hepatobiliary imaging, Radiology 146:181-184, Jan. 1983.

Kune, C.C., and others: Correlation of technetium-99m-DISIDA hepatobiliary studies with biopsies in liver transplant patients, J. Nucl. Med. 32(8):1545-1547, 1991. [Published erratum appears in J. Nucl. Med. 32(12):2214, 1991.

Leopold, G.R., Amberg, J., Gosnik, B.B., and Mittelstaedt, C.: Gray scale ultrasonic cholecystography: a comparison with conventional radiographic techniques, Radiology 121:445-448, 1976.

Loberg, M.D., Buddemeyer, E.V.: Application of pharmacokenetic modeling to the radiation dosimetry of hepatobiliary agents. In Third international radiopharmaceutical dosimetry symposium, FDA No. 81-8166, U.S. Department of Health and Human Services, Public Health Service, FDA, Bureau of Radiological Health, Rockville, Md., 1981, pp. 318-332.

Morrow, D.J., Thompson, J., Wilson, S.E.: Acute cholecystitis in the elderly, Arch. Surg. 113:1149-1152, 1978.

Mujahed, Z., Evans, J.A., and Whalen, J.P.: The non opacified gallbladder on oral cholecystography, Radiology 112:1-4, 1974.

Munster, A.M., and Brown, J.R.: Acalculous cholecystitis, Am. J. Surg. 113:730-734, 1967.

Noel, A.W., Velchik, M.G., and Alavi, A.: The "liver scan" appearance in cholescintigraphy, a sign of complete common bile duct obstruction, Clin. Nucl. Med. 10:264-268, 1985.

Ochsner, S.F.: Performance and reliability of cholecystography, South Med. J. 63:1268-1271, 1970.

Patch, G.G., and others: Naloxone reverses pattern of obstruction of the distal common bile duct induced by analgesic narcotics in hepatobiliary imaging, J. Nucl. Med. 32(6):1270-1272, 1991.

Pauwels, S., Piret, L., and Schoutens, A.: Tc-99m-diethyl-IDA Imaging: clinical evaluation in jaundiced patients, J. Nucl. Med. 21:1022-1028, 1980.

Rienzo, R.J., Tyler, G., and Morel, D.E.: Sonographic and scintigraphic detection of a bile leak in a post cholecystectomy patient, Clin. Nucl. Med. 8:480-482, 1983.

Rosenthall, L.: Cholescintigraphy in the presence of jaundice utilizing Tc-IDA, Semin. Nucl. Med. 12:53-63, 1982.

Samuels, B.I., Freitas, J.E., and Bree, R.L.: A comparison of radionuclide hepatobiliary imaging and real time ultrasound for the detection of acute cholecystitis, Radiology 147:207-210, 1983.

Scharschmidt, B.F., Goldberg, H.I., and Schmid, R.: Medical intelligence: current concepts in diagnosis, approach to the patient with cholestatic jaundice, N. Engl. J. Med. 308:1515-1519, 1983.

Schein, C.J.: Acute cholecystitis, New York, 1972, Harper & Row.

Scott-Smith, W., Raftery, A.T., Wraight, E.P., and Calne, R.Y.: Tc-

99m-labeled HIDA imaging in suspected biliary leaks after liver transplantation, Clin. Nucl. Med. 8:478-479, 1983.

Smith, R., Rosen, J.M., Gallo, L.N., and Anderson, P.O.: Pericholecystic hepatic activity in cholescintigraphy, Radiology 156:797-800, 1985.

Stadalnik, R.C., Matolo, N.M.: Radionuclide imaging of the biliary tree, Surg. Clin. North Am. 61:827-841, 1981.

Swayne, L.C., and Ginsberg, H.N.: Diagnosis of acute cholecystitis by cholescintigraphy: significance of pericholecystic hepatic uptake, Am. J. Roentgenol. 152(6):1211-1213, 1989.

Szlabick, R.E., Catto, J.A., Fink-Bennett, D., and Ventura, V.: Hepatobiliary scanning in the diagnosis of acute cholecystitis, Arch. Surg. 115:540-544, 1980.

Van Der Linden, W., and Sunzel, H.: Early verses delayed operation for acute cholecystitis, Am. J. Surg. 120:7-13, 1970.

Velchik, M.G., Makler, P.T., and Alavi, A.: Gallbladder carcinoma: another cause of the photon deficient gallbladder in cholescintigraphy, Clin. Nucl. Med. 9:137-138, 1984.

Weissmann, H.S., Chun, K.J., Frank, M.: Demonstration of Traumatic Bile Leakage with Cholescintigraphy and Ultrasonography. Radiology 133:843-847, 1979.

Weissmann, H.S., Rosenblatt, R.R., and Sugarman, L.A.: Early diagnosis of acute common bile duct obstruction by Tc-99m-IDA cholescintigraphy, J. Nucl. Med. 21:41, 1980 (abstract).

Weissmann, H.S., Frank, M.S., Berstein, L.H., and Freeman, L.M.: Rapid and accurate diagnosis of acute cholecystitis with Tc-99m-HIDA cholescintigraphy, Am. J. Roentgenol. 132:523-528, 1979.

Weissmann, H.S., Sugarman, L.A., Frank, M.S., and Freeman, L.M.: Serendipity in technetium-99m-dimethyl iminodiacetic acid cholescintigraphy, Radiology 135:449-454, 1980.

Weissmann, H.S., Badia, J., and Sugarman, L.A.: Spectrum of Tc-99m-IDA cholescintigraphic patterns in acute cholecystitis, Radiology 138:167-175, 1981.

Weissmann, H.S., Berkowitz, D., Fox, M.S.: The role of technetium 99m iminodiacetic acid (IDA) cholescintigraphy in acute acalculous cholecystitis, Radiology 146:177-180, 1983.

Worthen, N.J., Uszler, J.M., and Funamura, J.L.: Cholecystitis: prospective evaluation of sonography and Tc-99m-cholescintigraphy, Am. J. Roentgenol. 137:973-978, 1981.

Zeman, R.K., Burrell, M.I., and Cahow, C.E.: Diagnostic utility of cholescintigraphy and ultrasonography in acute cholecystitis, Am. J. Surg. 141:446, 1981.

Zeman, R.K., Lee, C.H., Stahl, R.: Strategy for the use of biliary scintigraphy in non-iatrogenic biliary trauma, Radiology 151:771-777, 1984.

Zeman, R.K., Segal, H.B., Caride, V.J.: Tc-99m-HIDA cholescintigraphy: the distended photon deficient gallbladder, J. Nucl. Med. 22:39-41, 1981.

Meckel's diverticulum imaging

Berquist, T.H., Nolan, N.G., Stephens, D.H., and Carlson, H.C.: Specificity of Tc-99m-pertechnetate in scintigraphic diagnosis of Meckel's diverticulum: review of 100 Cases, J. Nucl. Med. 17:465-469, 1976.

Diamond, R.H., Rothstein, R.D., and Alavi, A.: The role of cimetidine-enhanced technetium-99m-pertechnetate imaging for visualizing Meckel's diverticulum, J. Nucl. Med. 32:1422-1424, 1991.

Dixon, P.M., Nolan, D.J.: The diagnosis of Meckel's diverticulum: a continuing challenge, Clin. Radiol. 38:615-619, 1987.

Jewett, T.C., Duszynski, D.O., and Allen, J.E.: The visualization of Meckel's diverticulum with 99m-Tc-pertechnetate, Surgery 68:567-570, 1970.

Sfakianakis, G.N., and Conway, J.J.: Detection of ectopic gastric mucosa in Meckel's diverticulum and in other aberrations by scintigraphy: I—Pathophysiology and 10-year clinical experience. J. Nucl. Med. 22:647-654, 1981.

Sfakianakis, G.N., Conway, J.J.: Detection of ectopic gastric mucosa in Meckel's diverticulum and in other aberrations by scintigraphy: II. Indications and methods—A 10-year experience, J. Nucl. Med. 22:732-738, 1981.

GI bleeding imaging

Alavi, A., Dann, R.W., Baum, S., and Biery, D.N.: Scintigraphic detection of acute gastrointestinal bleeding, Radiology 124:753-756, 1977.

Alavi, A.: Detection of gastrointestinal bleeding with 99m-Tc sulfur colloid, Semin. Nucl. Med. 12:126-138, 1982.

Alavi, A., and Ring, E.J.: Localization of gastrointestinal bleeding: superiority of 99m-Tc sulfur colloid compared with angiography, Am. J. Roentgenol. 137:741-748, 1981.

Bunker, S.R., Brown, J.M., McAuley, R.J., and others: Detection of gastrointestinal bleeding sites: use of in vitro technetium Tc-99m-labeled RBC's, JAMA 247:789-792, 1982.

Maurer, A.H., Rodman, M.S., Vitti, R.A., and others: Gastrointestinal bleeding: improved localization with cine scintigraphy, Radiology 185:187-192, 1992.

Smith, R., Copely, D.J., and Bolen, F.H.: 99m-Tc RBC scintigraphy: correlation of gastrointestinal bleeding rates with scintigraphic findings, Am. J. Roentgenol. 148:869-874, 1987.

Thorne, D.A., Datz, F.L., Remley, K., and Christian, P.E.: Bleeding rates necessary for detecting acute gastrointestinal bleeding with technetium-99m-labeled red blood cells in an experimental model, J. Nucl. Med. 28:514-520, 1987.

Winn, M., Weissmann, H.S., Sprayregen, S., and Freeman, L.M.: The radionuclide detection of lower gastrointestinal bleeding sites, Clin. Nucl. Med. 8:389-395, 1983.

Winzelberg, G.G., McKusick, K.A., Froelich, J.W., and others: Detection of gastrointestinal bleeding with 99m-Tc-labeled red blood cells, Semin. Nucl. Med. 12:139-146, 1982.

Winzelberg, G.G., McKusick, K.A., Strauss, H.W., and others: Evaluation of gastrointestinal bleeding by red blood cells labeled in vivo with technetium-99m, J. Nucl. Med. 20:1080-1086, 1979.

Esophageal transit imaging

Holloway, R.H., Lange, R.C., Plankey, M.W., McCallum, R.W.: Detection of esophageal motor disorders by radionuclide transit studies: a reappraisal, Dig. Dis. Sci. 34:905-912, 1989.

Kazem, I.: A new scintigraphic technique for the study of the esophagus, Am. J. Roentgenol. Rad. Ther. Nucl. Med. 115:681-688, 1972.

Lichtenstein, G.R., and Alavi, A.: Esophageal scintigraphy in achalasia and achalasia-like disorders, J. Nucl. Med. 33:590-594, 1992.

Reilley, J.J., Malmud, L.S., Fisher, R.S., and others: Dynamic esophageal scintigraphy, J. Nucl. Med. Technol. 10:71-74, 1982.

Russell, C.O., Hill, L.D., Holmes, E.R., and others: Radionuclide transit: a sensitive screening test for esophageal dysfunction, Gastroenterology 80:887-892, 1981.

Taillefer, R., Jadliwalla, M., Pellerin, E., and others: Radionuclide esophageal transit study in detection of esophageal motor dysfunction: comparison with motility studies (manometry), J. Nucl. Med. 31:1921-1926, 1990.

Tolin, R.D., Malmud, L.S., Reilley, J., and Fisher, R.S.: Esophageal scintigraphy to quantitate esophageal transit (quantitation of esophageal transit), Gastroenterology 76:1402-1408, 1979.

Gastric emptying imaging

Christian, P.E., Datz, F.L., Sorenson, J.A., and Taylor, A.: Technical factors in gastric emptying studies, J. Nucl. Med. 24:264-268, 1983.

Christian, P.E., Moore, J.G., Sorenson, J.A., and others: Effects of meal size and correction technique on gastric emptying time: studies with two tracers and opposed detectors, J. Nucl. Med. 21:883-885, 1980.

Datz, F.L., Christian, P.E., Hutson, W.R., and others: Physiological and pharmacological interventions in radionuclide imaging of the tubular gastrointestinal tract, Semin. Nucl. Med. 16:140-152, 1991.

Griffith, G.H., Owen, G.M., Kirkman, S., and Shields, R.: Measurement of rate of gastric emptying using chromium-51, Lancet 1:1244-1245, 1966.

Heading, R.C., Tothill, P., McLoughlin, G.P., and Shearman, D.J.: Gastric emptying rate measurement in man: a dual isotope scanning technique for simultaneous study of liquid and solid components of a meal, Gastroenterology 71:45-50, 1976.

Knight, L.C., and Malmud, L.S.: Tc-99m ovalbumin labeled eggs: comparison with other solid food markers in vitro, J. Nucl. Med. 22:P28, 1981.

Kroop, H.S., Long, W.B., Alavi, A., and Hansell, J.R.: Effect of water and fat on gastric emptying of solid meals, Gastroenterology 77:997-1000, 1979.

Meyer, J.H., MacGregor, I.L., Gueller, R., and others: Tc-99m tagged chicken liver as a marker of solid food in the human stomach, Am. J. Dig. Dis. 21:296-304, 1976.

Velchik M.G., Reynolds J.C., and Alavi A.: The effect of meal energy content on gastric emptying, J. Nucl. Med. 30:1106-1110, 1989.

Gastroesophageal reflux imaging

Fisher, R.S., Malmud, L.S., Roberts, G.S., and Lobis, I.F.: Gastroesophageal (GE) scintiscanning to detect and quantitate GE reflux, Gastroenterology 70:301-308, 1976.

Heyman, S., Kirkpatrick, J.A., Winter, H.S., and Treves, S.: An improved radionuclide method for the diagnosis of gastroesophageal reflux and aspiration in children (milk scan), Radiology 131:479-482, 1979.

Malmud, L.S., Fisher, R.S.: Scintigraphic detection of gastroesophageal reflux. In Alavi, A., and Arger, P.H. (eds): Multiple Imaging Procedures: Abdomen, pp. 97-119, New York, 1980, Grune & Stratton.

Malmud, L.S., and Fisher, R.S.: The evaluation of gastroesophageal reflux before and after medical therapies, Semin. Nucl. Med. 11:205-215, 1981.

Rudd, T.G., and Christie, D.L.: Demonstration of gastroesophageal reflux in children by radionuclide gastroesophagography, Radiology 131:483-486, 1979.

LeVeen shunt patency imaging

Algeo, J.H., Powell, M., and Couacaud, J.: LeVeen shunt visualization without function using technetium-99m macroaggregated albumin, Clin. Nucl. Med. 12:741-743, 1987.

Kirchmer, N., and Hart, U.: Radionuclide assessment of LeVeen shunt patency, Ann. Surg. 185:145-146, 1977.

LeVeen, H.H., Christoudias, G., Ip, M., and others: Peritoneo-venous shunting for ascites, Ann. Surg. 180:580-591, 1974.

Rosenthall, L., Arzoumanian, A., Hampson, L.G., and Shennib, H.: Observations on the radionuclide assessment of peritoneovenous shunt patency, Clin. Nucl. Med. 9:227-235, 1984.

Singh, A., Grossman, Z.D., McAfee, J.G., and Thomas, F.D.: LeVeen shunt patency studies: clarification of scintigraphic findings, Clin. Nucl. Med. 5:106-108, 1980.

Barrett's esophagus imaging

Barrett, N.R.: Chronic peptic ulcer of the oesophagus and 'oesophagitis', Br. J. Surg. 38:175-182, 1950.

Berquist, T.H., Nolan, N.G., Carlson, H.C., and Stephens, D.H.: Diagnosis of Barrett's esophagus by pertechnetate scintigraphy, Mayo Clin. Proc. 48:276-279, 1973.

Gordon, F., Ramirez-Degollado, J., Munoz, R., and others: Diagnosis of Barrett's esophagus with radioisotopes, Am. J. Roentgenol. Rad. Ther. Nucl. Med. 121:716-719, 1974.

Kweka, E.L., O'Neill, M., Cooney, C., and O'Sullivan, G.: Imaging Barrett's oesophagus, Clin. Radiol. 38:415-418, 1987.

Retained antrum imaging

Lee, C., P'eng, F., and Yeh, P.H.: Sodium pertechnetate Tc-99m antral scan in the diagnosis of retained gastric antrum, Arch. Surg. 119:309-311, 1984.

Safaie-Shirazi, S., Chaudhuri, T.K., and Condon, R.E.: Visualization of isolated retained antrum by using technetium-99m, Surgery 73:278-283, 1973.

Sciarretta, G., Malaguti, P., Turba, E., and others: Retained gastric antrum syndrome diagnosed by 99m-Tc pertechnetate scintiphotography in man: hormonal and radioisotopic study of two cases, J. Nucl. Med. 19:377-380, 1978.

Chapter 21

THE SPLEEN

RICHARD P. SPENCER

■ ANATOMY (Fig. 21-1)

The spleen (Fig. 21-1), located in the posterior portion of the left upper abdomen, is usually seated below the left leaf of the diaphragm and beneath the left ninth, tenth, and eleventh ribs (and thus can be damaged by a fractured rib). The spleen is above and lateral to the left kidney; sometimes the organs are in such close proximity that their blood-pool images nearly merge. These anatomic relationships can be defined by means of a posterior image obtained with an intravascular agent such as ^{99m}Tc red blood cells (Fig. 21-2). The weight of the adult spleen falls from about 200 grams to 150 grams between the ages of 25 and 40 and then remains stable until about age 65 when a further decrease in size can be noted (this can be correlated with the overall loss of body weight).

The adult spleen is about 10 cm × 6 cm in size and 4 cm thick. It has a distinct curved appearance, very much like a baseball catcher's mitt. Unlike the liver, the spleen, which has no firm ligamentous attachments, can be more readily displaced (ptosis); it is also subject to twisting with embarrassment of the vascular supply (torsion). The spleen is surrounded by a fibrous capsule that does not contain muscle. The capsule extends into the spleen and forms distinct trabeculae, which subdivide the organ. Vessels, nerves, and lymphatics travel along the trabeculae. Major vessels enter and leave the spleen at a fissure that is usually located toward the medial side of the body; this part of the organ is referred to as the *hilum* of the spleen. The splenic mobility may rotate this upward, producing the "upside down" spleen.

Major blood supply to the spleen is via the splenic artery, a branch of the celiac axis that arises from the aorta. Frequently, small vessels enter the spleen from mesenteric and other abdominal arteries; thus splenic artery obstruction by clot, or following vessel ligation, does not necessarily mean that the entire organ will lose viability. Vascular drainage of the spleen is through the splenic vein, which is a contributor to the portal vein (the portal vein is actually often defined as beginning at the point at which the splenic and mesenteric veins join). Therefore, liver disease or portal vein obstruction can result in splenic disorders.

A cross section of the spleen reveals distinct white and red areas, referred to as the *white pulp* and the *red pulp*. The white pulp is composed largely of lymphocytes that have a role in the immune process. Subdivisions of the splenic artery can be surrounded by T lymphocytes (thymus-dependent), while follicles are largely composed of B lymphocytes. From the white pulp, small arteries enter red pulp cords and sinusoids. It is this region that acts as a sieve or filtration system for removing foreign particles as well as intraerythrocytic inclusions. Blood then passes outward to the splenic vein and the portal system.

The spleen thus can be understood as a vascular organ with filtration and immune functions, which is largely composed of reticuloendothelial (phagocytic) cells as well as lymphocytes.

■ PHYSIOLOGY

Multiple functions of the spleen can be divided into several categories:

A. Phagocytic ability of splenic cells.
    1. Small particulates: radiocolloids such as ^{99m}Tc colloid or ^{99m}Tc albumin colloid.
    2. Large formed blood elements: red blood cells tagged with ^{99m}Tc or with ^{51}Cr sodium chromate, and denatured.

B. Spleen as a site for sequestering formed blood elements: labeled but not denatured platelets, white blood cells, and red blood cells. Calculation of spleen/liver ratio.

C. Splenic blood pool: intravascular labels such as ^{99m}Tc-labeled red blood cells.

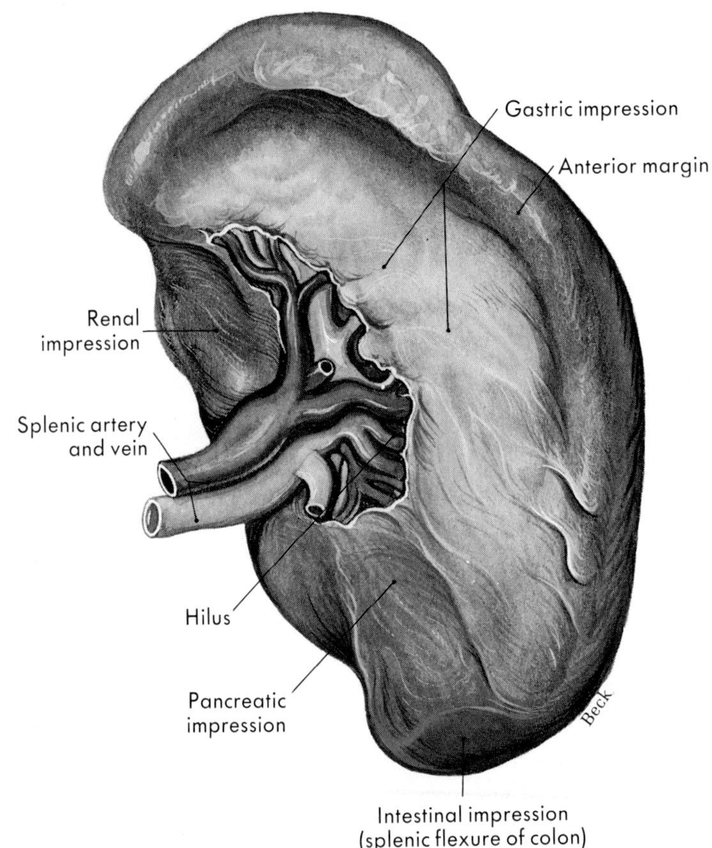

Fig. 21-1. Spleen, medial aspect. Arrangement of vessels at hilus is highly variable. (From Thibodeau, G.A.: Anatomy and physiology, St. Louis, 1987, Times Mirror/Mosby College Publishing.)

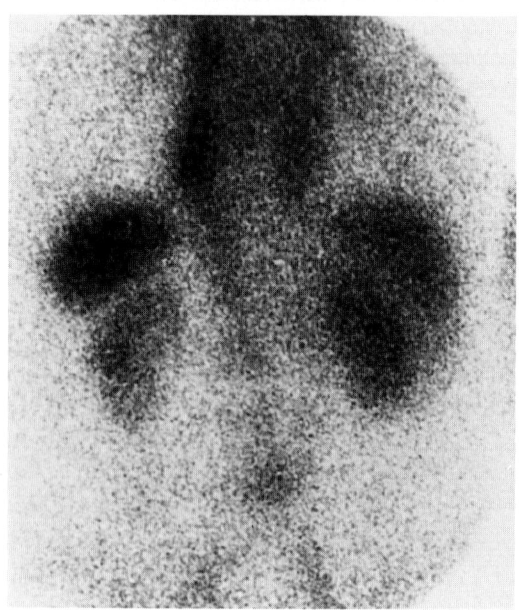

Fig. 21-2. Posterior gamma camera image in 77-year-old male. Red blood cells were labeled by means of stannous pyrophosphate and ^{99m}Tc pertechnetate. The image is of the lower thoracic and abdominal blood pools. The two kidneys can be seen and, to the viewer's left the spleen; the liver is on the right.

D. Spleen as a site of red blood cell production: use of radioiron salts.

The spleen is a "reservoir" for formed blood elements. Some of these leave the spleen on strenuous exercise (perhaps related to an anaerobic threshold and the need for additional oxygenation that can be provided by the red cells in the spleen; this can be studied by ^{99m}Tc red blood cells and following their concentration before, during, and after strenuous exercise). Splenic discharge of blood elements also follows epinephrine administration.

The spleen is involved in platelet handling. The organ can be a site of production of antiplatelet antibodies; this production can result in platelet damage and extraction by the spleen in idiopathic thrombocytopenic purpura, or ITP. In treated cases, if there is a recurrence, it is important to know if there is recurrent or accessory splenic tissue that is triggering the disease. Spleen images in such individuals are therefore a key component of the diagnostic process.

When the bone marrow fails to produce red blood cells, occasionally other sites can take over this function. This process of red cells being manufactured outside of the bone marrow cavity is referred to as *extramedullary hematopoiesis*. Here, radioiron is used as a tracer, and entry-plus discharge is monitored by surface counting over the spleen, liver, and other sites.

The spleen can be a site of sequestration of any of the formed blood elements (platelets, leukocytes, red blood cells). In hypersplenism, the circulating quantity of one or more of these elements is reduced not by a defect in production but by early and excessive trapping in the spleen. The individual components are radiolabeled (by ^{51}Cr sodium chromate or ^{111}In oxine) and the rate of disappearance from the blood followed as well as the sites of localization.

The spleen plays several roles in the processing of red blood cells. First, the spleen is a site of red cell elimination and destruction. However, in the normal individual (following splenectomy) this function can be assumed by other sites and there is little change in red-cell survival. The spleen is carrying out several activities on circulating red blood cells. Crosby has referred to this as "culling" and "pitting." That is, the spleen appears to cull red cells from the circulation if they have intraerythrocytic inclusions (such as Howell-Jolly bodies, which are remnants of the nucleus). It is probably through the sinusoid mechanism that the inclusions are "pinched off;" the "pitted" red cells (slightly smaller in size) continue circulating. Thus, the appearance of Howell-Jolly bodies in the red cells, on a smear of peripheral blood, suggests that the spleen is either absent or not functioning normally *(functional asplenia).* The spleen is also involved in repairing the red-cell membrane; in splenic absence or functional asplenia, red-cell pits or pocks appear in the membrane. Certain disorders such as sickle cell disease are frequently associated with functional asplenia, which is most likely related to splenic hypoxia due to obstruction of small vessels within the spleen. Early on (in the first year of life) this may be transiently reversible if nonsickled blood (non-SS) is transfused and the oxygen tension raised. Recent research has indicated that in sickle cell disease, selected medications can raise the circulating level of fetal hemoglobin (which has a high oxygen-carrying capacity); whether this is adequate to spare the spleen from hypoxia is currently unknown.

The spleen has the ability to filter out or trap particulates from the blood stream. Although only one cell type is likely involved, functionally it appears that two systems are operative. One involves small particles (such as ^{99m}Tc sulfur colloid, which is about 1 micron in diameter). The second removes larger particles such as labeled and denatured red blood cells (about 7 microns in diameter). This has formed the basis for relatively "spleen-specific" agents that can be used for searching for accessory splenic tissue, if ^{99m}Tc sulfur colloid is not revealing. Spleen-specific agents may be used when searching for accessory splenic tissue. These agents are:

A. ^{99m}Tc red cells labeled via the stannous ion, and then heat denatured.
B. ^{111}In-oxine white blood cells.
C. ^{111}In-oxine platelets.

In its various functions the spleen plays multiple roles in the immune process. It not only removes circulating particulates (as explained above); it also contains many lymphocytes that manufacture antibodies in response to foreign antigens. Thus in cases of absence of the spleen or its nonfunction, the patient is at increased risk for overwhelming infection, particularly by organisms such as the pneumococcus and meningococcus (which possess surface capsules). It is because of these vital roles in the immune process that efforts are made to save rather than sacrifice the spleen after trauma.

■ PATHOPHYSIOLOGY

The spleen can be affected not only by intrinsic disorders, but also by alterations in blood flow to the organ and from the spleen into the portal system. Indeed, congestion of the spleen as a result of disease of the liver and the portal venous system may be one of the most common causes of an enlarged spleen (splenomegaly). Throughout the world, the spleen can be involved in infectious disorders such as malaria. This particular disease causes significant enlargement of the spleen, but there is often a subsequent decrease in the size of the organ when the disease is treated. The spleen is not immune to infiltrative or malignant disease, and lymphomas frequently involve the organ. Loss of integrity of the spleen (disruption of the normal appearance of the border) can occur following trauma or when tumor invades the organ either from intrasplenic growth or from external tumor extending into the spleen. When a radioactive colloid is used for splenic studies, comments are made as to the "spleen/liver ratio" (as viewed posteriorly). A decreased ratio may indicate splenic dysfunction, while an increased ratio can follow from liver disease, with the spleen successfully competing for extraction of the radiocolloid. In some immunologic disorders, the spleen may also have increased uptake, perhaps related to increased function that is in turn related to trapping of immune complexes.

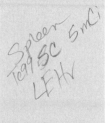

LABORATORY APPLICATION

64

SPLEEN IMAGING USING COLLOIDAL ^{99m}Tc

Purpose

Imaging of the spleen with colloidal ^{99m}Tc is a functional test that depends on an intact reticuloendothelial system within the organ to define its functional anatomy.

Indications

1. Does a palpable abdominal left upper quadrant mass correspond to the spleen?
2. Is the spleen functional (in terms of reticuloendothelial activity) in patients with disorders known to damage the organ, such as sickle cell disease, prior thorotrast (thorium dioxide) injection, abdominal radiation, or long-term use of multiple chemotherapeutic agents?
3. What is the integrity of the spleen following trauma, and if one or more defects are found, do these resolve with the passage of time?
4. Is the spleen involved in systemic diseases that may affect that structure, such as the lymphomas, polycythemia vera, and subacute bacterial endocarditis (in which septic emboli can bring bacteria to the spleen)?
5. Is the spleen functioning in individuals with major infections such as encapsulated bacteria?
6. Following splenectomy, has functional splenic tissue returned either through hypertrophy of an accessory spleen or the growth of splenic implants (splenosis)?
7. In the newborn with congenital defects, is the spleen involved such as in asplenia or polysplenia?
8. Are known intrasplenic defects such as infiltrates or tumor responding to therapy?

Procedure

Materials

1. Scintillation camera with low-energy, high-resolution collimator
2. Precalibrate the camera by using ^{99m}Tc markers 10 cm apart on absorbent paper. Example: if the image produced shows the markers to be 2 cm apart, the minification factor is $\frac{10}{2} = 5$. This will allow determination of actual spleen size from the images.
3. Angle sponge
4. Lead marker to determine location of last rib (about ⅛ inch thick, ½ inch wide and 12 inches long; since this is flexible, it should not be used to determine organ sizes).
5. 5 mCi (185 MBq) of technetium ^{99m}Tc sulfur colloid or technetium ^{99m}Tc albumin colloid, for adults.

Patient preparation

1. Explain the entire procedure to the patient and answer his/her questions.
2. Be certain that there is no metal such as buckles or pins in the field of view.

Technique

1. Set camera controls for ^{99m}Tc peak (140 keV).
2. Set proper intensity and orientation. First part of the study will be a posterior dynamic examination. That is, the camera is looking at the patient's back. This can be done with the patient lying on his or her abdomen and the camera viewing the back, or the patient lying on his or her back and the camera under the "see-through" plastic table.
3. Inject the ^{99m}Tc sulfur colloid intravenously. Press the start button for sequential images at approximately 3-second intervals for the first minute. The field of view should encompass the lower cardiac border, kidneys, spleen, and aorta.
4. At the completion of the dynamic sequence, reset the camera for static images. Wait 5 minutes. The first static image will be for 1,000,000 counts. After that image, observe the time that elapsed. All the other views must be for the same time (that is, set them for the number of seconds that were required for the first image).
5. For each image, have the gamma camera as close to the patient as possible, with a sheet separating the collimator surface from the patient.

6. If a large-field-of-view gamma camera is used, it may be possible to visualize both the liver and spleen on the anterior and posterior views. If not, be certain that the liver is included in additional views anteriorly and posteriorly (so that size and radiocolloid distribution can be compared).
7. Following the anterior spleen image, repeat with the lead marker on the last anterior left rib.
8. A complete spleen examination includes anterior and posterior images, as well as a left lateral, left anterior, and posterior oblique views (angulated 30 degrees with the spleen in the center of the field of view). Note the following:
   a. It may not be possible to turn the patient if he or she has been traumatized; in such instances do the best possible with camera rotation.
   b. On lateral and oblique views, angulate the patient to separate the liver fully from the spleen. If these are not separated, the images may tend to merge, producing a "gourd" effect (Fig. 21-3).

Interpretation

The radiocolloid images are a functional index, and certain facts must be reported.

1. Is a functional spleen noted? If not, there may have been surgical splenectomy, avulsion of the spleen as in severe trauma, or functional asplenia.
2. Is there more than one spleen noted (accessory spleen, splenosis, or other cause of ectopic activity such as a gastrointestinal bleed while the radiocolloid was circulating). In some newborns, polysplenia can occur, usually with other defects.
3. What is the location of the spleen? The organ may be ptotic, or it could be displaced by a mass or be in an ectopic location.
4. What is the size of the spleen? In adults, the spleen is 10 ± 1.5 cm in length. Thus a large spleen is 13 cm or more in length, and a small one is 7 cm or under in length. In children, the spleen is about 5 cm in length at birth and grows at a rate of 0.3 cm per year up to the age of 16.
5. What is the posterior distribution of radiocolloid? The spleen/liver ratio visually or by computer processing is about 1:1. A notable shift to the spleen represents either liver disease or excessive splenic trapping of radiocolloid.
6. Are there intrasplenic defects? These can occur in trauma, in the lymphomas and in infiltrative or infectious diseases.

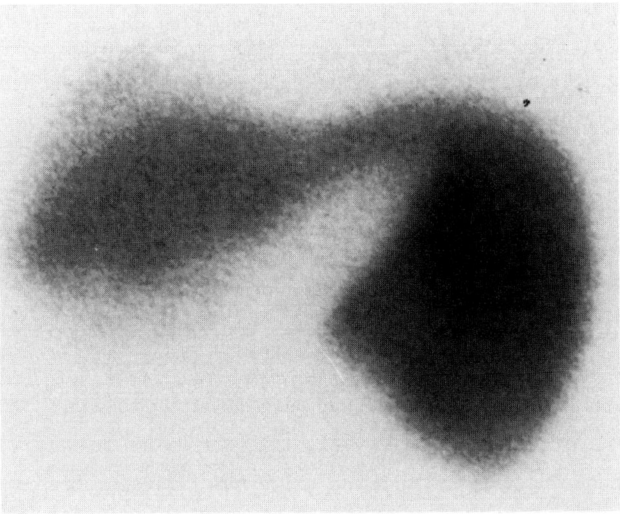

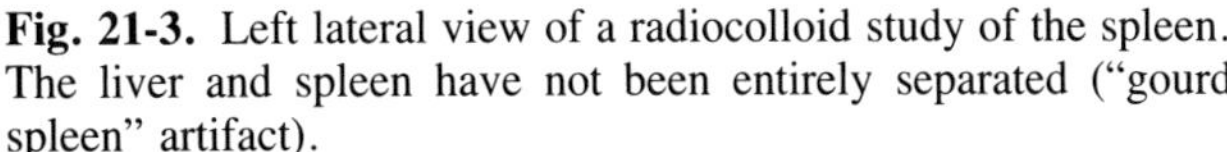

Fig. 21-3. Left lateral view of a radiocolloid study of the spleen. The liver and spleen have not been entirely separated ("gourd spleen" artifact).

Continued.

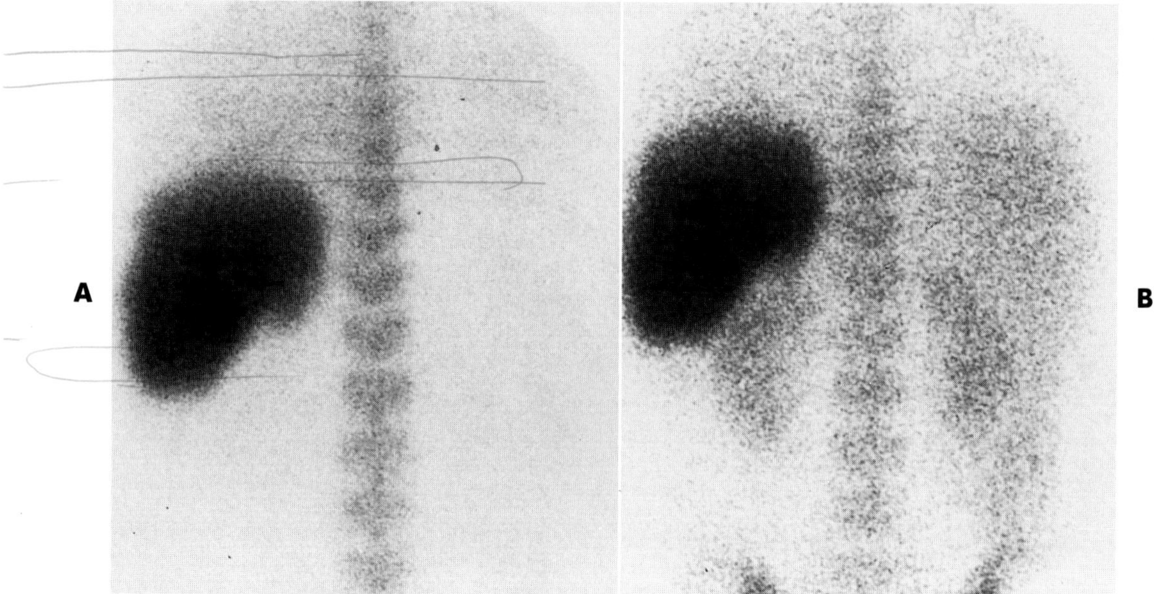

Fig. 21-4. A, Posterior image of the abdomen in a 36-year-old woman with liver failure. This ^{99m}Tc sulfur colloid image defines the spleen, vertebrae, and ribs. The liver is not clearly seen. **B,** A hepatobiliary agent (^{99m}Tc DISIDA) was administered intravenously, and this image was obtained. The liver as well as the kidneys can be faintly seen as well.

7. Comments should be made on a comparison of the spleen and liver (not only radiocolloid distribution as mentioned above, but also on organ sizes and uniformity of radiocolloid distribution) because an enlarged spleen may follow from liver disease, particularly cirrhosis with portal hypertension. (Fig. 21-4).

Diagnosis

Normally the splenic contour is smooth and the organ is in the left upper quadrant posteriorly. Only when there is splenic displacement by tumor or significant splenomegaly does the organ move anteriorly (Fig. 21-5). The spleen is mobile, and if there is liver/spleen overlap this can often be remedied by having the patient stand.

A discussion of the differential diagnosis of the most frequently encountered variants of the ^{99m}Tc colloid spleen scan follows.

Enlarged spleen

There is sufficient information now available to safely permit two statements, as follows:

1. The palpable spleen is not necessarily enlarged. There can be downward and anterior displacement of the spleen in several conditions.
2. Not all enlarged spleens are readily palpable. Body habitus (such as muscle mass and the presence of obesity) may "hide" an enlarged spleen.

Radionuclide techniques (dynamic and static spleen images) are thus of importance in determining the following:

1. Does a palpable left upper quadrant mass represent the functional spleen? For identification, note that the spleen must be both present and functional.
2. What is the size (usually reported as length) of the spleen?

These questions have particular relevance because of the following three statements, which have been verified on numerous occasions.

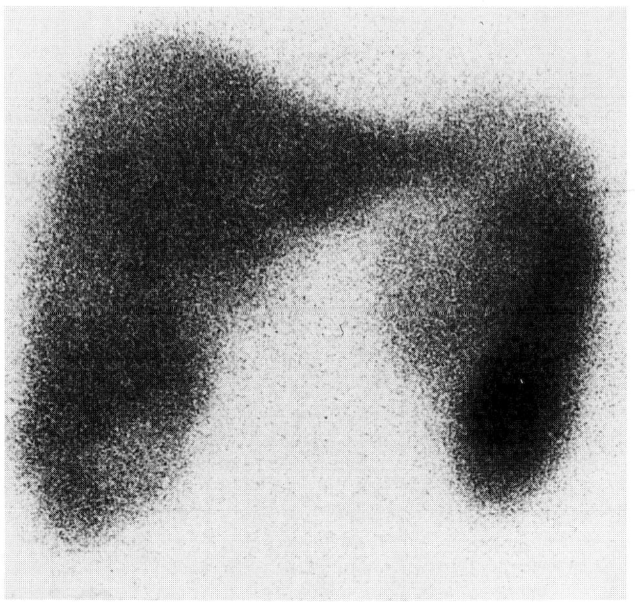

Fig. 21-5. Anterior radiocolloid image obtained in woman with sarcoid. The liver is enlarged (24 cm in length) and shows multiple defects. The spleen, measured posteriorly, is also enlarged, measuring 18 cm.

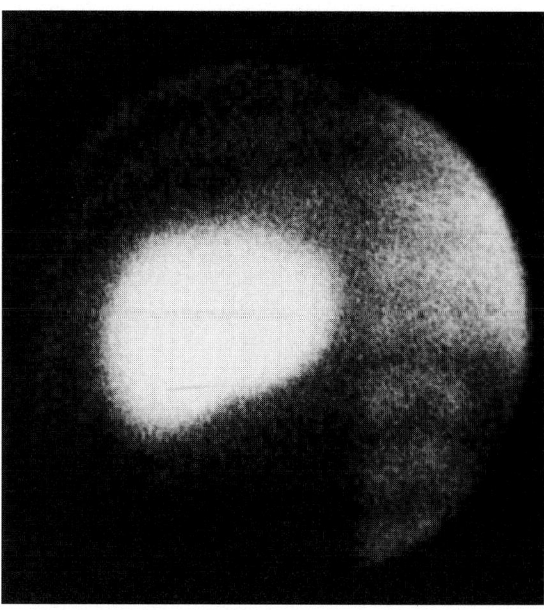

Fig. 21-6. Posterior view of the spleen in patient with severe liver disease. The vertebrae and ribs can also be delineated. The spleen/liver ratio is quite elevated.

1. Palpation of a left upper quadrant mass is often the starting point for an investigation of splenic size and function.
2. Splenic size is not fixed, but may change with exercise (transient) and with treatment such as radiation therapy.
3. The spleen may change its location and orientation.

Determination of splenic size (and that of the liver) is thus of importance because we routinely report on length of the organ as determined by liver/spleen radiocolloid imaging. For the liver, the length is defined as the distance from superior to inferior poles (parallel to the long axis of the body on the anterior view). Normal liver length is 17 ± 2 cm. Splenic length is measured from the posterior image, along the greatest axis of the organ. Use of the minification factor, as well as the gamma camera images, was previously discussed. The enlarged spleen in an adult (13 cm in length or more) can have many causes.

True splenic enlargement

- Secondary to liver disease (Fig. 21-6)
- Secondary to other causes of outflow tract obstruction, such as portal vein thrombosis or acute splenic vein thrombosis
- Infiltrates in the spleen (as in amyloid, sarcoid)
- In polycythemia vera (about two thirds of the cases)
- In myeloid metaplasia and extramedullary hematopoiesis (red cells being made outside of the bone marrow)
- In many hemoglobinopathies (perhaps representing sites of iron-compound deposition and extramedullary hematopoiesis)
- Containing tumor: Benign, such as vascular anomalies and hemangiomas
Malignant ("primary"), such as lymphomas
Malignant, metastatic

False splenic enlargement

- Hepatic tissue extending into the left upper quadrant and giving the impression of splenomegaly

Continued.

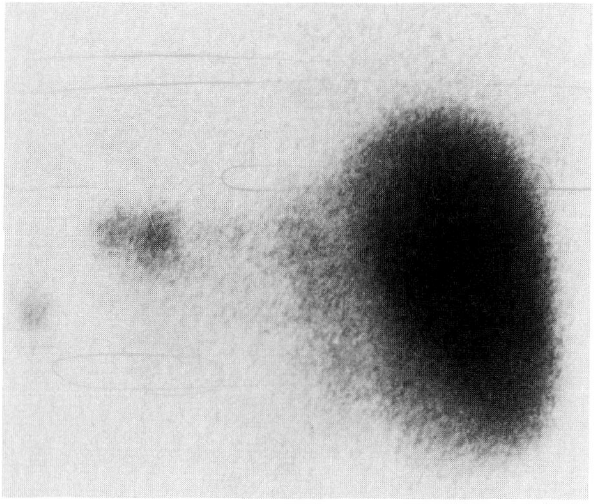

Fig. 21-7. In a woman who had a surgical splenectomy 5 years previously, this posterior radiocolloid image showed 3 small areas of uptake to the left. These likely represented regrowth of splenic tissue.

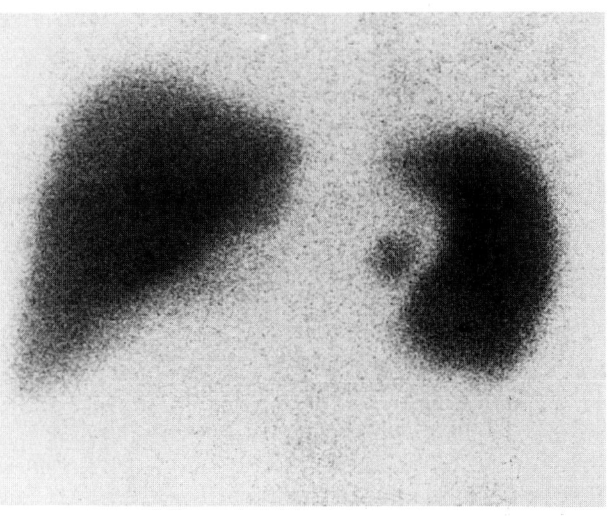

Fig. 21-8. Left posterior oblique radiocolloid image in a male. There is an accessory spleen medial to the principal organ. Finding of functional accessory splenic tissue is unusual unless there was prior splenectomy (Courtesy of Dr. John J. Sziklas, Hartford Hospital, Hartford, Conn.)

- Radioactivity from a prior study, such as gastric radioactivity in continuity with the spleen.
- Radiocolloid accumulation from a bleeding site, with overlap or approximation to the spleen

Small spleen

A small spleen in an adult is one that is two or more standard deviations below the mean value of 10 ± 1.5 cm. Thus an adult spleen that is 7 cm or smaller causes suspicion.

Physiologically small spleen

In children, an approximation to the age-dependence of splenic size (S, in cm) to age (A, in years) is as follows:

$$S = 5.7 + 0.31\ A$$

We report on actual splenic size in children.

Artifactual small spleen

Spleen absent:

1. "Splenosis" or growth of splenic remnants after surgery or trauma (Fig. 21-7)
2. Accessory spleen, which becomes apparent after splenectomy; in rare cases such tissue can be identified before splenectomy (Fig. 21-8)
3. Misidentification of other tissue as representing spleen

Spleen present:

1. Shielding of spleen by hematoma or prosthesis
2. Spleen partially involved by cyst or other process so that the functional area is small

Small spleen due to failure to grow or involution after growth

1. Failure to grow, such as in familial splenic hypoplasia, severe marasmus, and failure to thrive; congenital syndromes of "rapid aging"
2. Some growth, then involution: occlusion of splenic vessels external to the organ, occlusion of vessels within spleen (as in sickle cell disease, malabsorptive disorders such as celiac-sprue—possible immune response), and effects of external or internal irradiation

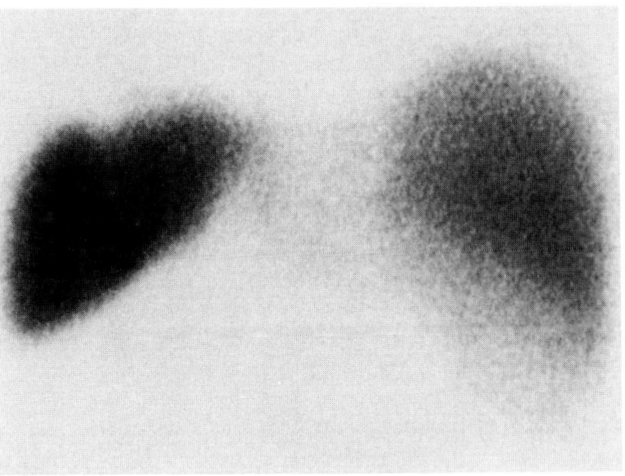

Fig. 21-9. On this posterior radiocolloid image, the spleen (14 cm in length) showed a superior notch or defect. The patient, a 56-year-old woman, had an essentially identical image 23 months previously. There was probably a splenic lobulation.

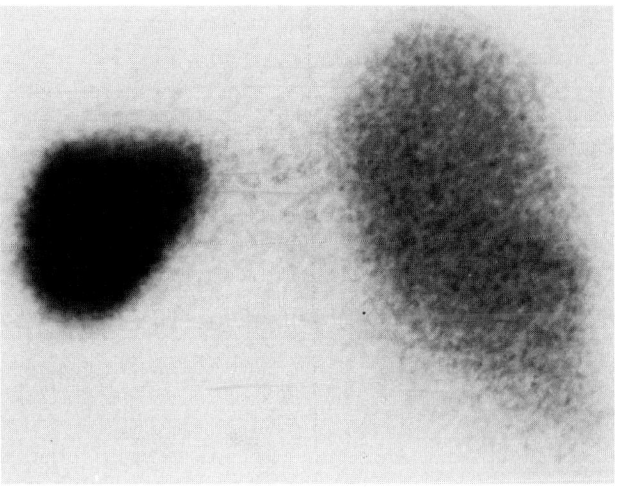

Fig. 21-10. This posterior radiocolloid image, in a 66-year-old woman, revealed the spleen to be displaced downward and rotated, with a major shift of radiocolloid. In some cases, the rotated splenic hilar area will give the appearance of a defect.

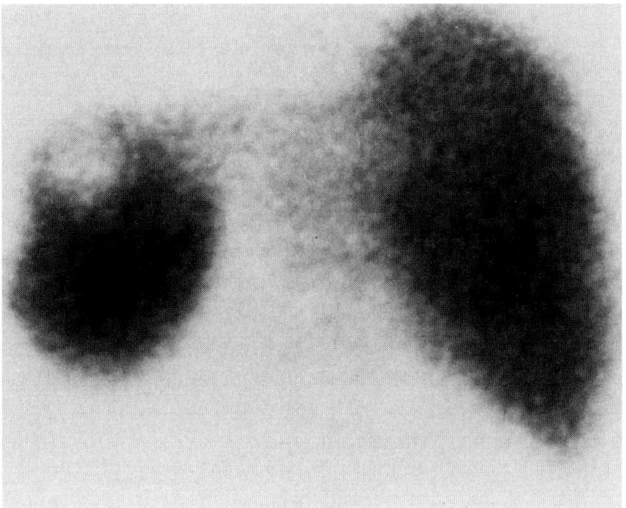

Fig. 21-11. Posterior radiocolloid image in a 74-year-old woman. She had known carcinoma of the lung. The splenic defect could represent a cyst or a metastatic malignancy.

Splenic defects

A splenic defect means a break in the continuity of radiotracer either within the substance of the spleen or along the periphery (near the capsule). There can be lobulations subdividing the spleen (Fig. 21-9). The spleen often can be rotated, bringing the hilar area out of its usual location and creating interpretive difficulties (Fig. 21-10). Defects in the spleen can have a variety of causes and a number of appearances. If the defect is near the periphery of the spleen, a subcapsular bleed or disruption of the organ should be considered. A rounded defect can represent a cyst, but small malignancies can sometimes produce a similar appearance (Fig. 21-11). Linear or band-like patterns can appear after trauma. A patchy distribution suggests an infiltrating disorder or multiple small emboli or vascular occlusions. Multiple defects in the spleen can occur in diffuse vascular disease as well as in tumors involving the organ (Fig. 21-12).

Continued.

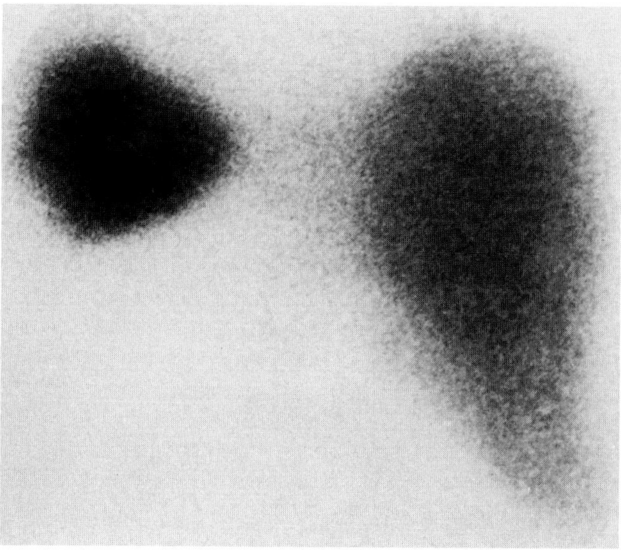

Fig. 21-12. On this posterior radiocolloid view, in a 46-year-old woman, multiple splenic defects can be seen. The patient had a diffuse vasculitis, and this could represent the results of interfering with the splenic blood supply.

The differential diagnosis of intrasplenic defects must include the following:

1. Artifactual, as a result of metal or other absorber overlying the spleen
2. Misinterpretation of the "gap" between the left hepatic lobe and the spleen
3. Extrinsic defect due to encasement of the spleen
4. Direct extension into the spleen (such as from gastric or pancreatic carcinoma or other tumors)
5. True intrasplenic
   a. Vascular occlusion (arterial, venous, capillary)
   b. Cysts
   c. Results of trauma, bleeding, tear
   d. Infiltrates (but often uniform decrease in activity)
   e. Infectious foci (can occur in subacute bacterial endocarditis)
   f. Tumors: benign, malignant, vascular anomalies
   g. Retained metallic fragments within the spleen
   h. Intrasplenic gas
   i. Significant congenital lobulations with apposition of lobes

Shift of radiocolloid to the spleen

On the posterior view, the normal colloidal ^{99m}Tc image reveals the liver and spleen to have about the same optical density. In some cases, particularly when the spleen is involved by a pathologic condition, the spleen/liver ratio of densities can be less than unity. More commonly, a variety of pathologic processes can result in the spleen having a posterior image optical density greater than that of the liver (spleen/liver ratio of greater than about 1.3); an example is shown in (Fig. 21-13). The analysis can also be made by computer processing of counts per units of area of liver and spleen. In the population that we see, the most frequent cause of the "shift of radiocolloid" is hepatic damage such as that due to ethanolism. However, this can occur in malignancies, diabetes (perhaps related to fatty infiltrates of the liver), and in some cases of severe anemia. In malignant melanoma, cases of radiocolloid shift to the spleen have been described (without tumor in the spleen), perhaps related to the trapping of immune complexes.

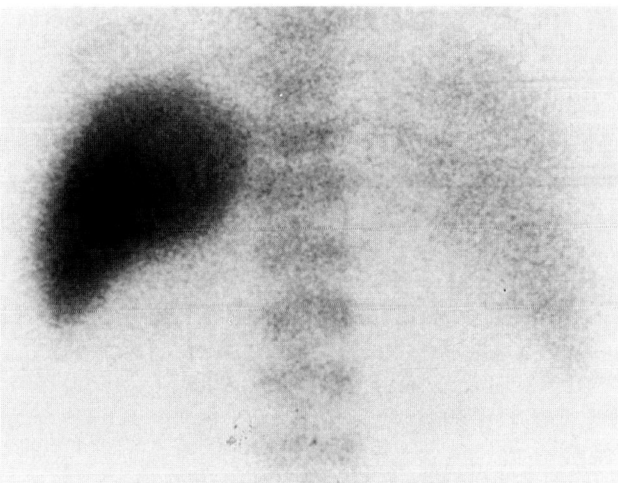

Fig. 21-13. Posterior radiocolloid image shows a significant shift of activity to the spleen and to the bone marrow of the vertebrae and ribs.

The differential diagnosis of an elevated posterior spleen/liver radiocolloid ratio must consider the following:

1. Major replacement or loss of liver function, such as tumor-displacing liver reticuloendothelial cells or metabolic changes such as after bowel bypass for morbid obesity
2. Hepatic damage from vessel obstruction, such as Budd-Chiari syndrome with blockade of the hepatic veins
3. Splenic or portal vein obstruction, which may have an associated elevated ratio
4. Probable immune mechanisms such as in malignant melanoma
5. Some cases of hypersplenism (although there is not a one-to-one correspondence between radiocolloid trapping and erythrocyte uptake)
6. Following medications, perhaps related to liver dysfunction
7. Artefactual
   a. Liver tissue overlying the spleen, giving falsely elevated splenic region counts
   b. Gastrointestinal (GI) bleed or other source of radioactivity overlying spleen
   c. Shielding of liver by hematoma or metal, on posterior view

No spleen visualized on radiocolloid images

On the posterior radiocolloid image, activity in the left upper quadrant is usually assumed to represent the spleen. Care has to be taken to distinguish this from hepatic tissue (and liver-specific agents such as ^{99m}Tc hepatobiliary compounds, or relatively spleen-specific substances such as ^{99m}Tc denatured red blood cells, which may have to be used). Principal causes of failure to appreciate the spleen on a radiocolloid image are as follows:

1. Congenital asplenia (with or without cardiac and other defects)
2. Reversible hyposplenia due to anoxia (often resembles congenital asplenia)
3. Surgical or traumatic splenectomy
4. Acquired asplenia due to vascular occlusion or tumor replacement
5. Functional asplenia

Absence of the spleen (anatomic absence or functional inactivity) can be associated with a number of hematologic markers (such as red cell pocks and intraerythrocytic inclusions such as Howell-Jolly bodies). However, if the splenic vasculature is acutely occluded, failure to take up radiocolloid can be shown to occur before Howell-Jolly bodies have an opportunity to appear in circulating erythrocytes. Most intriguing are cases in which the spleen, which has lost its ability to accumulate col-

Continued.

loidal ^{99m}Tc, later regains this function. A classification of the causes of such "reversible functional asplenia" has been presented.

Ectopic spleen (single)

If the spleen is not found in the left upper quadrant, then a search has to be made for the tissue in other locales. The differential diagnosis includes the following:

1. A spleen that is "high riding" under an elevated diaphragm, or one that is displaced downward by the diaphragm
2. Spleen displaced such as by gastric dilatation
3. Surgical implantation of the spleen into an ectopic site
4. Growth of an ectopic accessory spleen after splenectomy
5. Growth of surgically or traumatically "dropped" splenic tissue in an ectopic site after removal of the spleen (splenosis)
6. Congenital defective location (these are often accessory spleens such as in splenogonadal fusion; their function has not yet been determined)
7. Asplenia, but false localization such as radiocolloid leakage during GI bleeding, or uptake into rejecting tissue

Multiple splenic tissue

It is rare that uptake in more than one "spleen" is found. However, it does occur. The differential diagnosis includes several entities, as follows:

1. Congenital polysplenia (often with other anomalies)
2. Splenic trauma, with surviving fragments in proximity
3. Multiple splenic tissue ("splenosis") from surgery or trauma
4. Accessory spleens, particularly after removal of the major spleen
5. False positive causes of "multiple splenic tissue"
   a. More than one GI bleeding site at time of injection
   b. Foci of radiocolloid uptake around rejecting tissue
   c. Radioactivity from a prior study (as in stomach)

Unexpected left upper quadrant activity

While the spleen accumulates colloidal ^{99m}Tc, other radiopharmaceuticals may show little or no activity in the area. The spleen can usually be located by means of blood-pool imaging. After intravenous administration of hepatobiliary agents, activity usually clears rapidly from the bloodstream and from the splenic blood pool. There are several causes of unexpected left upper quadrant activity:

1. Splenic activity
   a. In splenic vasculature, as a result of delayed clearance
   b. Demonstration of splenic vasculature by agents that bind proteins in the bloodstream
   c. Unusual splenic uptake of radiopharmaceuticals. Examples include splenic activity from ^{99m}Tc MAA when a right-to-left cardiac shunt is present, and splenic accumulation of ^{99m}Tc phosphates in sickle cell disease
2. Nonsplenic uptake in the left upper quadrant
   a. Bowel activity, as during a ^{67}Ga gallium citrate study
   b. GI bleed during injection of colloidal ^{99m}Tc
   c. Stomach uptake, such as after ingesting a radionuclide, or after intravenous administration of ^{99m}Tc-pertechnetate.
   d. Renal activity, especially if displaced (the left kidney and spleen often are in continuity)
   e. Liver extending into the left upper quadrant
   f. Tumor uptake in the region
   g. Inflammatory mass in the left upper quadrant, with radioactivity concentration

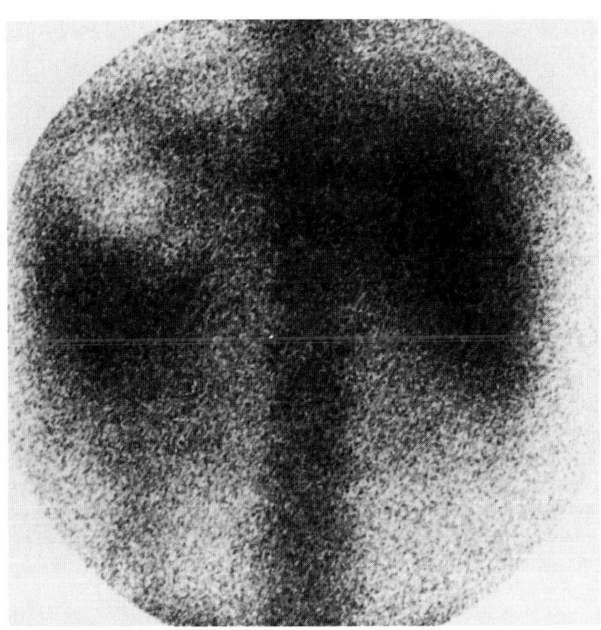

Fig. 21-14. Posterior image of a radiogallium study (^{67}Ga) in a 15-year-old boy. The prominent gastric "bubble" can be seen on the left (probably air, fluid, solids).

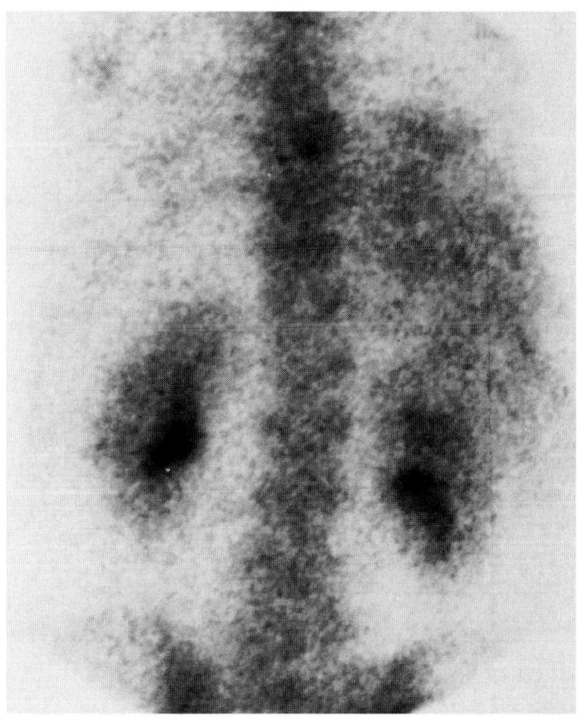

Fig. 21-16. ^{99m}Tc diphosphonate (MDP) uptake in the liver, but not the spleen. This can occur when metastatic disease is in the liver (there are other causes as well).

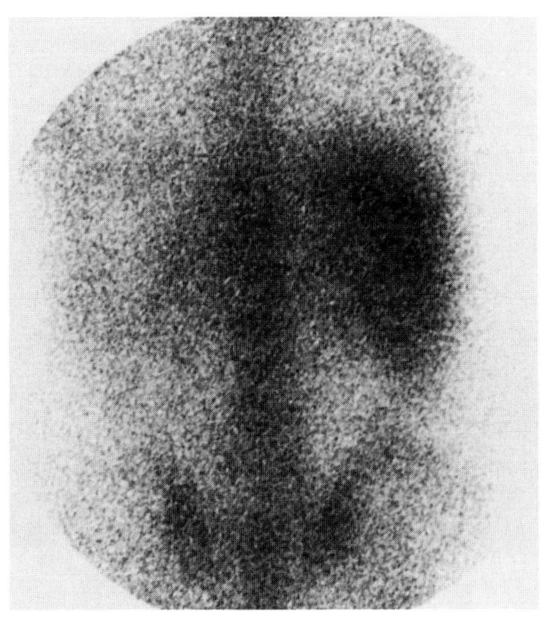

Fig. 21-15. Posterior radiogallium image, in a 12-year-old male, shows a relative "void" in the splenic area (prior splenectomy).

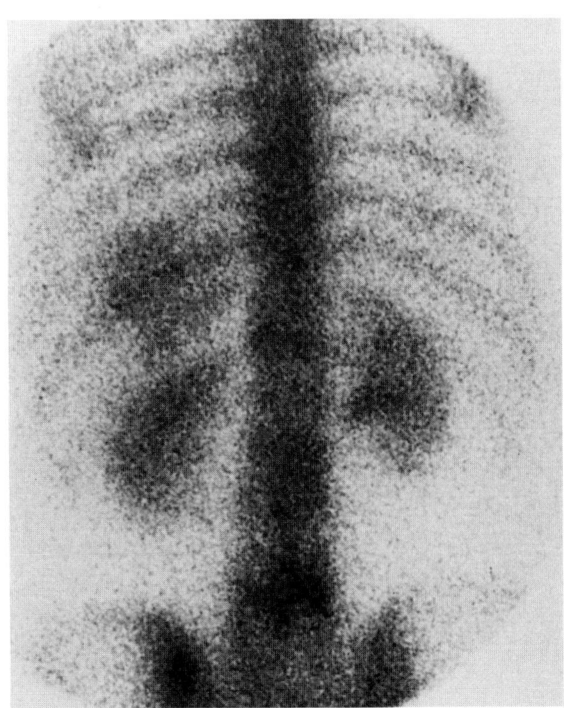

Fig. 21-17. This posterior ^{99m}Tc MDP image shows activity above the left kidney; the image represented the spleen in a case of lymphoma.

■ SPLENIC ACCUMULATION OF OTHER RADIOTRACERS

Page 535 lists the major splenic activities and the radiotracers used in their evaluation. ^{111}In-labeled white blood cells (used in evaluating possible infections) concentrate in the spleen; thus the organ has the highest radiation exposure during use of the indium-tagged white cells. The tagged cells can be used when searching for accessory splenic tissue.

The spleen usually only accumulates small amounts of ^{67}Ga gallium citrate. The quantity however can increase with intrasplenic tumors or infarcts. The gastric bubble of air/fluid/food just above the spleen (Fig. 21-14) can produce a complex image. The gastric bubble has to be distinguished from the "void" that can occur in the region after splenectomy (Fig. 21-15). During bone imaging with ^{99m}Tc-diphosphonates, the liver may occasionally be visualized (Fig. 21-16). The spleen can also accumulate the labeled diphosphonates (Fig. 21-17) perhaps related to splenic hypoxia.

BIBLIOGRAPHY

Antar, M.A., Kassamali, H., and Spencer, R.P.: Sequential loss of splenic and then hepatic function in a patient with thorotrast loading, Clin. Nucl. Med. 14:634-635, 1989.

Larson, S.M., Tuell, S.H., Moores, K.D., and Nelp, W.B.: Dimensions of the normal spleen and prediction of spleen weight, J. Nucl. Med. 11:341, 1970.

Levine, G.M., Cinti, D.C., Hawkins, H.B., and Spencer, R.P.: Left upper quadrant mass: radiocolloid study to differentiate spleen from a gastric leiomyosarcoma, NucCompact 22:115-116, 1991.

Negrin, J.A., Sziklas, J.J., Spencer, R.P., Levine, G.M., and Rosenberg, R.J.: "Resolving" splenic uptake of Tc-99m MDP in aplastic anemia, Clin. Nucl. Med. 16:944-945, 1991.

Pearson, H.A., Spencer, R.P., and Cornelius, E.A.: Functional asplenia in sickle-cell anemia, New Engl. J. Med. 281:923-926, 1969.

Perrine, S.P., Ginder, G.D, Faller, D.V., and others: A short-term trial of butyrate to stimulate fetal-globin-gene expression the β-globin disorders, New Engl. J. Med. 328:81-86, 1993.

Rodgers, G.P., Dover, G.J., Uyesaka, N., and others: Augmentation by erythropoietein of the fetal-hemoglobin response to hydroxyurea in sickle cell disease, New Engl. J. Med. 328:73-80, 1993.

Rosenberg, R.J., Sziklas, J.J., and Rich, D.A.: Dual radionuclide subtraction imaging of the spleen, Semin. Nucl. Med. 15:299-304, 1985.

Spencer, R.P., Grimmond, A.P., and Treschuk-Bahn, J.: Abdominal trauma with leukocytosis and Howell-Jolly bodies: idiopathic functional asplenia, Clin. Nucl. Med. 13:544, 1988.

Spencer, R.P., Sziklas, J.J., Rosenberg, R.J., and others: Splenic uptake of Tc-99m-MDP: possible relationship to hemosiderin, Clin. Nucl. Med. 15:582, 1990.

Spencer, R.P.: Compensatory splenic growth: role of functional indicators, J. Nucl. Med. 32:207-209, 1991.

Spencer, R.P., Sziklas, J.J., and Zubi, S.M.: Disassociation of splenic accumulation of Tc-99m MDP and radiocolloid, Clin. Nucl. Med. 16:747-749, 1991.

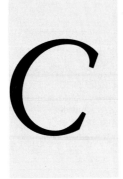

Chapter 22

ENTRAL NERVOUS SYSTEM

RICHARD A. HOLMES
KIMBERLY G. HOFFMAN

In spite of the nineties being designated as the "decade of the brain," scintigraphic imaging has not clinically expanded to challenge other techniques such as computed tomography (CT) or magnetic resonance imaging (MRI). Except in special instances, cerebral planar scintigraphy has been replaced by single-photon emission computed tomography (SPECT), which holds several advantages over the conventional technique. The anatomic description of the brain when topographically imaged not only provides a description of deep brain structures but allows comparisons or registration with the more popular radiographic techniques. The radiopharmaceuticals used for SPECT brain imaging differ dramatically from the planar imaging agents, providing information that reflects physiologic functions or dysfunctions. The generation of SPECT images employs modified routine scintillation cameras with interfaced computers and appropriate software. The clinical results with radiotracers that localize and concentrate in brain relative to blood perfusion have revealed new information for a variety of diseases and cognitive stimuli.

■ ANATOMY AND PHYSIOLOGY

The brain and spinal cord form the central nervous system. Brain tissue is composed of richly perfused gray matter possessing an abundance of neurons (nerve cells) and dendrites, as well as white matter containing myelinated axons. Anatomically the brain has paired cerebral hemispheres that make up seven eighths of total brain weight, filling the cranial vault with the cerebellum and the brain stem that extends caudally and extracranial as the spinal cord. The cerebral hemispheres are each divided into four lobes by deep sulci and fissures. The central sulcus (fissure of Rolando) divides the frontal lobe from the parietal lobes. The frontal lobe and proximal parietal lobes are separated from the temporal lobe by the lateral cerebral sulcus (fissure of Sylvius) A parietooccipital sulcus divides the parietal and occipital lobes, while the transverse fissure separates the cerebrum from the cerebellum (Fig. 22-1). Fig. 22-2 shows the topography of the functional lobes of the cerebral hemispheres. The *frontal lobe* contains memory and motor function, with each cerebral hemisphere controlling functions on the opposite (contralateral) side of the body. The *parietal lobe* controls sensory function and is concerned with the initial processing of tactile and proprioceptive information as well as orientation of the individual in space and time. Along with the temporal lobe, the parietal lobe is also involved in language function. The *temporal lobe* mediates hearing, emotional and visceral responses, learning, and memory recall. A part of the temporal lobe is responsible for language recognition and organization. The *occipital lobe* is concerned exclusively with visual function. The *cerebellum,* located in the cranial posterior fossa, is separated from the occipital lobes by the tentorium cerebelli and from the brain stem by the fourth ventricle. The cerebellum is subdivided into the narrow medial vermis and the larger paired lateral hemispheres. Cerebellar functions include the coordination of voluntary movement and posture adjustments to gravity. Structurally the *brain stem* includes the midbrain, the pons, and the medulla oblongata. Functionally it is divided into three general activities: conduit functions, cranial nerve function, and integrative functions. The brain stem with the hypothalamus controls the autonomic nervous system and many basic physiologic functions. The distal (caudal) brain stem exits the cranium through the foramen magnum and continues as the *spinal cord.* Thirty-one pairs of spinal nerves branch from the spinal cord; 8 cervical, 12 thoracic, 5 lumbar, 5 sacral, and a pair of coccygeal nerves. The spinal cord terminates as the cauda equina near the level of the first or second lumbar vertebrae. Within the brain is a series of communicating hollow spaces, the ventricular system. The two C-shaped lateral ventricles are located beneath the corpus callosum in each of the cerebral hemispheres. The lateral ventricles connect with the narrow, slit-shaped third ventricle of the diencephalon via the foramina of Monro. The fourth ventricle, located between the pons

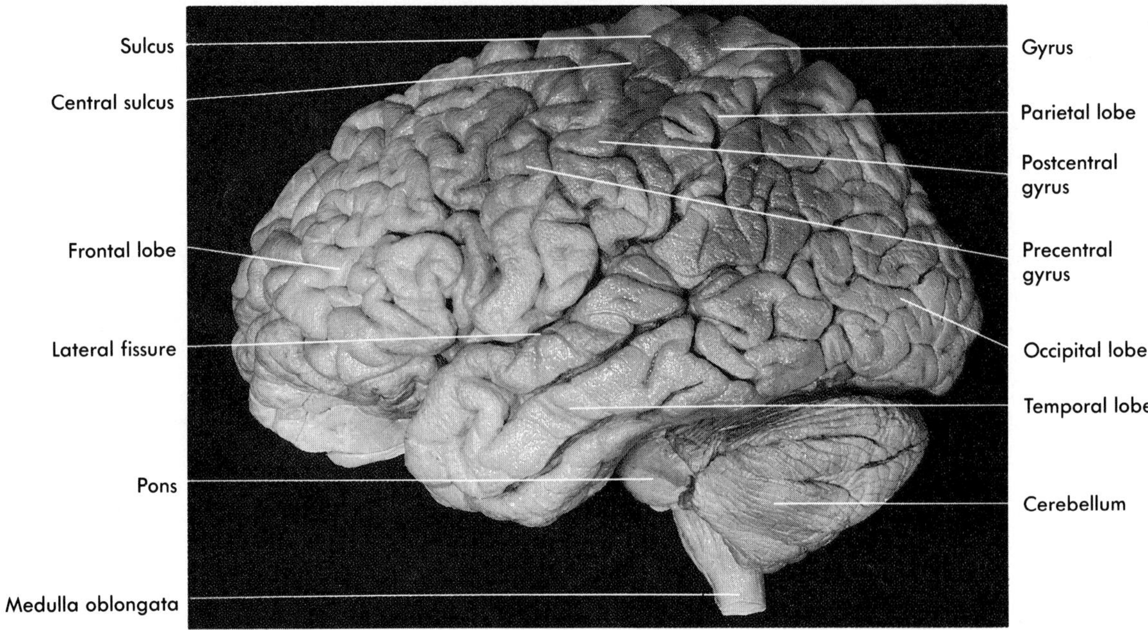

Fig. 22-1. Cerebral anatomy. (From Seeley, R.R., Stephens, T.D., and Tate, P.: Essentials of anatomy and physiology, St. Louis, 1991, Mosby–Year Book.)

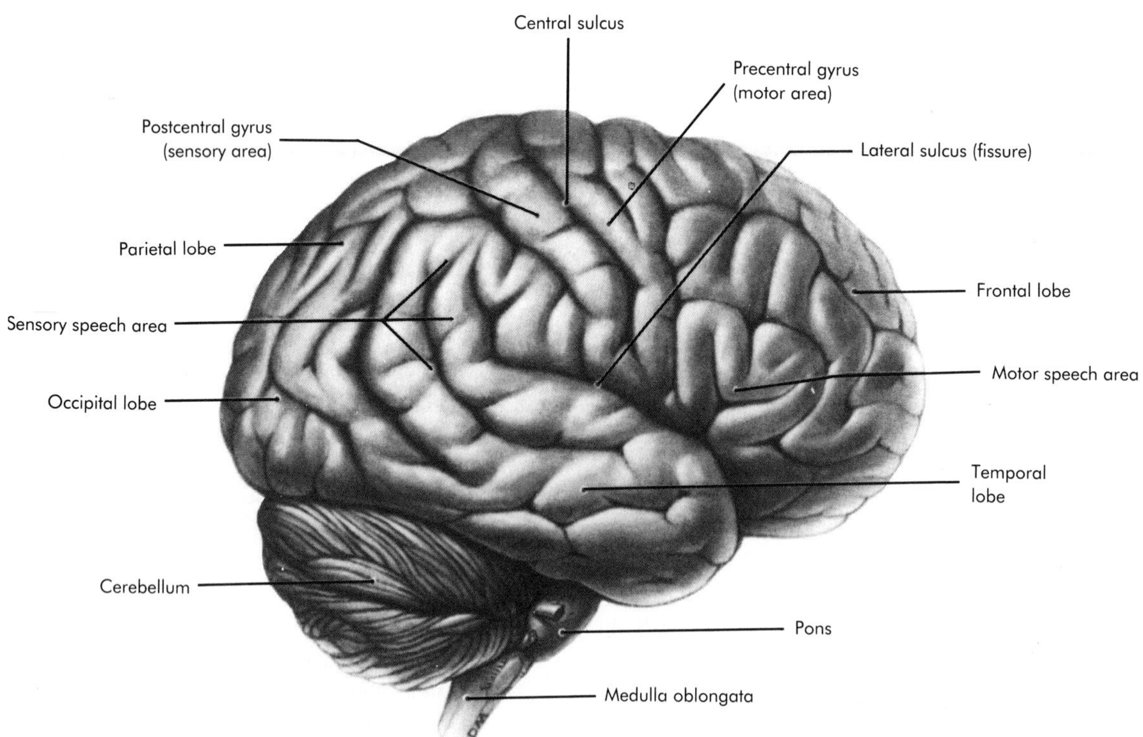

Fig. 22-2. Topography of major cortical regions. (From Bernier, D.R.: Nuclear medicine technology and techniques, ed 3, St. Louis, 1994, Mosby–Year Book.)

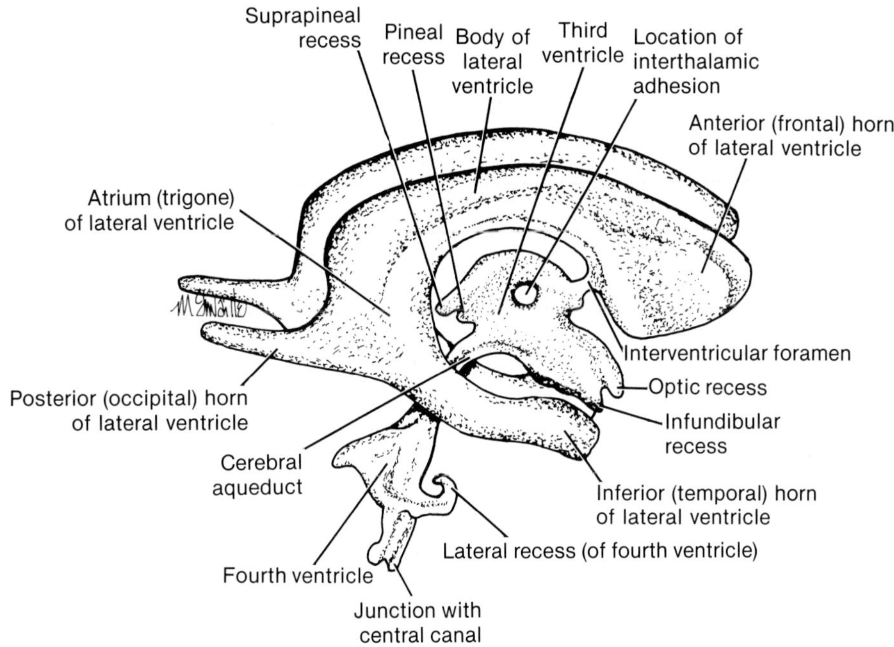

Fig. 22-3. Ventricular anatomy. (From Nolte, J.: The human brain, an introduction to its functional anatomy, ed 3, St. Louis, 1993, Mosby–Year Book.)

and rostral medulla, is connected to the third ventricle through the aqueduct of Sylvius (Fig. 22-3).

Brain tissue is very pliable and without some type of support would be unable to maintain its shape. Protection and support of the brain is provided by eight bones (frontal, two parietal, two temporal, an occipital, a sphenoid, and an ethmoid) making up the cranium and a series of membranous coverings called the *meninges*. The tough outermost layer of the meninges, the dura matter, adheres to the inner surface of the cranium and protrudes inward, toward the surface of the brain, in two principal reflections, the falx cerebri separating the two cerebral hemispheres, and the tentorium cerebelli separating the posterior cerebral hemispheres from the cerebellum. The second meninx, the arachnoid, is a thin avascular membrane adherent to the inner surface of the dura; it helps "suspend" the brain within the cranium. The pia mater is a thin vascular membrane that adheres to and follows the contours of the cerebrum, the cerebellum, and the brain stem. The meninges stabilizes the shape and position of nerve tissue during head and body movement.

The brain is further protected by the cushioning effect of cerebral spinal fluid (CSF) that is formed by the choroid plexus, a layer of vascular, membranous material located in the temporal horns of the lateral ventricles, the posterior portion of the third ventricle, and the roof of the fourth ventricle. The CSF is a colorless aqueous transudate of plasma with low levels of protein, potassium, and calcium, and high concentrations of sodium and magnesium. These concentrations are maintained at stable levels despite changes in plasma concentration. In a normal adult the choroid plexus produces approximately 500 ml of CSF each day. Cerebrospinal fluid travels from the lateral ventricles through the foramina of Monro to the third ventricle where additional CSF is added from the third ventricle's choroid plexus. The fluid continues through the aqueduct of Sylvius into the fourth ventricle, where more CSF is added from the choroid plexus in the roof of the fourth ventricle. The CSF passes through the foramen of Magendie (the median aperture) and the foramina of Luschka (two lateral apertures) into the subarachnoid space (cisterna magna). The CSF courses through the subarachnoid space, down the dorsal spinal cord and up the ventral spinal cord, into the basal and medial cisterns over the hemispheric free convexities to the vertex of the brain where it is gradually absorbed by arachnoid villi in the superior sagittal sinus. Functionally, the arachnoid villi act as one-way valves, allowing unidirectional flow from the subarachnoid space into venous blood. The total volume of CSF contained in the ventricular/subarachnoid space is approximately 135 ml in a normal 70-kg adult. The time required to complete the CSF transit from production to reabsorption is 6 to 36 hours. Normal pressure for CSF averages 130 mm water (10 mm Hg).

■ BLOOD SUPPLY

Although the brain constitutes 2% to 3% of total body weight, it requires 20% of total oxygen consumption and 15% of cardiac output. Normal cortical blood flow aver-

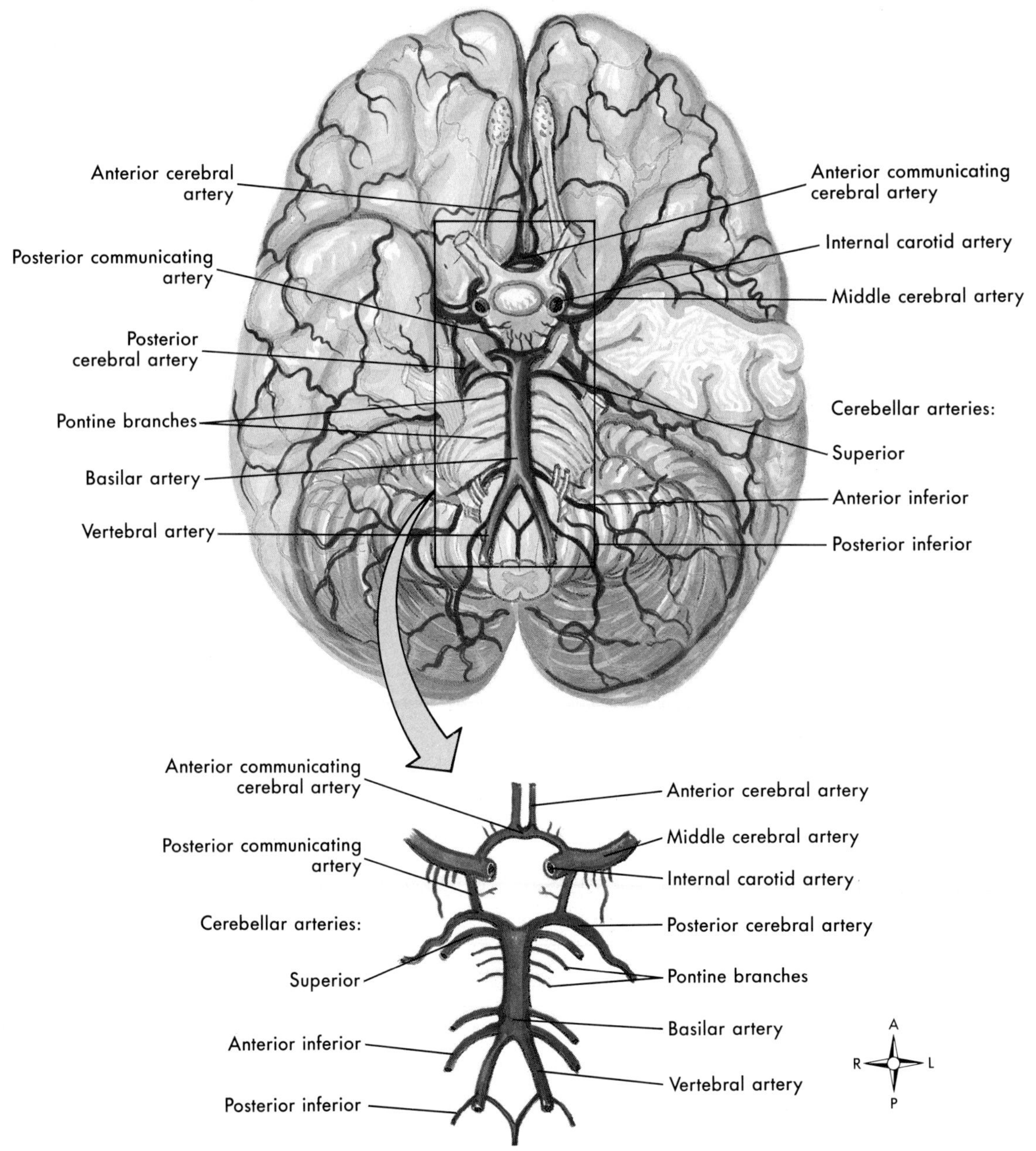

Fig. 22-4. Cerebral and cerebellar arterial anatomy. (From Thibodeau, G.A., Patton, K.T.: Anthony's textbook of anatomy and physiology, ed 14, St. Louis, 1994, Mosby–Year Book.)

ages 50 to 55 ml per minute per 100 g of brain. Blood is supplied to the brain through the right and left common carotid and vertebrobasilar arteries. The right common carotid artery is a branch of the right subclavian artery; at the level of the larynx it divides into the right internal and external carotid arteries. The left common carotid branches from the aortic arch into internal and external branches. The vertebral arteries branch from the aorta and anastomose at the base of the brain, forming the basilar artery. The basilar artery continues cephalad and bifurcates at its terminal end, into the right and left posterior cerebral arteries. The left and right internal carotids are anastomosed to the basilar artery by the posterior communicating and the anterior communicating arteries from the circle of Willis (Fig. 22-4). Brain blood flow is rigidly maintained by several control mechanisms. This autoregulation allows cerebral blood vessels to constrict in response to increased blood pressure and to relax with decreased pressure. The principal regulator of blood flow to the brain is the carbon dioxide concentrations and, to a lesser degree, diminished oxygen concentration. Excess carbon dioxide and diminished oxygen concentrations cause cerebral vasodilation. Autonomic nerves are of

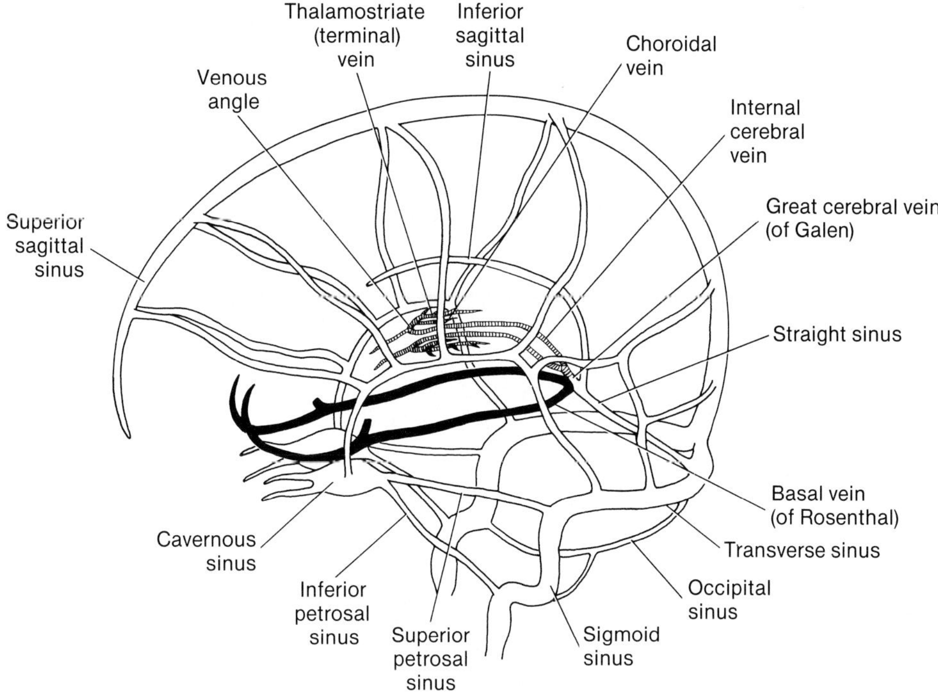

Fig. 22-5. Cerebral venous anatomy. Dural sinuses and superficial veins are white, deep veins are striped, and the basal vein and its tributaries are black, (From Nolte J.: The human brain, an introduction to its functional anatomy, ed 3, St. Louis, 1993, Mosby–Year Book.)

limited importance in regulating regional cerebral blood flow.

The cerebral cortex is drained by the superior sagittal, inferior sagittal, straight, and transverse dural sinus (Fig. 22-5). The sinuses drain through the internal jugular veins that exit the cranium through the jugular foramina.

■ Blood-brain barrier

The blood-brain barrier (BBB) is distinct to the central nervous system and refers to the anatomic and physiologic complex that controls the movement of substances from the vascular space to the brain's extracellular fluid. This barrier permits nutrients essential to brain tissue (e.g., glucose, oxygen, electrolytes, carbon dioxide) to readily cross the barrier while toxic and unwanted substances are restricted from passage. The barrier also prevents rapid changes in plasma concentrations of ions and other substrates from reaching lethal concentrations in the brain. Although conventional brain imaging relies on the localization of the radiopharmaceuticals in brain lesions due to the deterioration of the blood-brain barrier, newer radiopharmaceuticals have been developed that normally cross the intact blood-brain barrier. Examples of the latter include Xenon-133, *N*-isopropyl-*p* I-123-iodoamphetamine (^{123}I-IMP), (^{123}I-IMP is no longer commercially available in the United States) and Tc-99m-d,l-hexamethyl propylene amine oxime (^{99m}Tc-d,l-HMPAO).

■ CEREBRAL FUNCTION AND NEUROTRANSMISSION

The brain's nerve cell mass comprises nearly 40% of the total brain volume and has a high energy requirement. The axons and dendrites of the nerve cells require energy to transport intracellular material peripherally and centrally. Additional energy is needed for interneuronal communication to occur such as the release of excitatory and inhibitory neurotransmitters (e.g., acetylcholine, catecholamines, serotonin, dopamine) and their subsequent degradation and restoration of membrane polarization.

Neuronal metabolism consumes adenosine triphosphate (ATP) during work and the ensuing resynthesization of ATP from adenosine diphosphate (ADP). Glucose is the brain's sole energy substrate, except during ketosis. Ninety-five percent of normal brain energy requirements results from the oxidation of glucose to water and carbon dioxide. Only a limited reserve of glucose is found in the neuron, and the brain is critically dependent on blood supply to provide the glucose and oxygen it needs. If the oxygen supply is interrupted, tissue ATP drops to zero within 7 minutes and the damage is irreparable.

The neurons are specialized by the way they process impulses. Afferent neurons carry sensory impulses to the brain (centrally) while efferent neurons carry motor impulses to the body (peripherally). The transmission of impulses resides in the ability of neuron cell membranes to undergo electrical changes mediated by selective chemical neurotransmitters. Chemicals such as acetylcholine, catecholamines, serotonin, and dopamine each display characteristic inhibitory or excitatory effects on the neurons. These transmitters are located in axon clusters in specific regions of the brain. When an impulse from a sending neuron arrives at a receiver neuron, a sudden release of the chemical neurotransmitter occurs and the transmitter molecules diffuse across the fluid-filled space between the neurons (synapse), thus altering the electrical activity of the receiver neuron. This constant activity makes the brain the largest consumer of energy in the body.

The average rate of metabolic glucose consumption in the brain is approximately 60 ml/100 g/min and shows considerable regional variation, being four to five times greater in the superior midbrain than in the basilar midbrain. Oxygen is critical to brain integrity and energy production and is created solely by aerobic oxidation of glucose. Oxygen is used at an average rate of 6 ml/100 g/min in cortex (gray matter) and 2 ml/100 g/min in white matter. The regional variations in the metabolic rates of these substrates reflects variations in the density of neurons and their activity and is also influenced by the other cells (e.g., macroglia, microglia) that make up the remaining 60% of the cerebral volume.

■ BRAIN IMAGING

LABORATORY APPLICATION

65

PLANAR BRAIN IMAGING

Background

In the 1940s the detection of brain tumors using radionuclides was accomplished using beta emitting sodium ^{32}P phosphate and a hand-held Geiger-Mueller detector that was used to probe the brain. Following the development of the rectilinear scanner by Cassen in the early 1950s, the detection of brain tumors was first made by using ^{131}I-diiodofluorescein (a gamma-emitting photon radiotracer) and scanning over the surface of the head. Multicrystal sodium iodide scanners were eventually developed to decrease the scanning time while gamma-emitting, non–BBB-penetrating, high–photon-flux radiopharmaceuticals were developed to diminish scanning time and improve scan resolution and diagnostic accuracy. Discovery of the Anger scintillation camera, which because of its size allowed the imaging of composite areas of the head from various projections, subsequently added the perfusion or "flow" study to routine planar imaging.

Purpose

In the late 1960s and 1970s, before the discovery of x-ray computed tomography, planar brain imaging provided the only noninvasive means to evaluate brain diseases. This method was complemented by direct carotid artery contrast angiography, which provided exclusively anatomic information. Because of the radiopharmaceuticals' rate and degree of uptake in a variety of brain lesions, planar brain imaging not only provided anatomic information but assessed some degree of function as well. Functional imaging has become a mainstay of phase planar brain imaging and has added to its specificity.

Planar brain imaging is accomplished by collecting a sufficient number of gamma photons and using the Anger scintillation camera to form an image. A routine planar brain image is composed of a series of planar views (anterior, posterior, vertex and lateral projections) of the head. Lesions show as photon rich areas (hot spots) on the planar views due to local BBB disruption and radiopharmaceutical diffusion into the brain.

Radiopharmaceuticals

Two types of gamma-emitting photon radiopharmaceuticals are used to scintigraphically image the brain (Table 22-1). Those that do not cross (nonpenetrating) the BBB are used for planar brain imaging. The most commonly used include: ^{99m}Tc-pertechnetate, ^{99m}Tc-diethylenetriamine pentaacetic acid (DTPA) and ^{99m}Tc-glucoheptonate (GHA). Although all three give similar image results using the same dose, their optimum imaging times differ. ^{99m}Tc-pertechnetate requires the longest equilibration time, while ^{99m}Tc-DTPA clears the blood rapidly and has the shortest equilibration time. ^{99m}Tc-pertechnetate concentrates in the choroid plexus and the salivary glands. To eliminate this

Table 22-1. Gamma photon radiopharmaceuticals for brain imaging

Radiopharmaceutical	Photon energy keV	Physical half-life	Usual dose	Optimum imaging time	Comments
Non-BBB penetration					
^{99m}Tc-pertechnetate	140	6 hr	15-20 mCi (555-740 MBq)	2-4 hr	$KC10_4$, atropine
^{99m}Tc-DTPA	140	6 hr	15-20 mCi (555-740 MBq)	0.5-1 hr	Rapid uptake
^{99m}Tc-GHA	140	6 hr	15-20 mCi (555-740 MBq)	1-4 hr	—
^{99m}Tc-red cells (in vivo)	140	6 hr	15-20 mCi (555-740 MBq)	0.5-1 hr	Blood pool
^{99m}Tc-phosphonate (MDP,HDP)	140	6 hr	15-20 mCi (555-740 MBq)	2-4 hr	Infarcts
^{67}Ga-citrate	92, 187, 296	78 hr	3-6 mCi (111-222 MBq)	24-72 hr	Inflammation
^{201}Tl-chloride	68-80 135, 167	73 hr	2-3 mCi (74-111 MBq)	Immediately	Metastases
BBB penetration					
^{133}Xe (gas)	81	127 hr	0.5-10 mCi (18.5-370 MBq)	Immediately	rCBF
^{123}I-iodoamphetamine	159	13.3 hr	3-5 mCi (111-185 MBq)	0.5-1 hr	rCBF
^{99m}Tc-HMPAO	140	6 hr	20 mCi (740 MBq)	0.25-3 hr	rCBF
^{99m}Tc-ECD	140	6 hr	20 mCi (740 MBq)	2-3 hr	rCBF

unwanted uptake, pretreatment with potassium perchlorate ($KClO^4$), given orally 1 hour before the pertechnetate administration, is required. An adult dose of 0.75 to 1.0 g or a children's dose of 50 mg per year of age to a maximum of 750 mg, is usually administered. Neither of the ^{99m}Tc-labeled chelates, DTPA or GHA, concentrate in the choroid plexus and salivary glands; in addition, neither labels red blood cells in the presence of excess stannous ion in patients who received ^{99m}Tc labeled stannous phosphonate for a bone image before the administration of the ^{99m}Tc pertechnetate.

Although the ^{99m}Tc-labeled phosphonates have been used nearly exclusively for skeletal imaging, they have been shown to concentrate in cerebral infarcts. Thallous-201 chloride has demonstrated cerebral metastases and gallium-67 citrate has been used selectively to localize inflammatory and neoplastic brain lesions.

Indications

1. Screening of patients suspected of having primary and metastatic brain tumors.
2. Evaluation of patients with cerebrovascular accidents (CVA).
3. Evaluation of and monitoring cerebral infectious disease.
4. Evaluation of head trauma (i.e., subdural hematomas).
5. Evaluation of patients with suspected arteriovenous malformations (AVMs).
6. Following patients after neurosurgery, radiotherapy, or chemotherapy of brain lesions.
7. Evaluation of patients with unexplained neurologic symptoms.
8. Evaluation of intracerebral inflammatory/degenerative diseases (i.e., AIDS, multiple sclerosis, collagen diseases).

Procedure

Materials

1. Scintillation camera
2. Low-energy all-purpose collimator (LEAP)
3. Lead cape

Continued.

4. A suitable apparatus to deliver a radiopharmaceutical bolus injection followed by a rapid saline flush
5. Non–BBB-penetrating radiopharmaceutical (NOTE—The radiopharmaceutical should be in a small volume with a specific activity suitable for rapid administration).
6. Head-restraining device: a velcro band, head immobilizer, or tape

Patient preparation

1. Signed order for study.
2. Explain the entire procedure to the patient.
3. Allow for proper time lapse between imaging stages (Table 22-1).

Technique

1. Peak scintillation camera for technetium-99m.
2. Select proper camera orientation.
3. Determine proper intensity setting for the imager, or set up computer acquisition parameters.

Cerebral radionuclide angiogram (flow study)

4. Position the patient for the following:
   A. An *anterior* flow study with the patient's head at the collimator surface. Correct alignment is maintained if the canthomeatal line is perpendicular to the collimator face. Proper use of a head restraint device ensures that no movement occurs during the acquisition. Take care to eliminate side-to-side rotation of the head while positioning the patient.
   B. A *vertex* flow study with the patient either sitting or supine and the head hyperextended to reduce body background. Use a lead cape to further reduce the body and neck background in the image. Align the collimator so that the infraorbital meatal line is parallel to the collimator surface.
5. Inject the patient using a rapid bolus injection followed by a rapid saline flush. Begin imaging when the radioactivity first appears on the persistence scope.
6. Collect two seconds per frame preset timed images for 60 to 120 seconds on film and/or into a computer.
7. After completing the flow study, take a single static image (300,000-count) before releasing the patient.
8. Start the planar equilibrium images 20 minutes to 1 hour postinjection of the radiopharmaceutical (Table 22-1). Take images for 300,000 counts for a standard–field-of-view camera, and 500,000 counts for a large–field-of-view camera in each of the following projections. Images may also be acquired by collecting the anterior view and by acquiring additional equilibrium views for the time required to obtain the anterior image.

Anterior—Position the patient either sitting or supine with the forehead and nose at the face of the collimator, and the head flexed slightly in the anterior position. Take care to exclude as much facial activity as practical and to ensure that side-to-side rotation of the head does not occur. Appropriate use of a head immobilizer may accomplish this.

Posterior—Position the patient sitting or supine with the head flexed anteriorly and the median plane perpendicular to the collimator surface. Rotate the camera slightly anterior so that the posterior fossa is well visualized. Take care to minimize rotation of the head.

Right and left lateral—Position patient sitting or supine, with the patient's head flexed anteriorly to reduce as much facial activity as possible in the image. The sagittal plane of the patient's head is parallel with the detector surface.

Vertex—Position the patient sitting or supine with the collimator above the head and the canthomeatal line parallel to the collimator surface. Shield shoulder and neck activity with the lead cape. Position the patient's head with the canthomeatal line centered in the field of view and equal exposure of both cerebral hemispheres.

Special Views:

A. *Orbital*—Obtain the orbital view by positioning the patient with the forehead at the collimator surface and the canthomeatal line at a 25-degree angle to the vertical axis of the camera.

B. *Magnification*—Magnified images may be required in suspected posterior fossa lesions. This may be accomplished by positioning a pinhole collimator over the area of interest or by using the magnification features available with the newer-generation camera systems.

Interpretation

Disorders demonstrable by planar brain imaging may develop external from the scalp to the cerebral cortex. Changes in regional vascularity and local factors that affect the tissue binding of radiopharmaceuticals are important in their extracortical uptake, and usually their exact localization cannot be differentiated by imaging. Traumatic scalp lesions (cephalhematoma) are usually diagnosed by inspection and palpation, when seen on the brain image these will usually resolve in 10 to 14 days on a repeat brain image. Cranial lesions such as metastases, fibrous dysplasia, and Paget's disease may be differentiated from superficial cortical lesions by using bone-seeking radiopharmaceuticals (^{99m}Tc-MDP, ^{99m}Tc-HDP).

Of the brain tumors, high-grade gliomas (glioblastoma multiforme), meningiomas, and cerebral metastases are consistently detected by planar imaging because of their intense radiopharmaceutical uptake on both the radionuclide flow (perfusion) and equilibrium images. Because of the lesion variations in their blood supply, delayed imaging may be required to detect certain metastatic brain tumors (Fig. 22-6). Many low-grade gliomas, pituitary tumors, and brain-stem tumors go undetected by planar brain imaging even if longer equilibration is permitted. Brain tumors in children are frequently located in the posterior fossa with a predilection for the midline; these produce a characteristic pattern on the posterior and lateral equilibrium brain images.

Cerebrovascular diseases may be congenital, spontaneous, or traumatic. A congenital berry aneurysm can rupture, producing a catastrophic subarachnoid or intercerebral hemorrhage. The lesion is rarely detected by brain imaging. Arteriovenous malformation (AVM) in contrast produces a characteristic flow pattern while the equilibrium images may be normal or positive, depending on local cortical damage due to the leakage of red cells into surrounding brain tissue.

Spontaneous cerebral thrombosis is the pathogenesis of most strokes (65%) and usually involves the middle cerebral artery and its branches alone or in combination with other cerebral arteries in

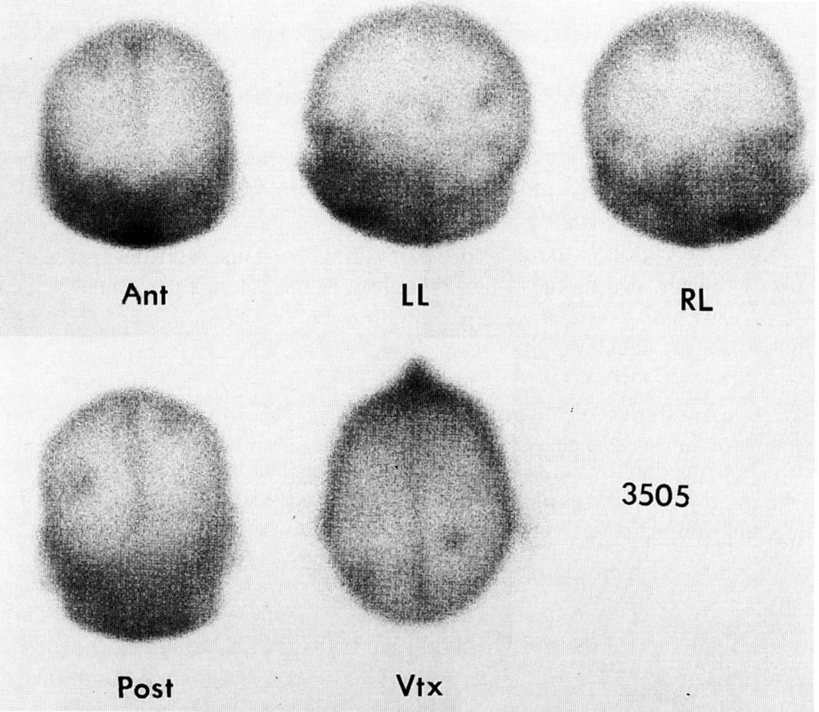

Fig. 22-6. Several irregularly shaped foci of increased uptake in both cerebral hemispheres of a patient with lung cancer. Cerebral metastases show variable intensities and locations.

Continued.

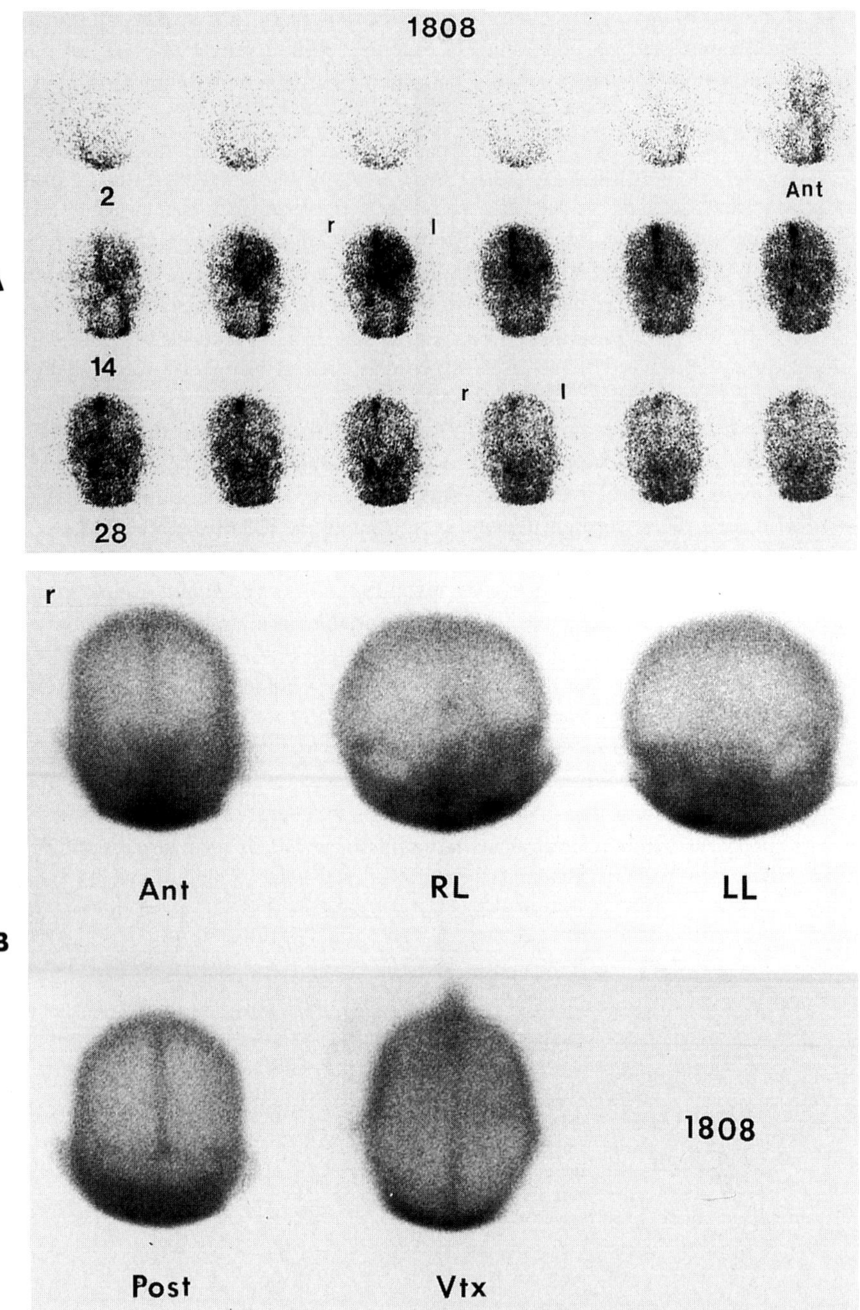

Fig. 22-7. A, Anterior 2 second sequential cerebral perfusion images of a patient with the recent (5 days) onset of left-sided hemiplegia. Initial decrease in right middle cerebral artery (RMCA) with subsequent "flip flop" indicating collateral flow. **B,** Equilibrium images (anterior, posterior, vertex, and laterals) of stroke patient demonstrate subtle increased activity in mid temporal region only on the right lateral view.

80% of the affected patients. The discordant finding of regional ischemia on the flow (perfusion) study and a normal multiview equilibrium brain image during the first 2 weeks following the insult is characteristic of a stroke (Fig. 22-7). Conversion of the equilibrium image to an abnormal image with regional increased uptake within a week or less of the insult suggests cerebral embolism as the pathogenesis.

The chronic subdural hematoma (more than 2 weeks old) is readily detected by planar brain imaging (greater than 83% detection accuracy). The neomembrane forms around the hemorrhage; it is the principal site of the radiopharmaceutical concentration and produces a crescent abnormality on the anterior and posterior brain-image views.

Of the inflammatory lesions, brain abscesses are the most consistently detected with planar brain imaging. Greater than 90% of brain abscesses are demonstrable by imaging and are more apt to be visualized when imaging is delayed for 3 hours or longer. A doughnut sign (lesion with central clearing) may be seen and when monitoring the effectiveness of therapy of an abscess with brain imaging, a 3- to 7-day lag in the image resolution may occur compared to the clinical improvement. Granulomas of the brain react like avascular tumors and usually go undetected on the delayed equilibrium planar brain image. Degenerative brain lesions such as those with multiple sclerosis may, even during an acute exacerbation, give a completely normal planar brain image; at other times, however, when clinical symptoms are absent the brain image is grossly abnormal. A similar paradox may occur following therapy. Cerebral atrophy or dementias such as Alzheimer's disease generally give normal planar brain images. Single-photon emission computed tomography (SPECT), positron emission tomography (PET), x-ray computed tomography (CT), and magnetic resonance imaging (MRI) have replaced planar brain images in these conditions.

Cystic lesions are demonstrated indirectly by planar brain imaging by producing "supernormal" negative defects, depending on their size. CT has replaced radionuclide brain imaging for detecting cystic lesions. In special circumstances such as in children with a Dandy-Walker cyst of the fourth ventricle, the brain image may have screening value since it produces an unusual tenting configuration of the torcular and the transverse sinuses (cyclops sign) on the posterior projection.

LABORATORY APPLICATION

66

SINGLE-PHOTON EMISSION COMPUTED TOMOGRAPHY (SPECT) BRAIN IMAGING (SINGLE-CRYSTAL)

Background

With the increasing clinical utility of CT and MRI, it has become essential to understand the tomographic anatomy of the brain. Tomography has now become such an integral part of radionuclide imaging in SPECT and PET that a brief review is in order. The tomographic anatomy of the brain is generally presented in one or more of three orthogonal planes; transverse, coronal, and sagittal (Fig. 22-8). Sections from the transverse plane begin at the anterior (facial) brain and proceed to the posterior (back of the head); they are perpendicular to the midline falx cerebri. The plane and angle it assumes (15-degree anterior-posterior tilt with CT; parallel with the orbitomeatal line in MRI, SPECT and PET) may vary but the orientation of the transverse projection appear as if one is looking up at the hemispheres from below. Therefore, on the SPECT and PET transverse section im-

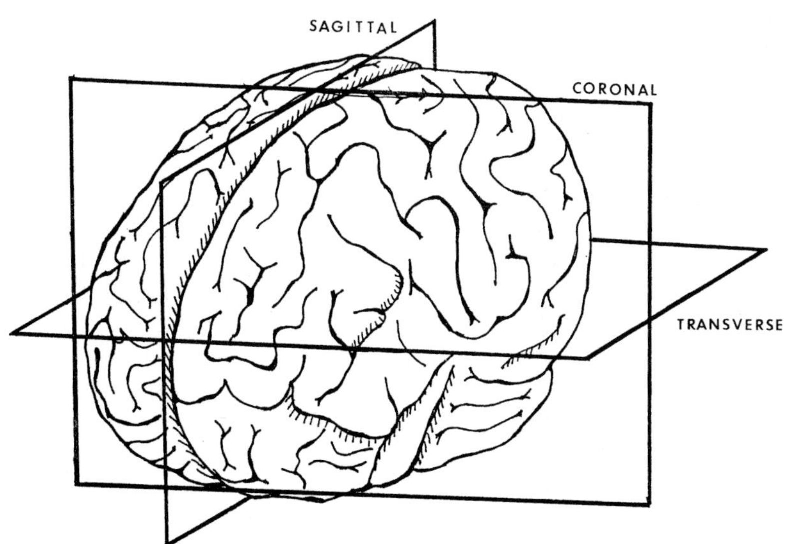

Fig. 22-8. Cerebral coronal, sagittal, and transverse planes.

Continued.

ages, the front (anterior) of the brain is at the top while the left side of the brain is on the viewer's right. The diencephalon and substructural anatomy of the hemispheres are well visualized in this plane; most clinical interpretations are made from the transverse sections.

The coronal plane sections the brain from the anterior to the posterior and from the apex (top) of the head to the base of the brain in a plane that is perpendicular to the transverse plane. The sections display the cortex in its short axis and encompass both hemispheres and the basilar brain structures on a single slice. It is probably the best plane to assess the symmetry of low hemisphere and basilar brain abnormalities.

The sagittal plane produces tomographic sections from the anterior to the posterior and from one side to the other across the midline. It is perpendicular to both the transverse and coronal planes and best describes the ventricular system in nearly its entirety parallel to the midline. The plane bisects the basilar structures near the midline and is the only view on the SPECT or PET images that evaluates the brain stem.

Purpose

Radiopharmaceuticals that normally diffuse into the brain obscure defects on routine planar imaging and require tomographic scintillation imaging to demonstrate brain structure. Commonly employed CT and MRI have exploited tomography and have increased the diagnostic accuracy in practically all neurologic diseases. The concomitant use of PET and SPECT has capitalized on their superior anatomic description by the registration (direct comparison) of the two types of images to the scintigraphic images.

Single-photon emission computed tomography images of the brain are produced from count data collected from an Anger camera, which rotates around the circumference of the patient's head. The 360-degree raw data are processed on a computer that reconstructs the data into three orthogonal planes. These planes display cerebral lesions in three dimension, increasing the sensitivity of the SPECT brain images over the planar images. A variety of SPECT imaging systems are available, from the single-head rotating Anger camera to the multihead rotating camera. Regardless of the imaging system employed, however, several data-collection parameters must be optimized to obtain high-quality tomographic brain images.

Radiopharmaceutical

The second type of gamma-emitting radiopharmaceuticals normally cross (penetrate) the intact blood-brain barrier and diffusely distribute throughout the cerebral cortex relative to regional cerebral blood flow (rCBF) (Table 22-1). Xenon-133 is an inert gas that, when dissolved in saline or breathed, is transported in the blood to the brain and quickly diffuses into the cerebral cortex. Once in the brain, it rapidly clears multiexponentially; its rate of clearance is used to calculate rCBF in ml/100 g/min. Its principal limitation is its low gamma photon energy (81 keV) that reduces its detection accuracy at depth. Specialized tomographic imaging equipment, however, has eliminated this problem.

Iodine-123 iodoamphetamine (IMP) and its analog ^{123}I-HIPDM give similar brain distributional patterns on SPECT imaging. Limitation in the pharmacokinetics of the iodine-123 iodoamphetamines are their relatively short brain retention (cortical clearance $t_{1/2}$ = 1.5 to 2.0 h) and redistribution. Redistribution appears to occur from the initial high lung uptake (about 30%) pool and may be a means to detect cerebral ischemia and image remaining viable metabolically intact cerebral tissue. Unfortunately, ^{123}I-IMP and ^{123}I-HIPDM are no longer commercially available in the United States. Tc-99m-d,l-hexamethyl propylene amine oxime (HMPAO or Ceretec™) is the first neutral-charged lipophilic ^{99m}Tc chelate with prolonged cortical retention ($t_{1/2}$ = > 6 h). It has been used successfully in clinical neuro-SPECT imaging. However, its major limitation is its in vitro instability. Significant decomposition of lipophilic ^{99m}Tc-HMPAO to a hydrophobic species occurs within 30 minutes following reconstitution; however, this can be avoided if the radiopharmaceutical is administered immediately after preparation. Recently, a cyclic diaminodithiol derivative labeled with ^{99m}Tc has been introduced as a rCBF radiotracer. Tc-99m-oxo-1,1-N,N′-ethylenediylbis-d,d-cysteinediethyl ester (^{99m}Tc-ECD) distributes intracerebrally similar to ^{99m}Tc-HMPAO but has shorter brain retention. It is a stable compound, and studies have indicated that it too may have excellent clinical utility. FDA approval of ECD (Neurolite™) for routine use is anticipated in the near future.

Indications

1. Evaluation of cerebrovascular diseases (i.e., infarction, hemorrhage, TIAs).
2. Evaluation of neuropsychiatric disorders including dementias.
3. Evaluation of head trauma (acute and chronic).
4. Evaluation of convulsive disorders.
5. Assessment of cognitive functions.

SPECT acquisition parameters

Exemplary quality-control procedures are essential for producing high-quality brain images. SPECT quality-control procedures have been previously discussed in Chapter 14 and will therefore only be highlighted in this discussion.

Several quality-control technical factors will influence the quality of SPECT brain images, whether they are obtained from a single-head system or a multihead system. First, small differences in regional nonuniformities, when amplified through the reconstruction process, can produce ring artifacts in the final brain images. Multiple-detector systems in particular require very careful calibration because uniformity should be matched for all heads.

Second, a shift in center of rotation will result in loss of resolution and may introduce artifacts in the final images.

Third, accurate calibration of pixel size is important for many of the commercially available attenuation correction packages.

Regardless of the camera system employed, quality control in advance of data collection is essential if reproducible, high-quality tomographic brain images are to be obtained. A rigorous quality-control program that includes the assessment of a SPECT phantom containing the radionuclide to be used clinically, as well as accurate measurements of uniformity and resolution, must be employed. Phantom data collection parameters that optimize resolution and still provide practical clinical application should be implemented. Patient images should be acquired with the same collimator used for the quality-control analysis. Point-source data may add in the determination of an adequate number of azmiths in the collection.

The collection of the SPECT brain image is characterized by a compromise between optimizing the technical acquisition components required to produce a high-quality image, and the comfort limitations and compliance of the patient being imaged. An important technical factor in the acquisition of high-resolution brain images is the pixel size of the collection matrix. Generally, increasing the size of the collection matrix will increase the resolution of the image, but it may also increase the statistical noise associated with each pixel if sufficient counts are not available in the acquisition process. Although large matrix sizes are certainly consistent with the spatial resolution of newer-generation gamma cameras, they may necessitate an increase in imaging times to collect sufficient data to keep statistical noise at an acceptable level. Typically 64 × 64 and 128 × 128 matrices have been used with most single-head imaging systems. While the 128 × 128 matrix provides smaller pixel size, it necessitates a fourfold increase in computer storage, an increase in processing time, and may reduce the statistical significance of the data in each pixel. Matrix selection should incorporate the most detail while allowing the least amount of noise to contribute to the image.

As an alternative, quality brain images may be obtained with a single-head SPECT system by collecting the raw data using a 64 × 64 magnified image that approximates a 128 × 128 pixel size. Typically the enhancement required to accomplish this approximation with a single-head system is on the order of 1.5 to 2.0 magnification. Using the smaller matrix reduces the need for computer storage and saves processing time while producing good image resolution with adequate count densities.

In multihead SPECT systems the count densities of the individual pixels may be less of an issue because of the increased number of counts collected without requiring an increase in the collection times. In these systems, larger matrices may be used to produce the desired higher resolution, without fear of statistical noise in the pixels. Magnification may also be employed to produce a desirable pixel size.

One could reason that the greater the number of angles sampled in a rotation the better the reconstruction. Patient tolerance for the imaging procedure and the number of counts required for each projection, however, limit the number of angles sampled. For the single-head systems, thirty-two

Continued.

angular samples are insufficient to obtain high-quality brain images; 128 angles may be unnecessary because of the statistics associated with the clinical data and the patient compliance time. Sixty-four projections per rotation provide adequate data, realistic acquisition time, and patient tolerance for single-head SPECT brain imaging. When using multihead systems, because of the increase in the total number of counts contributing to the final image, increases in the number of angles sampled *may* be obtained without compromising the count densities or increasing the total imaging time for the acquisition. Sixty-four angles, however, are usually sufficient to sample the brain.

As with planar imaging, the theory that the highest number of counts contributes to a high-quality final image applies to SPECT imaging. In the ideal situation, statistically abundant data would be collected at each projection, several practical aspects such as the radiopharmaceutical dosage (available count rate), patient comfort, and patient immobility must be considered. The evaluation of the patient endurance (in projected time) divided by the number of projections needed provides a general guide for brain SPECT acquisition determinations. This calculation must include a realistic assessment of the patient's ability to remain immobile and the optimum acquisition time calculated from the count rate, matrix size, angular sampling, and statistical significance.

Minimizing the source to detector distance is critical to the resolution of the final SPECT image. This distance creates a special problem in SPECT brain imaging because of the limits created by the patient's shoulder width. The shoulders can add as much as 10 cm to the orbit in a fixed-orbit, single-crystal system, which can have a deleterious effect on image resolution. In an attempt to reduce this distance and optimize the activity detected from the patient's head, a number of specialized detector/collimator designs have been introduced as alternatives for SPECT brain imaging. Among these alternatives are the 30-degree slant-hole collimator; the fanbeam collimator, which allows the camera to receive a greater number of counts from the head; and the camera systems in which a portion of the detector head is recessed to allow for closer patient alignment. With multihead systems, collimators with improved resolution and consequently decreased sensitivity may be used to produce high-quality images.

Imaging parameters may be further improved by using an imaging table with a narrow cephalic extension to accommodate the patient's head. A nonattenuating restraint placed over the forehead helps to ensure immobilization during the acquisition while minimizing discomfort. Care should be taken to position the head with reference to the planes of the reconstructed images; also, minimizing head rotation and chin tilt will be of benefit to the final image quality. Laser positioning is helpful for reproducibility of patient positioning.

Processing

Computer processing of the brain SPECT raw data depends not only on the imaging system but on the computer software used for data collection, and should be thoroughly evaluated on phantom data before clinical implementation. The three-dimensional images are constructed by employing a filtered backprojection technique to the raw data to produce quality, low-noise images. An infinite number of preprocessing, backprojection, and postprocessing filter combinations can be used to produce the final three-dimensional planes. Preprocessing filters apply a two-dimensional filter to the planar data acquired in each projection before the reconstruction; preprocessing filters produce a smoothing effect on the images. Reconstruction filters range from the simple backprojection techniques (e.g., ramp filter) that allow the contribution of high-frequency noise to the final image, to filters that drastically smooth the image and potentially mask defects. Postprocessing filters also smooth the images, but apply the filter in three dimensions to the reconstructed image.

Procedure single head SPECT

Materials

1. Rotating gamma camera
2. Low-energy, parallel-hole collimator, or special high-resolution brain collimator, as applicable
3. Dedicated computer system with software capable of single-photon emission computed tomography (SPECT) acquisition and reconstruction
4. BBB-penetrating and/or BBB-nonpenetrating radiopharmaceuticals
5. SPECT imaging table with head extension
6. Nonattenuating head restraint device such as a velcro strip or tape

Patient preparation

1. Signed order for study.
2. Explain the entire procedure to the patient.
3. Allow for a proper time lapse between this and other nuclear medicine procedures.
4. Inject the patient in a quiet, low-lit room. Start image acquisition 0.25 to 3.0 hours postinjection (Table 22-1).

Computer acquisition parameters

1. Use a 128 × 128 or 64 × 64 matrix with a magnification factor.
2. 64 projections per rotation acquisition
3. Allow sufficient time to acquire 200,000 counts per projection, or greater.
4. 360-degree rotation

Camera acquisition parameters

1. 64 projections per rotation (PPR) acquisition
2. 360 degree rotation. Acquisition may begin from several positions, but the most common starting acquisition site is the anterior or lateral view.
3. Magnification to approximate the 128 × 128 matrix as applicable. Note: Magnification may be accomplished through the camera or the computer.

Technique

1. Position the patient supine on the imaging table with the head toward the gantry.
2. Secure the patient's head with a nonattenuating substance such as a velcro restraint or bandage tape, making sure that no rotation of the head occurs.
3. Make the patient as comfortable as possible to ensure a minimum of movement during the procedure, and solicit the patient's cooperation.
4. Center the head in the field of view in the anterior, posterior, and lateral projections. The collimator should be positioned as close to the patient's head as possible. Complete a 360-degree test rotation to ensure adequate clearance of all structures by the collimator.
5. Begin the acquisition from the anterior or lateral projection. Complete a 360-degree acquisition.
6. Stay with the patient throughout the entire procedure to make sure that no movement occurs and that an appropriate distance between the collimator and all other objects is maintained.
7. Reconstruct the data according to a predetermined protocol supported by phantom data.

Multicrystal SPECT

Materials

1. Rotating multicrystal gamma camera
2. Low-energy, parallel-hole collimator, special high-resolution brain collimator, or fanbeam collimator, as available
3. Dedicated computer system with software capable of single-photon emission computed tomography (SPECT) acquisition and reconstruction
4. BBB penetrating and/or nonpenetrating radiopharmaceuticals
5. SPECT-imaging table with head extension
6. Nonattenuating head restraint device, such as a velcro strip or tape

Patient preparation

1. Signed order for study.
2. Explain the entire procedure to the patient.
3. Allow a proper time lapse between this and other nuclear medicine procedures.
4. Inject the patient in a quiet, low-lit room. Image acquisition is begun 0.25 to 3 hours postinjection (Table 22-1).

Computer acquisition parameters

1. Matrix size: 128 × 128 or 64 × 64 magnified as applicable to achieve appropriate pixel size
2. 64 projections per rotation acquisition

Continued.

3. Allow sufficient time to acquire adequate counting statistics.
4. 360-degree rotation

Camera acquisition parameters

1. 64 projections per rotation (PPR) acquisition
2. 360 degree rotation. Acquisition may begin from several positions, but the most common starting acquisition site is the anterior or lateral view.

Technique

1. Position the patient supine on the imaging table with the head toward the gantry.
2. Secure the patient's head with a nonattenuating substance such as a velcro restraint, ensuring that no rotation of the head occurs.
3. Make the patient as comfortable as possible to ensure a minimum of movement during the procedure, and solicit the patient's cooperation.
4. Center the head in the field of view in the anterior, posterior, and lateral projections. The collimator should be positioned as close to the patient's head as possible. Complete a 360-degree test rotation to ensure adequate clearance of all structures by the collimator. When employing a magnification, take care not to exclude any portion of the brain volume from the image.
5. Begin the acquisition from the anterior or lateral projection. Complete a 360-degree acquisition.
6. Stay with the patient throughout the entire procedure to make sure that no movement occurs and that an appropriate distance between the collimator and all other objects is maintained.
7. Reconstruct the data according to a predetermined protocol supported by phantom data.

Interpretation

Figure 22-9 is a 16-image sequence of the transverse tomographic sections of a normal ^{99m}Tc-HMPAO brain image. The basilar cuts demonstrate the cerebellum and inferior temporal lobes. Since gray matter has a higher rate of blood flow, it is well visualized while white matter, which has a low rate of flow, is not seen. The two hemispheres are relatively symmetrical as the sectioning continues to the top of the brain. Although many subcortical structures can be visualized, because of the rotating camera's limited resolution (1.4 cm) they are not sharply resolved. The coronal tomographic sections (Fig. 22-10) appear symmetrical from the anterior to the posterior aspect of the head. In

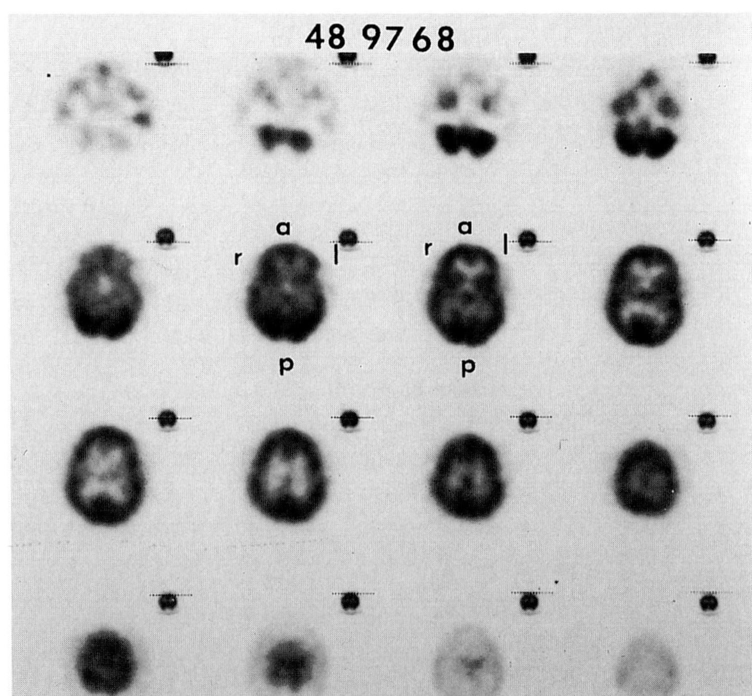

Fig. 22-9. Normal 2 pixel thick (6 mm) transverse tomographic slices of the ^{99m}Tc-HMPAO total brain volume of a patient with panic attacks. Grey matter with the highest flow shows the greatest activity and is generally symmetrical throughout the brain.

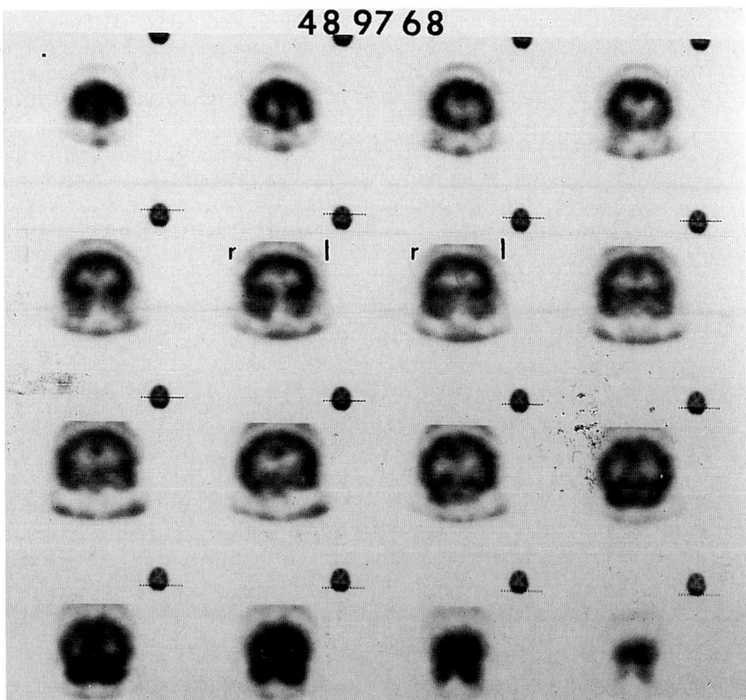

Fig. 22-10. Normal coronal tomographs of the ^{99m}Tc-HMPAO total brain volume demonstrating the cerebellum's higher activity.

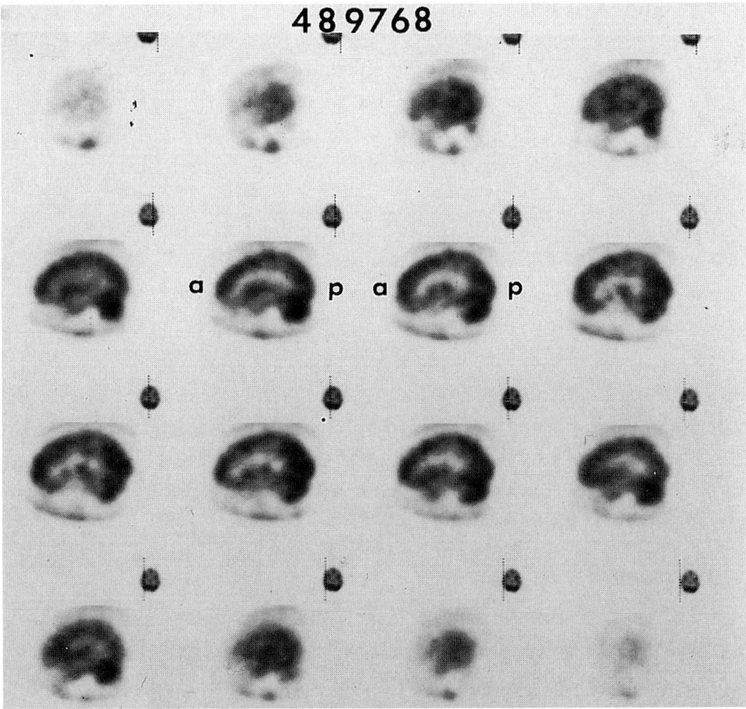

Fig. 22-11. Normal *sagittal* tomographs of the ^{99m}Tc-HMPAO total brain volume demonstrating the grey matter symmetry.

Continued.

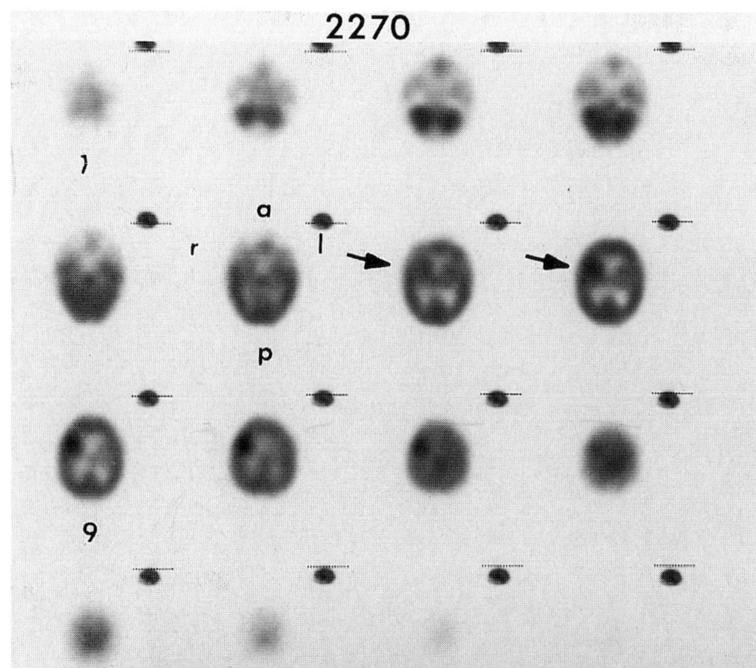

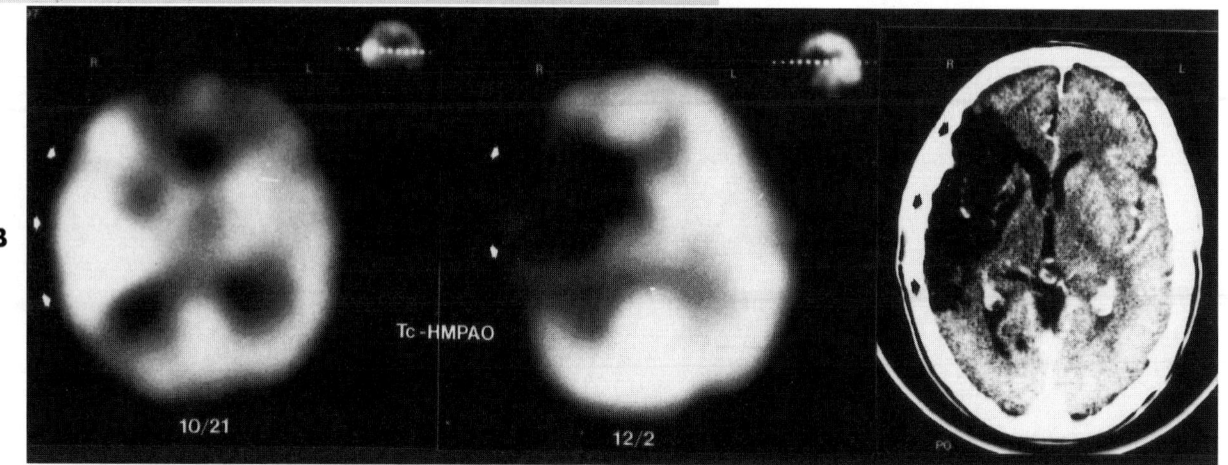

Fig. 22-12. **A,** Transverse tomographs of a patient with a right-sided hyperemic infarction and left-sided hemiparesis. **B,** Selected tomographs of the hyperemic infarct demonstrating its localization to the right anterotemporal region of the brain. The hyperemia converted to an ischemic infarct on repeat image 5 weeks later. (From Holmes, R.A.: Cerebral perfusion imaging, Curr. Opin. in Radiol. 2:863, 1990.)

addition to the hemispheres, both temporal lobes can be seen along with many basilar structures on the mid and caudal brain sections. In reconstructing the sagittal tomographic sections, we start from the left and progress to the right side (Fig. 22-11). The gray matter uptake on the sagittal section paramedially and at the midline assumes a spiraling configuration and also demonstrates the functional anatomy of the brain base.

Image diagnosis

Cerebrovascular disease has been the principal nervous system disorder studied with SPECT imaging and the newer lipophilic chelates. Early cerebral infarction is usually sharply demonstrated on the SPECT images while frequently going undetected or less well-defined on CT during the initial 2 weeks following the insult. Hyperemic infarction, "luxury perfusion," has consistently been demonstrated with SPECT brain imaging following infarction and appears to be quite common (Fig. 22-12). Transient ischemic attacks (TIAs) are frequently the forerunner of overt cerebral infarction (stroke); a method to detect it early on the regional cerebral blood flow (rCBF) study could more accurately predict the utility of neurovascular shunt surgery. To address the patient experiencing TIAs with a normal SPECT perfusion brain image, Diamox (acetazolamide), a potent cerebral va-

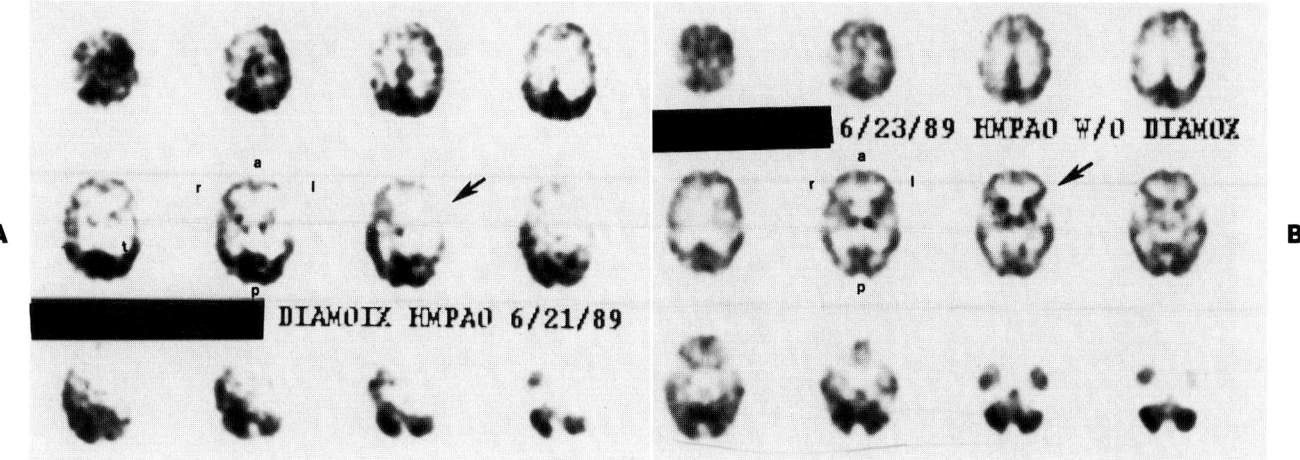

Fig. 22-13. A, A patient with TIA, normal bicarotid angiography and normal CT. Oral acetazolamide (Diamox) induced right and left hemisphere hypoperfusion with posterior brain shunting (reverse Robin Hood effect). **B,** Normal baseline HMPAO image of same patient. (From Holmes, R.A.: Cerebral perfusion imaging, Curr. Opin. Radiol. 2:863, 1990.)

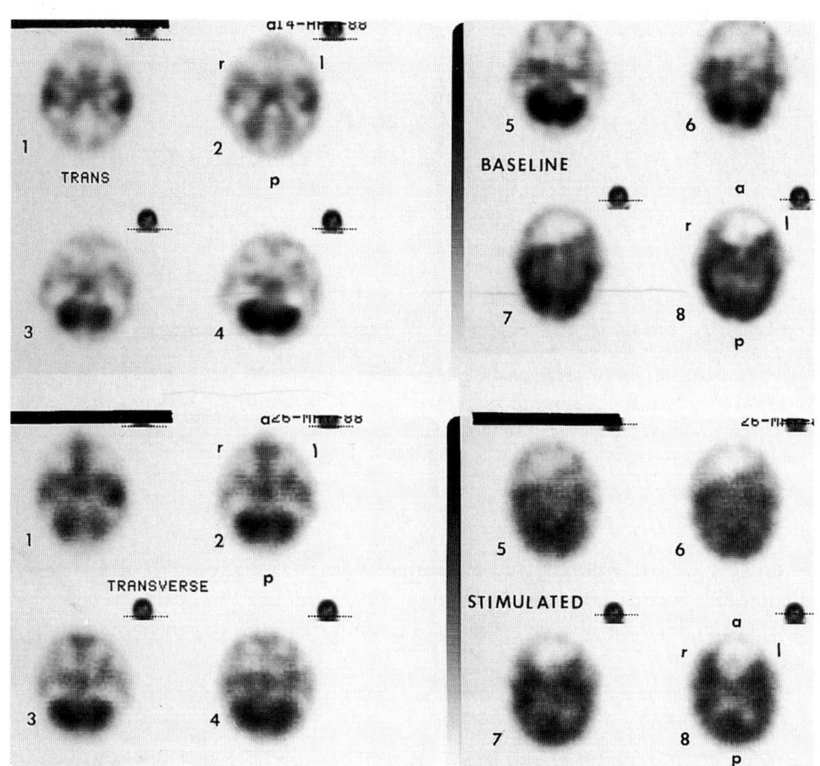

Fig 22-14. Partial frontal lobe symptoms. Baseline (*upper panel*) normal transverse tomographs using ^{99m}Tc-HMPAO. Following psychological stimulation (stress) midline frontal lobe activity is seen near the base of the brain (*lower panel*).

Continued.

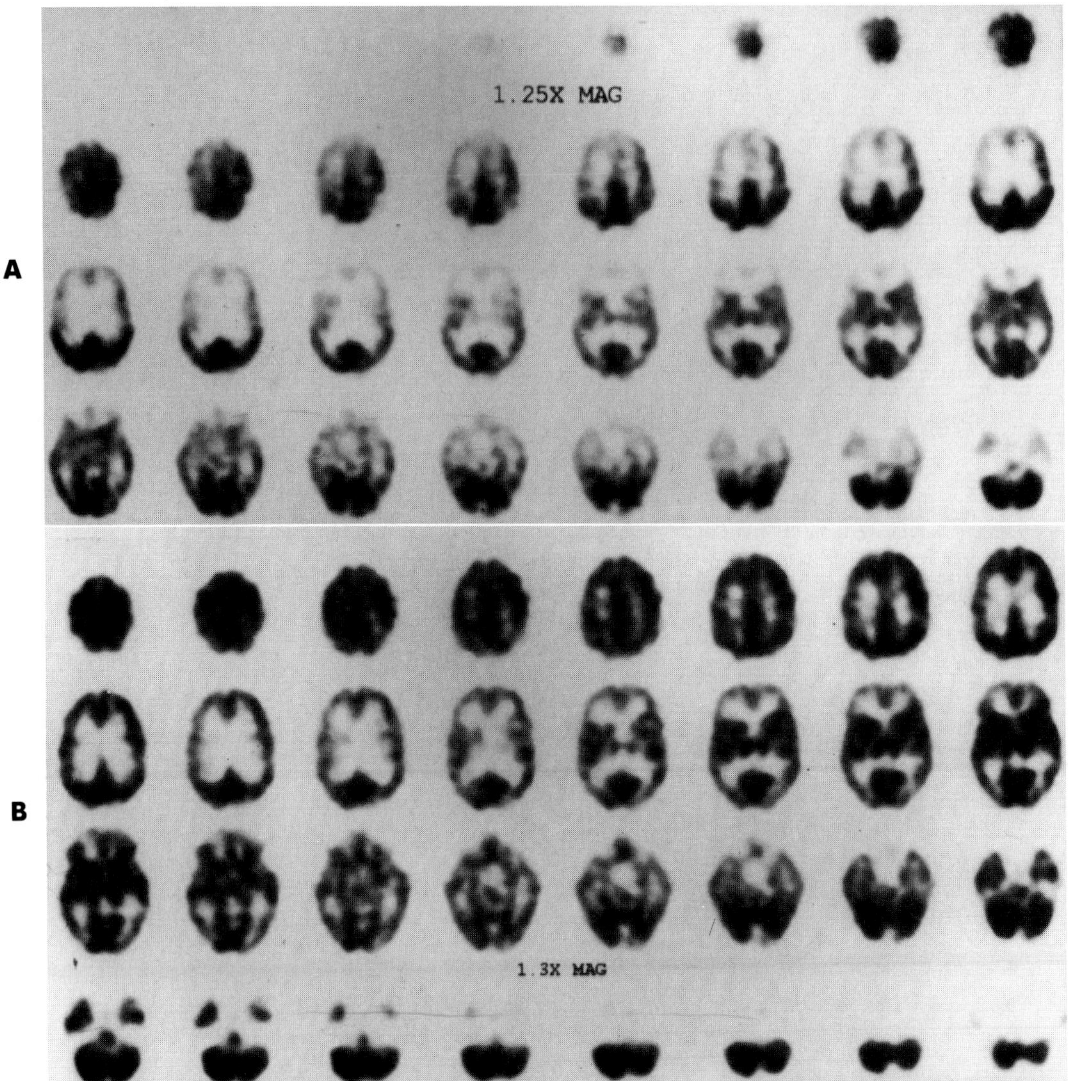

Fig. 22-15. A, Middle-aged, severely depressed patient demonstrating hypoperfusion of frontal lobes on Ceretec *transverse* SPECT images. **B,** After 6 weeks of amitriptyline therapy, mood improvement was accompanied by normal frontal lobes perfusion.

sodilator, can be administered to demonstrate the affected vascular area as regional decreased perfusion; the normal brain shows shunting and is referred to as the "reversed Robin Hood" effect (Fig. 22-13). Diamox can be given intravenously or orally (1.0 g) before the radiopharmaceutical is administered.

Alterations in rCBF have been seen on the SPECT brain image in acute head trauma. Although hemispheral lesions may be extensive, ultimate survival appears to rely on the maintenance of blood flow to the basilar brain and brain stem. The sagittal plane appears to be the most revealing view and has the greatest prognostic significance because it clearly shows the perfusion or lack of perfusion in the basilar brain structures. In chronic severe head trauma, patients may develop a posttraumatic syndrome that symptomatically mimics the "frontal lobe syndrome," and although the tomographic images are frequently normal, when the patient is psychologically stimulated hyperperfusion in the frontal lobe region has been observed (Fig. 22-14).

Other neuropsychiatric disorders (i.e., schizophrenia, manic depression, dementias) have been studied with neuro-SPECT with varying degrees of success. Depressive states frequently demonstrate frontal lobe hypoperfusion (Fig. 22-15). Differentiating dementias such as Alzheimer's dis-

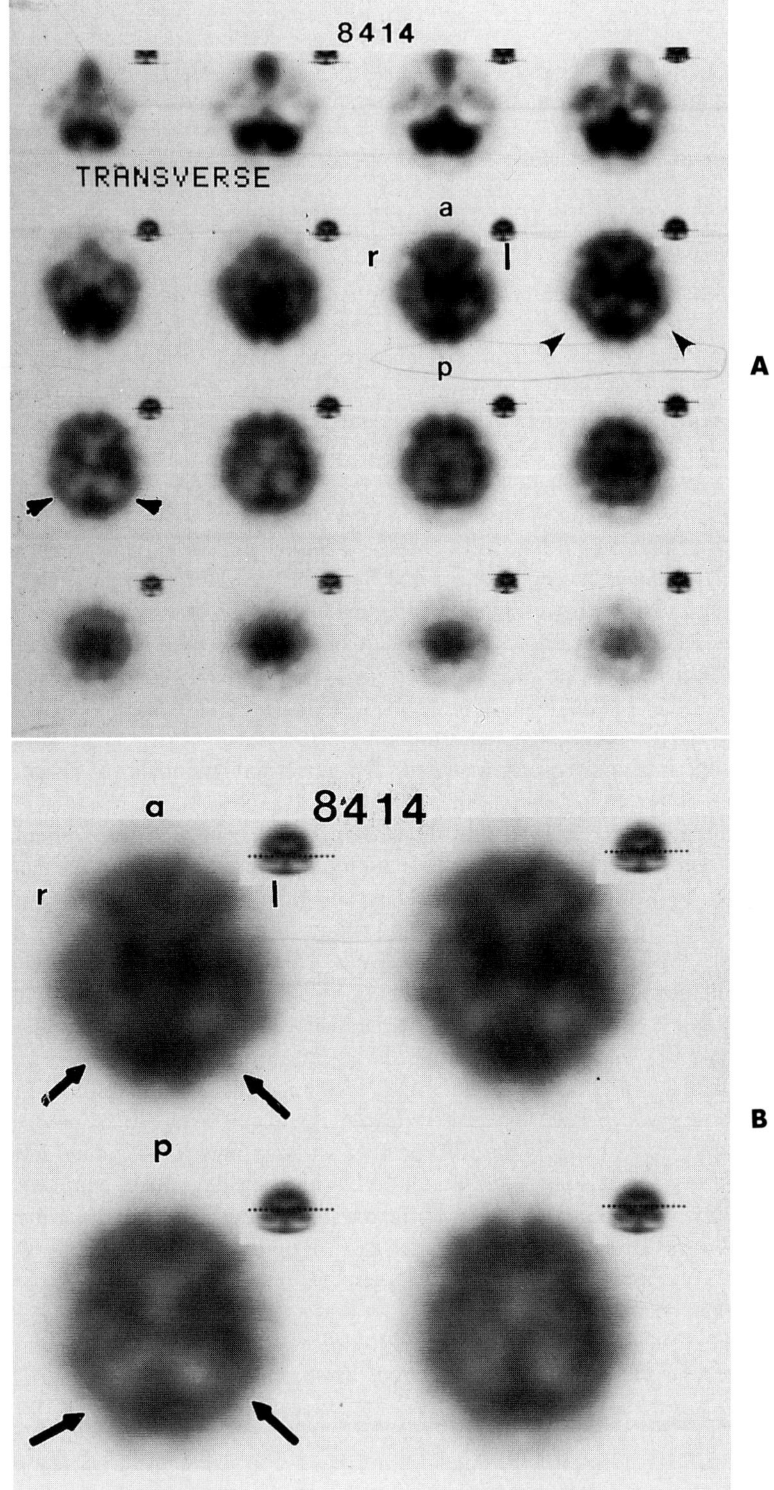

Fig. 22-16. A, Patient with documented Alzheimer's disease demonstrates a near-normal ^{99m}Tc-HMPAO transverse tomograph, except for decreased posterior lateral perfusion. **B,** Selected tomographic slices indicate the decreased perfusion is confined to the bitemporal-parietal areas.

Continued.

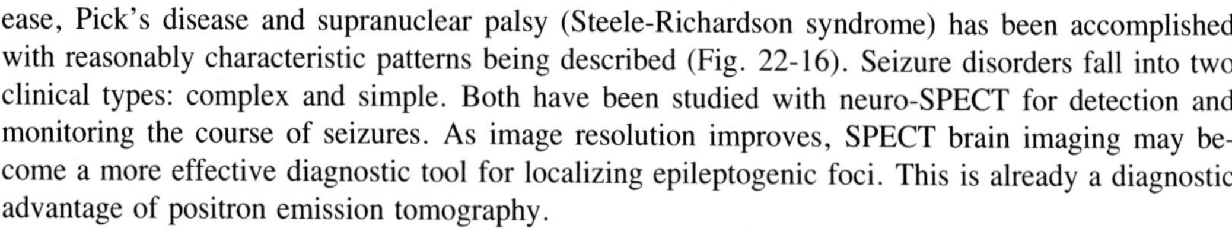
ease, Pick's disease and supranuclear palsy (Steele-Richardson syndrome) has been accomplished with reasonably characteristic patterns being described (Fig. 22-16). Seizure disorders fall into two clinical types: complex and simple. Both have been studied with neuro-SPECT for detection and monitoring the course of seizures. As image resolution improves, SPECT brain imaging may become a more effective diagnostic tool for localizing epileptogenic foci. This is already a diagnostic advantage of positron emission tomography.

LABORATORY APPLICATION

67

POSITRON EMISSION TOMOGRAPHY (PET)

Background

Although positron emission tomography is beyond the scope of routine clinical neuro imaging, the interest in PET imaging has increased to the point that a brief discussion is indicated. Positrons are cyclotron-produced radionuclides that decay by emitting a positively charged electron that interacts with a negatively charged electron in the tissue, forming two 511-keV gamma photons that travel in opposite directions (180 degrees). Four positron radionuclides—carbon-11, nitrogen-13, oxygen-15 and fluorine-18—are used as the radionuclide in most PET imaging studies. All have very short physical half-lives: C-11 – $t_{1/2}$ = 10.4m; N-13 – $t_{1/2}$ = 9.96m; 0-15 – $t_{1/2}$ = 124s; F-18 – $t_{1/2}$ = 109.9m, and require rapid radiosynthesis into compounds that can be used to evaluate a variety of physiologic functions. Since the majority of these compounds are identical to materials normally found in the body (e.g., 15-O_2-oxygen; 13-NH_4-ammonia; C-11-glucose), they give PET a distinct advantage over other imaging modalities. Because of its longer physical half-life, fluorine-18 is easier to synthesize into compounds and F-18-fluorodeoxyglucose (FDG), an analog of glucose, has been used extensively to assess regional cerebral glucose metabolism (CMR glu) because it is irreversibly trapped within the brain. O-15 as H_2 O-15 is used to measure rCBF while O_2-15 can be used to measure oxygen consumption.

PET imaging requires a source of positron radionuclides (an on-site cyclotron), a rapid synthesizer of positron radiopharmaceuticals, and a positron tomographic imaging system. Unlike the rotating-head SPECT camera, the PET imager is constructed in a circular array of scintillation crystals with coincidence electronics that eliminate the need for mechanical collimation to produce spatially high-resolution tomographic images. The patient's head is surrounded by the detectors; this results in greater sensitivity that is lacking in most SPECT systems. PET cameras are capable of producing images with 5- to 7-mm FWHM resolution. PET's accurate scatter correction allows absolute quantification of the image, giving PET a unique advantage over the relative quantitation that is possible with SPECT. The principal disadvantage of PET is its cost; the PET camera is priced in excess of 1 million dollars while the cyclotron and rapid radiopharmaceutical synthesizer cost an additional 1 to 2 million dollars. Less well appreciated is the million-dollar yearly cost for personnel and supplies to keep the center functioning. Until a means of patient payment for the studies is established, it is likely that PET studies will continue to be limited in number and clinical utility.

The principal diagnostic uses of PET imaging have been confined to assessing cerebral infarct metabolism and blood volume, differentiating depression from the dementias (e.g., multiinfarct, Alzheimer's disease), evaluating basal ganglia disorders (e.g., Parkinson's disease, Huntington's disease), pinpointing epileptogenic trigger sites in patients with intractable seizure disorders, determining the extent and recurrence of brain tumors, and quantifying the neuroreceptor binding of unique positron-labeled psycholeptic drugs to describe and monitor their therapeutic efficacy in mental disease. A variety of cognitive functions have also been described by PET imaging.

LABORATORY APPLICATION

68

CSF RADIONUCLIDE IMAGING

Purpose

Cerebrospinal fluid (CSF) is constantly produced by the choroid plexuses in the ventricular system of the brain, giving buoyancy to the brain. The hydrodynamics of CSF can only be assessed by determining its flow characteristics once isobaric and detectable compounds are instilled into the CSF and their course is mapped. Radionuclide cisternography is one of the most reliable techniques to assess CSF hydrodynamics, particularly in determining the patency of shunts or intraventricular blocks.

Radionuclide CSF imaging is accomplished by obtaining a series of planar views (anterior, posterior, and laterals) over several hours (routinely 2 to 48 hours). The radiopharmaceutical is administered by sterile, atraumatic, intrathecal injection. Appropriate radiopharmaceutical instillation is demonstrated by a short vertical line of activity in the spinal column immediately following the injection. The radiopharmaceutical is allowed to move with the cerebral spinal fluid, and the CSF dynamics are recorded by sequential planar image acquisition. Routine imaging times in the adult are at 2 hours, 6 hours, 24 hours, and 48 hours postinjection. Children are routinely imaged at 1 to 2 hours, 4 to 6 hours, 8 hours, and 24 hours postinjection. Slow movement may require imaging as long as 72 hours and even 96 hours postinstillation.

Radiopharmaceutical

The optimum CSF imaging radiopharmaceutical should: *(a)* not be metabolized while in the cerebrospinal fluid (CSF), *(b)* be lipid insoluble to prevent diffusion across tissue membranes, *(c)* clear rapidly from the blood, *(d)* be excreted primarily by the arachnoid villi, *(e)* be nonirritating, nonantigenic, and nonreactive when instilled intrathecally, *(f)* be molecularly diffusible throughout the CSF, *(g)* be easy to label with a gamma-photon–emitting radionuclide and *(h)* be nonpyrogenic and easy to sterilize. Although ^{99m}Tc human serum albumin is recommended for most shunt patency studies and in children in whom the CSF hydrodynamics are more rapid, its physical half-life of 6 hours discourages its use to no more than 24-hour imaging. ^{111}In-DTPA meets most of the criteria for the optimum agent and possesses an abundance of gamma photons at 173 and 247 keV with a 2.8d physical half-life. Since ytterbium (Yb)-169-DTPA is no longer commercially available, ^{111}In-DTPA is the preferred radiopharmaceutical for cisternography.

Indications

1. Assessment of normal and abnormal pathways of cerebral spinal fluid drainage.
2. Assessment of cerebral spinal fluid hydrodynamics.
3. Evaluation of shunting in hydrocephalus.
4. Assessment of shunt patency.
5. Diagnosis and localization of cerebral spinal fluid leaks such as in rhinorrhea and otorrhea.

Procedure

Materials

1. Scintillating camera
2. Medium-energy, parallel-hole collimator
3. Sterile lumbar puncture tray
4. 500 μCi (18.5 MBq) to 1 mCi (37 MBq) of ^{111}In-DTPA (adult)
5. Pledgets for diagnosis of CSF leaks, if appropriate

Patient preparation

1. Signed order for study.
2. Explain the entire procedure to the patient.
3. Allow a proper time lapse between nuclear medicine procedures.
4. Obtain a signed patient consent for intrathecal injection, this is required in most institutions.

Continued.

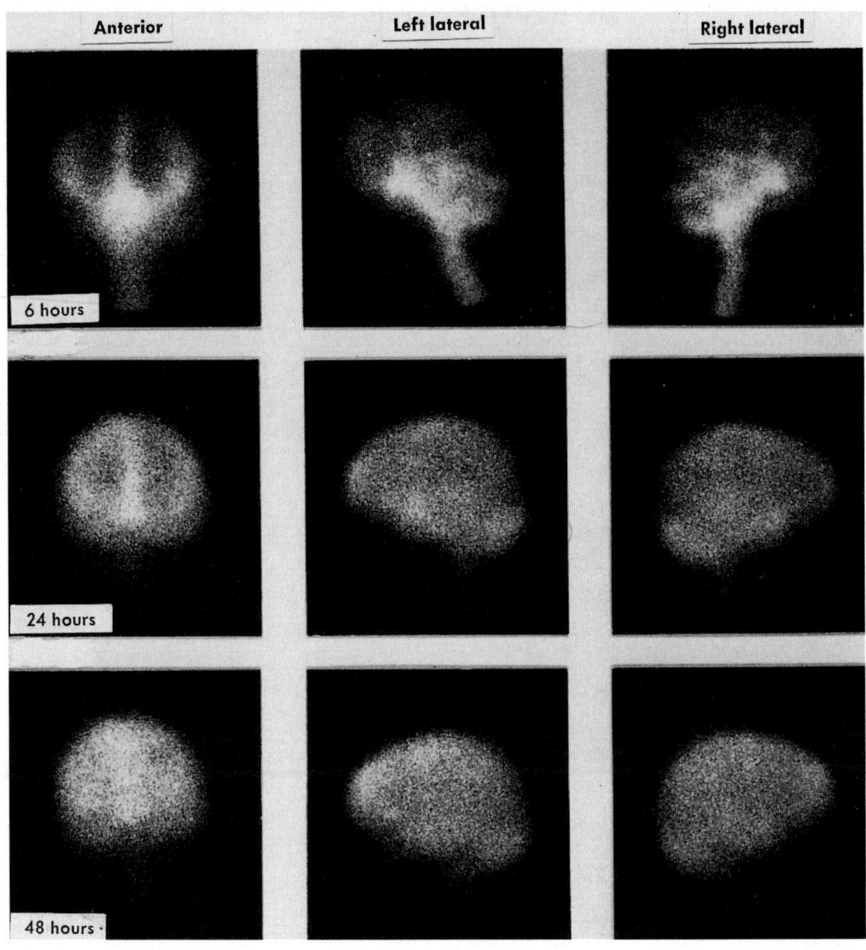

Fig. 22-17. Normal cisternography using In-111-DTPA. By 6 hours the agent has ascended into the basilar and middle cisterns without ventricular reflux. By 24 hours the agent begins to move over the free convexities. At 48 hours the agent starts to be absorbed at the superior sagittal sinus.

Technique

1. Position the patient in a supported fetal position. Under sterile preparation an atraumatic lumbar puncture is performed by the nuclear medicine physician (or he/she directly supervises its performance by qualified medical personnel).
2. Once the spinal needle is in place, attach a three-way stopcock to collect cerebrospinal fluid (CSF) samples, monitor the CSF pressure, and administer the radiopharmaceutical.
3. After delivering the radiopharmaceutical, remove, isolate, and shield the needle. Place a sterile Band-aid at the injection site.
4. Immediately after the radiopharmaceutical administration, obtain a 100,000-count image of the injection site to confirm the adequacy of the instillation.
5. The patient should remain recumbent, preferably supine, with the head positioned slightly lower than the hips for 1 to 2 hours postinjection.
6. In the adult, 100,000-count images (or 10 minutes per view) in the anterior, posterior, and both lateral views are routinely taken at 2, 6, 24, and 48 hours. Occasionally, images at 72 hours or longer may be required. Vertex views may be added at any time to clarify the findings. In children, routine images are taken between 1 and 2 hours, 4 and 6 hours, 8 hours, and 24 hours. Planar images are obtained using the same technique described previously for routine planar brain images. Cerebrospinal fluid leaks of the nose (rhinorrhea) and ear (otorrhea) may be evaluated by placing absorbent pledgets in the area suspected of leakage for an appropriate time period. The pledgets are removed and counted and compared with a pledget containing equal volume and weights of plasma sample. Such pledgets must be inserted by the physician before the radiopharmaceutical injection. Activity three to four times that of background indicates a significant leakage site.

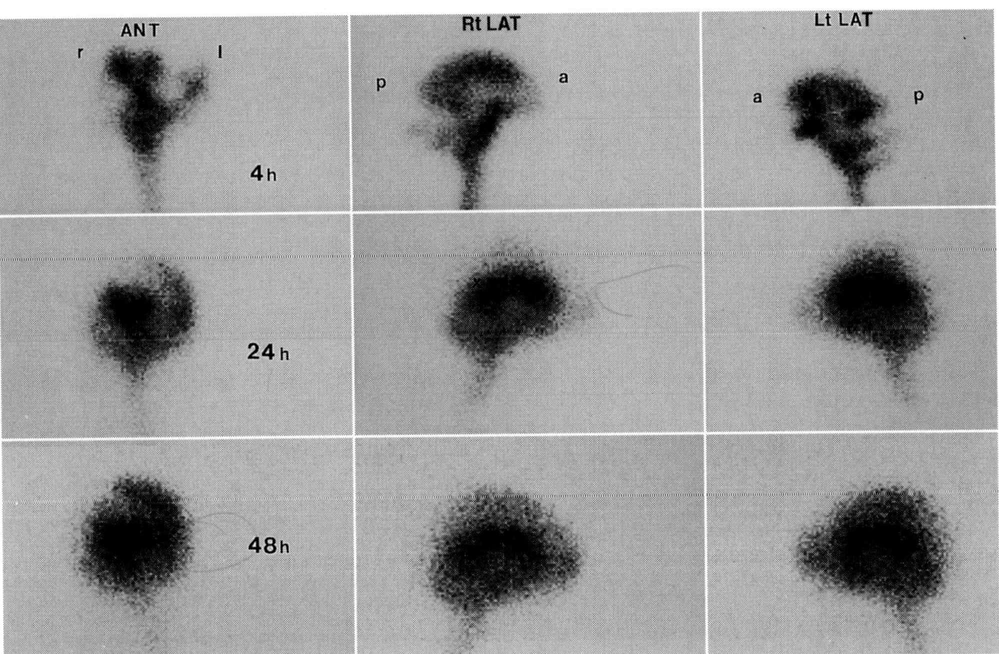

Fig. 22-18. A 60-year-old man with *normal pressure hydrocephalus* characterized by dystaxia, dementia, and urinary incontinence. The In-111-DTPA cisternogram demonstrates biventricular reflux and slow clearance over 48 hours.

Image diagnosis

Figure 22-17 is a normal multiview radionuclide cisternogram demonstrating the timed ascension of the lumbar-injected radiopharmaceutical. By 6 hours, the basilar and mid cisterns and temporal lobe activity are seen giving a "viking helmet" configuration on the anterior view. By 12 to 24 hours the activity extends over the free convexities of the hemispheres, and by 24 to 48 hours or longer it begins to cap along the superior sagittal sinus area. Besides the normal radionuclide cisternographic pattern, several others have been described: (1) slow CSF flow, (2) ventricular reflux (filling), (3) subarachnoid space blocks, (4) asymmetric CSF flow, and (5) focal CSF pooling. Slow CSF flow is frequently encountered with increasing age but is more evident with cerebral atrophy. Ventricular reflux is always abnormal in the adult and may be complete or incomplete with no or slow ventricular clearance. Subarachnoid blocks with or without pooling can occur anywhere along the spine, in the basal or mid cisterns, or over the cerebral convexities.

Hydrocephalus indicates a symmetric or asymmetric enlargement of the ventricles as a result of a pathologic increase in the volume of CSF with or without increased intracranial pressure. Hydrocephalus may be obstructive or nonobstructive. The obstructive forms are either communicating or noncommunicating while the nonobstructive forms, also called hydrocephalus *ex vacuo,* may be focal or generalized. A form of obstructive communicating hydrocephalus commonly occurring in middle-age males with normal CSF pressure and clinical dementia, ataxia, and urinary incontinence is of particular interest because an early diagnosis and shunting can correct the symptoms and restore the patient to normal. Figure 22-18 are the cisternographic images of a patient with normal pressure hydrocephalus (NPH) demonstrating retained ventricular reflux. The pathogenesis of NPH or the Hakim-Adams syndrome is unknown; however, many of those affected have had previous subarachnoid hemorrhage, head trauma, CNS infection, or a brain tumor.

To evaluate shunt patency, the radiopharmaceutical can be administered in a conventional manner or be instilled at either the source of the suspected obstruction or directly into the shunt reservoir. Appropriate timed images are then taken to determine the patency.

■ SPECIAL CENTRAL NERVOUS SYSTEM PROCEDURES

LABORATORY APPLICATION

69

BRAIN DEATH CONFIRMATION

Purpose

In cases in which a decision is needed to help confirm brain death of patients with unresponsive coma, fixed dilated pupils, apnea, absent cephalic reflexes, and/or isometric (silent) electroencephalogram, the intravenous bolus injection of ^{99m}Tc-pertechnetate or one of its analogs coupled with rapid sequential brain imaging can confirm absent cerebral perfusion and brain death.

Procedure

Materials

1. Venipuncture apparatus capable of delivering a rapid bolus injection
2. Low-energy, all-purpose collimator (LEAP)
3. Scintillation camera peaked for ^{99m}Tc
4. Radiopharmaceuticals that readily cross the intact blood-brain barrier.

Technique

1. Peak the scintillation camera for ^{99m}Tc and attach the LEAP collimator.
2. Select proper camera orientation. NOTE—This procedure is frequently performed at bedside; special attention should be made to the camera orientation selection).
3. Position the patient for the anterior view, with the patient head at the collimator surface. Correct alignment is maintained if the canthomeatal line is perpendicular to the collimator face. Take care to eliminate side-to-side rotation of the head while positioning the patient.
4. Inject the radiopharmaceutical as a bolus and obtain 2-second perfusion images for 90 seconds, both on film and in a 64 × 64 matrix, if available.
5. Collect images at about 15 to 20 minutes postinjection for 500,000 counts. Using the same positioning techniques as those described for the planar brain images, obtain views in the anterior, posterior, right lateral, left lateral, and vertex positions.
6. Take care to visualize the posterior fossa for cerebellar and brain-stem activity by acquiring both lateral and posterior projections. If the posterior view cannot be taken because of the patient's condition, the lateral view must be adequate to evaluate the posterior fossa.

Recent use of the ^{99m}Tc lipophilic chelate HMPAO (Ceretec™) has provided a more practical method to demonstrate cortical perfusion. Following the intravenous administration of Ceretec, the radiopharmaceutical rapidly diffuses into the brain tissue relative to cerebral blood flow (CBF). Absent or low cortical uptake can be planar imaged and confirms the state of perfusion and the state of "brain death." Posterior view and at least one lateral head view should be obtained to visualize the brain stem. Although SPECT imaging can be performed, it is not needed to generate the required image data.

Image diagnosis

Characteristically, patients with some cortical circulation show the cerebral dural sinuses on the early equilibrium images. In contrast, patients who are brain dead show no cortical flow and only the extracortical circulation is seen but never the dural sinuses (Fig. 22-19). If a tourniquet is placed around the head before the bolus injection and no or little cranial activity is seen, this confirms brain death. Since the procedure can easily be performed with the mobile camera, it has become a valuable confirmatory test to expedite the harvesting of transplantable organs.

When Ceretec is used to determine brain perfusion to confirm the state of brain death, the images can only be interpreted as cortical death if attempts to see the brain stem are unsuccessful.

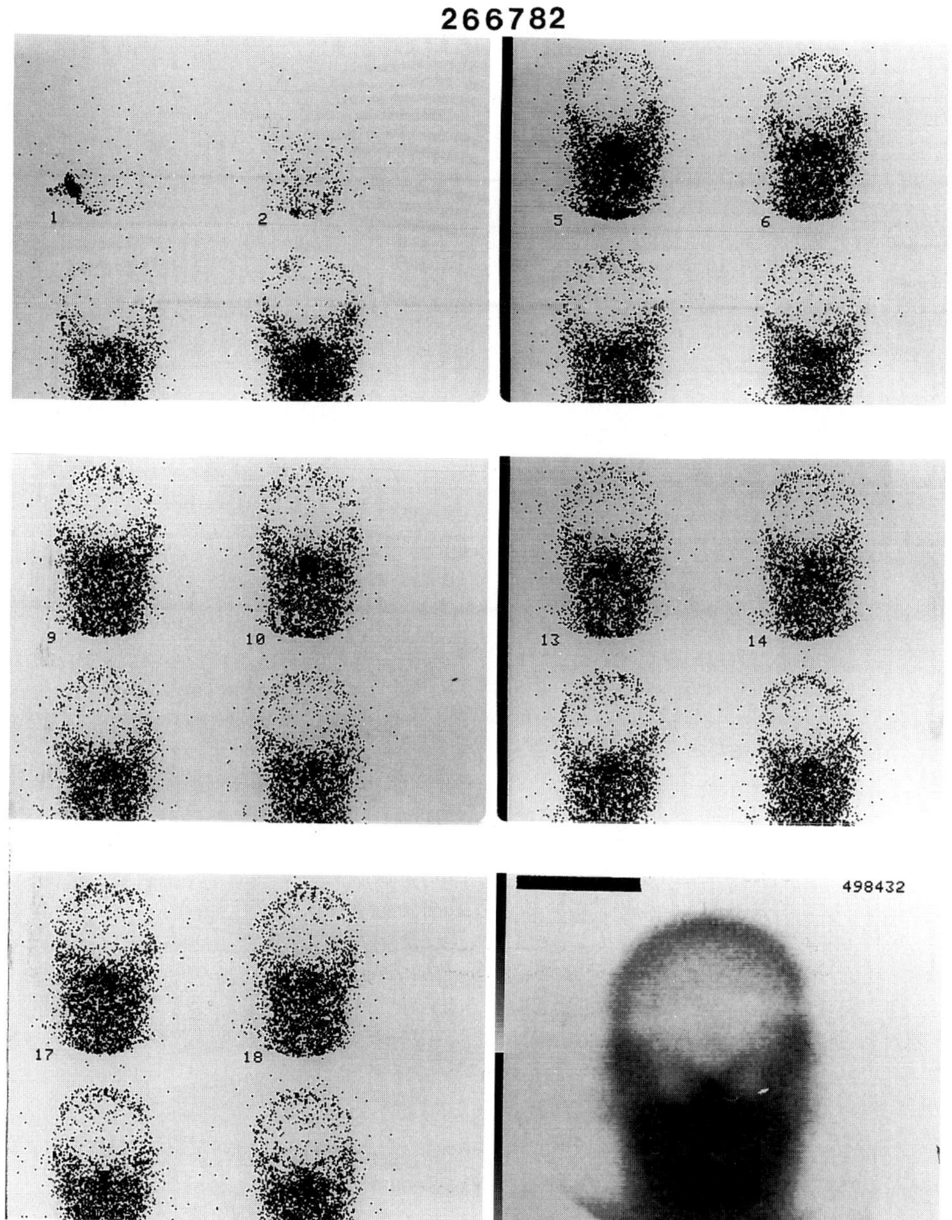

Fig. 22-19. A *brain dead* patient demonstrating no intracerebral blood flow. Only extracortical flow is recorded using ^{99m}Tc-DTPA.

LABORATORY APPLICATION

70

BLOOD-BRAIN BARRIER DISRUPTION

Purpose

As discussed earlier in the chapter, the blood-brain barrier (BBB) restricts the passage of all but essential compounds and ions from the blood to the brain substance. The BBB prevents adequate amounts of chemotherapeutic agents to reach that level of concentration in the brain to be therapeutically effective. By locally disrupting the BBB chemically with mannitol, a hyperosmolar sugar, the barrier is temporarily opened and chemotherapeutic agents like cytoxan, methotrexate, and others can readily diffuse through the site of disruption into the regional brain tissue. Figure 22-20 is the study of a patient with a malignant glioma that could not be totally removed at surgery and recurred on follow-up. The patient was given cytoxan orally and underwent BBB disruption through

Continued.

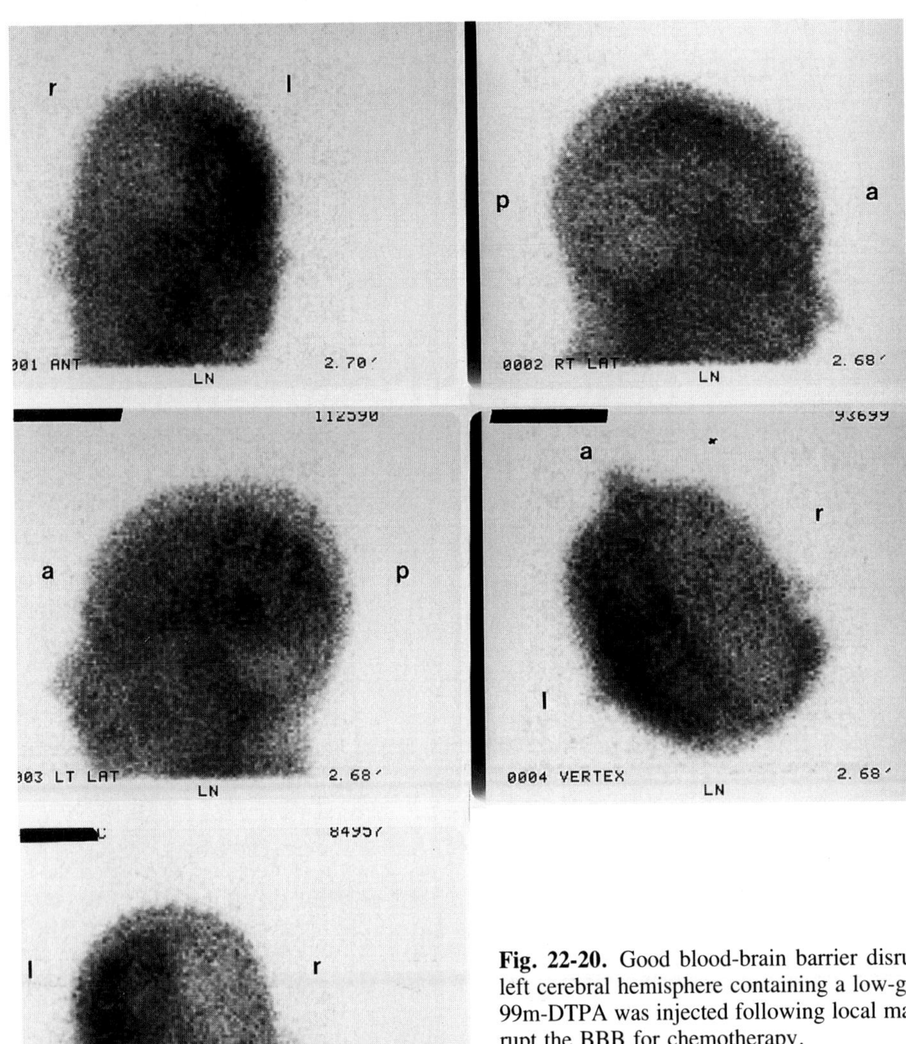

Fig. 22-20. Good blood-brain barrier disruption (BBBD) of the left cerebral hemisphere containing a low-grade astrocytoma. Tc-99m-DTPA was injected following local mannitol infusion to disrupt the BBB for chemotherapy.

an arterial catheter supply to the region of the brain tumor. ^{99m}Tc-DTPA (20 mCi, 740 MBq) were injected intravenously and imaged within 30 minutes of the injection to access the regional disruption.

Procedure
Materials

1. Scintillation camera peaked for ^{99m}Tc
2. Low-energy, all-purpose collimator (LEAP)
3. 20 mCi (740 MBq) ^{99m}Tc-DTPA

Technique

1. Once the blood-brain barrier has been chemically disrupted and the radiopharmaceutical injected images are taken in the anterior, posterior, laterals and vertex views as described in the planar section.
2. Images may be collected simultaneously on film and in a 64 × 64 computer matrix.

BIBLIOGRAPHY

Abdel-Dayem, H.M., El-Hilu, S., Sehwel, A., Higazi, E., Johan, S., Salkat, M., and Al-Mohanddi, S.: Cerebral perfusion changes in schizophrenic patients using Tc-99mm-hexamethylpropyleneamineoxime (HMPAO), Clin. Nucl. Med. 15:468-472, 1990.

Abdel-Dayem, H.M., Sadek, S.A., Kouris, K., Bahar, R.H., Higazi, I., Erikson, S., Englesson, S.H., Berntman, L., Sigurdsson, G.H., Ford, M., and others: Changes in cerebral perfusion after acute head injury: comparison of CT with Tc-99m-HM-PAO SPECT, Radiology 165:221-226, 1987.

Akluwalia, B.: Single-photon emission computed tomography (SPECT) imaging system and quality control. In Akluwalia, B.D., editor: *Tomographic method in nuclear medicine: physical principles, instruments and clinical applications,* Boca Raton, Fla., 1989, CRC Press, pp. 43-52.

Amori, D., and Basset, J.Y.: Diagnosis of cerebral metastases by thallium-201, Br. J. Radiology 53:443-445, 1980.

Berberich, A., Bucll, V., Eilles, A., Gerhards, W., Jaeger, A., Ferbert, A., Moser, E., and Krappel, W.: Tc-99m hexamethylpropyleneamine oxime (HM-PAO) SPECT in cerebrovascular disease (CVD)—a comparison to transmission CT, J. Nucl. Med. 27:888, 1986.

Berman, K.F., and Weinberger, D.R.: Cognitive and physiological factors that affect regional cerebral blood flow and other measures of brain function, In Diksic, M., and Reba, R.C., editors: *Radiopharmaceuticals and brain pathology studied with PET and SPECT,* Boca Raton, Fla., 1991, CRC Press, pp. 427-442.

Biersack, H.J., Stefan, H., Reichman, K., Hunermann, B., Kuhnen, K., Bockisch, A., Penin, H., Knapp, F.F., and Winckler, C.: Brain imaging with ^{99m}Tc-HMPAO SPECT, CT, and NMR results in epilepsy. J. Nucl. Med 27:1028, 1986.

Cassen, B., Curtis, L., and Reed, C.: Sensitive directional gamma-ray detector, *Nucleonics* 6:78-81, 1950.

Chandler, W.M., and Schuck, L.D.: Abnormal technetium-99m pertechnetate imaging following stannous pyrophosphate bone imaging, J. Nucl. Med. 16:518-519, 1975.

Conway, J.J., Yarzagaray, L., and Welch, D.: Radionuclide evaluation of Dandy-Walker malformation and congenital arachnoid cyst of the posterior fossa, Am. J. Roentgenol., Radium, Ther. Nucl. Med. 112:306-309, 1971.

Croft, B.Y.: *Single photon emission computed tomography,* Chicago, Ill., 1986, Year Book Medical Publishers, Inc.

DeLand, F.H.: *Cerebral radionuclide angiography,* Philadelphia, Pa., 1976, W.B. Saunders Co.

Devous, M.D., Raese, J.D., Herman, J.H., Paulman, R.G., Gregory, R.R., Rush, A.J., Chekali, H.H., and Bonte, F.J.: SPECT determination of regional cerebral blood flow in schizophrenic patients at rest and during a mental task, J. Nucl. Med. 27:734, 1986.

Dierckx, R., Dobbeleir, A., and Martin, J.J.: Tc-99m-HMPAO tomography using a three-headed SPECT system equipped with lead fanbeam collimators, Clin. Nucl. Med. 18(6):532-594, 1993.

Eisner, R.L.: Principles of instrumentation in SPECT, J. Nucl. Med. Technol. 13:1-25, 1985.

English, R.J., and Brown, S.E.: Single photon emission computed tomography: a premier, New York, 1986, Soc. of Nucl. Med.

Esser, P.D., Alderson, P.O., Mitnick, R.J., and Arliss, J.J.: Angled collimator SPECT (A-SPECT): an improved approach to cranial single photon emission tomography, J. Nucl. Med. 25:805-809, 1984.

Frackowiak, R.S., Jones, T., Lenzi, G.I., and Health, J.D.: Regional cerebral oxygen utilization and blood flow in normal man using oxygen-15 and positron emission tomography, Acta Neurol. Scand. 62:336-344, 1980.

Frackowiak, R.S.J., Lenzi, G.I., Jones, T., and Heather, J.D.: Quantitative measurement of regional cerebral blood flow and oxygen metabolism in man using O-15 and positron emission tomography: theory, procedure and normal values, J. Comput. Assist. Tomogr. 4:727-736, 1980.

Gelmers, H.T.: *Regional cerebral blood flow regulation, measurement and changes with diseases,* Netherlands, 1978, Van Gorcum. Assen.

Genna, S., and Smith, A.: The development of ASPECT, an annular single crystal brain camera for high efficiency SPECT, IEEE Trans. Nucl. Sci. NS-35:654, 1988.

Greer, K., Jaszczak, R.J., Harris, C., and Coleman, R.E.: Quality control in SPECT, J. Nucl. Med. Technol. 13:76-85, 1985.

Guyton, A.C.: *Textbook of medical physiology,* ed. 3, Philadelphia, Pa., 1966, W.B. Saunders Company, pp. 322, 324-326, 459-462.

Hakim, S., and Adams, R.D.: Special clinical problems of symptomatic hydrocephalus with normal cerebrospinal fluid pressure observation on cerebrospinal fluid hydrodynamics, J. Neurol. Sci. 2:307-312, 1965.

Hauser, W., Atkins, H.L., Nelson, K.G., and Richards, P.: Technetium-99m-DTPA: a new radiopharmaceutical for brain and kidney scanning, Radiology 94:679-683, 1970.

Hill, T.C., Holman, B.L., and Magistrotti, P.L.: Emission-computed tomography of the brain with radiolabeled amines, In Ell, P.J., and Holman, B.L., editors: *Computed emission tomography,* New York, 1982, Oxford University Press, Chapter 15.

Holman, B.L., and Hill, T.C.: Functional imaging of the brain with SPECT, Appl. Radiol. 13(6):21-27, 1984.

Holman, B.L., and Hill, T.C.: Perfusion imaging with single-photon emission computed tomography, In Wood, J.H., editor: *Cerebral blood flow,* New York, 1987, McGraw-Hill, Inc., pp. 247-252.

Holmes, R.A.: Cerebral perfusion imaging, Curr. Opin. Radiol. 2:860-867, 1990.

Holmes, R.A.: The central nervous system. Section I, Conventional brain imaging. In Freeman, L., and Johnson, S., editors: *Clinical radionuclide imaging,* ed. 3, New York, 1984, Grune & Stratton, Inc., pp. 630-640, 648, 651-660.

Holmes, R.A., Gini, A., and Logan, K.W.: Demonstration of cerebral infarct hyperemia with Tc-99m-HM-PAO, J. Nucl. Med. 28:633, 1987.

Holmes, R.A., and Staab, E.V.: The central nervous system. In Freeman, L., and Johnson, P.M., editors: *Clinical scintillation imaging,* New York, 1975, Grune & Stratton, Inc., pp. 247-325.

Iverson, L.L.: The chemistry of the brain, Sci. Amer. 241:134-141, 1979.

Jaggi, J.L., and Obrist, W.D.: Regional cerebral blood flow determined by xenon-133 clearance. In Wood, J.H., editor: *Cerebral blood flow,* New York, 1987, McGraw-Hill Book Co., pp. 189-219.

Jaszczak, R.J.: SPECT: state-of-the-art scanners and reconstruction strategies. In Diksic, M., and Reba, R.C., editors: *Radiopharmaceuticals and brain pathology studied with PET and SPECT,* Boca Raton, Fla., 1990, CRC Press, pp. 93-118.

Jaszczak, R.J.: SPECT: state-of-the art scanners and reconstruction strategies. In Diksic, M., and Reba, R.C., editors: *Radiopharmaceuticals and brain pathology studied with PET and SPECT,* Boca Raton, Fla., 1991, CRC Press, pp. 94-115.

Kim, K.I., and Lim, C.B.: High sensitivity resolution brain SPECT imaging with rectangular gamma cameras by fan beam projection data collection, J. Nucl. Med. 26:99, 1985.

Kuhl, D.E., Barrio, J.R., Huang, S.C., Selin, C., Ackerman, R.F., Lear, J.L., Wu, J.L., Lin, T.H., and Phelps, M.E.: Quantifying local cerebral blood flow by N-isopropyl-p[^{123}I]iodoamphetamine (IMP) tomography, J. Nucl. Med. 23:196-203, 1982.

Kung, H.F.: New technetium 99m-labeled brain perfusion imaging agents, Semin. Nucl. Med. 20:150-158, 1990.

Larsson, S.A.: Gamma camera emission tomography, Acta Radiol. (suppl.) 363:1-75, 1980.

Lassen, N.A.: The luxury-perfusion syndrome and its possible relationship to acute metabolic acidosis localized within the brain, Lancet 2:1113-1115, 1966.

Lee, K.: Computers in nuclear medicine, a practical approach, Soc. of Nucl. Med., 1991.

Links, J.M.: Multidetector single-photon emission tomography: are two (or three or four) heads really better than one? Eur. J. Nucl. Med. 20(5):440-447, 1993.

Logan, K.W., and Holmes, R.A.: Missouri University multi-plane imager (MUMPI): a high sensitivity rapid dynamic ECT brain imager, J. Nucl. Med. 25:105, 1984.

Mishkin, F.S.: Determination of cerebral death by radionuclide angiography, Radiology 115:135-137, 1975.

Moore, G.E.: Use of radioactive diiodofluorescein in the diagnosis and localization of brain tumors, Science 107:569-573, 1971.

Nagle, C.E.: Use of immediate static scans in combination with radionuclide cerebral angiography as a confirmatory test in the diagnosis of brain death, Clin. Nucl. Med. 5:152-153, 1980.

Neary, D., Snowden, J.S., Shields, R.A., Burjan, A.W.I., Northen, B., MacDermott, N., Prescott, M.C., and Testa, H.J.: Single photon emission tomography using ^{99m}Tc-HM-PAO in the investigation of dementia, J. Neurol. Neurosurg. Psychiatry 50:1101-1109, 1987.

Neirinckx, R.D., Canning, L.R., Piper, I.M., Nowotnik, D.P., Pickett, R.D., Holmes, R.A., Volkert, W.A., Forster, A.M., Weisner, P.S., Marriott, J.A., and Chaplin, S.B.: Technetium-99m-d,l-HMPAO: a new radiopharmaceutical for SPECT imaging or regional cerebral blood perfusion, J. Nucl. Med. 28:191-198, 1990.

Nolte, J.: *The human brain: an introduction to its functional anatomy,* St. Louis, Mo., 1981, C.V. Mosby Co., pp. 59, 107.

Podreka, I., Suess, E., Goldenberg, G., Steiner, M., Brucke, T., Muller, C., Lang, W., Neirinckx, R.D., and Deecke, L.: Initial experience with technetium-99m HM-PAO brain SPECT, J. Nucl. Med. 28:1657-1666, 1987.

Reivich, M., Kuhl, D., Wolf, A., Greenberg, J., Phelps, M., Ido, T., Casella, V., Fowler, J., Hoffman, E., Alavi, A., Som, P., and Sokoloff, L.: The [^{18}F]fluoro-deoxyglucose method for the measurement of local cerebral glucose utilization in man, Circ. Res. 44:127-135, 1979.

Siesjo, B.K.: Cerebral circulation and metabolism, J. Neurosurg. 60:883-908, 1981.

Stokely, E.M., Sveinsdattir, E., Lassen, N.A., and Rommer, P.: A single photon dynamic computer assisted tomograph (DCTA) for imaging brain function in multiple cross sections, J. Assist. Tomogr. 4:230-240, 1980.

Testa, H.J., Snowden, J.S., Neary, D., Shields, R.A., Burjan, A.W., Prescott, M.C., Northen, B., and Goulding, P.: The use of [^{99m}Tc]-HM-PAO in the diagnosis of primary degenerative dementia, J. Cereb. Blood Flow Metab. 8:S123-S126, 1988.

Tortora, G.J.: *Principles of human anatomy,* ed. 2, 1980, Harper & Row, p. 396.

Tsui, B.M.L.O., Gullberg, G.T., Edgerton, E.R., Gilland, D.R., Rho, T., Johnston, R.E., Perry, J.R., and McCartney, W.H.: High resolution SPECT imaging of the brain using fan beam collimators, J. Nucl. Med. 28:5, 1989.

Tuscan, M.J., Roger, W.L., Juni, J.E., and Clinthorne, V.H.: Analysis of gamma camera detector stability and its effect on uniformity correction for SPECT, J. Nucl. Med. Technol. 13:1-4, 1985.

Vallabhajosula, S., Zimmerman, R.E., Pickard, M., Strizke, P., Mena, I., Hellman, R.S., Tikofsky, R.S., Stabin, M.G., Morgan, R.A., and Goldsmith, S.J.: Technetium-99m ethylcysteinate: a new brain imaging agent; *in vivo* kinetics and biodistribution studies in normal subjects, J. Nucl. Med. 30:599-604, 1989.

Wagner, H.N.: Positron emission tomography (PET) imaging of neuroreceptors in mental illness. In Diksic, M., and Reba, R.C., editors: Radiopharmaceuticals and brain pathology studied with PET and SPECT, Boca Raton, Fla., 1991, CRC Press, pp. 381-387.

Waxman, A.D., Lee, G., Wolfstein, R., and Sienisen, J.K.: Differential diagnosis of brain lesions by gallium scanning, J. Nucl. Med. 14:903-908, 1973.

Wilhelm, K.R., Schroeder, J., Henningsen, H., Saver, H., and George, P.: ^{99m}Tc-HMPAO-SPECT studies in endogenous psychoses, Nucklear Medizin 28:88-91, 1989.

Witcofski, R.L., Janeway, R., Maynard, D.C., Bearden, E.K., and Schultz, J.L.: Visualization of the choroid plexus on the technetium-99m brain scan—clinical significance and blocking by potassium perchlorate, Arch. Neurol. 16:282-286, 1967.

Yatsu, F.M., Pettigrew, L.C., and Grotta, J.C.: Medical therapies for acute ischemic stroke. In Wood, J.H., editor: *Cerebral blood flow,* New York, 1987, McGraw-Hill Book Co., p. 605.

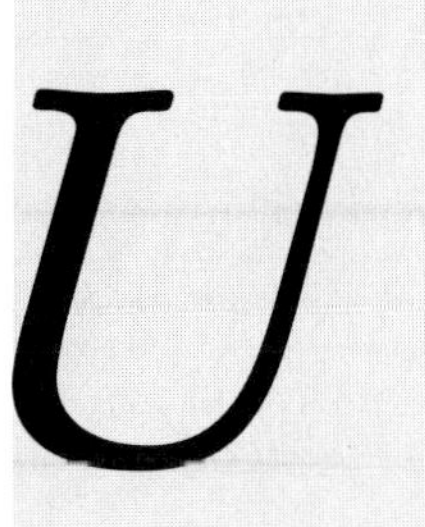

Chapter 23

RINARY TRACT

ANDREW TAYLOR, JR.
JACK ZIFFER

■ ANATOMY

The urinary tract is comprised of two kidneys, two ureters, the urinary bladder and the urethra (Fig. 23-1). The kidneys' principal function is urine formation. The urine collects in the renal pelvis and is transported via the ureter to the urinary bladder secondary to the effects of gravity, a pressure gradient between the renal pelvis and the bladder and ureteral peristalsis. Urine exits the bladder by way of the urethra.

The kidneys are bilateral retroperitoneal organs, located between the twelfth thoracic and third lumbar vertebrae, with the left kidney usually 1 to 2 cm superior to the right. The kidneys are each about 11 cm in length, 6 cm in width, and 3 cm in thickness; they are each semilunar in shape with the concave aspect of the organ lying medially. The long axis of the kidney is more lateral in its inferior extent. An abnormal location of a kidney may raise the question of adjacent space-occupying mass.

The renal capsule surrounds the kidney parenchyma; this capsule is surrounded by fatty tissue that is enveloped by connective tissue called *Gerota's fascia*. The adrenal glands lie within *Gerota's fascia* but are extrinsic to the renal capsule. The kidney itself may be divided into three portions: the cortex, the medulla, and the hilum (Fig. 23-2). The cortex is 1 to 2 cm in thickness and contains the glomeruli. The renal medulla is more centrally located and consists of radially striated cones called *renal pyramids;* these pyramids consist of renal tubules that converge into papillae emptying into minor calyces which, in turn, drain into the renal pelvis. Portions of the renal cortex penetrate between the pyramids; these cortical penetrations are known as *columns of Bertin*. The hilum of the kidney is medially located and contains the central urine reservoir, the renal pelvis. The blood vessels, lymphatic vessels, and ureter converge in each renal hilum.

The proximal ureters are retroperitoneal structures that originate at the uretero-pelvic junction and are located laterally and slightly anteriorly to the aorta. The ureters course inferiorly and then laterally to enter the posterior urinary bladder at the ureterovesicle junction, which normally only permits the flow of urine in an antegrade direction. The ureters enter the bladder's posterior aspect at the *trigone*. The urethra originates at the inferior margin of the bladder and exits the patient at the external urethral meatus.

There is frequent variation in the anatomy of the urinary tract; this may be related to its complex embryological origin. Variants include single, ectopic, and horseshoe-shaped kidneys, and aberrently located or duplicated collecting systems and ureters. These variations may be of no clinical significance, however, in regard to function.

The functional unit of the kidney is the *nephron* (Fig. 23-3). The nephron consists of the microscopic spherical Bowman's capsule and a capillary tuft known as the glomerulus. The glomerulus and Bowman's capsule make up the renal corpuscle, or *malpighian body*. There are more than 1 million corpuscles in each kidney, and each is supplied with an *afferent* and an *efferant* arteriole. The renal corpuscle continues as the renal tubule, which is composed of a proximal convoluted portion, a U-shaped midportion called the *loop of Henle,* a distal convoluted segment, and a collecting tubule which terminates at the papilla and drains into the renal calyces.

The kidneys receive about 20% of the cardiac output via the renal arteries, which are branches of the abdominal aorta. As the renal artery enters the hilum of the kidney, it divides into segmental branches and subsequently the interlobar arteries. As these arteries reach the zone between the cortex and the medulla, they divide and form the arcuate arteries. These arteries branch into interlobular arteries, which penetrate the renal cortex and further subdivide into the afferent arterioles supplying the glomeruli. The glomerular capillaries converge into the *efferent* arteriole,

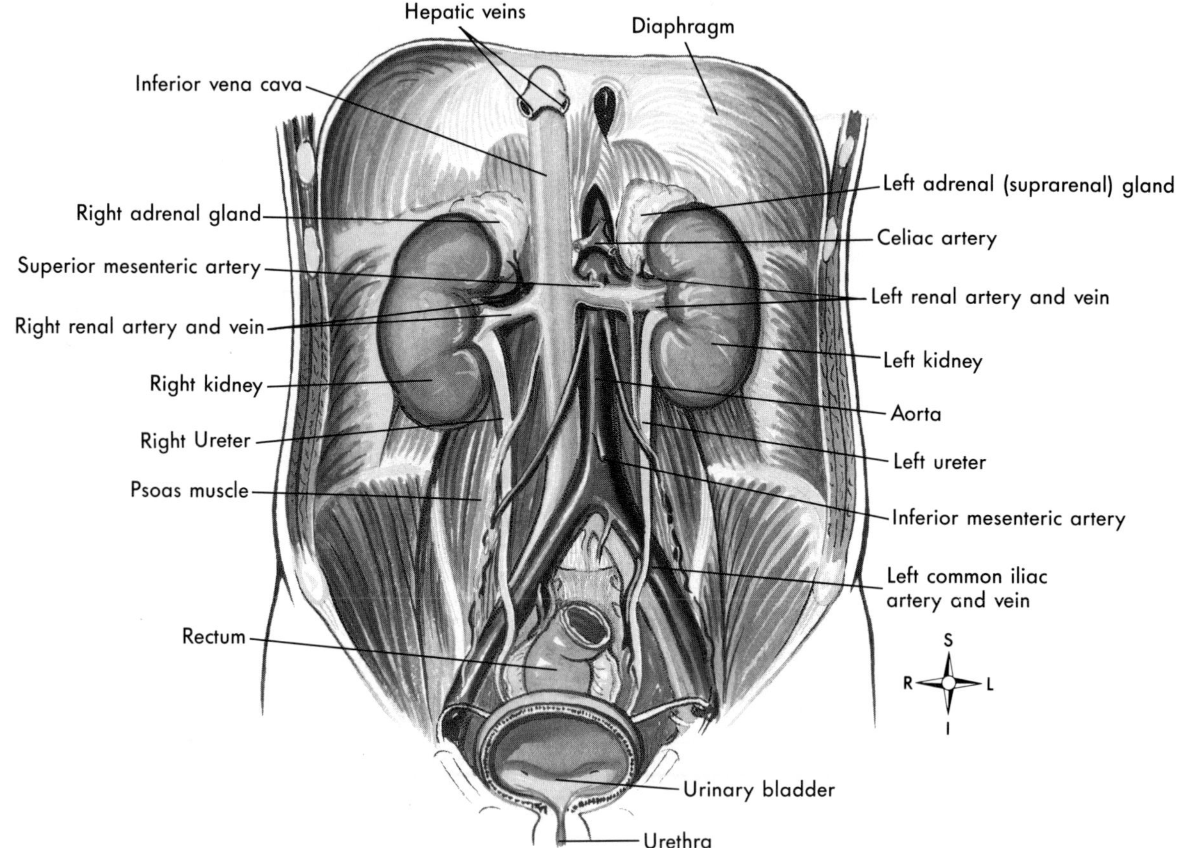

Fig. 23-1. Urinary system. (From Thibodeau, G.A. and Patton, K.T.: Anatomy and physiology, St. Louis, 1993, ed. 2, Mosby–Year Book.)

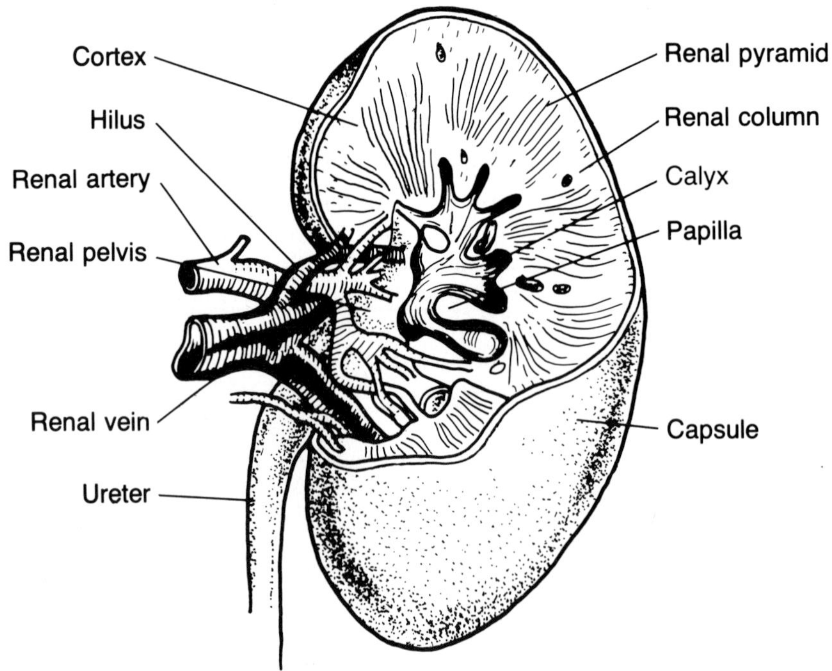

Fig. 23-2. Intrarenal anatomy. (From Austrin, M.G. and Austrin, H.R.: Learning medical terminology: a worktext, ed. 7, St. Louis, 1991, Mosby–Year Book, Inc.)

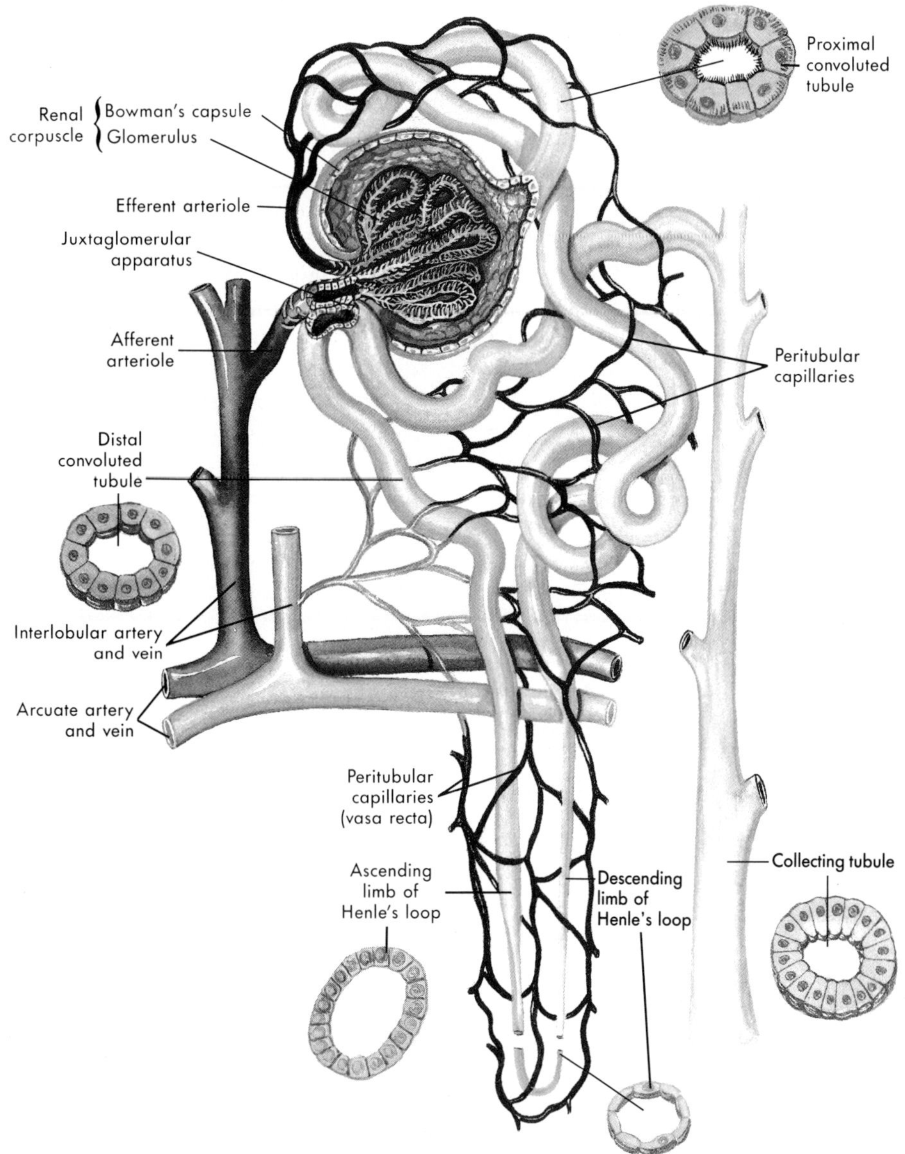

Fig. 23-3. Anatomy of the nephron. (From Thibodeau, G.A. and Patton, K.T.: Anatomy and physiology, St. Louis, 1993, ed. 2, Mosby–Year Book.)

which is adjacent to the *afferent* arteriole. The efferent arteriole subsequently forms a meshwork of capillaries in close approximation to the convoluted tubules and the loop of Henle. These capillaries then converge into the interlobular, arcuate, interlobar, and main renal veins that are adjacent to the correspondingly named arteries. Each renal vein empties into the inferior vena cava.

The juxtaglomerular apparatus lies adjacent to the afferent and efferent arterioles. This is a baroreceptor system containing specialized cells called the *juxtaglomerular cells,* which produce renin when stimulated by decreased arterial blood pressure. The *macula densa* is an area of specialized tubular cells in the distal convoluted tubule. When hyponaturia is present, these cells release renin.

■ PHYSIOLOGY

The kidneys are endocrine and exocrine glands. The endocrine functions include regulation of blood pressure via renin secretion, regulation of red blood cell production via erythropoetin synthesis, and calcium homeostasis via 1-hydroxylation of 25-hydroxy cholecalciferol (production of the active form of vitamin D,1, 25-$(OH)_2$vitamin D_3. The kidneys also contain sites of prostaglandin synthesis; prostaglandins and renin act to modulate renal blood flow and glomerular filtration.

The exocrine function of the kidneys regulates the volume and composition of plasma and extracellular fluid. Renal control of sodium chloride excretion is the principal determinant of extracellular fluid volume. The kidneys also participate in the regulation of the plasma concentrations of bicarbonate (acid-base balance), phosphate, potassium, and calcium. Finally, the kidneys eliminate metabolic waste products, mainly urea.

■ Urine formation

Glomerular filtration is the first step in urine formation. As blood flows through the glomerular capillaries, water and solutes are filtered out of the blood into Bowman's capsule. The glomerular endothelium has many pores in it and is more permeable than tissue capillary endothelium. The efferent arteriole, which carries blood out of the glomerulus, is smaller in diameter than the afferent arteriole that brings blood into it. The increased resistance to flow as a result of the decreased lumen size of the efferent arteriole increases the hydrostatic pressure in the glomeruli, which facilitates movement of fluid and solutes from the glomeruli into Bowman's capsule. The ultrafiltrate reaching the proximal tubule is similar to plasma, but it lacks protein above the molecular weight of albumin, which is 70,000 daltons. Resorption of the nutrients, sodium, and 60% to 70% of the filtered water takes place in the proximal convoluted tubules by both passive and active transport mechanisms. The transfer of sodium across the cell membrane into the interstitial fluid is primarily an active reabsorptive process, while the passage of nutrients such as glucose and water from the tubule into the interstitial space is largely passive. Other actively absorbed substances include ascorbic acid, acetoacetic acids, basic amino acids, sulfates, small proteins, and most iodinated radiographic contrast agents. In addition to glomerular filtration, a number of substances are removed from the peritubular fluid by the renal tubular cells and transferred to the tubule lumen by an active secretory process. These substances include organic acids such as paraaminohippuric acid, ortho-iodohippuric acid (OIH) and ^{99m}Tc mercaptoacetyltriglycine (MAG_3); the latter two are radiopharmaceuticals for determining function and imaging the kidneys.

Additional salt and water reabsorption takes place in the loops of Henle as they course through the medulla of the kidney. The distal tubules are the site of action of antidiuretic hormone secreted by the posterior pituitary. If antidiuretic hormone is not present in the cellular membrane of the distal and collecting tubules, the tubules are impermeable to water and no additional reabsorption of water takes place. When antidiuretic hormone is present, the distal and collecting tubules are extremely permeable to water, which passes from the tubular space into the hypertonic interstitial fluid, allowing excretion of a concentrated urine.

The kidney tubules also have a primary role in regulation of acid base balance and in urine acidification. The enzyme carbonic anhydrase is present in the tubular cells and catalyzes the hydration of CO_2 to produce H_2CO_3, which dissociates into H^+ and HCO_3^-. The hydrogen ion is exchanged for the sodium ion in both proximal and distal tubules. Aldosterone, deoxycorticosterone, corticosterone, cortisol and synthetic steroids all facilitate reabsorption of sodium and sodium exchange for potassium and hydrogen ions in the distal renal tubule and collecting ducts, permitting further acidification of the urine.

About half the solute excreted in the urine is urea, a metabolic product of ammonia, which is removed continuously as it is formed. About 1 to 2 g of creatinine are excreted daily into the urine. The amount excreted by a given individual is proportional to muscle mass and is relatively constant. Therefore, a measurement of urine creatinine can be used as an indirect measurement to determine if a 24-hour urine sample was completely collected. Creatinine is formed from creatine and creatine phosphate of muscle. These latter products are not usually found in the urine. Ammonia is produced by the tubular cells primarily from glutamine. Since ammonia is uncharged and lipid-soluble, it diffuses into the urine where it combines with secreted H^+ ions to form NH_4^+. The net effect is removal of acid from the body and conservation of sodium. Uric acids are also found in the urine and are derived from foods containing purine, such as meat.

■ PATHOPHYSIOLOGY

■ Protein in the urine (proteinuria)

Proteinuria is a common finding in renal disease. Glomerular ultrafiltration excludes all but the smallest plasma proteins from entry into Bowman's capsular space. The barrier discrimination between molecules is based on size, shape, and net molecular charge. The fixed negative (anionic) charge on the glomerular membrane provides an electrostatic barrier to negatively charged proteins. Normally the few low molecular weight proteins that are filtered at the glomerulus are resorbed by the proximal tubular cells, but loss of glomerular-fixed negative charge can predispose an individual to proteinuria consisting largely of albumin and other intermediate-sized macromolecular proteins. Proteinuria may also occur when the proximal tubules fail to reabsorb small amounts of normally filtered small proteins, including lysozyme and beta$_2$-microglobulin (MW = 17,000 and 12,000 daltons, respectively). These diseases are known as tubular-interstitial nephritides. Thus diseases that affect either the glomerulus or the tubule can be associated with proteinuria. High–molecular-weight proteinuria is generally secondary to glomerular disease, while low–molecular-weight proteinuria is generally secondary to proximal tubular dysfunction.

■ Nephrotic syndrome

Normal urinary protein content is less than 150 mg per day. Protein excretion exceeding 2 to 3 g per day results in the nephrotic syndrome, a clinical entity characterized by proteinuria, hypoalbuminemia, edema, hyperlipidemia, and lipiduria. The heavy loss of protein in the urine leads to a reduction in serum proteins accompanied by a loss of plasma colloid oncotic pressure. As fluid diffuses from plasma to the extracellular fluid space, the kidneys are stimulated to retain sodium and water. The retained intravascular fluid cannot be held in the plasma compartment because of low colloid oncotic pressure, and edema results. Patients with nephrotic syndrome are susceptible to infections because immunoglobulins are lost through the kidney. These patients are prone to develop thromboembolism and abnormal vitamin D metabolism. Drugs that are normally protein-bound have to be monitored carefully because these patients have an increased concentration of free drug in the serum.

■ Blood in the urine (hematuria)

Hematuria, or blood in the urine, is usually an index of renal disease but may originate from any point along the nephron or in the genitourinary tract and may be caused by hematologic, traumatic, or neoplastic disease. When disease such as poststreptococcal glomerulonephritis involves the glomerulus, red cells entering the tubules become compacted in a red-cell–protein matrix and are excreted as cylindrical casts. The presence of these red cell casts indicates upper urinary tract disease.

■ White cells in the urine (pyuria) and cylindruria

The presence of leukocytes in the urine (pyuria) usually indicates inflammatory disease of the kidneys or of the genitourinary (GU) tract. White cells are most indicative of bacterial infection, but their presence may occur in other forms of inflammatory disease or in chemical insults to the GU tract. White cell casts indicate upper urinary tract disease.

Microscopic casts (cylindruria) in the urine may also be composed of protein derived from renal tubular epithelium; these casts are indicative of nephrons that are still functional but damaged.

■ Renal disorders

The many diseases that affect the kidney may be classified loosely by their specific target area in the nephron.

Primary glomerulopathies. Glomerular inflammatory diseases are associated with hematuria, generalized edema, and proteinuria. Causes include group A poststreptococcal glomerulonephritis, which may occur 1 to 3 weeks after infection. The acute syndrome has a rapid course with recovery of renal function usually within a few weeks. Microscopically, subendothelial deposits are found in the periphery of the glomerular basement membrane. The etiology of the other forms of proliferative glomerulonephritis are not as clear-cut as the poststreptococcal form of the disease. Some of this large group of patients progress to chronic glomerular nephritis, significant proteinuria, nephrotic syndrome, and a progressive decline in renal function. Membranous glomerular nephropathy may be induced by drugs, infection, or neoplasm. Systemic diseases such as lupus erythematosis and diabetes mellitus are also associated with glomerular disease.

Tubular-interstitial nephritis. A large group of diverse renal disorders that damage the interstitium and tubules of the kidney and alter tubular function are called *tubular-interstitial nephritic disease processes*. These diseases are associated with interstitial edema and cellular infiltrates of inflammatory cells. As the diseases become chronic, interstitial fibrosis, tubular atrophy, and inflammatory and connective cellular infiltrates are seen. This disease state is mediated primarily by the toxic effects of drugs on the kidney (aminoglycoside antibiotics), toxins (chronic cadmium poisoning), and by metabolic disturbances (elevated blood uric acid, heat stroke, and eclampsia). The disease may occur secondary to autoimmune disorders or neoplastic processes, or it may be idiopathic.

Urinary tract infection. A urinary tract infection can be acute or chronic with localization to the upper or lower urinary tract. Infections of the renal parenchyma are commonly associated with fever, dysuria (pain on urination), and pain in the region of the kidney. Bacteriuria and pyuria are often present. Pain in the suprapubic area may be caused by infection of the lower urinary tract. Chronic infection may be asymptomatic.

Ureterovesical reflux. Ureterovesical reflux occurs most commonly in children and refers to abnormal reflux of urine from the bladder into the ureters. Children with ureterovesical reflux are predisposed to chronic infection and renal scarring. Ureterovesical reflux can lead to chronic renal failure.

Nephrolithiasis (kidney stones). Stones that form within the urinary tract promote infection and are commonly found in patients with hypercalcemia or hyperuricemia. Urinary infections resulting from Proteus, Pseudomonas, or Staphyloccus bacteria increase the likelihood of stone formation because these bacteria form urease, which promotes urate stone formation. Also, calculi may cause obstruction of urinary outflow.

Hypertension. Chronic or severe hypertension may produce profound abnormalities in the kidney usually resulting from induced renal ischemia with activation of the renin angiotension system (renin being produced by the juxtaglomerular apparatus) and expansion of the extracellular fluid volume resulting from a failure to excrete sodium. Hypertension also causes vascular intimal connective tissue proliferation and peripheral pruning of the arterial supply of the kidney, known as *nephrosclerosis*. The ischemic regions of the kidney are a milieu for superimposed renal infection.

Renovascular stenosis is an uncommon but correctable cause of hypertension. The decreased arterial pressure distal to the stenosis results in increased renin and aldosterone production and systemic hypertension. When unilateral, the normal contralateral kidney can develop nephrosclerosis while the involved kidney may suffer from prolonged ischemia, further decreasing global renal function. Renovascular stenosis may be corrected by percutaneous transluminal angioplasty or surgery. Renovascular stenosis, however, does not always result in hypertension; the most common type of hypertension is known as *essential hypertension*.

Essential hypertension is treatable but it is currently not correctable by surgery.

Obstruction of the urinary collecting system. Obstruction may be complete or incomplete. For example, a calculus in the ureter may permit the passage of some urine, but hydrostatic pressure proximal to the obstruction is elevated. Following ureteral obstruction, tubular concentrating ability is the first function to be lost, followed by a reduced ability to excrete acid. Glomerular filtration rate (GFR) falls as a result of a drop in the transglomerular pressure gradient, and renal blood flow decreases thereafter. Pressure within the nephron gradually rises, and the tubules become increasingly permeable to urinary solutes. Long-standing obstruction results in tubular atrophy and interstitial fibrosis. Progressive dilatation of the pelvocalyceal system and superimposed infection lead to loss of renal parenchyma, beginning in the deeper cortical nephrons and extending to the outer cortex. Urinary stasis increases the likelihood of infection.

Renal failure. A sudden decrease in renal function is usually termed *acute renal failure* and is characterized by azotemia (the elevation of blood urea nitrogen), elevation of the plasma creatinine, and decreased urinary output. In an otherwise healthy person, a rapid decrease in renal function implies involvement of both kidneys. Causes include glomerulonephritis, urinary-tract obstruction, renal arterial or venous thrombosis, embolism, severe bilateral renal artery stenosis, and profound hypotension.

Acute tubular necrosis is usually secondary to a sudden drop in blood pressure, prolonged hypoxemia, or renal toxins. Nephrotoxic drugs such as gentamicin, the antineoplastic drug *cis*-platinum, or cyclosporine may produce renal failure. Radiographic contrast media may also cause acute renal failure, usually in elderly or diabetic patients, or in patients with prior compromised renal function.

Benign and malignant lesions of the kidney. Renal cysts are the most common benign lesions of the kidney. Cysts may be solitary, multiple, unilateral, or bilateral. Only the most severe forms of cystic disease of the kidney cause abnormal renal function. An autosomal dominant process, adult polycystic renal disease, is a frequent cause of chronic renal failure in young adults. The most common malignancy of the kidney is renal cell carcinoma (also known as hypernephroma) and comprises 85% of the malignancies found in the kidney. These tumors may grow silently to a large size and frequently invade venous spaces, including the vena cava. They commonly metastasize to bone and lung.

Renal transplantation. A successful kidney transplantation is the therapy of choice for patients with extended chronic renal failure. The transplant is usually anastomosed to the iliac vascular system and is located anteriorly, usually in the right iliac fossa. Patients are chosen when histocompatible donors are found. A cadaveric kidney may be used, but the kidney must still be histocompatible with the patient's tissues. Rejection of the kidney, the most common cause of graft failure, involves both a vascular and interstitial immune response. The donor kidney may be rejected almost immediately if the patient has a preformed circulating antibody against the transplanted kidney cell surface antigens. Chronic rejection may occur months to years after implantation of the kidney, and patients may present with chronic renal failure. In addition, particularly with cadaveric transplants, the prolonged ischemia occurring before revascularization can result in acute tubular necrosis. Other potential complications include arterial, venous or ureteral occlusion, and development of perinepheric fluid (urine, lymph, blood, pus). Parenchymal dysfunction secondary to the nephrotoxic effect of drugs designed to combat rejection (cyclosporine) is not uncommon.

LABORATORY APPLICATION

71

RENAL FUNCTION STUDIES

Purpose

Radionuclide imaging studies of the kidneys provide sensitive indices of relative renal blood flow, glomerular filtration, tubular function, and urinary excretion (Table 23-1 and Fig. 23-4). ^{99m}Tc-DTPA has a clearance comparable to inulin and iothalamate and may be used to measure glomerular filtration. Since 5% to 10% of ^{99m}Tc-DTPA is protein-bound, GFR measurements can be improved by correcting for protein binding; this, however, is rarely done for routine clinical studies. Orthoiodohippurate (OIH) is cleared similarly to paraaminohippuric acid (PAH) and provides a measure of effective renal plasma flow and tubular function. Approximately 60% to 80% of OIH entering the kidneys is extracted with each pass; a small percentage (5% to 15%) is cleared by glomerular filtration while the remainder is removed by the tubules. In normal conditions, the rate of OIH clearance by the kidneys is dependent on renal blood flow; in certain disease states, the extraction fraction may fall and OIH clearance is no longer a measure of renal plasma flow. ^{99m}Tc dimercaptosuccinic acid (DMSA) has an extraction efficiency of 4% to 8%, binds to the cortical tubules, and is considered to

Table 23-1. Radiopharmaceuticals used in renal imaging

Radiopharmaceutical	IV dosage	Mechanism of excretion
^{99m}Tc DTPA	3-10 mCi (111-370 MBq)	Glomerular filtration
^{99m}Tc DMSA	1-5 mCi (37-185 MBq)	Glomerular filtration and tubular extraction with 40%-50% tubular binding
^{99m}Tc glucoheptomate	10 mCi (370 MBq)	Glomerular filtration with 5%-10% tubular binding
^{99m}Tc mercaptoacetyltriglycine (MAG_3)	3-10 mCi (111-370 MBq)	Tubular secretion
^{131}I hippuran	150 uCi (5.55 MBq)/kidney	Tubular (80%-90%) Glomerular (10%-20%)
^{123}I hippuran	250 uCi (9.25 MBq)/kidney	Tubular (80%-90%) Glomerular (10%-20%)

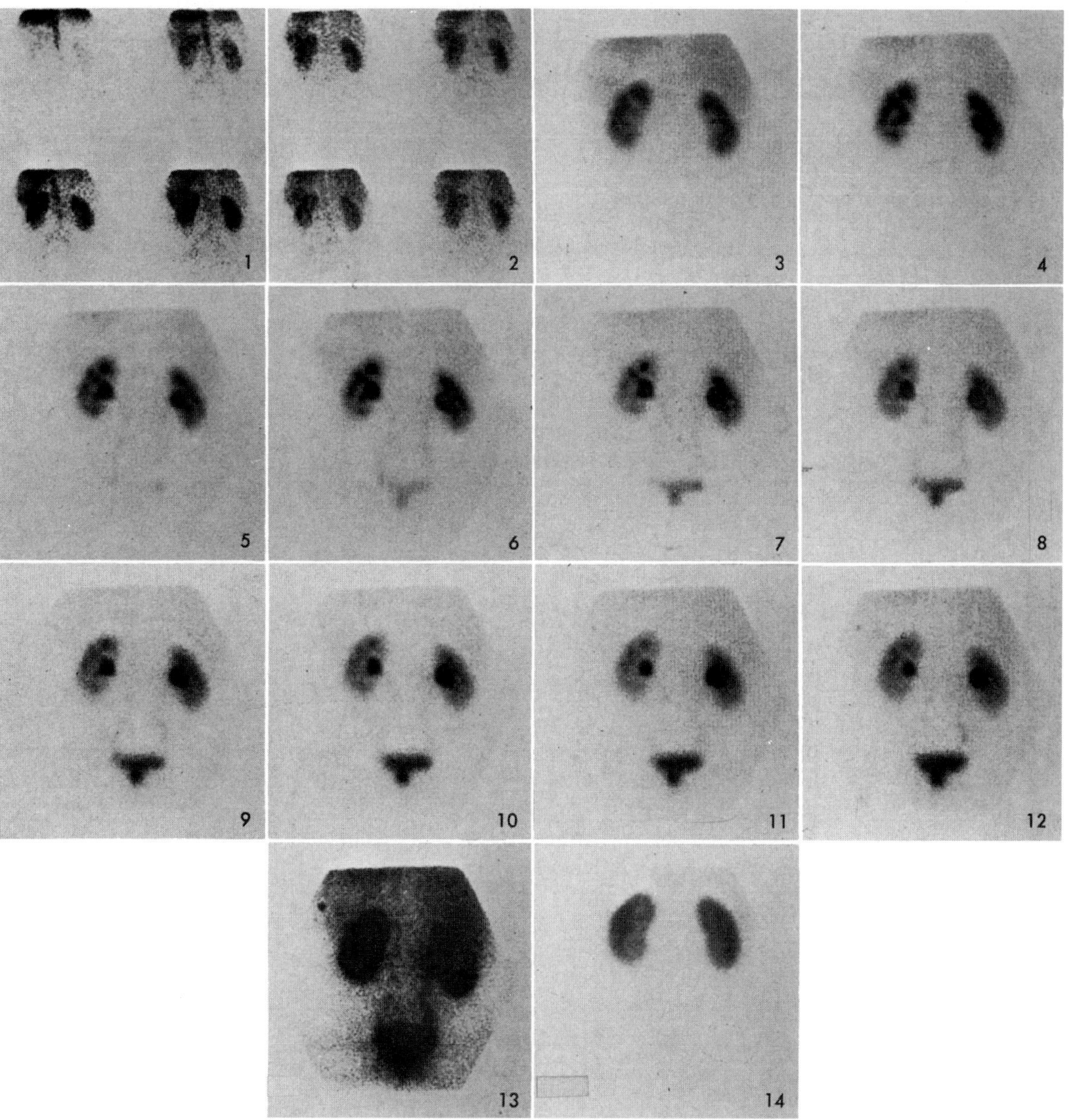

Fig. 23-4. Normal renal flow studies performed with 15 mCi (555 MBq) of ^{99m}Tc glucoheptonate. *1* and *2*, Four-second interval renal perfusion study reveals symmetric perfusion of both kidneys. Sequential 1-minute images. *3*, Immediate 1-minute static image revealing even distribution throughout normal renal cortices. *4*, Visualization of calyces and pelves bilaterally. *5* to *12*, Continued increased visualization of renal excretory system. *13*, Image enhanced to bring out ureters. *14*, Five-hour delayed image of renal tubular retention of nuclide.

Continued.

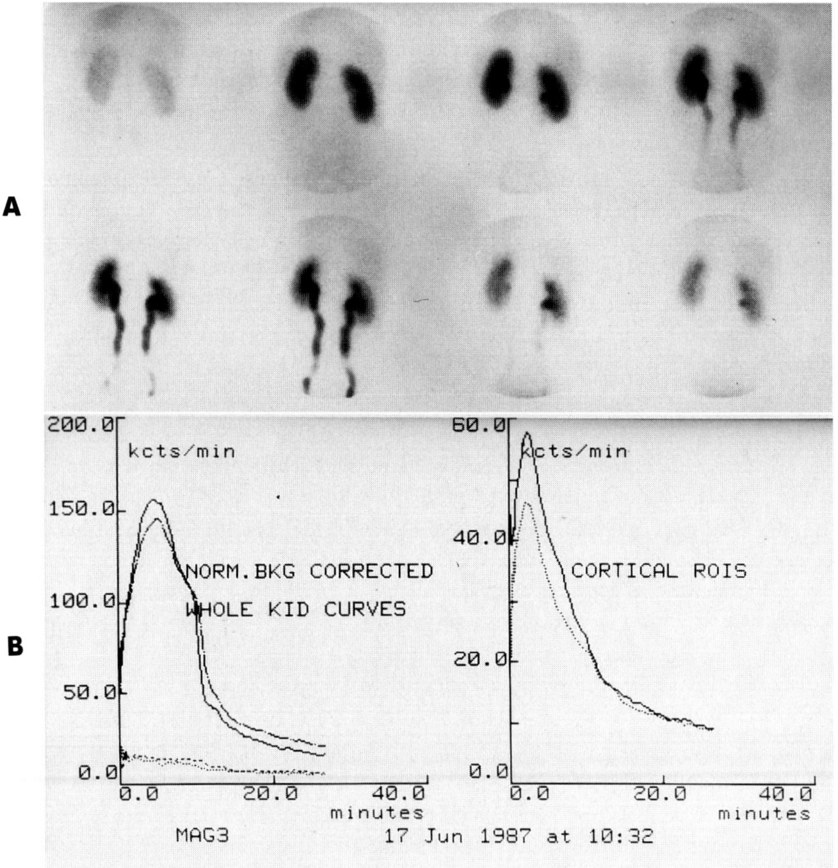

Fig. 23-5. A, Normal renal image with 10 mCi (370 MBq) ^{99m}Tc-MAG_3 2-minute images demonstrate prompt symmetric renal uptake and excretion into the collecting system, with subsequent clearance from the collecting system into the bladder (not visualized) **B,** Whole kidney and cortical renogram time-activity curves.

represent functioning tubular mass. ^{99m}Tc DMSA reaches the tubules via the glomerular filtrate as well as tubular extraction from the peritubular capillaries. About 50% of the injected dose accumulates in the cortex within 1 hour of injection and remains in the kidneys for 24 hours. Thirty percent of the injected dose is excreted in the urine in the first 12 hours, allowing better renal definition with delayed images. Delayed imaging can also significantly improve the images in patients with renal failure. ^{99m}Tc glucoheptonate is primarily cleared by glomerular filtration, but a small tubular component is present and about 10% remains bound to the cortical tubules (Fig. 23-4). The ^{99m}Tc bone-imaging agents are cleared primarily by glomerular filtration and can also be used to image the kidneys in conjunction with routine bone scanning. Thallium-201 uptake in the kidneys is proportional to perfusion, and renal abnormalities may occasionally be detected in images obtained during routine cardiac evaluation.

^{99m}Tc mercaptoacetyltriglycine (MAG_3) is a new ^{99m}Tc radiopharmaceutical with properties similar to those of OIH (Fig. 23-5). The clearance of ^{99m}Tc MAG_3 ranges from 50% to 60% that of OIH; however, its clearance, proportional to OIH clearance, can be used as an independent measure of renal function. The clearance of ^{99m}Tc MAG_3 can be calculated based on the dose injected and a single sample obtained 43 minutes postinjection. ^{99m}Tc MAG_3 is highly protein-bound, is transported by the proximal renal tubules, and is not retained in the parenchyma of normal kidneys. Despite the fact that the clearance of ^{99m}Tc MAG_3 is less than the clearance of OIH, the renogram curves and the rate at which the two tracers appear in the urine are almost identical. These results can be explained by several factors. ^{99m}Tc MAG_3 is more highly protein-bound than is OIH, and a greater percentage of the injected dose is retained in the intravascular compartment. In addition, OIH enters the red cell, where it is less available for renal extraction. In contrast, little if any ^{99m}Tc MAG_3 enters the red cell, and consequently a higher percentage of the injected dose of ^{99m}Tc MAG_3 is available for renal extraction. These factors compensate for the lower clearance, and the 30-minute urine excretion of the two agents is essentially identical.

The image quality of ^{99m}Tc MAG_3 is routinely superior to that obtained by using ^{131}I OIH. The image quality of ^{99m}Tc MAG_3 is also superior to that obtained with ^{99m}Tc DTPA in patients with impaired renal function. The high count rate and superior target-to-background ratio provided by ^{99m}Tc MAG_3 should provide greater accuracy and precision for camera-based measurements of renal function. Preliminary results using the approach described by Gates for DTPA are promising, and an optimized approach that uses a superior depth correction formula and includes corrections for infiltration and table attenuation has recently been developed.

Indications

1. Differential diagnosis of renal enlargement and abdominal masses
2. Evaluation of renal parenchyma when kidney is not visualized by intravenous pyelography
3. Evaluation of renal parenchyma when blood urea nitrogen is above 30 mg/100 ml
4. Evaluation of renal parenchyma when patient has allergy to iodine-containing substances
5. Screening of patients with suspected unilateral renal hypertension
6. Investigation of obstructive uropathy
7. Differentiation of primary renal tumor and renal cyst
8. Evaluation in follow-up of patients with parenchymal renal disease
9. Differentiation in patients with solitary cysts or multicystic disease
10. Follow-up of patients with pelvic carcinoma to rule out ureteral involvement
11. Evaluation of possible renal infarct resulting from thrombosis or embolic phenomenon
12. Assessment of the function of renal transplantation
13. Evaluation of patients with suspected renal trauma

Procedure for MAG_3 Clearance: Camera-Based and Single-Sample Imaging

Materials

1. Scintillation camera with a large field of view and a low-energy, parallel-hole collimator
2. Computer for data acquisition and manipulation
3. ^{99m}Tc MAG_3 3 to 10 mCi (111 to 370 MBq)

Patient preparation

1. No special patient preparation is required.
2. Explain the entire procedure to the patient.

Technique

1. Place the patient in a supine position, centering the kidney(s) in the field of view. Kidney transplant patients should be imaged anteriorly with the kidney and bladder centered in the field of view. Native kidneys should be imaged in the posterior projection.
2. Using a ^{99m}Tc window (140 keV), obtain and record a preinjection syringe count on the gamma camera (see comments).
3. Prepare photographic unit for obtaining continuous rapid sequential images.
4. Inject 3 to 10 mCi (111-370 MBq) of ^{99m}Tc MAG_3 intravenously; start acquisition immediately.
5. Start acquisition immediately after intravenous injection and continue for 20 to 30 minutes postinjection, collecting in 20- to 120-second intervals.
6. For single-sample MAG_3 clearance (nonimaging), a 43-minute postinjection blood sample is obtained. Calculate ERPF as described.
7. The optimized imaging technique has not been described in detail. A simplified technique has been reported by Taylor and Arroyo.

Continued.

Procedure for Calculation of Glomerular Filtration Rate: Camera-Based (Gates) Study

Materials

1. Scintillation camera with a large field of view and a low-energy, parallel-hole collimator
2. Computer for data acquisition and manipulation
3. ^{99m}Tc DTPA (Sn) 3 to 10 mCi (111 to 370 MBq).

Patient preparation

1. No special patient preparation is required.
2. Explain the entire procedure to the patient.

Technique

1. Using a ^{99m}Tc window (140 keV), obtain and record a preinjection syringe count on the gamma camera (see comments).
2. Prepare photographic unit for obtaining continuous rapid sequential images.
3. Inject 3 to 10 mCi of ^{99m}Tc DTPA intravenously; start acquisition immediately and continue for 6 minutes.
4. Obtain and record a postinjection syringe 1-minute count and follow procedure as described in the text and references.

Key points

1. Some institutions prefer to use a larger dose (5 to 10 mCi [185 to 370 MBq]) to obtain a better quality perfusion study. A larger dose can be used as long as the count rate is linear with increasing dose. A standardized lead shield can be placed between the syringe and the face of the camera if the higher dose produces dead time losses in step 1 under Technique.
2. Careful attention to detail is required before reliable results can be expected.

Procedure for Renography Using ^{123}I- or ^{131}I-Hippuran

Materials

1. Scintillation gamma camera with a large field of view and a high-energy collimator when using ^{131}I hippuran, or low-energy parallel-hole collimator when using ^{123}I
2. Computer for data acquisition and data manipulation
3. ^{131}I or ^{123}I hippuran, 150 μCi (4.55 MBq) or 250 μCi (9.25 MBq) per kidney, respectively

Patient preparation

1. No special patient preparation is required.
2. Explain the entire procedure to the patient.

Technique

1. Place patient in supine position, with the kidney(s) and bladder centered in the field of view. Posterior imaging is performed for native kidneys; anterior imaging is performed for transplant kidneys.
2. Set camera controls for ^{123}I (159 keV) or ^{131}I (364 keV).
3. Administer hippuran intravenously.
4. Start data acquisition immediately and continue for 20 to 30 minutes postinjection, displaying images at 2-minute intervals.
5. Using regions of interest, generate curves according to the system's computer software.

Interpretation

Measurement of renal plasma flow

The most accurate method of calculating ERPF following bolus injection is to draw multiple blood samples and apply an open two-compartment model to the plasma disappearance curve. This method is cumbersome and is thus rarely used in routine clinical practice, however. A simple and popular method of determining ERPF is based on the fact that radioiodinated iodohippurate sodium concentration in a single postinjection plasma sample is inversely related to the total effective renal plasma flow. The exact relationship between the ERPF and the plasma concentration of radioiodinated iodohippurate sodium is empirical, and the best results are obtained by applying a regression equation to the 45-minute postinjection plasma sample.

$$\text{ERPF (ml/min)} = -51.1 + (8.21X) - (0.019X^2) \text{ in ml/min}$$

where X = dosage injected (counts/sec) divided by counts/sec/liter of plasma from a blood specimen obtained 45 minutes postinjection. This method has been validated by several institutions, but it requires extremely careful attention to detail and meticulous technique.

A second method introduced by Schlegel and Hamway is based on the premise that the renal uptake of ^{131}I hippuran in the 1- to 2-minute postinjection period is proportional to the total effective renal plasma flow to each kidney. This method does not depend on venous sampling and is included in some commercial software packages. The amount of radioactivity detected in the kidney during the 1- to 2-minute postinjection period depends on the injected activity, the uptake of OIH by the kidneys, the attenuation factor, and the distance of the kidneys from the camera. The first of these variables is determined using a gamma camera and computer-assisted regions of interest over the kidneys. A simple formula based on height and weight is used to estimate renal depth. The kidney depth in centimeters is:

Right kidney $= 13.3X + 0.7$
Left kidney $= 13.2X + 0.7$

where X = weight in kg/height (cm).

The renal uptake of OIH is corrected for dosage and depth using the following formula:

$$\text{Renal uptake of OIH} = \frac{\text{1- to 2-min background corrected kidney counts} \times Y^2 \times 100}{\text{1 min count of radionuclide injected}}$$

where Y = kidney depth (cm).

The attenuation factor for ^{131}I is not included in the calculation and was apparently assumed to equal the square of the kidney depth:

$$\text{Total uptake} = \text{left uptake} + \text{right uptake}$$

The 1- to 2-minute uptake of hippuran correlated with the 30-minute OIH urine excretion multiplied by the body surface area (BSA); this value was proportional to the PAH clearance and was used to develop an empirical regression equation to convert the total corrected OIH uptake to effective renal plasma flow. A number of commercial vendors supply the software to support this technique.

Significant errors can be introduced when a low kidney-to-background ratio is present, such as occurs in patients with azotemia. When the background is relatively high, an error in selecting the appropriate background correction can easily change the relative or absolute measurement of ERPF; this problem is compounded when either the liver or spleen are partially superimposed on the kidney. Correction for renal depth based on the height and weight formula may not give accurate results in a given patient. The depth correction factor for ^{123}I OIH will be different than for ^{131}I OIH and the Schlegel nomogram cannot be expected to provide accurate results for ^{123}I OIH. Nevertheless, the method appears to give an acceptable estimate of ERPF and can be particularly useful in following the same patient over a period of time in which the absolute ERPF may be less important than determining whether ERPF is changing. If this method is used to follow a patient over a period of time, the background correction needs to be performed in standardized fashion. As with other quantitative measurements, careful attention to detail and technique are required to optimize results.

Continued.

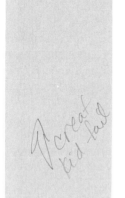

Miyamori and others have introduced a modification of the Schlegel formula that has theoretical advantages. This group has also shown that there is good correlation between OIH and PAH clearance.

Measurement of the glomerular filtration rate

Accurate measurement of the glomerular filtration (GFR) requires an agent that meets the following requirements: (1) completely filtered by the glomerulus, (2) neither synthesized, destroyed, reabsorbed or secreted by the renal tubular cells, (3) physically inert, and (4) not bound to serum proteins. Inulin, a fructose polysaccharide, satisfies these requirements and has served as the standard to measure glomerular filtration, but this technique is too laborious for a routine clinical procedure.

The creatinine clearance is commonly used to estimate the glomerular filtration rate (GFR), but the technique is dependent on complete urine collection during the 24 hours usually chosen to complete the study. Furthermore, creatinine is partially secreted by the renal tubular cells; in pathologic states the amount of creatinine secreted by the tubular cells increases, leading the creatinine clearance to overestimate GFR. A further limitation of the creatinine clearance is the inability to determine the GFR for each individual kidney unless selective ureteral catheterization is performed.

A number of radioactive tracers have been shown to be suitable for determining glomerular filtration rate including ^{14}C inulin, ^{51}Cr EDTA, ^{125}I iothalamate, ^{113m}In diethylenetriamine pentaacetic acid (DPTA) and ^{99m}Tc DTPA. ^{99m}Tc DTPA satisfies the requirements for measuring GFR, with the exception of the fact that about 5% to 10% of the injected dosage is protein-bound.

The relative GFR can be determined from the net activity that accumulates in the kidneys during the 1- to 2 or 2- to 3-minute postinjection period. Since the relative uptake of ^{99m}Tc-DTPA by the kidneys is proportional to the GFR, measurement of renal activity before excretion of the radiopharmaceutical into the ureters or bladder provides a measure of differential GFR of the two kidneys. The technique is similar to that employed for radioiodinated iodohippurate sodium (OIH).

Several different techniques are available to measure the total GFR using technetium-DTPA. These include: (1) calculation of a two-compartment clearance curve constructed from multiple venous or capillary blood samples, (2) a single exponential curve fitted to several plasma samples, (3) a modification of Tauxe's OIH method in which the counts in a single plasma sample are correlated with a GFR nomogram, and (4) a modification of Schlegel's OIH technique recently introduced by Gates.

Gates measured the uptake of DTPA by the kidneys in the 2- to 3-minute postinjection period as a percent of injected dosage and correlated this value with the creatinine clearance in a large group of patients with widely varying renal function. Gates used approximately 3 mCi (111 MBq) of ^{99m}Tc-DTPA and measured the dosage in the syringe by counting it 20 cm from the face of a gamma camera before and following injection. Renal uptake during the 2- to 3-minute postinjection period was determined and background corrected. These data were used to construct a nomogram relating the renal uptake of DTPA to the creatinine clearance.

$$\%\text{ renal uptake of }^{99m}\text{Tc-DTPA} = \frac{\dfrac{(\text{R kidney cts} - \text{Bkgd})}{e^{-ux}} + \dfrac{(\text{L kidney cts} = \text{Bkgd})}{e^{-ux}}}{\text{Preinjection counts} - \text{Postinjection counts}}$$

where x is the kidney depth in centimeters based on the formula previously described, and u is 0.153, the linear attenuation coefficient of ^{99m}Tc in soft tissue.

$$\text{GFR} = (\%\text{ renal uptake of }^{99m}\text{Tc-DTPA})\ (9.81270) - (6.82519)$$

This method produces reasonably good results and can be used to follow a patient serially. As with other camera-based techniques, problems can be encountered in patients with poor renal function because of the difficulty of accurately correcting for background. An additional problem may arise from the fact that the nomogram relates DTPA uptake to creatinine clearance and the creatinine clearance overestimates the GFR in patient with renal failure. The degree of protein-binding of ^{99m}Tc-DTPA may vary slightly between manufacturers, and for that reason it is best to use the same preparation if serial studies are anticipated. Quality-control data should be obtained from the nuclear

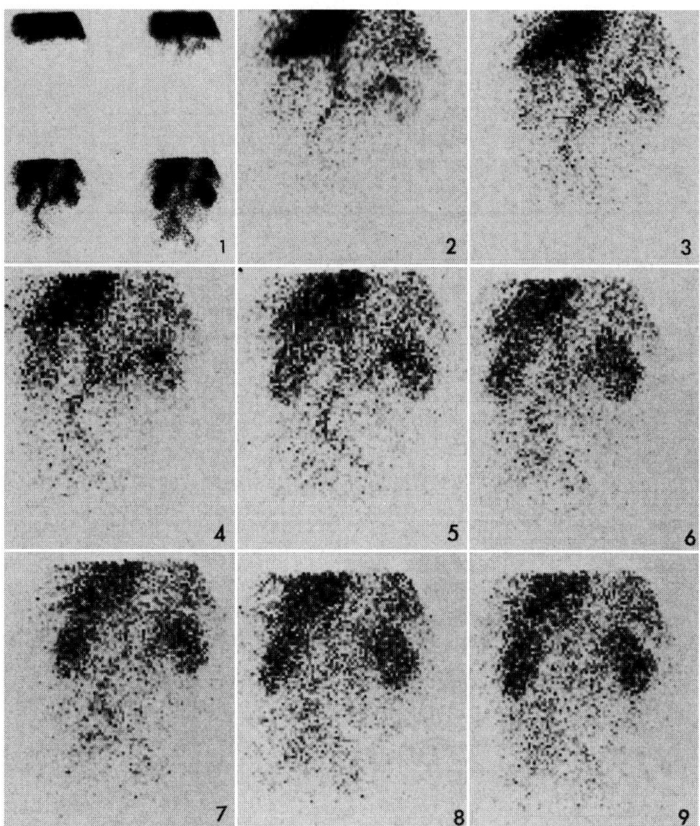

Fig. 23-6. Small renal AV fistula with dilation of renal artery. *1,* Computer-assisted, 4-second images. Note early visualization of right renal artery with increased concentration visualized in hilum of kidney. *2* to *9,* 1-second computer-assisted images. Note early visualization of activity on right side. Normal renal artery should not be visualized; therefore this is dilated renal artery. Note that increased concentration visualized in hilum of right kidney disappears in venous phase, which is compatible with AV fistula.

pharmacist when total GFR is being quantitated because a significant percentage of unbound ^{99m}Tc will invalidate the measurement. Too large a dosage of ^{99m}Tc-DTPA may result in an inaccurate preinjection syringe count because of saturation and dead-time losses of the camera. If the clinician wants to use a larger dosage than 3 mCi (111 MBq), a lead shield may be placed between the syringe and the face of the camera. Before instituting this technique, the investigator should verify that a linear relationship exists between the dosage to be administered and counts obtained by the camera/computer system. Finally, the method should be used with caution as a means to follow pediatric patients because renal depth may change during growth.

The majority of renal radiopharmaceutical applications involve a perfusion study with data collected at 1- to 2-second intervals following an intravenous bolus (Figs. 23-4 and 23-6) and subsequent images obtained and recorded on a computer at 2-minute intervals for 20 minutes. The exceptions are ^{131}I- or ^{123}I-OIH, with which the low count rate does not permit a perfusion study, and ^{99m}Tc-DMSA, with which static images are obtained immediately postinjection (blood pool) and at 1 or more hours postinjection.

LABORATORY APPLICATION

72

RENAL IMAGING

Purpose

Radionuclide imaging studies of the kidneys are sensitive indexes of relative renal blood flow, tubular function, and urinary excretion. Specific radionuclides are used as their mode of excretion isolates certain elements of renal function.

Indications

1. Determination of relative renal function.
2. Determination of the glomerular filtration rate.
3. Determination of the effective renal plasma flow.
4. Detection of possible ureteral obstruction.
5. Distinguishing nonobstructed dilatation of the renal pelvis from dilatation as a result of mechanical obstruction.
6. Quick and noninvasive evaluation of the vascular supply to the kidneys in patients with renal trauma, dissecting aneurysm, etc.
7. Distinguishing a renal column of Bertin from a true mass.
8. Determination of renal morphology and function in patients with idiosyncratic reactions to x-ray contrast media.
9. Evaluation of patients with suspected renovascular hypertension.
10. Determination of functional recovery and prognosis following renal injury, GU surgery, or vascular repair.
11. Evaluation of renal transplant function.
12. Follow-up and quantification of renal function in patients with parenchymal renal disease.
13. Detection of bacterial nephritis.
14. Detection and quantitation of ureteral reflux in pediatric patients or patients with neurogenic bladder.
15. Determination of postvoid volume.

Procedure for Renal Perfusion and Sequential Imaging Using ^{99m}Tc-DTPA, ^{99m}Tc-MAG_3 and ^{99m}Tc-Glucoheptonate

Materials

1. Scintillation gamma camera with a large field of view and a low-energy, medium-resolution collimator
2. ^{99m}Tc-DTPA (Sn), 10 mCi (370 MBq) or ^{99m}Tc-glucoheptonate, 10 mCi (370 MBq) for perfusion study and imaging

Patient preparation

1. No special patient preparation is required.
2. Explain the entire procedure to the patient.

Technique

1. Using ^{99m}Tc window (140 keV), place the patient supine centering the kidney(s) in the field of view.
2. Set camera controls for dynamic 1- to 2-second timed exposures.
3. Prepare photographic unit for obtaining continuous, rapid sequential images.
4. Inject a bolus dose of 10 mCi (370 MBq) of ^{99m}Tc-DTPA (Sn), ^{99m}Tc-MAG_3 or ^{99m}Tc-glucoheptonate intravenously.
5. Start acquisition immediately and continue at 1- to 2-second intervals for about 1 minute.
6. Immediately change camera controls to obtain 1-million-count sequential static images for about 20 to 30 minutes at 2- to 5-minute intervals.
7. A 3- to 4-minute image of kidneys and bladder using a slightly higher intensity setting will better demonstrate ureters.

8. Using regions of interest, generate curves according to the system's computer software.
9. If obstruction is a consideration based on images, for DTPA or MAG_3 administer furosemide intravenously and continue imaging for 30 minutes using similar technique.
10. For glucoheptonate, perform a 1-million count posterior image of the kidneys at 4 to 6 hours after administration of dose.

Procedure for Renal Imaging and Sequential Imaging Using ^{99m}Tc-DMSA

Materials

1. Scintillation gamma camera with a large field of view, or a low-energy, high-resolution collimator. Parallel-hole and either converging or pin-hole collimators are desired.
2. ^{99m}Tc-DMSA, 1 to 5 mCi (37 to 185 MBq) (this radiopharmaceutical should be administered within 30 minutes after preparation, and air should not be introduced into the reaction vial).

Patient preparation

1. No special preparation is required.
2. Explain the entire procedure to the patient.

Technique

1. A perfusion study may be performed using methodology described for DTPA if 5 mCi (185 MBq) are administered.
2. Using a ^{99m}Tc window (140 keV), place the patient in a supine position centering the kidney(s) in the field of view, with imaging performed about 2 hours postinjection.
3. Start data acquisition, collecting 1 million counts.
4. Differential uptake can be calculated using computer-generated regions of interest with appropriate background subtraction when a parallel-hole collimator is used.
5. Magnified images may be obtained using converging or pin-hole collimators for better detail. Differential function should not be derived from magnified images in that sensitivity will vary with renal depth.

Diagnosis

Hydronephrosis or possible obstruction (Fig. 23-7 to 23-9)

Hydronephrosis, the dilatation of the renal pelvis and/or collecting system, is often a result of obstruction. The intravenous urogram (IVU), the CT scan, and ultrasonography suggest that presence of obstruction based on pelvic or ureteral dilatation. If obstruction is present, an intervention is usually indicated. It is well recognized, however, that the ureters and renal pelves may be dilated in patients with no obstruction to urine flow. Dilatation can occur in patients with congenital anomalies, previous obstruction, and prior urinary tract surgery. The diuretic augmented renogram is an excellent test for distinguishing nonobstructive versus obstructive dilatation of the renal pelvis. The test can also be used to determine if surgery has been successful in relieving a known obstruction.

The study is usually performed with 10 mCi (370 MBq) of ^{99m}Tc-MAG_3 or ^{99m}Tc-DTPA because they allow good visualization of the pelvocalyceal system, but ^{123}I-OIH can also be used. ^{99m}Tc-MAG_3 or ^{123}I-OIH is preferred for patients with impaired renal function because of the decreased extraction efficiency of DTPA in those patients. ^{131}I-OIH may deliver a substantial radiation dose to an obstructed kidney. If there is prompt renal uptake and spontaneous clearance of the radiopharmaceutical from the collecting system in 20 to 30 minutes, there is no obstruction. If there is notable retention, the patient should be asked to stand up and void. If retention persists, the patient is given intravenous furosemide (usually 0.3 to 0.5 mg/kg for an adult, or 0.3 to 1.0 mg/kg for a child).

Following furosemide injection, imaging is continued for about 20 minutes and the data recorded on the computer. Prompt clearance of the radioactivity from the pelvis is the normal response. If the radioactivity in the pelvis increases, obstruction is present. The method is not valid if the kidney under evaluation is severely damaged because a poorly functioning kidney may not be able to respond to furosemide. In patients with impaired renal function, it may be advantageous to substan-

Continued.

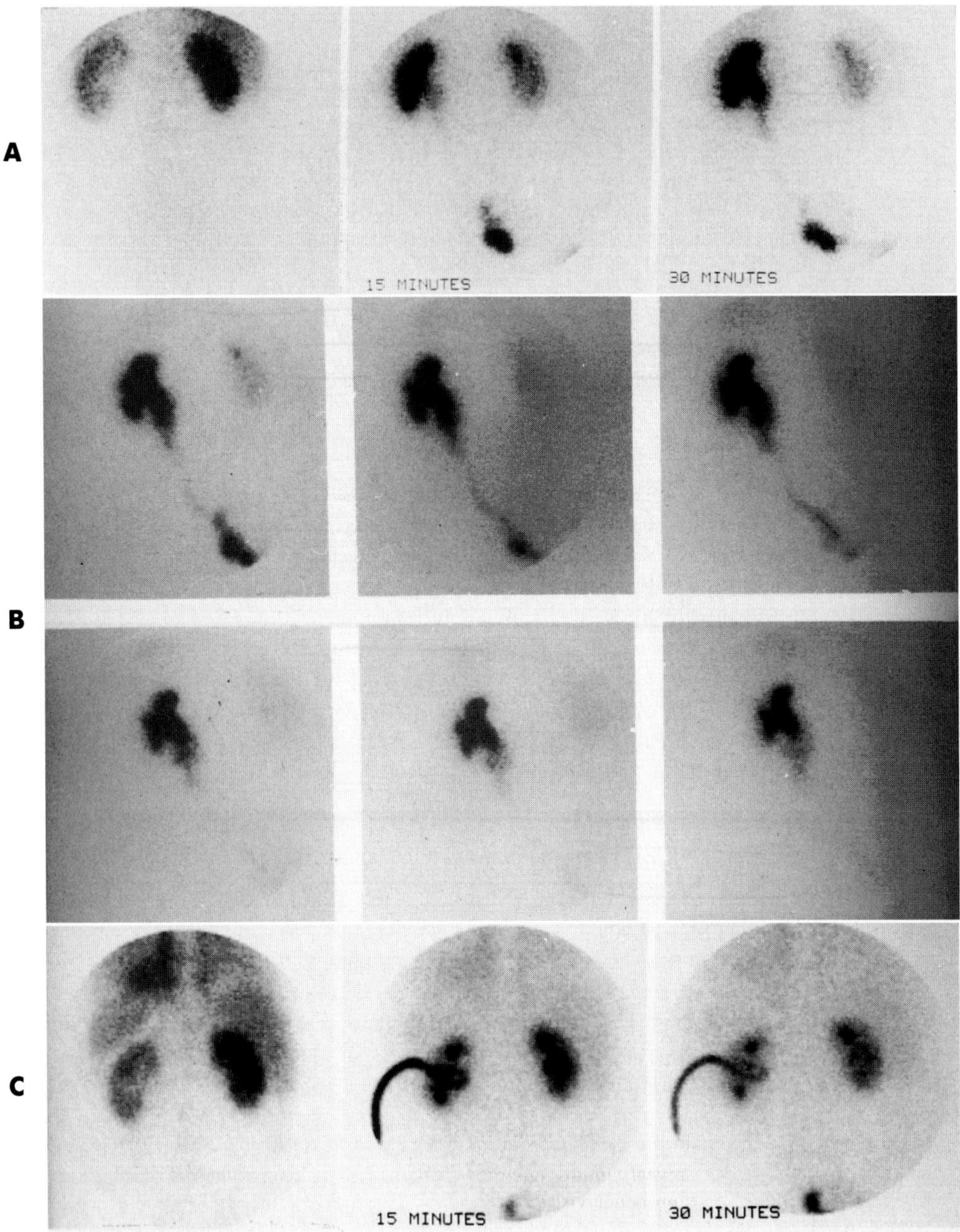

Fig. 23-7. Renal obstruction, status post left ureteral right ureterostomy with left obstruction. **A,** DTPA sequential images reveal accumulating activity in the left kidney and collecting system to the level of the bladder. **B,** Continued imaging in 8-minute intervals following the IV administration of furosemide, demonstrating marked delayed and decreased clearance of tracer from the collecting system. **C,** Repeat DTPA study with left nephrostomy decompressing obstructed distal left ureter.

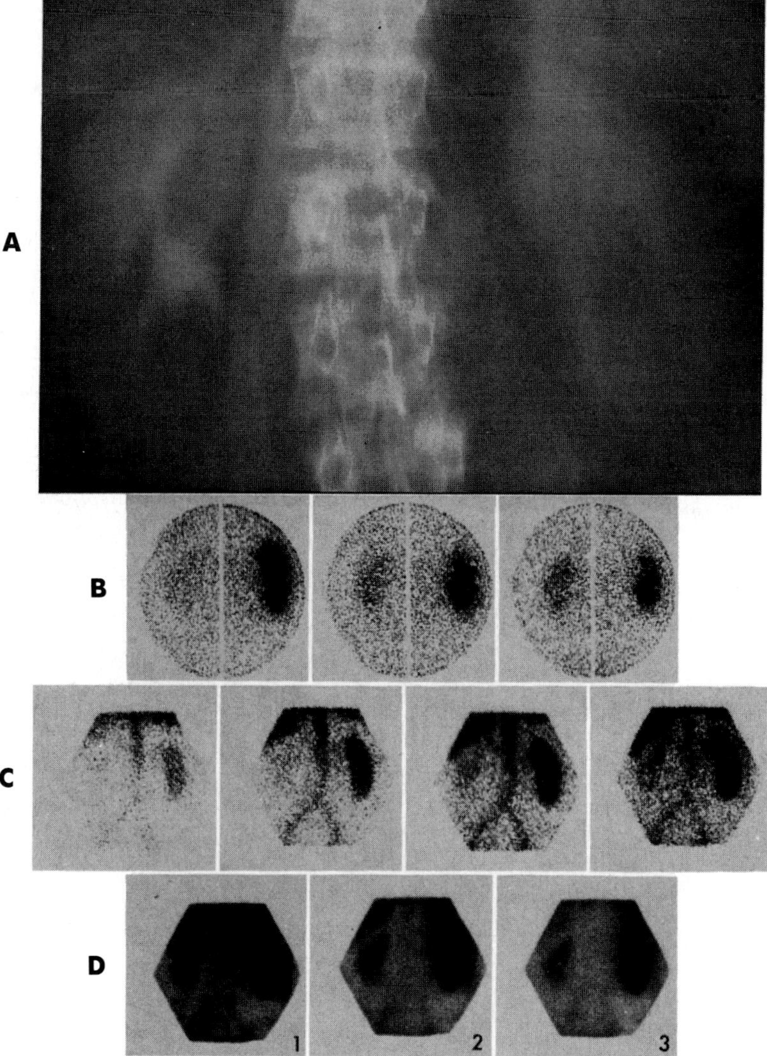

Fig. 23-8. A, Intravenous pyelogram (30 minutes after injection) with laminagraphy. **B,** Hippuran 2-minute sequential images reveal slightly enlarged right cortical volume with prolonged transit time and small left kidney with better visualization of cortex with time. There is no evidence of excretion. **C,** Glucoheptonate renal perfusion study reveals delayed and decreased perfusion of small left kidney. **D,** Static views reveal pelvis and ureter to be visualized on right side 4 minutes after administration of dose. There was grossly decreased left cortical volume without visualization of excretory system throughout 15-minute study. Comment: at surgery "nonfunctional" left kidney was removed. Cause was radiopaque calculus.

Continued.

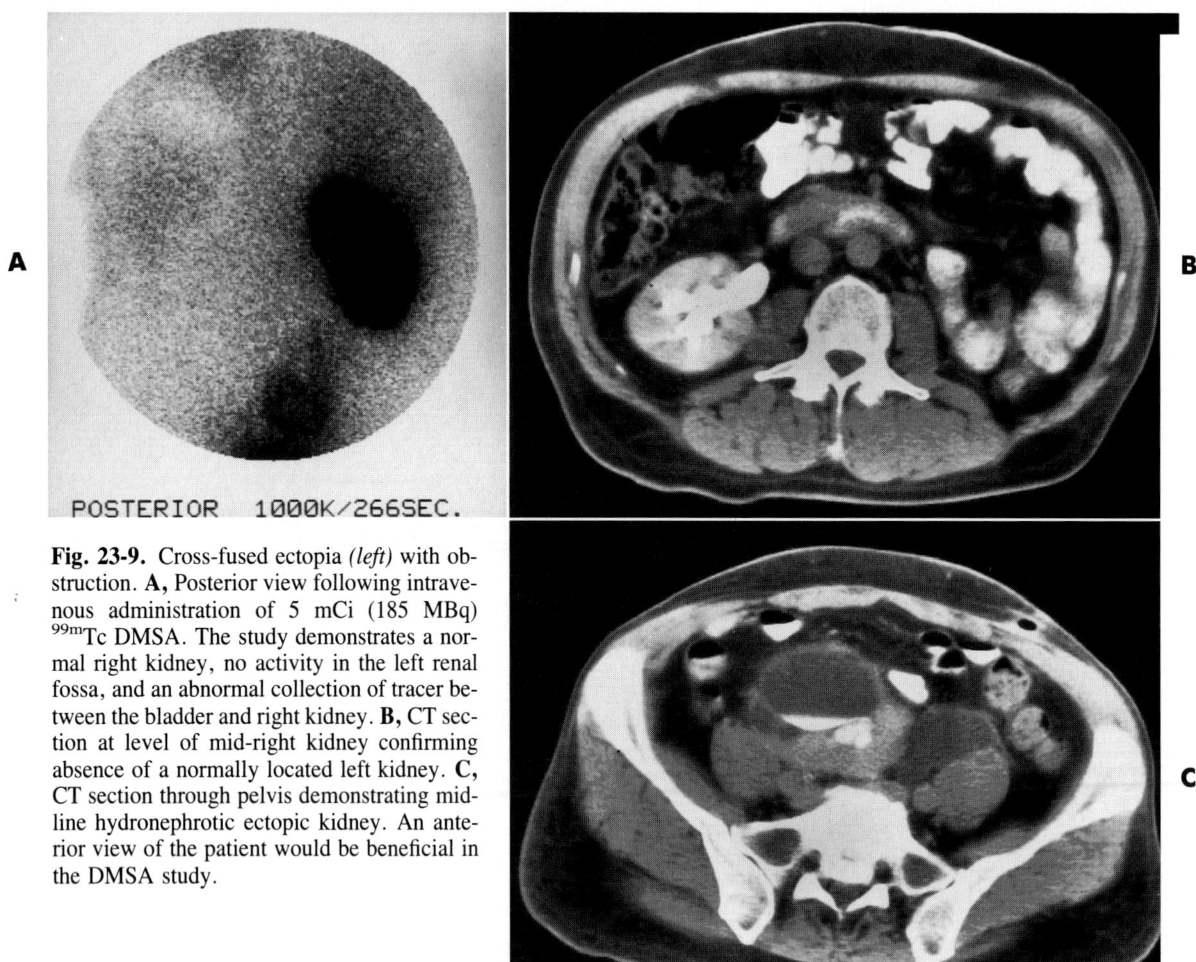

Fig. 23-9. Cross-fused ectopia *(left)* with obstruction. **A,** Posterior view following intravenous administration of 5 mCi (185 MBq) ^{99m}Tc DMSA. The study demonstrates a normal right kidney, no activity in the left renal fossa, and an abnormal collection of tracer between the bladder and right kidney. **B,** CT section at level of mid-right kidney confirming absence of a normally located left kidney. **C,** CT section through pelvis demonstrating midline hydronephrotic ectopic kidney. An anterior view of the patient would be beneficial in the DMSA study.

tially increase the amount of furosemide administered; the appropriate dose can be best determined by consulting the referring physician.

Kreuger and others (1980) measured the washout rates in pediatric patients following furosemide administration and reported that there was no obstruction if the time to half maximal counts ($T_{1/2}$) was less than 10 minutes; a $T_{1/2}$ greater than 20 minutes usually indicated obstruction, and a $T_{1/2}$ between 10 and 20 minutes was indeterminate. A certain number of studies will be difficult to interpret because of an intermediate response or slow washout of the radiopharmaceutical from the renal pelvis. It may be possible to minimize this problem by infusing normal saline (360 ml/M^2) over 30 minutes before imaging. It is also important to recognize that a furosemide washout study in a normal kidney with no pelvocalyceal retention will give a $T_{1/2}$ greater than 20 minutes. For this reason, and the fact that a normal image with normal washout excludes obstruction, the study should not be performed unless there is pelvocalyceal or ureteral retention of the radiopharmaceutical.

Some DTPA will still be circulating in the blood at the time for furosemide administration and will be entering the kidney at the same time radiopharmaceutical washout from the renal pelvis is being measured. This problem is compounded in neonates and patients with diminished GFR and can lead to an indeterminate study. Only 20% of the DTPA entering the kidney is extracted with each pass, compared with an extraction fraction of about 60% to 80% for OIH and 40% to 50% for MAG_3. For that reason, at a given time before furosemide administration, a greater percentage of OIH and MAG_3 will be in the kidney and bladder as compared with DTPA, and there will be less of

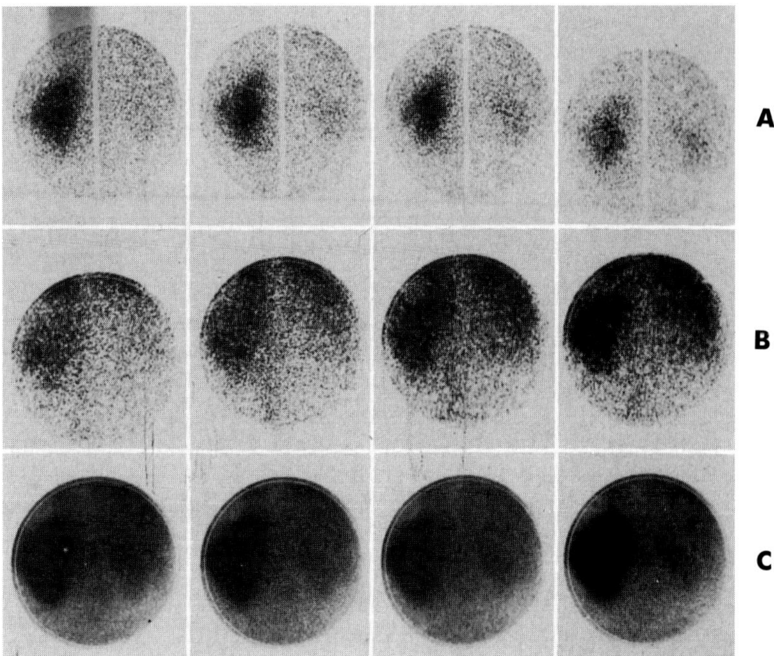

Fig. 23-10. Thrombosis renal artery graft. **A,** Hippuran study. The 2-minute accumulation view reveals increased left tubular volume. The 6-minute view (second frame) reveals normal left renal secretion, pelvis visualization beginning, and faint visualization of small right kidney. Third frame (approximately 10 minutes) reveals continued normal left renal function and faint visualization of small right kidney. Fourth frame reveals continued normal left renal function and faint visualization of small right kidney. **B,** Glucoheptonate renal perfusion study. The 4-second sequential images reveal normal perfusion, enlarged left kidney, and faint perfusion of rim of small right kidney. **C,** Increased cortical volume of left kidney and atrophic right kidney are revealed. Arteriography showed no visualization of right renal artery. Surgery revealed right renal artery graft to be thrombosed.

these tracers at the time of furosemide injection. Because of the optimal photon energy, low radiation dose, and high renal extraction efficiency, ^{99m}Tc-MAG$_3$ and ^{123}I-OIH are the agents of choice for diuretic renography, especially in patients with impaired renal function.

As in radiographic urography, delayed images (2 to 24 hours postinjection) may be of value when significant decreased excretory function is present. The delayed images may define a level of obstruction or aid in discriminating between parenchymal or vascular disease and obstruction.

Renal trauma

Renal trauma includes contusion, intrarenal hemorrhage, hemorrhage into the perirenal or retroperitoneal space, ruptured urinary bladder, and renal vascular pedical laceration or avulsion.

The spleen is often traumatized when the left kidney is injured. While renovascular imaging does not give the same anatomic detail as urography, it is both sensitive and specific for detecting traumatic injuries and in some institutions is the procedure of choice following physical examination, history, urinalysis, and skeletal chest and abdominal radiographs. Imaging has an advantage over urography because of its lower radiation, the possibility of detecting active intraperitoneal or retroperitoneal hemorrhage, freedom of interference from intestinal gas patterns, and no risk of contrast medium reaction. Abdominal and pelvic CT scanning, however, is gradually replacing contrast urography and nuclear imaging because of its superior anatomic detail and capability of evaluating the entire viscera.

Ideally, the trauma study should be performed using 15 to 20 mCi (555 to 740 MBq) of ^{99m}Tc-glucoheptonate with the patient in the supine position and the camera positioned beneath the patient. A dynamic study is obtained followed by static imaging until there is complete visualization of the upper urinary tract and bladder. Dynamic renal imaging will rapidly assess perfusion to both the kidneys and the spleen if it is included in the field of view. Excretory function can be evaluated in a few minutes, and delayed images can be obtained at 1 hour to evaluate renal morphology. Differences in renal size or position on the posterior image can represent a kidney displaced anteriorly by a retroperitoneal hemorrhage; in this setting, the lateral and anterior views may be helpful. For an example of a thrombosed renal artery, see Fig. 23-10.

Continued.

Renal masses (Figs. 23-11 to 23-16)

The majority of renal masses are identified in patients who have presented with painless hematuria; many are identified as incidental abnormalities when patients have undergone imaging for nonrenal indications. While nuclear imaging no longer has a direct role in evaluating patients presenting with suspected masses, it may be of significant value in defining differential renal function preoperatively. In addition, nuclear renal imaging may occasionally identify occult masses; when indicated, these should be evaluated with other imaging modalities such as ultrasound, CT, or MRI. Perinephric mass should also be suspected when, on a nuclear study, a kidney has an abnormal location or orientation not ascribable to congenital or anatomic variation.

Renal masses include cysts (simple cysts, complex cysts, polycystic disease), benign neoplasms (angiomyolipoma, mesoblastic nephroma), malignant neoplasms (renal cell carcinoma, lymphoma, Wilms tumor, transitional cell carcinoma), and inflammatory processes (abscess, lobar nephronia). The vast majority of masses are photopenic in delayed images with technetium-99m–based tracers. The cystic lesions are hypovascular on dynamic flow images; however, this is by no means specific. Most renal cell carcinomas are hypervascular on flow studies; this finding should raise a strong index of suspicion for malignancy.

Renal bacterial infection (see p. 614) (Figs. 23-15, 23-16, and 23-22)

Renal columns of Bertin

A renal column of Bertin is composed of normal cortical tissue, but it can appear as a questionable mass on radiographic studies such as an intravenous urogram. The presence of normal cortical tissue can be demonstrated by renal imaging when a cortical agent such as ^{99m}Tc-DMSA shows concentration of the radiopharmaceutical corresponding to the questionable area on the intravenous urogram. Photopenia in the region of abnormality is not compatible with normal cortical tissue and is usually secondary to a space-occupying lesion.

Renovascular hypertension (Figs. 23-17 and 23-18)

About 20% of adults in the United States are hypertensive, but the vast majority have essential hypertension; in fact, the prevalence of renovascular hypertension (RVH) in the general hyperten-

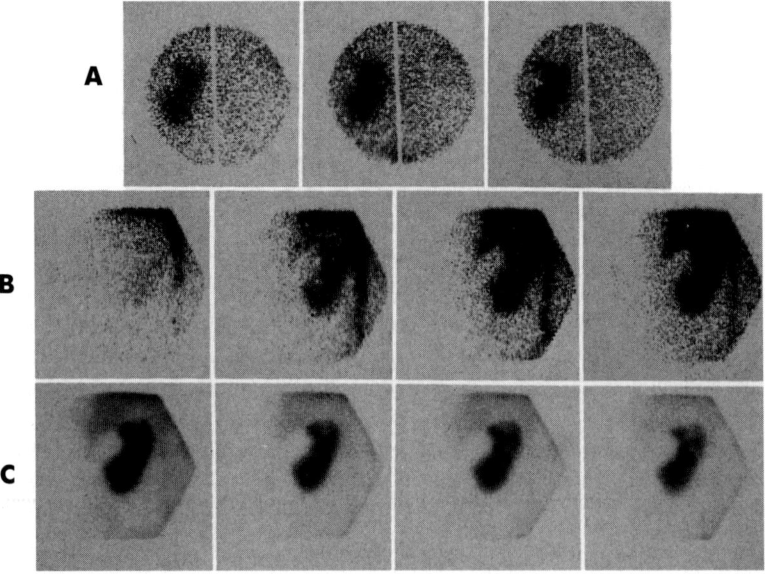

Fig. 23-11. Renal cyst; absent right kidney. Intravenous pyelogram showed lesion displacing left calyceal system. **A,** Hippuran sequential images reveal lateral left renal space-occupying lesion with retention of normal left renal function. Right renal tissue is absent. **B,** Glucoheptonate renal perfusion study reveals sharply defined left space-occupying lesion with absent perfusion. **C,** Static 1-minute images reveal calyceal and pelvic filling 3 minutes after administration of dose. Space-occupying lesion has sharply defined smooth edges.

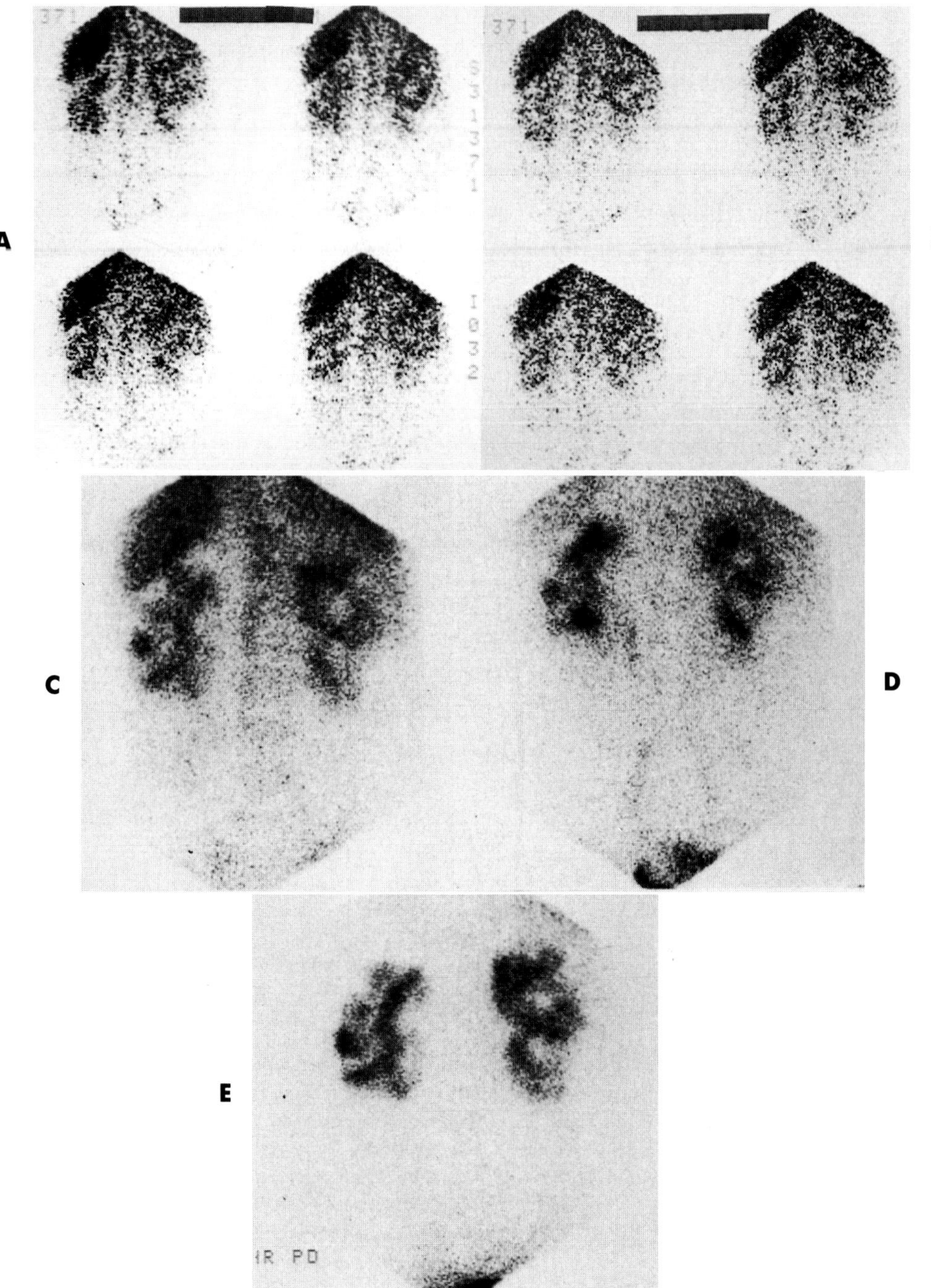

Fig. 23-12. Polycystic disease. Sequential images following intravenous administration of 15 mCi (555 MBq) ^{99m}Tc glucoheptonate reveal at, **A,** 32 seconds, and **B,** at 48 seconds, grossly distorted renal perfusion with multiple round areas of absent perfusion in enlarged kidneys. GFR is symmetrically decreased bilaterally. **C,** 1-minute and, **D,** 8-minute images reveal cortical pattern to be distorted. There is prompt clearance with visualization of normal sized ureters. There is delayed distorted calyceal emptying. **E,** 4-hour delayed tubular views reveal approximately bilaterally 50% decrease in functional tubular volume with tubular pattern of bilateral polycystic kidneys.

Continued.

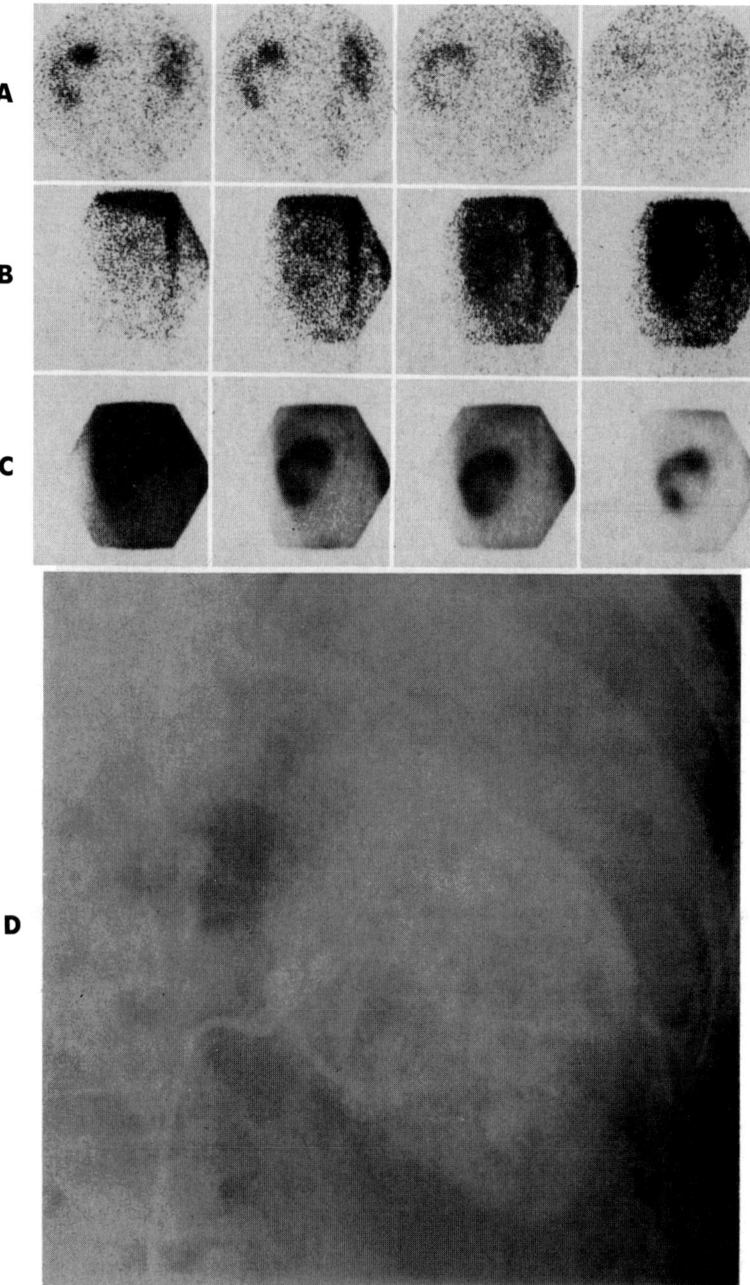

Fig. 23-13. Hypernephroma. Intravenous pyelogram revealed space-occupying lesion of left kidney interpreted as probable cyst. Hippuran renogram revealed delay in fall of excretory curve of left kidney interpreted as probable cyst.51Hippuran renogram revealed delay in fall of excretory curve of left kidney (not illustrated). **A,** Hippuran sequential images reveal central left renal space-occupying lesion with partial obstruction of superior calyceal system. **B,** Glucoheptonate renal perfusion study (centered over left kidney) reveals early vascularization of the left upper pole, abnormal vascularity of central kidney and upper pole, apparent distortion and stretching of inferior and superior intrarenal arteries, and small areas of increased perfusion throughout kidney. **C,** Static images 1 minute after administration of dose (1-minute sequential images) reveal large irregular space-occupying lesion of left kidney. **D,** Selective left renal arteriogram reveals abnormal neovascularity and areas of tumor blush.

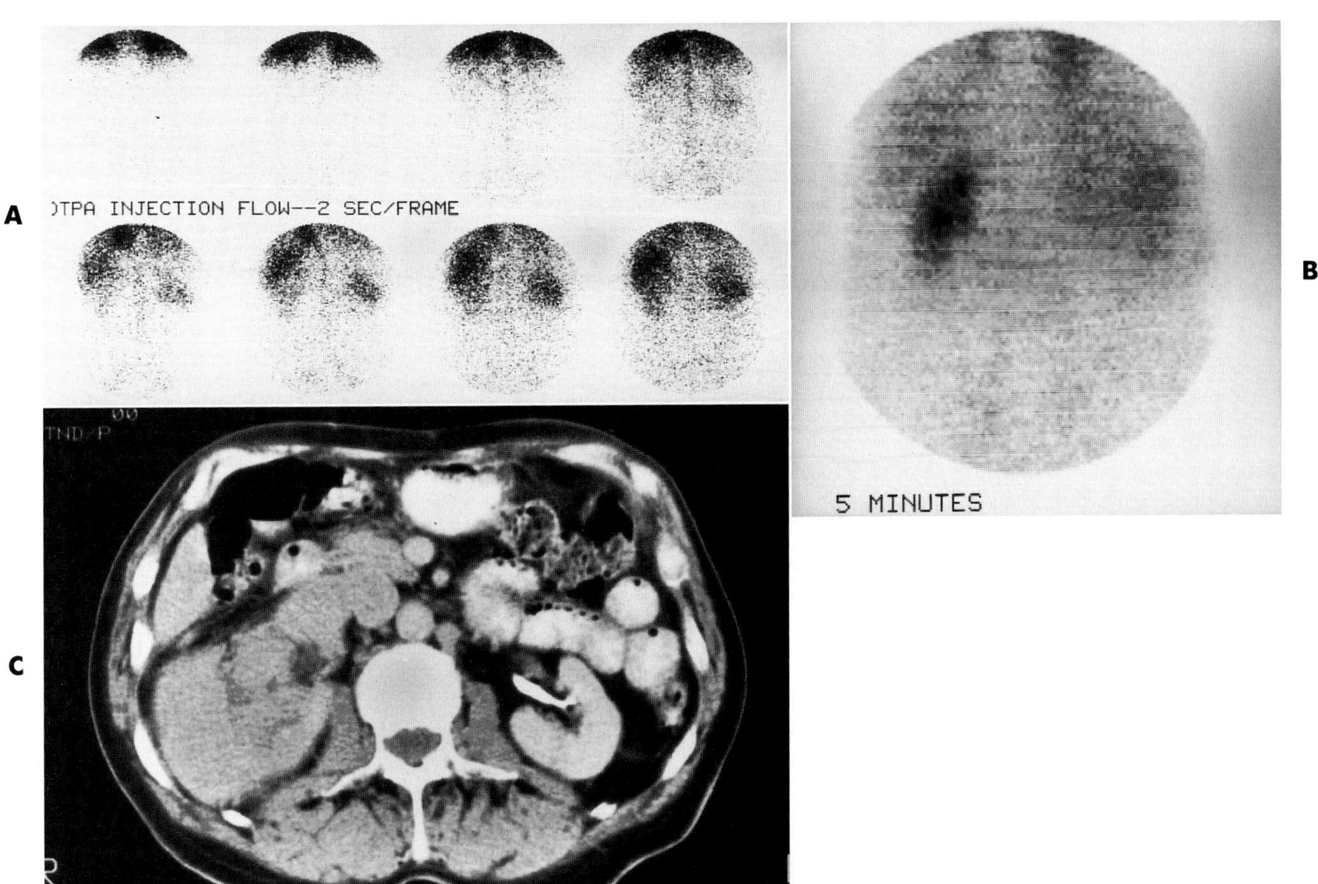

Fig. 23-14. Renal cell carcinoma (hypernephroma). Sequential images following intravenous administration of 10 mCi (370 MBq) ^{99m}Tc DTPA. **A,** Flow study demonstrates hyperemic distorted right kidney. **B,** Static image demonstrating decreased and inhomogeneous activity in the right kidney. **C,** CT section demonstrating mass in right kidney with perirenal adenopathy.

Continued.

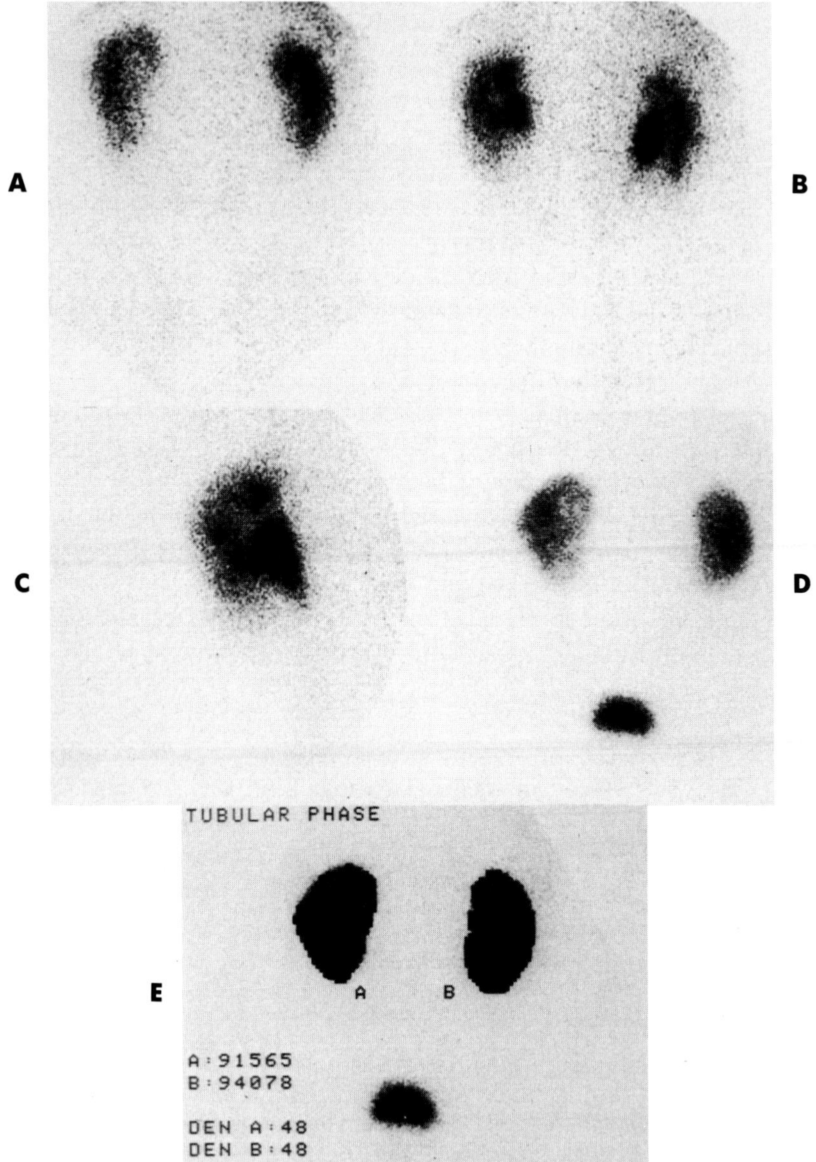

Fig. 23-15. Abscess. Sequential images performed following intravenous administration of 15 mCi (555 MBq) ^{99m}Tc glucoheptonate. **A,** 2-minute; **B,** 7-minute; and **C,** 13-minute images demonstrate persistent 1.5 cm defect. **D** and **E,** 4-hour delay reveal deep medullary, 1.5 cm lesion between superior and medial calyces of left kidney.

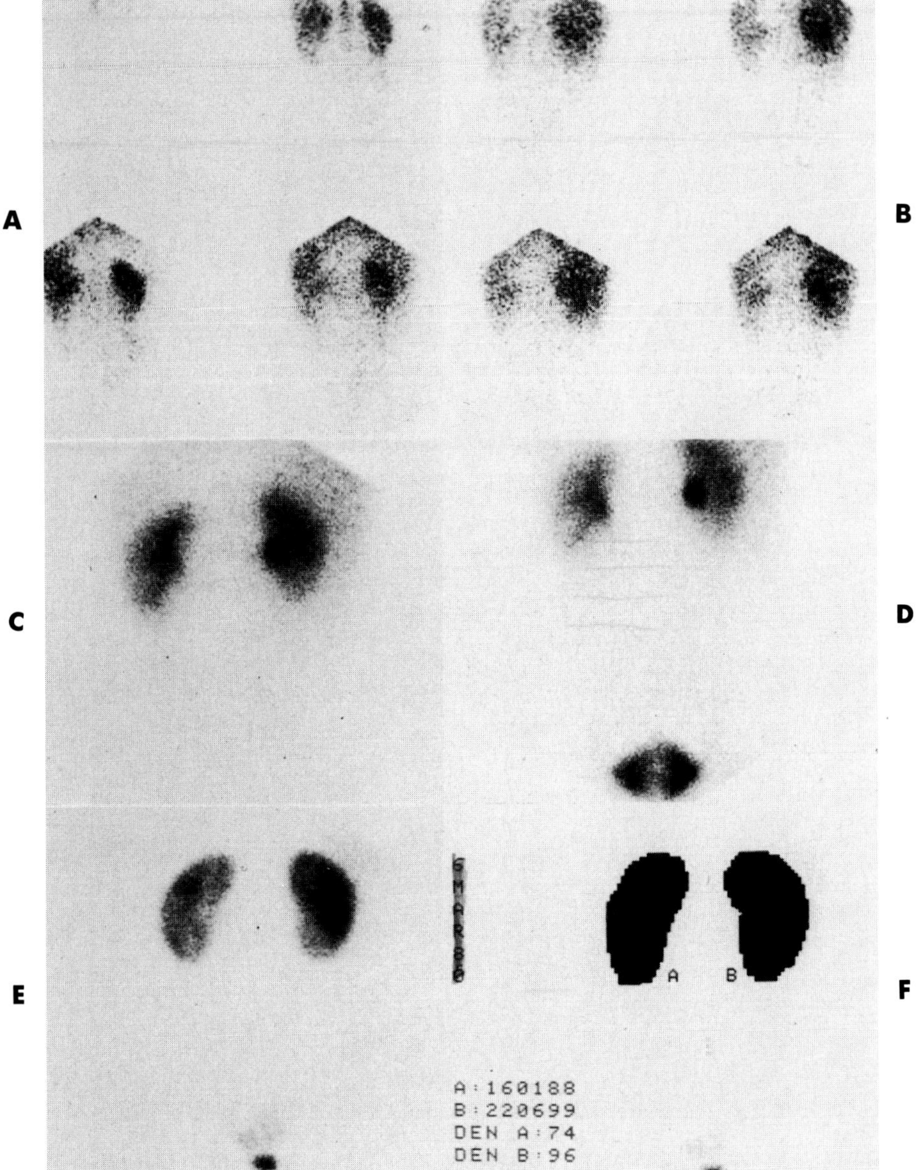

Fig. 23-16. Left acute pyelonephritis with possible small medullary abscess. Sequential images following intravenous administration of 15 mCi (555 MBq) ^{99m}Tc glucoheptonate reveal at **A,** 16 seconds and **B,** 32 seconds decreased perfusion of entire left kidney with greatest decrease in lower half. At **C,** 3 minutes and **D,** 8 minutes, the left kidney is of normal size with decreased concentration in cortex, primarily lower half. Right cortical visualization is normal. Apparent splaying of left renal calyces with rounded impression of 2-cm lower renal medullary lesion. Ureters are bilaterally normal. **E,** 4-hour delay and **F,** 4-hour delay tubular phase quantitation reveal mottled decreased function tubular volume in normal sized left kidney. Right kidney is normal.

Continued.

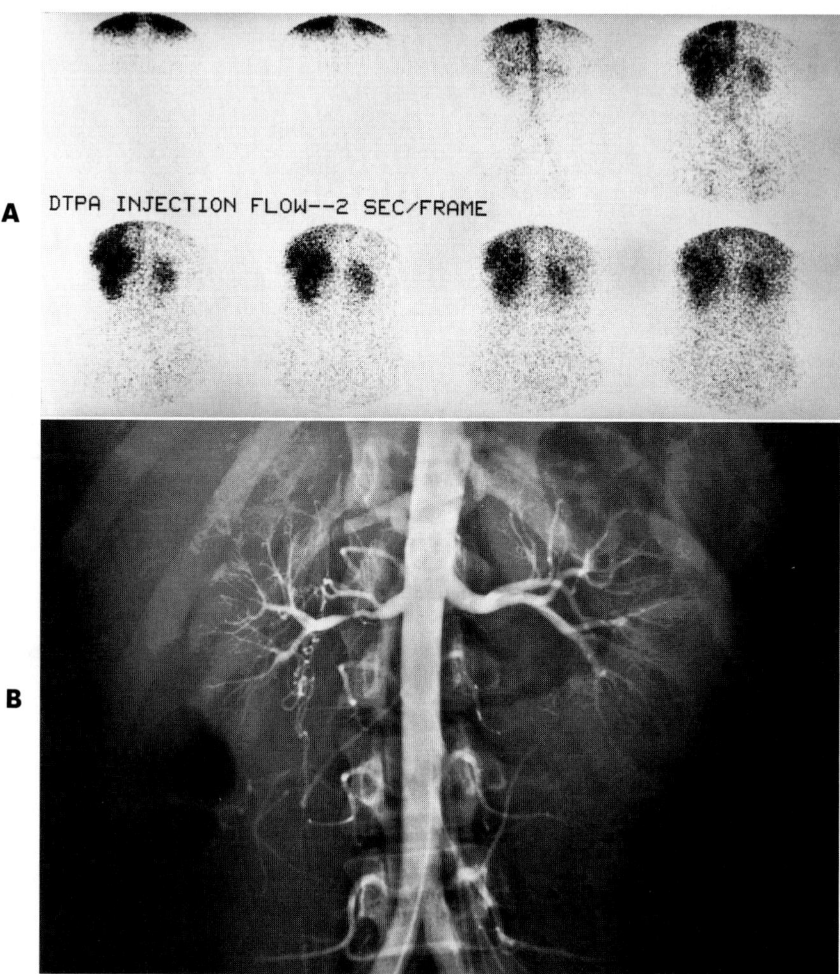

Fig. 23-17. A, Flow study following intravenous bolus injection of 10 mCi (370 MBq) ^{99m}Tc DTPA demonstrating a small hypoperfused right kidney. The findings could be due to several diseases, including renovascular or parenchymal disease. **B,** Aortogram revealing stenotic right renal artery with a somewhat shrunken, nephrosclerotic right kidney.

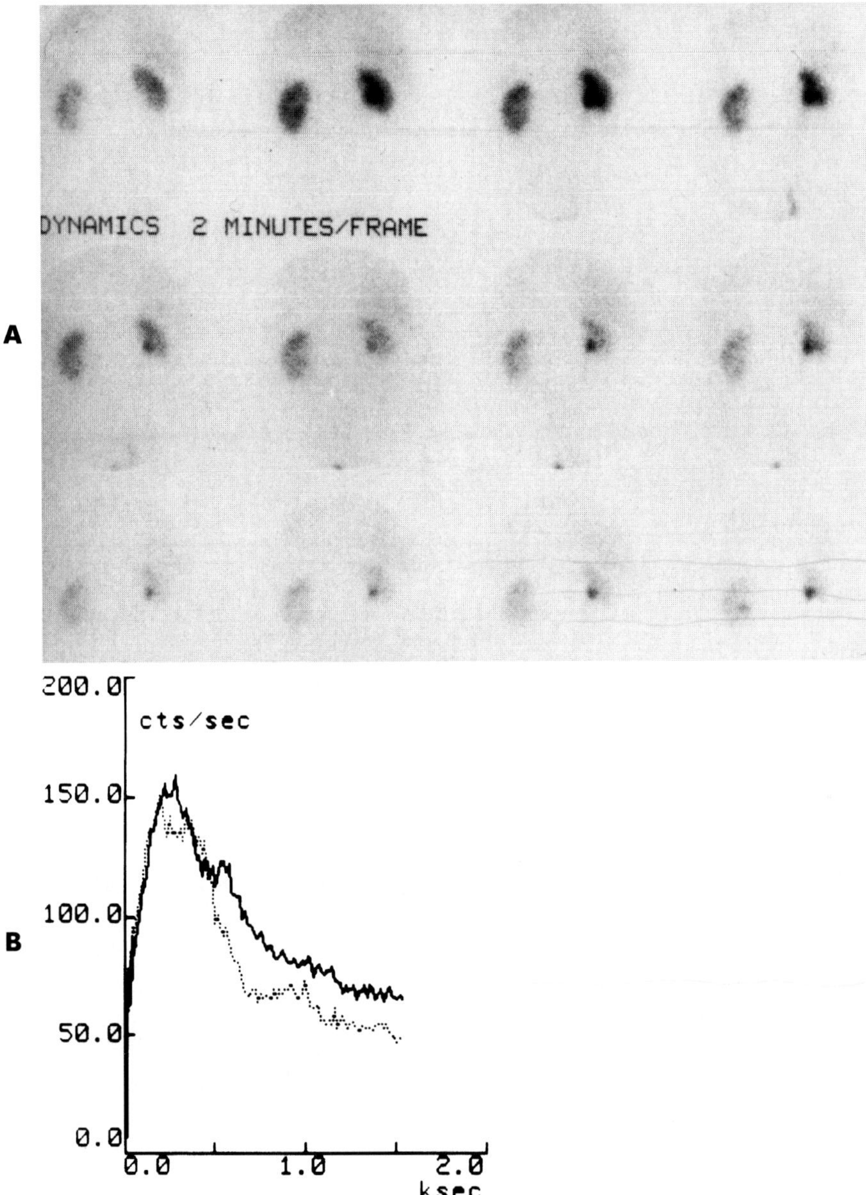

Fig. 23-18. A, A 78-year-old man presented with dizziness and was found to have a blood pressure of 230/120. He was treated with clonidine, triamterene/hydrochlorothiazide, and nifedipine and referred for angiography and renal scintigraphy. At the time of study, his creatinine was 1.7 mg/dL. He underwent baseline scintigraphy with 1.2 mCi of ^{99m}Tc-MAG$_3$. Images were obtained at 2-min intervals for 24 min. The relative uptake at 2 to 3 min was 52% in the right kidney and 48% in the left kidney and the sequential 2-min images are normal. **B,** Time-activity renogram curves for the baseline are also normal. *Continued.*

Continued.

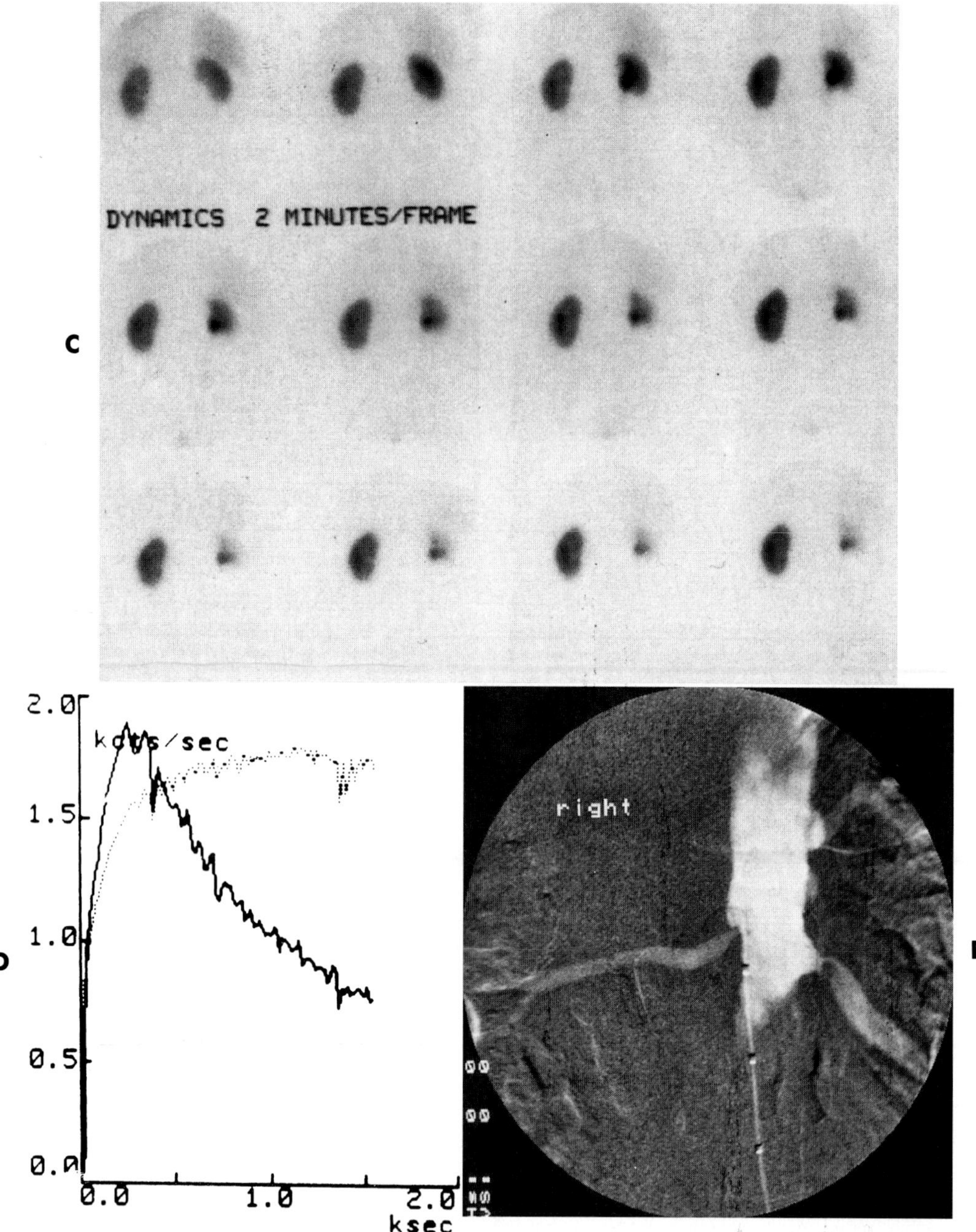

Fig. 23-18, cont'd. C, Following completion of the baseline study, the patient was given 50 mg of captopril. The tablet was crushed and administered with water. Approximately 1.5 h later, ^{99m}Tc-MAG$_3$ scintigraphy was performed with 9.3 mCi. Blood pressure fell from 190/80 at baseline to its lowest value of 140/68 following captopril administration. The sequential 2-min images show marked cortical retention in the left kidney; the right kidney remained normal. **D,** The renogram curve of the left kidney is also markedly abnormal. **E,** Angiography demonstrated bilateral renal artery stenosis. Renin secretion may have been suppressed in the right kidney[25] or the stenosis of the right renal artery may not have resulted in renovascular hypertension. Alternatively, the study may have been falsely negative for the right kidney. (From Taylor, A. and Martin L.G.: The utility of ^{99m}Tc-mercaptoacetyltriglycine in captopril renography, Amer. J. Hypertension, 4:731S-736S, 1991.)

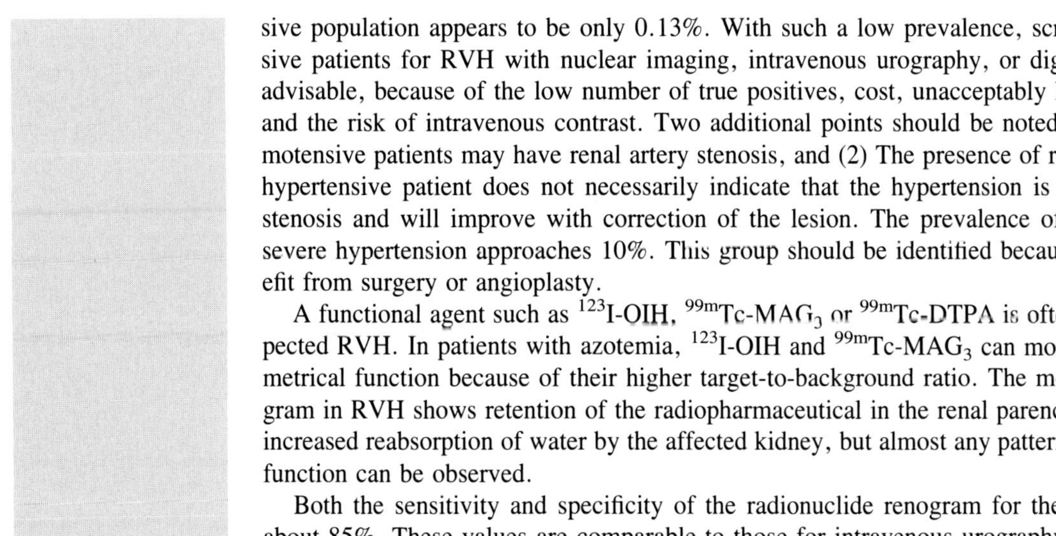

sive population appears to be only 0.13%. With such a low prevalence, screening of all hypertensive patients for RVH with nuclear imaging, intravenous urography, or digital angiography is not advisable, because of the low number of true positives, cost, unacceptably high false positive rate, and the risk of intravenous contrast. Two additional points should be noted: (1) A number of normotensive patients may have renal artery stenosis, and (2) The presence of renal artery stenosis in a hypertensive patient does not necessarily indicate that the hypertension is due to the renal artery stenosis and will improve with correction of the lesion. The prevalence of RVH in patients with severe hypertension approaches 10%. This group should be identified because of the potential benefit from surgery or angioplasty.

A functional agent such as ^{123}I-OIH, ^{99m}Tc-MAG$_3$ or ^{99m}Tc-DTPA is often used to evaluate suspected RVH. In patients with azotemia, ^{123}I-OIH and ^{99m}Tc-MAG$_3$ can more reliably detect asymmetrical function because of their higher target-to-background ratio. The most characteristic scintigram in RVH shows retention of the radiopharmaceutical in the renal parenchyma as a result of the increased reabsorption of water by the affected kidney, but almost any pattern indicating asymmetric function can be observed.

Both the sensitivity and specificity of the radionuclide renogram for the detection of RVH are about 85%. These values are comparable to those for intravenous urography. In a thorough review of the role of nuclear medicine in evaluating the hypertensive patient, Fine and others outline an initial screening procedure for evaluating hypertensive patients. Their protocol includes history, physical examination, laboratory studies (CBC, electrolytes, creatinine, BUN, cholesterol, uric acid, and urinalysis), chest x-ray examination, and electrocardiogram. Patients with a normal screen and an abdominal bruit of grade 3 or 4, hypertensive retinopathy, renal dysfunction, or severe diastolic hypertension (diastolic pressure ≥130 mm/Hg) have a 30% probability of having RVH.

■ ACE INHIBITOR RENOGRAPHY

Captopril is an angiotensin-converting enzyme (ACE) inhibitor that blocks the formation of angiotensin II. Angiotensin II is a potent vasoconstrictor; it preferentially causes vasoconstriction of the efferent glomerular arteriole. In significant renal artery stenosis, blood flow to the kidney is reduced. Decreased renal blood flow stimulates the release of renin; this catalyzes the production of angiotensin I leading to angiotensin II. Angiotensin II causes arterial constriction and sodium retention, increasing both systemic arterial pressure and blood flow to the stenotic kidney.

Transcapillary pressure in the glomerulus is a major factor in determining the glomerular filtration rate. A fall in the renal perfusion pressure lowers the transcapillary pressure gradient but efferent glomerular arteriole constriction induced by angiotensin II increases the glomerular pressure gradient and can maintain GFR in the face of decreased renal perfusion pressure. Captopril blocks formation of angiotensin II and can lead to a fall in GFR in kidneys with renal artery stenosis.

Wenting and others took advantage of the pharmacologic action of captopril to image a patient with unilateral renal artery stenosis. A baseline DTPA (GFR) scan showed essentially equal function. The patient was placed on captopril, and the DTPA uptake of the stenotic kidney fell dramatically. Captopril was discontinued, and the DTPA uptake of the stenotic kidney returned to its baseline level. Subsequent studies have confirmed the utility of ACE inhibitor renography in the detection of renovascular hypertension. ^{99m}Tc-DTPA is excreted purely by the glomerulus, whereas MAG$_3$ and OIH are primarily extracted by the proximal tubular cells and secreted into the tubular lumen. In patients with renovascular hypertension, the relative renal radiopharmaceutical uptake may remain equal because of compensatory mechanisms within the affected kidney. However, if the GFR is reduced by the administration of an ACE inhibitor, the relative uptake of a purely glomerular agent such as DTPA will fall. Since blood flow may be unchanged, the relative uptake of agents such as MAG$_3$ and OIH may remain the same as the cells of the proximal tubule continue to accumulate the tracer. However, washout of OIH and MAG$_3$ from the tubular cell and the tubular lumen are delayed because of the decreased glomerular filtration and decreased flow rate of the glomerular filtrate within the proximal tubule. The delayed washout results in cortical retention of the tracer, which can be quantitated by measuring the 20-minute-to-peak–activity ratio. Sfakianakis and his colleagues report that OIH and MAG$_3$ renography show greater promise than DTPA for the diagnosis of renovascular hypertension after ACE inhibition, particularly in patients with azotemia.

The protocols and criteria for a positive test often vary from center to center. The lack of standardization coupled with the fact that many reported studies use renal artery stenosis as the end point (not blood pressure response to revascularization) make it difficult to formulate precise guidelines. The guidelines discussed below are based on the recommendations of the consensus panel on ACE inhibitor renography, which were published in the *American Journal of Hypertension* by Black in 1991 and by Nally in 1992. Captopril (25- to 50-mg tablet crushed and administered orally with 250 ml of water) has been used in the majority of published studies. A 25-mg tablet is sufficient unless there is delayed gastric emptying or poor absorbtion from the GI tract. Food can interfere with the absorption of captopril; patients should not eat the morning of the study before captopril scintigraphy. It is important, however, for patients to be well hydrated. The peak activity of captopril does not occur until about 60 minutes after ingestion; for this reason the tracer is usually not injected until 60 to 90 minutes after captopril administration. Limitations of captopril scintigraphy include the time delay between administering the captopril and the tracer, and the possibility that delayed gastric emptying or poor absorption may result in a false negative test.

A second approach is to administer enalaprilat (40 μg/kg given intravenously over 3 to 5 minutes), wait 10 minutes, and inject the MAG_3; the total dose of enalapril should not exceed 2.5 mg. This procedure improves patient throughput, obviates the necessity of monitoring the patient for hypotension during the 60-minute period after captopril is administered, and avoids problems of delayed gastric emptying or poor absorption. A limitation of enalaprilat is the fact that it has not been as widely used as captopril; results using the two drugs, however, should be similar.

Blood pressure must be monitored. ACE inhibitors can result in a major hypotensive episode. The hypotension can usually be reversed by placing the patient supine, raising his or her legs, and infusing normal saline. The risk of hypotension can be minimized by having the patient well hydrated. If possible, diuretics should be stopped for several days before the study. The patient should be instructed to arrive well hydrated and should be further hydrated orally (up to 10 mL/kg) immediately on arrival in the department.

Ideally, all antihypertensive drugs should be discontinued 48 hrs before the study. In practice, this is usually not acceptable to the referring physician. Sometimes it is possible to discontinue diuretics and beta blockers; this will help decrease the risk of a hypotensive episode. ACE inhibitors should be discontinued for several days before the test. Failure to stop ACE inhibitors may decrease the sensitivity of the test.

A normal captopril or enalaprilat renogram obviates the need for a baseline study. For this reason many centers begin with the ACE inhibition renogram. If the study is abnormal, the specificity can be improved by obtaining a baseline renogram, particularly if the patient has azotemia. The baseline renogram cannot be performed after an ACE inhibitor has already been administered; the patient will have to return for the baseline study another day.

A second approach is to perform a baseline study with 1 mCi of ^{99m}Tc-MAG_3 or ^{99m}Tc-DTPA, administer the ACE inhibitor, and perform a second renogram with 10 mCi of MAG_3 or DTPA. This protocol requires two renograms on the same day and therefore requires the patient to spend a longer period of time in the department; there is no need, however, for the patient to return. The first approach is less expensive if the time required for a patient to return on a second day for a baseline test is not factored into the calculation.

Some centers advocate a furosemide-augmented captopril or enalaprilat renogram for the detection of renovascular hypertension. The diagnosis of renovascular hypertension is partially based on cortical retention of the tracer. Retention of the tracer in the calyces can distort both the visual and quantitative analysis of cortical retention (time to T_{max} and the 3- to 20-min/maximal activity ratio). Since furosemide is a loop diuretic and acts distally to the glomerulus and proximal tubules, a furosemide induced diuresis can wash tracer out of the calyces and pelvis but it does not affect cortical retention of MAG_3, OIH, or DTPA. A disadvantage of furosemide is volume depletion and a greater risk of severe hypotension. If furosemide is used, an intravenous line should be established for supplemental hydration; a protocol for furosemide and intravenous hydration is described by Erbsloh-Müller.

The Consensus Panel on renovascular hypertension recommends that the test be interpreted as high, low, or indeterminate probability. A high probability study requires a significant deterioration in relative function or the shape of the renogram curve following ACE inhibition, compared with the baseline study. Indeterminate scans include the group of patients with an abnormal baseline renogram but no change in the renogram following ACE inhibition. These also include the hypertensive patient with a small, poorly functioning kidney. Published results vary in this patient population; further studies along with standardized protocols may reduce the number of indeterminate studies. A normal ACE inhibition renogram is low probability for RVH.

■ RENAL TRANSPLANTATION (Figs. 23-19 to 23-21)

Complications of renal transplantation include parenchymal failure due to acute tubular necrosis (ATN), cyclosporine toxicity, infection, mechanical failure due to injury of the renal artery or vein, partial or complete ureteral obstruction, and a tear in the collecting system that results in urine extravasation. Acute renal vessel occlusion, poor parenchymal function, ureteral obstruction, and extravasation can usually be detected by renal imaging; a normal image following transplantation excludes these complications. There are a number of mathematical techniques for quantitating perfusion and parenchymal transit, but currently none appear to be specific enough to reliably distinguish between ATN, rejection, and cyclosporin toxicity. In general, however, poor perfusion with poor excretory function is more likely to be associated with rejection, while good perfusion associated with poor excretory function is more likely to be associated with acute tubular necrosis.

Fig. 23-19. Acute rejection. The patient demonstrated a deterioration in renal function two weeks following transplantation. Sequential images, anterior view, following the bolus intravenous administration of 10 mCi (370 MBq) of ^{99m}Tc DTPA. **A,** Flow study demonstrating delayed perfusion to the transplanted kidney in the right hemipelvis. Normally, the kidney should temporally appear isoactive with the iliac artery in the arterial phase. **B,** Static images demonstrating normal function of the transplant.

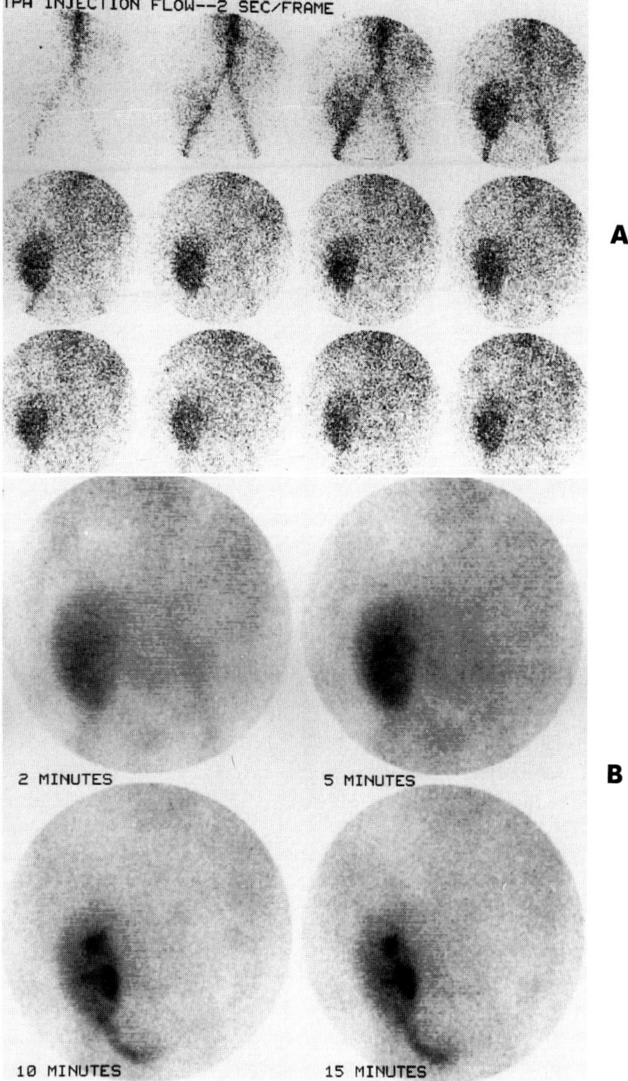

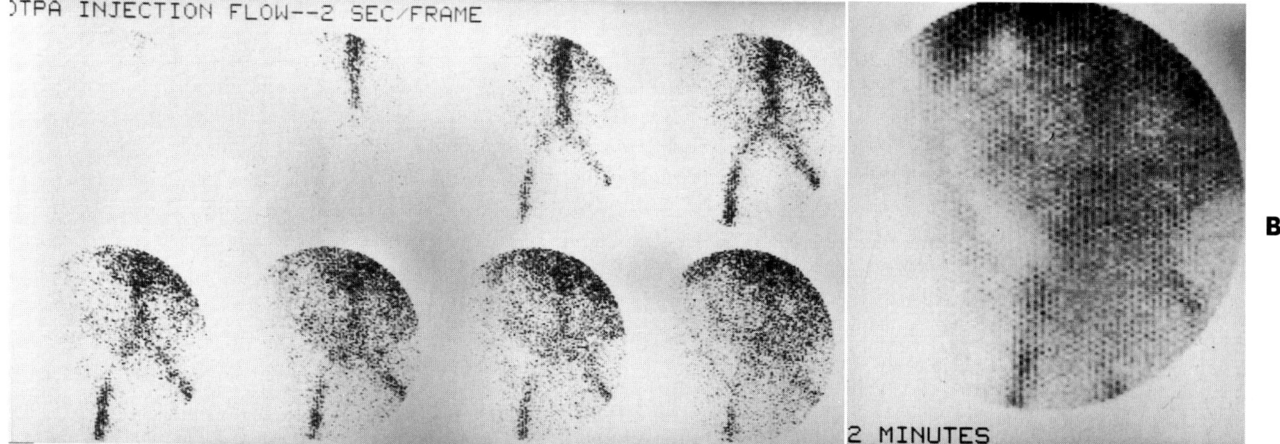

Fig. 23-20. Post-operative acute tubular necrosis (cadaveric renal transplant). A renal image was obtained one day following transplantation. Sequential images, anterior view, following the bolus intravenous administration of 10 mCi (370 MBq) of ^{99m}Tc DTPA. **A,** Flow study demonstrating preserved flow to the transplanted kidney. **B,** Static images demonstrating diminished function with marked background activity. Diagnosis: Post operative acute tubular necrosis (cadaveric renal transplant).

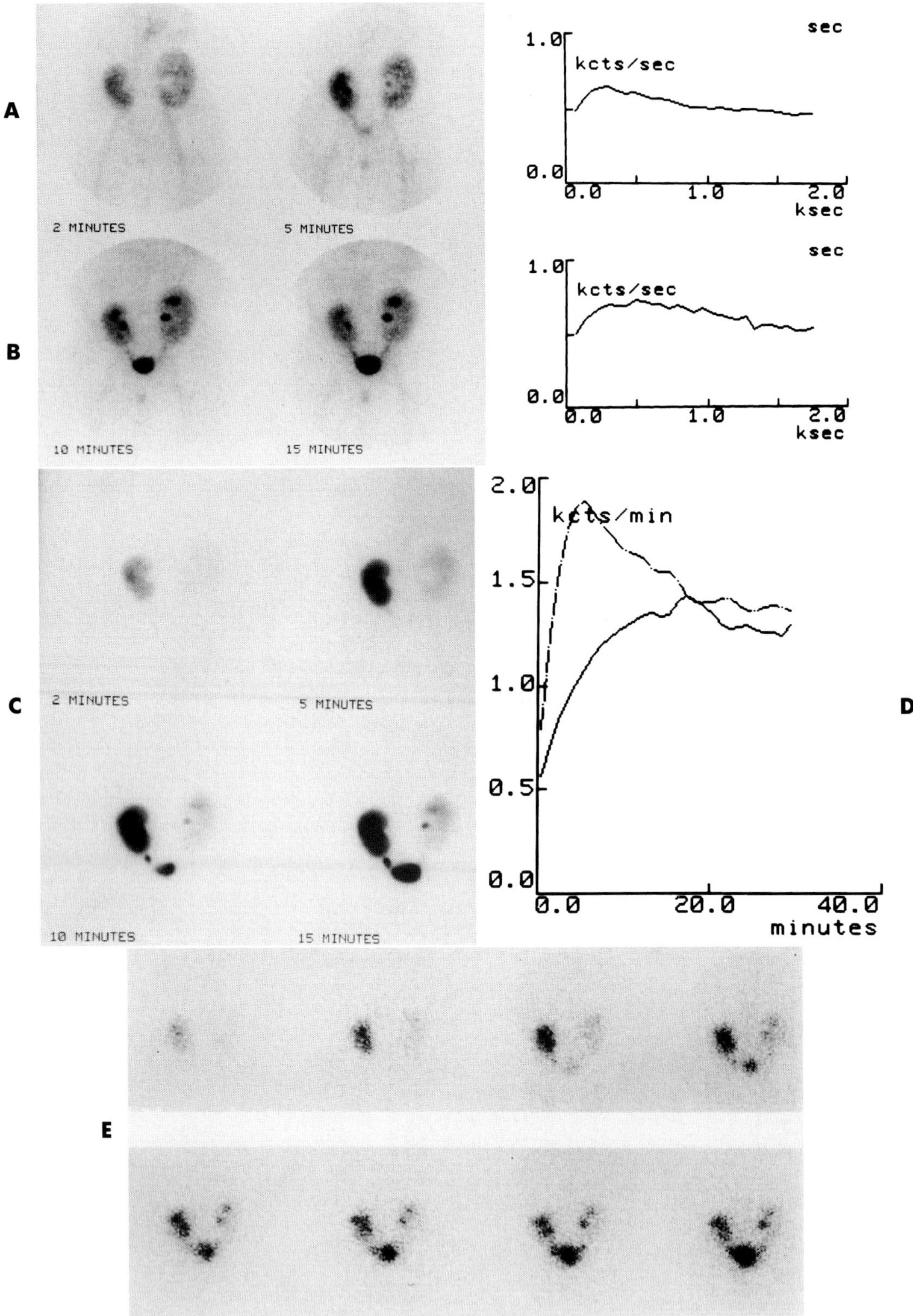

Fig. 23-21. A, The Tc-99m DTPA (10 mCi) study suggests relatively equal function (2-3 min uptake: L = 47%, R = 53%) in a patient with a serum creatinine of 2.9 mg/dl, a failed left hemipelvic transplant and a recent right hemipelvic transplant. **B,** The Tc-99m DTPA renogram curves for the two kidneys are almost identical. **C,** The Tc-99m MAG_3 (7.7 mCi) study obtained the following day gives results similar to the OIH study (2-3 min uptake: L = 27%, R = 73%). **D,** In contrast to the Tc-99m DTPA study, the Tc-99m MAG_3 renogram curves clearly demonstrate the abnormal right kidney. **E,** OIH (150 μCi) images obtained the same day are displayed in 2-minute increments and clearly distinguish between the functioning right hemipelvic transplant and the rejected left hemipelvic transplant (1-2 min uptake: L = 29%, R = 71%). (From Taylor, A., Ziffer, J.A., and Eshima, D.: Comparison of Tc-99m MAG_3 and Tc-99m DTPA in renal transplant patients with impaired renal function, Clin. Nucl. Med. 15(6), June 1990.)

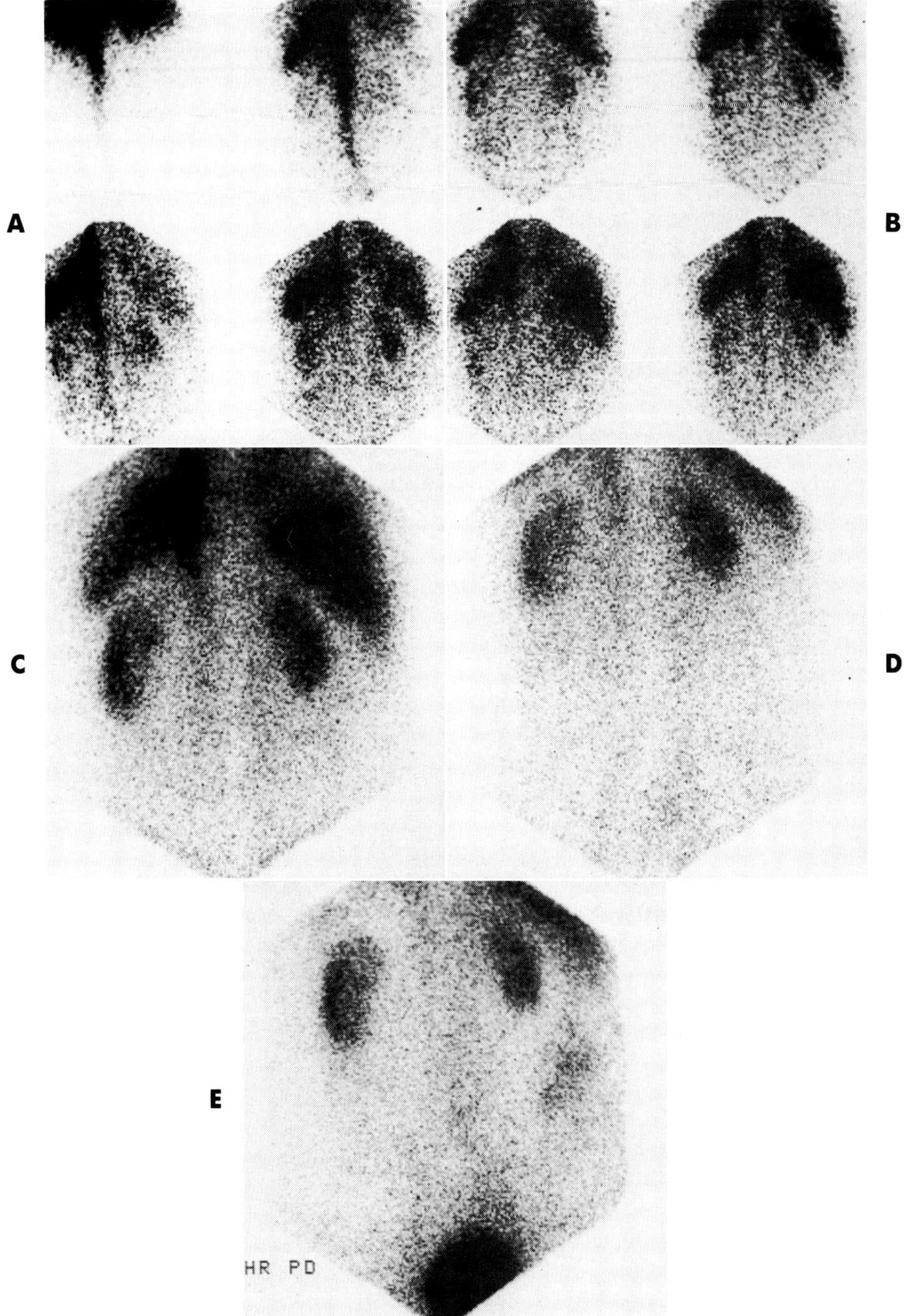

Fig. 23-22. Chronic pyelonephritis. Sequential images following intravenous administration of 15 mCi ^{99}Tc glucoheptonate reveal at **A,** 16 seconds; **B,** 32 seconds; **C,** 1 minute; and **D,** 3 minutes bilaterally decreased renal perfusion. Bilateral symmetric decreased cortical volumes with normal appearance time of collecting structures and ureters. There is a 3-cm rounded defect in bladder. **E,** 4-hour delay reveals approximate 75% symmetric decrease in tubular volumes.

Dubovsky (1985) has published a table based on the ERPF and excretory index (EI). This is helpful in discriminating between acute rejection, chronic rejection, acute tubular necrosis, and incomplete obstruction. In general, normal posttransplant kidneys have an ERPF of 270 to 450 ml/min and an excretory index (EI) of 0.8 to 1.2. With acute rejection, both ERPF (100 to 270) and EI (0.2 to 0.7) are decreased. With chronic rejection, the principal abnormality is decreased ERPF (30 to 270) with a more normal excretory index unless ERPF is severely decreased. ATN results in profound decrease in EI (less than 0.2) with ERPF ranging from 50 to 300 ml/min. In incomplete obstruction, ERPF is normal (300 to 400), while EI is moderately decreased (0.5 to 0.7). Recent data suggest that the ratio of the renal activity at 19 to 20 minutes to the maximal or 2- to 3-minute activity may be able to substitute for the excretory index.

Posttransplant renal artery stenosis can develop, usually at the anastomotic site of the donor artery and recipient internal iliac artery. It has an insidious onset accompanied by gradually rising blood pressure and decreasing ERPF. It therefore mimics chronic rejection in nuclear imaging procedures.

Other nuclear procedures have been used to detect rejection; these are based on the fact that the vascular inflammatory response in rejection may result in endothelial damage and local thrombosis. The procedures include imaging with ^{111}In platelets, ^{125}I- or ^{131}I-labeled fibrinogen, ^{99m}Tc sulfur colloid and ^{67}Ga citrate. In general, these procedures have had less widespread application, because of variable results. Furthermore, these techniques do not detect other pathologic states including ATN or obstruction. ^{67}Ga citrate and ^{111}In-labeled white cells, however, may be of benefit in assessing whether infection is present, particularly in perinephric fluid collections (although needle aspiration is usually preferred). ^{111}In-labeled white cells may accumulate in a normally functioning transplant.

Serial images using ^{99m}Tc-MAG$_3$, ^{99m}Tc-OIH, or ^{99m}Tc-DTPA obtained during the first 1 to 2 weeks posttransplantation are useful in monitoring recovery from posttransplantation ATN and may also detect a deterioration in function 24 to 48 hours before an increasing BUN or serum creatinine. Quantitative as well as qualitative data should be obtained to facilitate comparison of sequential studies.

■ Determination of functional recovery and prognosis

An acutely injured kidney (trauma, obstruction, ischemia, etc.) that demonstrates good function on renal scintigraphy is likely to maintain that level of function or improve. Normal cortical renograms are a further indication of a good prognosis in patients with obstruction. It should be remembered that renal imaging evaluates renal function at the time the study is performed, and the poor function should not be used to exclude the possibility of recovery in acute renal injury.

■ URETEROCYSTOGRAPHY

LABORATORY APPLICATION

73

RADIONUCLIDE CYSTOGRAPHY

Purpose and indications

Radionuclide studies are routinely used in the management of vesicoureteral reflux and can serve as a prognostic indicator to predict which patients will have spontaneous resolution of their reflux. The radiation dose to the gonads from radiographic techniques ranges from 130 millirads to several rads and is much higher than direct radionuclide cystography, which results in less than 30 mrad to the female gonads and less than 5 mrad to the male gonads. Moreover, the radionuclide cystogram is more sensitive and less subjective than x-ray cystography in the detection of vesicoureteral reflux.

There are two radionuclide techniques for detecting vesicoureteral reflux: direct and indirect cystography. The direct method involves introduction of the radiopharmaceutical via catheter into the urinary bladder. With the indirect technique, the radiopharmaceutical (^{99m}Tc-DTPA or ^{99m}Tc-MAG$_3$) is injected intravenously. When the radiopharmaceutical has cleared the kidney and filled the bladder, the patient is asked to void. The kidneys, ureters, and bladder are monitored using a gamma camera interfaced to a computer. The diagnosis of reflux is based on a significant increase in activity in the upper urinary tracts during or after voiding. The indirect technique is simple but unfortunately has several limitations. The sensitivity of the test will decrease in patients with impaired renal function, because of higher background activity. The technique best evaluates reflux associated with elevated bladder pressures that occur during voiding, yet reflux often occurs at low pressures and low volume. Because the radiopharmaceutical is injected intravenously, the radiation dose is higher and it is difficult to quantitate results for comparative studies. In spite of the fact that bladder catheterization is not necessary, the indirect technique has major limitations; therefore, direct radionuclide cystography is preferred.

The bladder volume at which reflux occurs is an important prognostic factor in predicting which patients will experience spontaneous resolution of their vesicoureteral reflux. Children who reflux at progressively larger volumes on subsequent studies tend to have spontaneous resolution of their reflux and can often be spared surgery. For this reason, it is important to study all aspects of bladder filling and emptying. Direct radionuclide cystography serves an important role in the management of patients with reflux or suspected reflux in that the prognostic information can be used to avoid surgery or indicate early intervention to prevent subsequent impairment of renal function due to reflux.

Procedure: adult

Materials

1. ^{99m}Tc pertechnetate or ^{99m}Tc sulfur colloid, 1 mCi (37 MBq)
2. Normal saline solution, 50 to 1500 ml, depending on the size of the patient
3. Scintillation camera with a low-energy, high-sensitivity or general all-purpose collimator
4. Computer for data acquisition
5. Infusion set with Foley catheter

Patient preparation

1. Have the patient void completely before the examination.
2. Insert the Foley catheter into the patient's bladder, using sterile technique.
3. Explain the entire procedure to the patient.

Technique

1. Inject radiopharmaceutical directly into bladder via puncture of infusion tubing.
2. Position the patient with the dome of the bladder above the lower edge of the field of view. The posterior view is best with the patient in a supine position and the camera placed under the patient. Data should be recorded continuously and stored on the computer for subsequent review.
3. Fill the bladder with normal saline solution. Complete filling is indicated by the patient's urgency, leakage around the catheter, or cessation of flow into the bladder from the infusion bottle.
4. Monitor a persistence scope for evidence of reflux. At the time of reflux, note volume instilled into the bladder.
5. When bladder is full, obtain 2-minute images in the posterior and in both oblique positions. Use a high-intensity image to visualize small amounts of reflux. Note count rate in straight posterior view.
6. Obtain a 2-minute posterior image of the bladder at a low-intensity setting.
7. Rotate camera head 90 degrees. Position patient with back to camera (lateral decubitus).
8. Instruct patient to void into urinal or bedpan, obtain an image while patient is voiding. Determine volume voided. Use urine volume and activity to determine bladder retention.

$$\text{Bladder retention (ml)} = \frac{\text{Postvoid cpm} \times \text{volume of urine (ml)}}{(\text{Prevoid cpm} - \text{Postvoid cpm})}$$

9. Obtain a 2-minute postvoid image.
10. Review dynamic data recorded by computer.

Key points

Ureteral reflux and residual volume measurements can also be performed after intravenous injection of ^{99m}Tc-DTPA or ^{99m}Tc-MAG$_3$, using the bladder-imaging procedure described above and in the text and quantitating bladder residual volume as outlined under renal perfusion and imaging procedure. This method has reduced sensitivity, is better suited to study of adult patients, and is not recommended if significant renal dysfunction is present.

Procedure: radionuclide cystography: pediatric

Before beginning the study, the procedure should be discussed with the child and parents to relieve anxiety and improve compliance. A Foley catheter is preferred because it has less tendency to

Continued.

slip out, although a number 5 or 8 infant feeding tube is usually required in boys under one year of age because of the small diameter of the meatus. A number 8 Foley catheter can be used in most boys 1 to 3 years of age. In girls, one can usually use a number 8 Foley catheter for patients under age 1, a number 10 Foley catheter between ages 1 and 3, and a number 12 Foley catheter for older girls. If there is no urine returned through the catheter, its position should be evaluated by instilling a small amount of saline.

Conway uses a double lumen catheter attached to a pressure transducer and recording device. He has found that pressure measurements concurrent with bladder filling are especially useful in evaluating patients with reflux, particularly those with abnormalities such as spinal cord injury or myelomeningocele. This procedure should be considered in institutions with large numbers of reflux studies.

Once it is determined that the catheter is in the bladder, 1 mCi (37 MBq) of ^{99m}Tc-pertechnetate is instilled into the tubing and allowed to flow into the bladder; this is followed by saline that has been warmed to body temperature. Mixing the ^{99m}Tc pertechnetate with the saline may not allow enough activity to enter the bladder of patients with a small bladder capacity. The bladder should be filled and the expected capacity can be estimated from the following formula:

$$\text{Expected bladder capacity (oz)} = \text{age (in years)} + 2$$

The gamma camera should be positioned posteriorly and fitted with the high-sensitivity, parallel-hole collimator, but a general all-purpose collimater can be used. Reflux can be monitored by watching the persistence scope, but sequential images acquired on the computer at 30-second intervals and displayed in a cine format to maximize sensitivity are preferred. Once a full bladder is achieved (reaching predicted volume, the patient complains, voiding around the catheter, cessation of passive flow into the bladder), the patient sits on a bedpan with the camera positioned posteriorly over the genitourinary tract; the catheter is removed as the patient voids.

Residual volume can be determined and the urinary tract capacity calculated based on the sum of the residual volume and voided volume. The bladder volume at which reflux occurs should be noted, this may be a useful prognostic factor. Reflux at progressively higher bladder volumes carries a favorable prognosis. For more detail, the reader is referred to a recent review article by Conway (1985).

Determination of residual volume

Residual volume can be easily determined using nuclear medicine techniques. The test is noninvasive and there is no increased risk of infection. At the conclusion of the study, the gamma camera is placed anteriorly over the bladder, data are recorded on the computer, a computer-assisted region of interest is placed over the bladder, and bladder activity is determined for a specific time interval before and immediately after voiding. The voided urine is collected for volume measurement. Residual volume is calculated from the following formula:

$$\text{Residual volume} = \frac{\text{Voided volume} \times \text{Postvoid counts}}{\text{Prevoid counts} - \text{Postvoid counts}}$$

This method gives results comparable to those obtained at catheterization.

Diagnosis

Renal bacterial infection (Figs. 23-15, 23-16, and 23-22)

Patients with bacterial infection of the kidney may present with fever, leukocytosis, and bacteremia, but these findings do not distinguish between upper and lower urinary tract infection. Since parenchymal involvement is much more serious than a lower urinary tract infection, it is important to make this distinction quickly. Furthermore, patients with bacterial nephritis may present with only fever and leukocytosis, with little to indicate the kidney as the site of infection. Conway and others (1984) evaluated 38 children with suspected urinary tract infection with scintigraphy (gallium-67 citrate or ^{99m}Tc glucoheptonate), ultrasonography, and intravenous urography. Intravenous urography was "notably ineffective," and ultrasonography was little better. The authors concluded that radionuclide imaging is the most efficacious modality to detect acute bacterial nephritis. Cortical scans with glucoheptonate or DMSA can be used to diagnose pyelonephritis, to follow its resolution, and to evaluate the return of function. There may also be a complementary role for cortical agents, which

localize in normal renal parenchyma, and radiopharmaceuticals such as gallium-67 citrate and ^{111}In leukocytes, which localize in infection. When ^{67}Ga or ^{111}In leukocytes accumulate in a cortical defect, the probability that infection is the cause of that cortical abnormality substantially increases.

Gallium-67 imaging alone has an 86% accuracy in distinguishing upper tract infection from lower tract infection. In pyelonephritis, the gallium image is often abnormal by 24 hours and can be recognized by focal, asymmetrical renal uptake. Minimal diffuse bilateral uptake may be seen in normal individuals, and more intense diffuse bilateral renal uptake can occur in liver failure, ATN, and vasculitis. If a cortical image is equivocal or confirmatory data are needed, gallium-67 can be injected after the ^{99m}Tc cortical images are obtained, and the patient can be reimaged the following day. ^{111}In leukocyte imaging also appears to be quite useful in the setting of acute pyelonephritis.

BIBLIOGRAPHY

Arroyo, A.J. Effective renal plasma flow determination using technetium-99m MAG_3: comparison of two camera techniques with the Tauxe method, J. Nucl. Med. Technol. 1993, 21:162-166.

Bedont, R., Cook, P., Taylor, A., and others: Diuretic radionuclide renography to evaluate suspected ureteral obstruction on bone scans, Radiology 153:825, 1984.

Berg, B.C., Jr.: Nuclear medicine and complementary modalities in renal trauma, Semin. Nucl. Med. 12:280-300, 1982.

Berger, R.M., Maizels, J., Moran, G.G., and others: Bladder capacity (ounces) = age (years) + 2 predicts normal bladder capacity and aids diagnosis of abnormal voiding patterns, J. Urol. 129:347-349, 1983.

Black, H.R., Bourgoignie, J.J., Pickering, T., and others: Report of the working party group for patient selection and preparation, Am. J. Hypertension 4:745S-146S, 1991.

Blaufox, M.D., Iloreta, F., Heller, S., and others: Evaluation of renal functional reserve with cortical regions of interest, J. Nucl. Med. 20:620, 1979.

Blaufox, M.D., Potchen, E.J., and Merrill, J.P.: Measurement of effective renal plasma flow in man by external counting methods, J. Nucl. Med. 8:77-85, 1967.

Chachati, A., Meyers, A., Godon, J.P., Rigo, P.: Rapid method for the measurement of differential renal function: validation, J. Nucl. Med. 28:829-836, 1987.

Conway, J.J.: Radionuclide cystography. In Tauxe, W.N., and Dubovsky, E.V., editors: Nuclear medicine in clinical urology and nephrology, Norwalk, Conn., 1985, Appleton Century Crofts, pp. 305-320.

Conway, J.J., King, L.R., Belman, A.B., and others: Detection of vesicoureteral reflux with radionuclide cystography: a comparison study with roentgenographic cystography, AJR Am. J. Roentgenol. 115:720-727, 1972.

Conway, J.J., Weiss, S.C., Skolnik, A., and others: Radionuclide scintigraphy of bacterial nephritis, J. Nucl. Med. 25:76, 1984.

Conway, J.J., "Well-tempered" diuresis renography: its historical development, physiological and technical pitfalls, and standardized technique protocol, Semin. Nucl. Med. 22:74-84, 1992.

Dondi, M., Tanti, S., DeFebritiis, A., and others: Prognostic value of captopril renal scintigraphy in renovascular hypertension, J. Nucl. Med. 33:2040-2044, 1992.

Dubovsky, E.V.: Renal transplantation. In Tauxe, W.N., and Dubovsky, E.V.: Nuclear medicine in clinical urology and nephrology, Norwalk, Conn., 1985, Appleton Century Crofts, pp. 233-278.

Dubovsky, E.V., and Russell, C.D.: Quantitation of renal function with glomerular and tubular agents, Semin. Nucl. Med. 12:308-329, 1982.

Eckelman, W., and Richards, P.: Instant 99m Tc-DTPA, J. Nucl. Med. 11:761, 1970.

Eshima, D., Taylor, Jr., A.: Technetium-99m (99mTc) mercaptoacetyltriglycine: Update on the new 99m Tc renal tubular function agent, Semin. Nucl. Med. 22:61-73, 1992.

Fawcett, H.D., Goodwin, D.A., and Lantieri, R.L.: In-111 leukocyte scanning in inflammatory renal disease, Clin. Nucl. Med. 6:237-241, 1981.

Fine, E.J., Scharf, S.C., and Blaufox, M.D.: The role of nuclear medicine in evaluating the hypertensive patient. In Freeman, L.M., and Weissman, H.S., editors: Nuclear medicine annual, New York, 1984, Raven Press, pp. 23-79.

Fommei, E., Ghione, S., Ferrai, M., and others: Captopril scintingraphy in arterial hypertension: evaluation of scintigraphic results in relation to blood pressure and renin response, J. Hypertension 4(S):282-284, 1986.

Fommei, E., Ghione, S., Hilson, A.J.W., and others: Captopril radionuclide test in renovascular hypertension: a European multicentre study, Eur. J. Nucl. Med. 20:617-623, 1993.

Gates, G.F.: Split renal function testing using Tc-99m DTPA: a rapid technique for determining differential glomerular filtration, Clin. Nucl. Med. 8:400-407, 1983.

Geyskes, G., Oei, H., Puylaert, C.B., and others: Renovascular hypertension identified by captopril-induced changes in the renogram, Hypertension 9:451-458, 1987.

Geyskes, G.G., and deBruyn, J.G.: Captopril renography and the effect of percutaneous transluminal angioplasty on blood pressure in 94 patients with renal artery stenosis, Am. J. Hypertension 4:685S-689S, 1991.

Handmaker, H.: Nuclear renal imaging in acute pyelonephritis, Semin. Nucl. Med. 12:246-253, 1982.

Howman-Giles, R., Uren, R., Roy, L.P., and others: Volume expansion diuretic renal scan in urinary tract obstruction, J. Nucl. Med. 28:824-828, 1987.

Hurwitz, S.R., Kessler, W.O., Alazraki, N.P., and others: Gallium-67 imaging to localize urinary-tract infections, Br. J. Radiol. 499:156-160, 1976.

Kirchner, P.T., and Rosenthall, L.: Renal transplant evaluation, Semin. Nucl. Med. 12:370-378, 1982.

Klopper, J.F., Hauser, W., Atkins, H.L., and others: Evaluation of Tc-99m DTPA for the measurement of glomerular filtration rate, J. Nucl. Med. 13:107-110, 1972.

Krueger, R.P., Ash, J.M., Silver, M.M., and others: Primary hydronephrosis: assessment of diuretic renography, pelvis perfusion pressure, operative findings, and renal and ureteral histology, Urol. Clin. North Am. 7(2):231-242, 1980.

Lee, H.B., and Blaufox, M.D.: Mechanism of renal concentration of technetium-99 glucoheptonate, J. Nucl. Med. 26:1308-1313, 1985.

Maizels, M., Weiss, S., Conway, J.J., and others: The cystometric nuclear cystogram, J. Urol. 121:203-205, 1979.

Mann, S.J., Pickering, T.G.: Detection of renovascular hypertension: state of the art: 1992, Ann. Intern. Med. 117:845-853, 1992.

McNeil, B.J., Varady, P.D., Burrows, B.B., and others: Measures of clinical efficacy: cost effectiveness calculations in the diagnosis and treatment of hypertensive renovascular disease, N. Engl. J. Med. 293:216-221, 1975.

Miyamori, J., Yashura, S., Takeda, Y., and others: Effects of converting enzyme inhibition on split renal function in renovascular hypertension, Hypertension 8:415-421, 1986.

Müller-Suur, R., Bois-Svensson, I., and Meskol: A comparative study of renal scintigraphy and clearance with technetium-99m-MAG_3 and iodine-123-hippurate in patients with renal disorders, J. Nucl. Med. 31:1811-1817, 1990.

Nally, J.W., Jr., Chen, C., Fine, E., and others: Diagnostic criteria of renovascular hypertension with captopril renography, Am. J. Hypertension 4:749S-752S, 1992.

Nasrallah, P.F., Conway, J.J., King, L.R., and others: Quantitative nuclear cystogram: an aid in determining spontaneous resolution of vesicoureteral reflux, Urology 12:654-658, 1978.

Nissenkorn, I., Gil, I., Servadio, C., and Lubin, E.: Radionuclide cystography: the significance of retention time of the refluxed radioisotope, J. Urol. 126:448-451, 1981.

O'Reilly, P.H., Lawson, R.S., Shields, R.A., and others: Idiopathic hydronephrosis the diuresis renogram: a new non-invasive method of assessing equivocal pelviureteral junction obstruction, J. Urol. 121:153-155, 1979.

O'Reilly, P.H.: Diuresis renography: recent advances and recommended protocols, Br. J. Urol. 69:113-120, 1992.

Powers, T.A., Stone, W.J., Grove, B., and others: Radionuclide measurement of differential glomerular filtration rate, Invest. Radiol. 16:59-64, 1981.

Russell, C.D., Bischoff, P.G., Kontzen, F.N., and others: Measurement of glomerular filtration rate: single injection plasma clearance method without urine collection, J. Nucl. Med. 26:1243-1247, 1985.

Russell, C.D., Rowell, K., and Scott, J.W.: Quality control of technetium-99m DTPA: correlation of analytic tests with in vivo protein binding in man, J. Nucl. Med. 27:560-562, 1986.

Schlegel, J.U., Halikiopoulos, H.L., and Prima, R.: Determination of filtration fraction using the gamma scintillation camera, J. Urol. 122:447-450, 1979.

Schlegel, J.U., Hamway, S.A.: Individual renal plasma flow determination in 2 minutes, J. Urol. 116:282-285, 1976.

Setaro, J.F., Saddler, M.C., Chen, C.C., and others: Simplified captopril renography in diagnosis and treatment of renal artery stenosis, Hypertension 18:289-298, 1991.

Sfakianakis, G.N., Bourgoignie, J.J., Georgiou, M., and Guerra, J.J.: Diagnosis of renovascular hypertension with ace inhibition scintigraphy, Radiologic Clin. North Am. 31:831-848, 1993.

Stabin, M., Taylor, A., Eshima, D., and Wooten, W.: Radiation dosimetry for technetium-99m-MAG_3 technetium-99m-DTPA, and iodine-131-OIH based on human biodistribution studies, J. Nucl. Med. 33:33-40, 1992.

Strauss, B.S., and Blaufox, M.D.: Estimation of residual urine and urine flow rates without urethral catheterization, J. Nucl. Med. 11:81-84, 1970.

Strauss, H.W., Harrison, K., and Pitt, B.: Thallium-201: noninvasive determination of the regional distribution of cardiac output, J. Nucl. Med. 18:1167-1170, 1977.

Talner, L.B., Sokoloff, J., Halpert, S.E., and Taylor, A.: Limitations of renal function scanning in acute obstruction, Int. J. Nucl. Med. Biol. 9:181-187, 1982.

Tauxe, W.N., Maher, F.T., and Taylor, W.F.: Effective renal plasma flow: estimation from theoretical volumes of distribution of intravenously injected I-131 orthoiodohippurate, Mayo Clin. Proc. 46:524-531, 1971.

Tauxe, W.N., Dubovsky, E.V., Kidd, T., and others: New formulas for the calculation of effective renal plasma flow, Eur. J. Nucl. Med. 7:51-54, 1982.

Taylor, A.T., Jr.: Quantitative renal function scanning: a historical and current status report on renal radiopharmaceuticals. In Freeman, L., and Weissman, H.S., editors: Nuclear medicine annual 1980, New York, 1980, Raven Press, pp. 303-340.

Taylor, A.: Quantitation of renal function with static imaging agents, Semin. Nucl. Med. 12:330-344, 1982.

Taylor, A., Eshima, D., Christian, P.E., and others: Evaluation of Tc-99m mercaptoacetyltriglycine in patients with impaired renal function, Radiology 162:365-370, 1987.

Taylor, A., Eshima, D., Christian, P.E., and others: A technetium-99m MAG_3 kit formulation: preliminary results in normal volunteers and patients with renal failure, J. Nucl. Med. 29:616-622, 1988.

Taylor, A., and Eshima, D.: Effects of altered physiologic states on clearance and biodistribution of technetium-99m MAG_3, iodine-131 OIH and iodine-125 iothalamate, J. Nucl. Med. 29:669-675, 1988.

Taylor, A., Jr., Corrigan, P., Eshima, D., and Folks, R.: Prospective validation of a single sample technique to determine technetium-99m-MAG_3 clearance, J. Nucl. Med. 433:1620-1622, 1992.

Taylor, A., Garcia, E., Jones, M., and others: An optimized camera based technique to calculate Tc-99m MAG_3 clearance, J. Nucl. Med. 33:948(521), 1992 (abstract).

Taylor, A., Halkar, R.K., Garcia, E., and others: A camera-based method to calculate Tc-99m MAG_3 clearance, J. Nucl. Med. 32:953, 1991 (abstract).

Taylor, A., Lewis, C., Giacometti, A., and others: Improved formulas for the estimation of renal depth in adults, J. Nucl. Med. 34:1766-1769, 1993.

Thakore, K., Folks, R., and Taylor, A.: The effect of different ROIs for background correction on relative renal function in patients with unilateral nephrectomy, J. Nucl. Med. 34(5):87P, 1993 (abstract).

Thrall, J.H., Koff, S.A., and Keyes, J.W.: Diuretic radionuclide urography in the differential diagnosis of hydroureteronephrosis, Semin. Nucl. Med., 11:89-104, 1981.

Van Luyk, W.H.J., Ensing, G.J., and Piers, D.A.: Low renal uptake of Tc-99m DMSA in patients with proximal tubular dysfunction, Eur. J. Nucl. Med. 8:404-405, 1983.

Wenting, G.L., Tan-Tijiong, H.L., Derkx, F.H.M., and others: Split renal function after captopril in unilateral renal artery stenosis, Br. Med. J. 288:886-890, 1984.

Yee, C.A., Lee, H.B., and Blaufox, M.D.: Tc-99m DMSA renal uptake: influence of biomechanical and physiologic factors, J. Nucl. Med. 22:1054-1058, 1981.

Ziffer, J.A., Alazraki, N.P., and Fajman, W.A.: Thallium renal imaging in patients undergoing stress cardiac evaluation, J. Nucl. Med. 24:910(2b), 1988.

Chapter 24

THYROID

JAMES C. SISSON

Some of the earliest nuclear medicine procedures were designed to evaluate the physiology and the diseases of the thyroid gland. Iodine is the key to thyroid hormonogenesis, and with availability and relative safety of the radionuclide ^{131}I, thyroidology became a firm component in the foundation of nuclear medicine. Multiple radionuclides and radiopharmaceuticals are now brought to bear on the diagnosis of thyroid diseases, and the expanding knowledge in the field makes thyroidology an essential and continually challenging part of the practice of nuclear medicine.

■ ANATOMY

Forming a butterfly configuration, the two lobes of the thyroid gland are joined by an isthmus, which crosses the trachea just below the cricoid cartilage. In an adult human subject, the gland weighs between 15 and 25 g. The lobes constitute most of the volume; the isthmus is generally thin and, in some people, may contain very few thyroid cells (Fig. 24-1). During ontogenesis, the thyroid anlage descends from the base of the tongue, and a tract containing a variable number of thyroid cells remains in the adult, in some individuals creating a pyramidal lobe (arising from the isthmus or the medial aspect of one lobe) and a thyroglossal duct remnant. The thyroid cells in this tract can participate in and give rise to diseases of the thyroid gland.

Because the isthmus of the thyroid varies in thickness, it may or may not appear on scintigraphic images of the thyroid and be visible on deglutition during clinical inspection. Although the isthmus and a thread-like thyroglossal duct remnant may be palpable, the thyroid lobes, despite containing most of the thyroid tissue, are normally neither visible nor readily defined by palpation; they are distinguishable only by a vague fullness in the neck. As individuals become older, the neck structures tend to descend toward the thorax, partly because of a kyphosis of aging. In some elderly patients, the thyroid cartilage resides just above the suprasternal notch, and therefore for these individuals the thyroid glands, normal and abnormal, rest in substernal positions.

There is a natural tendency for thyroid glands to develop lobulation and nodules over many years (Mazzaferri, 1993). How much heterogeneity of the thyroid gland should be considered normal is uncertain, but palpable, discrete nodules are abnormal. Lymph nodes draining the thyroid gland reside in the jugular chains, which occasionally extend to the carotid bifurcation in the regions immediately superior to the gland, as well as in the upper mediastinum.

■ PHYSIOLOGY

Epithelial cells arranged in follicles of varying size make up functional units of the thyroid gland. Thyroid cells, or thyrocytes, are committed to thyroid hormone synthesis, storage, and release. Since iodine constitutes a large and integral part of the two thyroid hormones, thyroxine or T_4 (from the four iodine atoms) and triiodothyronine or T_3 (from the three iodine atoms) (Larsen, 1987), the metabolism of the iodine provides an index of the courses of thyroid biochemistry and physiology (Fig. 24-2). Ingested iodide, including radioiodide, is readily absorbed into the bloodstream and then concentrated by the thyroid gland in a gradient of 20:1; the concentrating process is called "trapping." Iodine is then oxidized and organified to produce iodotyrosines, a process catalyzed by the thyroperoxidase (TPO) enzyme and occurring just outside the apex of the cell in the follicular space. Filling the follicular spaces is colloid, material that is composed of thyroglobulin, large molecules of glycoprotein, within which the iodotyrosines can be efficiently synthesized and then coupled to produce T_4 and T_3 in a reaction also catalyzed by TPO (Sugawara, 1985). Thyroglobulin not only serves as a matrix for the synthesis of hormones, but it also enables storage of substantial quantities (as much as 10 mg) of thyroid hormones that are released to the circulation by a controlled proteol-

The author is indebted to Mrs. Karen Grahl for expert typing and tireless efforts in the preparation of this chapter.

ysis of this biologic structure. Most of the stored and secreted hormone is in the form of T_4.

On entry into the bloodstream, both T_4 and T_3 are avidly bound to plasma proteins, particularly to thyroid-binding globulin or TBG. Thyroxine is also bound to prealbumin and albumin but with lesser affinities than it is to TBG. Protein-bound T_4 and T_3 are in equilibrium with the free hormones, free T_4 and free T_3, respectively. Although the free hormones make up small fractions—less than 0.1%—of the total thyroid hormones in the circulation, the concentrations of free hormones effect the physiologic and, in disease states, the pathologic responses from tissues in the body. Nevertheless, many of the commonly used assays of T_4 and T_3 in serum measure the total quantity of the hormones, which reflects the protein-bound hormones and not the active or free forms.

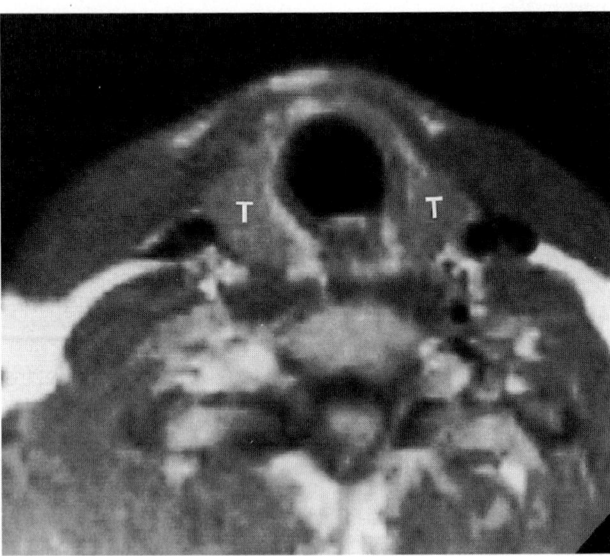

Fig. 24-1. Cross-sectional magnetic resonance image of a normal neck. Thyroid lobes (T) are on either side of the trachea; isthmus of the thyroid is the thin region on the anterior of the trachea. Internal jugular vein and carotid artery are dark regions lateral to the thyroid lobes, and a vertebra is seen behind. (Reproduced from Mountz, J.M., et al: J. Comp. Assist. Tomogr. 11:612-619, 1987, with permission.)

Current theory holds that most, if not all, of the effects of thyroid hormones in tissues are exerted through T_3 (Fig. 24-3). Thyroxine then acts as a prohormone that is deiodinated in numerous tissues of the body to yield T_3 (3,5,3′-triiodothyronine), the physiologic hormone, and reverse T_3 (3,3′,5′-triiodothyronine), an inert derivative, and other products with little or no physiologic action (Fig. 24-3). Most of the secreted hormone is in the form of T_4, and the majority (70% to 90%) of T_3 is derived from deiodination of T_4 in extrathyroidal tissues. Two T_4 deiodinases of importance have been identified: type I resides in most nonneural tissues, but particularly in the liver, and type II is found in neural-type cells, most prominently in the anterior pituitary. Several differences distinguish these two deiodinases (Itagaki, 1990; Mandel, 1992), but of interest are two: (1) the type II deiodinase appears to produce T_3 for use only in the pituitary gland, and thus influences of thyroid hormones on pituitary function are predominantly controlled by the prevailing T_4 levels while type I deiodinase gives rise to T_3, which enters the circulation and may act anywhere in the body; and (2) propylthiouracil inhibits type I, but not type II deiodinase, creating discrepancies in tissue responses to thyroxine during antithyroid drug treatment of hyperthyroidism. The remainder of the iodine within T_4 and T_3 is ultimately stripped away and appears in the urine as iodide. To bring about metabolic effects, T_3 is bound to cell membranes and then is transported to the nucleus within the cell where anabolic and thermogenic actions are initiated (Oppenheimer, 1987). Most likely T_3 can produce effects at the cell membrane, but the response in the nucleus is the best documented. The nuclear receptors for T_3 are closely associated with those for glucocorticoids, estrogens, and other hormones, yet the effect of each hor-

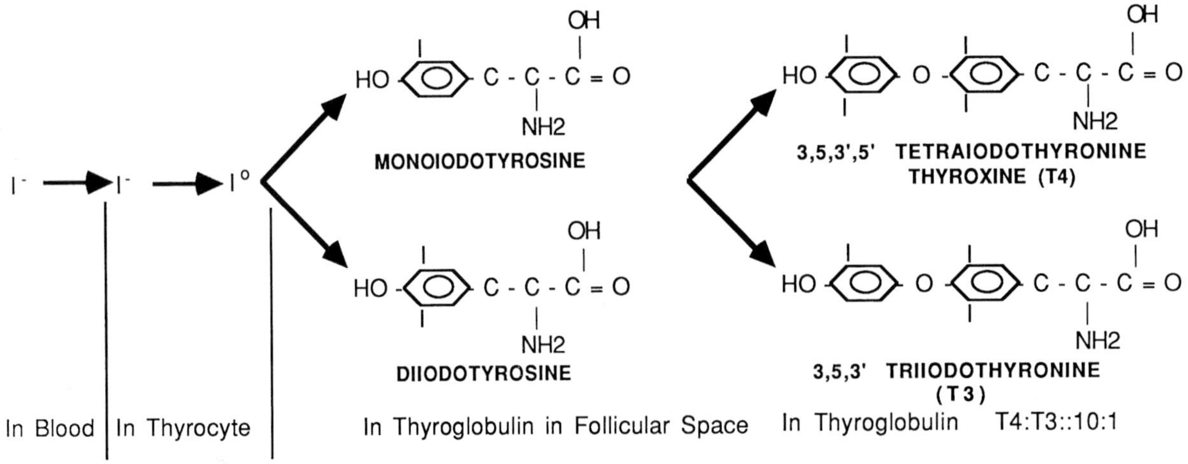

Fig. 24-2. Synthetic pathway of thyroid hormones.

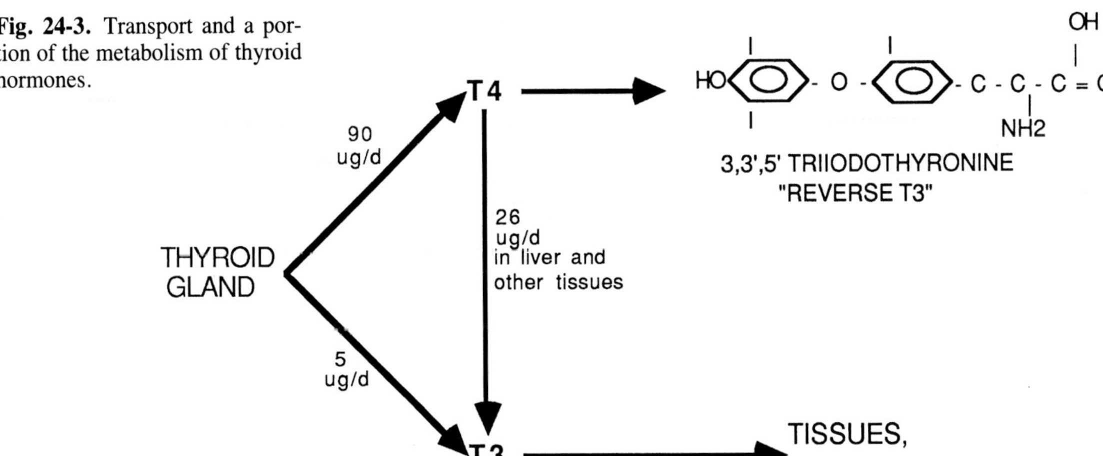

Fig. 24-3. Transport and a portion of the metabolism of thyroid hormones.

mone is distinct (Evans, 1988; Usala, 1991). The action of T_3 appears to remove repression of gene function; however, the protein products of the gene response to T_3 are still of an uncertain nature.

Ingested iodide that is not sequestered by the thyroid gland can be trapped temporarily by the salivary glands and by the gastric mucosa, and these organs, along with iodide propelled into the remainder of the gut, will appear on images made with a radioactive iodine. Excretion of iodide, which is almost entirely via the kidney, correlates closely with the glomerular filtration rate.

Function within the thyroid gland is controlled primarily by thyroid stimulating hormone (TSH), or thyrotropin, which is secreted by the thyrotroph cells in the pituitary gland (Fig. 24-4). The feedback controls between the pituitary and thyroid gland are finely regulated, and thus a measurement of circulating TSH is a sensitive index of the effect of thyroid hormones on tissues. The hypothalamus secretes thyrotropin-releasing hormone (TRH), which stimulates the synthesis and release of TSH by the pituitary gland (Fig. 24-4) (Utiger, 1987). TRH synthesis and probably secretion are also inhibited by increases in thyroid hormone concentration (Koller, 1987). Although overall physiologic regulation is not fully defined, two physiologic principles are well established: (1) TRH is essential for the normal function of the thyrotrophs in the pituitary, and (2) inhibition by thyroid hormones is exerted primarily at the pituitary thyrotroph level. Dopamine also inhibits TSH secretion.

The receptors for TSH found on thyroid cells appear to have components that stimulate growth and function of the thyroid glands. It is possible that under some circumstances these two components of the receptors can be separated. Functional responses to TSH can be observed in terms of increased concentration of iodide and enhanced release of hormones. A mechanism of autoregulation has also been identified in the thyroid gland (Ingbar, 1972). Excessive levels of circulating iodides will cause a temporary reduc-

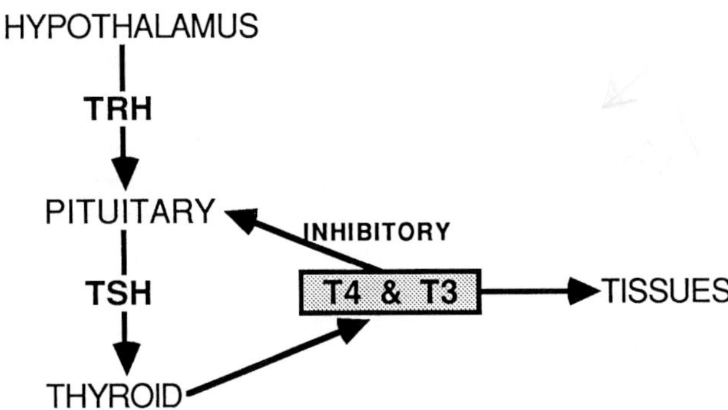

Fig. 24-4. Physiologic control thyroid gland function.

tion in thyroid gland function, but through events unrelated to TSH activity, autoregulation eventually permits hormonogenesis to resume.

The thyroid gland also harbors parafollicular cells, which secrete the hormone calcitonin. The release of calcitonin is increased by rises in circulating concentrations of calcium and gastrin (Gharib, 1987b), but the parafollicular cells are not influenced by TSH or iodide.

■ PATHOPHYSIOLOGY OF THYROID DISEASE

■ Hyperthyroidism

Hyperthyroidism is the state in which the tissues of the body are responding to excessive thyroid hormone. It is important to recognize that hyperthyroidism is a metabolic disorder of tissues and organs because tests for hyperthyroidism, although precise for what they measure, usually give evidence of events removed from tissue metabolism. For example, concentrations of hormones in sera and radioiodine uptakes are strongly correlated with the presence of hyperthyroidism, but in some circumstances the values of these tests will relate to factors other than the metabolic state of the patient (Wenzel, 1981; Borst, 1983).

Several different pathogenic mechanisms can give rise

to hyperthyroidism, and the consequential clinical disorders are distinguished with the help of nuclear medicine techniques (Table 24-1).

Graves' disease. Circulating antibodies, thyroid-stimulating immunoglobulins (TSI), directed at the TSH receptor (the antigen) on thyrocytes stimulate thyroid function by activating the receptor. Graves' disease is an autoimmune malady in which the immunoglobulins increase the function of the target organ rather than act destructively (Burman, 1985). The excessive secretion of thyroid hormones leads to hyperthyroidism. In addition, extrathyroidal tissues may manifest fundamental features of Graves' disease unrelated to thyroid hormone effects. About 50% of patients exhibit an ophthalmopathy in which exophthalmos may be a prominent component. The diagnosis of Graves' disease is usually made by recognition of the clinical features. However, standard practice requires diagnostic support from the laboratory to establish the presence of hyperthyroidism. A suppressed concentration of circulating TSH will invariably be found in patients who have hyperthyroidism from Graves' disease. Levels of serum T_4 and T_3 may also be necessary to define fully the status of the patient. A scintigraphic image is almost never needed to conclude the presence of Graves' disease, which regularly presents with a diffusely hyperplastic goiter that is readily defined by palpation. In special circumstances, the nature of the disorder may be further delineated by assays of antibodies against the TSH receptor that are present in the sera of virtually every patient with hyperthyroidism of Graves' disease. Algorithms of approaches to patients suspected of having Graves' hyperthyroidism are recorded below under the section Tests of Thyroid Diseases.

Toxic nodular goiter. Single thyroid nodules can, through autonomous function, secrete sufficient thyroid hormone to cause hyperthyroidism. These nodules generally must be greater than 3 cm in diameter to be capable of this level of function (Hamburger, 1980). Hyperfunction may also arise in a gland containing multiple nodules (Peter, 1982); the secretion of hormone can be from nodules that are assumed to be autonomous or from the internodular parenchyma, which may be an expression of Graves disease in an otherwise nodular goiter. The term *Plummer's disease* has been used to designate hyperthyroidism in glands with both single and multiple nodules.

Table 24-1. Types of hyperthyroidism

High thyroidal uptake values

(Require intervention at the thyroid gland level or elsewhere)
- Graves' disease
- Toxic nodular goiter:
  - Single nodule
  - Multiple nodules
- TSH-induced
- Tumor-secreted stimulators

Low thyroidal values

(Require attention away from thyroid gland, observation for spontaneous remission, or withdrawal of agents)
- Ectopic secretion of thyroid hormone (rare thyroid cancers; teratomas)
- Injury to thyroid (hormone release):
  - Subacute thyroiditis
  - Autoimmune thyroiditis
- Ingested (or injected) thyroid hormone
- Iodine-induced hyperthyroidism (Jod-Basedow disease)

TSH secretion. In rare cases, hyperthyroidism arises from stimulation of the thyroid gland by TSH. Thyrotropin can be secreted in abnormally regulated quantities by pituitary thyrotrophs that exhibit a resistance to inhibition by thyroid hormones either by inherent nature or as part of an autonomous adenoma. This type of hyperthyroidism can be recognized by the presence of measurable levels of TSH, in addition to which the patients would not manifest Graves' eye disease. Although an uncommon disorder, hyperthyroidism from TSH secretion should be considered because, if present, it may be associated with a pituitary tumor, and because the associated laboratory values resemble those seen in euthyroid patients in whom both pituitary gland and other body tissues are resistant to the effects of thyroid hormone. (See the section Generalized Thyroid Enlargement, below).

TSH-like hormonal stimulation. Tumors of gonadal or chorion origin, such as choriocarcinoma and hydatidiform mole, have been found to secrete a TSH-like substance that is not identified in assays of TSH. The hyperthyroidism produced by this means is generally mild but can be severe. The offending tumors are usually discovered by clinical examination. Diagnosis of this type of hyperthyroidism will be made by a careful appraisal of the whole patient accompanied by measurement of the serum level of human chorionic gonadotropin, which is usually elevated.

Ectopic secretion of thyroid hormone. The only tumors that are sufficiently differentiated to synthesize large amounts of thyroid hormone are teratomas (e.g., struma ovarii), which are exceptionally rare, and a few follicular thyroid cancers.

In each case, examination of the patient's neck should be a guide to the diagnosis; there should be no abnormality of the thyroid in the presence of teratomas, and either a primary tumor or thyroidectomy scar will be present when thyroid cancer is the cause of hyperthyroidism. Scintigraphic images should locate the source(s) of hormone production.

Injury to the thyroid gland. Since the thyroid gland stores a substantial quantity of thyroid hormone, release of this hormone to the circulation can produce hyperthyroidism. Thyroiditis of two types can injure the gland sufficiently to bring on hyperthyroidism: (1) subacute thyroiditis, presumably caused by a viral infection and manifest as a painful, tender gland; and (2) a painless thyroiditis of autoimmune origin, one form of which frequently follows pregnancy. The hyperthyroidism in each case is transient, lasting no longer than a few weeks (until the excessive hormone spilled into the circulation is dissipated); it is followed by a recovery phase that may include temporary hypothyroidism. Episodes may recur. The injury to the thyroid gland causes an inability of the thyrocytes to take up iodine, and consequently the radioiodine uptake as a percent of the dose is close to zero in these patients. A rise in the radioiodine uptake value usually heralds the recovery phase.

Ingestion of thyroid hormone. Although the human body has mechanisms that buffer against the effects of excessive thyroid hormone especially when administered acutely, it is possible to induce hyperthyroidism by ingestion of either thyroxine or triiodothyronine. A careful investigation will be necessary to disclose the surreptitious ingestion of thyroid hormone. However, the iatrogenic prescription of thyroid hormone in doses that are only moderately in excess of the patient's needs is a more common cause of hyperthyroidism of this type. Unless there is concomitant autonomous function, the uptake of iodide by the thyroid gland is suppressed.

Iodide-induced hyperthyroidism (Jod-Basedow's disease). The thyroid gland's adaptation to the increased availability of iodine occasionally fails, and the iodine is incorporated into hormone, which upon release evokes hyperthyroid responses in tissues. The frequency of this type of hyperthyroidism is unknown, but given the ubiquity of iodine in the hospital environment, the potential is appreciable. Generally, the patient will give a history of a preexisting goiter and receipt of large amounts of iodine. Here, too, a valuable clue to the diagnosis is a low radioiodine uptake value (in this case from dilution of the radioiodine by the large quantity of acquired stable iodide).

■ Hypothyroidism

Hypothyroidism, defined as the opposite of hyperthyroidism, is the state in which tissues of the body are responding to diminished thyroid hormone. Although in the classic presentation the clinical features should point to the diagnosis, many patients have atypical symptoms and signs, and therefore laboratory assessment will be necessary to confirm the diagnosis. Nevertheless, the proper uses of laboratory tests are contingent on some reasonable probability of hypothyroidism derived from examination of the patient.

Primary hypothyroidism. In over 95% of hypothyroid patients, the disorder arises within the thyroid gland; the gland is then unable to secrete sufficient hormone. For all patients so afflicted, the concentration of TSH in the serum gives evidence of a tissue's response to diminished thyroid hormone.

Autoimmune thyroiditis or Hashimoto's disease is the most common cause of spontaneous hypothyroidism in the adult patient and in children over 2 years of age. Two clinical forms of autoimmune thyroiditis are recognized. In the goitrous form, the thyroid gland exhibits generalized albeit often irregular enlargement; a valuable diagnostic clue is the notable firmness of the gland. Inefficient use of iodine in the impaired homonogenesis may lead to normal or high radioiodine uptakes values. The atrophic form of autoimmune thyroiditis differs from the goitrous form in the absence of a thyroid enlargement and the usually more profound hypothyroidism. Antibodies that block the TSH receptor appear to be a function of the pathogenic mechanism.

Iatrogenic hypothyroidism frequently follows thyroidectomy, treatment with radioiodine, and therapeutic external beam radiation to the neck. A careful history lays the foundation for these diagnoses.

Iodine-induced hypothyroidism may be the result of either of two opposite conditions. Prolonged iodine deficiency is a long recognized cause of hypothyroidism, but this state is now observed in only a few areas of the world. In a few susceptible individuals, iodine in large doses over many days will inhibit thyroid hormonogenesis, an impairment of function that persists as long as the iodine is given. A goiter develops as a compensatory mechanism and usually precedes the hypothyroidism.

Congenital and other acquired abnormalities that impair thyroid function are rare but still common enough to warrant neonatal screening programs for thyroid dysfunction. The thyroid gland may be absent or malformed (as in cases of lingual thyroid tissue that failed to descend into the neck in ontogenesis), or it may manifest biochemical abnormalities in the pathway of hormone synthesis. Absence of a thyroid gland or thyroid tissue in an ectopic site signifies a permanent hypothyroid disorder. On the other hand, the hypothyroidism occurring from a normally situated gland may be a result of either an irreversible enzyme defect in hormonogenesis or a transient interference in the synthesis of T_4 and T_3; a later trial of cessation of thyroxine therapy will differentiate between the two possibilities. Scintigraphic imaging of the thyroid gland region in a hypothyroid infant will then help to determine if thyroid hormone treatment should continue unabated or be assessed at some future time.

Uncommon causes of acquired hypothyroidism are drugs or other compounds that interfere with thyroid function. Lithium and amiodarone are examples of prescribed pharmaceuticals that can induce hypothyroidism.

Pituitary disease. When the pituitary gland is damaged, the secretion of TSH will be reduced and hypothyroidism will ensue. In some patients with pituitary disease, a few thyrotrophs remain to respond to stimulation, and a small rise in TSH in response to injected TRH does not exclude a pituitary cause of hypothyroidism. Most patients who have pituitary disease manifest abnormalities in other trophic hormones; a thorough examination of the patient will lead to a proper clinical conclusion.

Hypothalamic disease. The considerations cited above

for pituitary disease pertain to patients with hypothalamic disease.

■ Thyroiditis

The thyroiditides are also discussed in other sections of this chapter.

Autoimmune thyroiditis. The most frequent type of thyroiditis is the autoimmune disorder usually termed *Hashimoto's disease*. Autoimmune thyroiditis, described under the section Hypothyroidism, often presents as spontaneous hypothyroidism. However, the enlargement of the thyroid gland, which is a common manifestation of Hashimoto's disease, may be sufficient to compensate for the impaired hormonogenesis, and the patient then will be euthyroid. In this instance, the clinical character of the thyroid gland and titers of antibodies against thyroid microsomes (TPO is now recognized as the antigen) and thyroglobulin will establish the diagnosis. The autoimmune thyroiditis that appears as an injury type of hyperthyroidism is described in the section Hyperthyroidism.

Subacute thyroiditis. This type of thyroiditis appears in a broad clinical spectrum: at one extreme, a subclinical form; and at the other, a classic presentation of an acute illness as an injury-type hyperthyroidism described in the section Hyperthyroidism. Although subacute thyroiditis is probably caused by a virus, the etiologic agent is usually not discovered. Occasionally the disease is first observed when only one lobe is involved and before the disease is spread to the other lobe, in which case the radioiodine uptake may not be very low and the scintigraphic image will portray a lack of function in only one lobe.

Riedel's thyroiditis. Although Riedel's thyroiditis is always included in lists of thyroiditis, it is so rare that large institutions are able to record only a few such cases. From the nuclear medicine point of view, the appearance may simulate Hashimoto's disease. The fibrous growth makes the gland adherent to surrounding structures in the neck, indicating that Riedel's thyroiditis may be part of a more generalized fibrosis.

■ Euthyroid gland enlargement other than thyroiditis and neoplasm

Three types of forces may cause generalized enlargement of the thyroid gland: thyrotropin, usually stimulating the gland because hormonogenesis has been subnormal; autoimmune stimulators of growth; and intrinsic or autonomous forces, some of which are associated with age. The enlargement of the thyroid gland may be asymmetric.

Inefficient hormonogenesis by the thyroid gland. The types of thyroid enlargement related to insufficient hormonogenesis and consequently to TSH stimulation have been discussed in previous sections; iodine-induced goiter, effects of goitrogens, and congenital defects within the thyroid gland are found in the section Hypothyroidism. However, in each type the compensatory enlargement of the gland may be sufficient to maintain euthyroidism.

Resistance to thyroid hormone effects. The congenital defect in tissues that is manifest as a generalized resistance to thyroid hormone is now seen with sufficient frequency to warrant the attention of the nuclear medicine specialist. When sufficient historical data were obtained on patients with generalized resistance to thyroid hormone, it was found that the inheritance pattern was the autosomal dominant type, except in one family. The disorder is a syndrome in which there are variations in expression; however, resistance to thyroid hormone is observed in both peripheral tissues and the pituitary thyrotrophs so that the result is increased secretion of TSH, which induces the thyroid gland to make more than normal amounts of thyroid hormone to overcome the resistance. In a compensated equilibrium, the thyroid gland is enlarged, all circulating thyroid hormone levels (including those of the free hormones) are elevated to thyrotoxic levels, and the serum TSH concentration is inappropriately normal or elevated; the patient, however, is euthyroid. For such patients, euthyroidism must be determined by careful clinical appraisal. Clues to the disorder are the measurable level of TSH and the lack of clinical features of hyperthyroidism; in addition, hyperactivity with attention deficit is a manifestation commonly detected in affected children.

Autoimmune stimulators of thyroid growth. The TSH-receptor on thyroid cells may have the capacity to transmit stimulations separately to function and growth. Immune globulins have been reported to selectively enhance growth on the thyroid gland. In these cases, thyroid function remains normal and, since function is modulated through the pituitary-thyroid axis, TSH is normally suppressed by administered thyroid hormone. Yet, suppressive doses of thyroid hormone will not inhibit growth of the gland. It is controversial whether such immune stimulators are a frequent cause of euthyroid goiter.

Intrinsic changes in the thyroid gland. When the cause of generalized enlargement of the thyroid gland is unknown, through ignorance we usually attribute the change to intrinsic factors. Nevertheless, there is a tendency for the thyroid gland to enlarge with age, and subclinical nodules appear to be an expression of the aging process as well. As expected in a disorder of uncertain mechanism, no laboratory tests give clues or special insights as to the diagnosis.

■ Thyroid nodules and thyroid cancer

Thyroid nodules. On discovery of a thyroid nodule in a patient, a major concern is whether the nodule is benign or malignant. A few general rules apply, as follows:

1. Most cancers present as a single or dominant nodule within a nodular gland. Exceptions are seen in patients who: (a) have received therapeutic radiation to the neck (several nodules may be carcinomas), (b) inherited multiple endocrine neoplasia type 2A or 2B (the component medullary carcinomas will be multi-

centric), or (c) developed a lymphoma (which may involve both lobes, often intermingled with Hashimoto's disease).

2. Most nodules are benign; in aspiration cytology less than 10% are malignant.
3. The function of a cancer, even a well-differentiated thyroid neoplasm, is almost always less than that of the adjacent normal thyroid tissue, so that scintigraphic images will portray a malignant nodule as hypofunctioning or nonfunctioning. However, on removal of the normal thyroid tissue and especially with increasing stimulation by TSH, many well-differentiated cancers can be shown to concentrate radioiodine by imaging techniques. This of course is the basis for treatment of thyroid cancers with ^{131}I.
4. Probably less than 10% of thyroid nodules concentrate one of the radiotracers to levels greater than that of surrounding normal tissue. However, since nodules with this level of function are virtually always benign, inferences of nonmalignancy may be drawn from scintigraphic images in some patients.

Thyroid cancers. Papillary carcinoma, also called papillary-follicular cancer because the neoplasm contains both papillary and follicular elements, is the most common thyroid malignancy. Papillary tumors grow slowly, and enlargement is perceived only over many years. Spread is first to regional lymph nodes and then, in a few patients, to lungs and bone. Follicular thyroid cancer is less common but more aggressive than the papillary type, and these carcinomas metastasize by the hematogenous rather than by the lymphogenous route.

The other thyroid cancers sequester little or no radioiodine (as iodide) and consequently are of less interest to the nuclear medicine specialist. However, in some instances, scintigraphy is applied to medullary and undifferentiated cancers; the methods for this purpose are recorded in the section Tests of Thyroid Diseases.

LABORATORY APPLICATION

74

IN VITRO TESTS OF THYROID FUNCTION AND THYROID DISEASES

Purpose

In vitro tests of thyroid function serve as the major laboratory methods of detecting thyroid dysfunction (i.e., hyperthyroidism and hypothyroidism) in patients. Certain in vitro tests are also of diagnostic value for other thyroid disorders. These tests must be preceded by a careful clinical evaluation of the patient to define the problem and to establish a probability of diagnosis. The reliability of a laboratory test result is contingent on the *a priori* probability of disease (obtained from the clinical data), and the meaning of the result must be put into perspective by the circumstances of the given patient. Except in the search for hypothyroidism in neonates and in subjects at risk for multiple endocrine neoplasia type 2A, screening of patients for thyroid disorders without regard to clinical status is not warranted.

Indications

In the process of concluding that there is a reasonable probability (even 10%) that hyperthyroidism, hypothyroidism or some other disease exists in a patient, one or two tests will generally suffice to make clear the presence or absence of the suspected disorder. In only a small fraction of patients should it be necessary to obtain multiple tests or a panel of thyroid tests to establish a diagnosis with the degree of confidence necessary to institute therapy. Indications will be refined in discussions of interpretation of each test.

Procedures

Materials

The materials for the in vitro tests of thyroid function are available in commercial kits that frequently make use of small quantities of radiolabeled hormones, including those of radioimmunoassays. However, markers other than radionuclides have proved to be of value in some assays, and chemoluminometric technology has enabled accurate measurements of very low concentrations of hormones, particularly TSH (Spencer, 1990; Nicoloff, 1990). Nuclear medicine specialists and clinicians should be aware that in vitro testing advances have been and are likely to be frequent. For the ex vivo types of testing, thyrotropin-releasing hormone, pentagastrin, and calcium chloride may be obtained in pharmacies.

Continued.

Patient preparation

Patient preparation is unnecessary. Although some thyroid and thyroid-related hormones exhibit diurnal changes (such as TSH), the variations with such factors as time and meals are insufficient to affect interpretations of results of serum. However, T_3 assays will be influenced by recent ingestion or injection of that hormone. It is best that patients receiving injections for the ex vivo tests be fasting.

Techniques

The techniques are defined by the kits used for in vitro assays. Techniques for the free T_4 indices and for ex vivo tests require more explanation.

Free T_4 concentrations can be estimated from the T_4 concentration (the total T_4) in serum and a test using resin, now called the *thyroid hormone binding ratio,* to give an index of the binding of T_4 to serum proteins (actually the reciprocal of the open binding sites on these proteins). The following equations explain the relationship.

$$(T_4)\ (TBG) = K\ (T_4 \times TBG)$$

where

T_4 = Concentration of free T_4,
TBG = Concentration of open binding sites on thyroid binding proteins or TBG,
K = A constant, and
$T_4 \times$ TBG = Concentration of T_4 bound to TBG

Since ($T_4 \times$ TBG) contains almost all of the circulating T_4, it is equivalent to the total T_4 concentration. The thyroid-hormone-binding ratio is the reciprocal of the open binding sites on TBG, or 1/(TBG).

Rearranging the original equation, the relationship is as follows:

$$T_4 = K\ (T_4 \times TBG) \times 1/(TBG);$$

Substituting as follows:

$$T_4 = K \times \text{total } T_4 \times \text{thyroid hormone binding ratio}$$

where T_4 is proportional to total $T_4 \times$ thyroid-hormone-binding ratio.

Then, the product of total T_4 and thyroid-hormone-binding ratio gives an index (not the actual value) of the free T_4 concentration. Kits have been developed to give a more direct assessment of free T_4 levels in serum (Melmed, 1982; Surks, 1988), but many clinicians still prefer to see the total T_4 value to give perspective on the binding protein events in a given patient.

The TRH-TSH test is performed by giving an intravenous dose of TRH, such as 200 μg, that gives a submaximal rise in the serum TSH concentration. Blood samples are obtained for measurement of TSH at the following times:

- Before the TRH injection
- 30 minutes after the TRH injection
- In patients suspected of pituitary or hypothalamic disease, 60 minutes after the TRH injection

The patient is recumbent throughout the test and should be observed for symptoms. Toxic reactions are rare, but the patient should be warned about nausea and flushing. Blood pressure and heart rate should be recorded for reference before the test.

To stimulate calcitonin secretion, pentagastrin, 0.5 μg/kg is given intravenously over no more than 10 seconds. Blood samples are obtained (and put on ice) for measurement of calcitonin before, and at 2 and 5 minutes after the injection. The patient should be warned that cramping in the abdomen and lower chest, as well as nausea, are almost inevitable accompaniments of a pentagastrin injection, but the symptoms will last only about 2 minutes. Calcium chloride can be injected or infused as a substitute for the pentagastrin stimulation of calcitonin secretion, but this approach is not popular.

Interpretation

Results in patients suspected of having hyperthyroidism

A measurement of *serum TSH* should be considered an essential initial test to establish hyperthyroidism as a diagnosis. Third-generation assays using chemoluminometric technology reliably detect levels of TSH as low as 0.01 μU/ml. A fourth-generation procedure with functional accuracy at even lower concentrations, 0.001 μU/ml, has recently been developed.

Individuals with clinical features of hyperthyroidism from Graves' disease and toxic nodular goiter will invariably exhibit TSH concentrations below 0.05 μU/ml. In patients who exhibit typical clinical manifestations of hyperthyroidism, only those rare subjects whose excessive thyroid hormones have been provoked by increased secretions of thyrotropin (see above) will have TSH levels above 0.05 μU/ml. (In fact, these patients usually have normal or slightly elevated TSH values.) Depending on the doses administered, treatments with more than maintenance quantities of thyroxine can suppress TSH concentrations to any subnormal level. In the presence of thyroxine therapy, suppressed TSH values including those between 0.05 μU/ml and the normal range have been correlated with accelerated bone loss over many years. However, other clinical manifestations of hyperthyroidism are most uncommon when TSH values are above 0.05 μU/ml. Euthyroid subjects who develop a severe nonthyroidal illness or who receive drugs (such as glucocorticoids and dopamine) that interfere with TSH secretion may have subnormal levels of TSH, but a proportion of individuals will have values above 0.05 μU/ml. These subjects usually can be allocated to a category of patients in whom symptoms are unlikely to be caused by hyperthyroidism.

Thus, a measurement of TSH gives an exceedingly sensitive and highly specific index of hyperthyroidism. It is invaluable in determining the diagnosis when the clinical presentation leaves some doubt. There are experts who believe that the serum TSH should be measured in all patients in whom the diagnosis of hyperthyroidism is established so that the pathogenesis of hyperthyroidism in those rare individuals with normal-to-high TSH can be uncovered. The cost-effectiveness of this approach is uncertain. It is possible to omit the assay of TSH in patients for whom the clinical symptoms and signs give an unequivocal diagnosis, and the physician wishes to use the T_4 level as an index of response to therapy because important but incomplete improvement would not be reflected in TSH concentrations that are undetectable as long as any hyperthyroidism persists.

Injections of thyrotropin-releasing hormone (TRH) will provoke measurable rises in serum TSH values in normal subjects, but in patients with hyperthyroidism there is a notable inhibition of pituitary thyrotroph function and no response to TRH can be elicited. Although the results of TRH-TSH testing are sensitive and specific for hyperthyroidism, the procedure is no longer necessary to establish that diagnosis. Values of serum TSH obtained with third-generation TSH assays distinguish between hyperthyroidism and euthyroidism as well as the TRH-TSH test results.

A long-used measurement of thyroid function has been the *T_4 concentration* in serum, an assay of the total T_4 level. Because metabolic events relate to the free T_4 concentration and because over 99% of circulating T_4 is in the protein-bound form, changes in the binding of T_4 by proteins affect the total T_4 level while not altering the metabolism of the patient. Moreover, alterations in the binding of T_4 occur relatively commonly in clinical practice. On the other hand, the free T_4 concentration generally indicates the clinical status of the patient with respect to thyroid function. Measurements of free T_4 by each of several different methods have been validated. The free T_4 level was elevated in over 90% of patients with hyperthyroidism, and an elevated value in the proper clinical context was highly specific. As noted above, the test result is of particular value: (1) in confirming the presence of hyperthyroidism when the TSH concentration and clinical data are insufficient, and (2) if an index of response to therapy of hyperthyroidism is desired.

Of course, there will be patients for whom the above laboratory data appear equivocal or the clinical suspicion of hyperthyroidism remains in spite of a normal free T_4 level; then it is prudent to search for the so-called T_3 thyrotoxicosis. For subjects suspected of this diagnosis, measurement of the *T_3 concentration* in serum is an essential next step. The concentration of free T_3 is more likely to correlate with the diagnosis of hyperthyroidism than is the concentration of total T_3, for the same

Continued.

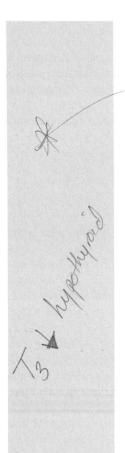

reasons that were applied to free T_4 and total T_4. Measurements of free T_3 are not as readily available as those of free T_4, but additional tests and thyroid-hormone-binding ratio (see above), along with the total T_4 results, will indicate whether binding of total T_3 is likely increased, decreased, or normal.

A *radioiodine uptake* test can also provide confirming evidence of hyperthyroidism, but this test is usually performed for other reasons; it is also described in the section on In Vivo Tests of Thyroid Function. Similarly, the suppression test that employs the radioiodine uptake as the indicator will be discussed below under the same section.

Results in patients suspected of having hypothyroidism

When the clinical question is the presence or absence of primary hypothyroidism, the answer is obtained simply and directly from the serum *TSH concentration.*

For patients in whom hypothyroidism could arise from pituitary or hypothalamic disease, an estimate of the *free T_4 level* is also essential. Such patients must be carefully evaluated for other disturbances including clinical, hormonal, and anatomic manifestations in the pituitary and hypothalamic regions. A *TRH-TSH test result* may provide valuable information in that the absence of thyrotrophs will give an abnormal response, but in some patients thyrotrophs remain and release varying quantities of immunoreactive TSH. Knowledge of the probable pituitary and/or hypothalamic disorder must guide the interpretation of results.

Hypothyroidism caused by pituitary or hypothalamic disease is usually associated with a diminution in concentrations of all hormones associated with thyroid function. Such a constellation of findings must be distinguished from those of severe nonthyroidal illness. In the presence of severe nonthyroidal illness, all the above described assessments of thyroid function may be reduced. The T_3 (and free T_3) concentrations are the first to fall (a decline may be seen even after a moderate degree of stress such as weight loss), but with more severe disease the free T_4 and TSH levels may also become subnormal. In contrast, the *reverse T_3 concentration* may then be elevated in nonthyroidal illness, becoming a helpful guide to distinguish hypothyroidism of pituitary or hypothalamic origin from the effects of severe nonthyroidal illness. However, clinical judgment will generally be sufficient to allow this distinction.

Results in patients suspected of having Graves' disease

Since the hyperthyroidism of Graves' disease is brought about by stimulating antibodies, *thyroid stimulating immunoglobulins (TSI)* are detectable in almost every patient with Graves' hyperthyroidism. However, the clinical usefulness of the test is limited. A high titer of TSI in a pregnant woman gives a reasonable probability that hyperthyroidism will develop in the fetus and be present at birth. Knowledge of this probability is important because prenatal and neonatal hyperthyroidism will require special treatment.

It would seem that a decline in TSI titer would herald a permanent remission in hyperthyroidism for the patient under treatment with antithyroid drugs. Unfortunately, the changes in TSI titers have not been as accurate in this prediction as had been hoped; thus permanent remissions in hyperthyroidism are best determined by observation of the patient after stopping the treatment.

The most commonly used test for presence of autoimmune disease is that of a *titer of antibody* against the microsomal fraction of thyroid cells (thyroperoxidase or TPO is the antigen) and thyroglobulin. The presence of these antibodies in significant titer give strong evidence of autoimmune disease. Detection of antibodies directed against TPO is the more sensitive assay. Usually, the diagnosis of autoimmune thyroiditis or Hashimoto's disease can be established without resort to antibody titers, but such assays will help to define the nature of the disease in the occasional patient who exhibits a goiter that otherwise defies ready classification from clinical data.

Antibody titers are also elevated in most patients with Graves' disease. Some euthyroid patients present eye signs that could be manifestations of Graves' disease (euthyroid Graves' disease); in these individuals, the presence of antibody titers gives evidence of autoimmune thyroid disease, and by inference, of Graves' ophthalmopathy.

Results in patients suspected of having thyroid cancer

In patients with well-differentiated thyroid cancer, a rise in the *thyroglobulin concentration* is an indicator that predicts growth of the cancer. Thyroglobulin is released to the circulation by normal thyroid tissue and by papillary and follicular carcinomas. The cancers appear to discharge thyroglobulin at greater rates per cell than do normal thyrocytes. After a total or near-total thyroidectomy, changes in the thyroglobulin level predict growth of thyroid tissue that most likely will be neoplastic. Treatment with thyroid hormone reduces the function of normal thyroid tissue and that of the thyroid-hormone-dependent neoplasms. Thus, thyroglobulin "secretions" and the consequential serum thyroglobulin concentrations are generally lower in the euthyroid state than when the patient is hypothyroid. Since a thyroglobulin concentration is less than perfect as an indicator of residual thyroid cancer, the relative roles of both this test and thyroid imaging with ^{131}I in the periodic evaluations of patients remain uncertain.

Thyroglobulin levels may also help in the diagnosis of thyrotoxicosis factitia.

Proper standards of thyroglobulin are necessary to attain meaningful results, but no standard has attained widespread approval.

Concentrations of both *calcitonin* and of *carcinoembryonic antigen* are used as indices of medullary thyroid cancer. When a patient suspected of the diagnosis of medullary cancer of the thyroid has a normal basal calcitonin concentration, a stimulation test is performed to gain sensitivity. This has been of particular importance in testing individuals at risk for multiple endocrine neoplasia type 2A, a syndrome inherited by an autosomal dominant mode wherein medullary thyroid cancer is almost always expressed. If the test result is abnormal, it should be confirmed by repetition before thyroidectomy is prescribed. Avoidance of pitfalls in measurements of calcitonin and in interpretation of results of stimulation tests will require knowledge of both the methodology and the patients being tested. Genetic testing has made progress, and when the gene is cloned this approach will replace the ex vivo stimulation tests.

Calcitonin levels may be used to follow progression of medullary thyroid cancer in patients who exhibit familial or sporadic disease, and serial assays of carcinoembryonic antigen may also be a useful adjunct in determining the prognosis of affected individuals.

LABORATORY APPLICATION

IN VIVO TESTS OF THYROID FUNCTION

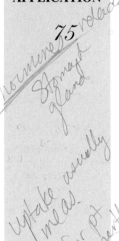

Purpose

Each of the in vivo tests of thyroid function makes use of an uptake measurement. Reflecting early phases of thyroid hormonogenesis, uptake values give information that relates to overall thyroid gland function. This information will differ at times from the data obtained by in vitro tests, which generally indicate the prevailing serum levels of hormones released from the gland or absorbed from the gut.

Indications

Thyroid uptake of ^{131}I-, ^{123}I- or ^{99m}Tc-pertechnetate

A high uptake value can help confirm or refute the diagnosis of either hyperthyroidism of Graves' disease or toxic nodular goiter. In addition, low uptake values point to other types of hyperthyroidism. Thus, the types of hyperthyroidism can be classified into low and high uptake categories (Table 24-1), a distinction that is necessary when considering treatments since the patients with low uptake values should have agents withdrawn or be observed for spontaneous remission. Most often the uptake result is used as a factor in calculating the dose of ^{131}I for treating a patient with hyperthyroidism.

Suppression test: suppression of uptake by thyroid hormone

The suppression test is used as an additional test of thyroid function to help determine if thyroid function is under physiologic control (by suppressing TSH) or is arising from aberrant stimulation or autonomous activity. Generally, assays of TSH concentrations will demonstrate if the prevailing func-

Continued.

tion has any physiologic control. If the TSH level is suppressed, then excessive thyroid hormone beyond the influence normal regulation is present (see above). If the TSH level is normal, then results of a suppression test would indicate whether a proportion of function is not under physiologic control. A suppression test in the presence of a normal TSH concentration is not usually undertaken except in conjunction with thyroid images, wherein the sites of uncontrolled function are revealed.

Stimulation test: stimulation of uptake by injected TSH

Although the stimulation test will help to determine the presence and sufficiency of residual thyroid tissue, it is now rarely used because the only form of TSH available, bovine, has potential to cause unfavorable reactions. Recombinant human TSH will soon be available; this agent may be used to prepare a patient with thyroid cancer for ^{131}I therapy by stimulating the residual cancer to increased function. Whether the procedure will have value in determining the presence of normal thyroid function in the face of thyroid hormone treatment remains to be determined.

Perchlorate washout test

This procedure is so rarely used that it should now be classified as a research tool.

Procedures: thyroid uptakes and suppression test

Materials: thyroid uptakes

1. A scintillation probe that has a pulse-height analyzer, a flat field of view (it may be too difficult to aim collimated probes accurately), and a sensitivity that will give statistically valid counts when 7% (lower limit of normal uptake) or less of a 0.01 mCi (0.37 MBq) dose of ^{131}I is assayed at a distance of 25 cm for 2 minutes. ^{99m}Tc may be best measured by a gamma camera using a parallel-hole collimator and defining regions of interest that circumscribe the thyroid gland and an appropriate background area in the neck.
2. Tracer doses of ^{131}I are usually 0.005 to .010 mCi (0.185 to 0.37 MBq), but the dose may be higher, 2 to 5 mCi (74 to 185 MBq) when given as part of imaging procedures in patients with thyroid cancer; or ^{123}I, usually 0.10 to 0.25 mCi (0.185 to 0.46 MBq); or ^{99m}Tc-pertechnetate, 2 to 5 mCi (74 to 85 MBq). See Table 24-2.
3. Standards are prepared from the radiopharmaceutical doses to a volume of 10 to 20 ml; these should be in a container that will fit into an appropriate neck phantom (Hine, 1967).
4. A method for counting background is required. Usually background is determined by counting with a lead shield to selectively reduce the radioactivity emanating from the thyroid gland; much less preferably, counts of radioactivity are measured in the patient's thigh (Schneider, 1979).

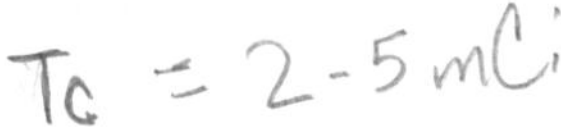

Table 24-2. Dosimetry in imaging thyroid tissue adult subjects

	^{99m}Tc-pertechnetate	^{123}I-Iodide	^{131}I-Iodide	^{201}Tl-thallous chloride
Administered doses[a], mCI (MBq)	5 (185)	0.3 (10.5)[b]	2 (74)[c]	2 (74)
Absorbed doses, rad (cGy):				
Thyroid gland[d]	0.43	2.1[e]	1550	1.9
Whole body	0.65	0.008[e]	0.48	0.42
Ovaries	0.19	0.013[e]	0.32	0.88
Testes	0.05	0.006[e]	0.20	4.2

[a]Commonly prescribed administered doses.
[b]May be given in 5 to 10 mCi (185 to 370 MBq) to patients with thyroid cancer.
[c]Dose for patients with thyroid cancer. Doses of 1 to 10 mCi (37 to 370 mBq) have been used.
[d]Assumes a 15% uptake of radioiodine at 24 hours.
[e]Contaminants of ^{124}I or ^{125}I will increase the absorbed doses (Ziessman and others, 1986).
Radiation dose to patients from radiopharmaceuticals. In Annals of ICRP, New York, 1988, Pergamon Press, pp. 199, 264, 276, 373.

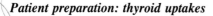

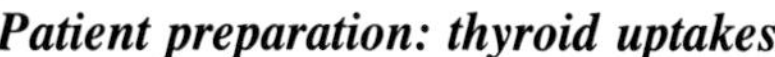

Patient preparation: thyroid uptakes

1. Review the indication for uptake test.
2. Inquire about medications and other materials that could interfere in uptake tests, particularly iodine-containing medications including topical substances, thyroid hormones, antithyroid drugs, and recent radiopharmaceuticals. (It is helpful to have the patient review a prepared list of medications that are known to interfere with uptake tests).
3. Measure the quantity of any prior radioactivity in the patient before administering the radiopharmaceutical dosage, both in thyroid and in the designated background region. The probe is aimed at the patient's cricoid cartilage with the crystal 25 cm from the skin.

Technique: thyroid uptakes

1. Administer the selected dose. ^{131}I and ^{123}I are ingested (usually as a capsule), but ^{99m}Tc is injected intravenously.
2. Select energy settings as follows: 30% window centered on 364 keV for ^{131}I; 20% window centered on 159 keV for ^{123}I (special precautions should be taken to ensure stable voltage) (Chervu, 1982); and 20% window centered on 140 keV for ^{99m}Tc.
3. Obtain thyroid uptakes over 2 minutes and background radioactivity over 2 to 5 minutes.
4. Measure the uptakes after administering the radiopharmaceutical, as follows:
   a. At 24 hours and possibly 6 hours for ^{131}I and ^{123}I, and
   b. At 20 minutes for ^{99m}Tc
5. Perform calculations, as follows:

$$\frac{\text{Thyroid cpm} - \text{Thyroid background cpm} \times 100 = \text{\% uptake}}{\text{Standard cpm} - \text{Standard background cpm}}$$

If prior radioactivity is present, it is recorded as follows:

$$\text{Prior thyroid cpm} - \text{Prior background cpm}$$

Without measured values to the contrary, the decay rate of this prior radioactivity is generally estimated to be that derived from physical half-life of the radionuclide present; the resulting value is subtracted from the net thyroid cpm in the equation shown above.

Modifications for suppression test

Usually the uptake tests in this procedure are performed at 24 hours after the dose administration; therefore, either ^{131}I or ^{123}I is used. The suppression test is performed using two uptake tests: the first gives the baseline value and the second follows treatment with thyroid hormone. Either triiodothyronine 25 μg/d four times per day for 7 days (the second tracer dose is given on the seventh day), or thyroxine 0.2 mg/d for 21 days may be used, but the latter protocol more closely stimulates the effects of thyroid hormone treatment in the patient.

Interpretation: thyroid uptakes and suppression test

Thyroid uptakes: support for the diagnosis of hyperthyroidism

Although separation of normal from hyperthyroid uptake values may be statistically better at times earlier than 24 hours after the tracer dose is given, in practice adequate information is usually obtained at 24 hours. Some hyperthyroid glands turn over radioiodine more rapidly than others, but none has exhibited a biologic half-life of radioiodine less than 2 days, and the mean is about 20 days. Thus, the effective half-life of ^{131}I in the gland usually is 5.4 to 6.4 days. Therefore, even in the most extreme circumstances, a relatively small amount of radioiodine will be lost from a hyperthyroid gland between 6 and 24 hours. Normal ranges should be established for each laboratory especially since the dietary iodine of populations may vary. Some general guides for ^{131}I and ^{123}I values are as follows: at 6 hours, normal up to 12%; at 24 hours, normal between 7% and 30%. The ^{99m}Tc uptake normal range is as follows: at 20 to 30 minutes, up to 4%.

Continued.

Thyroid uptakes: classifying patients with hyperthyroidism

See under Indications (above) and Table 24-1. Since treatment varies with the different types of hyperthyroidism, it is important to classify a patient's disease with an uptake value unless the distinction can otherwise be made.

Thyroid uptakes: calculating a treatment dosage of ^{131}I

The uptake value, usually obtained at 24 hours, is used in formulas for prescribing ^{131}I therapy for patients with hyperthyroidism to give microcuries retained in the thyroid gland per gram of tissue. Uptakes measured at earlier times have been shown to correlate with the 24-hour value, and the use of these values in calculating the therapy dose would assist in the determination of the diagnostic uptake value and the administration of treatment for a single day. Formulas for calculating doses may be more elaborate than those using the uptake value and an estimate of gland volume, but there is little evidence they add precision to the predicted outcome.

Suppression test

Except in unusual cases, hyperthyroidism is not mediated by TSH; therefore, the function of the hyperthyroid gland is unaffected by administered thyroid hormone, which modulates thyroid function only through inhibition of TSH secretion. Generally, when the suppressed uptake levels are less than 50% of the baseline value, the suppression test result is normal. This range allows for variation in uptake values from time to time. It is virtually impossible for hyperthyroidism to exist in the presence of a normal response to suppression. Hyperthyroidism is also unlikely when TSH levels are normal. However, it should be remembered that the suppression test and the TSH concentration do not measure the same functional abnormality. For instance, it would be possible for a patient who had Graves' hyperthyroidism treated to the point of euthyroidism to have a normal TSH level but still exhibit unsuppressibility in the suppression test because residual thyroid function was only partially sustained by TSH.

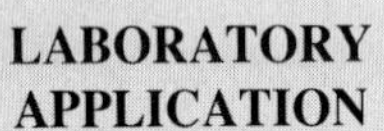

LABORATORY APPLICATION

THYROID IMAGING

Purpose

Two general purposes guide the imaging of thyroid tissue. The first is to determine the relative function in different regions within the thyroid gland with a special emphasis on the function of nodules compared with that of the rest of the gland. The second is to determine the presence and site of thyroid tissue, either within the bed of an incompletely excised gland or in other locations such as normal tissue in the sublingual region, or metastases of thyroid cancer almost anywhere.

Indications

1. To define functioning benign thyroid tissue to:
   - help distinguish benign from malignant nodules
   - indicate possible autonomy of function of a nodule
   - demonstrate heterogeneity of function within a hyperthyroid gland (typical of a toxic nodular goiter)
   - detect benign thyroid tissue in unusual locations such as in lingual and substernal sites
2. To detect the presence and locations of metastases from thyroid cancer, including:
   - papillary and follicular carcinomas (with ^{131}I-iodide or ^{123}I-iodide)
   - medullary carcinomas (with ^{201}Tl-thallous chloride or ^{131}I- or ^{123}I- metaiodobenzylguanidine [mIBG], ^{99m}Tc [V] dimercaptosuccnic acid [DMSA])
   - undifferentiated carcinomas (with ^{201}Tl-thallous chloride)

Procedures

Materials

1. Scintillation camera
2. A variety of collimators (that will be used for different indications) as follows:
   a. Pinhole of 3 or 6 mm, particularly of value in using ^{99m}Tc and ^{123}I for abnormalities within the thyroid gland
   b. High-energy, parallel-hole for a high-energy radionuclide (^{131}I)
   c. Low-energy, high-resolution parallel-hole for low-energy radionuclides (^{99m}Tc, ^{123}I, ^{201}T1) in examining large fields of view
3. Radiopharmaceuticals (see Table 24-2 for comparisons)
   a. To examine the thyroid gland and adjacent regions:
      (1) ^{99m}Tc-pertechnetate, 5 mCi (185 MBq) to be injected IV, *or*
      (2) ^{123}I-iodide, 0.15 to 0.30 mCi (5.55 to 11.1 MBq) to be swallowed, *or*
      (3) ^{131}I-iodide, 0.03 to 0.05 mCi (1.11 to 1.85 MBq) to be swallowed, but this radiopharmaceutical is not recommended because of the relatively high absorbed radiation and poor counting statistics
   b. To search for residual or recurrent thyroid cancer:
      (1) ^{131}I-iodide, 1 to 10 mCi (37 to 370 MBq) to be swallowed, but there is concern for the absorbed radiation and possible "stunning" effects (Park, 1992) of the larger doses; 2 mCi is preferred
      (2) ^{123}I-iodide up to 20 mCi (740 MBq) can be given but imaging must be limited to about 24 hours
      (3) ^{201}T1-thallous chloride, 2 mCi (74 MBq) to be injected IV
      (4) ^{131}I-mIBG, 0.5 mCi (18.5 MBq) or ^{123}I-mIBG 5 to 10 mCi (185 to 370 MBq) to be injected IV, *or*
      (5) ^{99m}Tc [V]-DMSA, 8-12 mCi (296-444 MBq), to be injected IV

Patient preparation

1. Review the indication for imaging.
2. Explain the entire procedure to the patient.
3. Inquire about medications and other materials that may alter the distribution of the selected radiopharmaceutical. For the types of interfering agents of most concern when using ^{99m}Tc-pertechnetate, ^{123}I-iodide and ^{131}I-iodide, see the section Patient Preparation for Uptake Tests. mIBG uptake into tissues such as medullary thyroid cancer will be reduced by inhibitors of the adrenergic uptake-1 system (such as tricyclic antidepressants, cocaine, labetolol) and sympathomimetics (such as pseudoephedrine, phenylpropanolomine).
4. Special approaches are necessary for two of the imaging procedures:
   a. When examining for residual or recurrent papillary or follicular thyroid cancer with ^{131}I-iodide, one relies on endogenous TSH to stimulate thyroid tissue to a point of optimum uptake function. Such a functional state is confirmed by recording an elevated serum TSH concentration (usually >50 μU/ml) and is attained by discontinuing thyroxine for a 6-week period, or triiodothyronine for 3 weeks. If superphysiologic doses of hormone (e.g., 0.3 mg per day of thyroxine) have been given, longer periods of abstinence may be required to disinhibit pituitary secretion of TSH. A low-iodine diet (>25 μg per day) for 1 week may also increase the uptake of ^{131}I by residual cancer, but it may also prolong retention of ^{131}I in the body.
   b. Even though the uptake of ^{201}Tl by well-differentiated thyroid cancers are less affected by TSH than is the uptake of radioiodine, the optimal imaging of these neoplasms even by a "flow agent" such as ^{201}Tl will probably require stimulation by TSH, a condition attained by cessation of thyroid hormone therapy as described above.
   c. When using ^{131}I-mIBG or ^{123}I-mIBG to search for residual or recurrent medullary thyroid cancer, the uptake function of any normal thyroid tissue should be reduced by the ingestion of iodides, such as one drop of saturated solution of potassium iodide three times a day beginning the day before the injection of the radiolabeled mIBG.

Continued.

5. Immediately before becoming recumbent, the patient should swallow a few ounces of water to clear the esophagus of any radioactivity.
6. Position the patient with neck extended and mark on the skin the desired anatomic reference points (such as suprasternal notch, thyroid cartilage notch, and any nodules).

Techniques using ^{99m}Tc

1. Center a 20% window on 140 keV.
2. Begin 20 minutes after injection of the tracer.
3. The thyroid gland and any associated concentration of radioactivity (excluding the salivary glands and mouth) should take up about 75% of the image space.
4. Collect 100,000 counts in the anterior view.
5. With camera and collimator still positioned in the anterior view, be sure that the anatomic marks still correspond to the previously identified anatomic structures; then tape ^{57}Co markers to these sites. Also, two ^{57}Co markers 5 cm apart may be taped to the skin to give a reference for anatomic distance. The image is repeated with the markers in place to give anatomic reference points on a comparable image.
6. Obtain two additional views, 100,000 counts each as follows:
   a. Right anterior oblique 45°
   b. Left anterior oblique 45°

Technique: using ^{123}I-iodide

1. Center a 20% window on 159 keV.
2. The best images may be obtained 5 to 6 hours after the dosage, but images up to 24 hours should contain sufficient counts to be of high quality.
3. The remainder of the procedure is as for imaging with ^{99m}Tc-pertechnetate. However, caution is advised because of contaminations of ^{124}I in preparations of ^{123}I made by the *p, 2n* method. Moreover, care must be given to the reconstruction algorithm if artifacts are to be avoided when single-photon emission tomography is used to portray the distributions of ^{123}I.

Technique: using ^{131}I-iodide

This technique is recommended only to locate residual or recurrent thyroid cancer.

1. Center a 30% window on 364 keV.
2. Images can be obtained at 24 hours, but images at 48 and 72 hours may exhibit greater tumor/background ratios and, by demonstrating retention of the ^{131}I by cancer over days, may be useful in decisions on therapy.
3. Make anterior images of 100,000 counts of each of the neck and chest to include the xiphoid, abdomen, pelvis and upper thighs, upper arms, and any other region that may be suspicious from prior data; posterior images particularly should be considered for selected areas of the spine or skull.
4. Dual-head cameras will allow simultaneous acquisition of anterior and posterior views and will add to the sensitivity of the technique. ^{57}Co markers should be used in the same or separate views to identify landmarks for anatomic orientation.

NOTE—^{123}I-iodide may be used to locate well-differentiated thyroid cancer. Doses are usually 5 to 10 mCi. Instrumentation is as described above for this radionuclide in imaging benign thyroid disease, but the fields of view will be the same as when ^{131}I-iodide is used. Images of most value will be made 24 hours after the dosage.

Technique: using ^{201}Tl-thallous chloride

1. Center a 20% window on 80 keV.
2. Obtain images beginning 20 minutes after the tracer.
3. In the initial image, include the neck and chest. (Images of other regions of the body are difficult to interpret). Images of regions within the neck and chest and of any suspicious re-

gion of the body should be obtained to identify more certainly the presence and position of abnormal foci of radioactivity.

4. Use ^{57}Co markers liberally to enable foci of radioactivity to be related to anatomic structures.

Technique: using ^{131}I-mIBG and ^{123}I-mIBG

The protocols used for locating pheochromocytomas with this radiopharmaceutical should be used, but with an emphasis on the neck and chest.

Technique: using ^{99m}Tc [V] DMSA

The DMSA must be prepared by a special method to attain the pentavalent form. Inject intravenously and obtain images 2 hours later.

Interpretation

Histologic character of thyroid nodules

The preferred diagnostic algorithm for the single or dominant thyroid nodule is first to aspirate for cytology. Only if the cytology leaves some uncertainty of diagnosis are images obtained to add to the diagnostic data.

On the other hand, if the cytology is benign and thyroid hormone therapy is contemplated (a controversial approach), then an image demonstrating a functioning and possibly autonomous nodule would be dissuasive. Most nodules, including those of benign histology, are hypofunctioning (Fig. 24-5, *B*) and cannot be distinguished from malignant nodules by nuclear imaging. However, if a nodule exhibits unequivocal function in the ^{99m}Tc-pertechnetate image (Fig. 24-5, *C* and *D*), there is high probability that it is histologically benign. A few cancers have the ability to trap iodine and technetium, but they cannot organify iodine. These nodules will give evidence of function only in the first few hours after administration of a radiotracer, after which they appear to be hypofunctioning. However, the occurrence of cancer in nodules that function on ^{99m}Tc images is so rare that it is questionable whether it is necessary to follow such images with one made with radioiodine to ensure that the nodule can organify iodine and is therefore more likely to be benign. A nodule that concentrates either ^{123}I- or ^{131}I-iodide as well or better than the surrounding gland must contain most or all of the synthetic mechanisms of normal thyroid tissue; such a functioning nodule is benign with a probability of 99.5% to 99.9%.

There is another variation in the functioning nodule. If on an image made with any of the tracers a nodule is associated with little or no function in the rest of the gland (Fig. 24-5, *D*), one can conclude that the nodule is producing sufficient hormone to suppress TSH secretion, and possibly enough to produce hyperthyroidism. A nodule that functions on an image such as in Fig. 24-5, *C*, may be autonomous, and one that appears as in Fig. 24-5, *D*, is almost certainly autonomous in function. Patients with such nodules should not be given thyroid hormone.

Images of normal thyroid glands (Fig. 24-5, *A*) may have a broad range of configurations. Hypofunctioning nodules (Fig. 24-5, *B*) are of uncertain histology, only 6% to 10% contain cancer. Hypofunction should be assumed for any nodule in which the concentration of the radiopharmaceutical in the nodule is uncertain when compared with that in the rest of the gland; over 90% of thyroid nodules will be of the hypofunctioning type. Because ^{99m}Tc-pertechnetate imparts the least radiation to the thyroid gland while creating highly resolved images, this radiopharmaceutical is usually chosen for the initial image of a thyroid gland that contains nodule(s). A comparison of images made with ^{99m}Tc and ^{123}I has been published (Ryo, 1983).

Heterogeneity of function in hyperthyroid gland

A common experience has been that hyperthyroidism associated with nodules and heterogeneity of function within the gland is more resistant to treatment with ^{131}I. Occasionally, a thyroid gland feels lobular, and on clinical examination it is difficult to conclude whether nodules are present. In such cases, a thyroid image made with either of the two tracers (^{99m}Tc-pertechnetate or ^{123}I) will reveal whether there is heterogenous function within the gland (Fig. 24-5, *E*) and thus give indication for a larger than usual dose of ^{131}I for treating the hyperthyroidism.

Continued.

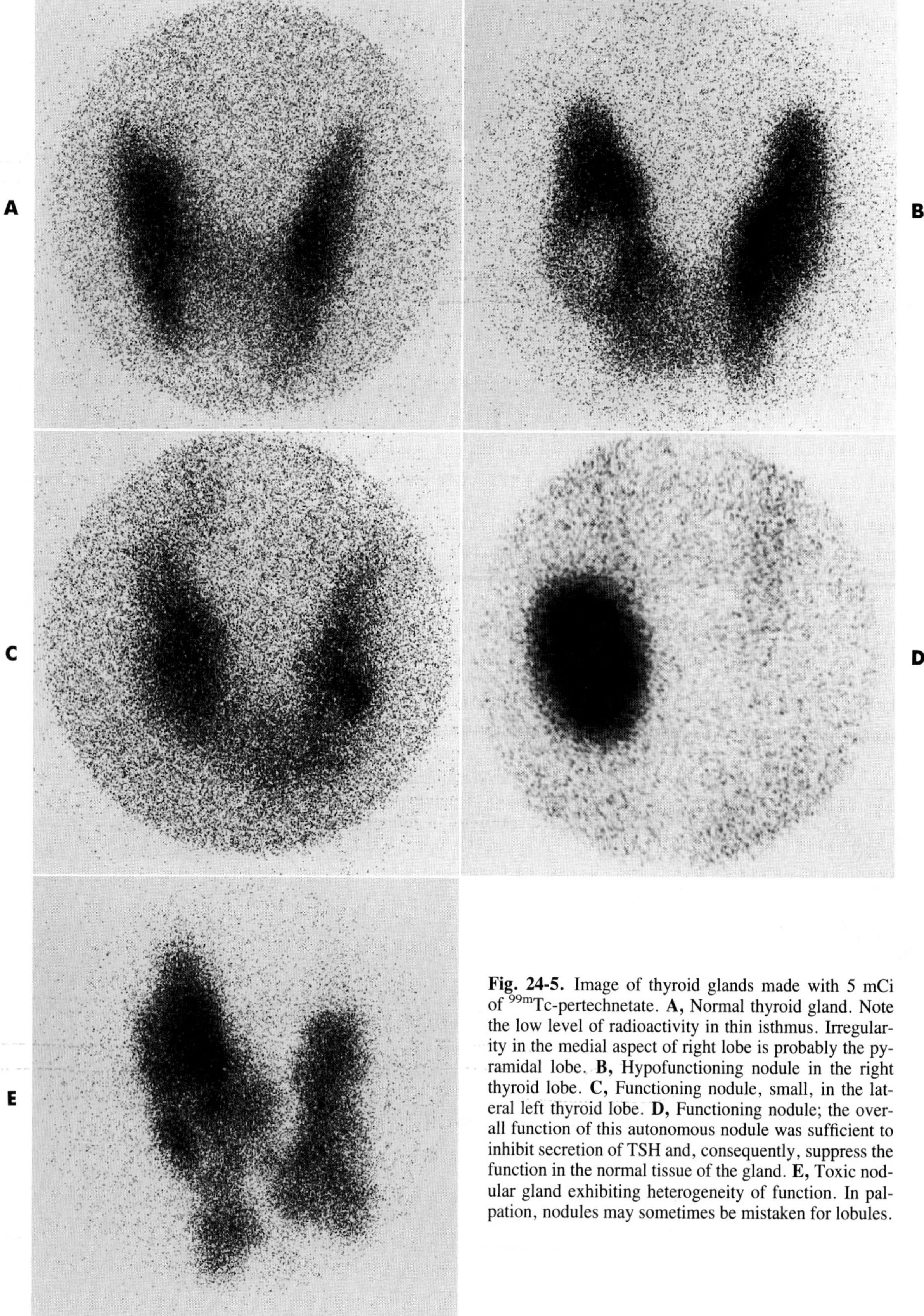

Fig. 24-5. Image of thyroid glands made with 5 mCi of ^{99m}Tc-pertechnetate. **A,** Normal thyroid gland. Note the low level of radioactivity in thin isthmus. Irregularity in the medial aspect of right lobe is probably the pyramidal lobe. **B,** Hypofunctioning nodule in the right thyroid lobe. **C,** Functioning nodule, small, in the lateral left thyroid lobe. **D,** Functioning nodule; the overall function of this autonomous nodule was sufficient to inhibit secretion of TSH and, consequently, suppress the function in the normal tissue of the gland. **E,** Toxic nodular gland exhibiting heterogeneity of function. In palpation, nodules may sometimes be mistaken for lobules.

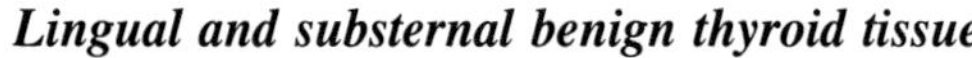

Lingual and substernal benign thyroid tissue

Primary hypothyroidism in infants may be associated with an apparent absence of the thyroid gland. In some cases, the descent of thyroid anlage from the base of the tongue to the neck may be abnormal, and aberrant thyroid tissue, usually functioning less than normally, may be present in the sublingual region. Although ^{99m}Tc and the ^{123}I are concentrated in saliva within the mouth, either of these tracers will still reveal sublingual thyroid tissue as a midline structure when the patient's head is extended. Because of its low radiation dose and relatively low background activity, ^{123}I has been preferred for this purpose, but ^{99m}Tc is probably adequate. In a similar manner, thyroid tissue can be identified in thyroglossal duct remnants, which are often slightly off the midline. Thyroglossal duct cysts may or may not contain functioning thyroid cells.

If a chest x-ray examination of a patient reveals an anterior mediastinal tumor, scintigraphy may aid in determining the nature of the abnormality. Concentration of ^{99m}Tc-pertechnetate, ^{123}I, or ^{131}I in a substernal region corresponding to the tumor seen on x-ray makes it very likely that the anterior mediastinal abnormality is thyroid tissue and a substernal goiter.

Presence and location of well-differentiated thyroid cancer with radioiodine

The structures that normally concentrate ^{131}I must be recognized. These are the salivary glands and saliva in the mouth; gastric mucosa and its secretions extending into the intestine; and the urinary bladder. Virtually all other concentrations of ^{131}I in scintigraphic images will reflect sites of thyroid tissue. Foci of ^{131}I activity outside the thyroid bed region can then be considered to represent metastatic tumor at least in patients who are known to have had primary thyroid carcinomas (Fig. 24-6, *A and B*). Nonthyroid cancer diseases only rarely concentrate ^{131}I. However, contaminations from saliva and urine may show up as localizations on images; care should be taken to repeat images after removal of clothing, washing of skin, and swallowing water.

The sensitivity of the method is uncertain. Most papillary and follicular carcinomas will sequester ^{131}I. On the other hand, some metastatic deposits that are small but treatable may elude even the most careful scintigraphic searches; such tumors may be visualized only after therapeutic doses of ^{131}I. Presumably these elusive cancers would also be detected over time by a rising serum thyroglobulin concentration and/or repeated diagnostic scintigraphy. Foci of radioactivity appearing on an image using a parallel-hold collimator can be resolved for more accurate identification on an image made over a longer period with a pinhole collimator.

How frequently scintigraphic images should be repeated in patients with cancer is a controversial matter. Patients should have images made after the last therapy, usually by 6 weeks or possibly a few months after thyroidectomy and within 1 year after therapy with radioiodine. Subsequent images of patients with low-risk papillary or follicular cancers can probably be deferred until (if ever) there is a clinical abnormality (such as a tumor in the neck) or the thyroglobulin concentration is rising. Patients with higher risk neoplasms should be reimaged as indicated by their course and probably not less often than every 5 years.

Presence and location of thyroid cancer detected by ^{201}Tl

Generally, scintigraphic searches with ^{201}Tl are confined to the neck and chest because the normal background activity of the radiopharmaceutical is high in the abdomen. Concentrations of ^{201}Tl are nonspecific, and radioactivity in normal structures, including residual thyroid tissue, must be distinguished from that in the cancers. Thallous-201 chloride has been of value in detecting regional metastases of medullary carcinoma (Fig. 24-7, *A*) and may be useful in defining the extent of undifferentiated cancers. Another flow agent, ^{99m}Tc-sestamibi, may also detect thyroid cancers of different types through the same mechanism.

Presence and location of medullary carcinoma

The concentrations of ^{131}I-mIBG or ^{123}I-mIBG in medullary cancers are frequently of low magnitude; this modest uptake limits the usefulness of the radiopharmaceutical in searches for this neoplasm (Fig. 24-7, *B*). Also, some of the ^{131}I is metabolized from ^{131}I-mIBG and, in spite of iodide treatment, may appear in normal thyroid tissue. Therefore, any foci of ^{131}I in the neck should be put into perspective by a prior ^{99m}Tc-pertechnetate image, which will define normal thyroid residuals.

Continued.

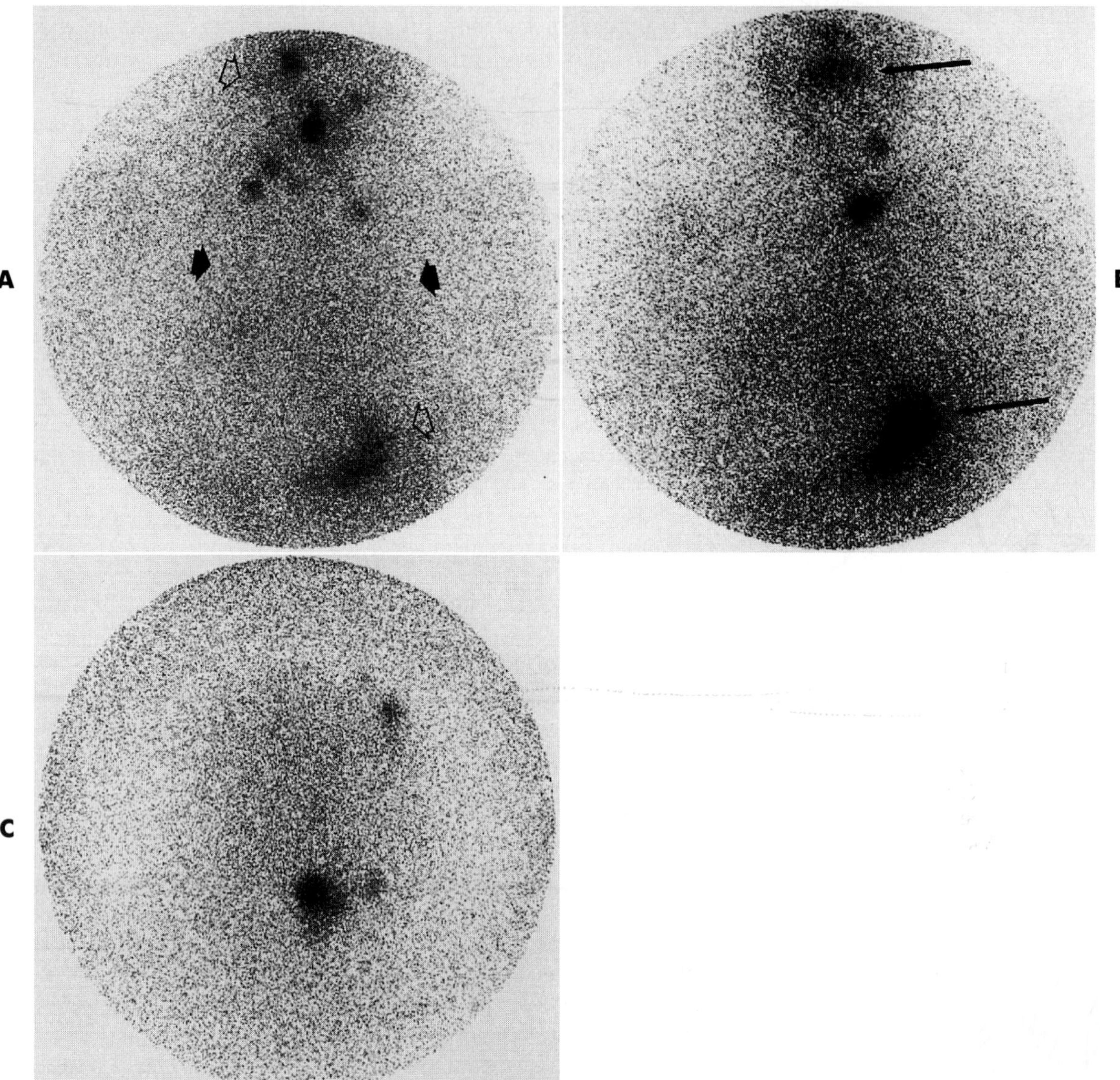

Fig. 24-6. Images made 24 hours after the administration of 2 mCi of ^{131}I. **A,** Focal concentrations of radioactivity are readily seen on the neck region of this male patient who had undergone a total thyroidectomy 6 weeks previously for papillary carcinoma. The multiple foci almost certainly represent regional lymph-node metastases of the cancer. There is faint concentration of radioactivity in the lung regions *(closed arrows)* which, in this patient, was demonstrated more vividly on an image obtained after treatment with ^{131}I. This lung radioactivity represents the most subtle evidence for pulmonary metastases; his chest x-ray was normal. This image should be compared with that in **B.** Radioactivity is also seen in normal structures: the mouth and stomach regions *(open arrows)*. The radioactivity may extend into the intestine in some patients. **B,** Focal concentrations of radioactivity are seen in the neck region *(no arrows)* of a female patient who had a total or near-total thyroidectomy for papillary carcinoma 6 weeks previously. These concentrations represent thyroid tissue of uncertain nature. Radioactivity is also seen in the region of the lower lungs but, in this case, and in contrast to the image in **A,** the concentrations were in the breasts. A lateral view may be necessary to define the location of radioactivity within the chest. Radioactivity is also seen in normal structures: the mouth and stomach *(arrows)*. This image was made with a parallel-hole collimator. For an additional image, see **C. C,** Concentrations of radioactivity in the neck of the patient shown in **B.** The radioactivity is now resolved into additional foci by a pinhole collimator. At least some of the multiple foci must represent lymph-node metastases.

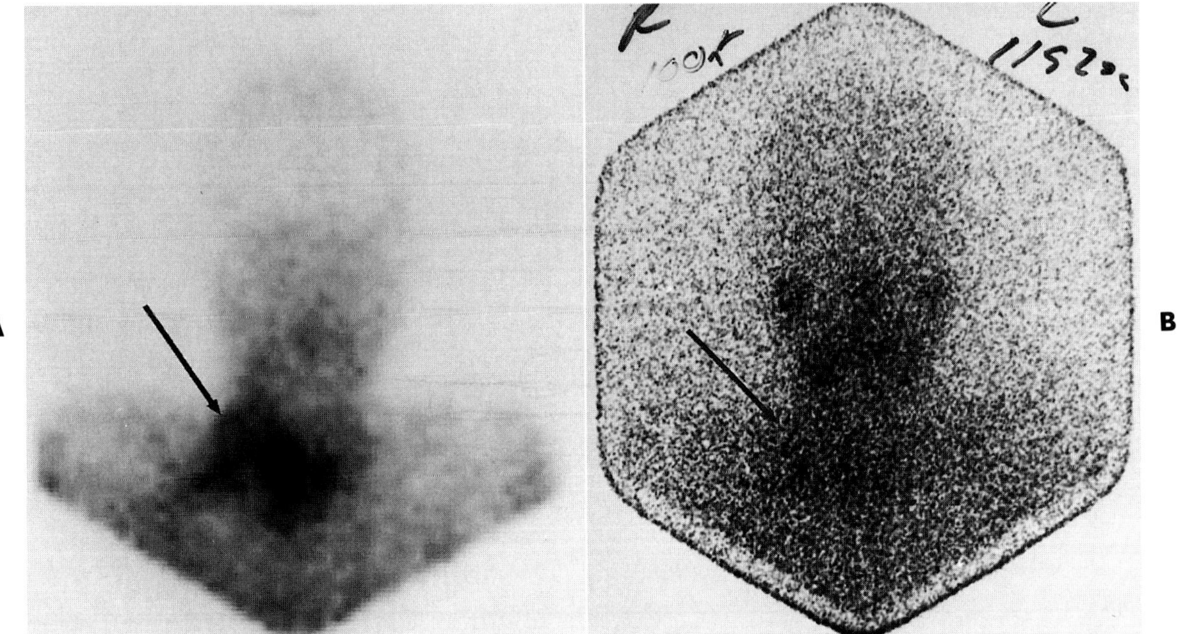

Fig. 24-7. A, Image of the anterior neck and upper chest made 30 minutes after 3 mCi of ^{201}Tl in a patient with multiple endocrine neoplasia type 2B. The concentrations of ^{201}Tl corresponded to nodules in the right lobe and isthmus of the thyroid gland and to nearby lymph nodes in the right jugular region *(arrow)*. The abnormalities were shown to be medullary cancer of the thyroid. This image should be compared with that in **B. B,** Same patient as in **A.** Image of the anterior neck and upper mediastinum was made 1 day after administration of 0.5 mCi of ^{131}I-mIBG. The concentration of this radiopharmaceutical in the medullary cancer is vague *(arrow)* and less than that of ^{201}Tl as shown in **A.** The salivary glands are readily seen. (From Yobbagy, J.J., and others: Scintigraphic portrayal of the syndrome of multiple endocrine neoplasia type-2B, Clin. Nucl. Med. 13:433-437, 1988, with permission.)

Also, concentrations of ^{131}I-mIBG in other tumors, including pheochromocytomas that may develop in a variety of sites, must be differentiated from those in medullary cancer.

^{99m}Tc [V] DMSA appears to have a higher affinity for medullary carcinoma than does mIBG. This agent has not been available in the United States, and its full potential for diagnosis of medullary cancer has not been defined.

REFERENCES

Arnstein, N.B., Carey, J.E., Spaulding, S.A., and Sisson, J.C.: Determination of iodine-131 diagnostic dose for imaging metastac thyroid cancer, J. Nucl. Med. 27:1764-1769, 1986.

Bacci, V., Schussler, G.C., and Kaplan, T.B.: The relationship between serum triiodothyronine and thyrotropin during systemic illness, J. Clin. Endocrinal. Metab. 54:1229-1235, 1982.

Bigsby, R.J., Lepp, E.K., and Litwin, D.E.M., Wilkinson, A.A., and Matte, G.G.: Technetium 99m pentavalent dimercaptosuccinic acid and thallium 201 in detecting recurrent medullary carcinoma of the thyroid, Can. J. Surg. 75:388-392, 1992.

Borst, G.C., Eil, C., and Burman, K.D.: Euthyroid hyperthyroxinemia, Ann. Intern. Med. 98:366-378, 1983.

Burman, K.D., Anderson, J.H., Wartofsky, L., Mong, D.P., and Jelinek, J.J.: Management of patients with thyroid carcinoma: application of thallium-201 scintigraphy and magnetic resonance imaging, J. Nucl. Med. 31:1958-1964, 1990.

Burman, K.D., and Baker, J.R., Jr: Immune mechanisms in Graves' disease, Endocrinol. Rev. 6:183-232, 1985.

Busnardo, B., Girelli, M.E., Simioni, N., Nacamulli, D., and Busetto, E.: Nonparallel patterns of calcitonin and carcinoembryonic antigen levels in the follow-up of medullary thyroid carcinoma, Cancer 53:278-285, 1984.

Cady, B., and Rossi, R.: An expanded view of risk-group definition in differentiated thyroid carcinoma, Surgery 104:947-953, 1988.

Charkes, N.D., Vitti, R.A., and Brooks, K.: Thallium-201 SPECT increases detectability of thyroid cancer metastases, J. Nucl. Med. 31:147-153, 1990.

Chervu, S., Chervu, L.R., Goodwin, P.N., and Blaufox, M.D.: Thyroid uptake measurements with I-123: problems and pitfalls: concise communication, J. Nucl. Med. 23:667-670, 1982.

Chiovato, L., Vitti, P., Santini, F., and others: Incidence of antibodies blocking thyrotropin effect in vitro in patients with euthyroid or hypothyroid autoimmune thyroiditis, J. Clin. Endocrinol. Metab. 71:40-45, 1990.

Chopra, I.J.: Thyroid function in nonthyroidal illnesses, Ann. Intern. Med. 98:946-957, 1983.

Connell, J.M.C., Hilditch, T.E., Robertson, J., Coghill, G., and Alexander, W.D.: Radioprotective action of carbimazole in radioiodine therapy for thyrotoxicosis—influence of the drug on iodine kinetics, Eur. J. Nucl. Med. 13:358-361, 1987.

Dussault, J.H., and Morissette, J.: Higher sensitivity of primary thyrotropin in screening for congenital hypothyroidism: a myth? J. Clin. Endocrinol. Metab. 56:849-852, 1983.

Evans, R.M.: The steroid and thyroid hormone receptor superfamily, Science 240:889-895, 1988.

Fisher, D.A., and Klein, A.H.: Thyroid development and disorders of thyroid function in the newborn, N. Engl. J. Med. 304:702-712, 1981.

Gagel, R.F., Robinson, M.F., Donovan, D.T., and Alford, B.R.: Clinical review 44, Medullary thyroid carcinoma: recent progress, J. Clin. Endocrinol. Metab. 76:809-814, 1993.

Gagel, R.F., Tashjian, A.H., Jr, Cummings, T., and others: The clinical outcome of prospective screening for multiple endocrine neoplasia type 2a, N. Engl. J. Med. 318:478-484, 1988.

Gharib, H., and Goellner, J.R.: Fine-needle aspiration biopsy of the thyroid: an appraisal, Ann. Intern. Med. 118:282-289, 1993.

Gharib, H., James, E.M., Charboneau, J.W., Naessens, J.M., Offord, K.P., and Gorman, C.A.: Suppressive therapy with levothyroxine for solitary thyroid nodules: a double-blind controlled clinical study, N. Engl. J. Med. 317:70-75, 1987a.

Gharib, H., Kao, P.C., and Heath, H. III: Determination of silica-purified plasma calcitonin for the detection and management of medullary thyroid carcinoma: comparison of two provocative tests, Mayo Clin. Proc. 62:373-378, 1987b.

Gharib, H., and Klee, G.G.: Familial euthyroid hyperthyroxinemia secondary to pituitary and peripheral resistance to thyroid hormones, Mayo Clin. Proc. 60:9-15, 1985.

Gilland, D.R., Jaszczak, R.J., Greer, K.L., and Coleman, R.E., Quantitative SPECT reconstruction of iodine-123 data, J. Nucl. Med. 32:527-533, 1991.

Girelli, M.E., Busnardo, B., Amerio, R., Casara, D., Betterle, C., and Piccolo, M.: Critical evaluation of serum thyroglobulin (Tg) levels during thyroid hormone suppression therapy versus Tg levels after hormone withdrawal and total body scan: results in 291 patients with thyroid cancer, Eur. J. Nucl. Med. 11:333-335, 1986.

Goldman, J.M., Line, B.R., Aamodt, R.L., and Robbins, J.: Influence of triiodothyronine withdrawl time on ^{131}I uptake post-thyroidectomy for thyroid cancer, J. Clin. Endocrinol. Metab. 50:734-739, 1980.

Graham, S.M., Genel, M., Touloukian, R.J., Barwick, K.W., Gertner, J.M., and Torony, C.: Provocative testing for occult medullary carcinoma of the thyroid: findings in seven children with multiple endocrine neoplasia type IIa, J. Pediatr. Surg. 22:501-503, 1987.

Guilloteau, D., Perdrisot, R., Calmettes, C., and others: Diagnosis of medullary carcinoma of the thyroid (MCT) by calcitonin assay using monoclonal antibodies: criteria for the pentagastrin stimulation test in hereditary MCT, J. Clin. Endocrinol. Metab. 71:1064-1067, 1990.

Hamburger, J.I.: Evolution of toxicity in solitary nontoxic autonomously functioning thyroid nodules, J. Clin. Endocrinol. Metab. 50:1089-1093, 1980.

Hauser, P., Zametkin, A.J., and Martinez, P. and others: Attention deficit-hyperactivity disorder in people with generalized resistance to thyroid hormone, N. Engl. J. Med. 328:997-1001, 1993.

Hay, I.D.: Papillary thyroid carcinoma, Endocrinol. Metab. Clin. North Am. 19:545-576, 1990.

Hayes, A.A., Akre, C.M., and Gorman, C.A.: Iodine-131 treatment of Graves' disease using modified early iodine-131 uptake measurements in therapy dose calculations, J. Nucl. Med. 31:519-522, 1990.

Heyman, S., Crigler, J.F., Jr, and Treves, S.: Congenital hypothyroidism: ^{123}I thyroidal uptake and scintigraphy, J. Pediatr. 101:571-574, 1982.

Hilts, S.V., Hellman, D., Anderson, J., Woolfenden, J., Van Antwerp, J., and Patton, D.: Serial TSH determination after T_3 withdrawal or thyroidectomy in the therapy of thyroid carcinoma, J. Nucl. Med. 20:928-932, 1979.

Hine, G.J., and Williams, J.B.: Thyroid radioiodine uptake measurements. In Hine, G.J., editor: Instrumentation in nuclear medicine, vol. 1, New York, 1967, Academic Press, pp. 330-331.

Hopwood, N.J., Sauder, S.E., Shapiro, B., and Sisson, J.C.: Familial partial peripheral and pituitary resistance to thyroid hormone: a frequently missed diagnosis? Pediatrics 78:1114-1122, 1986.

Iida, Y., Hidaka, A., Hatabu, H., Kasagi, K., and Konishi, J.: Follow-up study of postoperative patients with thyroid cancer by thallium-201 scintigraphy and serum thyroglobulin measurement, J. Nucl. Med. 32:2098-2100, 1991.

Iida, Y., Konishi, J., Kasagi, K., and others: Inhibition of thyrotropin-induced growth of rat thyroid cells, FRTL-5, by immunoglobulin G from patients with primary myxedema, J. Clin. Endocrinol. Metab. 64:124-130, 1987.

Ingbar, S.H.: Autoregulation of the thyroid: response to iodide excess and depletion, Mayo Clin. Proc. 47:814-823, 1972.

Itagaki, Y., Yoshida, K., Ikeda, H., and others: Thyroxine 5′-deiodinase in human anterior pituitary tumors, J. Clin. Endocrinol. Metab. 71:340-344, 1990.

Kashiwai, T., Ichihara, K., Endo, Y., Tamaki, H., Amino, N., and Miyai, K.: Immunological and biological characteristics of recombinant human thyrotropin, J. Immunol. Methods 143:25-30, 1991.

Koller, K.J., Wolff, R.S., Warden, M.K., and Zoeller, R.T.: Thyroid hormones regulate levels of thyrotropin-releasing hormone RNA in the paraventricular nucleus, Proc. Natl. Acad. Sci. USA 84:7329-7333, 1987.

Kusic, Z., Becker, D.V., Saenger, E.L., and others: Comparison of technetium-99m and iodine-123 imaging of thyroid nodules: correlation with pathologic findings, J. Nucl. Med. 31:393-399, 1990.

Larsen, P.R., Alexander, N.M., Chopra, I.J., and others: Revised nomenclature for tests of thyroid hormones and thyroid-related proteins in serum, J. Clin. Endocrinol. Metab. 64:1089-1094, 1987.

Lichter, J.B., Wu, J., Genel, M., and others: Presymptomatic testing using DNA markers for individuals at risk for familial multiple endocrine neoplasia 2A, J. Clin. Endocrinol Metab. 745:368-373, 1992.

Lips, C.J.M., Leo, J.R., Berends, M.J.H., and others: Thyroid C-cell hyperplasia and micronodules in close relatives of MEN-2A patients: pitfalls in early diagnosis and reevaluation of criteria for surgery, Henry Ford Hosp. Med. J. 35:133-138, 1987.

Lombardi, A., Martino, E., and Bravermann, L.E.: Amiodarone and the thyroid, Thyroid Today 13:1-7, 1990.

Maldonado, L.S., Murata, G.H., Hershman, J.M., and Braunstein, G.D.: Do thyroid function tests independently predict survival in the critically ill? Thyroid 2:119-123, 1992.

Mandel, S.J., Berry, M.J., Kieffer, J.D., Harney, J.W., Warne, R.L., and Larsen, P.R.: Cloning and in vitro expression of the human selenoprotein, type I iodothyronine deiodinase, J. Clin. Endocrinol. Metab. 75:1133-1139, 1992.

Mariotti, S., Caturegli, P., Piccolo, P., Barbesino, G., and Pinchera, A.: Antithyroid peroxidase autoantibodies in thyroid diseases, J. Clin. Endocrinol. Metab. 71:661-669, 1990.

Mariotti, S., Martino, E., Cupini, C., and others: Low serum thyroglobulin as a clue to the diagnosis of thyrotoxicosis factitia, N. Engl. J. Med. 307:410-412, 1982.

Martino, E., Aghini-Lombardi, F., Lippi, F., and others: Twenty-four hour radioactive iodine uptake in 35 patients with amiodarone associated thyrotoxicosis, J. Nucl. Med. 26:1402-1407, 1985.

Maruca, J., Santner, S., Miller, K., and Santen, R.J.: Prolonged iodine clearance with a depletion regimen for thyroid carcinoma: concise communication, J. Nucl. Med. 25:1089-1093, 1984.

Mashiter, K., Von Noorden, S., Fahlbusch, R., Fill, H., and Skrabal, K.: Hyperthyroidism due to a TSH secreting pituitary adenoma: case report, treatment and evidence for adenoma TSH by morphological and cell culture studies, Clin. Endocrinol. 18:473-483, 1983.

Maxon, H.R., and Smith, H.S.: Radioiodine-131 in the diagnosis and treatment of metastatic well differentiated thyroid cancer, Endocrinol. Metab. Clin. N. Am. 19:685-718, 1990.

Mazzaferri, E.L.: Management of a solitary thyroid nodule, N. Engl. J. Med. 328:553-559, 1993.

Mclmed, S., Geola, F.L., Reed, A.W., Pekary, A.E., Park, J., and Hershman, J.M.: A comparison of methods for assessing thyroid function in nonthyroidal illness, J. Clin. Endocrinol. Metab. 54:300-306, 1982.

Mendelsohn, G., Wells, S.A., and Baylin, S.B.: Relationship of tissue carcinoembryonic antigen and calcitonin to tumor virulence in medullary thyroid carcinoma; an immunohistochemical study in early, localized, and virulent disseminated stages of disease, Cancer 54:657-662, 1984.

Mojiminiyi, O.A., Udelsman, R., Soper, N.D.W., Shepstone, B.J., and Dudley, N.E.: Pentavalent Tc-99m DMSA scintigraphy prospective evaluation of its role in the management of patients with medullary carcinoma of the thyroid, Clin. Nucl. Med. 16:259-262, 1991.

Mountz, J.M., Glazer, G.M., Dmuchowski, C., and Sisson, J.C.: MR imaging of the thyroid: comparison with scintigraphy in the normal and diseased gland, J. Comp. Assist. Tomogr. 11:612-619, 1987.

Nicoloff, J.T., and Spencer, C.A.: The use and misuse of the sensitive thyrotropin assays, J. Clin. Endocrinol. Metab. 71:553-558, 1990.

Nikolai, T.F., Coombs, G.J., McKenzie, A.K., Miller, R.W., and Weir, J., Jr.: Treatment of lymphocytic thyroiditis with spontaneously resolving hyperthyroidism (silent thyroiditis), Arch. Intern. Med. 142:2281-2283, 1982.

Oppenheimer, J.H., Schwartz, H.L., Mariash, C.N., Kinlaw, W.B., Wong, N.C.W., and Freake, H.C.: Advances in our understanding of thyroid hormone action at the cellular level, Endocrinol. Rev. 8:288-308, 1987.

Park, H.M.: Stunned thyroid after high-dose I-131 imaging, Clin. Nucl. Med. 17:501-502, 1992.

Paul, S.J., and Sisson, J.C.: Thyrotoxicosis caused by thyroid cancer, Endocrinol. Metab. Clin. North Am. 19:593-612, 1990.

Peter, H.J., Studer, H., Forster, R., and Gerber, H.: The pathogenesis of "hot" and "cold" follicles in multinodular goiters, J. Clin. Endocrinol. Metab. 55:941-946, 1982.

Polak, J.F., English, R.J., and Holman, B.L.: Performance of collimators used for tomographic imaging of I-123 contaminated with I-124, J. Nucl. Med. 24:1065-1069, 1983.

Ramanathan, P., Patel, R.B., Subrahmanyam, N., Nayak, U.N., Sachdev, S.S., and Ramamoorthy, N.: Visualization of suppressed thyroid tissue by technetium-99m-tertiary butyl isonitrile: an alternative to post-TSH stimulation scanning, J. Nucl. Med. 31:1163-1165, 1990.

Ramanna, L., Waxman, A., and Braunstein, G.: Thallium-201 scintigraphy in differentiated thyroid cancer: comparison with radioiodine scintigraphy and serum thyroglobulin determinations, J. Nucl. Med. 32:441-446, 1991.

Rapoport, B., and Ingbar, S.H.: Production of triiodothyronine in normal human subjects and in patients with hyperthyroidism: contribution of intrathyroid iodine analysis, Am. J. Med. 56:586-591, 1974.

Robbins, J., Merino, M.J., Boice, J.D., Jr., and others: Thyroid cancer: a lethal endocrine neoplasm, Ann. Intern. Med. 115:133-147, 1991.

Ronga, G., Fiorentino, A., Paserio, E., and others: Can iodine-131 whole-body scan be replaced by thyroglobulin measurement in the post-surgical follow-up of differential thyroid carcinoma? J. Nucl. Med. 31:1766-1771, 1990.

Ruiz-Garcia, J., Ruiz de Almodóvar, M., Olea, N., and Pedraza, V.: Thyroglobulin level as a predictive factor of tumoral recurrence in differentiated thyroid cancer, J. Nucl. Med. 32:395-398, 1991.

Ryo, U.Y., Vaidya, P.V., Schneider, A.B., Bekerman, C., and Pinsky, S.M.: Thyroid imaging agents: a comparison of I-123 and Tc-99m pertechnetate, Radiology 148:819-822, 1983.

Salata, R., and Klein, I.: Effects of lithium on the endocrine system: a review, J. Lab. Clin. Med. 110:130-136, 1987.

Schlumberger, M., Arcangioli, O., Piekarski, J.D., Tubiana, M., and Parmentier, C.: Detection and treatment of lung metastases of differentiated thyroid carcinoma in patients with normal chest x-rays, J. Nucl. Med. 29:1790-1794, 1988.

Schneider, P.B.: Simple, rapid thyroid function testing with ^{99m}Tc-pertechnetate thyroid uptake ratio and neck/thigh ratio, A.J.R. Am. J. Roentgenol. 132:249-253, 1979.

Seto, P., Hirayu, H., Magnusson, R.P., and others: Isolation of a complementary DNA clone for the microsomal antigen: hcmology with the gene for thyroid peroxidase, J. Clin. Invest. 80:1205-1208, 1987.

Singer, P.A., and Gorsky, J.E.: Familial postpartum transient hyperthyroidism, Arch. Intern. Med. 145:240-242, 1985.

Sisson, J.C., Gross, M.D., Frietas, J.E., Jackson, C.E., and England, B.G.: Combining provocative agents of calcitonin to detect medullary carcinoma of the thyroid, Henry Ford Hosp. Med. J. 29:75-80, 1981.

Sobol, H., Narod, S.A., Yusuke, N., and others: Screening for multiple endocrine neoplasia type 2a with DNA-polymorphism analysis, N. Engl. J. Med. 321:996-1001, 1989.

Soutter, W.P., Norman, R., and Green-Thompson R.W.: The management of choriocarcinoma causing severe thyrotoxicosis: two case reports, Br. J. Obstet. Gynaecol. 88:938-943, 1981.

Spencer, C.A., LoPresti, J.S., Patel, A., and others: Applications of a new chemiluminometric thyrotropin assay to subnormal measurement, J. Clin. Endocrinol. Metab. 70:453-460, 1990.

Spencer, C.A., Schwarzbein, D., Guttler, R.B., LoPresti, J.S., Nicoloff, J.T.: Thyrotropin (TSH)-releasing hormone stimulation test responses employing third and fourth generation TSH assays, J. Clin. Endocrinol. Metab. 76:494-498, 1993.

Stall, G.M., Harris, S., Sokoll, L.J., and Dawson-Hughes, B.: Accelerated bone loss in hypothyroid patients overtreated with L-thyroxine, Ann. Intern. Med. 113:265-269, 1990.

Sugawara, M.: Coupling of iodotyrosine catalyzed by human thyroid peroxidase in vitro, J. Clin. Endocrinol. Metab. 60:1069-1075, 1985.

Surks, M.I., Hupart, K.H., Pan, C., and Shapiro, L.E.: Normal free thyroxine in critical nonthyroidal illnesses measured by ultrafiltration of undiluted serum and equilibrium dialysis, J. Clin. Endocrinol. Metab. 67:1031-1039, 1988.

Telander, R.L., Zimmerman, D., van Heerden, J.A., and Sizemore, G.W.: Results of early thyroidectomy for medullary thyroid carcinoma in children with multiple endocrine neoplasia type 2, J. Pediatr. Surg. 21:1190-1194, 1986.

Usala, S.J.: Molecular diagnosis and characterization of thyroid hormone resistance syndromes, Thyroid 1:361-387, 1991.

Utiger, R.D.: Thyrotropin-releasing hormone and thyrotropin secretion, J. Lab. Clin. Med. 109:327-335, 1987.

van Heerden, J.A., Grant, C.S., Gharib, H., Hay, I.D., and Ilstrup, D.M.: Long-term course of patients with persistent hypercalcitoninemia after apparent curative primary surgery for medullary thyroid carcinoma, Ann. Surg. 212:395-410, 1990.

Van Herle, A.J., Van Herle, I.S., and Greipel, M.A.: An international cooperative study evaluating serum thyroglobulin standards, J. Clin. Endocrinol. Metab. 60:338-343, 1985.

Vassart, G., and Dumont, J.E.: The thyrotropin receptor and the regulation of thyrocyte function and growth, Endocrinol. Rev. 13:596-611, 1992.

Von Moll, L., McEwan, A.J., Shapiro, B., and others: Iodine-131 MIBG scintigraphy of neuroendocrine tumors other than pheochromocytoma and neuroblastoma, J. Nucl. Med. 28:979-988, 1987.

Weetman, A.P., and McGregor, A.M.: Autoimmune thyroid disease: developments in our understanding, Endocrinol. Rev. 5:309-355, 1984.

Wenzel, K.W.: Pharmacological interference with in vitro tests of thyroid function, Metabolism 30:717-732, 1981.

Woolner, L.B.: Thyroid carcinoma: pathologic classificaiton with data on prognosis, Semin. Nucl. Med. 1:481-502, 1971.

Yobbagy, J.J., Levatter, R., Sisson, J.C., Shulkin, B.L., and Polley, T.: Scintigraphic portrayal of the syndrome of multiple endocrine neoplasia type-2B, Clin. Nucl. Med. 13:433-437, 1988.

Yokoyama, N., Taurog, A. Dorris, M.L., and Klee, G.G.: Studies with purified human thyroid peroxidase and thyroid microsomal autoantibodies, J. Clin. Endocrinol. Metab. 70:758-765, 1990.

Zakarija, M., McKenzie, J.M., and Hoffman, W.H.: Prediction and therapy of intrauterine and late-onset neonatal hyperthyroidism, J. Clin. Endocrinol. Metab. 62:368-371, 1986.

Zakarija, M., and McKenzie, J.M.: Do thyroid growth-promoting immunoglobulin exist? J. Clin. Endocrinol. Metab. 70:308-310, 1990.

Ziessman, H.A., Fahey, F.H., and Gochoco, J.M.: Impact of radiocontaminants in commercially available iodine-123: dosimetric evaluation, J. Nucl. Med. 27:428-432, 1986.

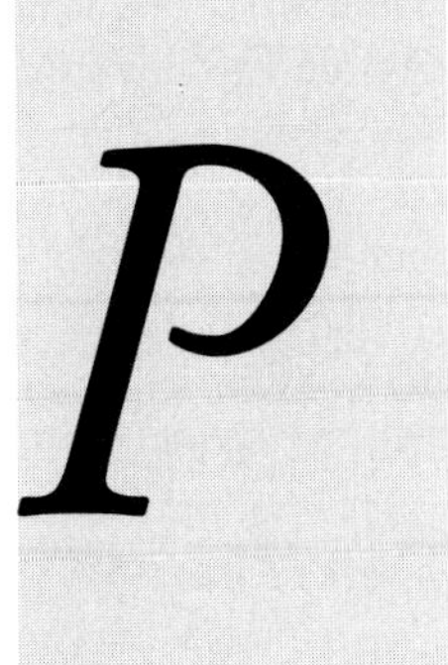

Chapter 25

ARATHYROID GLAND

DAVID C. PRICE
MICHAEL D. OKERLUND

Imaging of the parathyroid glands has been an important challenge in the last several decades, one first approached by nuclear medicine in the 1960s and investigated further in recent years by ultrasound (US), computed tomography (CT), and most recently, magnetic resonance imaging (MRI). In spite of the impressive technical advances of the latter three modalities, nuclear medicine techniques have remained prominent and have continued to evolve. This chapter will outline this evolution and describe the current methodology. For detailed information, the reader is referred to three recent books by Sandler and others (1986), Eisenberg (1991), and Sandler and others (1992).

■ ANATOMY

Most humans have two superior and two inferior parathyroid glands, each about 1 × 3 × 5 mm in dimensions and 40 to 48 mg in weight. They are usually oval, bean-shaped, or spherical in configuration, but can vary considerably in shape. The two superior parathyroids arise with the lateral thyroid complex from the fourth pharyngeal pouch and migrate inferiorly in the second month of gestation to rest customarily behind the upper pole of each thyroid lobe, between the upper one third and lower two thirds of the lobe. The inferior parathyroids arise from the third pharyngeal pouch with the thymus gland, and migrate inferiorly to settle customarily just at or below the lower pole of each thyroid lobe. In 2% to 3% of humans, one or more parathyroids may fail to descend completely; this results in an ectopic location above the superior pole of the thyroid or posteriorly near the esophagus or pharynx. In an additional 2% of humans, the parathyroid gland may over-descend, lying in the superior mediastinum with the thymus in the case of an inferior parathyroid, or less commonly in the posterior mediastinum in the case of a superior parathyroid. In 0.2% of humans, one or more parathyroids will actually be imbedded in the thyroid gland. A small number of humans, perhaps 1% to 3%, have only three parathyroids. Much more commonly, however, in as many as 13% of individuals, there will be supernumerary parathyroids, most often five or six but sometimes as many as 12 or 13. In such instances, ectopic locations are common. It is important to be familiar with the spectrum of locations and numbers of parathyroid glands when imaging scintigraphically, particularly because ectopic locations will be the more likely sites for additional parathyroid glands in a patient who has undergone prior parathyroidectomy for hyperparathyroidism.

■ PHYSIOLOGY

The function of the parathyroid glands is to regulate calcium ion concentration in interstitial fluid, and therefore in plasma, by synthesis and release of parathyroid hormone (PTH). Lower-than-normal interstitial calcium concentration stimulates PTH synthesis and release by the parathyroids, with resultant mobilization of calcium from the skeleton, the GI tract by absorption, and from renal retention. Plasma calcium and phosphates usually maintain an inverse relationship such that disorders with low serum calcium will have a high serum phosphate level, and vice versa. Nevertheless, the effect of PTH is primarily on calcium ion concentration itself, and only secondarily on phosphorus metabolism. The parathyroid glands are fundamentally different from the thyroid gland in that PTH is not stored within the parathyroids but is synthesized and released directly on stimulation by low interstitial calcium concentrations. In addition, the parathyroids respond directly to interstitial calcium, without control from another endocrine organ (such as is the case with the thyroid, under the control of the pituitary and hypothalamus).

PTH is an 84-amino-acid polypeptide which, once released into circulation, is rapidly cleaved into a physiologically active amino-terminal fragment with a rapid blood disappearance half-time of 3 to 5 minutes and an inactive carboxy-terminal fragment with a long blood disappearance half-time of several hours. There are radioimmunoassays, and now enzyme immunoassays, for the whole PTH molecule as well as for these two fragments. Assay of the slower-clearing carboxy-terminal fragment in plasma is important in the primary diagnosis of hyperparathyroidism because this component will accumulate in circulation. However, it is essential to assay the rapidly disappearing amino-terminal fragment in situations such as selective venous catheterization in which one is attempting to identify the specific anatomic location of increased PTH synthesis.

■ PATHOPHYSIOLOGY

The two important clinical disorders of parathyroid function are hypoparathyroidism and hyperparathyroidism. Hypoparathyroidism results from low PTH synthesis and secretion by the parathyroids, with consequent fall in plasma calcium levels and rise in inorganic phosphates. The disease may occur spontaneously, but it is most commonly the result of unexpected removal of all parathyroid tissue at the time of thyroidectomy. It is readily resolved by therapy with PTH and calcium. There is no place for parathyroid imaging in the diagnosis and management of hypoparathyroidism.

Hyperparathyroidism is a disorder characterized by increased PTH synthesis and release, with consequent rise in serum calcium and drop in inorganic phosphates. The elevated plasma calcium levels can predispose to kidney stone formation; in extreme instances these elevated levels can cause calcification of a variety of soft tissues. In addition, the mobilization of calcium from the skeleton by PTH results in severe and progressive osteoporosis leading to bone pain, fractures, cystic bone changes, brown tumors of bone, and in the extreme, a skeletal disorder termed *osteitis fibrosa cystica generalisata*. In addition to formation of kidney stones, hyperparathyroidism can result in recurrent kidney infections and deposition of calcium within the renal cortex itself, ultimately producing chronic renal insufficiency. Although hyperparathyroidism was thought several decades ago to be a rather rare disease, with a prevalence on the order of 1 in 10,000, the development of multitest automatic chemistry panels in the 1960s resulted in a much more frequent detection of the disorder, such that its current prevalence is considered to be on the order of 1 in 1000. Because such patients are now detected at a very early stage in their disease, fewer than 50% will develop significant symptoms. Hyperparathyroidism may be divided into a primary form, which develops spontaneously and idiopathically; a secondary form in which the parathyroid glands hypertrophy in response to chronic low serum calcium levels (e.g., chronic renal insufficiency); and a tertiary form in which long-standing secondary hyperparathyroidism has become completely autonomous. In patients with primary hyperparathyroidism, the cause will be a single parathyroid adenoma in 80% to 86% of cases, two or more adenomas in 1% to 4%, multiglandular hyperplasia in 12% to 15%, and functioning parathyroid carcinoma in 1% to 3%. The disease is much more common in females, with a female-to-male ratio of 3:1. The disease generally peaks in the fifth decade of life. Although the cause of primary hyperparathyroidism is generally unknown, it should be noted that, as with thyroid disorders, there is an increased incidence of hyperparathyroidism in patients who have a previous history of head and neck radiation (on the order of 200 to 600 rad exposure). Anywhere from 6% to 29% of hyperparathyroid patients will give a history of prior head and neck radiation, depending on the reported series.

There are three hereditary disorders that can predispose an individual to hyperparathyroidism. These include multiple endocrine neoplasia type I (MEN I), MEN IIa, and familial hypocalciuric hyperparathyroidism (FHH). The former two diseases are the association of parathyroid adenomas with a variety of other endocrine neoplasms, and the latter is a hereditary form of the disorder with hypercalcemia, reduced kidney secretion of calcium and magnesium, and multiglandular hyperparathyroidism. Although these three disorders are rare, they are important to recognize because they commonly result in failure of initial surgery and often lead to repeated surgeries for recurrent hyperparathyroidism.

The current diagnostic approach to hyperparathyroidism consists initially of a thorough history and physical examination, confirmation of the presence of hypercalcemia (and elimination of the nonhyperparathyroid causes thereof, such as the hypercalcemia of widespread metastatic disease), documentation of elevated levels of circulating parathyroid hormone, and finally, an attempt at localization of the suspected parathyroid tumor or tumors before surgical intervention. It is important to note, however, that an experienced parathyroid surgeon operating on a patient with primary hyperparathyroidism will be successful 95% of the time, so that a diagnostic test carrying 80% sensitivity and considerable cost will be of relatively little value. The most important application of parathyroid imaging is in the patient with persistent or recurrent hyperparathyroidism following one or more previous surgeries, in which case all the customary normal locations of parathyroids have been explored and there is a high likelihood of an ectopic adenoma. In this situation the surgical success rate is only 50% to 60% without prior imaging, and these surgeries are more extensive and risky for the patient. Consequently presurgical localization can be of great help to the surgeon and can shorten the surgery time with consequent reduced risk to the patient.

■ PARATHYROID GLAND IMAGING

LABORATORY APPLICATION

77

LOCALIZATION AND EVALUATION OF PARATHYROID TUMORS

Purpose and historical background

Early attempts at parathyroid imaging in the 1960s explored the use of ^{75}Se-selenomethionine, an amino acid precursor to many polypeptides, and ^{57}Co-cyanocobalamin, a tracer empirically found to concentrate in parathyroids. At this time imaging was performed with rectilinear scanners, and the uptake of both tracers in the parathyroids was sufficiently poor that image quality was also quite poor. Success rate with the tracers ranged from 20% to 60%, most frequently at the lower end of this range, so that gradually parathyroid scintigraphy fell completely out of use.

In 1979, Fukunaga and others first noted imageable uptake of ^{201}Tl in a functioning parathyroid adenoma. This led to subsequent development by Ferlin and others of a standardized technique using ^{201}Tl for its uptake in parathyroid and thyroid tissue, then computer-subtraction of the thyroid component of thallium using ^{99m}Tc pertechnetate. The uptake of thallium by parathyroids is entirely nonspecific, because thallium is a potassium analog that goes to all tissues with high cellularity and high blood flow. This is why the thyroid, customarily a 20-g organ, labels so well with thallium and is such a problem in parathyroid identification. Since the average parathyroid is only 40 mg in size, it is not possible to see normal parathyroids by the thallium/technetium subtraction technique, even under optimum imaging conditions. For parathyroid adenomas below 500 mg, the sensitivity of detection falls off significantly. Nevertheless, a large proportion of patients with functioning parathyroid adenomas have tumors that are greater than 500 mg in size, with consequent imaging detection rates in the range of 80% to 90%.

Radiopharmaceuticals

Thallium-201 is a radionuclide that decays by electron capture with a 74-hour half-life and with emission of gamma rays of 135 keV (2% abundance) and 167 keV (8% abundance), but fortunately with the coincident emission of 69 to 83 keV characteristic x-rays (98% abundance) from the stable daughter isotope, mercury-201. Thus, one can image the characteristic x-rays alone, or using dual-peak energies one can image the x-rays with the 167-keV gamma ray simultaneously. Thallium disappears from the blood with a half-time of 5.0 minutes, so that peak uptake occurs in the parathyroids at 5 to 10 minutes after injection. It is important to image the parathyroids within 10 to 15 minutes of the thallium injection because activity falls to 50% of the 10-minute peak by 30 minutes after injection.

Because of the dominant uptake of thallium in the 20-g thyroid, a subsequent intravenous injection of ^{99m}Tc pertechnetate permits labeling of thyroid alone and consequently discrimination of parathyroid tissue from thyroid by either visual examination of unprocessed analog images, computer-subtraction in progressive increments of the technetium thyroid image from the thallium dual image until only parathyroid remains, or use of a color-ratio–computed technique (which colors thallium red and technetium blue, so that excess of thallium in a parathyroid adenoma will appear red in the magenta thyroid background).

There has been recent interest in other radiopharmaceutical approaches to the parathyroids. Zwas and others (1987) reported the use of ^{131}I-labeled toluidine blue (RTB) for parathyroid imaging. This tracer labels the parathyroids selectively and therefore does not require technetium subtraction. Although these authors found their technique demonstrated a 93% sensitivity and 80% specificity in patients with hyperparathyroidism, there have been no other groups exploring the technique and no apparent commercial interest in making the radiopharmaceutical available. Several published abstracts have indicated that ^{99m}Tc sestamibi, introduced recently for myocardial imaging like thallium, has significant advantages for parathyroid scintigraphy. Initial images during the first 5 to 10 minutes demonstrate combined uptake in both thyroid and parathyroid tissue, but serial imaging thereafter up to 2 or 3 hours will demonstrate progressive clearance of thyroid activity with persistence of activity in enlarged parathyroid glands. It appears that sestamibi will achieve the sensitivity and specificity of the thallium/technetium subtraction technique, and will have the advantages of single isotope injection and avoidance of computer processing.

Continued.

Indications

1. To identify single adenomas, multiple adenomas, or glandular hyperplasia in patients with newly diagnosed hypercalcemia and elevated PTH levels.
2. To shorten the operating time in acutely ill patients by providing localization information before surgery.
3. To localize the parathyroid tissue in patients with persistent or recurrent hyperparathyroidism after one or more previous surgical explorations.

Procedure

Materials

1. 2 to 3 mCi (74 to 111 MBq) ^{201}Tl chloride
2. 5 to 10 mCi (185 to 370 MBq) ^{99m}Tc pertechnetate
3. Scintillation camera/computer
4. Pinhole collimator

Patient preparation

1. Explain the entire procedure to the patient.

Technique

1. Biochemically document the presence of hyperparathyroidism (elevated serum calcium and parathyroid hormone).
2. Palpate the neck for evidence of a pathologic parathyroid (or thyroid) condition.
3. Position the patient comfortably supine under the scintillation camera with pinhole collimator.
4. Comfortably immobilize the patient's head.
5. Establish intravenous access through an indwelling butterfly cannula in the forearm.
6. Inject 2 to 3 mCi (74 to 111 MBq) ^{201}Tl chloride intravenously.
7. Obtain a 5-minute image of the mediastinum between the heart and the thyroid by positioning the pinhole collimator/camera centered over the upper mediastinum; look for any evidence of focal uptake between these two structures. Begin this image no later than 2 to 3 minutes after thallium injection.
8. Immediately at completion of the upper mediastinal image, move the pinhole collimator up to the neck and closer to the patient and obtain a 15-minute image with the thyroid centered and one thyroid length visible above and below.
9. At completion of the 15-minute ^{201}Tl neck image, inject 5 to 10 mCi (185 to 370 MBq) ^{99m}Tc pertechnetate intravenously.
10. Wait 5 minutes for thyroid uptake of the technetium, then obtain an image to the same total count as the 15-minute ^{201}Tl image, making sure that there is no patient motion between these images. Both of these thyroid-region images should be computer-acquired in either a $128 \times 128 \times 8$ or a $64 \times 64 \times 16$ matrix.
11. Visually inspect the analog images of ^{201}Tl and ^{99m}Tc for areas of excess thallium.
12. Computer-process the images by serial subtraction of 10% increments of the technetium image from the thallium image until the entire thyroid is removed, or by color-ratio processing as described by O'Connell.

NOTE:

1. It is important to carefully select patients with biochemically documented hyperparathyroidism.
2. It is important to carefully immobilize the patient between thallium and technetium injections, and to be certain to visualize appropriate areas of the mediastinum and the entire neck around the thyroid so that the likelihood of overlooking ectopic parathyroid glands is minimized.

Table 25-1. Sensitivity and false positive rate of parathyroid scintigraphy in 52 recently reviewed publications (Price, 1990)

	No. of publications	No. of patients	Sensitivity	False positive rate
Primary hyperparathyroidism:				
• Adenoma	41	834	80.2% (673/839)	8.9% (49/552)
• Hyperplasia	17	97	45.5% (118/260)	14.3% (5/35)
Secondary hyperparathyroidism	15	123	47.1% (212/450)	6.0% (3/50)
Parathyroid carcinoma	8	15	80.0% (12/15)	— —
Persistent or recurrent hyperparathyroidism	17	280	41.4% (115/278)	11.1% (24/216)
Totals	52	1349	61.4% (1130/1842)	9.5% (81/853)

Interpretation

Sensitivity

In their original report, Ferlin and others reported successful localization of 17 of 19 parathyroid adenomas (89%) using the thallium/technetium imaging technique and a rectilinear scanner. Okerlund and others reported localization of 40 of 50 consecutive parathyroid adenomas (80%) using scintillation camera and pinhole collimator images of thallium/technetium and visual interpretation of unprocessed analog images. They found an increase in sensitivity to 88% when computerized color-ratio images were used; this finding emphasizes the importance of computer processing. Table 25-1 summarizes a large number of scintigraphic parathyroid localization publications (as reviewed by Price, 1990), comparing parathyroid adenomas with hyperplasia and carcinoma in primary hyperparathyroidism, and in patients with persistent or recurrent hyperparathyroidism. The detected hyperplastic or adenomatous parathyroids reported in the literature have ranged from as little as 60 mg in size to as large as 19 g in size, with sensitivity generally falling off as the size diminishes below 500 g. As noted in Table 25-1, sensitivity in general is lower for glandular hyperplasia (45%) than for adenomas (80%). The sensitivity for carcinoma of the parathyroid is 80%. Not indicated in this summary table is the fact that parathyroids located away from the thyroid gland are detected with greater sensitivity than those lying behind or within the thyroid, with the possible exception of mediastinal parathyroids. In a separate study of primary and secondary parathyroid hyperplasia, Okerlund and others reported localization of 12 of 23 glands in six patients with the secondary disorder (a sensitivity of only 52%) by visual assessment of the scintigrams with an additional seven glands localized by examination of color-processed images, raising sensitivity to 83%. In 10 patients with primary hyperplasia, a total of 9 of 29 total glands were localized in analog images (31% sensitivity), with 10 additional glands localized by color comparison for a total glandular sensitivity of 66% in this group of patients. Once again, computer processing substantially improves the sensitivity. In regard to secondary parathyroid hyperplasia, it is important to recognize that although a few patients have all hyperplastic glands identified by scintigraphy, the demonstration of even two abnormal glands strongly suggests parathyroid hyperplasia because "double adenoma" is exceedingly infrequent by comparison.

Significance of a positive imaging test

A single parathyroid area found to have focal uptake of ^{201}Tl out of proportion to ^{99m}Tc in a biochemically documented case of hyperparathyroidism is almost always going to be a single parathyroid adenoma. It is very unlikely that it will represent one hyperplastic gland in a patient in whom the other hyperplastic glands do not visualize successfully, and even less likely to represent a parathyroid carcinoma of which only 120 cases have been reported in the world literature up to 1987. The finding of two sites of ^{201}Tl excess strongly suggests the presence of parathyroid hyperplasia, with larger glands tending to occur in secondary hyperparathyroidism (particularly those cases due to renal failure) and smaller degrees of glandular enlargement in primary parathyroid hyperplasia. The presence of two or more adenomas, as mentioned previously, is quite rare, occurring in only

Continued.

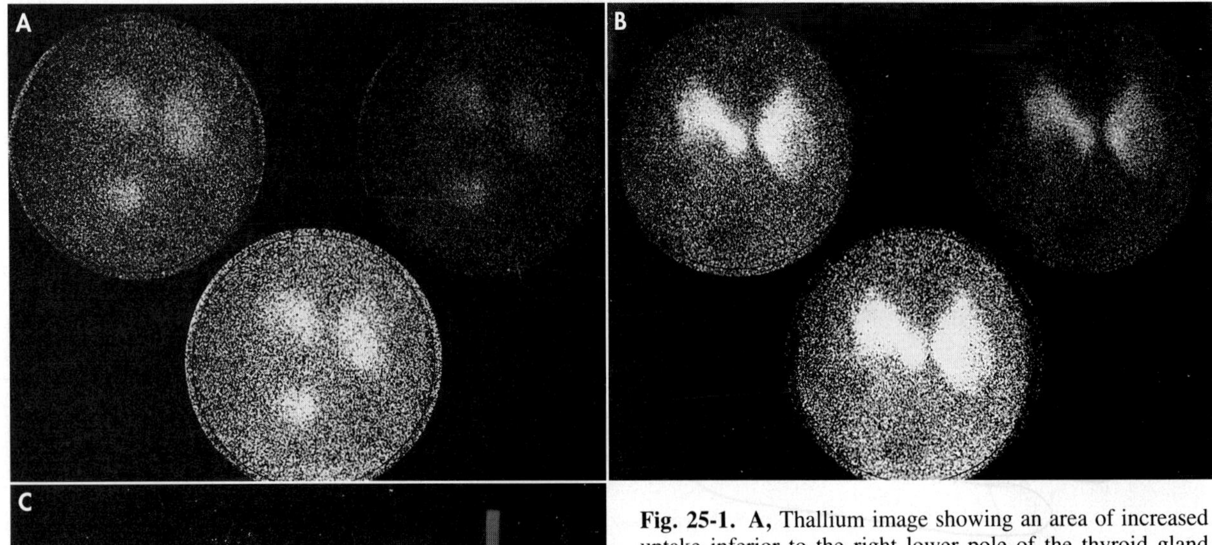

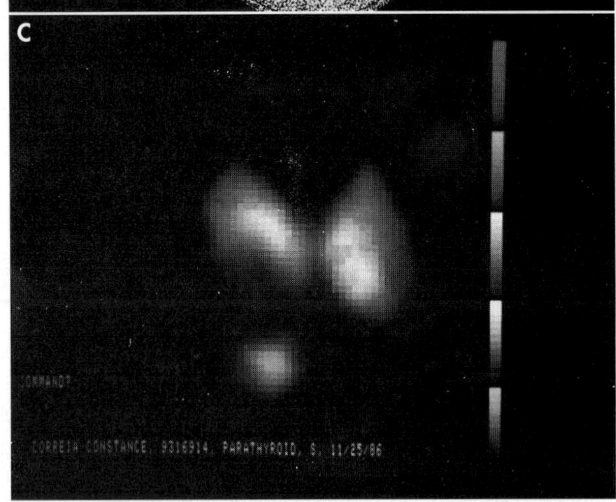

Fig. 25-1. A, Thallium image showing an area of increased uptake inferior to the right lower pole of the thyroid gland and a lesser area of increased uptake closely related to the left lower pole of the thyroid proper. **B,** Absence of pertechnetate uptake below the right lower pole and decreased pertechnetate uptake in the infero-lateral aspect of the left thyroid lobe. **C,** Color-comparison image showing definite lesion compatible with a parathyroid adenoma inferior to the right thyroid lobe and a less definite lesion related to the left lower thyroid lobe area. Surgery showed the extremely rare situation of bilateral parathyroid adenomas. The other two parathyroids were normal by appearance and on biopsy. (This illustration was generated in color and reproduced in black and white.)

1% to 4% of patients with hyperparathyroidism (Fig. 25-1). Visualization of normal parathyroid glands by scintigraphy does not occur, presumably because of their small size and perhaps because of a relative lack of avidity for ^{201}Tl. In addition, presence of a functioning adenoma will result in suppression of nontumorous normal glands (Figs. 25-2, 25-3, 25-4).

It is problematic that parathyroid scintigraphy is a planar technology with two-dimensional images and little ability to discern the actual depth of the tumor. Consequently, correlation with US or MRI can be of great assistance to the surgeon. In general, location of the adenoma (right or left, superior or inferior) does not affect sensitivity of detection, and in spite of the low energy of the x-rays associated with ^{201}Tl decay, the procedure has proved quite sensitive for substernal parathyroid adenomas. In cases of primary or secondary parathyroid hyperplasia, it is common for one parathyroid to appear larger than the others; this can be somewhat confusing in the process of deciding if the patient truly has hyperplasia.

False positive studies

The commonest cause of false positive thallium/technetium parathyroid scintigraphy is thyroid pathology, including thyroid adenomas, multinodular goiters, and much less frequently, thyroid carcinomas (Fig. 25-5). This is unfortunate, because there is reportedly a high incidence (40%) of thyroid disease in patients with hyperparathyroidism. Since many pathologic thyroid conditions are readily detectable by careful palpation of the neck, the physical examination is an important part of parathyroid evaluation, at least in identifying the fact that a pathologic thyroid condition is present. Thyroid disease is also a common cause of false positive studies for US, CT, or MRI, so this provides no particular advantage to these other imaging modalities. The second most common cause of

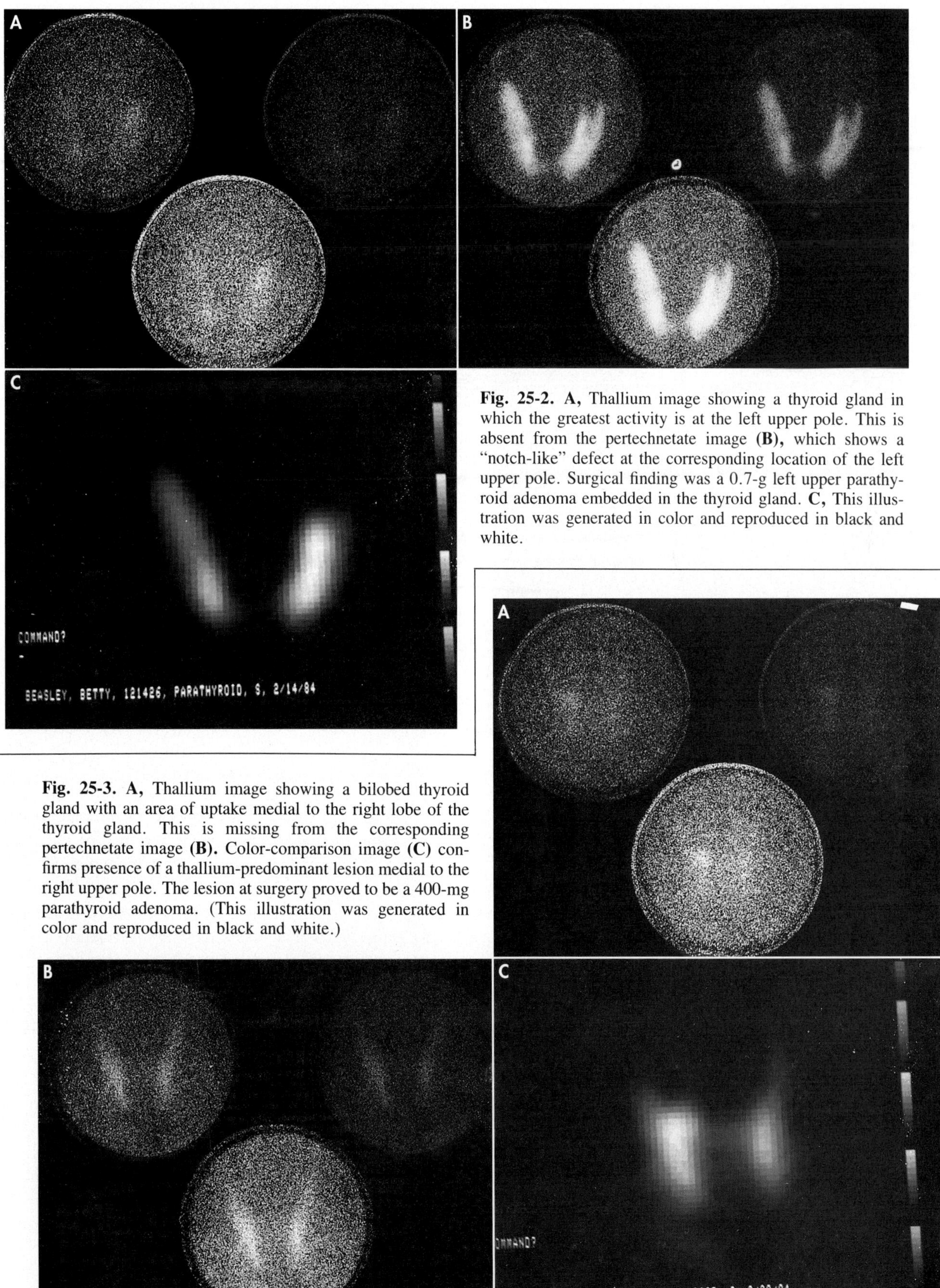

Fig. 25-2. A, Thallium image showing a thyroid gland in which the greatest activity is at the left upper pole. This is absent from the pertechnetate image **(B),** which shows a "notch-like" defect at the corresponding location of the left upper pole. Surgical finding was a 0.7-g left upper parathyroid adenoma embedded in the thyroid gland. **C,** This illustration was generated in color and reproduced in black and white.

Fig. 25-3. A, Thallium image showing a bilobed thyroid gland with an area of uptake medial to the right lobe of the thyroid gland. This is missing from the corresponding pertechnetate image **(B).** Color-comparison image **(C)** confirms presence of a thallium-predominant lesion medial to the right upper pole. The lesion at surgery proved to be a 400-mg parathyroid adenoma. (This illustration was generated in color and reproduced in black and white.)

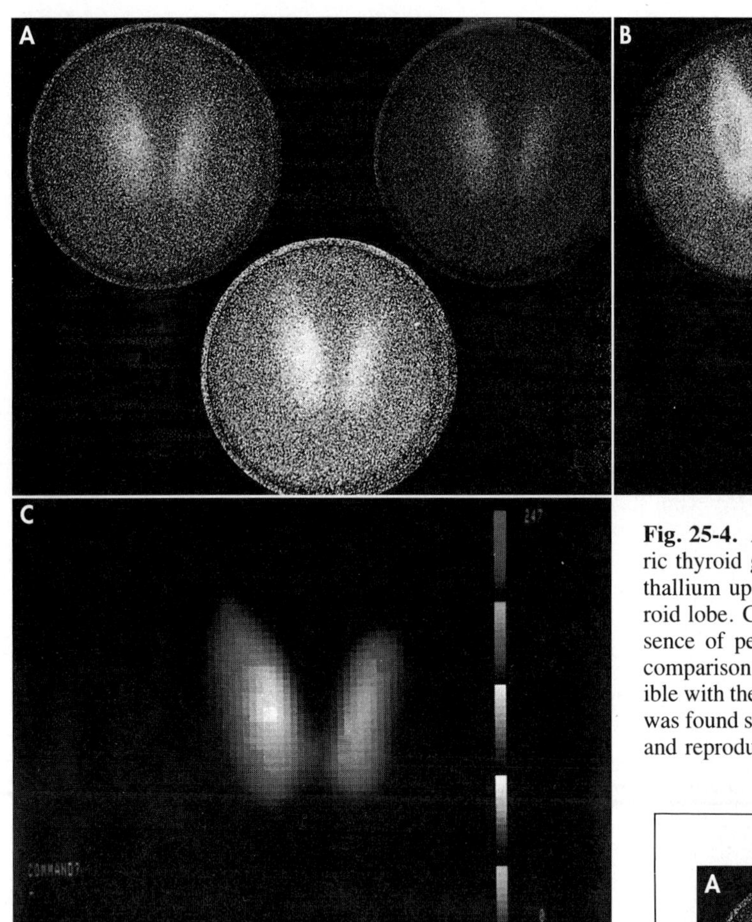

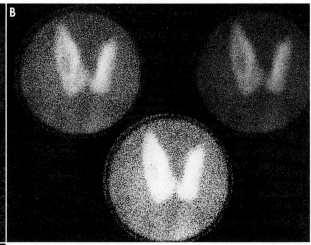

Fig. 25-4. A, Thallium image indicating a slightly asymmetric thyroid gland in which there may be a subtle increase of thallium uptake at the medial aspect of the right upper thyroid lobe. Corresponding pertechnetate image **(B)** shows absence of pertechnetate uptake at a similar location. Color-comparison image **(C)** shows thallium predominance compatible with the 0.5-g intrathyroidal parathyroid adenoma, which was found surgically. (This illustration was generated in color and reproduced in black and white.)

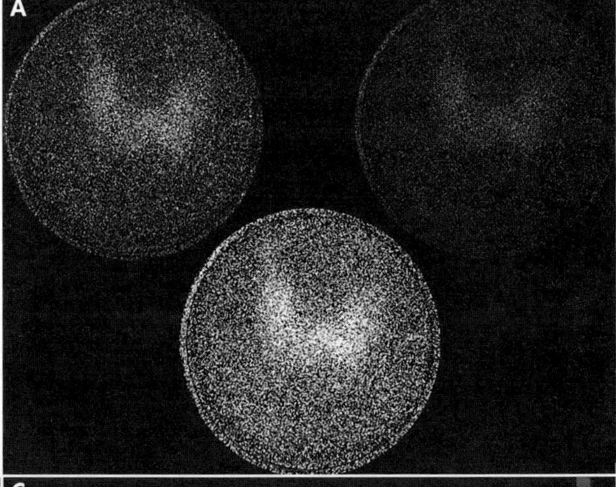

Fig. 25-5. A, Thallium image with an area of thallium uptake at the superior aspect of the junction of the isthmus and left lobe of thyroid. This is absent from the pertechnetate image **(B).** The latter also shows an intense area of pertechnetate uptake in the supero-lateral aspect of the left thyroid lobe. Color-comparison image **(C)** shows a thallium predominant lesion at the junction of the isthmus and left lobe that is compatible with a parathyroid tumor and a pertechnetate-predominant lesion in the left thyroid lobe that is compatible with a functioning thyroid nodule. The findings were conformed surgically, the parathyroid adenoma weighing 0.7 g. (This illustration was generated in color and reproduced in black and white.)

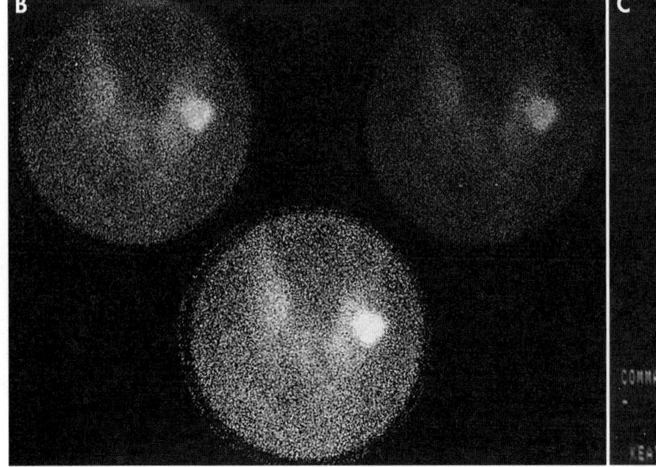

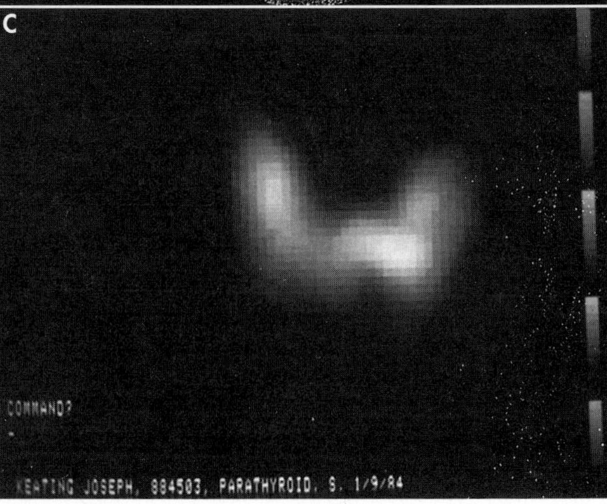

false positive studies with parathyroid imaging is patient movement; therefore, careful attention to keeping the patient still is essential. Other causes of false positive parathyroid scintigraphic findings include neoplastic adenopathy in the cervical region (lymphomas, melanomas, and other metastatic tumors from breast or lung), sarcoidosis, and granulomatous cervical lymph nodes.

False negative studies

The most common cause of a false negative parathyroid scintigraphic examination is a small parathyroid adenoma. As mentioned before, sensitivity drops off significantly with adenomas smaller than 500 mg, although it is curious and unexplained that there are a small number of very large adenomas reported as false negatives in the literature. Other causes of false negative studies include multinodular goiters, ectopic glands (particularly deep in the neck or mediastinum), and one reported case of ^{99m}Tc uptake in a true parathyroid adenoma.

Because of the importance of ^{99m}Tc thyroid subtraction, both false positive and false negative findings can arise from interference with thyroid imageability. This problem occurs with patients with hypothyroidism, patients on suppressive doses of thyroid hormones, and patients with low thyroid radionuclide uptake due to recent iodide administration. In such cases, the problem is the presence of sufficient thyroid tissue to pick up thallium in the face of reduced or absent technetium uptake. In general, patients who have undergone prior total thyroidectomy do not present problems unless there is a small amount of residual thyroid tissue remaining. When the thyroid can be induced to recover from the problem (such as in patients whose thyroid medication can be discontinued or in whom the plasma iodide level can be allowed to fall over some weeks), the study can be repeated several weeks later.

As mentioned previously, thallium uptake reaches its peak in the parathyroids at 5 to 10 minutes after injection and has fallen to half peak by 30 minutes. Thus it generally becomes unrewarding to attempt to continue imaging beyond 30 minutes in a patient whose study up to that point has been negative. It is particularly important that the initial mediastinal image be appropriately centered between heart and thyroid. The thyroid pinhole image should include an area bordered by the salivary glands, the neck area lateral to the thyroid lobes and the suprasternal notch. Occasionally with a completely negative study and high clinical suspicion for parathyroid adenoma, it is worth repeating the study 1 to 2 weeks later using a parallel-hole collimator and imaging from the heart up to the salivary glands, accumulating a 15-minute picture beginning 5 minutes after thallium injection. In such a case, since attention had been directed previously to the thyroid area itself with technetium subtraction, this need only be an analog image of thallium distribution to look for an ectopic location such as the mediastinum.

Recurrent or persistent hyperparathyroidism

Hyperparathyroidism that has persisted or recurred after previous parathyroid surgery is a challenging diagnostic and therapeutic problem. Surgical success without presurgical localization is only 60%, but this success rate can be increased to 80% to 90% by using various techniques of presurgical localization. With recurrent or persistent hyperparathyroidism, parathyroid imaging has the dual advantage of increasing the effectiveness of the surgery and decreasing the surgical time for the surgeon, who then knows exactly where to explore. Scintigraphy has an additional advantage over US, CT, and MRI in that surgical scars do not show up as confusing information and possible causes of false positive studies. Finally, it is important to recognize that ectopic locations of parathyroids are much more common in patients with recurrent or persistent hyperparathyroidism, generally because the normal locations have been surgically evaluated and the findable glands have been removed. For example, the normal incidence of mediastinal parathyroids ranges from 0% to 8% in a variety of surgical and pathological publications, whereas in patients with recurrent or persistent hyperparathyroidism, mediastinal adenomas are found in 15% to 52% of patients. This again emphasizes the importance of looking actively for ectopic sites in patients who have undergone previous surgery. This is particularly true for patients with supernumerary glands, who have had four or more glands removed at primary surgery and therefore are most likely to have an ectopic location for the remaining adenomatous gland.

Continued.

Parathyroid localization by other modalities

Localization of parathyroid adenomas or hyperplastic glands can also be achieved successfully with US, CT, and MRI, with sensitivities and specificities that tend to be rather similar to those of scintigraphy, as reviewed by Price in 1990. Arteriography is used much less frequently for this purpose, and selective venous catheterization is a highly specific but somewhat insensitive localization technique that is tremendously invasive and used by a relatively small number of surgeons in academic centers. US achieves its greatest sensitivity with superficial lesions using a 7.5- or 10-MHz transducer. Because of the physical characteristics of ultrasound, sensitivity is significantly reduced in areas deep in the neck or in the substernal region. It should be noted, however, that US sensitivity is highly dependent on the availability of a skilled radiologist who has had considerable experience with the technique. Although almost as sensitive as US, CT has largely fallen out of use in the last several years for parathyroid localization. There is considerable interest in the use of MRI, but the published experience to date has not been sufficient to develop certainty of its true sensitivity and specificity. For a surgeon, the clear high-resolution anatomic images of MRI are highly advantageous in decisions concerning surgical approach.

■ SPECIAL APPLICATIONS OF PARATHYROID IMAGING

■ Evaluation of parathyroid forearm transplants

In recent years, subtotal parathyroidectomy has become increasingly recognized as the preferable treatment for parathyroid hyperplasia. Many surgeons accomplish this by autotransplanting all or part of one parathyroid gland into the patient's forearm, providing both protection against hypoparathyroidism and a known location for the residual parathyroid gland in case further surgery is necessary. Should hyperparathyroidism recur, the transplanted gland can easily be partially or totally removed. It has been observed that parathyroid glands transplanted into the forearm do not show significant uptake of ^{201}Tl above background levels in patients with normal calcium and PTH levels. Consequently, in patients with persistent or recurrent hyperparathyroidism, if the forearm gland is the only one visualizable it is therefore the offending hyperplastic or adenomatous gland, whereas if the forearm gland is nonvisualized and a hot spot is found in the neck, the surgeon can be certain that further neck surgery is necessary. Thus, forearm imaging followed by neck imaging frequently provides an absolute answer for the surgeon.

■ Rapid differentiation between hyperparathyroidism and the hypercalcium of malignancy

There are some cases in which there are two contending diagnoses: hyperparathyroidism and the hypercalcemia of malignancy. These patients are generally elderly and frail, admitted to the hospital with severe hypercalcemia, dehydration, and obtundation. Immunoassays of parathyroid hormone in human serum require time and often repeated determinations or repeat assays in serial dilutions, whereas a scintigraphic parathyroid study may provide definitive information on such a patient in as little time as 1 hour. Hyperparathyroidism of sufficient severity to produce profound hypercalcemia is generally produced by a very large parathyroid tumor, often several grams or more in weight. These are usually identified rapidly and easily by scintigraphy and can then be targeted for rapid removal. Patients with hypercalcemia of malignancy will have functionally suppressed thyroid glands, however, with a negative scintigraphic study.

Nuclear parathyroid imaging continues to play a prominent role in the evaluation of hyperparathyroidism, particularly in patients with recurrent or persistent forms of the disease following prior surgery. In such cases the surgical success rate is only 50% to 60% without preoperative localization procedures; the success rate increases to 80% with presurgical localization. Scintigraphy and US, having similar sensitivities and specificities, are the two most frequently used parathyroid imaging modalities, with many surgeons first employing US because of its lower cost. MRI appears to have an important future in parathyroid imaging, but at considerable increase in cost. Currently the predominant scintigraphic technique is that of thallium/technetium–computer-processed subtraction or color-ratio imaging, but recent early experience with ^{99m}Tc-sestamibi appears quite promising.

BIBLIOGRAPHY

Atkins, H.L., Budinger, T.F., Lebowitz, E., and others: Thallium-201 for medical use. Part 3: Human distribution and physical imaging properties, J. Nucl. Med. 18:133-140, 1977.

Bekerman, C., Schulak, J.A., Kaplan, E.L., and others: Parathyroid adenoma imaged by Ga-67 citrate scintigraphy: case report, J. Nucl. Med. 18:1096-1098, 1977.

Carnavale, N., Samson, R., and Bennett, B.P.: Multiple parathyroid adenomas, J.A.M.A. 246:1332-1334, 1981.

Digulio, W., and Beierwaltes, W.H.: Parathyroid scanning with selenium-75-labeled methionine, J. Nucl. Med. 5:417-427, 1964.

Dufour, D.R., and Wilkerson, S.Y.: Factors related to parathyroid weight in normal persons, Arch. Pathol. Lab. Med. 107:167-172, 1983.

Edis, A.J., Sheehy, P.F., Bearhs, O.H., and van Heerden, J.A.: Results of reoperation for hyperparathyroidism, with evaluation of preoperative localization studies, Surgery 84:384-391, 1978.

Eisenberg, B., editor: Imaging of the thyroid and parathyroid glands: a practical guide, New York, 1991, Churchill Livingstone, p. 209.

Ferlin, G., Conte, N., Borsato, N., and others: Parathyroid scintigraphy with 131-Cs and 201-T1, J. Nucl. Med. Allied Sci. 25:119-123, 1981.

Ferlin, G., Borsato, N., Perelli, R., and others: Technetium-thallium subtraction scan: a new method in the localization of parathyroid enlargement, Eur. J. Nucl. Med. 6:A12, 1981.

Ferlin, G., Borsato, N., Camerani, M., and others: Parathyroid scintigraphy with a new double-tracer (99m-Tc-T1) technique, J. Endocrinol. Invest. 5.101, 1982.

Ferlin, G., Camerani, M., Conte, N., and Zoth, D.: New perspectives in localizing enlarged parathyroids by technetium-thallium subtraction scan, J. Nucl. Med. 24:438-441, 1983.

Fukunaga, M., Morita, R., Yonekura, Y., and others: Accumulation of 201-T1-Chloride in a parathyroid adenoma, Clin. Nucl. Med. 4:229-230, 1979.

Gilmour, J.R.: The gross anatomy of the parathyroid gland, J. Pathol. Bacteriol. 46:133-149, 1938.

Harness, J.K., Ramsburg, S.R., Nishiyama, R.H., and Thompson, N.W.: Multiple adenomas of the parathyroids: do they exist? Arch. Surg. 114:468-474, 1976.

Ito, Y., Muranika, A., Harada, T., and others: Experimental study on tumor affinity of 201-T1-chloride, Eur. J. Nucl. Med. 3:81-86, 1978.

Mikiuchi, M., Miyakawa, M., Sugermoya, A., and others: Diagnostic usefulness of 201-T1-chloride scintigraphy for localization of parathyroid tumor, Jpn. J. Surg. 11:162-166, 1981.

Narmann, E., Rootwell, K., Solheim, D., and Sdae, G.: Use of 131-I-toluidine blue in radionuclide imaging of enlarged parathyroid glands, Ann. Chir. Gynecol. 65:249-252, 1976.

O'Connell, J.W., Faulkner, D.B., Ortendahl, D.A., and others: Color composites: display of two independent parameters in a single functional image. In Emission computed tomography, current trends, 13th Annual Symposium on the Sharing of Computer Programs and Technology in Nuclear Medicine, New York, 1983, Society of Nuclear Medicine, pp. 275-287.

O'Doherty, M.J., and others: Parathyroid imaging with technetium-99m-sestambi: preoperative localization and tissue uptake studies, J. Nucl. Med. 33:313-318, 1992.

Okerlund, M.D., Sheldon, K., Corpuz, S., and others: A new method with high sensitivity and specificity for localization of abnormal parathyroid glands, Ann. Surg. 200:381-388, 1984.

Palmer, J.A., and Sutton, F.R.: Importance of the fifth parathyroid gland in the surgical treatment of hyperparathyroidism, Can. J. Surg. 21:350-351, 1978.

Percival, R.C., Balke, G.M., Urwin, G.H., and others: Assessment of thallium-pertechnetate subtraction scintigraphy in hyperparathyroidism, Br. J. Radiol. 58:131-135, 1985.

Potchen, E.J., and Sodee, D.B.: Selective isotopic labeling of the human parathyroid: a preliminary report, J. Clin. Endocrin. 24:1125-1128, 1964.

Price, D.C.: Parathyroid imaging: effectiveness of different methodologies. In Gooding, C.A., editor: Diagnostic radiology 1990, University of California, San Francisco, 1990, Radiology Research and Education Foundation, pp. 489-502.

Russell, C.F., Grant, C.S., and van Heerden, J.A.: Hyperfunctioning supernumerary parathyroid glands: an occasional cause of hyperparathyroidism, Mayo Clin. Proc. 57:121-125, 1982.

Sandler, M.P., Patton, J.A., and Partain, C.L.: Thyroid and parathyroid imaging, Norwalk, 1986, Appleton-Century-Crofts, p. 379.

Sandler, M.P., Patton, J.A., Gross, M.D., and others: Endocrine imaging, Norwalk, 1992, Appleton & Lange, p. 461.

Satava, R.M., Bearhs, O.H., and Scholz, D.A.: Success rate of cervical exploration for hyperparathyroidism, Arch. Surg. 110:625-627, 1975.

Sisson, J.C., and Beierwaltes, W.H.: Radiocyanocobolamine ($Co^{57}B_{12}$) concentration in parathyroid glands, J. Nucl. Med. 3:160-166, 1962.

Skibber, J.M., Reynolds, J.C., Spiegel, A.M., and others: Computerized technetium/thallium scans and parathyroid reoperation, Surgery 98: 1077-1082, 1985.

Strauss, H.W., Harrison, K., and Pitt, B.: Thallium-201 non-invasive determination of the regional distribution of cardiac output, J. Nucl. Med. 18:1167-1170, 1977.

Taillefer, R., and others: Detection and localization of parathyroid adenomas in patients with hyperparathroidism using a single radionuclide imaging procedure with technetium-99m-sestamibi (double-phase study), J. Nucl. Med. 33:1801-1807, 1992.

Wang, C.A.: The anatomic basis of parathyroid surgery, Ann. Surg. 183:271-275, 1976.

Wang, C.A., Mahaffy, J.E., Axelrod, L., and Perlman, J.A.: Hyperfunctioning supernumerary parathyroid glands, Surg. Gynecol. Obstet. 148:711-714, 1979.

Wheeler, M.H., Harrison, B.S., French, A.P., and others: Preliminary results of thallium-201 and technetium-99m subtraction of parathyroid glands, Surgery 96:1978-1081, 1984.

Winzelberg, G.G., Hydovitz, J.D., O'Hara, K.R., and others: Parathyroid adenomas evaluated by T1-201/Tc-99m pertechnetate subtraction scintigraphy and high-resolution ultrasonography, Radiology 155:231-235, 1985.

Young, A.E., Gaunt, J.I., Croft, D.N., and others: Localization of parathyroid adenomas by thallium-201 and technetium-99m subtraction scanning, Br. Med. J. 286:1384-1385, 1983.

Zwas, S.T., Czerniak, A., Boruchowsky, S., and others: Preoperative parathyroid localization by superimposed iodine-131 toluidine blue and technetium-99m pertechnetate imaging, J. Nucl. Med. 28:298-307, 1987.

Chapter 26

ADRENAL GLAND

H. L. MALINOFF
MILTON D. GROSS
BRAHM SHAPIRO

■ ANATOMY (Fig. 26-1)

The adrenal (suprarenal) glands are paired structures that sit atop the kidneys. Normally, each gland weighs about 5 grams; in conditions of adrenocorticotrophic hormone (ACTH) excess they may enlarge to 4 times this weight. The outer portion, or adrenal cortex, accounts for 80% of the gland's weight in the adult. The adrenal glands have their own fascial support, so they do not descend with the kidneys when these are displaced. The right adrenal gland occupies a slightly higher and more lateral position than does the left (Fig. 26-1).

The adrenals have a rich vascular supply. Arterial blood reaches the adrenals from the aorta directly, as well as from renal, phrenic, and lumbar arteries. Venous drainage usually occurs via a single cortical vein into the inferior vena cava on the right, and the renal vein on the left (Fig. 26-1). The adult adrenal gland consists of two major divisions, the cortex and the medulla. The adrenal cortex is further divided into three functional, histologic segments. The cortex is derived from mesodermal tissue, while the medulla develops from neuroectoderm. In the fifth to sixth week of gestation the cortical portion of each adrenal begins as a proliferation of cells of the peritoneal epithelium near the cranial end of the mesonephros. These cells then penetrate the retroperitoneal mesenchyme to become the primitive cortex. By 8 weeks of gestation, the primitive cortex has become wrapped in a layer of cells that later forms the permanent cortex, which is located near the poles of the primitive kidneys. At birth, the primitive or fetal cortex constitutes the bulk of the adrenal. This primitive cortex then undergoes involution as the permanent cortex proliferates and differentiates. Full development of the permanent cortex into the three adult zones is not complete until the third year after birth. The adrenal medulla is derived from ectodermal cells of the neural crest. In addition to forming sympathetic neurons of the autonomic nervous system, some of these cells become endocrine, or chromaffin, cells—designated thus because they stain brown with chromic acid. During the seventh week of gestation, masses of migrating chromaffin cells come in contact with the developing adrenal cortex. The primitive medulla elements migrate through the cortex and ultimately occupy a central position within the adrenal gland (Fig. 26-2).

Pathologic conditions of both the adrenal cortex and the medulla often raise the question of the presence of accessory adrenal tissues. Although true accessory adrenal glands (cortex and medulla) are rare, many sites in the abdomen and pelvis may harbor ectopic adrenal cortical tissues. Accessory, separate cortical or medulla tissues may occur in the spleen, retroperitoneum along the aorta, or in the pelvis. Extra-adrenal chromaffin cells may also be found in aorto-sympathetic, intravagal, branchiomeric or visceral autonomic ganglia (Table 26-1).

■ PHYSIOLOGY

The adrenal gland is a two-part structure consisting of the outer cortex and the inner medulla; each is composed from functionally distinct embryonic tissues. The adrenal cortex consists of mesenchymal cells arranged in three concentric zones: an outer zona glomerulosa, a middle zona fasciculata, and an inner zona reticularis (Fig. 26-3). These three zones, respectively, are the sites of production of three

We wish to thank Phoenix Memorial Laboratories for the use of their radiochemistry facilities, as well as Ms. Leann C. Beird for her expert secretarial assistance.
This work was supported in part by NIAMDD 5P60 AM-20575, NIAMDD R01 AM 214767, NCI T32 CA 09015 HIW 3 M01 RR-0042 SICLR NIH R01-CA-43300-01; The Veterans Administration Research Service; and the Nuclear Medicine Research Fund, Division of Nuclear Medicine at the University of Michigan Medical Center.

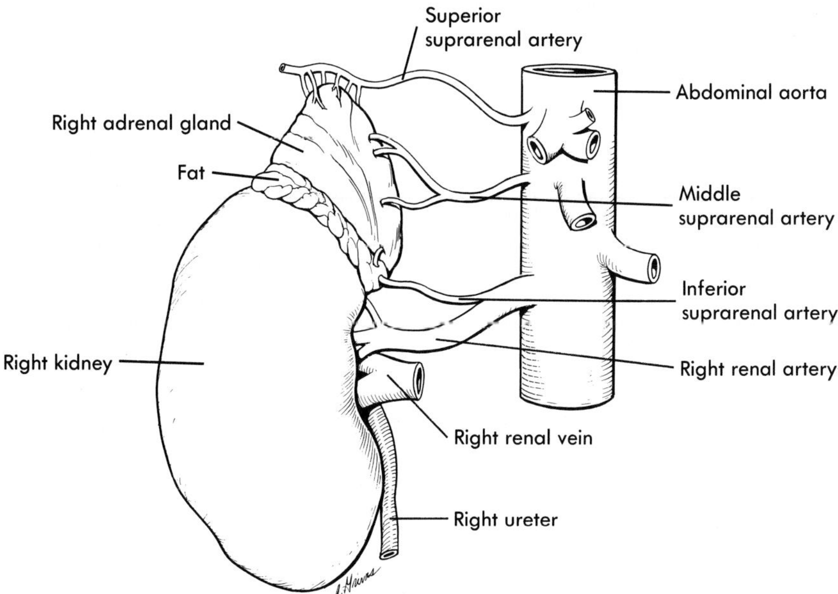

Fig. 26-1. Adrenal gland anatomy. (From Seeley, and others: Anatomy & physiology, ed. 2, St. Louis, 1991, Mosby–Year Book.)

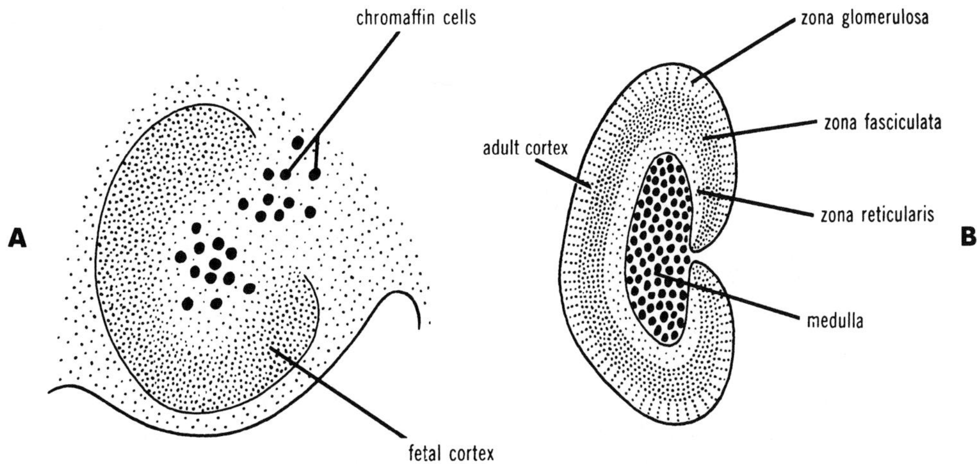

Fig. 26-2. Primitive adrenal cortex. **A,** Invasion by migrating cells from neural crest to form the primitive adrenal medulla. **B,** Anatomic relationship between adrenal cortex and medulla at birth. (From Langman, J.: Medical embryology, Baltimore, 1969, Williams & Wilkins.)

Table 26-1. Potential sites of ectopic adrenal tissues

Composite (cortex + medulla)	Cortex only	Nonadrenal medulla (Chromaffin-tissues)
Coeliac ganglion	Spleen	*(a)* **Branchiomeric**
Renal cortex	Retroperitoneum	jugular ganglion
	Pelvis	auricular br. X nerve
	Spermatic cord	tympanic
	Ovary	tympanic br. IX nerve
	Broad ligament	intercarotid
		subclavian
		laryngeal
		coronary
		aorticopulmonary
		(b) **Intravagal**
		perineurium X nerve
		(c) **Aorticosympathetic**
		(d) **Visceral-autonomic**
		pericardium
		cardiac atria
		intraatrial septum
		hepatic hilum
		bladder wall
		mesenteric vessels
		duodenum

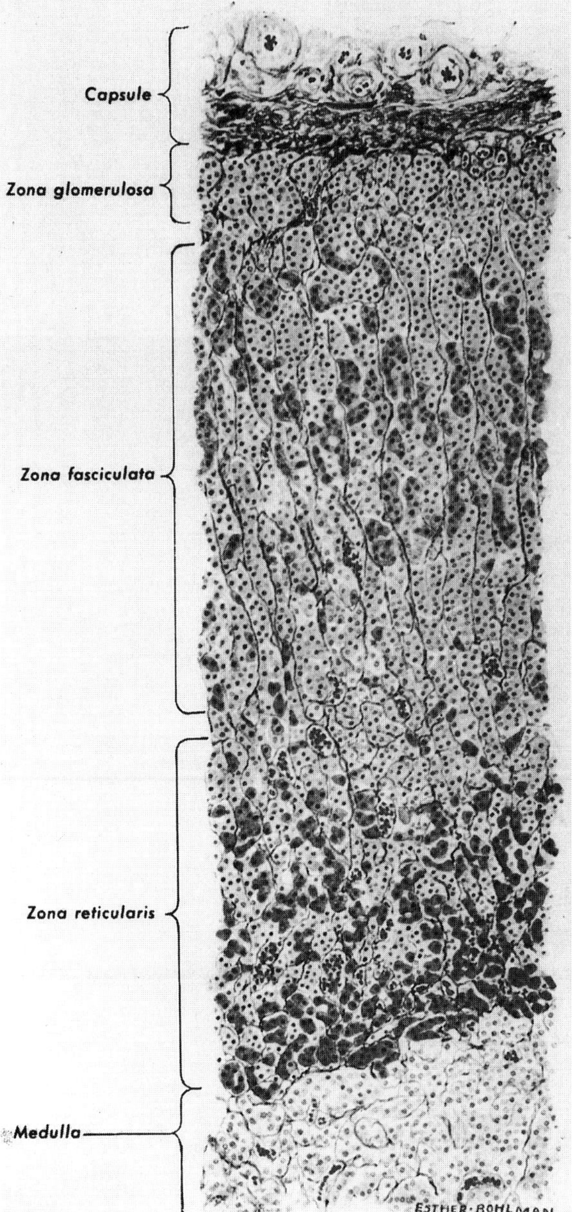

Fig. 26-3. Histology of the adrenal gland. (From Nelson, D.H.: The adrenal gland. In Williams textbook of endocrinology, Philadelphia, 1976, W.B. Saunders Co.)

major types of steroid hormones—mineralocorticoids, glucocorticoids, and androgens. The cells in the zona glomerulosa produce the mineralocorticoids aldosterone and (to a lesser degree) deoxycorticosterone. Aldosterone, the major mineralocorticoid in humans, is secreted in response to a complex interplay of signals between the adrenal, kidney, and lung (Fig. 26-4). Specialized cells in the renal glomerulus, the juxtaglomerular cells (JGA), produce renin, an enzyme. JGA cells are in contact with a special portion of the afferent glomerular arteriole (macula densa), which acts as a monitor of renal perfusion and glomerular filtration. Decrements in these parameters result in a rise in renin secretion by the JGA. Angiotensin I is formed from angiotensinogen substrate by the action of the enzyme renin. Angiotensin I is in turn converted to the octapeptide angiotensin II in the lung by converting enzyme (ACE). Angiotensin, in addition to being a potent vasoconstrictor, interacts directly with specific receptors on cells of the zona glomerulosa to stimulate the secretion of aldosterone. Aldosterone then acts on the tubular epithelium of the distal nephron and promotes the exchange of Na^+ for K^+ and H^+. Aldosterone secretion is further affected by hyperkalemia, drug therapy (e.g., β-adrenergic blockade), and changes in posture. These effects are mediated via the renin-angiotensin system and are important in identifying and evaluating zona glomerulosa function. In addition, pituitary ACTH plays a role in aldosterone secretion.

Cortisol and the adrenal androgens are synthesized and secreted by the inner zones of the adrenal cortex. Cortisol, the major glucocorticoid hormone, is secreted by cells in the zona fasciculata and has multiple effects on intermediary metabolism. Adrenal androgens, responsible for secondary sex characteristics, are produced in the zona reticularis. The only known control mechanism for cortisol and androgen secretion is by means of ACTH. This hormone is produced by enzymatic cleavage of the larger promelanocortin (POMC), in the anterior pituitary in response to hypothalamic-corticotrophic–releasing factor (CRF). ACTH not only stimulates the secretion of cortisol and androgens from the adrenals, it is an important mediator of steroid biosynthesis and adrenal cortical growth.

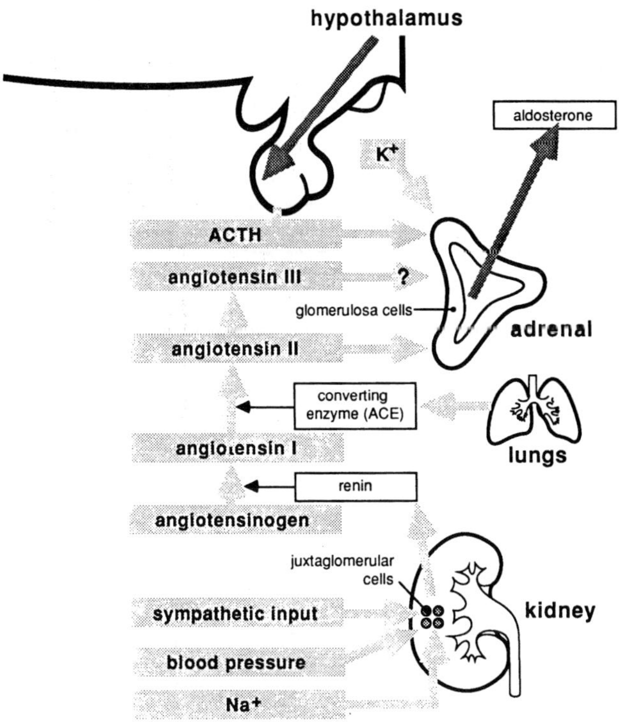

Fig. 26-4. Renin-angiotensin-aldosterone axis. (From Besser, B.M., and Cudworth, A.G.: Clinical endocrinology, Philadelphia, 1987, J.B. Lippincott Co.)

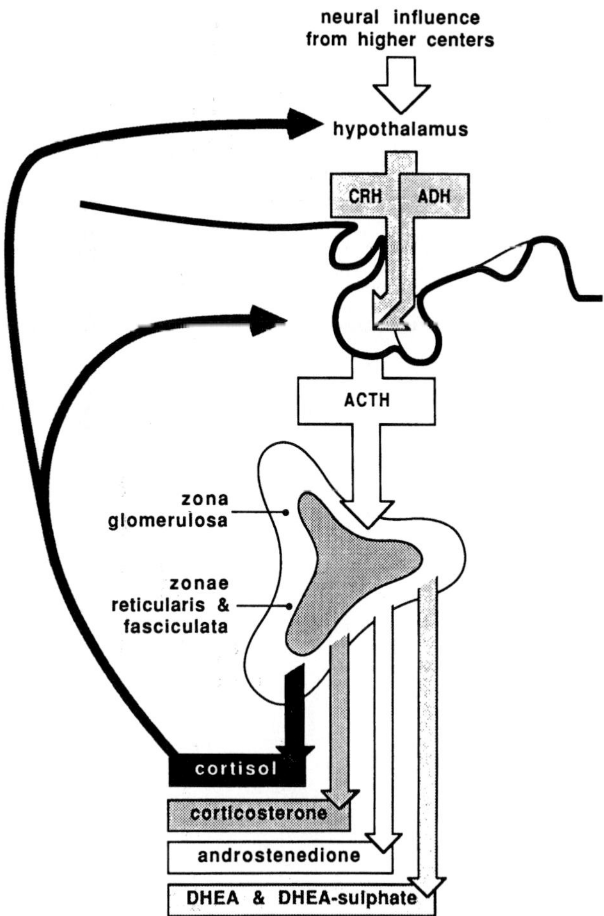

Fig. 26-5. Neuroendocrine control of cortisol secretion from adrenal cortex (hypothalamic-pituitary-adrenal axis). (From Besser, B.M., and Cudworth, A.G.: Clinical endocrinology, Philadelphia, 1987, J.B. Lippincott Co.)

ACTH acts as part of a negative feedback loop that links the hypothalamus, pituitary, and adrenal glands (Fig. 26-5). Biochemical and scintigraphic evaluation of zona fasciculata and reticularis function rely on the relationship between ACTH and plasma cortisol levels.

All adrenocortical hormones are derived from cholesterol, which is transported to the adrenal cortex via a receptor mediated pathway for low-density lipoproteins (although intracellular biosynthesis of cholesterol from acetate also occurs). The overall scheme of steroid biosynthesis is shown in Fig. 26-6. Although the synthesis of aldosterone, cortisol, and the androgens initially follow common paths, specificity is achieved by the differential distribution of receptors for ACTH and angiotensin, and by the sequestration of specific enzymes. Thus glomerulosa cells lack the 17α-hydroxylase enzyme and cannot synthesize cortisol or androgens. Conversely, reticularis and fasiculata cells lack 18-hydroxylase, and cannot synthesize aldosterone.

The principal catecholamine hormone secreted by the adrenal medulla is epinephrine, which is synthesized from tyrosine (Fig. 26-7). Other catecholamine-secreting tissues in the body (e.g., sympathetic ganglia) lack the enzyme necessary for the conversion of norepinephrine (NE—a neurotransmitter) to epinephrine (E—a hormone) by the specific enzyme phenyl ethanolamine-N-methyl transferase. This enzyme requires as a cofactor a high ambient concentration of cortisol, which is present in the adrenal medulla. The central nervous system controls E secretion by way of the splanchnic nerves and the neurotransmitter acetylcholine. Stimulation of the adrenal medulla may occur in response to hypoglycemia, hypovolemia, hypotension, hypoxia, hypercapnea, acidosis, pain, anxiety, and hemorrhage. Various drugs (Table 26-2) may suppress adrenal medulla secretion of E by reducing splanchnic nerve tone.

■ PATHOPHYSIOLOGY

The adrenocortical hormones produce distinct patterns of signs and symptoms when secreted in excess, as does hypercatecholaminemia from adrenal medulla or other catecholamine (E and NE)-secreting tissues. These patterns will be considered separately.

■ Primary aldosteronism

Hypertension, hypokalemia, hypernatremia and metabolic alkalosis may result from excessive secretion of the

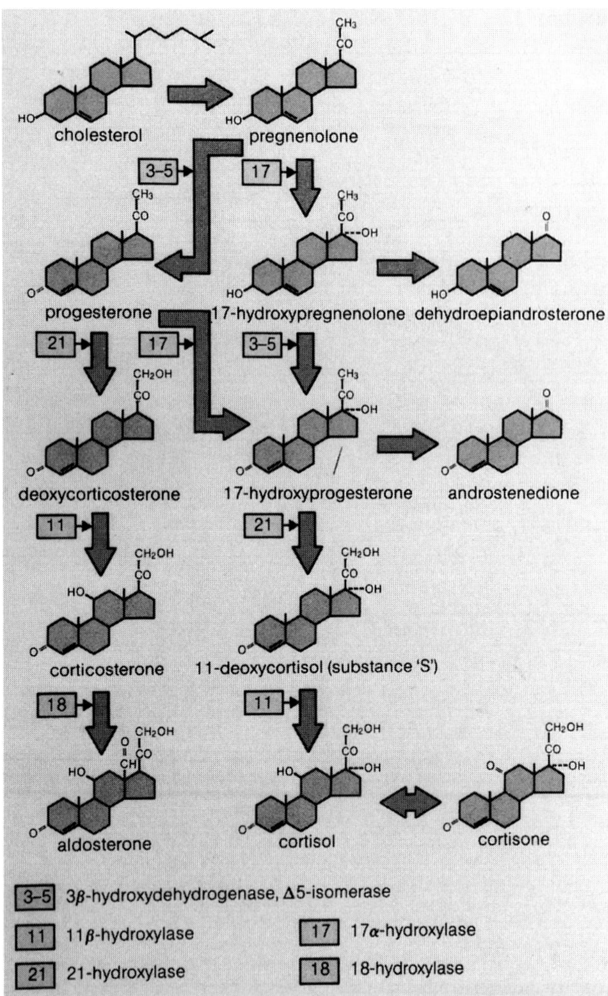

Fig. 26-6. Steroid biosynthesis in adrenal cortex from precursor cholesterol. (From Besser, B.M., and Cudworth, A.G.: Clinical endocrinology, Philadelphia, 1987, J.B. Lippincott Co.)

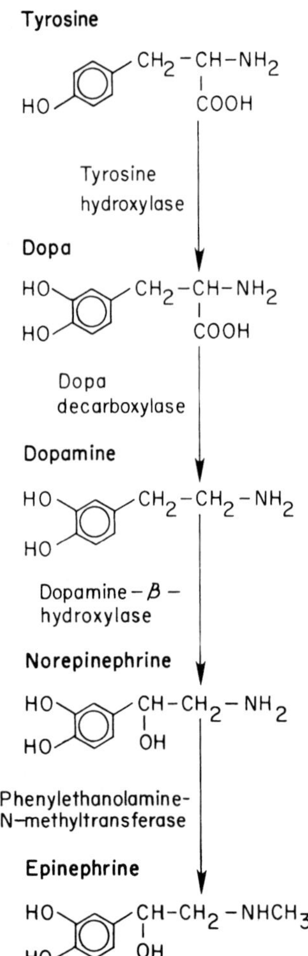

Fig. 26-7. Biosynthesis of the catecholamine epinephrine from tyrosine within the adrenal medulla.

mineralocorticoid hormone aldosterone. Serum and urinary aldosterone levels are elevated, and plasma renin activity is suppressed. This disorder results from an autonomous (and virtually always benign) tumor of zona glomerulosa cells in two thirds of cases, and from bilateral zona glomerulosa hyperplasia in the remaining one third. The successful treatment of primary aldosteronism depends on distinguishing between adenoma and hyperplasia because surgery is required for the former and contraindicated for the latter.

■ Cushing's syndrome

Cushing's syndrome (CS) is a symptom complex, the manifestations of which result from excessive and inappropriate exposure to glucocorticoids. The major clinical features of CS include central obesity, muscle wasting, hyperglycemia, vascular fragility, hirsutism, hypertension, emotional lability and osteoporosis. Apart from the iatrogenic administration of either corticosteroids or ACTH, the main causes of CS are listed in Table 26-3. Most commonly CS results from a pituitary ACTH-secreting tumor (Cushing's disease). Excessive levels of ACTH may also be caused by tumors of endocrine and nonendocrine origin (ectopic ACTH syndrome); the result is frank and often severe CS. Intrinsic adrenal cortical disease—either adenoma, bilateral nodular hyperplasia, or carcinoma—may result in CS. The most severe clinical manifestations of CS are seen in these cases. The intrinsic adrenal causes of CS are usually treated by adrenal resection and thus must be distinguished from bilateral hyperplasia due to ACTH excess.

■ Adrenal hyperandrogenism

The zona reticularis of the adrenal cortex secretes the weak androgens dihydroepiandrosterone and androstenedione as their principal hormones. If secreted in excess in women, these may lead to oligomenorrhea or amenorrhea, temporal balding, clitoromegaly, and other features of virilization. This may be a result of autonomous tumors (ad-

Table 26-2. Drugs that alter function and adrenal scintigraphic imaging[1]

	Effect	Mechanism	Scan appearance
Adrenal cortex			
Zona fasiculata-reticularis			
Adrenocorticoids:	Cortisol	CRF	↓ Uptake
Dexamethasone	Androgens	ACTH	
Metabolic inhibitors:			
Aminoglutethimide	Cortisol synthesis		
Metyrapone	Adrenal cholesterol uptake	ACTH	↓ Uptake
Op DDD	Cortisol-ACTH	Adrenal pituitary suppression	↓ Uptake
Exogenous ACTH	Direct adrenal stimulation		↓ Uptake
Zona glomerulosa			
Antihypertensives:			
Propanolol	Plasma renin activity	β-receptor blockade	↓ Uptake
Antagonists:			
Spironolactone	Aldosterone	Adrenal suppression	↓ Uptake(?)
Diuretics: all	Serum sodium	Plasma renin activity	↓ Uptake
	Plasma volume		↓ Uptake
Oral contraceptives: all	Plasma renin activity	Cortisol secretion rate	↑ Uptake
Excessive salt intake	Aldosterone	Plasma renin activity	↓ Uptake
General			
Cholesterol-lowering agents	Serum cholesterol	(?) Cholesterol pool effect	↓ Uptake
4-Aminopyrazolopyrimidine	Serum cholesterol	LDL-receptor activity	↓ Uptake
Hypercholesterolemia	Serum cholesterol	(?) Cholesterol pool effect	↓ Uptake
Adrenal medulla			
Tricyclic antidepressants:	Catecholamines	Adrenal catecholamine reuptake	↑ Uptake
Reserpine	Catecholamines	Block catecholamine release/reuptake	↓ Uptake
Clonidine	Catecholamines	Central sympathetic suppression of catecholamines	↓ Uptake (?)
Alphamethylparatyrosine	Catecholamines	Suppress catecholamine biosynthesis	No change in uptake
Radiation therapy	Catecholamines	Suppress catecholamine biosynthesis	↓ Uptake (?)
Cocaine	Discharges catecholamines	Suppress catecholamine biosynthesis	↑ Uptake
Phenylpropranolamine	Discharges catecholamines	Suppress catecholamine biosynthesis	↓ Uptake

[1]Modified from Gross, M.D., and Shapiro, B.: Scintigraphic studies in adrenal hypertension, Semin. Nucl. Med. 11(2):146, 1981.

enomas or carcinoma) or hyperplasia due to inborn or acquired errors of adrenocortical hormone biosynthesis. The polycystic ovary syndrome (PCO) is also associated with ovarian and adrenal hypersecretion of androgens, varying degrees of virilization (usually hirsutism), and menstrual abnormalities. Rational therapy thus requires the identification of the site(s) of androgen hypersecretion.

■ Pheochromocytoma

Hypertension is the most common clinical feature associated with pheochromocytoma. The hypertension is most often labile and associated with episodes of symptoms such as palpitation, headache, flushing or pallor, anxiety, and diaphoresis. About two thirds of patients will have some degree of concomitant orthostatic hypotension. In 10% of cases these tumors may be associated with neurofibromatosis, von Hipple Landau disease, and familial endocrine neoplasia syndromes (MEN). Most pheochromocytomas are unilateral, but about 10% will be multiple, extra-adrenal, metastatic, or familial. Tumors secreting catecholamines may arise throughout the sympathetic nervous system from the glomus jugulare at the base of the skull to the adrenergic plexus of the urinary bladder; these are variously termed *functional paragangliomas* or *extra-adrenal pheochromocytomas* (Fig. 26-8).

Table 26-3. Etiologies of Cushing's syndrome

ACTH-dependent	ACTH-independent
Pituitary ACTH	Adrenal
Adenoma	Adenoma
Nontumoral (hypothalamic)	Carcinoma
	Bilateral nodular hyperplasia
Ectopic ACTH syndrome	
Iatrogenic	Iatrogenic

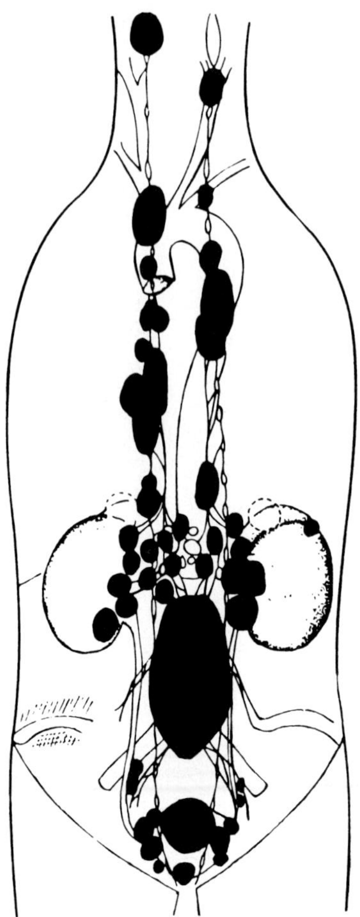

Fig. 26-8. Multiple sites of catecholamine-secreting tissue. (From Manger, W., and Gifford, R.W., Jr.: Pheochromocytoma, New York, 1977, Springer-Verlag.)

■ ADRENAL IMAGING

LABORATORY APPLICATION

78

ADRENOCORTICAL IMAGING USING NP-59

Purpose

Adrenal scintigraphy provides an effective, noninvasive, functional method for identifying and localizing both adrenocortical and sympathomedulla disease. Considerable information not available by other anatomic imaging techniques (i.e., CT, MRI, angiography, or US) may be obtained. Adrenal scintigraphic images provide both functional and anatomic assessment of the adrenal glands; this method is complementary to CT, MRI, and other anatomic imaging techniques.

Radiopharmaceutical preparation

The imaging agent of choice for adrenal cortical scintigraphy is ^{131}I-6β iodomethylnorcholesterol (NP-59) (Fig. 26-9). This compound demonstrates a high affinity for the adrenal cortex and has replaced other iodinated cholesterol analogs (e.g., 19-iodocholesterol). The introduction of ^{131}I-, and more recently ^{123}I-metaiodobenzylguanidine (mIBG) (Fig. 26-10), and the demonstration of its affinity for catecholamine-secreting tissues, provides a new and effective approach to the detection of pheochromocytoma, neuroblastoma, and other related neoplasms.

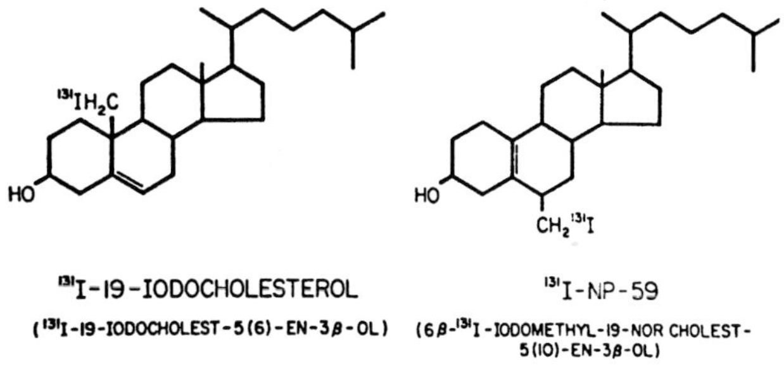

Fig. 26-9. Structures of ^{131}I-19-iodocholesterol and NP-59.

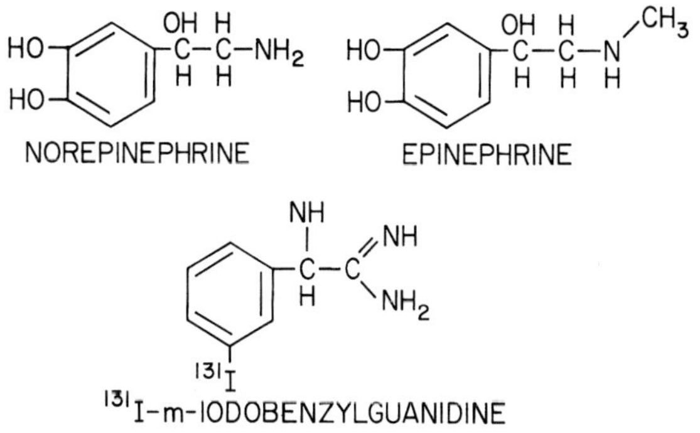

Fig. 26-10. Structure of ^{131}I-mIBG compared with that of the neurotransmitters norepinephrine and epinephrine.

Table 26-4. Dosimetry of the radiocholesterols*

	^{131}I-19-iodocholesterol (NM-145)	^{131}I-6β-iodomethyl-norcholesterol (NP-59)	^{75}Se-selenomethyl-norcholesterol (Scintadren)
Total body	1.8	1.2	1.4
Adrenals	60	26	6.1
Ovaries	6	8.0	1.9
Testes	7	2.3	
Liver	2.3	2.4	3.5

*Rads/mCi

(From Gross, M.D., and others: The scintigraphic imaging of endocrine organs, Endocrinol. Rev. 5:249, 1984.)

A critical factor that should precede any adrenal scintigraphic procedure is the precise biochemical identification of adrenocortical or sympathomedulla dysfunction. This is necessary if successful identification, localization, and treatment of these disorders is to occur. Also, numerous drugs have profound effects on adrenocortical and adrenomedullary hormone secretion and NP-59/mIBG accumulation, respectively. Successful adrenal scintigraphy depends on a complete knowledge of medications taken by patients before and during the imaging procedures. Table 26-2 lists medications known to affect either adrenocortical NP-59 or sympathomedulla ^{131}I-mIBG uptake.

Adrenal gland exposure during NP-59 scintigraphy ranges from 12 to 39 rads/mCi with an average dose of about 25 rad/mCi (Table 26-4), while studies performed with dexamethasone suppression (in patients with primary aldosteronism and adrenal hyperandrogenism) result in adrenal exposure that is about half this dose. ^{131}I-mIBG scintigraphy results in adrenal exposures of 4 to 8 rads/mCi and total body exposures of 0.2 rads/mCi (Table 26-5). More recently, ^{123}I-mIBG has demonstrated more favorable dosimetry, reflecting the shorter half-life of ^{123}I (Table 26-5). In any case, the radiation dose received is in the range of a comprehensive CT examination or from other more invasive roentgenographic procedures such as adrenal arteriography or venography.

Indications

1. In cases of documented primary hyperaldosteronism.
2. For identifying and localizing abnormal adrenal function in ACTH-independent Cushing's syndrome.
3. In cases of virilization/amenorrhea secondary to suspected adrenal hyperandrogenism.
4. To evaluate the nature of incidentally discovered adrenal lesions seen on other imaging techniques (CT, MRI, US).

Continued.

Table 26-5. Dosimetry of ^{131}I- and ^{123}I-metaiodobenzylguanidine (mIBG)

Organ	0.5 mCl ^{131}I-mIBG* (in rads)	10 mCi ^{123}I mIBG† (in rads)
Thyroid (blocked)	0.66	<0.33
Adrenal medulla	50†	8-28
Myocardium	0.35	0.4
Liver	0.2	0.5
Spleen	0.8	1.5
Ovary	0.5	0.7
Total body	0.1	0.2

*From human data
†From canine data
(From Swanson, D.P., and others: Proceedings of the Third International Radiopharmaceutical Dosimetry Symposium, Oak Ridge, Tenn., HHS Publication FDA 81-8166, Bethesda, Md., 1981, pp. 213-224.)

Procedure

Materials

1. Scintillation camera equipped with a high-energy, parallel-hole collimator interfaced to a minicomputer
2. 1 mCi NP-59 per 1.75 m^2 body surface area for IV administration*

Patient preparation

1. Select patient(s) for reasonable probability of the presence of a defined adrenocortical disorder on the basis of history, physical examination, and biochemistry.
2. Obtain a careful medication history to identify interfering medications (see Table 26-2).
3. Lugol's solution or SSKI, started 24 to 48 hours before NP-59 administration to prevent thyroid uptake of free ^{131}I.
4. Studies requiring suppression of adrenal cortex-dexamethasone (4 mg daily in divided doses) is started 7 days before and continued throughout a 5-day postinjection-imaging interval NP-59 injection.
5. ACTH augmentation: 50 IU IV given daily 2 days before NP-59 administration.
6. Dulcolax® (bisacodyl) 10 mg PO BID × 3 days before imaging to diminish colonic activity (occasionally enemas may be required).
7. Explain the entire procedure to the patient and obtain signed informed consent.

Technique

1. Inject NP-59 slowly over a period of 2 to 3 minutes (more rapid injection may lead to local skin reaction secondary to the presence of Tween 80 in the preparation).
2. To image, use a wide–field-of-view camera with a high-energy, parallel-hole collimator.
3. For nondexamethasone-suppressed imaging, begin on Day 5 following NP-59 injection with repeat imaging on Days 6 and 7, if required.
4. For dexamethasone-suppression studies, image on Day 3 or 4 (preferably the latter), with re-imaging on Days 5 and 6.
5. Position the patient for a posterior projection with the collimator centered over the 12th rib.
6. Collect at least 100K image with minicomputer interface.
7. When quantitative adrenal uptake is required, collect a lateral image of the area for depth definition (for estimation of NP-59 uptake using an appropriately validated adrenal uptake program).

*NP-59 is available from the Nuclear Pharmacy, Division of Nuclear Medicine, University of Michigan Medical Center (requires modified physician sponsored investigational New Drug Application approval from the FDA).

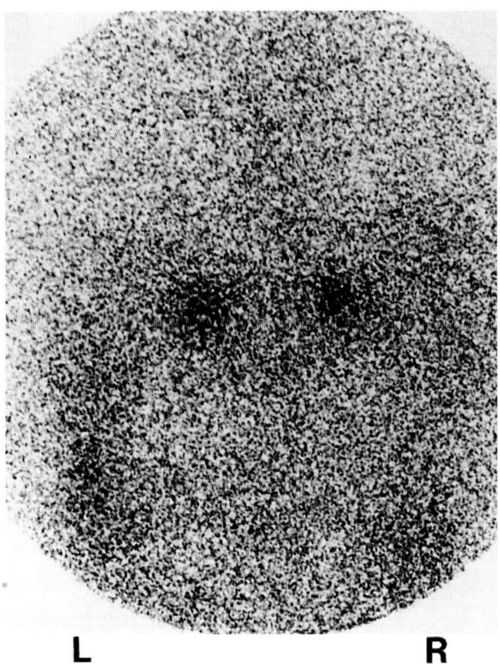

Fig. 26-11. Normal posterior NP-59 scintiscan. Note asymmetric shape of adrenal glands.

Diagnosis

Normal image pattern

Under normal conditions, image patterns correlate well with standard anatomic features on the posterior image. The right adrenal is slightly superior to the left (Fig. 26-11). The right gland is usually more circular, while the left tends to be vertically ovoid or oblong. On posterior imaging, the intensity of uptake in the right adrenal is greater than left in about two thirds of normal subjects. This is due to the depth-related asymmetry of adrenal gland anatomy: the left is partially shielded by the superior aspect of the left kidney. The right adrenal is slightly superior to (and not shielded by) the right kidney. The liver displays significant radioactivity; however, the right adrenal appears medial and can usually be clearly identified. In contrast, gallbladder activity may be problematic on posterior images. Gallbladder (an anterior abdominal structure) activity, because of the excretion of NP-59 and its metabolites in bile, may be distinguished from right adrenal (a posterior abdominal structure) by obtaining a lateral view or by obtaining single-photon emission tomography (SPECT). In this situation gallbladder activity, apparent in anterior views, gives way to the right adrenal gland on posterior images. An alternative approach is reimaging after administration of a fatty meal or cholecystokinin.

Normally, dexamethasone will suppress that fraction of adrenal uptake of NP-59 which is ACTH-dependent (about 50% of basal). Scintigraphic studies in normals will show only faint visualization by day 5 or bilateral nonvisualization. The adrenal glands may subsequently image 24 to 48 hours after dexamethasone is discontinued.

Adrenal cortical dysfunction

Cushing's syndrome—The hallmark of Cushing's syndrome (CS) is the excessive secretion of cortisol and excretion of glucocorticoid hormone metabolites. The clinical picture is well characterized and consists in most cases of obesity, hyperglycemia, vascular fragility, hypertension, amenorrhea, hirsutism, weight gain, and osteoporosis. The laboratory abnormalities accompanying CS are elevated serum cortisol, elevated urinary free cortisol, and the loss of normal diurnal variation in

Continued.

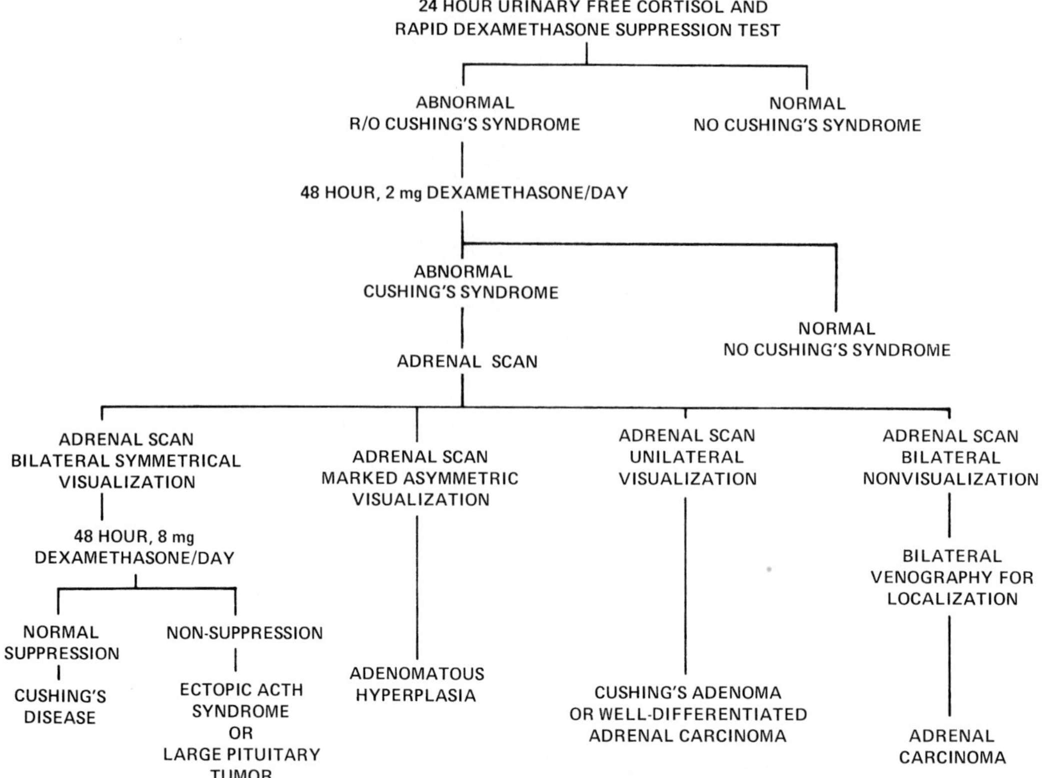

Fig. 26-12. An algorithm for the evaluation of Cushing's syndrome.

Table 26-6. Patterns of imaging in Cushing's syndrome

Scintigraphic pattern	Form of Cushing's syndrome
Bilateral symmetrical	ACTH-dependent hypothalamic pituitary ectopic ACTH syndrome
Bilateral asymmetric	ACTH-independent nodular hyperplasia
Unilateral	Adrenal adenoma Adrenal remnant (ectopic adrenocortical tissue)
Bilateral nonvisualization	Adrenal carcinoma (functioning tumor suppresses contralateral gland)

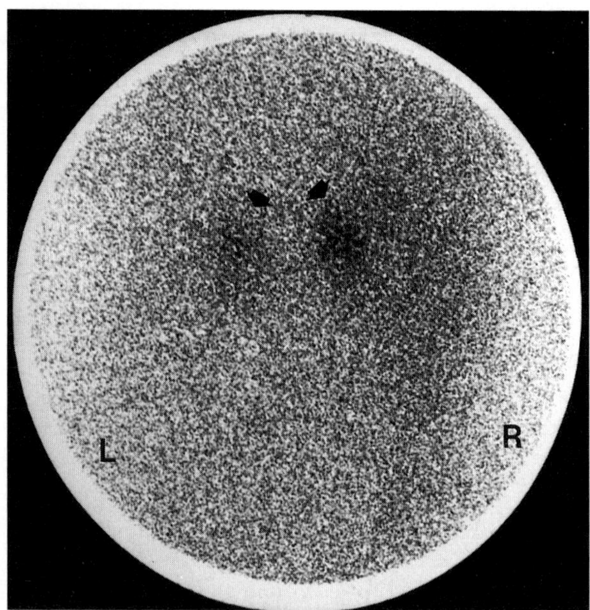

Fig. 26-13. Posterior NP-59 adrenal scintiscan in ACTH-dependent bilateral adrenal hyperplasia due to a pituitary adenoma. Uptake in adrenals is symmetric.

Fig. 26-14. Posterior NP-59 scintiscan in ACTH-independent bilateral nodular hyperplasia. **A,** Posterior view. Note intense asymmetric uptake. **B,** Lateral view with body surface marker *(arrows).*

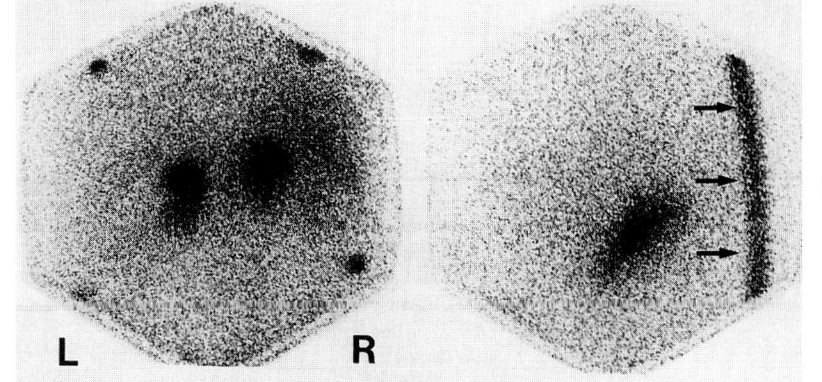

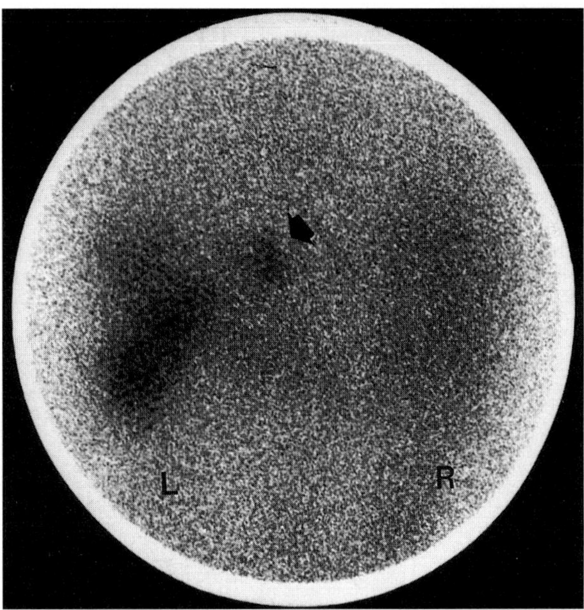

Fig. 26-15. Posterior NP-59 adrenal scintiscan of a left sided adrenal adenoma *(arrow).* The contralateral cortex does not image, because of suppression of pituitary ACTH.

both cortisol and ACTH levels, as well as a failure of cortisol levels to suppress in response to dexamethasone. The proper therapy of CS depends on the ability to accurately localize the site of disease. Identifying the biochemical abnormalities in CS may suggest the presence of either pituitary, adrenal, or ectopic etiologies. Fig. 26-12 shows a suggested algorithm for the clinical evaluation of suspected CS.

The scintigraphic patterns seen on NP-59 imaging in CS are a reflection of the underlying pathophysiologic process involved. Four distinct adrenal imaging patterns are possible: (1) symmetric bilateral increased adrenal uptake, (2) asymmetric bilateral increased uptake, (3) unilateral uptake, and (4) bilateral nonvisualization (Table 26-6).

The pattern of symmetric bilateral adrenal uptake results from the excessive ACTH secretion seen in pituitary CS (Cushing's disease) and extra-pituitary ACTH-secreting tumors (ectopic ACTH syndrome) (Fig. 26-13). The presence of asymmetric, bilateral, intense NP-59 uptake suggests autonomous, ACTH-independent cortical nodular hyperplasia (Fig. 26-14).

The presence of unilateral, intense NP-59 uptake in the biochemical setting of CS is highly suggestive of adrenal cortical adenoma (Fig. 26-15). Unusual cases of functioning (usually well differentiated) adrenal cortical carcinomas have also produced this scintigraphic pattern, but the unilateral

Continued.

Table 26-7. Localization of ACTH-independent Cushing's syndrome with computed tomography

Reference		Adenoma	Carcinoma	CNH
Sample	(1978)	3/3[a]	—	0/1
Reynes	(1979)	6/6	—	—
Korobkin	(1979)	2/2	1/1	—
Dunnick	(1979)	4/4	5/5	—
Eghbari	(1980)	5/5	3/3	—
Dunnick	(1982)	6/6	1/1	—
Baba	(1982)	5/5	—	3/4
Joffe	(1983)	—	—	1/3
Guerin	(1983)	4/4	1/1	0/1
Huebner	(1984)	14/14	4/4	?[b]
VanBurkhout	(1986)	—	—	0/2
Sarkar	(1987)	7/7	—	0/4
Wulffraat	(1988)	—	—	0/5
Fig	(1988)	14/14	4/4	1/4
Totals		**70/70**	**19/19**	**5/24**[c]

[a]Correctly localized/total studied

[b]Does not distinguish ACTH-dependent vs. ACTH-independent hyperplasia

[c]Five of 24 with CNH interpreted as unilateral adrenal mass; 15 of 24 considered normal

(Modified from Fig, L.M., and others: Adrenal localization in the adrenocorticotropic hormone-independent Cushing syndrome, Ann. Intern. Med. 109:547-553, 1988.)

Table 26-8. Scintigraphic localization in ACTH-independent Cushing's syndrome

Reference		Agent	Adenoma	Carcinoma*	CNH
Moses	(1974)	19-IC[b]	8/8[c]	2/2	—
Kehlet	(1976)	19-IC	5/5	1/1	—
Dige-Petersen	(1976)	19/IC	3/3	1/1	—
Ryo	(1976)	19-IC/NP-59	7/7	—	—
Sarkar	(1977)	NP-59	3/3	—	—
Wahner	(1977)	19-IC	3/3	4/4	—
Barliev	(1979)	19-IC	3/3	2/2	2/2
Dunnick	(1979)	NP-59	3/3	—	—
Miles	(1979)	NP-59	2/2	—	1/1
Ortega	(1980)	19-IC	5/5	—	—
Troncone	(1980)	19-IC	5/5	2/2	—
Leger	(1981)	75-Se	7/7	3/3	—
Shapiro	(1981)	19-IC	5/5	3/3	1/1
Skalkeas	(1982)	19-IC	2/2	1/1	1/1
Shapiro	(1982)	75-Se[d]	—	—	1/1
Baba	(1982)	19-IC/NP-59	5/5	—	4/4
Guerin	(1983)	19-IC/NP-59	6/6	5/5	—
Joffe	(1983)	75-Se	—	—	2/2
Watson	(1985)	75-Se	6/6	—	—
Lindberg	(1985)	19-IC	10/10	3/3	—
Sudell	(1985)	75-Se	—	3/3	2/2
VanBerkhout	(1986)	19-IC	—	—	2/2
Sarkar	(1987)	NP-59	7/7	—	4/4
Wulffraat	(1988)	NP-59	—	—	5/5
Fig	(1988)	NP-59	14/14	4/4	6/6
Reschini	(1991)	75-Se	11/12[e]	2/4[f]	3/3
Totals			**122/123**	**36/38**	**34/34**

[a]Characteristic pattern of bilateral nonvisualization in a patient with an adrenal mass

[b]19-IC = 19-iodocholesterol

[c]Correctly localized/total studied

[d]75-Se = 75-Se-selenomethylnorcholesterol

[e]One nonimaging "black adenoma"

*Two of four imaging adrenal carcinomas

(Modified from Fig, L.M., and others: Adrenal localization in ACTH-independent Cushing's syndrome, Ann. Intern. Med. 109:547, 1988.)

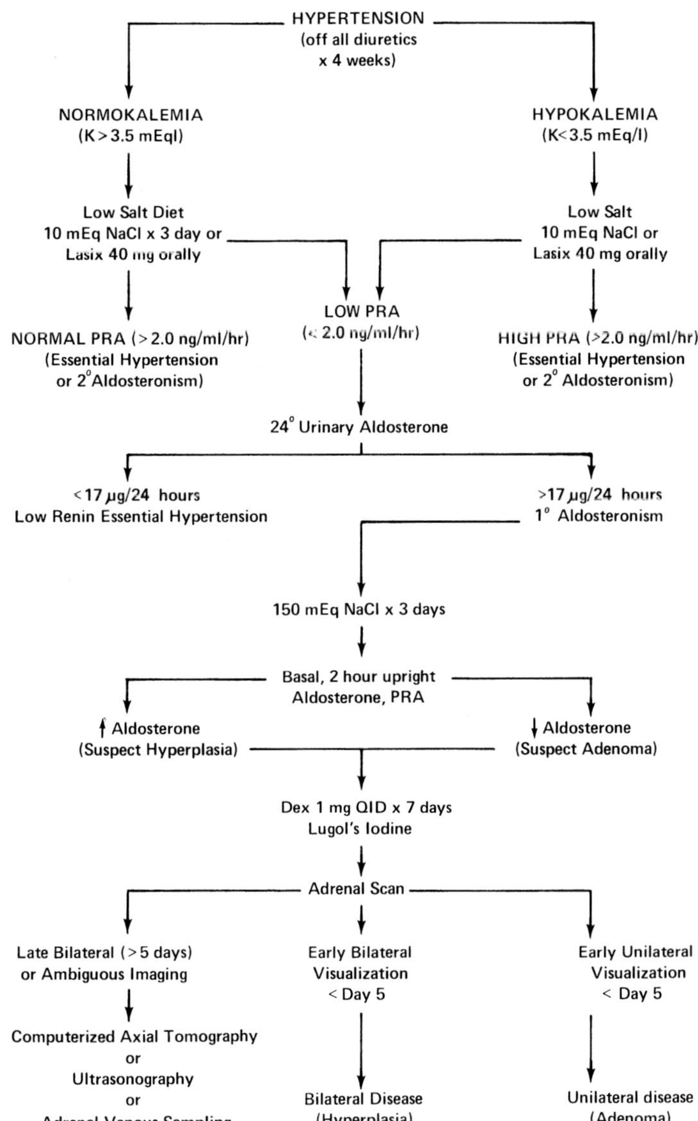

Fig. 26-16. An investigative algorithm for PA. (From H. Weissman and L. Freeman, editors: Nuclear medicine annual, New York, 1980, Raven Press.)

uptake is not as intense as in adenoma. Most commonly, an adrenal carcinoma will not image with NP-59 but will secrete sufficient cortisol to suppress the normal contralateral adrenal gland, causing only very faint visualization or (most frequently) bilateral nonvisualization. The diagnostic accuracy of scintigraphy and other anatomic imaging modalities in identifying the cause of ACTH-independent CS has been recently compared (Tables 26-7, 26-8).

Primary aldosteronism

Patients with primary hyperaldosteronism (PA) develop hypertension, hypokalemia, hypernatremia, and metabolic alkalosis. Serum and urinary aldosterone levels are elevated, and plasma renin activity is suppressed. PA results from an aldosterone-secreting adenoma in two thirds of cases, and bilateral adrenocortical hyperplasia in one third. The former is best treated surgically, while the latter may require medical management. Thus, the NP-59 scintiscan assumes pivotal importance in this differential diagnosis. Figure 26-16 lists a suggested algorithm for the biochemical and imaging approach to PA. Imaging techniques (CT, MRI) are often suboptimal in PA because adenomas are often small (5 to 10 mm), and bilateral hyperplasia may not distort adrenal gland contours sufficient to be recognized by high-resolution, multi-thin slice CT.

NP-59 imaging in PA is facilitated by the oral administration of dexamethasone before and during imaging. Dexamethasone will suppress pituitary ACTH secretion, thus accentuating NP-59 up-

Continued.

Table 26-9. Etiologies of primary aldosteronism

Scintigraphy pattern	Form of primary aldosteronism
Unilateral early (<5 days)	Adenoma Carcinoma
Bilateral early (<5 days)	Bilateral hyperplasia
Bilateral late (>5 days)	Dexamethasone suppressible hyperplasia

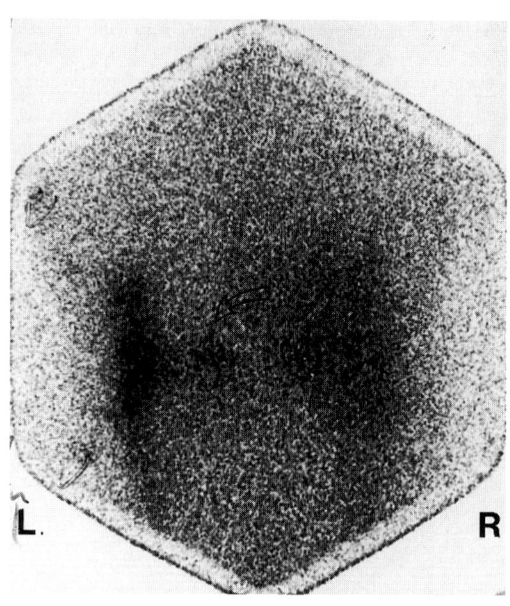

Fig. 26-18. Posterior NP-59 dexamethasone suppression scintiscan demonstrating an autonomously functioning L adrenal cortical adenoma resulting in PA.

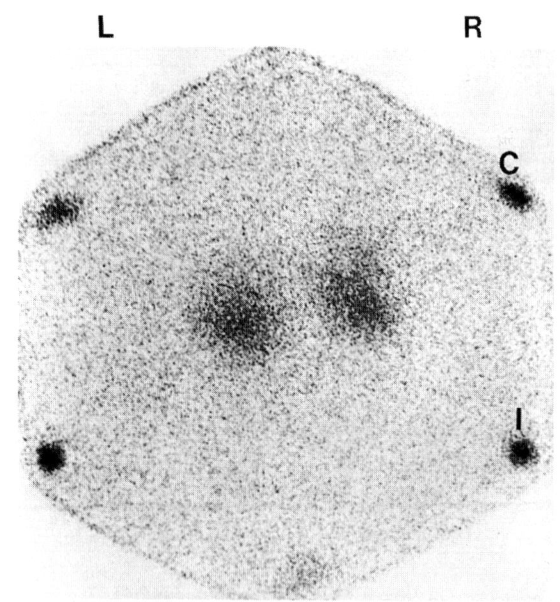

Fig. 26-17. Posterior NP-59 dexamethasone suppression scintiscan demonstrating early, intense, bilateral adrenal gland uptake of tracer in a patient with PA. Diagnosis is bilateral zona glomerulosa hyperplasia. Markers identify costal margin *(C)* and iliac crest *(I)*.

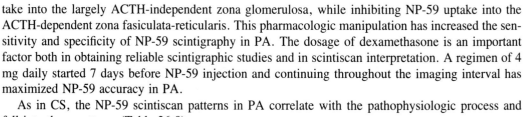

take into the largely ACTH-independent zona glomerulosa, while inhibiting NP-59 uptake into the ACTH-dependent zona fasiculata-reticularis. This pharmacologic manipulation has increased the sensitivity and specificity of NP-59 scintigraphy in PA. The dosage of dexamethasone is an important factor both in obtaining reliable scintigraphic studies and in scintiscan interpretation. A regimen of 4 mg daily started 7 days before NP-59 injection and continuing throughout the imaging interval has maximized NP-59 accuracy in PA.

As in CS, the NP-59 scintiscan patterns in PA correlate with the pathophysiologic process and fall into three patterns (Table 26-9):

- Bilateral early visualization. Both adrenal glands are visualized prior to 5 days after the time of NP-59 injection (Fig. 26-17). This scan pattern is compatible with bilateral adrenocortical hyperplasia.
- Unilateral visualization. A single adrenal gland is imaged within 5 days of injection of NP-59. After 5 days the contralateral gland becomes visible, but NP-59 uptake is much less intense. The scintigraphic image suggests an aldosterone-secreting adenoma (Conn's tumor) in the early visualized gland (Fig. 26-18).
- Bilateral late or nonvisualization. The failure to visualize either adrenal within 5 days of NP-59 imaging is generally considered "nondiagnostic." In some cases the adrenals may only be faintly imaged by day 7 or 10, while in others images may not be obtained until dexamethasone is discontinued. This pattern may suggest bilateral dexamethasone suppressible aldosteronism; it may also imply an incorrect prescan diagnosis (e.g., low renin hypertension). In these cases repeat biochemical tests of zona glomerulosa function on dexamethasone will make this dis-

Table 26-10. Computed tomography in primary aldosteronism

Authors		Total scans	Adenoma	Hyperplasia	Localization*	Specificity**
Linde	1979	9	4	—	4 (44%)	—
Korobkin	1979	22	12	10	9 (75%)	10/13 (76%)*
Reynes	1979	3	3	—	1 (33%)	—
White	1980	22	16	6	12 (75%)	6/7 (85%)
Goldman	1982	3	3	—	3 (100%)	—
Dunnick	1984	28	18	4	11 (61%)	4/11 (36%)†
Geisinger	1983	29	23	6	16 (70%)	3/8 (37%)§
Guerin	1983	32	14	18	12 (85%)	17/18 (94%)†
Total		**148**	**93**	**44**	**68%**	**66%**

*Total number of adrenal cortical adenomas localized/total number of adrenal cortical adenomas.
**Total number of bilateral adrenal hyperplasias localized/total number of bilateral adrenal hyperplasias plus total number of normal scanning results in patients with adrenal cortical adenoma.
†The absence of a unilateral enlarged adrenal and biochemical evidence of primary aldosteronism were considered consistent with a diagnosis of hyperplasia.
§Three of six patients with proven hyperplasia were found to have normal adrenal glands by computed tomography.
(From Gross, M.D., and others: Scintigraphic localization of adrenal lesions in primary aldosteronism, Am. J. Med. 77:839, 1984, by permission.)

Table 26-11. Scintigraphic localization in primary aldosteronism

Authors		Total scans	Adenoma	Hyperplasia	Localization*	Specificity**
Dige-Peterson	1975	4	3	1	3 (100%)	1/1 (100%)
Conn	1976	37	25	12	21 (84%)	11/12 (92%)
Trancone	1980	8	7	—	7 (87%)	—
Ryo	1978	7	5	2	5 (100%)	2/2 (100%)
Freitas	1979	20	10	10	9 (90%)	9/10 (90%)
Weinberger	1979	18	13	5	6 (47%)	2/7 (28%)
Miles	1979	17	9	8	9 (100%)	8/8 (100%)
Herf	1979	11	8	3	8 (100%)	3/3 (100%)
Leger	1981	42	22	20	17 (77%)	19/19 (100%)
Hoefnagels	1981	10	9	—	8 (89%)	—
Guerin	1983	44	18	26	15 (83%)	24/26 (92%)
Gross	1984	87	50	37	48 (96%)	35/37 (94%)
Reschini	1991	33	19	14	16 (84%)	14/17 (82%)
Total		**338**	**198**	**138**	**87%**	**89%**

*Total number of adrenal cortical adenomas localized/total number of adrenal cortical adenomas.
**Total number of bilateral adrenal hyperplasia patterns/total number of bilateral adrenal hyperplasia plus false positive results.
(From Gross, M.D., and others: Scintigraphic localization of adrenal lesions in primary aldosteronism, Am. J. Med. 77:839, 1984, by permission).

tinction. The accuracy of scintigraphic localization of AP compares favorably with other imaging techniques (Tables 26-9, 26-10, 26-11).

Adrenal hyperandrogenism

Patients with clinical evidence of adrenal hirsutism or virilization should have biochemical confirmation before NP-59 scintigraphy. A suggested algorithm for the clinical detection of adrenal hyperandrogenism is shown in Fig. 26-19. As in PA, patients with suspected adrenal hyperandrogenism are optimally studied using dexamethasone suppression NP-59 scintigraphy. Androgen secretion is a partially ACTH-independent process, and as such, hyperfunction of the zona reticularis has little effect on the hypothalamic, pituitary adrenal axis. Thus, dexamethasone suppression of the cortisol-secreting zona fasiculata makes abnormalities of androgen secretion more evident and detectable.

Continued.

FLOW DIAGRAM FOR SUSPECTED ADRENAL HYPERANDROGENISM

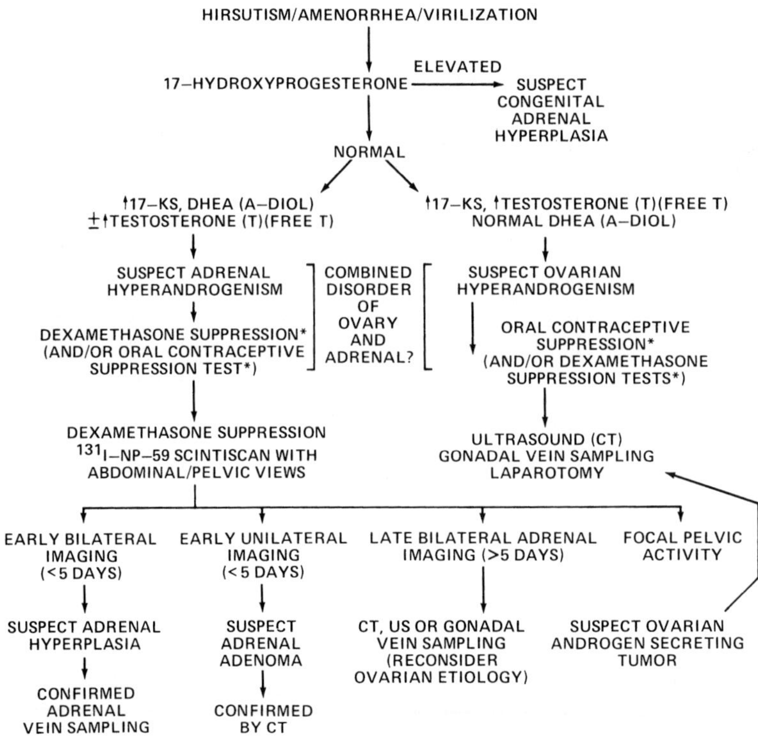

Fig. 26-19. An investigative algorithm for hyperandrogenism.

Table 26-12. Etiologies of hyperandrogenism

Scintigraphic pattern	Form of hyperandrogenism
Unilateral (early) imaging	Adrenal adenoma
Bilateral (early) imaging	Adrenal hyperplasia
Bilateral (late) imaging	Polycystic ovary disease
	Congenital adrenal hyperplasia (CAH)
Early nonvisualization	Ovarian and/or peripheral HA

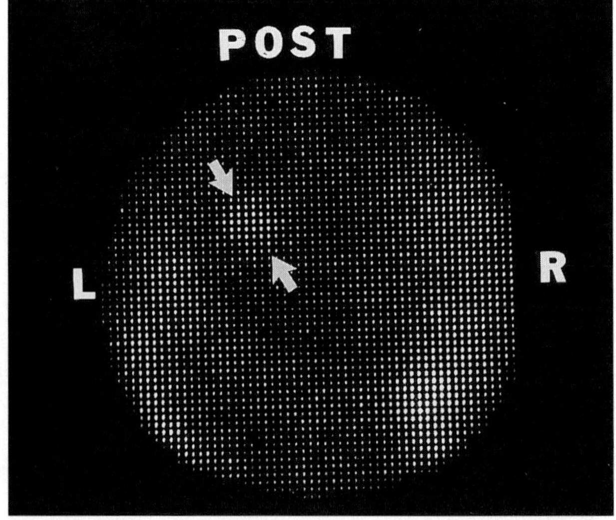

Fig. 26-20. Posterior NP-59 dexamethasone suppression scintiscan demonstrating an autonomously functioning left adrenal adenoma causing HA *(arrows)*. (From Gross, M.D., and others: Dexamethasone-supression adrenal scintigraphy in hyperandizogenism, J. Nucl. Med. 22:12, 1981.)

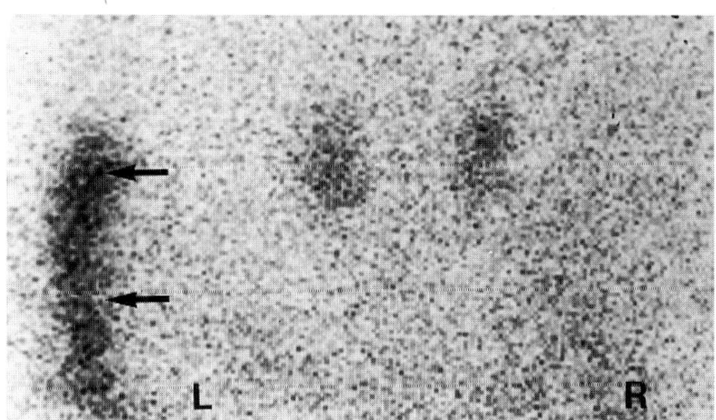

Fig. 26-21. Posterior NP-59 dexamethasone suppression scintiscan demonstrating early (day 5) visualization of both adrenal glands in a patient with hyperandrogenism. Colonic radioactivity is identified *(arrows)*.

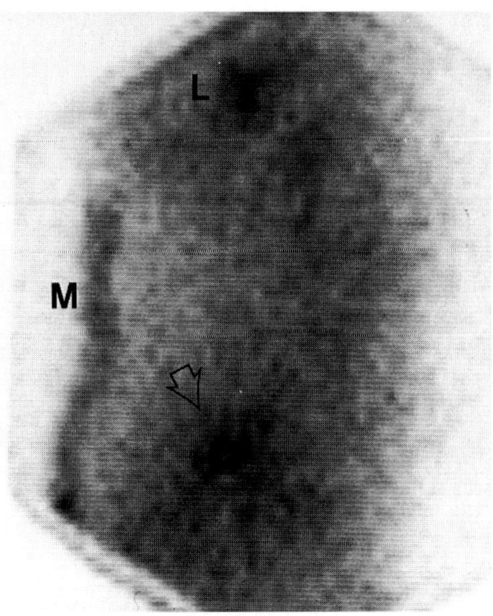

Fig. 26-22. Anterior NP-59 dexamethasone suppression scintiscan demonstrating subtle uptake in the pelvis. Body surface marker *(M)* and liver *(L)* help define anatomy. Patient had an ovarian tumor resulting in virilization.

Four imaging patterns in adrenal hyperandrogenism may be found in Table 26-12. Imaging of adenomas (Fig. 26-20) and bilateral adrenal hyperplasia (Fig. 26-21) usually is accomplished by the fifth day following injection of NP-59. Late visualization (after day 7) suggests polycystic ovary syndrome or congenital adrenal hyperplasia. Bilateral nonvisualization suggests an ovarian or other nonadrenal (exogenous) source of HA. The diagnosis of congenital adrenal hyperplasia is usually based on finding elevated levels of serum and urine 17-hydroxyprogesterone as well as other androgen precursors. The scans in congenital adrenal hyperplasia (CAH) are less useful because dexamethasone suppression of ACTH will result in bilateral nonvisualization.

Ovarian hyperandrogenism

NP-59 uptake by virilizing tumors of the ovary have been reported, and scintigraphic evaluation of the pelvis may be indicated in those women in whom no adrenal abnormality can be identified with other anatomic imaging methods (Fig. 26-22). The pelvic scintigraphy must be preceded by meticulous bowel preparation.

Incidentally discovered (nonhyperfunctioning) adrenal mass lesions

Patients without known adrenal disease may undergo CT, MRI or US examination for other reasons, with the incidental discovery of an adrenal mass lesion. These patients generally, but not always, lack clinical or biochemical evidence of disease of the adrenal cortex or medulla. A critical consideration in this context is whether an incidental mass lesion in an adrenal is malignant (e.g., metastasis) or benign (i.e., adenoma). Imaging with NP-59 may be a useful diagnostic tool in this regard, although it is still under investigation. Increased NP-59 uptake on the same side as the adrenal enlargement noted on CT or MRI suggests a benign nonhyperfunctioning adenoma (Fig. 26-23). Reduced, distorted, or absent NP-59 uptake on the same side as the adrenal lesions suggests a destructive lesion (e.g., adrenal carcinoma, metastatic tumor, hemorrhage, or infarction) (Fig. 26-24, *A* and *B*). Small lesions (less than 1.5 cm) may not result in sufficient functional differences to be identified using NP-59 scintigraphy.

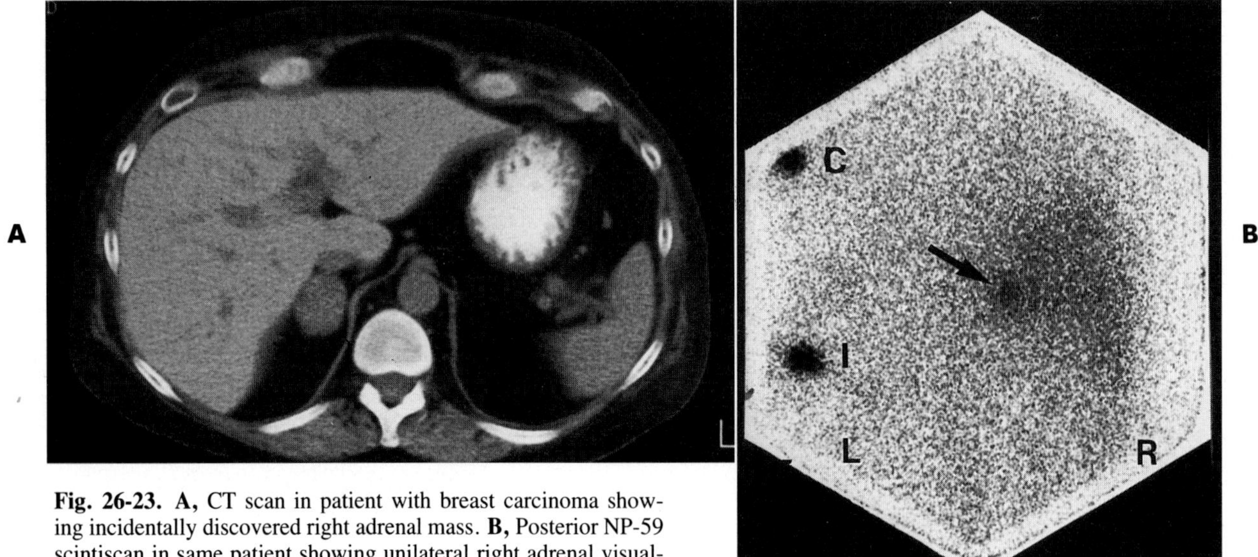

Fig. 26-23. **A,** CT scan in patient with breast carcinoma showing incidentally discovered right adrenal mass. **B,** Posterior NP-59 scintiscan in same patient showing unilateral right adrenal visualization *(arrow)*. Markers identify left costal margin *(C)* and iliac crest *(I)*. Biopsy showed benign adenoma.

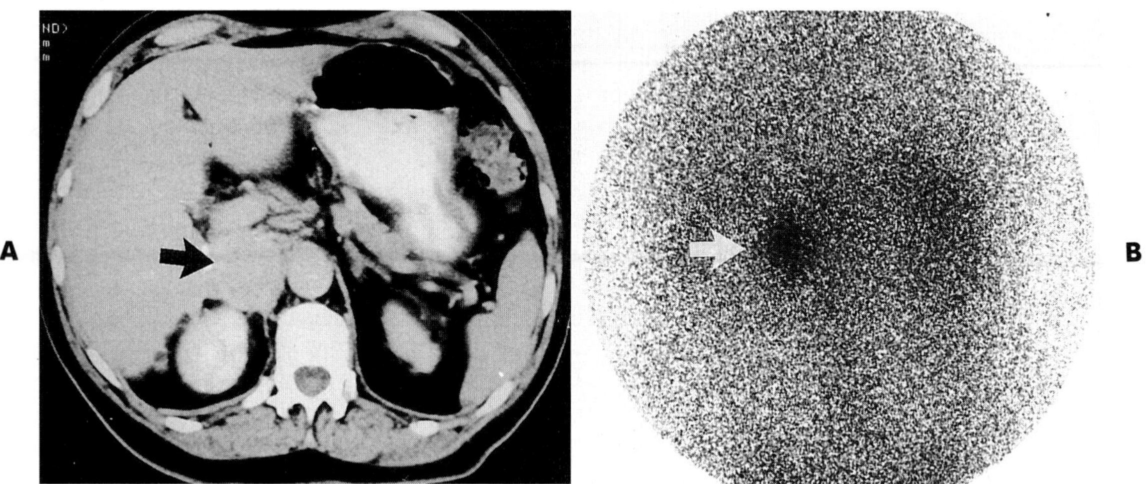

Fig. 26-24. **A,** CT scan in patient with adenocarcinoma undergoing preoperative staging. Right adrenal mass *(arrow)* is identified. **B,** Posterior NP-59 scintiscan in same patient. Uptake in left adrenal alone *(arrow)* identified. Biopsy of right adrenal showed adenocarcinoma.

LABORATORY APPLICATION

79

SYMPATHOMEDULLA IMAGING WITH ^{131}I-mIBG

Purpose

The demonstration that (^{123}I) ^{131}I-mIBG could visualize the canine and primate adrenal medullae opened the way for this agent to be used in demonstrating the presence of adrenal pheochromocytoma, as well as extra-adrenal metastatic deposits, and other catecholamine-secreting tumors in humans. ^{131}I-mIBG scintigraphy has been found especially useful in situations in which other anatomic localizing techniques may fail, such as extra-adrenal lesions, recurrent or metastatic tumors, and in patients in whom previous surgery may alter anatomic planes and/or the placement of metallic clips and may thus interfere with accurate CT or MRI diagnosis (Table 26-13). ^{131}I-mIBG has

Table 26-13. Results of ^{131}I-mIBG scintigraphy for suspected pheochromocytoma by cases (1980 to 1988)

	Total	True positive	True negative	False positive	False negative
Sporadic intraadrenal pheochromocytoma	47	44	0	0	3
Sporadic extraadrenal abdominal pheochromocytoma	15	13	0	0	2
Sporadic extraadrenal thoracic pheochromocytoma	11	11	0	0	0
Sporadic extraadrenal cervical pheochromocytoma	3	2	0	0	1
Sporadic malignant pheochromocytoma	71	64	0	0	7
Familial syndromes:					
MEN 2a and 2b	39 (2 malig)	23	15	0	1
Neurofibromatosis	17 (1 malig)	9	8	0	1
von Hippel-Lindau Disease	4 (1 malig)	3	0	0	1
Simple familial	10 (5 malig)	5	4	0	1
Unknown site	6	0	0	0	1
"False positive"*	4	0	0	4	0
Pheochromocytoma excluded†	700	0	700	0	0
Totals	**927**	**174**	**727**	**4**	**22**

*Suspected pheochromocytoma with positive scan. These were subsequently shown to have been due to one case each of retroperitoneal secretory granule containing atypical schwannoma, metastatic choriocarcinoma, and probable dilated renal pelvis.

†Nondiagnostically elevated catecholamines but negative radiology and follow-up or negative scan and entirely normal biochemistry.

(From Shapiro, B., and others: Radiochemical diagnosis of adrenal diseases, Crit. Rev. Clin. Lab. Sci. 27:280, 1989.)

also proved useful in imaging primary and metastatic neuroblastoma and in the identification of other tumors of neuroectodermal origin (Table 26-14).

Radiopharmaceutical preparation

1. See page 658 and Table 26-5.

Indications

1. To localize pheochromocytoma suspected on the basis of both clinical features and biochemical abnormalities. See Fig. 24-25 for a suggested investigational algorithm for pheochromocytoma.
2. To aid in the identification of metastatic deposits from a previously diagnosed pheochromocytoma.
3. To evaluate patients with neuroblastoma and other neuroendocrine tumors (e.g., carcinoids, nonfunctioning paragangliomas, medullary thyroid carcinoma, and Merkel cell tumors).

Procedure

Materials

1. ^{131}I-mIBG[2] 0.5 mCi (18.5 MBq) per 1.7 m^2 body-weight surface area. A larger dosage of 1 mCi (37 MBq) is recommended for patients with suspected metastatic pheochromocytoma.
2. ^{123}I-mIBG dosage is 3 to 10 mCi (111 to 370 MBq) (in United States, requires in-house synthesis; commercial preparations may be available outside the United States).
3. Scintillation camera with high-energy collimator (low-energy if ^{123}I is used) interfaced to a digital minicomputer
4. Photographic device or data storage system

[2]MIBG is available from the Nuclear Pharmacy, Division of Nuclear Medicine, University of Michigan Medical Center (requires modified, physician-sponsored Investigational New Drug application approval from the Federal Drug Administration [FDA]).

Continued.

Table 26-14. Results of ^{131}I-mIBG scintigraphy in neuroendocrine tumors other than pheochromocytomas and neuroblastoma (1980 to 1988)

Tumor type	Total number studied	^{131}I-mIBG positive	^{131}I-mIBG Positive (%)
Carcinoids	10	4	40
Nonsecretory paraganglioma	3	3	100
Chemodectoma (carotid body tumor)	5	2	40
Sporadic MCT[a]	7	1	14
Multiple endocrine neoplasia			
Types 2a and 2b associated MCT*			
(*a*) Cases with elevated calcitonin	12	1	8
(*b*) Cases with normal calcitonin	8	0	0
(*c*) Cases with unavailable calcitonin	6	0	0
Oat-cell carcinoma of lung	4	0	100
Metastatic choriocarcinoma	1	1	100
Atypical schwannoma†	1	1	100
Merkel cell skin cancer	1	1	100
Islet-cell tumor of pancreas	4	1**	25
Undifferential neuroendocrine tumors	2	0	0
Totals	**64**	**15**	**23**

*MCT = medullary carcinoma of the thyroid
†Tumor contained neurosecretory granules
**Case of insulinoma studies in collaboration with Dr. O. Geatti, Udine, Italy
(From Shapiro, B., and others: Radiochemical diagnosis of adrenal disease, Crit. Rev. Clin. Lab. Sci., 27:280, 1989.)

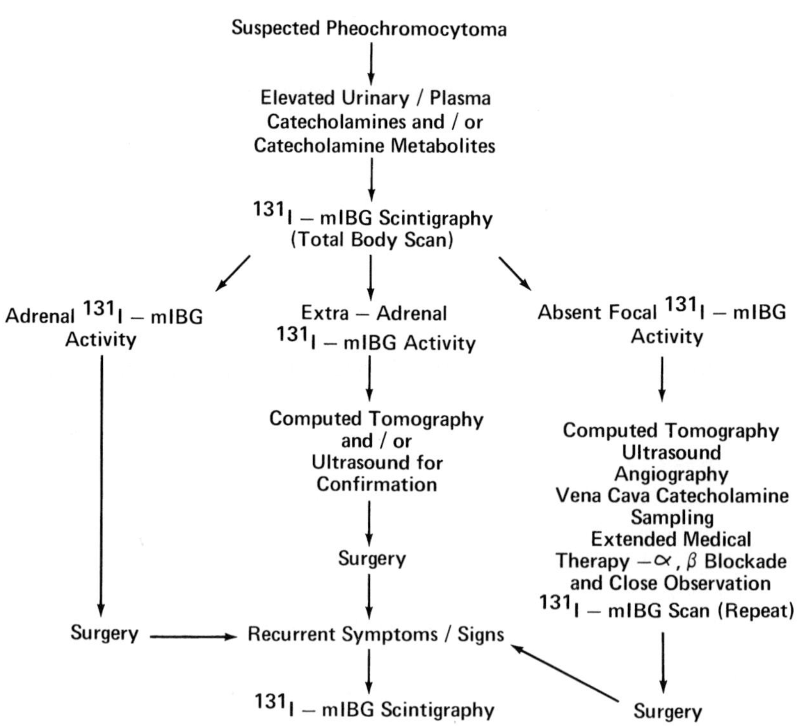

Fig. 26-25. An investigative algorithm for pheochromocytoma.

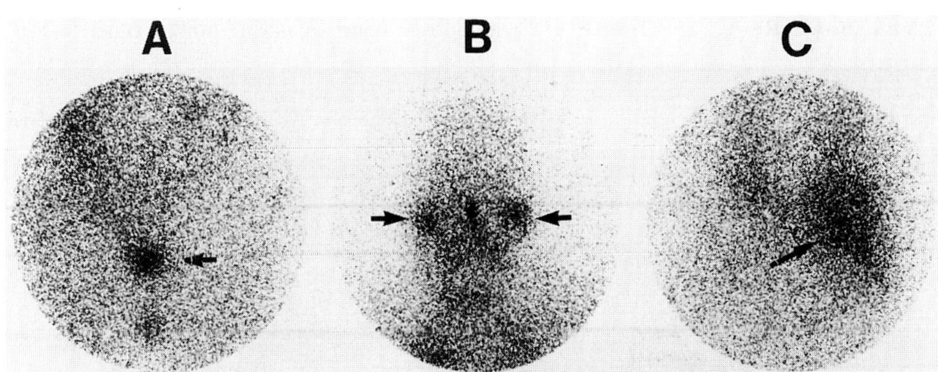

Fig. 26-26. Normal distribution of ^{131}I-mIBG. **A,** Anteriorabdomen and pelvis. Note normal uptake in bladder *(arrow)*. **B,** Anterior skull. Note uptake in salivary glands *(arrows)*. **C,** Posterior chest and abdomen. Note uptake in liver *(arrow)*.

Patient preparation

1. Explain the entire procedure to the patient and obtain signed informed consent.
2. Uptake of free ^{131}I by thyroid is prevented by administration of SSKI or Lugol's solution, 1 drop TID beginning 1 day before mIBG administration and continuing for 6 days after injection (perchlorate may be used when iodides are contraindicated).
3. Be sure that a careful medication history is taken. Many drugs either interfere with or promote mIBG uptake, and this could seriously alter the scintiscan findings (Table 26-2). Ideally, the patient should not be receiving any medications for 2 to 3 week interval before mIBG imaging.

Technique

1. Use a 30% window centered on 364 keV (^{131}I) or 30% window at 140 keV (^{123}I).
2. Administer mIBG by intravenous injection over 15 seconds.
3. Obtain routine images at 24, 48, and 72 hours following ^{131}I-mIBG injection, and at 3, 18, and 40 hours following ^{123}I-mIBG injection. Images at 72 hours may be useful if 48-hour images are weakly positive or equivocal.
4. Scan the entire patient from top of skull to the pelvis for abnormal foci of ^{131}I-mIBG uptake. Images of anterior pelvis and lower abdomen, anterior skull and thorax, and posterior abdomen and chest should be obtained with radioactive markers placed on lateral iliac crests, axillae, and lateral lower costal margins. In patients evaluated for metastatic pheochromocytoma, an additional view of mid and proximal femurs should be obtained. The pelvis should be imaged after the bladder has been emptied, as metastatic pheochromocytoma may rarely present as abnormal bladder uptake. Lateral views of areas of abnormal uptake are helpful for purposes of localization.
5. Images following ^{131}I-mIBG are acquired for at least 100K counts or 20-minute imaging time and displayed in an analog or digital form on film. Moderate background subtraction is helpful. At least 500K counts per image should be acquired if ^{123}I-mIBG is used. The latter radiopharmaceutical permits the performance of SPECT, which can then be presented as a rotating image and transaxial, sagittal, and coronal sections.

Diagnosis

Normal image pattern

The normal distribution of ^{131}I-mIBG includes uptake in salivary glands, liver, and spleen in all cases (Fig. 26-26). The heart is often visualized in patients with normal catecholamine levels, but it is seldom visualized if levels are elevated. The colon is less frequently visualized. In contrast, normal adrenal medulla is seldom visualized (2% of cases at 24 hours and 16% of cases at 48 hours after ^{131}I-mIBG administration). Areas of normal uptake tend to diminish in intensity with time, but pheochromocytoma usually demonstrates scintigraphic activity that increases over time. ^{123}I-mIBG permits a more clear visualization of the heart and of the adrenal medulla in most cases.

Continued.

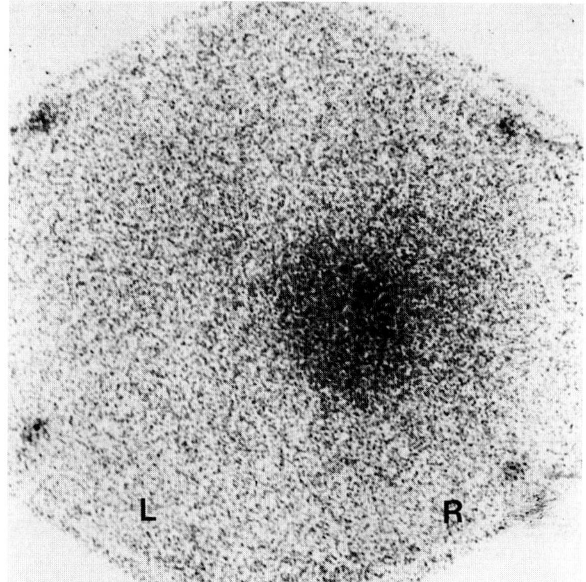

Fig. 26-27. Posterior ^{131}I-mIBG scintiscan of a large sporadic pheochromocytoma.

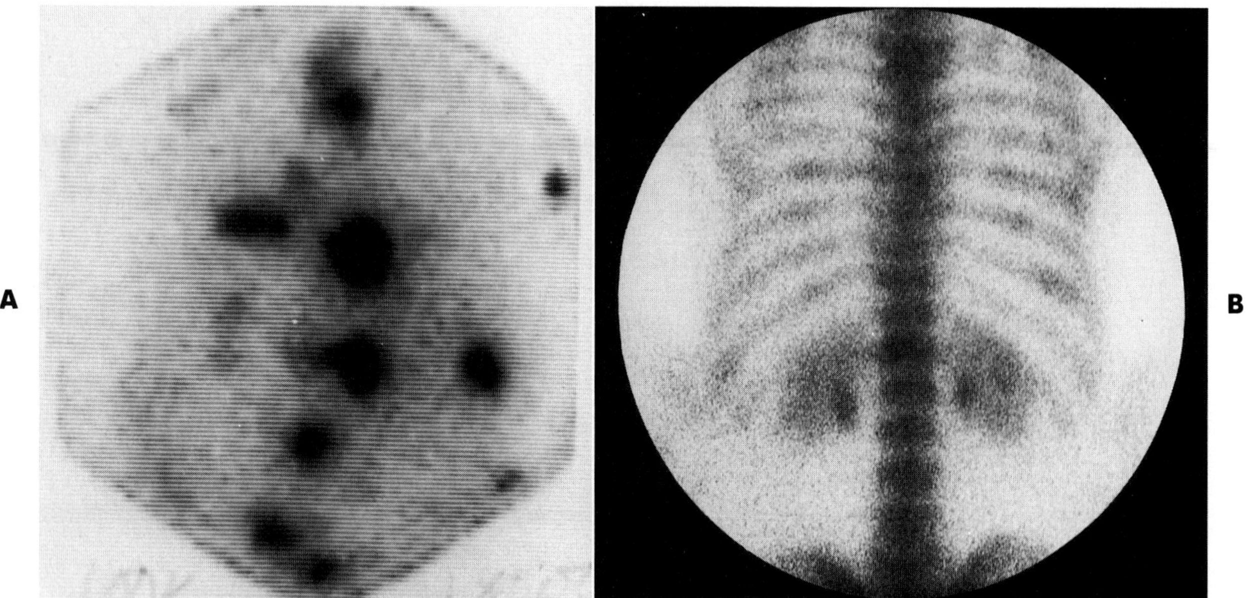

Fig. 26-28. Metastatic pheochromocytoma: **A,** Anterior chest ^{131}I-mIBG scintiscan showing multiple sites of ^{131}I-mIBG accumulation in ribs and spine, including some areas not appreciated on bone scan shown in **B.**

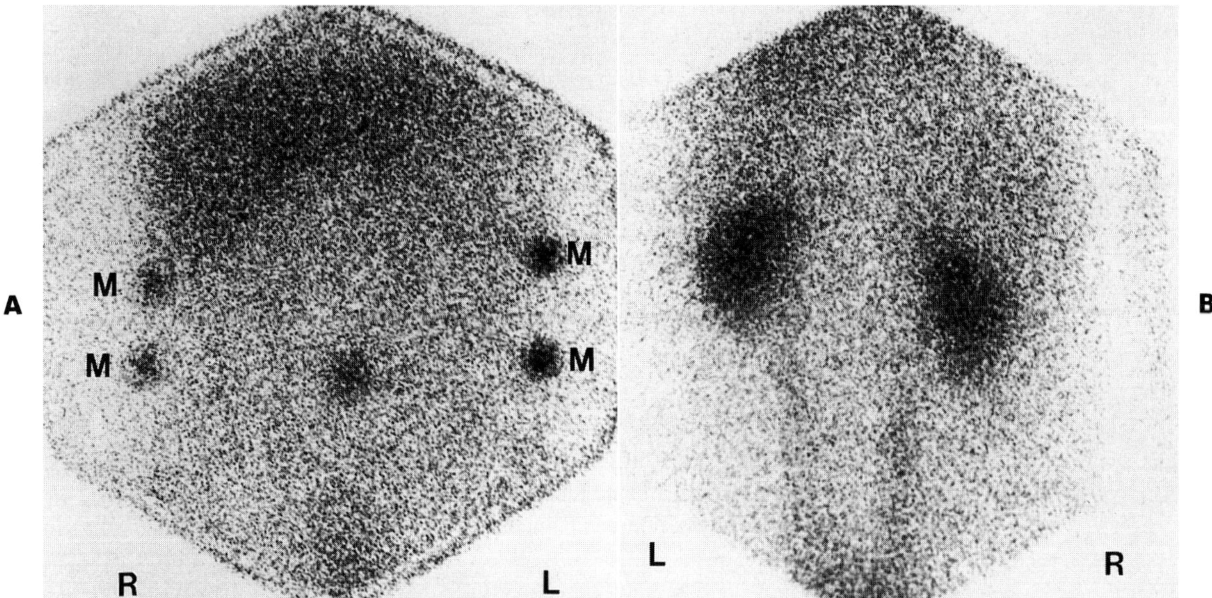

Fig. 26-29. A, Anterior abdominal ^{131}I-mIBG scintiscan of an extraadrenal pheochromocytoma showing ^{131}I-mIBG activity at aortic bifurcation markers *(M)* used to aid localization. **B,** ^{99m}Tc-DTPA renal scan aids in localization of ^{131}I-mIBG activity.

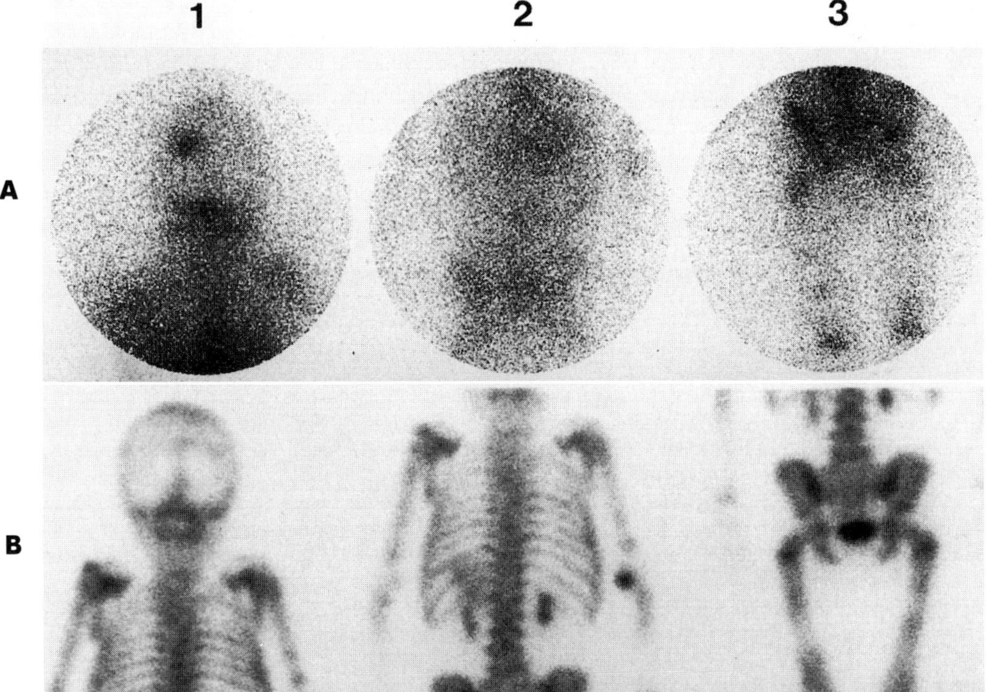

Fig. 26-30. A, ^{123}I-mIBG scintiscan in a child with neuroblastoma with *(1)* anterior skull, *(2)* anterior chest and abdomen, and *(3)* anterior pelvis and lower extremity views. Note both diffuse and focal areas of uptake. **B,** Bone scan in same child shows diffuse increased uptake especially in extremities. Bone-marrow biopsy was positive.

^{131}I-mIBG imaging of adrenergic dysfunction

Pheochromocytoma—^{131}I-mIBG scintigraphy demonstrates high sensitivity and specificity in the localization of pheochromocytoma (Table 26-13). It is reliable in the detection of lesions originating either intraadrenally or extraadrenally, benign or malignant lesions, and in cases of familial syndromes (MEN IIa, neurofibromatosis, von Hipple-Lindau disease, and familial pheochromocytoma). The scintigraphic pattern depends on the localization of the pheochromocytoma(s). Sporadic, unilateral tumors show focal intense ^{131}I-mIBG uptake (Figs. 26-27). Metastatic disease is usually visualized in the axial skeleton, lung, and liver (Fig. 26-28, *A* and *B*). Recurrent and/or metastatic pheochromocytomas are accurately localized. Superimposition or subtraction of ^{131}I-mIBG scans on bone scans (^{99m}Tc MDP), kidneys (^{99m}Tc DTPA), blood pool (^{99m}Tc RBCs), liver and spleen (^{99m}TcSC), and myocardium (^{201}Tl) may be helpful in accurately locating the site(s) of abnormal foci of ^{131}I-mIBG uptake (Fig. 26-29, *A* and *B*).

Recently ^{123}I-mIBG has been used in adrenomedullary scintigraphy. Its favorable dosimetry (Table 26-5), photon flux, and ability to use SPECT has increased the sensitivity of mIBG scintigraphy. Lesions not demonstrable by ^{131}I-mIBG may be disclosed by ^{123}I-mIBG, which, when available, should be considered the radiopharmaceutical of choice.

Neuroblastoma—This highly malignant tumor is the most common extracranial solid tumor of childhood. Neuroblastoma is of neural crest origin and may arise in any location of sympathetic nervous system tissue. The most common presentation is an abdominal mass. The tumor tends to metastasize early, favoring bone and bone marrow. ^{131}I-mIBG scintigraphy has demonstrated utility in the diagnosis, staging, monitoring, and (potentially) in the therapy of neuroblastoma. The ^{131}I-mIBG scintiscan in neuroblastoma is complementary to other imaging modalities (CT, MRI, bone scan) (Fig. 26-30) and may provide information not obtainable by other means. The presence of mIBG uptake may be used as one criteria in distinguishing neuroblastoma from a non-neuroendocrine tumor, e.g. Ewing's sarcoma, lymphoma, and other small round cell tumors. The sensitivity and specificity of ^{131}I-mIBG scintigraphy in neuroblastoma is similar to that for pheochromocytoma.

Other neuroendocrine tumors—Like the catecholamine-secreting tumors, several other types of tumors share the property of amine precursor uptake in decarboxylation (APUD) and may accumulate ^{131}I-mIBG. These include carcinoid, medullary carcinoma of the thyroid, paraganglioma, schwannoma, small-cell lung carcinoma, and Merkel cell tumors. While at this time studies are preliminary, ^{131}I-mIBG scintigraphy is less efficacious in the localization of these neoplasms than in pheochromocytoma and neuroblastoma, although the overall clinical experience is limited (Table 26-14).

BIBLIOGRAPHY

Barbarino, A., and others: Evaluation of steroid laboratory tests and adrenal gland imaging with radiocholesterol in the etiological diagnosis of Cushing's syndrome, Clin. Endocrinol. 10:107, 1979.

Basmadjian, G.P., and others: Synthesis of a new adrenal cortex imaging agent 6B ^{131}I-iodomethyl-19-norcholest-5(10)-en-3B-ol (NP-59), J. Lab. Comp. Radiopharmacol. 11:427, 1975.

Besser, G.M., and Cudworth, A.G., editors: Clinical endocrinology, Philadelphia, 1987, J.B. Lippincott Co.

Carpenter, B.C., and others: Demonstration of steroid producing gonadal tumors by external scanning with the use of NP-59, Mayo Clin. Proc. 54:332, 1979.

Carey, J.E., and others: Absorbed dose of the human adrenal from iodomethyl-norcholesterol (^{131}I) "NP-59", J. Nucl. Med. 20:60, 1979.

Elias, H., and Pauly, J.E.: The structure of the human adrenal cortex, Endocrinology 58:714, 1956.

Engelman, K.: Pheochromocytoma, Clin. Endocrinol. 6:769, 1977.

Fig, L.M., and others: Adrenal localization in the adrenocorticotropic hormone-independent Cushing syndrome, Ann. Intern. Med. 109:547-553, 1988.

Freitas, J.E., and others: Normal adrenal asymmetry: explanation and interpretation, J. Nucl. Med. 19:149, 1978.

Frietas, J.E., and others: Adrenal imaging with ^{131}I NP-59 in primary aldosteronism, J. Nucl. Med. 20:7, 1979.

Givens, J.R.: Hirsutism and hyperandrogenism, Adv. Intern. Med. 1:227, 1976.

Glazer, H.S., and others: Nonfunctioning adrenal masses: incidental discovery on computed tomography, AJR 139:81, 1982.

Grekin, R.J., and Gross, M.D.: Endocrine hypertension, Comput. Ther. 9:65, 1983.

Gross, M.D., and others: Dexamethasone suppression adrenal scintigraphy in hyperandrogenism, J. Nucl. Med. 20:1131, 1979.

Gross, M.D., and others: The relationship of ^{131}I-6β-iodomethyl-19-norcholesterol (NP-59) adrenal cortical uptake to indices of androgen secretion in women with hyperandrogenism, Clin. Nucl. Med. 9:264, 1984.

Gross, M.D., and others: Scintigraphic localization of adrenal lesions in primary aldosteronism, Am. J. Med. 77:839, 1984.

Gross, M.D., and others: The relationship of adrenal iodocholesterol uptake to adrenal zona glomerulosa function, J. Clin. Endocrinol. Metab. 52:612, 1981.

Gross, M.D., and others: The role of pharmacologic manipulation in adrenal cortical scintigraphy, Semin. Nucl. Med. 9:128, 1981.

Hogan, M.J., and others: Location of aldosterone producing adenomas with ^{131}I-19-iodocholesterol, N. Engl. J. Med. 294:410, 1976.

Innes, I.R., and Nickerson, M.: Drugs acting on post-ganglion adrenergic nerve endings and structures innervated by them (sympathomimetic drugs). In L.S. Goodman and A. Gilman, editors: The pharmacologic basis of therapeutics, London, 1970, MacMillan Co., p. 478.

Jeffcoate, W.J., and Edwards, C.D.S.: Cushing's syndrome: pathogenesis, diagnosis, and treatment. In V.H.T. James, editor: The adrenal gland, New York, 1979, Raven Press, p. 165.

Liddle, G.W., and others: Normal and abnormal regulation of corticotropin secretion in man, Rec. Prog. Horm. Res.

Lightman, S.: Adrenal medulla. In V.H.T. James, editor: The adrenal gland, New York, 1979, Raven Press, p. 283.

Nakajo, M., and others: The normal and abnormal distribution of the adrenomedullary imaging agent ^{131}I-metiodobenzylguanadine (^{131}I-mIBG) in man, J. Nucl. Med. 24:672, 1983.

Nelson, D.H.: The adrenal cortex: physiological function and disease, Philadelphia, 1980, W.B. Saunders Co., p. 197.

Reschini, E., and Catania, A.: Clinical experience with the adrenal scanning agents iodine-131-19-iodocholesterol and selenium-75-selenomethylcholesterol, Eur. J. Nucl. Med. 18:817, 1991.

Sarkar, S.D., and others: A new and superior adrenal imaging agent ^{131}I-6B-iodomethyl-19-norcholesterol (NP-59). Evaluation in humans, J. Clin. Endocrinol. Metab. 45:353, 1977.

Shima, S., and others: Effects of ACTH on cholesterol dynamics in rat adrenal tissue, Endocrinology 90:808, 1972.

Schteingart, D.E., and others: Iodocholesterol: adrenal tissue uptake and imaging in adrenal neoplasms, J. Clin. Endocrinol. Metab. 52:1152, 1981.

Shapiro, B., and others: ^{131}I-metaiodobenzylguanadine for the locating of suspected pheochromocytoma: experience in 400 cases (441 studies), J. Nucl. Med. 26:576, 1984.

Shapiro, B., and others: ^{131}I-metiodobenzylguanidine (mIBG) adrenal medullary scintigraphy: interventional studies. In R.P. Spencer, editor: Interventional nuclear medicine, New York, 1984, Grune & Stratton, p. 451.

Sisson, J.C., and others: Scintigraphic localization of pheochromocytoma, N. Engl. J. Med. 305:12, 1981.

Sisson, J.C., and others: Scintigraphy with ^{131}I-mIBG as an aid to treatment of pheochromocytoma in patients with MEN-2 syndromes, Henry Ford Med. J. 32:254, 1984.

Sizemore, G.W., and others: Multiple endocrine neoplasia, Clin. Endocrinol. Metab. 9:299, 1980.

Skeggs, L.T., and others: The biochemistry of the renin-angiotensin system and its role in hypertension, Am. J. Med. 60:737, 1976.

Stokigt, J.R.: Mineralocorticoid excess. In V.H.T. James, editor: The adrenal gland, New York, 1979, Raven Press, p. 197.

Thrall, J.H., and others: Adrenal scintigraph, J. Nucl. Med. 8:23, 1978.

Weinberger, M.H., and others: Primary aldosteronism: diagnosis, localization, and treatment, Ann. Intern. Med. 90:386, 1979.

Weiss, E.R., and others: Evaluation of stimulation and suppression tests in the etiological diagnosis of Cushing's syndrome, Ann. Intern. Med. 71:941, 1969.

Williams, R.H.: Textbook of endocrinology, Philadelphia, 1974, W.B. Saunders Co., p. 322.

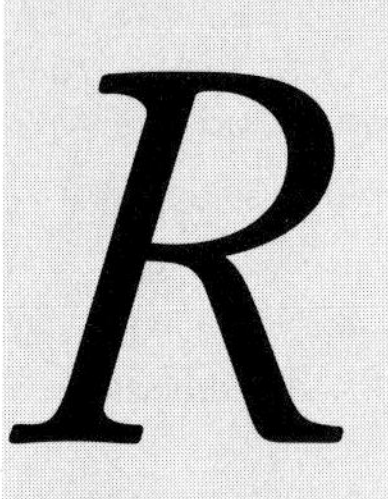

Chapter 27

ADIOLABELED MONOCLONAL ANTIBODIES

RICHARD L. WAHL

The high specificity of antibodies for the antigens they recognize has been used to substantial advantage in nuclear medicine over the past decades in the area of radioimmunoassay (RIA). The radioimmunoassay approach is an in vitro procedure, discussed elsewhere in this text, which involves the use of a highly specific antibody, often a polyclonal antibody, to detect a very small quantity of an antigen present in a human body fluid, generally in the serum. In this approach antigen is radiolabeled, and unlabeled antibody is used to competitively bind the radiolabeled and unlabeled antigen for counting and quantitation. The monoclonal antibody imaging and therapy approach is one in which rather than labeling the antigen, the antibody (often monoclonal) itself is labeled and injected into patients in an effort to either image cancer and other diseases or treat the cancer. While this radioantibody approach has been applied to a variety of diseases, to date routine clinical utility has been demonstrated only in selected situations. The concept of using antibody specificity to detect or fight disease has existed since Ehrlich proposed the concept of the "magic bullet" or targeted treatment in the early part of the 20th century. Unfortunately, few specific potentially "magic bullets" have existed until recently to test this theory, until monoclonal antibodies were developed.

■ MONOCLONAL ANTIBODIES

Monoclonal antibodies are the most recent candidate molecules for the role of "magic bullet." While monoclonal antibodies are quite new, antibodies have been known about for many years. Since the time of Edward Jenner it has been known that it was possible to make an individual immune to a disease. In Jenner's studies, cowpox antigenically cross-reacted with smallpox, and patient immunization with cowpox imparted immunity to smallpox. As vaccination is now practiced to prevent measles, for example, this immunity is generally humoral or antibody in nature. The antibodies formed by the body following immunization, however, are "polyclonal" antibodies. These polyclonal antibodies are a spectrum of antibodies from different B-cell parents which are reactive with different sites on the immunizing antigen(s). These individual sites to which the antibodies bind to are known as epitopes of the antigen. Polyclonal antibodies cross-reactive with tumors were used to study tumor localization about 40 years ago, but this approach only proceeded slowly because of several difficulties with polyclonal antibodies. For example, even if a tumor antigen can be defined and completely purified, this pure antigen, when given as an immunogen to a small animal in an effort to produce antibodies, will result in a large spectrum of antibodies being produced. This is illustrated in Fig. 27-1 in which a wide range of antibodies is produced by immunization, even using pure antigen. These polyclonal antibodies can be quite useful, but their spectrum of reactivity is highly varied and they are not replicable from day to day (i.e., if the animal producing the antibody is bled on a given day to remove antibody from the blood and then sampled weeks later, the antibody will be different a few days or weeks later). This limited supply and nonreproducibility is of particular concern for a diagnostic or therapeutic agent.

The field of antibody imaging and therapy gained momentum in the late 1970s with the discovery of a method to produce large quantities of highly pure and uniform antibody that did not vary from day to day. This was the Nobel-Prize–winning monoclonal antibody approach as defined and developed by Kohler and Milstein. The monoclonal antibodies are made when an animal is immunized with antigen and then specific immune B-cells are taken from the immunized animal's spleen or lymphoid tissue and fused with malignant myeloma cells. Malignant myeloma cells have the property of an unlimited life span (they are malignant, in contrast to normal B-cells); with proper selection techniques, the characteristics of unlimited life span of the myeloma can be combined with the characteristics

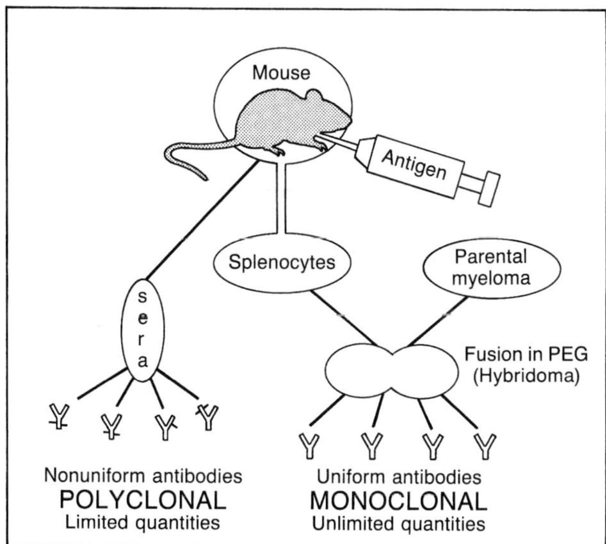

Fig. 27-1. Schematic illustration of the difference between polyclonal and monoclonal antibodies. When the mouse is immunized with a pure antigen, a mixture of nonuniform antibodies appears in the serum. These antibodies are reactive with different sites on the antigen (epitopes), and they vary in their affinity and specificity. In addition, the cells producing them do not have an unlimited life span (i.e., they are mortal). In contrast, if these same antibody-producing cells are immortalized by fusion of them with malignant antibody-producing cells (myelomas), they will have an unlimited life span and can be plated out and produced in unlimited quantities (monoclonal antibodies). The availability of large quantities of the antibodies through the monoclonal method has been key to the success of this area of work. (From Wahl, R.L.: Radiolabeled monoclonal antibody imaging, Radiology Report 1(3):347-361, 1989.)

of antibody production of the parental B-cell. If such a fusion can be achieved, the offspring hybridoma will make large quantities of an antibody that is specific for a given antigen. Moreover, the antibody will be uniform and the cell line producing antibody can be used to make enough of the antibody so that it could be manufactured, purified, and widely disseminated, as is necessary for a drug. Most monoclonal antibodies are still initially made in mice, as human myeloma fusion partners (to produce human rather than mouse antibodies) have been difficult to come by. Immunizing humans is also difficult, at least with tumor antigens. As will be discussed later, if necessary these murine antibody-producing cells can be genetically altered to become more like a human antibody. Thus it is now possible to make substantial quantities of antibody reactive with antigens. This raises the question of whether there are, in fact, antigens that are specific to tumors.

■ Tumor antigens

Tumor-specific antigens have been very difficult to identify in humans. Unfortunately, except for a few lymphomas and myelomas, tumors that actually produce an antibody-like molecule that in itself can be antigenic (tidiotypic), rarely are there tumor-specific antigens and as a result, rarely are there tumor-specific antibodies. There are a large number of antigens that are expressed on the surface of tumor cells to a much greater extent than on normal tissues; these are tumor-associated antigens. These often may be normal antigens, but they are normally expressed in very low levels on normal tissues. Thus, if there is a quantitative difference of the expression of antigen between tumor and normal tissues, this difference in antigen density may be sufficient for the radioimmunoimaging or therapy approach to be conducted.

Perhaps the most studied of the tumor-associated antigens has been the "onco-fetal antigen" carcinoembryonic antigen (CEA). This approximately 200-KD (molecular weight) glycoprotein is present in substantial levels in the mid-gut of developing humans, but it is expressed in much lower levels in the mature human colon. CEA antigen is expressed on the large majority of colorectal carcinomas; this relative excess in expression in colorectal carcinoma versus normal tissues is sufficient to allow for targeting of anti-CEA antibodies to CEA-producing tumors, as will be discussed later. A similar situation exists for the transferrin receptor antigen, which is associated with rapid tumor growth, though it is present in lesser quantity or normal tissues. The epidermal growth-factor receptor antigen and alphafeto protein (AFP) (the latter which is expressed on hepatomas to a much greater extent than normal liver at least in adults) are also antigenic targets. Ideally, tumor-associated antigens are bound to the surface of the tumor cell as membrane antigens so that the antibody is delivered directly to the cell membrane surface. However, this is not always achieved, and some of the antigens chosen for radioimmunoimaging studies are actually shed. Other tumor-associated antigens do exist; these include glycoproteins that are expressed in excessive amounts in certain adenocarcinomas, such as the high–molecular-weight TAG-72 antigen on colorectal and breast cancers, the human milk-fat globule-associated proteins seen on breast cancers, and other tumor-associated glycoproteins. These have been acceptable targets for tumor imaging.

Some diseases that are not histologically malignant but can be lethal can also be imaged using radiolabeled antibodies. These diseases also have excessive display of certain antigens as a result of alterations in the physiology of the cells. An example is the imaging of cardiac myosin using anti-myosin antibodies. This sort of approach can detect myocardial infarctions and transplant rejection. Myosin, a normal antigen present in high quantities in myocardial cells is normally inaccessible; it becomes accessible because of cell death and the increased permeability of the cell membrane. Other antigens, such as those on granulocytes, can be used to image infection. Another example represents the imaging of fibrin or fibrin-associated products to detect thrombosis. These approaches benefit from the fact that the antigens are well defined and quantitatively occasionally present in larger amount than are tumor-associated antigens.

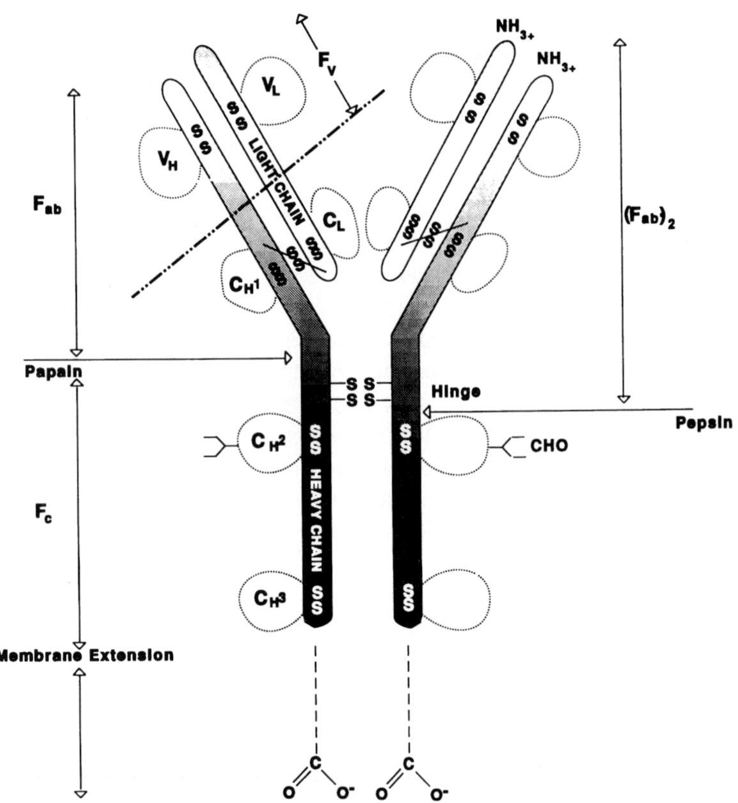

Fig. 27-2. Two-dimensional diagram of the structure of IgG, the most commonly used antibody class in imaging/therapy studies to date. Note that the antibody is bivalent but can be cleaved to bivalent $F(ab')_2$ fragments by pepsin or to monovalent Fab fragments by treatment with papain. Recombinant DNA techniques are allowing for the engineering of antibodies to be partly mouse and partly human, or nearly entirely human in structure. In addition, these techniques are allowing for the production of such smaller fragments of the binding area as Fv fragments. (From Wahl, R.L.: Radiolabeled monoclonal antibody imaging, Radiology Report 1(3):347-361, 1989.)

An area of importance is the identification, before studies in humans, of antibodies that do not cross-react with normal tissues. Cross-reactivity with normal tissues is a potential and sometimes real problem. If an antibody cross-reacts with an antigen present on a normal tissue, the antibody may localize to that tissue and damage it, or at least not reach the desired target. Cross-reactivity may be acceptable in imaging studies in which low doses of radioactivity are given; if therapy is considered, however, this cross-reactivity can cause toxicity to the normal tissue that receives excessive radiation. Another more common potential cross-reactivity that should be assessed is cross-reactivity with circulating white cells. In this situation, if cross-reactive antibodies are given in large quantity, toxicity can result. It should be noted, however, that at low doses of protein some level of cross-reactivity may be acceptable and that these agents could safely be used for imaging. Thus cross-reactivity with normal tissues is a relative and not an absolute contraindication to the choice of an antibody for imaging. Currently, a variety of methods exists to screen antibodies for cross-reactivity with normal tissues; these include flow cytometry, immunofluorescence, and immunoperoxidase staining. These are laborious techniques but generally are performed before antibodies are initially given to humans.

The immunohistochemical technique can also help assess the problem of tumor antigenic heterogeneity that affects both antibody imaging and treatment. Some tumor cells may express large quantities of an antigen and may be well suited for targeting with the antibody, but other tumor cells may completely lack them. The problem of heterogeneity may, in some instances, be addressed by using cocktails of antibodies that are reactive with more than one antigen or with radioactive labels with long enough path lengths to target multiple cells. The use of antibody cocktails over the use of a single antibody following intravenous delivery does not definitely result in superior tumor-to-background ratios, though it may result in more uniform antibody uptake within tumors on a microscopic level. These issues remain under study though in general a single antibody is currently used in imaging studies.

■ Fragments and antibody-like molecules

Assuming an appropriate antigen identifying the tumor or other disease process can be found, one can potentially produce and evaluate several different classes of antibodies. As mentioned earlier, in humans there are five major classes of antibody: IgA, IgD, IgG, and IgM. In the mouse, the major classes are IgG, IgA, and IgM. There are several subclasses of mouse IgG in: IgG1, IgG2a, IgG2b, and IgG3. In general, IgGs have been used for antibody imaging. The IgG molecule (Fig. 27-2) is composed of two heavy and two light chains. There are two active antigen-binding sites composed of variable protein regions with tails on both the light and heavy chains that are quite constant in composition and which define the antibody as mouse or human in structure.

Thus the antigen-binding function is at one end of the

molecule while the opposite F-C end is for interaction with effector cells. IgM antibodies have also been used for tumor imaging; however, IgMs weigh about 5 to 6 times more than do the 160-KD IgGs. This larger molecular weight can potentially result in lesser diffusion of the antibody. This can present particular problems for radio antibody therapy because of nonuniform delivery of antibody dose.

While intact antibodies weighing 150,000 daltons are often used in antibody imaging and therapy studies, antibody fragments are also commonly used. The two most commonly used antibody fragments (Fig. 27-2) are the $F(ab')_2$, which weighs approximately 100,000 daltons and which is a product of pepsin cleavage, and the Fab fragment of papain digestion, which weighs roughly 50,000 daltons. These fragments are cleared more rapidly from the blood than intact antibody, and they do not have the F-C tail of intact antibody that can interact with hepatic receptors and immobilized macrophages. Furthermore, these fragments do not fix-complement and appear to have less normal hepatic uptake than intact IgG. These also have higher vascular permeability. The fact that they diffuse better into tumors, bind less well to normal tissues, and have more rapid clearance from the body means that tumor-to-background ratios are generally higher with antibody fragments at early time points postintravenous injection than they are with intact antibody. Unfortunately, these antibody fragments accumulate to tumors to a lesser fractional extent than do intact antibodies. It is variable as to whether Fab fragments will always represent an improvement over intact antibody; however, $F(ab')_2$ fragments generally do represent an improvement. It appears that affinity of binding to antigen may have a substantial role in determining the utility of Fab fragments. This may vary from antibody to antibody, so it is not always possible to state that mono and bivalent fragments are superior to intact antibody for imaging; most would agree, however, that this is commonly the case.

As alluded to earlier, recombinant DNA techniques can be used to produce monoclonal antibodies in which the mouse constant region is replaced by the human constant regions (Fig. 27-2). This renders the antibodies less immunogenic than mouse antibodies because there is a larger amount of commonality between these human-mouse chimeric antibodies than between mouse antibodies and humans when they are given to humans. Humans appear to be less likely to mount an immune response to these chimeric antibodies.

It should also be noted that within the past several years it has become possible to produce antibodies and antibody-like molecules with a somewhat different approach to bacteria that uses recombinant DNA techniques and thus does not require the use of mice or plasma cells at all. This is a promising approach, but it is too early to assess its utility. In addition, it is possible to use recombinant DNA techniques to produce single-chain variable region antibodies. In this approach, a Fab-like molecule (or shorter molecule) is produced instead of the intact molecule. Both approaches have potential, but each will require extensive further evaluation. These very short antibody fragments have been referred to as single-chain antibody (SCA) and can achieve rapid tumor targeting.

■ MONOCLONAL ANTIBODY IMAGING

■ Tumor pathophysiology related to antibody localization

The anatomy and physiology of tumor and normal tissues are important to the absolute concentration of antibody labeled with a radionuclide in tissue. Molecules circulate through organs having different ranges of blood flow and vascular architecture. The liver receives 0.5 ml of blood per minute per gram of tissue and has sinusoids that allow penetration of large molecules. The bowel has a high blood flow and will allow large molecules through its capillaries. The kidney has close integrity of its capillary endothelium and receives 3 ml of blood per gram of tissue per minute.

Tumors get only about 0.2 ml of blood flow per gram of tumor per minute. As tumors increase in volume, their blood flow per gram decreases; as the tumor grows in size the distribution of blood flow within the tumor will vary considerably. Because of arteriovenous shunting, blood delivered to the tumor may not perfuse the tumor. Tumor capillaries usually are more easily penetrated by large molecular weight proteins; however, if the intratumor capillaries have integrity, a small amount of high molecular weight proteins crosses into the tumor interstitial fluid space. Antibodies that flow into the interstitium of the tumor cross the interstitial space. The antibodies travel through this space by convection currents and move between the tumor cells, attaching to cells close to the capillary endothelium. The larger immunoreactive molecule will have a shorter migration distance from the capillary wall.

Venous outflow of tumors is poor. As tumors grow, the venous architecture becomes chaotic and flow becomes more sluggish. There are no lymphatics in tumors. Poor venous outflow and absence of lymphatics in tumors will cause some nonspecific antibodies to concentrate in tumor tissue.

■ Physiology of antibody localization

Initial studies of antibody imaging were performed in rodent models of human cancer. These studies demonstrated that intact antibodies will localize to xenografts of tumors. For example, as seen in Fig. 27-3, when an intact antibody is injected with this ^{131}I-labeled (anti-CEA) into a Syrian hamster bearing a GW-39 human colon cancer, there is considerable blood-pool activity when imaging is performed 2 days postinjection. By 6 days postinjection, the blood-pool activity has substantially cleared and the tumor is more visible. By 11 days postinjection, further blood-pool clearance and more clear visualization of the tumor is seen. Thus, background activity clears more rapidly than does tumor activity with intact antitumor antibodies, though it can take some time from the injection of intact antibodies until op-

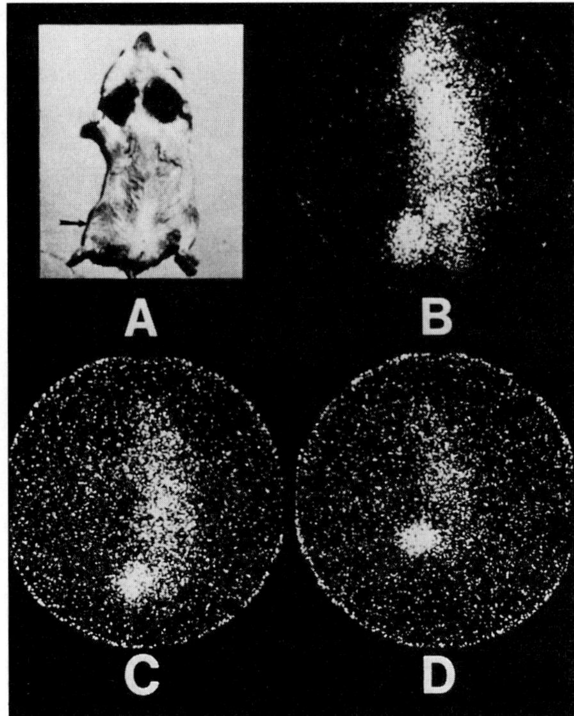

Fig. 27-3. Gamma-camera images of the biodistribution of ^{131}I intact anti-CEA monoclonal antibody following I.V. injection into a Syrian hamster with GW39 human colorectal carcinoma xenograft in the thigh. Note that at 2, 6, and 11 days post-antibody injection there is a gradual decrease in radioantibody levels in the blood, with relative retention in tumor, resulting in improved target-to-background ratios and consequent tumor visualization. (From Wahl, R.L., and others: Improved radioimaging and tumor localization with monoclonal $F(ab')_2$, J. Nucl. Med. 24:316, 1983.)

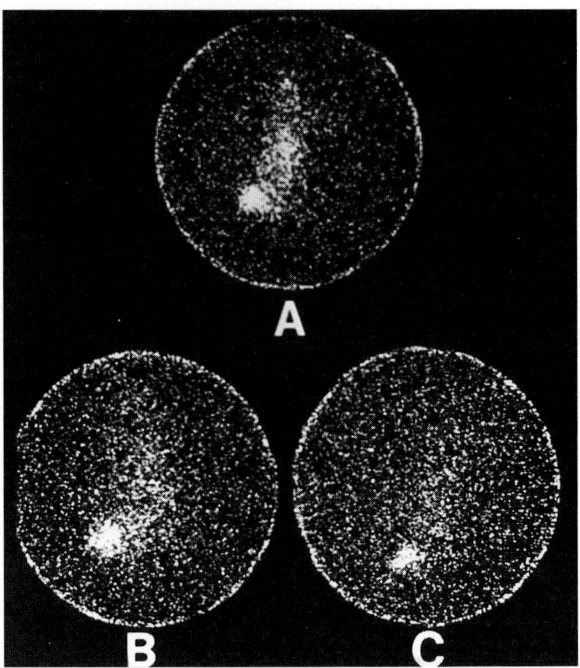

Fig. 27-4. Gamma camera images of the biodistribution of ^{131}I $F(ab')_2$ fragments of anti-CEA monoclonal antibody following I.V. injection into a Syrian hamster with GW39 human colon cancer in the thigh. Note that at 1, 2, and 4 days postinjection, there is more rapid clearance of blood background activity with consequent visualization of the tumor at earlier time points than with the intact monoclonal antibody. (From Wahl, R.L., and others: Improved radioimaging and tumor localization with monoclonal $F(ab')_2$, J. Nucl. Med. 24:316, 1983.)

timal tumor imaging occurs. As will be seen in the discussion that follows, this can result in the necessity for image enhancement techniques to remove background activity. By using antibody fragments, imaging can be successful at earlier time points. Fig. 27-4 illustrates that the $F(ab')_2$ of the same antibody was injected and distinct tumor uptake was seen at much earlier times with less background activity in images at 2, 3, and 4 days postinjection. In addition to earlier imaging, the tumor-to-background ratios are more superior with $F(ab')_2$ than with the intact antibody. Nonetheless, not all antibodies can be successfully fragmented to $F(ab')_2$, and background activity in the bloodstream and elsewhere exists even with fragments. For this reason, background subtraction image-enhancement techniques have been explored. Background subtraction can be used to avoid the problem of the low photon flux that may be present at the 5 to 7 days or more following antibody injection when the tumor-to-background ratios are best. Thus, photon flux is superior early postinjection at a time when there is relatively suboptimal tumor targeting. By using two radioisotopes, background subtraction methods attempt to extract the antibody-specific signal from the background activity caused by residual blood-pool and extracellular-fluid activity. One radioisotope is attached to the specifically labeled antibody; the other radioisotope is attached to a nonspecific protein such as albumin. Generally, the patient is injected with an ^{131}I-labeled specific antibody; then, 1 or 2 days later, the patient is injected with technetium-99m–labeled albumin or red cells that mimic background blood-pool activity. Then using modern gamma cameras and computers, it is possible to simultaneously obtain images of both specific and nonspecific isotopes (by imaging on the ^{99m}Tc and ^{131}I photopeaks) and to then subtract the nonspecific activity from the specific activity. This is a theoretically appealing approach that must be addressed empirically because the antibodies and the albumin are of different molecular size and are injected at different times. Thus only an approximation of background activity is indicated. It is possible to use computer methods to enhance this currently empirical approach. Artifacts can occur, however, if there is excessive excretion of one tracer versus another. For example, excessive iodine excretion in the gut can cause apparent "false positive foci" of uptake that can mimic tumor (Fig. 27-5). For these reasons, as well as dif-

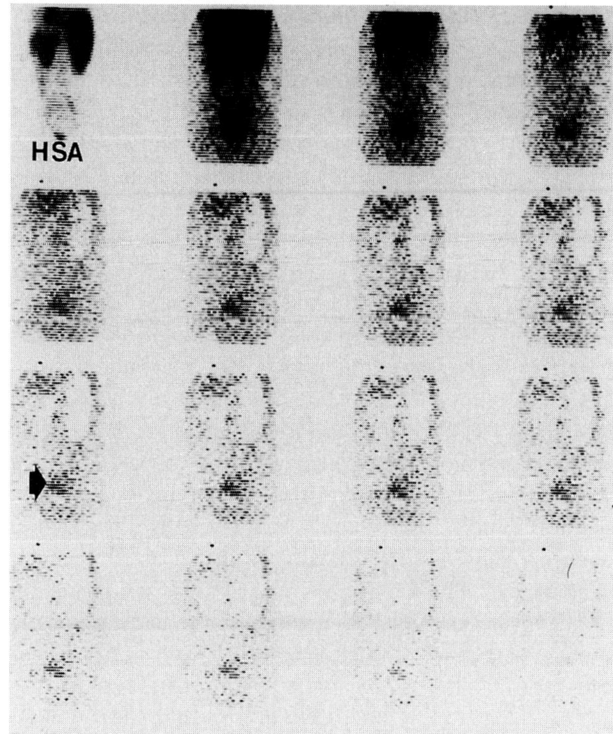

Fig. 27-5. Sequence of background subtraction images of the abdomen of a patient with a history of choriocarcinoma. ^{131}I-labeled monoclonal antibody 5F9.3 was injected I.V. and then ^{99m}Tc human serum albumin. Images of the biodistribution of both photopeaks radioactivity were then obtained. Sequential images show subtraction of varying levels of ^{99m}Tc radioactivity from the ^{131}I image. Increased visualization of activity in the mid abdomen *(arrow)* is seen. In this case, this was excreted iodine activity that was not in tumor but rather in dilated bowel loops. This illustrates that caution must be exercised in the interpretation of dual-isotope images. (From Wahl, R.L.: Radiolabeled monoclonal antibody imaging, Radiology Report 1(3):347-361, 1989.)

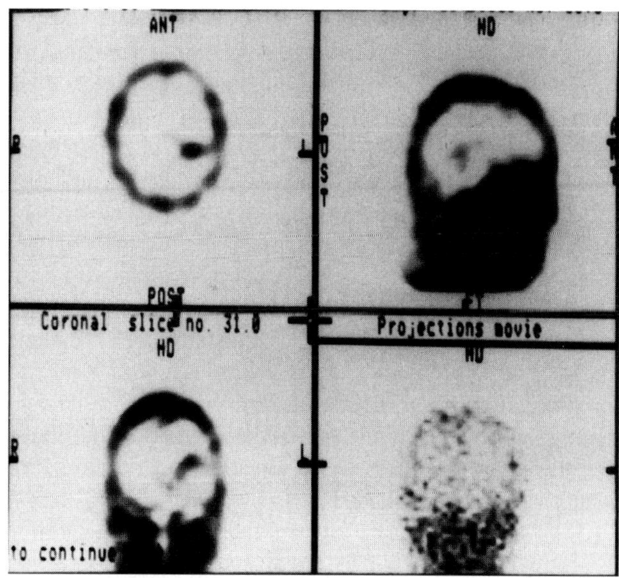

Fig. 27-6. SPECT images at 7 hours after the I.V. injection of ^{99m}Tc Fab anti-melanoma fragments. Clockwise from upper left: transverse, sagittal, anterior projection, and coronal images demonstrating focal antibody uptake in cerebral metastasis of melanoma. (From Wahl, R.L.: Radiolabeled monoclonal antibody imaging, Radiology Report 1(3):347-361, 1989.)

ficulty in implementation, background subtraction is only infrequently performed with current tracers.

Another display system for antibody studies is single-photon emission computer tomography (SPECT) (Fig. 27-6), which is much more commonly applied than is background subtraction. SPECT has the capability of removing overlying background activity through the multiple projections that are obtained. With higher photon flux isotopes such as ^{111}In and ^{99m}Tc now available, it is usually more possible to perform SPECT with labeled antibodies. SPECT appears, in some instances, to be able to better localize foci of tumor uptake, but SPECT can also result in artifacts. In addition, it is somewhat time-consuming to perform SPECT imaging of the entire body. With the availability of "triple-head" gamma cameras, SPECT has proved quite useful if diverted to specific areas of cancer. Although antibodies have been labeled with positron emitters, for the foreseeable future PET is unlikely to contribute substantially to the clinical process of radioimmunodiagnosis (though it represents an interesting area for research) because of the expense of PET cameras. Thus, most antibody imaging is currently performed using either planar or SPECT imaging techniques.

■ ANTIBODY RADIOLABELING

A key aspect of antibody imaging and treatment is the labeling of the antibody. Radiolabeling, for imaging purposes, uses a radionuclide whose gamma energy is suitable for gamma camera detection. Ideally, this radionuclide is lacking in particulate irradiation, and the energy of the radionuclide is appropriate for SPECT imaging. Recent work has suggested that it may be possible to use positron emitters to label antibodies. Regardless of the radiolabeling method, it is essential that the immunoreactivity of the antibody be preserved following radiolabeling. Immunoreactivity is how well the antibody binds to the target antigen before and after labeling. The radiolabeled antibody should bind to the antigen as well, or nearly as well, as the intact antibody did before radiolabeling.

The largest experience in radiolabeling antibodies exists with the use of radioactive iodine. The most common method of radiolabeling is probably the chloramine-T method, in which iodine is oxidized and then electrophilically attacks electron rich rings present on tyrosine or histidine residues. Several other chemical agents can be used to cause oxidation reaction, including iodogen. Iodogen is plated onto the reaction vessel, whereas chloramine-T is soluble and is dissolved in the reaction mixture. The solubility of chloramine-T probably results in superior labeling efficiency, but the sparingly soluble chloramine-T analog, iodogen, has the advantage that separation of unbound iodogen from the reaction mixture is not essential. Other radioiodination methods have also been used, including the Bolton-Hunter method or the lactoperoxidase method. These alternate methods are not used as commonly in radiolabeling antibodies, however. It should be noted that the Bolton-Hunter method attacks amino acid residues other than tyrosine and histidine, particularly reacting with epsilon amino acids such as lysine. In addition, two other methods in which the epsilon amino acids are labeled include the ATE and PIP methods. These latter methods appear to be less vulnerable to deiodination than the more standard iodination methods. Some animal data suggest that this may result in delivery of iodine and retention superior to that of standard iodination methods.

It should be realized that radioiodine bound to tyrosine is somewhat susceptible to deiodination. This deiodination can cause radioiodine to accumulate in the thyroid or to be excreted via the urinary tract. Similarly, gastric excretion will result in gut activity. This nontarget-iodine activity may make tumor detection more difficult, especially if tumor is in the region of these sites. In addition, the methods described for iodination are "randon methods" in that they place radioactivity at random on the antibody molecule. If the label is placed in the region of the antibody binding site, this may cause the loss of antibody activity. This is particularly likely to occur when a large number of iodine molecules are added to the antibody. For many antibodies, radiolabeling with specific activity levels of over 20 mCi (740 MBq)/mg may result in loss of immunoreactivity; this can be highly variable from antibody to antibody, however.

A potential way to avoid loss of immunoreactivity may be through the use of site-specific labeling, although this appealing concept has not been fully evaluated. Site-specific labeling is a method in which a radiolabel is attached to a specific area of the antibody, at some distance from the antigen-combining site. This distance of the radioactive molecule from the antigen-combining region should result in less steric inhibition of antibody combination with antigen. One of these site-directed approaches involves the use of radiobiotin, which binds (via a iodoacetyl linkage) to the sulfhydryl residues on partially reduced antibodies. If the antibody is partially reduced, this can be site-specifically targeted to the heavy-chain, hinge-region antibodies; this may be dependent on the antibody, however. Another method has been recently described, in which site-specific labeling can be achieved through the use of equilibrium transfer alkylation and coupling reagents (ETAC), which bind to the disulfide bond of molecules and preserve the integrity of the antibody molecule by reannealing at the SH bond. Neither of these approaches have been fully investigated in humans. The ^{131}I-biotin/avidin approach has an additional potential advantage in that it may be possible to preadminister the antitumor antibody, allow it time to localize to the tumor, and subsequently administer the radiolabel on the streptavidin or biotin ligand, depending on what the antibody is labeled with. This has been tried in experimental animals and more recently in patients. ^{131}I has a 364-keV gamma ray, a beta emission and an 8-day half-life. In addition, it is not an optimal imaging agent. ^{123}I has a 159-keV gamma ray, a lower radiation dose, and a 13-hour half-life. It is also a better physical match for the short life of antibody fragments, as compared with intact antibody. Unfortunately, despite these advantages, ^{123}I is expensive in the United States and in short supply in many parts of the world. This has limited its use, though in clinical trials it has been quite useful. Its 159-keV energy is also suitable for SPECT, though there can be some contamination of some iodine preparations with ^{124}I, which seriously degrades image quality. ^{124}I, a positron emitter with roughly a 3-day half-life, has been proposed and has been recently evaluated as an agent for imaging with PET.

^{111}In is a radiometal commonly used in nuclear imaging studies, particularly for the labeling of white cells. It has a half-life of 67 hours and gamma-photon energies of 173 and 247 keV that can be imaged with a medium-energy collimator on a gamma camera. Indium can be attached to antibody molecules through use of chelating molecules such as DTPA or related compounds such as benzyl EDTA or "DOTA" (Fig. 27-7). The latter, along with other, more stable ligands under development may be superior chelates. It was initially believed that these labels were firmly attached to antibodies, because the whole-body clearance rate of the radiometal labeled antibody was much slower with iodinated antibodies in general and because the circulating indium activity was only found in the form of antibody bound to indium. Further studies, however, suggest that there is often increased uptake of ^{111}In in the liver, as compared with ^{131}I label when antibodies are given intravenously. Much of the ^{111}In activity seen in the liver is not directly bound to intact antibody but is rather in lower molecular-weight forms. Thus ^{111}In is detached from the whole antibody and stored in the liver as small molecular-weight complexes of ^{111}In bound to chelate and are retained. Species with the molecular weight of intact antibody, indium transferrin, and in the weight range of free indium of ^{111}In-DTPA are present on extracts of radioisotope removed from the liver of rodents. Thus, there is catabolism of the antibody and/or loss of indium from the chelate. Of interest is a recent report indicating that indium is associated with metal chelate when excreted in the urine, suggesting that the phenomenon seen in the liver is due to storage of both indium and low-molecular-weight antibody protein catabolic products. In the kidneys, a similar phenomenon occurs. The retention of radiolabel does not happen with ^{131}I, because ^{131}I activity is only found associated with antibody in the kidneys and liver on tissue extracts. Apparently, ^{131}I that is removed by deiodinase enzymes is

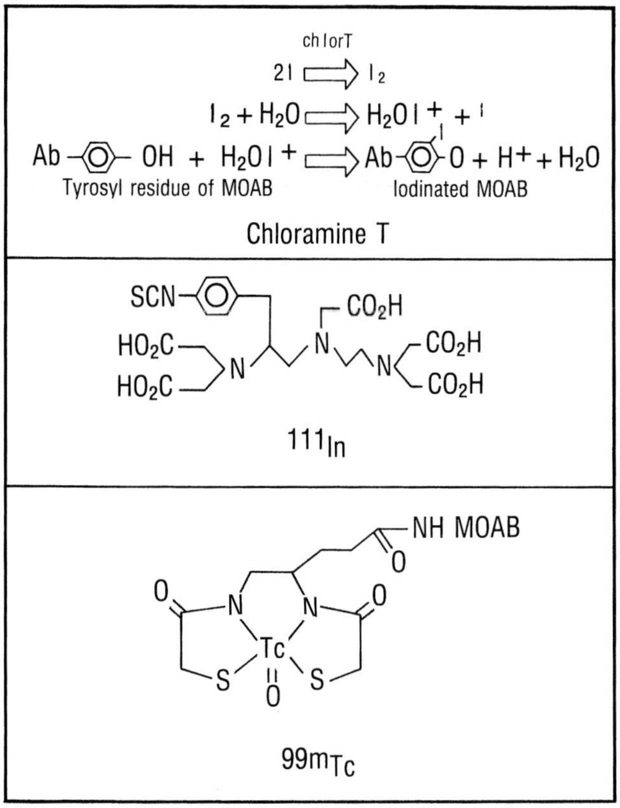

Tyrosyl residue of MOAB

Iodinated MOAB

Chloramine T

^{111}In

NH MOAB

^{99m}Tc

Fig. 27-7. Diagnostic radiolabeling is usually performed with either 123 or 131 iodine, ^{111}In, or ^{99m}Tc. The chloramine T method is probably the most common iodination method, though 131 iodine is not an optimal imaging isotope. ^{111}In can be chelated to antibodies by a molecule such as SCN benzyl DTPA, which generally would be attached to lysyl residues on the antibody molecule. ^{99m}Tc can be attached to antibodies using several approaches; however, coupling via the N2S2 ligand and antibody epsilon amino groups has been studied extensively in the United States in the past several years. (From Wahl, R.L.: Radiolabeled monoclonal antibody imaging, Radiology Report 1(3):347-361, 1989.)

rapidly excreted. Thus this instability of ^{131}I may in some ways be advantageous. Recently, efforts have been made to make ^{111}In behave somewhat more like iodine by having a cleavable linkage present between the indium chelator and the antibody molecule, to facilitate excretion. It should also be noted that there is some hepatic and gut excretion of the indium isotope. With ^{111}In, uptake in the kidneys is also particularly substantial when fragments are used. Although there are problems with indium, particularly the intense liver uptake, image quality with ^{111}In-labeled antibodies is often superior to iodine, except in the liver (because of the high background liver activities). ^{111}In has been shown in patients to be clearly superior to iodine in imaging T-cell lymphoma. It has also been used successfully in the imaging of colon cancer as well as other diseases using anti-CEA antibodies.

Technetium-99m is the most frequently used radioisotope in nuclear medicine because its 140-keV gamma energy, 6hr $T_{1/2}$, and photon flux, are excellent for imaging. The 6-hour half-life of ^{99m}Tc is not well matched, however, to the biologic behavior of intact antibodies; in general, ^{99m}Tc is used with antibody fragments, particularly the shorter-lived Fab fragments. There are several methods for labeling with ^{99m}Tc. One of the methods involves using the N_2S_2 method in which a chelate is formed (Fig. 27-7). This method can produce excellent images, but there is substantial excretion of the ^{99m}Tc activity via the gut; this can make evaluation of the midabdomen difficult. Another method involves the direct attachment of technetium to the sulfhydryl region following partial reduction of the antibody. This approach may result in the formation of smaller antibody fragments, but it appears to cause less hepatic and gut activity than do other methods. Obviously, if antibody fragments are used, there will be more uptake of the antibody in the kidneys and bladder than there will be of intact antibody, because these represent routes of excretion. ^{99m}Tc-labeled antibodies, however, do generally have less background activity in the normal liver than do ^{111}In-labeled antibodies. This property tends to make visualization of isolated liver lesions more possible with ^{99m}Tc than with ^{111}In-labeled antibodies. ^{123}I, ^{111}In, and ^{99m}Tc, unlike ^{131}I, are also well suited to SPECT imaging because of their superior photon flux and dosimetry. Therapy with radioantibodies has generally used ^{131}I or ^{90}Y, though rhenium 86 and rhenium 88 are also under investigation.

■ CLINICAL IMAGING STUDIES

Though most human tumors have been studied in the nude mouse as xenografts or in other animal models, many of the systems in which excellent tumor imaging has been seen in animals have not provided equally good imaging in humans. This may be because of the artificiality of these model systems in which the antibody may be mouse in origin; the host mouse and the tumor human. This and the small volume of blood in rodents stacks the cards in favor of successful imaging in small animals. Though they will not be discussed in this chapter, several key articles on antibody localization in experimental tumors appear in the reference list, which focuses on human applications. Following is a discussion of the clinical applications in which antibody imaging or therapy has been used and appears to be promising.

■ Colon cancer (Fig. 27-8)

Colon cancer is one of the most common malignancies in the Western hemisphere. This tumor has several antigenic determinants associated with it. One of the first recognized was carcinoembryonic antigen (CEA). As discussed earlier, anti-CEA antibodies were used to image colon cancer in mice and hamsters in the early 1970s. Polyclonal antibodies to CEA were used to image colon cancer with excellent success. Most studies have involved the use of monoclonal antibodies; results have generally improved

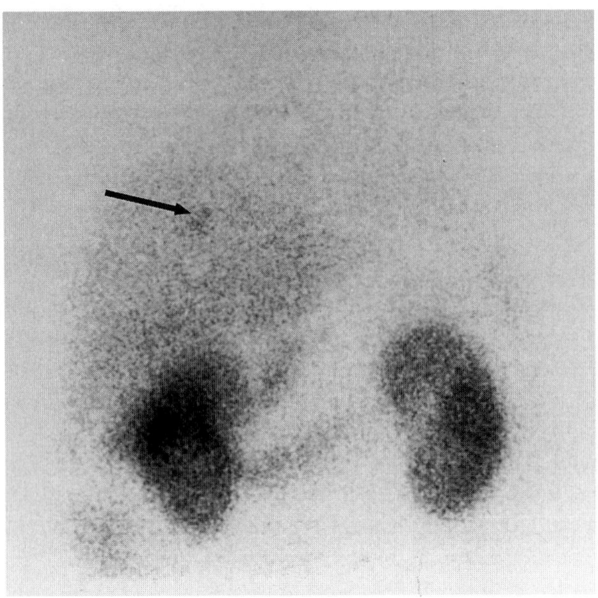

Fig. 27-8. ^{99m}Tc Fab′ anti-colorectal carcinoma imaging study demonstrates focal uptake in a known colorectal cancer.

versus studies with polyclonal antibodies. Successful imaging of colon cancer has now been achieved by numerous groups. Generally it has been shown that anti-CEA Fab or $F(ab')_2$ fragment and ^{123}I label give better results than do polyclonal antibodies with sensitivity of greater than 90%. Several different antibodies have been used labeled with ^{99m}Tc. In Europe, the BW 431/26 intact antibody has been labeled with ^{99m}Tc and used in several studies, with varying results. There are limitations to the use of the ^{99m}Tc intact Mab in imaging, including high blood-pool activity and nonspecific bowel uptake. Focused application of the method to patients with a known diagnosis of tumor and elevated CEA level has been recommended. Haseman and others have reported on an ^{111}In-labeled Mab reactive with CEA, evaluated in the setting of rising CEA level in 146 patients with rising CEA levels, and equivocal or negative CT scans. In this study Mab scanning complemented CT.

While much colorectal cancer imaging has been performed with anti-CEA antibodies, other tumor markers are expressed on colorectal cancers. B72.3 Mab is a murine IgG high-molecular-weight, glycoprotein (MW greater than 1 million) that binds to 90% of colonic, gastric, and ovarian cancers and does not react with normal adult tissue (with the exception of secretory endometrium). The monoclonal antibody B72.3-GYK-DTPA ^{111}In is known as ^{111}In CYT 103 or Oncoscint CR-OV. Recently ^{111}In-labeled B72.3 was approved for clinical use in the United States.

Abdel-Nabi, Doerr, and Collier summarize results from 227 imaged patients suspected of having primary or secondary colorectal cancer. Antibody imaging detected occult tumor lesions in 11 of 92 patients with confirmed adenocarcinoma; the method accurately diagnosed 7 of 10 patients with elevated serum CEA levels and negative presurgical work-ups. Antibody imaging confirmed the absence of distant disease in 18 of 22 patients with isolated recurrences. This study has been recommended in postsurgical patients before second-look surgical procedures and in patients who have questionable nondiagnostic CT scans of the abdomen postsurgery.

In 155 of 169 patients with proven cancer, the Mab scan was 69% sensitive, comparable to CT results, and 77% specific. Computed tomography was more sensitive in detecting liver metastases, as might be expected, but the Mab scan was significantly more sensitive in the anatomic pelvis and the abdomen than was CT.

In another group of patients, one focus of tumor was identified on imaging in 75 to 95 patients shown to have cancer on follow-up, with 79% sensitivity and 84% specificity. Less than 5% of the images were technically inadequate. In the false-positive group of patients, localization was seen primarily in lymph nodes that were positive for CEA by immunohistochemistry. These nodes were in the drainage pathway of the primary tumor.

It has been suggested that aggressive surgical resection of metastatic colon cancer is a means of improving the life span of patients with colon cancer. Five-year survival rates of 33% have been obtained after surgery for local recurrence. Mab staging may be performed before such surgery.

A 39% incidence of human antimouse antibodies (HAMA) has been found in patients who have been imaged with this monoclonal antibody. It is therefore suggested that patients not be reinjected with this antibody until further controlled studies have been completed, though preliminary results suggest that re-injection is safe if there is no HAMA.

■ Melanoma

Melanoma has been a relatively infrequent cutaneous neoplasm, but it is increasing in frequency. When it is diagnosed early, it generally can be cured surgically. Unfortunately, when it disseminates systemically, it is nearly always lethal. Melanoma has been studied extensively using monoclonal antibodies. A variety of antigens that are expressed to a greater extent on melanomas than on normal cells have been defined. The three major antigens are the high–molecular-weight, melanoma-associated antigen, a chondroitin sulfate proteoglycan antigen quite restricted to melanomas and present on about 90% of them; the transferrin receptor antigen, an antigen expressed on rapidly growing cells and found in substantial quantity on many melanomas (also found in substantial quantity on the normal liver); and ganglioside antigens GD-2 and GD-3, found on melanomas and other tumors (such as neuroblastoma) that are somewhat restricted to them. Though the detection rate in the lymph nodes and liver metastases is encouraging, considerable gut uptake of the radioactivity was seen, presumably because of excretion by the hepatobiliary system. For this reason, an evaluation of the central abdomen was made difficult. This probably would make the detection of metastases to bowel difficult. In our study, lung background activity was noticeable, and in the multicenter study the detection of pulmonary metastases was somewhat difficult. Results with ^{111}In-labeled antibodies have been relatively similar, except that the detection of liver metastases did not appear to be as accurate. How antimelanoma antibodies will optimally fit into the management of melanoma patients remains unclear, though such antibodies have been approved for clinical use in parts of Europe. The importance of antimelanoma antibodies is illustrated by the following:

1. Unlike colon cancer, complete resection of isolated melanoma metastases is less often successful, making the optimal initial surgical excision crucial. In this regard, the study by Blend and others using ^{99m}Tc Fab fragments in preoperative staging with a 95% positive predictive value and a 91% sensitivity appears promising. These data suggest preoperative staging and surgical decision-making are a clinical possibility in the melanoma patient.
2. The high detection sensitivity for lymph node metastases is encouraging, but we do not know if antibodies can be used to guide the surgical removal of melanoma metastases before they are clinically apparent (i.e., prophylactic lymphadenectomy).
3. An alternative approach has been used in this situation using subcutaneous antibody delivery (Fig. 27-9). Note that nodal metastases are clearly delineated. Substantial nonspecific background tracer accumulation also occurs in known non–tumor-involved lymph nodes, particularly with ^{111}In as a label or at early times postinjection. Our approach in using an ^{131}I-labeled antimelanoma antibody cocktail (225.28S and 763.24T) administered subcutaneously has been encouraging, with tumor visualization seen. In this setting, we have seen 24 times greater uptake in the tumor-involved nodes than in the noninvolved nodes with 17 patients and over 500 lymph nodes studied, respectively. Controlled trials are necessary before such methodologies could be recommended for adaptation or routine clinical practice. The detection of melanomas involving the eye is also possible using antibodies, though the role of this in managing pigmented eye lesions is as yet not fully established. A recent report on 101 patients with possible ocular melanoma showed a 78% sensitivity and a 94% specificity of immunoscintigraphy with ^{99m}Tc F(ab′)$_2$ 225.28S. It seems apparent that antibody imaging may have a role in the management of melanoma, but this role may be limited to guiding the initial operation until treatment options in melanoma become better.

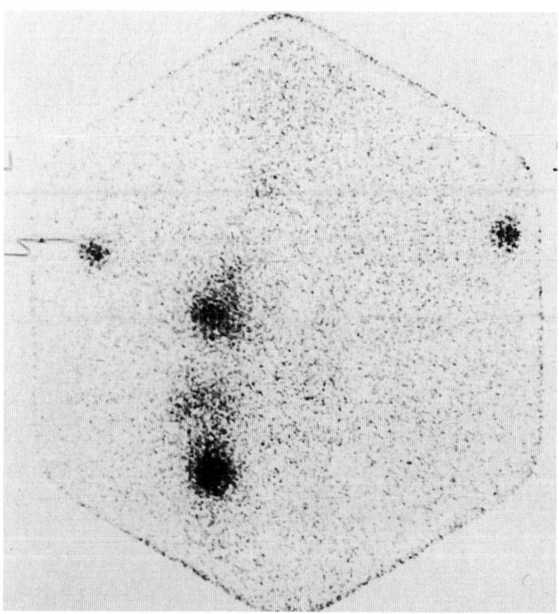

Fig. 27-9. Focal uptake of antimelanoma antibody cocktail, labeled with ^{131}I, in the inguinal lymph nodes of a patient with metastatic melanoma to these nodes. The antibody was injected subcutaneously into the skin of the thigh, below the nodal group. Note the high target-to-background ratio achieved by subcutaneous antibody delivery. (From Wahl, R.L., and others: Lymphoscintigraphy in melanoma: initial evaluation of a low protein dose monoclonal antibody cocktail, Cancer Res. (suppl) 50:941s-948s, 1 Feb. 1990.)

■ Ovarian carcinoma

Ovarian carcinoma, like melanoma, is increasing in frequency. Ovarian carcinoma is highly lethal if it presents as stage three or four disease (extending out of the pelvis). Other diagnostic tests, such as CT scan, are quite insensitive for the detection of ovarian carcinoma, with some studies suggesting that CT scanning is only 40% sensitive in this disease. Ovarian cancer has successfully been imaged using anti-CEA antibodies and background subtraction with polyclonal anti-CEA antibodies. Granowska has demonstrated with ^{123}I-labeled antibody HMFG-2 positive scan patterns in 19 or 20 patients with ovarian cancer and in 5 of 10 without cancer. Thus the technique was sensitive but not specific in their study. Another trial in 16 patients imaged with up to 1 mCi (37 MBq) of ^{131}I antibody showed sensitivity in the 80% range. Imaging with ^{111}In OC-125 F(ab′)$_2$ fragments all showed comparable sensitivities. Since ovarian carcinoma is poorly imaged by CT scanning, particularly in cases of early recurrences when CA-125 antigen levels are increased in the blood, it may be possible that an imperfect test (i.e., one that may be 70% to 80% sensitive for ovarian cancer detection) may still be clinically useful. ^{111}In-labeled antibody B72.3, reactive with the TAG-72 antigen, was recently approved for routine clinical use in ovarian cancer imaging in the United States by

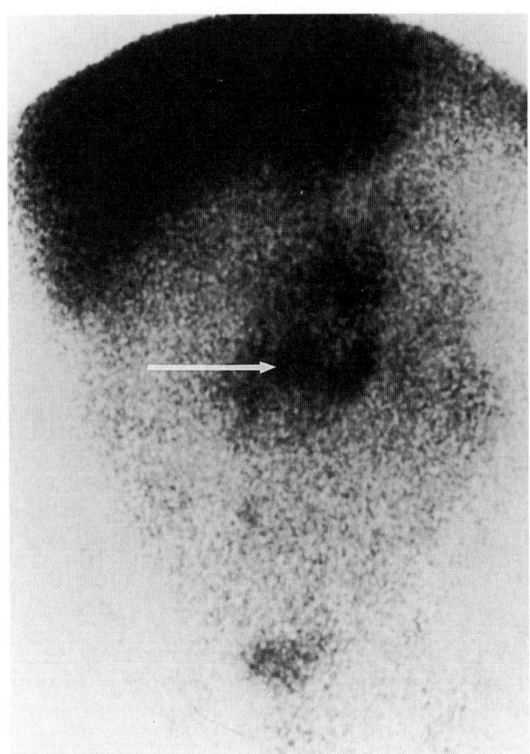

Fig. 27-10. Focal uptake of ^{111}In B72.3 antibody in an intraperitoneal focus of ovarian cancer. Note as well the uptake of the ^{111}In antibody in the normal liver. (Courtesy Cytogen Corp., Princeton, N.J.)

the FDA. The agent was 68% sensitive for ovarian cancer on a per patient basis, but it appears more sensitive than CT, which was 44% sensitive in a series of 103 patients. The alternative to an imaging procedure for evaluation is a diagnostic surgical reexploration. Thus, antibody scanning may have a role in the management of disease by reducing or eliminating the need for reexploration following chemotherapy. An example of an antibody scan in ovarian cancer is seen in Fig. 27-10. Ovarian cancer can also be imaged by the intraperitoneal injection of monoclonal antibodies, because this route of delivery offers substantially more exposure of accessible tumor cells to the therapeutic agent than does intravenous delivery. Several antibodies have also been assessed for therapeutic potential in ovarian cancer.

■ Neuroblastoma

As the most common solid extracranial neoplasm of children, neuroblastoma is an uncommon but disproportionally important disease. This tumor is imaged well using monoclonal antibodies. The antibody 3F8 reactive with the GD-2 antigens has produced excellent images of neuroblastoma. Recent data suggests that the ^{131}I radioantibody is better at lesion detection than is ^{131}I mIBG when given at roughly equivalent patient rad doses. Although the injected doses administered are not comparable, and ^{123}I mIBG is probably a preferable agent, this study suggests that antibodies may be at least as sensitive as mIBG and perhaps more sensitive in the detection of foci of neuroblastoma. Obviously, knowing the exact stage of the disease is important to therapy because these tumors are responsive to treatment. Recently, ^{124}I has been used as a label in these imaging studies because of its excellent characteristics as a positron emitter for the imaging of neuroblastoma. These antibodies to neuroblastoma eventually may assume a role in the clinical management of this infrequent though important tumor; however, more study is necessary. This antibody also has therapeutic potential.

■ Choriocarcinoma

This is also an infrequent tumor, yet it is another of the diseases in which antibody scanning may have a clinical impact. Human chorionic gonadotropin is produced by germ-cell tumors, most commonly by choriocarcinomas; it was used as a target for the localization of an ^{131}I anti-HCG polyclonal antibody as early as 1971 when Quinones and Beierwaltes showed that this antibody localization approach was feasible in hamsters. Several investigators have used anti-HCG antibodies to localize choriocarcinomas in patients who have rising serum HCG levels, with only scars or no known morphologic evidence of the disease recurrence. Although the technique is certainly imperfect, Begent reported on 18 patients in whom the serum HCG level was elevated than in which the site of tumor occurrence was not known to be present. Of the nearly half of the patients (8) with positive antibody scans in whom resection was attempted surgically, 5 had a complete response for up to 5 years of follow-up. There were also two false positive cases in this series, and five false negatives. Similarly antibody uptake in tumor or suspected sites of apparent fibrosis or scar was found when elevated HCG levels are present (Fig. 27-11). Thus, as in colon cancer and ovarian cancer, it appears that with a rising serum marker in a case of choriocarcinoma, an antibody scan may, in some instances, reveal the focus of recurrent disease before other methods. This approach remains under development, however.

■ Lymphomas

Lymphomas are abnormal proliferations of T or B lymphocytes. ^{111}In T101 has been effective in imaging T-cell lymphoma. Similarly, several groups have used ^{131}I MB-1 (anti–CD-37, anti–B-1, anti–CD-20) and other pan B-cell antibodies to image lymphoma (Fig. 27-12). Currently, although imaging these tumors is possible, there is not conclusive evidence that antibody imaging is superior to other methods for disease detection. Lesion detection sensitivities have ranged from 42% to 100% for lesions of $\geq$2 cm in size. Goldenberg and colleagues have recently reported good imaging results in B-cell lymphoma with the ^{131}I- or ^{99m}Tc-labeled LL-2 antibody. Because of their initial nodal involvement, lymphomas (at least T-cell type) can also be

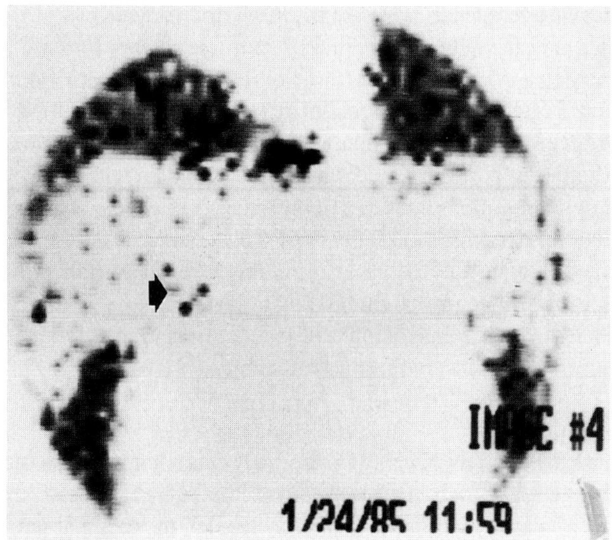

Fig. 27-11. Focal increased uptake of ^{131}I 5F9.3 monoclonal antibody into biopsy-proven choriocarcinoma focus in the upper lung. This tumor is best visualized through the use of the background subtraction technique. This lesion was believed to have represented before scanning a focus of upper lung scarring. (From Wahl, R.L., and others: Dynamic variable background subtraction: a simple means of displaying radiolabeled monoclonal antibody scintigrams, J. Nucl. Med. 27:545-548, 1986.)

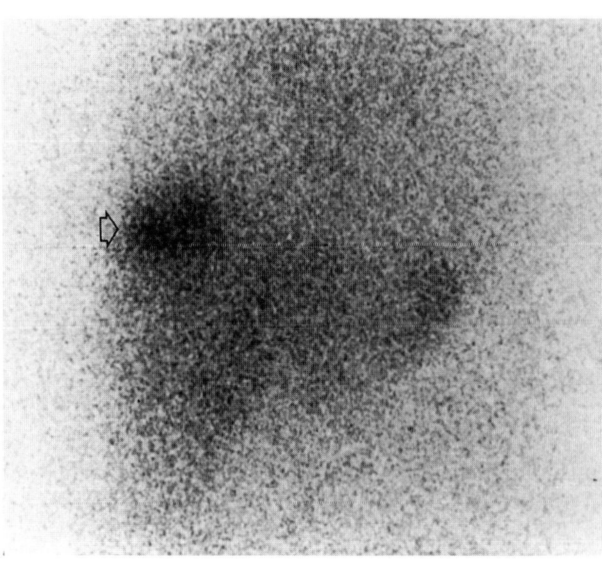

Fig. 27-12. Gamma-camera image of the right upper abdomen of a patient with known focal lymphomatous infiltration of the liver (B-cell lymphoma). The ^{131}I MB-1 antibody had been injected 5 days before this scan. In contrast to indium antibodies, iodinated antibodies tend to have focal increased activity in liver tumors, though higher tumor than liver uptake can also occur with In-labeled antibodies. (From Wahl, R.L.: Radiolabeled monoclonal antibody imaging, Radiology Report 1(3):347-361, 1989.)

imaged by regional antibody delivery; this has been reported by Keenan and others. Recently, Hodgkin's disease and non-Hodgkin's lymphoma have been detected with an ^{111}In antibody to eosinophil peroxidase. The subject of monoclonal antibody use in lymphoma and leukemia is under intense investigation at this time, because in addition to imaging there has been recent progress in the radioantibody treatment of this disease.

■ Breast cancer

Breast cancer is one of the most common of human malignancies. To date, attempts at visualizing breast cancer by intravenous antibody imaging can be met with variable success. ^{131}I antibodies reactive with CEA have been used with success in early studies. ^{111}In B72.3 has also been used, as well as antihuman milk fat globule antibodies and anti-EMA. These studies demonstrate that it is possible to image breast cancers, but they also demonstrate instances in which no tumor visualization is seen. A recent report by Kramer was more encouraging, with 80% lesion detection sensitivity using the Br E-3 antibody. An example of positive tumor visualization using the ^{111}In 103 D2 $F(ab')_2$ antibody appears in Fig. 27-13. When ^{111}In is the label, the same problems seen with other ^{111}In labels remain, especially high liver uptake of the radioantibody. One of the important clinical problems in breast cancer is knowing whether axillary nodes are involved with tumor or not, because this can considerably alter the prognosis of the patient. Specifically, if tumor is present, more aggressive tu-

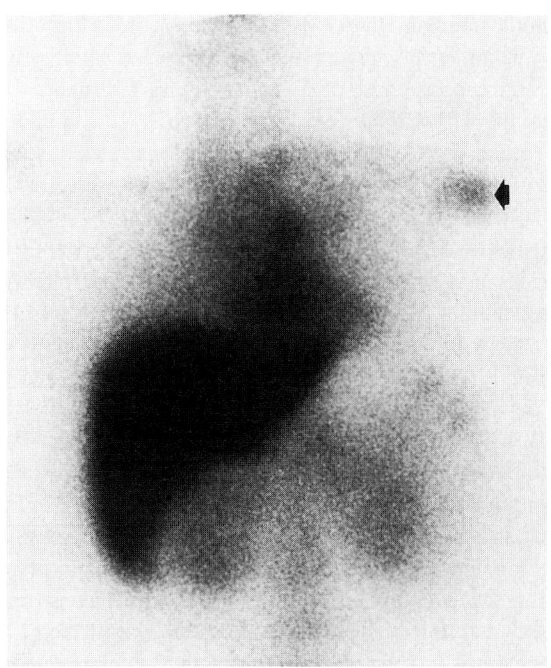

Fig. 27-13. Breast cancer can also be imaged in some cases with ^{111}In antibodies. Here, a brachial plexus metastasis is seen clearly at 2 days following the IV injection of the 103D2 nomoclonal antibody $F(ab')_2$ fragment. (From Wahl, R.L.: Radiolabeled monoclonal antibody imaging, Radiology Report 1(3):347-361, 1989.)

mor therapy such as aggressive adjuvant treatment may be undertaken early in the course of management of the patient. Several attempts have been made to use anti–breast-carcinoma-associated antibodies to image axillary nodal metastases of breast carcinoma, including regional delivery. These approaches have been met with variable degrees of success, but the preliminary data are somewhat more encouraging than are data of intravenous delivery of such antibodies. For instance, subcutaneously injected antibodies have shown increased retention in tumor-involved axillary lymph nodes as compared with normal axillary lymph nodes. Unfortunately, breast carcinoma is an antigenically heterogenous condition, and so far it has been difficult to identify a single antibody that reacts with all breast cancers. Preliminary studies are underway evaluating the C-ErB B-2 gene product as an antigen for breast cancer imaging. In addition, those reagents that do react with all breast cancers tend to react with only a limited percentage of cells from the breast cancer. Thus, finding optimal antibodies for this disease will be very important for antibody imaging to make further progress.

■ Lung cancer

Computed tomography (CT) scanning has recently been shown to be only about 50% to 60% accurate in staging non–small-cell lung cancer. Recently, several results from antibody imaging studies have been presented; these indicate that antibody imaging may have some advantages over CT. Vansant reported on 33 patients with 150 tumor sites using the ^{99m}Tc Fab fragment of NR-LU-10, a murine IgG2b. He showed 100% detection of primary lesions, with 78% of metastases detected. Additional tumor sites not seen on CT were identified in 11 patients. Thus non–small-cell lung cancer may represent a condition in which antibody scanning may offer an improvement over existing methods. Mab scanning has also been studied in small-cell lung cancer, where an overall disease staging accuracy of 88% was seen in 17 patients. Results with antibodies other than this one have been variable, including anti-CEA antibodies and the B72.3 antibody. For example, in 63 patients an ^{111}In–anti-CEA antibody was only about 62% sensitive for detecting mediastinal metastases. For example, using ^{111}In or ^{99m}Tc as a label, only 50% to 62% of tumor sites of small-cell lung cancer were detected. This is also an area of continuing investigation; in the meantime, direct comparison trials of varying Mabs are lacking. The data of Biggi and others are of interest because they show a higher accuracy with anti-CEA in primary lung cancer.

■ Prostatic and renal carcinoma

Prostatic carcinoma is a common cancer that has been successfully imaged in some instances using monoclonal antibodies. Several groups have reported these findings using several reagents. Unfortunately, as with many antibody studies, the detection efficiency is about 70%. Several important diagnostic issues are only partly answered in prostate cancer, including staging the primary staging for lymph nodes involvement with disease to determine operability and to evaluate the response of bony metastases to treatment. Monoclonal antibody lymphoscintigraphy using antibodies to prostate cancer has been undertaken with encouraging preliminary results; more study is necessary, however, to determine the efficacy of the technique. At this time the clinical utility of an ^{111}In antibody reactive with prostate cancer is under extensive clinical trial in the United States. Such reagents, if sufficiently sensitive, could be quite helpful in guiding prostatectomy.

■ Other tumors

Rhabdomyosarcoma is uncommon carcinoma that more frequently affects the young. This tumor has successfully been imaged with the use of radiolabeled monoclonal antibodies reactive with myosin. Apparently, myosin antigenic sites are exposed in this condition, and some nonspecific uptake of the antibody is present. Nonetheless, these tumors can be imaged using monoclonal antibodies, though the role of this technique needs further study in management. Sarcomas have also been imaged with a Mab 19-24, with detection of tumor in 83% of patients. Similarly head and neck cancers have been imaged with Tc-labeled anti-EGFR in 10 patients; preliminary results were good in imaging malignant lesions.

■ Imaging of "nonmalignant" diseases

Radiolabeled antibody imaging of diseases that have antigenically unique phenotypes that are not tumors is feasible and practical. Examples of this include several histologically benign diseases that are medically lethal, such as myocardial infarction. Khaw and collaborators have demonstrated the feasibility of imaging myocardial infarcts using antimyosin antibodies as previously discussed. Myosin becomes exposed when myocardial cells are injured. Their results have suggested that ^{111}In and ^{99m}Tc are both good labels for this study (^{111}In antimyosin is available commercially in Europe). Imaging is generally performed at a day or two after antibody injection. Blood-pool activity can be problematic, but background subtraction and SPECT techniques have been used to allow for earlier imaging. In addition, waiting longer from injection for imaging can be useful. These antimyosin antibodies given intravenously have been reported to have sensitivities for the detection of myocardial infarcts of over 90% with excellent specificity (Fig. 27-14). The agents compare well with ^{99m}Tc pyrophosphate; ^{99m}Tc pyrophosphate can be repeatedly injected. Infarcts are detected as areas of increased focal uptake of antimyosin. It should be noted, however, that the incidence of anti-myosin–antibody responses to the antimyosin antibody have been reported to be quite low. Thus, readministration has been possible with relatively little difficulty in most patients. A potential area of difficulty with antimyo-

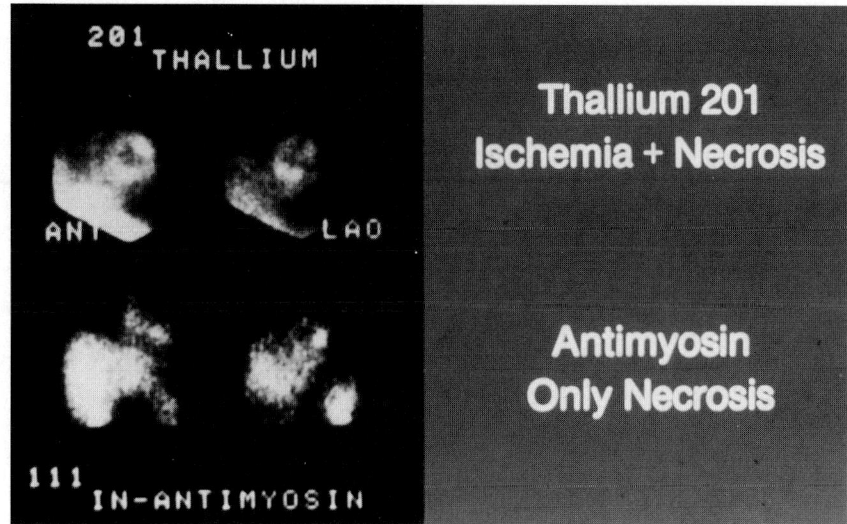

Fig. 27-14. ^{111}In anti-myosin scan of a myocardial infarct. Note focal increased uptake in the infarction. (Courtesy Centocor, Inc., Malvern, Pa.)

sin antibody imaging is that the inferior portion of the heart near the liver can be somewhat more difficult to evaluate than the other walls because of the uptake of radiolabel in the normal liver. An excellent correlation has been observed between ^{111}In anti-myosin–infarct imaging and infarct size. In addition, this antimyosin antibody appears capable of detecting myocardial transplant rejection and chemotherapy drug toxicity. Because the rejection is ongoing damage of heart muscle, there apparently can be increased accessibility of the myosin in rejecting versus nonrejecting hearts. Thus, quantitatively different myocardial uptake values are seen in the rejecting versus nonrejecting patients, at least in groups. This myocyte necrosis is one of the histologic findings used to diagnose rejection and antimyosin scanning; it thus seems to be a rational technique. Thus, the antimyosin scanning technique has potential but requires further study. It appears clear that antimyosin antibodies will have at least a limited role in the clinical practice of nuclear cardiology. It may be that the indium antimyosin scans will be used to evaluate patients whose chest pain has appeared a day or more before the patient arrives at the emergency room for admission, or to evaluate patients in whom other findings are equivocal. The scan may also be used in the transplant patients to follow their myocardial myosin uptake sequentially.

■ Antileukocyte and anticlot antibodies

The production of polyclonal and monoclonal antibodies that bind to fibrin but not fibrinogen has allowed for the imaging of blood clots. A similar approach has also been used imaging platelets that are activated. Rosenbrough and Knight have both shown that a monoclonal antibody reacted with NH_2 terminus of human fibrin could be used to image fresh and older venous thrombi in dogs. This approach is now being tested in human venous thrombosis; the utility in this study is uncertain, however, and it needs further evaluation. This is well reviewed in the reference by these authors. If this technique is effective, it could obviously be very useful, though additional study is clearly necessary. One physiologic advantage in imaging fibrin as opposed to imaging tumors is that the blood flow may be somewhat better in vessels and the access to antigen may be somewhat better for imaging fibrin than it is for tumor detection with antibodies. The area of clot imaging is under intense study, and much progress is expected.

Antibodies reactive with white cells have been used to localize the white cell accumulation in vivo in transplant rejection and more recently in infection. Of interest is that clinical studies with ^{123}I- and ^{99m}Tc-labeled antileukocyte antibodies have shown a sensitivity for lesion or infection detection comparable to that of ^{111}In WBCs. The dosimetry of antibodies with ^{123}I labeling is superior to that with the ^{111}In. It is of interest that an approach using nonspecific human immunoglobulin has shown results that have been almost as good, though it is somewhat difficult to assess how much of the activity in infected lesions is actually due to antibody-specific binding or to altered vascular permeability.

LABORATORY APPLICATION

80

IMAGING: COLORECTAL AND OVARIAN CANCER

Purpose

This new imaging procedure is used to help in determining the location and extent of extrahepatic malignant disease in patients with a known diagnosis of colorectal or ovarian carcinoma.

Indications

1. Elevation of serum CEA or CA-125 with no radiologic evidence of recurrence.
2. Establishment of the sites of localized recurrent disease in patients who are surgical candidates.
3. Evaluation of possible presurgical or postsurgical recurrence of adenocarcinoma with equivocal CT/MRI studies.

Procedure

Materials

1. 5 mCi (185 MBq) ^{111}In chloride, to be administered intravenously
2. OncoScint kit
3. Blood pressure and EKG monitoring equipment
4. Gamma camera with medium-energy collimator
5. 1-mg dose of epinephrine (to treat anaphylaxis)
6. Crash cart
7. 1 mCi (37 MBq) ^{99m}Tc sulfur colloid (optional)
8. Intercath
9. Fleet kit
10. GoLYTELY® (Braintree Laboratories, Inc., Braintree, Mass.) or appropriate cathartic

Patient preparation

1. Explain the entire procedure to the patient. Include a discussion of the potential allergic reactions and other risks of injecting a foreign protein.
2. Obtain a detailed history of allergies and previous exposure murine antibodies (i.e., previous antibody imaging or immune therapy).
3. Record baseline vital signs (temperature, pulse rate, respiratory rate, and blood pressure).
4. Have a 1-mg dose of epinephrine available to treat anaphylaxis.
5. Have a crash cart ready and a physician available at the time of injection.
6. Slowly inject intravenously through an intercath between 4.5 and 5.5 mCi (166 to 203.5 MBq) of ^{111}In Chlor-CYT-103. The entire dose should be injected over 5 minutes.
7. Obtain vital signs at 5, 15, 30, and 60 minutes postinjection.
8. The patient is given a Fleet Kit to use the night before the examination at 72 hours and 96 hours.
9. GoLYTELY® or appropriate cathartic is given the day before imaging (e.g., at 48 hours and following 72 hour images completion).

Technique for planar images

1. The patient is imaged at 72 hours and 96 to 120 hours after 5 mCi ^{111}In OncoScint administration.
2. Set pulse height analyzer (PHA) for indium photopeaks (173 and 247 keV) with a 15 to 20% window.
3. Use medium energy collimator.
4. 128 x 128 matrix
5. Acquisition time 10 minutes.
6. Perform static acquisitions of the chest, abdomen and pelvis (anterior and posterior views).

Technique for SPECT acquisition

1. Image 72 hours post ^{111}In OncoScint administration.
2. Set pulse height analyzer for indium photopeak (173 and 247 keV) with a 15 to 20% window.
3. Use medium energy collimator.
4. 128 x 128 matrix
5. Magnification can be applied as a matter of preference and as determined by patient size, detector size, count density, etc.
6. Acquisition techniques will vary with type of SPECT camera (single, double, or triple head). Suggest under 6° between stops and approximately 40 seconds per stop.

Technique for whole-body acquisition

1. Acquire anterior/posterior images for 30 minutes per image.

Technique for SPECT acquisition (^{99m}Tc sulfur colloid subtraction) (optional)

1. Administer 1 mCi (37 MBq) ^{99m}Tc sulfur colloid.
2. Set PHA at 140 keV (15% window), and a second PHA at 173 and 247 keV with a 15 to 20% window.
3. Follow Steps 3 to 6 in SPECT acquisition.

Technique for processing

1. Reconstruct transverse, coronal and sagittal slices. Change slice thickness to 2. This will improve statistics while providing an acceptable slice thickness for the 128 x 128 acquisition. Type of filter, filter parametrics and sequencing of filter steps are a matter of personal preference.
2. A low pass filter such as a Butterworth with 0.4 Nyquist cutoff and order 7 has produced acceptable images. It is suggested that, in initial attempts, low, intermediate, and high pass filters be utilized on the same data, observing the effects on the final image.
3. When reconstructing ^{99m}Tc sulfur colloid and indium image take care to ensure that slices are matching before subtraction. As determined by your computer system incorporate the processes that will subtract indium or technetium data for the finished image. (optional)
4. Display all images.

Preparation and quality control of ^{111}In-OncoScint Kit Preparation (From package insert, Cytogen Corporation, Princeton, N.J.)

1. One-half hour before the labeling procedure, take the OncoScint kit out of the refrigerator and bring to room temperature.
2. Add 0.5 ml sodium acetate to the ^{111}In-chloride vial. Mix carefully.
3. Inject between 5 and 6 mCi (185 to 222 MBq) of the buffered ^{111}In-chloride into the OncoScint vial. Mix and incubate at room temperature for 30 minutes.
4. Filter the solution with a 0.22-μm filter by attaching the filter to a 10-ml syringe and drawing up the contents of the reaction vial.

Quality control (From Cytogen Corporation, Princeton, N.J.)

1. Materials: ITLC paper, 0.9% sodium chloride, and 0.05 molar DTPA
2. Mix 75 μL of the ^{111}In-OncoScint with 75 μL of 0.05 molar DTPA. Allow to stand at room temperature for 1 minute.
3. Fill a test tube with 0.9% sodium chloride solution to a depth of about 0.5 cm.

Continued.

4. Spot a small drop of the DTPA-treated product onto an ITLC strip 1 cm from the bottom (origin).
5. Place the spotted strip in the solvent.
6. Allow the saline front to migrate 10 cm from the origin (approximately 2 to 4 minutes).
7. Remove the strip and cut in half. Count each half-strip in a gamma counter.
8. Radiochemical purity = [cpm in bottom/(cpm in bottom + cpm in tip)] × 100.
9. To be acceptable for injection, radiochemical purity of the preparation must be greater than 95%.

Key points

With the computer the whole body and upper abdomen SPECT ^{99m}Tc and ^{111}In images are subtracted. ^{99m}Tc sulfur colloid is taken up by the hepatic reticuloendothelial system, which is displaced by metastatic invasion. The ^{111}In Mab and free indium will be concentrated in the entire liver, including the metastatic disease. Subtraction images will reveal the metastatic lesions (^{111}In concentrations or even identify cysts—absent ^{111}In and ^{99m}Tc). The SPECT resolution of a lesion is less than a centimeter; therefore, lesions can be imaged, but CT will always have better resolution than will SPECT. Because ^{111} In Mab is inferior to CT in defining metastatic disease in the liver, the use of ^{99m}Tc sulfur colloid is viewed as optional if additional evaluation of the liver is necessary.

Interpretation and image diagnosis

On 72-hour whole-body and abdominal SPECT images, normal vascularity containing background ^{111}In activity will be visualized (i.e., heart, IVC, portal venous system, and the iliac veins). Residual colon background as well as a left upper quadrant blush (omentum vascularity) may be seen. On 96 to 120 hour images, vascular background activity will diminish as will the left upper quadrant blush.

The liver on the 72 and 96 to 120 hour images will have high concentration. Hepatic metastases will usually have far less concentration of indium than will normal tissue. The relative differences are accentuated on subtraction whole-body and upper abdominal SPECT images, which will define >1-cm hepatic lesions.

Focal abnormal malignant concentrations will be better visualized on 96 to 120 hour images. The peritoneal spread of metastatic disease of colon and ovary will produce a generalized increase in concentration of ^{111}In throughout the lower abdomen.

Nonimaging "probe" studies

Small hand-held radiation-detection probes have been developed and are being increasingly applied to antibody detection at the time of surgery. These probes are more sensitive to low levels of radiation than are gamma cameras. The most extensive studies have been performed by Martin and his colleagues from Ohio State University. They evaluated B72.3 and CC-49, two antibodies reactive with colorectal-cancer–associated antigen TAG 72, mainly in the setting of surgery for primary or suspected recurrence of colorectal cancer. They found the probe to be much more sensitive than the gamma camera, and in recent studies they have detected primary and metastatic lesions with over 85% sensitivity. The surgical approach has been reported to be changed in 30% to 50% of cases based on probe data. False positive results can occur with shed antigen and perhaps in other settings, however, which means appropriate caution must be used in interpreting a positive signal. This same kind of approach has been applied in a pilot fashion in 10 studies to patients with prostate cancer, when a better definition of the location of the tumor in the prostate was possible using an anti-TAG 72 Mab labeled with ^{125}I and the probe. If ^{99m}Tc, and not ^{125}I, is the label, radiation exposure to the surgeon should be monitored in such procedures.

Therapy with monoclonal antibodies

Treatment with radiolabeled antibodies has been reported in several diseases with somewhat encouraging results. The results have been dramatic in lymphoma. In hepatoma, ^{131}I antiferritin antibody has been used to treat hepatomas. Order and his collaborators have detected elevated ferritin levels within hepatomas. They have been treating these tumors with antiferritin antibodies. While the antibody treatment has in many instances been combined with other forms of treatment, it appears that ^{131}I antiferritin antibody can have a beneficial effect on these tumors. Since hepatomas are of the more common tumors worldwide, this methodology has considerable potential significance. Follow-up studies by Sitzmann have shown that radioimmunotherapy plus chemotherapy, radiation therapy, and surgery improves the survival of patients with hepatoma. Just as hepatomas express increased levels of ferritin, so do certain lymphomas such as Hodgkin's disease. This disease has been treated in a limited number of patients using the ^{131}I- and ^{90}Y-labeled antiferritin antibodies. Recent data in cases in which patients received ^{90}Y antiferritin, chemotherapy, and bone marrow transplant have been encouraging.

Several groups have recently investigated the possibility of treating lymphomas using Pan B- or Pan T-cell antibodies. T-cell lymphomas are much less frequent than are B-cell lymphomas. The Pan T-cell antibody T101 labeled with 100 to 150 mCi (3700 to 5550 MBq) of ^{131}I has been used by Rosen and collaborators to treat five patients with cutaneous T-cell lymphoma. Substantial remission of skin and nodal lesions using this technique were introduced, but the remissions were of very short duration (3 weeks to 3 months), and most of the patients developed human-antimouse antibodies. Retreatments were difficult even when plasmapheresis was used in three patients. Nonetheless, very impressive but transient results were obtained. Extensive cell-kill has also been seen in leukemia treatment.

^{131}I antibody to B-cell lymphoma treatment has been used by several groups. DeNardo and others have reported on 18 patients who have received repeated low doses of ^{131}I Lym-1. These low doses can be in the range of 30 mCi (1110 MBq) per dose. They reported that 10 patients had either partial or complete responses. In contrast, an alternative and much more aggressive approach has been taken by investigators at the University of Washington, where very high protein and radioactivity doses of the MB-1 antibody are administered. These doses are followed by bone-marrow transplantation, because the amount of ^{131}I MB-1 antibody given often is myelotoxic. Complete responses in 4 out of 5 patients were seen. We have recently reported our preliminary experience in treating lymphoma with ^{131}I MB-1 antibody at lower doses that are not designed to result in bone marrow aplasia or severe hypoplasia. These data indicate that partial or complete remissions of nonHodgkin's lymphomas are possible with the ^{131}I MB-1 antibody at doses to the whole body of 50 cGy or less. An example of a response to ^{131}I MB-1 treatment is shown in Fig. 27-15. We recently have reported much better clinical results with the ^{131}I anti-CD-20 Mab anti B-1 in 9 patients with nonHodgkin's lymphoma. Six of nine patients had responses; four were complete responses. No toxicity was seen. The treatment of other diseases with radiolabeled antibodies has been less investigated, with results that are less dramatic to date. Intraperitoneal therapy of ovarian cancer has been reported by several

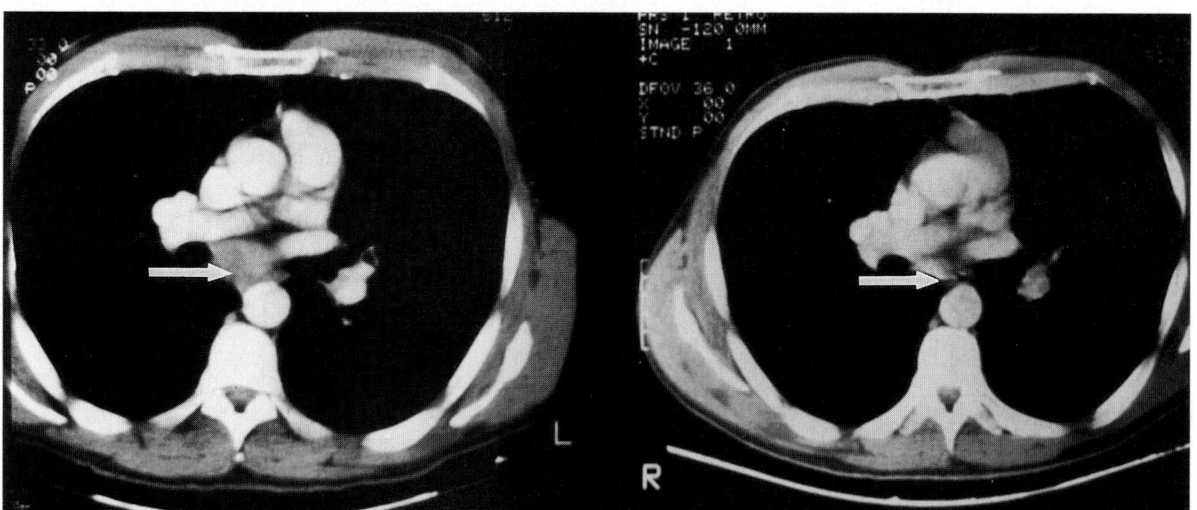

Fig. 27-15. NonHodgkin's lymphoma of the mediastinal lymph nodes before and after treatment with 67 mCi of the I MB-1 antibody. Note the near total disappearance of the subcarinal lymphadenopathy with radioantibody treatment. (From Wahl, R.L.: Radiolabeled antibodies: from research to clinical tool, Decisions in Imag. Econ. 5(4), Fall 1992.)

Continued.

groups, with Stewart and others (1989) having significant experience. They reported on 36 patients treated with ^{131}I Mabs to tumor antigen. Five responses were se with three complete responses in patients with microscopic disease and two partial responses in patients with small nodules. There were no responses in patients with bulk disease. Toxicity with marrow suppression at doses over 120 mCi (4440 MBq) Muto and others observed similar types of toxicity in their study of intraperitoneal therapy in 29 women treated with ^{131}I OC-125 Mab. These studies suggest high-bulk ovarian cancer is very difficult to treat by radioimmunotherapy, but they show some promise for low-bulk disease. Similarly, treatment of melanoma with ^{131}I Fab fragments has not been very successful. Recently, treatment of brain tumor has been performed by regional injection of radioantibody. Papanastassiou and others reported the technique to be safe and possibly effective in seven patients treated with ^{131}I ERIC1 anti-NCAM Mab. Riva studied 10 similar patients, treating them with ^{131}I antitenascin Mab. Three of the patients responded. This is a promising area of research. Very limited data now exists to suggest that some breast cancers can respond to radioimmunotherapy. This area needs much more study, however. The basic problem in antibody treatment is similar to that in antibody imaging: the absolute amount of antibody reaching tumors is low at 0.001 to 0.01% of the injected dose per gram. This low absorbed dose of the tumor, along with relatively high doses to other organs, results in a relatively low therapeutic advantage for the intravenous antibody delivery. Thus far it appears this technique is working in the more radiosensitive tumors of lymphoma/leukemia at surprisingly low radiation-absorbed doses per gram of tumor. Radioimmunotherapy will be a growing area of nuclear medicine research and practice in the next few years.

Conclusion

Antibody imaging is now a clinical reality, but as a clinical technique it still faces several difficulties. The amount of injected intravenously activity that reaches tumors is low. The amount of antibody in background organs is substantial. Thus relatively low target-to-background ratios are present, making detecting small lesions difficult. Second, none of the currently available antibody labels is perfect, with nonspecific accumulation of radioactivity in nontarget organs a problem. Third, tumor antigens are not as tumor-specific as one would like in most instances. And fourth, tumors are difficult to reach by intravenous delivery with antibodies because of the antibody size, relatively poor blood supply, and the limited diffusion into tumors. Despite these concerns, tumor imaging with monoclonal antibodies is not only feasible but appears clinically useful in several situations. As outlined previously, in colon carcinoma, ovarian cancer, melanoma, lung cancer, and choriocarcinoma, antibody scanning may be of great help in selected clinical cases. There certainly are instances in which the scan is the only test positive. This is an extremely difficult clinical situation; it is also possible that antibody scanning will be used before any major surgical procedure being undertaken, as in the case of colon cancer. Whether routine staging with antibodies will become possible (such as staging lymph nodes of breast, lung, or melanoma to determine operability) is still speculative. Additional clinical studies are necessary to evaluate these issues and improve accuracy of antibody scanning in these situations. Radionuclide therapy of tumors using antibodies is now being practiced and may become a routine clinical application in lymphoma. It is also encouraging that imaging of clots is now possible using several different antibodies and that anti-myosin and infection-detecting antibodies appear to be useful imaging tools. The role of these new agents in the routine management of patients with a disease potentially imaged by the agents is not fully resolved. Determining the best use for these agents will take years of study and will depend on the efforts of readers of this text. Similarly, more study of the safety and efficacy of repeat Mab studies if HAMA is present will be of great relevance.

In summary, it appears that monoclonal antibodies have a definite role in the practice of nuclear medicine for the diagnosis of malignant and nonmalignant conditions, as well as for the treatment of radiosensitive cancers. It is expected that this role will expand in the next few years.

REFERENCES

Abdel-Nabi, H., and others: Monoclonal antibodies and radioimmunoconjugates in the diagnosis and treatment of prostate and cancer, Semin. Urol. 10(1):45-54, 1992 (published erratum appears in Semin. Urol. 10(2):139, 1992).

Abdel-Nabi, H.H., and Doerr, R.J.: Multicenter clinical trials of monoclonal antibody B72.3-GYK-DTPA ^{111}In (^{111}In-CYT-103; OncoScint CR103) in patients with colorectal carcinoma. In Maguire, R.T., and Van Nostrand, D., editors: Diagnosis of colorectal and ovarian carcinoma-application of immunoscintigraphic technology, New York, 1992, Marcel Dekker, Inc., pp. 73-88.

Allan, S.M., and others: Radioimmunolocalisation in breast cancer using the gene product of c-erbB2 as the target antigen, Br. J. Cancer 67(4):706-712, 1993.

Andres, R.Y., Schubiger, P.A., Tiefenauer, L., Seybold, K., Locher, J.T., Mach, J.P., and Buchegger, F.: Immunoscintigraphic localization of inflammatory lesions: concept, radiolabelling and in vitro testing of a granulocyte specific antibody, Eur. J. Nucl. Med. 13(11):582-586, 1988.

Arnold, M.W., and others: Intraoperative detection of colorectal cancer with radioimmunoguided surgery and CC49, a second-generation monoclonal antibody, Ann. Surg. 216(6):627-632, 1992.

Arnold, M.W., and others: Radioimmunoguided surgery challenges traditional decision making in patients with primary colorectal cancer, Surgery 112(4):624-629, 1992.

Babaian, R.J., and Lamki, L.M.: Radioimmunoscintigraphy of prostate cancer, Semin. Nucl. Med. 19(4):309-321, Oct. 1989.

Badalament, R.A., and others: Radioimmunoguided radical prostatectomy and lymphadenectomy, Cancer 71(7):2268-2275, 1993.

Balaban, E.P., and others: Detection and staging of small cell lung carcinoma with a technetium-labeled monoclonal antibody: a comparison with standard staging methods, Clin. Nucl. Med. 17(6):439-445, 1992.

Ballou, B., Reiland, J., Levine, G., Knowles, B., and Hakala, T.R.: Tumor location using F(ab')2 mu from a monoclonal IgM antibody: pharmacokinetics, J. Nucl. Med. 26(3):283-292, 1985.

Bares, R., and others: The radiation dose to surgical personnel during intraoperative radioimmunoscintimetry, Eur. J. Nucl. Med. 19(2):110-112, 1992.

Begent, R.H., Bagshawe, K.D., Green, A.J., and Searle, F.: The clinical value of imaging with antibody to human chorionic gonadotrophin in the detection of residual choriocarcinoma, Br. J. Cancer 55(6):657-660, 1987.

Berche, C., Mach, J.P., Lumbroso, J.D., Langlais, C., Aubry, F., Buchegger, F., Carrel, S., Rougier, P., Parmentier, C., and Tubiana, M.: Tomoscintigraphy for detecting gastrointestinal and medullary thyroid cancers: first clinical results using radiolabelled monoclonal antibodies against carcinoembryonic antigen, Br. Med. J. Clin Res. 285(6353:1447-1451, 1982.

Bier, O.G.: Antibodies (Chapter 4). In Bier, Dias da Silva, Gotze, and Mota, editors: Fundamentals of immunology, ed. 2, 1986, Springer-Verlag, pp. 73-114.

Bierman, P.M., and others: Yttrium 90-labeled antiferritin followed by high-dose chemotherapy and autologous bone marrow transplantation for poor-prognosis Hodgkin's disease, J. Clin. Oncol. 11(4):698-703, 1993.

Biersack, H.J., and others: Tc-99m labeled monoclonal antibodies against granulocytes (BW 250/183) in the detection of appendicitis, Clin. Nucl. Med. 18(5):371-376, 1993.

Biggi, A., and others: Detection of suspected primary lung cancer by scintigraphy with indium-111-anti-carcinoembryonic antigen monoclonal antibodies (type FO23C5), J. Nucl. Med. 32(11):2064-2068, 1991.

Blend, M.J., and others: Role of technetium 99m-labeled monoclonal antibody in the management of melanoma patients, J. Clin. Oncol. 10(8):1330-1337, 1992.

Bolton, A.E., and Hunter, W.M.: The labeling of proteins to high specific radioactivities by conjugation to a I-125-containing acylating agent, Biochem. J. 133:529-539, 1973.

Breitz, H.B., Sullivan, J., and Nelp, W.B.: Imaging lung cancer with radiolabeled antibodies, Semin. Nucl. Med. 23(2):127-132, 1993.

Brown, B.A., Davis, G.L., Saltzgaber-Muller, J., Simon, P., Ho, M.K., Shaw, P.S., Stone, B.A., Sands, H., and Moore, G.P.: Tumor-specific genetically engineered murine/human chimeric monoclonal antibody, Cancer Res 47(13):3577-3583, 1987.

Buchegger, F., Haskell, C.M., Schreyer, M., Scazziga, B.R., Randin, S., Carrel, S., and March, J.: Radiolabeled fragments of monoclonal antibodies against carcinoembryonic antigen for localization of human colon carcinoma grafted into nude mice, J. Exp. Med. 158:413-427, 1983.

Buccheri, G., and others: Imaging lung cancer by scintigraphy with indium 111-labeled F(ab')2 fragments of the anticarcinoembryonic antigen monoclonal antibody FO23C5, Cancer 15(4):749-759, 1992.

Carrasquillo, J.A., Mulshine, J.L., Bunn, P.A., Jr., Reynolds, J.C., Foon, K.A., Schroff, R.W., Perentesis, P., Steis, R.G., Keenan, A.M., Horowitz, M., and others: Indium-111 T101 monoclonal antibody is superior to iodine-131 T101 in imaging of cutaneous T-cell lymphoma, J. Nucl. Med. 28(3):281-287, 1987.

Carrio, I., Berna, L., Ballester, M., Obradoe, D., Cladellas, M., Abadal, L., and Ginjaume, M.: Indium-111 antimyosin scintigraphy to assess myocardial damage in patients with suspected myocarditis and cardiac rejection, J. Nucl. Med. 29(12):1893-1900, 1988.

Carrio, I., and others: Assessment of anthracycline-induced myocardial damage by quantitative indium 111 myosin-specific monoclonal antibody studies, Eur. J. Nucl. Med. 18(10):806-812, 1991.

Chao, H., Peiper, S.C., and Philpott, G.W., and others: Selective uptake of specifically purified antibodies to carcinoembryonic antigen of human adenocarcinoma, Res. Commun. Chem. Pathol. Pharmacol. 9:749-761, 1974.

Colcher, D., Zalutsky, M., Kaplan, W., and others: Radiolocalization of human mammary tumors in athymic mice by a monoclonal antibody, Cancer Res. 43:736-742, 1983.

Collier, D.B., and others: Immunoscintigraphy performed with In-111-labeled CYT-103 in the management of colorectal cancer: comparison with CT, Radiology 185(1):179-186, 1992.

Collier, B.D., and others: A practical approach to planar and SPECT imaging of ^{111}In-CYT-102 in diagnosis of colorectal and ovarian carcinoma—application of immunoscintigraphic technology, edited by Maguire, R.T., and Van Nostrand, D., New York, 1992, Marcel Dekker, Inc., pp. 191-210.

Corstens, F.H., Oyen, W.J., and Becker, W.S.: Radioimmunoconjugates in the detection of infection and inflammation, Semin. Nucl. Med. 23(2):148-164, 1993.

del Rosario, R.B., and Wahl, R.L.: Site-specific radiolabeling of monoclonal antibodies with biotin/avidin, Nucl. Med. Biol. 16(5):525-529, 1989.

Delaloye, B., Bischof-Delaloye, A., Buchegger, F., von-Fliedner, V., Grob, J.P., Volant, J.C., Pettavel, J., and Mach, J.P.: Detection of colorectal carcinoma by emission-computerized tomography after injection of I-123-labeled Fab or F(ab')2 fragments from monoclonal anticarcinoembryonic antigen antibodies, J. Clin. Invest. 77(1):301-311, 1986.

DeLand, F.H., Kim, E.E., Primuas, F.J., Dine, M.E., and Goldenberg, D.M.: In vivo radioimmunodetection of occult recurrent colonic carcinoma, Am. Roentgenol. Ray Society 138:145-148, 1982.

DeLand, F.H., Goldenberg, D.M.: In vivo radioimmunological lymphoscintigraphy in cancer: the implications of positive findings, J. Can. Assoc. Radiol. 33(1):4-9, March 1982.

DeNardo, S.J., DeNardo, G.L., O'Grady, L.F., Macey, D.J., Mills, S.L., Epstein, A.L., Peng, J.S., and McGahan, J.P.: Treatment of a patient with B-cell lymphoma by I-131 LYM-1 monoclonal antibodies, Int. J. Biol. Markers 2(1):49-53, 1987.

DeNardo, G.L., and others: Fractionated radioimmunotherapy of B-cell malignancies with ^{131}I-Lym-1, Cancer Res. 1:50(3 suppl):1014S-1016S, 1990.

Deshpande, S.V., Subramanian, R., McCall, M.J., DeNardo, S.J., DeNardo, G.L., and Meares, C.F.: Metabolism of indium chelates attached to monoclonal antibody: minimal transchelation of indium from benzyl-EDTA chelate in vivo, J. Nucl. Med. 31(2):218-224, 1990.

Dillman, R.O., Beauregard, J.C., Sobol, R.E., Royston, I., Bartholomew, R.M., Hagan, P.S., and Halpern, S.E.: Lack of radioimmunodetection and complications associated with monoclonal anticarcinoembryonic antigen antibody: cross-reactivity with an antigen on circulating cells, Cancer Res. 44:2213-2218, 1984.

Ehrlich, P.: The collected papers of Paul Ehrlich. In Himmelweit, F., editor: Immunology and cancer research, vol. 2, London, 1957, Pergammon Press.

Engelstad, B.L., Spitler, L.E., Del-Rio, M.J., Ramos, E.C., Rosendorf, L.L., Reinhold, C.E., Khentigan, A., Huberty, J.P., Corpuz, S.W., Lee, H.M., and others: Phase 1 immunolymphoscintigraphy with an In-111-labeled antimelanoma monoclonal antibody, Radiology 161(2):419-422, 1986.

Fig, L.M., Von Moll, L., Brown, R., and others: Noninvasive diagnosis of axillary node metastases with monoclonal antibody lymphoscintigraphy, Radiology (P)173:419, November 1989.

Fotiou, S., Skarlos, D., Tserkezoglou, A., Aravantinos, G., Malamitsi, J., and Koutoulidis, K.: Monoclonal antibodies in ovarian tumor imaging, Eur. J. Gynaecol. Oncol. 9(4):304-307, 1988.

Fraker, P.J., and Speck, J.C.: Protein and cell membrane iodinations with a sparingly soluble chloroamide, 1,3,4,6-tetrachloro-3, 6-diphenylglycoluril, Biochem. Biophys. Res. Commun. 80:849-857, 1978.

Fritzberg, A.R., Abrams, P.G., Beaumier, P.L., Kasina, S., Morgan, A.C., Rao, T.N., Reno, J.M., Sanderson, J.A., Srinivasan, A., Wilbur, D.E., and others: Specific and stable labeling of antibodies with technetium-99m with a diamide dithiolate chelating agent, Proc. Natl. Acad. Sci. USA 85(11):4025-4029, 1988.

Gallup, D.G.: Multicenter clinical trial of ^{111}In-CYT-103 in patients with ovarian cancer. In Maguire, R.T., and Van Nostrand, D., editors: Diagnosis of colorectal and ovarian carcinoma-application of immunoscintigraphic technology, New York, 1992, Marcel Dekker, Inc., pp. 111-124.

Gold, P., and Freedman, S.O.: Specific carcinoembryonic antigens of the human digestive system, J. Exp. Med. 122:467+, 1965.

Goldenberg, D.M., DeLand, F.H., Kim, E.E., and others: Use of radiolabelled antibodies to a carcinoembryonic antigen for the detection and localization of diverse cancers by external photoscanning, N. Engl. J. Med. 298:1384-1388, 1978.

Goldenberg, D.M., Kim, E.E., DeLand, F., and others: Clinical studies on the radioimmunodetection of tumors containing alpha-fetoprotein, Cancer 45(10):2500-2505, 1980.

Goldenberg, D.M., Kim, E.E., DeLand, F.H., van Nagell, J.R., and Javadpour, N.: Clinical radioimmunodetection of cancer with radioactive antibodies to human chorionic gonadotropin, Science 208:1284-1286, 1980.

Goldenberg, D.M., Kim, E.E., DeLand, F.H., Bennett, S., and Primus, F.J.: Radioimmunodetection of cancer with radioactive antibodies to carcinoembryonic antigen, Cancer Res. 40(8 Pt 2):2984-2992, Aug. 1980.

Goldenberg, D.M., DeLand, F.H., Bennett, S.J., and others: Radioimmunodetection of prostatic cancer: in vivo use of radioactive antibodies against prostatic acid phosphatase for diagnosis and detection of prostatic cancer by nuclear imaging, JAMA 250(5):630-635, Aug 5 1983.

Goldenberg, D.M., and others: Clinical studies of cancer radioimmunodetection with carcinoembryonic antigen monoclonal antibody fragments labeled with ^{123}I or ^{99m}Tc, Cancer Res. 1:50(3 suppl):909S-921S, 1990.

Goldenberg, D.M., and others: Targeting, dosimetry, and radioimmunotherapy of B-cell lymphomas with iodine-131-labeled LL2 monoclonal antibody, J. Clin. Oncol. 9(4):548-564, 1991.

Goodwin, D.A.: Pharamockinetics and antibodies, J. Nucl. Med. 28:1358-1362, 1987.

Granowska, M., Britton, K.E., Shepherd, J.H., Nimmon, C.C., Mather, S., Ward, B., Osborne, R.J., and Slevin, M.L.: A prospective study of I-123 labeled monoclonal antibody imaging in ovarian cancer, J. Clin. Oncol. 4(5):730-736, 1986.

Greager, J.A., and others: Localization of human sarcoma with radiolabeled monoclonal antibody—a follow-up report, Cancer Immunol. Immunother. 33(5):341-345, 1991.

Haber, E.: In vivo diagnostic and therapeutic uses of monoclonal antibodies in cardiology, Ann. Rev. Med. 37:249-261, 1986.

Hach, A., and others: The clinical relevance of anti-CEA immunoscintigraphy with the ^{99m}Tc-labelled monoclonal antibody BW 431/26: a critical assessment after 119 studies, Rofo. Fortschr. Geb. Rontgenstr. Neuev. Bildget. Berfahr. 157(1):3-10, 1992.

Halpern, S.E., Haindl, W., Beauregard, J., Hagan, P., Clutter, M., Amox, D., Merchant, B., Unger, M., Mongovi, C., Bartholomew, R., and others: Scintigraphy with In-111-labeled monoclonal antitumor antibodies: kinetics, biodistribution, and tumor detection, Radiology 168(2):529-536, 1988.

Haseman, M.K., and others: Radioimmunodetection of occult carcinoembryonic antigen-producing cancer, J. Nucl. Med. 33(10):1750-1756, 1992.

Hatch, K.D., Mann, W.J., Boots, L.R., Tauxe, W.N., Shingleton, H.M., and Buchina, E.S.: Localization of choriocarcinoma by I-131-HCG antibody, Gynecol. Oncol. 10:253-261, 1980.

Hellstrom, K.E., and Helstrom, I.: Monoclonal anti-melanoma antibodies and their possible clinical use. (Chapter 2). In Balwin, R.W., and Byers, V.S., editors: Monoclonal antibodies for cancer detection and therapy, 1985, Academic Press, pp. 17-51.

Herlyn, D., Powe, J., Alavi, A., Mattis, J.A., Herlyn, M., Ernst, C., Vaum, R., and Koprowski, H.: Radioimmunodetection of human tumor xenografts by monoclonal antibodies, Cancer Res. 43(6):2731-2735, 1983.

Himmelsbach, M., and Wahl, R.L.: Sizing chromatographic evaluation of the in vivo fate of In-111 antibodies: preliminary evaluation, J. Nucl. Med. 29(5):923, 1988.

Hnatowich, D.J., Childs, R.L., Lanteigne, D., and Najafi, A.: The preparation of DTPA-coupled antibodies radiolabeled with metallic radionuclides: an improved method, J. Immunol. Method. 65:147-157, 1983.

Hnatowich, D.J., Virzi, F., and Ruschowski, M.: Investigations of avidin and biotin for imaging applications, J. Nucl. Med. 28:1294-1302, 1987.

Hoffer, P.G., Lathrup, K., and Bekerman, G.: Use of I-131-CEA antibody as a tumor scanning agent, J. Nucl. Med. 15:323-327, 1974.

Hsu, S.M., Raine, L., and Fanger, H.: A comparative study of the peroxidase-antiperoxidase method and an avidin-biotin complex method for studying polypeptide hormones with radioimmunoassay antibodies, Am. J. Clin. Pathol. 75(5):734-738, 1981.

Hunter, W.M., and Greenwood, F.C.: Preparation of iodine-131 labelled growth hormone of high specific activity, Nature 194:494-496, 1962.

Huse, W.D., Sastry, L., Iverson, S.A., and others: Generation of a large combinational library of the immunoglobulin repertoire in phage lambda, Science 246(4935):1275-1281, 1989.

Kalofonos, H.P., Pawlikowska, T.R., Hemingway, A., and others: Antibody guided diagnosis and therapy of brain gliomas using radiolabeled monoclonal antibodies against epidermal growth factor receptor and placental alkaline phosphatase, J. Nucl. Med. 30(10):1636-1645, 1989.

Kairemo, K.J.: Immunolymphoscintigraphy with ^{99m}Tc-labeled monoclonal antibody (BW 431/26) reacting with carcinoembryonic antigen in breast cancer, Cancer Res. 50(3 suppl):949S-954S, 1990.

Kairemo, K.J., Wiklund, T.A., Liewendahl, K., and others: Imaging of soft-tissue sarcomas with indium-111-labeled monoclonal antimyosin Fab fragments, J. Nucl. Med. 31(1):23-31, 1990.

Kaminski, M.S., and others: Imaging, dosimetry, and radioimmunotherapy with iodine 131-labeled anti-CD37 antibody in B-cell lymphomas, J. Clin. Oncol. 10(11):1696-1711, 1992.

Kaminski, M.S., and others: Radioimmunotherapy of B-cell lymphoma with ^{131}I anti-B1 (anti-CD20) antibody, N. Engl. J. Med. 329(7):459-465, 1993.

Keenan, A.M.: Immunolymphoscintigraphy, Semin. Nucl. Med. 19(4): 322-331, 1989.

Keenan, A.M., Weinstein, J.N., Carrasquillo, J.A., Bunn, P.A., Jr., Reynolds, J.C., Foon, K.A., Smarte, N.C., Ghosh, B., Fejka, R.M., Larson, S.M., and others: Immunolymphoscintigraphy and the dose dependence of In-111 labeled T-101 monoclonal antibody in patients with cutaneous T-cell lymphoma, Cancer Res. 47(22):6093-6099, 1987.

Khaw, B.A., Beller, G.A., Haber, E., and Smith, T.W.: Localization of cardiac myosin-specific antibody in myocardial infarction, J. Clin. Invest. 58:439-446, 1976.

Khaw, B.A., Yasuda, T., Gold, H.K., Leinbach, R.C., Johns, J.A., Kane, M., Bariai-Kovach, M., Strauss, H.W., and Haber, E.: Acute myocardial infarct imaging with indium-111 labeled monoclonal antimyosin Fab, J. Nucl. Med. 28(11):1671-1678, 1987.

Kilbourn, M.R., Dence, C.S., Welch, M.J., and Mathias, C.J.: Flourine-18 labeling of proteins, J. Nucl. Med. 28(4):462-470, April 1987.

Knight, L.C., Maurer, A.H., Ammar, I.A., Shealy, D.J., and Mattis, J.A.: Evaluation of indium-111 labeled anti-fibrin antibody for imaging vascular thrombi, J. Nucl. Med. 29(4):494-502, 1988.

Kohler, G., and Milstein, C.: Continuous cultures of fused cells secreting antibody of predefined specificity, Nature 256(5517:495-497, 1975.

Kozak, R.W., Waldman, T.A., Atcher, R.W., and Gansow, O.A.: Radionuclide-conjugated monoclonal antibodies: a synthesis of immunology, inorganic chemistry and nuclear science, Trends Biotechnol. 4(10):259-264, 1985.

Kramer, E.L., and others: Radioimmunolocalization of metastatic breast carcinoma using indium-111-methyl benzyl DTPA BrE-3 monoclonal antibody: phase I study, J. Nucl. Med. 34(7):1067-1074, 1993.

Krejcarek, G.E., and Tucker, K.L.: Covalent attachment of chelating groups to macromolecules, Biochem. Biophys. Res. Commun. 77(2):581-585, 1977.

Krishnamurthy, S., Krishnamurthy, G.T., Morris, J.M., and others: Concentration of In-111 anti CEA ZCE 025 monoclonal antibody by primary lung cancer, J. Nucl. Med. 30(5):905, 1989.

Krizan, Z., Murray, J.L., Hersh, E.M., Rosenblum, M.G., Glenn, H.J., Gschwind, C.R., and Carlo, D.J.: Increased labeling of human melanoma cells in vitro using combinations of monoclonal antibodies recognizing separate cell surface antigenic determinants, Cancer Res. 45(10):4904-4909, 1985.

Lan, M.S., Bast, R.C., Jr., Colnaghi, M.I., and others: Co-expression of human cancer-associated epitopes on mucin molecules, Int. J. Cancer 39(1):68-72, 1987.

Larson, S.M., Brown, J.P., Wright, P.W., Carrasquillo, J.A., Hellstrom, I., and Hellstrom, K.E.: Imaging of melanoma with I-131-labeled monoclonal antibodies, J. Nucl. Med. 24(2):123-129, 1983.

Larson, S.M., Carrasquillo, J.A., Krohn, K.A., Brown, J.P., McGuffin, R.W., Ferens, J.M., Graham, M.M., Hill, L.D., Beaumier, P.L., Hellstrom, K.E., and others: Localization of I-131-labeled p97-specific Fab fragments in human melanoma as a basis for radiotherapy, J. Clin. Invest. 72(6):2101-2114, 1983.

Larson, S.M., and others: PET scanning of iodine-124-3F9 as an approach to tumor dosimetry during treatment planning for radioimmunotherapy in a child with neuroblastoma, J. Nucl. Med. 33(11):2020-2023, 1992.

Leroy, M., Teillac, P., Rain, J.D., Saccavini, J.C., Le Duc, A., and Najean, Y.: Radioimmunodetection of lymph node invasion in prostatic cancer: the use of iodine 123 (^{123}I)-labeled monoclonal anti-prostatic acid phosphatse (PAP) 227 A F(ab')2 antibody fragments in vivo, Cancer 64(1):1-5, July 1, 1989.

Liebert, M., Laino, L., and Wahl, R.L.: A semi-automated fluorescent (SAF) assay using viable, whole cells for screening hybridomas supernatants, J. Immunol. Method. 101:85-90, 1987.

Lloyd, K.O.: Human tumor antigens: targets for mouse monoclonal antibodies. In Vogel, C.W., editor: Immunoconjugates Antibody Conjugates in Radioimaging and Therapy of Cancer, New York, 1987, Oxford University Press, pp. 8-27.

Locher, J.T., Seybold, K., Andres, R.Y., Schubiger, P.A., Mach, J.P., and Buchegger, F.: Imaging of inflammatory and infectious lesions after injection of radioiodinated monoclonal anti-granulocytes antibodies, Nucl. Med. Commun. 7(9):659-670, Sept. 1986.

Mach, J.P., Carrel, S., Merenda, C., and Sordat, B.: In vivo localization of radiolabeled antibodies to carcinoembryonic antigen in human colon carcinoma grafted into nude mice, Nature 248:704-706, 1974.

Mach, J.P., Carrel, S., Forni, M., Ritschard, J., Donath, A., and Alberto, P.: Tumor localization of radiolabeled antibodies against carcinoembryonic antigen in patients with carcinoma, N. Engl. J. Med. 303:5-10, 1980.

Macmillan, C.H., and others: Immunoscintigraphy of small-cell lung cancer: a study using technetium and indium labelled anti-carcinoembryonic antigen monoclonal antibody preparations, Br. J. Cancer 67(6):1391-1394, 1993.

Mandeville, R., Pateisky, N., Phillipp, K., Kubista, E., Dumas, F., and Grouix, B.: Immunolymphoscintigraphy of axillary lymph node metastases in breast cancer patients using monoclonal antibodies: first clinical findings, Anticancer Res. 6(6):1257-1263, Nov.-Dec. 1986.

Manspeaker, P., Weisman, H.F., and Schaible, T.F.: Cardiovascular applications: current status of immunoscintigraphy in the detection of myocardial necrosis using antimyosin (R11D10) and deep venous thrombosis using antifibrin (T2GIs), Semin. Nucl. Med. 23(2):133-147, 1993.

Martin, D.T., and others: Intraoperative radioimmunodetection of colorectal tumor with a hand-held radiation detector, Am. J. Surg. 150(6):672-675, 1985.

McLoud, T.C., Kosiuk, J.P., Templeton, P.A., and others: CT in the staging of bronchogenic carcinoma: update of analysis by correlative lymph node mapping and sampling, Radiology 173(P):69, 1989.

Meares, C.F.: Chelating agents for the binding of metal ions to antibodies, Nucl. Med. Biol. 13(4):311-318, 1985.

Miraldi, F.D., Nelson, A.D., Kraly, C., Ellery, S., Landmeier, B., Coccia, P.F., Standjord, S.E., Cheung, N.K.: Diagnostic imaging of human neuroblastoma with radiolabeled antibody, Radiology 161(2):413-418, 1986.

Murray, J.L., Rosenblum, M.G., Lamki, L., Glenn, H.J., Krizan, Z., and others: Clinical parameters related to optimal tumor localization of Indium-111-labeled mouse antimelanoma monoclonal antibody ZME-018, J. Nucl. Med. 28(1):25-33, 1987.

Murthy, S., and others: Lymphoma imaging with a new technetium-99m labelled antibody, LL2, Eur. J. Nucl. Med. 19(6):394-401, 1992.

Muto, M.G., and others: Intraperitoneal radioiummunotherapy of refractory ovarian carcinoma utilizing iodine-131-labeled monoclonal antibody OC125, Gynecol. Oncol. 45(3):265-272, 1992.

Muxi, A., and others: Radioimmunoscintigraphy of colorectal carcinoma with a ^{99m}Tc-labelled anti-CEA monoclonal antibody (BW 431/26), Nucl. Med. Commun. 13(4):261-270, 1992.

Nelp, W.B., Eary, J.F., Jones, R.F., Hellstrom, K.E., Hellstrom, I., Beaumier, P.L., and Krohn, K.A.: Preliminary studies of monoclonal antibody lymphoscintigraphy in malignant melanoma, J. Nucl. Med. 28(1):34-41, 1987.

Nisonoff, A., Markus, G., Iwssler, F.C., and others: Separation of univalent fragments of rabbit antibody by reduction of disulfide bonds, Arch. Biochem. 89:230-244, 1960.

Oosterwijk, E., and others: Antibody localization in human renal cell carcinoma I study of monoclonal antibody G250, J. Clin. Oncol. 11(4):738-750, 1993.

Order, S.E., Klein, J.L., Leichner, P.K., Ettinger, D.S., Kopher, K., Finney, K., Surdyke, M., and Leibel, S.A.: Radiolabeled antibody in the treatment of primary and metastatic liver malignancies, Recent Results Cancer Res. 100:307-314, 1986.

Oredipe, O.A., and others: Limits of sensitivity for the radioimmunodetection of colon cancer by means of a hand held gamma probe, Int. J. Rad. Appl. Instrum. (b) 15(6):595-603, 1988.

Oyen, W.J., and others: Diagnosis of bone, joint, and joint prosthesis infections with In-111-labeled nonspecific human immunoglobulin G scintigraphy, Radiology 182(1):195-199, 1992.

Paik, C.H., Quadri, S.M., and Reba, R.C.: Interposition of different chemical likages between antibody and ^{111}In-DTPA to accelerate clearance from non-target organs and blood, Int. J. Rad. Appl. Instrum. 16(5):475-481, 1989.

Papanastassiou, V., and others: Treatment of recurrent and cystic malignant gliomas by a single intracavity injection of ^{131}I monoclonal antibody: feasibility, pharmacokinetics and dosimetry, Br. J. Cancer 67(1):144-151, 1993.

Peltier, P., and others: Correlative imaging study in the diagnosis of ovarian cancer recurrences, The INSERM Research Newwork (Nantes, Rennes, Reims, Villejuif, Saclay), France, Eur. J. Nucl. Med. 19(12):1006-1010, 1992.

Planting, A., and others: Radioimmunodetection in rhabdo- and leiomyosarcoma with ^{111}In-anti-myosin monoclonal antibody complex, Cancer Res. 1:50(3 suppl):955S-957S, 1990.

Porter, R.R.: The hydrolysis of rabbit gamma globulin and antibodies with crystalline papain, Biochem. J. 73:119, 1959.

Powe, J., Pak, K.Y., Paik, C.H., Steplewski, Z., Ebbert, M.A., Herlyn, D., Ernst, C., Alavi, A., Eckelman, W.C., Reba, R.C., and others: Labeling monoclonal antibodies and F(ab')2 fragments with (In-111) Indium using cyclic DTPA anhydride and their in vivo behavior in mice bearing human tumor xenografts, Cancer Drug Deliv. 1(2):125-135, 1984.

Powers, T., Johnson, D., McCook, B., and others: Staging of carcinoma of the lung with Tc-99m-labeled NR-LU-10 monoclonal antibody, Radiology 173(P):418, 1989.

Press, O.W., Eary, J.F., Badger, C.C., and others: Treatment of refractory non-Hodgkin's lymphoma with radiolabeled MB-1 (anti-CD37) antibody, J. Clin. Oncol. 7(8):1027-1038, Aug 1989.

Pressman, D., and Korngold, L.: The in vivo localization of anti-Wagner-osteogenic sarcoma antibodies, Cancer 6:619-623, 1953.

Primus, F.J., Wang, R.M., Goldenberg, D.M., and others: Localization of human GW-39 tumors in hamsters by radiolabeled heterospecific antibody to carcino-embryonic antigen, Cancer Res. 33:2977-2983, 1973.

Quinones, J., Mizejewski, G., and Beierwaltes, W.H.: Choriocarcinoma scanning using radiolabeled antibody to chorionic gonadotrophin, J. Nucl. Med. 12:69-75, 1971.

Real, F.X., Houghton, A.N., Albino, A.P., Cordon-Cardo, C., Melamed, M.R., Oettgen, H.F., and Old, L.J.: Surface antigens of melanomas and melanocytes defined by mouse monoclonal antibodies: specificity analysis and comparison of antigen expression in cultured cells and tissues, Cancer Res. 45(9):4401-4411, 1985.

Riva, P., and others: Treatment of intracranial human glioblastoma by direct intratumoral administration of ^{131}I-labeled anti-tenascin monoclonal antibody BC-2, Int. J. Cancer 22:51(2):7-13, 1992.

Rosen, S.T., and others: Radioimmunodetection and radioimmunotherapy of cutaneous T cell lymphomas using an ^{131}I-labeled monoclonal antibody: an Illinois Cancer Council study, J. Clin. Oncol. 5(4):562-573, 1987.

Rosebrough, S.F., Grossman, Z.D., McAfee, J.G., Kudryk, B.J., Subramanian, G., Ritter-Hrncirik, C.A., Witanowski, L.S., Tillapaugh-Fay, G., Urrutia, E., and Zapf-Longo, C.: Thrombus imaging with indium-111 and iodine-131-labeled fibrin specific monoclonal antibody and its F(ab')2 and Fab fragments, J. Nucl. Med. 29(7):1212-1222, 1988.

Rubin, R.H., Fischman, A.J., Needleman, M., and others: Radiolabeled, nonspecific, polyclonal human immunoglobulin in the detection of focal inflammation by scintigraphy: comparison with gallium-67 citrate and technetium-99m-labeled albumin, J. Nucl. Med. 30(3):385-389, March 1989.

Salk, D.: Technetium-labeled monoclonal antibodies for imaging metastatic melanoma: results of a multicenter clinical study, Semin. Oncol. 15(6):608-618, 1988.

Samoszuk, M.K., and others: Radioimmunodetection of Hodgkin's disease and non-Hodgkin's lymphomas with monoclonal antibody to eosinophil peroxidase, J. Nucl. Med. 34(8):1246-1253, 1993.

Sands, H.: Radioimmunoconjugates: an overview of problems and promises, Antibody, Immunoconjugates and Radiopharmaceuticals 1(3):213-226, 1988.

Scheidhauer, K., Markl, A., Leinsinger, G., Moser, E., Scheiffarth, O.F., and others: Immunoscintigraphy in intraocular malignant melanoma, Nucl. Med. Commun. 9:669-679, 1988.

Scheidler, J., and others: Immunoimaging of choroidal melanoma: assessment of its diagnostic accuracy and limitations in 101 cases, Br. J. Ophthalmol. 76(8):457-460, 1992.

Schwartz, M.A., and others: Dose-escalation trial of M195 labeled with iodine 131 for cytoreduction and marrow ablation in relapsed or refractory myeloid leukemias, J. Clin. Oncol. 11(2):294-303, 1993.

Shaw, D.R., Khazaeli, M.B., and LoBuglio, A.F.: Mouse/human chimeric antibodies to a tumor-associate antigens biologic activity of the four human IgG subclasses, J. Natl. Cancer Inst. 80(19):1553-1559, 1988.

Siccardi, A.G., Buraggi, G.L., Callegaro, L., Mariani, G., Natali, P.G., and others: Multicenter study of immunoscintigraphy with radiolabeled monoclonal antibodies in patients with melanoma, Cancer Res. 46(9):4817-4822, 1986.

Silverman, P.M., Osborne, M., Dunnick, N.R., and Bandy, L.C.: CT prior to second-look operation in ovarian cancer, Am. J. Roentgenol. 150(4):829-832, 1988.

Sitzman, J.V., Order, S.E., Klein, J.L., Leichner, P.K., Fishman, E.K., and Smith, G.W.: Conversion by new treatment modalities of nonresectable to resectable hepatocellular cancer, J. Clin. Oncol. 5(10):1655-1573, 1987.

Sitzmann, J.V., and Abrams, R.: Improved survival for hepatocellular cancer with combination surgery and multimodality treatment, Ann. Surg. 217(2):149-154, 1993.

Stein, R., and others: Haematological effects of radioimmunotherapy in cancer patients, Br. J. Haematol. 80(1):69-76, 1992.

Stephens, A.D., Punja, U., and Sugarbaker, P.H.: False-positive lymph nodes by radioimmunoguided surgery: report of a patient and analysis of the problem, J. Nucl. Med. 34(5):804-808, 1993.

Stewart, J.S., Hird, V., Sullivan, M., Snook, D., and Epenetos, A.A.: Intraperitoneal radioimmunotherapy for ovarian cancer, Br. J. Obstet. Gynaecol. 96(5):529-536, May 1989.

Stewart, J.S., and others: Intraperitoneal radioimmunotherapy for ovarian cancer: pharmacokinetics, toxicity, and efficacy of I-131 labeled monoclonal antibodies, Int. J. Radiat. Oncol. Biol. Phys. 16(2):405-413, 1989.

Stya, M., Wahl, R.L., and Beierwaltes, W.H.: Dot-based Elisa and RIA: two rapid assays that screen hybridoma supernatants against whole live cells, J. Immunol. Method. 73:75-81, 1984.

Surwit, E.A., and others: Clinical assessment of ^{111}In-CYT-103 immunoscintigraphy in ovarian cancer, Gynecol. Oncol. 48(3):285-292, 1993.

Taylor, J.L., and others: Radioimmunoscintigraphy of metastatic breast carcinoma, Eur. J. Surg. Oncol. 18(1):57-63, 1992.

Thompson, C.H., Lichtenstein, M., Stacker, S.A., Leyden, M.J., Salehi, N., Andrew, J.T., and McKenzie, I.F.: Immunoscintigraphy for detection of lymph node metastases from breast cancer, Lancet 2(8414):1245-1247, 1984.

van Dongen, G.A., and others: Radioimmunoscintigraphy of head and neck cancer using ^{99m}Tc-labeled monoclonal antibody E48 F(ab')2, Cancer Res. 52(9):2569-2574, 1992.

van Nagell, J.R., Kim, E., Casper, S., Primus, F.J., Bennett, S., DeLand, F.H., and Goldenberg, D.M.: Radioimmunodetection of primary and metastatic ovarian cancer using radiolabeled antibodies to carcinoembryonic antigen, Cancer Res. 40:502-506, 1980.

Vansant, J.P., and others: Staging lung carcinoma with a Tc-99m labeled monoclonal antibody, Clin. Nucl. Med. 17(6):431-438, 1992.

Verhoeyen, M., Milstein, C., and Winter, G.: Reshaping human antibodies: grafting an antilysozyme activity, Science 239(4847):1534-1536, 1988.

Vieira, M.R., and others: Immunoscintigraphy with ^{99m}Tc-labelled anti-CEA monoclonal antibody in colorectal carcinoma, Eur. J. Surg. Oncol. 19(3):294-299, 1993.

Wahl, R.L., Parker, C.W., and Philpott, G.W.: Improved radioimaging and tumor localization with monoclonal F(ab')2, J. Nucl. Med. 24:316-325, 1983.

Wahl, R.L., and Parker, C.W.: Monoclonal antibody radioimmunodetection of transplant rejection, Transplantation 40(4):451-454, 1985.

Wahl, R.L., Liebert, M., and Wilson, B.S.: The influence of radiolabeled monoclonal antibody dose on tumor uptake of radiolabeled antibody, Cancer Drug Del. 3(4):243-249, 1986.

Wahl, R.L., Tuscan, M.J., and Botti, J.M.: Dynamic variable background subtraction: a simple means of displaying radiolabeled monoclonal antibody scintigraphy, J. Nucl. Med. 27:545-548, 1986.

Wahl, R.L., Khazaeli, M.B., LoBuglio, A.F., Patillo, R.A., Tuscan, M.J., and Beierwaltes, W.H.: Radioimmunodetection of occult gestational choriocarcinoma, Am. J. Obstet. Gynecol. 156:108-111, 1987.

Wahl, R.L., Barrett, J., Geatti, O., Liebert, M., Wilson, B.S., Fisher, S., and Wagner, J.G.: The intraperitoneal delivery of radiolabeled monoclonal antibodies: studies on the regional delivery advantage, Cancer Immunol. Immunother. 26(3):187-201, 1988.

Wahl, R.L., Johnson, J.W., Mallette, S., Natale, R., and Petry, N.A.: Clinical experience with Tc-99m anti-melanoma fragments and SPECT, J. Nucl. Med. 29(5):812, 1988.

Wahl, R.L., Liebert, M., Headington, J., and others: Lymphoscintigraphy in melanoma: initial evaluation of a low protein dose monoclonal antibody cocktail, Cancer Res. (suppl) 50:941S-948S, Feb. 1, 1990.

Wahl, R.L., and others: Clinical experience with Tc-99m labeled (N2S2) anti-melanoma antibody fragments and single photon emission computer tomography, Am. J. Physiol. Imaging 7(2):48-58, April-June 1992.

Wilbur, D.S., Hadley, S.W., Hylarides, M.D., and others: Development of a stable radioiodinating reagent to label monoclonal antibodies for radiotherapy of cancer, J. Nucl. Med. 30(2):216-226, 1989.

Yeh, S.D.J., Kushner, B., Sullivan, M., and Cheung, N.K.: Potentials for neuroblastoma imaging and target radiotherapy: a comparison between I-131 3F8 and I-131 mIBG, J. Nucl. Med. 29(5):846, 1988.

Zalutsky, M.R., and Narule, A.S.: A method for the radiohalogenation of proteins resulting in decreased thyroid uptake of radioiodine, Int. J. Rad. Appl. Instrum. 38(12):1051-1055, 1987.

Zimmer, A.M., Kazikiewicz, J.M., Rosen, S.T., and Spies, S.M.: Pharmacokinetics of ^{99m}Tc(Sn)- and ^{131}I-labeled anti-carcinoembryonic antigen monoclonal antibody fragments in nude mice, Cancer Res. 47: 1691-1694, 1987.

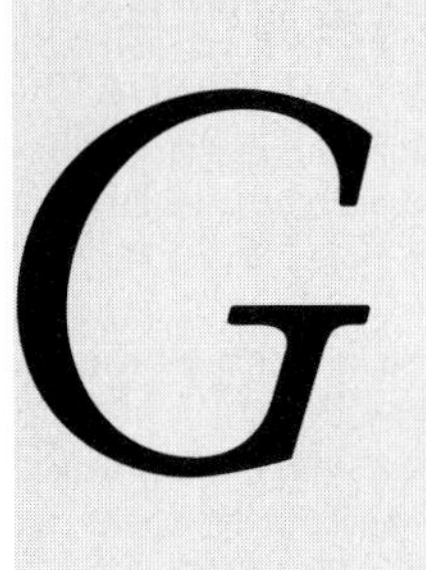

Chapter 28

ALLIUM-67 IMAGING IN INFECTION

NAOMI P. ALAZRAKI

"It is quite remarkable that such a simple substance is involved in so many physiological processes. Indeed, one might conjecture that gallium radionuclides may ultimately find their greatest use as tracers for biological processes rather than as agents for the detection of cancer of inflammatory lesions." When Hayes prefaced this remark with the comment that there are many unanswered questions, he stated the obvious about gallium interactions in biologic systems. Nonetheless, we have accumulated a body of data and experience with in vivo imaging of ^{67}Ga in patients with inflammatory infection and tumor. This chapter summarizes some of this data and clinical experiences.

■ PHYSIOLOGY OF GALLIUM-67 LOCALIZATION

Gallium-67 citrate binds rapidly to circulating transferrin in patients following intravenous administration. Gallium is usually administered in a carrier-free form; presence of carrier may alter the body distribution. Normally, gallium localizes within the liver, bowel, kidneys, bone marrow, and spleen. Within the first 24 hours following administration, about 10% to 20% of the administered dose is excreted through the kidneys and an additional similar amount through the bowel. Therefore, imaging within 24 hours will normally show gallium uptake in the kidneys, reflecting normal renal excretion. If imaging is performed later, for example at 72 hours, normally there is insufficient gallium remaining for renal excretion visualization on images; if the kidneys are imaged at 72 hours, infection or inflammatory renal disease or severe hepatocellular disease is present. The dose of gallium used may affect the degree of kidney uptake imageable at 24 hours, or even at 48 hours in the absence of disease. The higher the administered dose, the longer we can expect to see normal renal excretion in the kidneys.

Electron microscopy studies have shown intracellular localization of gallium-67 in lysozomes or lysozome-like granules. In some tumors (hepatomas and lymphosarcomas), gallium-67 has also been found in association with smaller cellular particulars such as endoplasmic reticulum and electron dense granules. Some investigators have shown gallium-67 in soluble fractions and bound to nuclear, mitochondrial, and microsomal cell components. The mechanism of gallium uptake in inflammatory tissue and in tumors is probably different. Hypotheses for tumor uptake of gallium include the "transferrin-receptor" hypothesis, whereby the tumor-cell–transferrin receptor facilitates gallium uptake in certain tumor types; endocytosis of protein-bound gallium by tumor cells; diffusion across hyperpermeable tumor cell and plasma membranes; and exchange of transferrin-bound gallium with lactoferrin.

As a transition metal, similar to ferric ion in atomic charge, radius, and types of inorganic complexes into which it is incorporated, gallium binds avidly to transferrin, lactoferrin, ferritin, and siderophores. Ferritin and siderophores are low–molecular-weight compounds that mediate incorporation of iron into bacteria. In infection, gallium has been identified in association with leukocytes, as well as with microorganisms, cell debris, and bacterial debris. The phenomenon of increased gallium accumulation at sites of bacterial concentration in agranulocytic animals can be explained by the affinity of gallium to ferritin and siderophores, and therefore bacteria, obviating dependence on the presence of leukocytes. The affinity of indium-111 leukocytes to sites of infection is completely dependent on migration of white blood cells (polymorphonuclear leukocytes) to the infection site. The high concentration of lactoferrin in neutrophilic leukocytes and in abscess fluids has been noted by Hoffer, who has suggested that lactoferrin is a major player in the mechanism of accumulation of gallium in the abscesses.

Radiation-absorbed doses from ^{67}Ga calculated by the MIRD Dose Estimate Committee of the Society of Nuclear Medicine are 0.90 r/mCi to the colon, 0.58 r/mCi to the marrow, 0.53 r/mCi to the spleen, 0.46 r/mCi to the liver, and 0.26 r/mCi to the gonads. These levels compare very favorably to levels quoted for ^{111}In leukocytes in cases in which the critical organ, the spleen, may get 19 rad for a 500-mCi injected dosage, while individual cells get many thousands of rad.

A comparison of ^{111}In leukocyte uptake and ^{67}Ga uptake in inflammatory tissue or infection has suggested that ^{111}In leukocytes are more sensitive for acute inflammatory lesions and ^{67}Ga is superior for localization in chronic inflammatory lesions. Better understanding of this observation is facilitated by a brief review of microscopic findings in inflammation of the acute and chronic types. Acutely inflamed tissue shows vasodilation (a reflection of augmented vascular permeability), expansion of the extracellular space, and increased concentrations of leukocytes. Both ^{67}Ga and ^{111}In leukocytes accumulate at sites of acute inflammation. In contrast, chronic inflammation is characterized by a predominate mononuclear cell infiltration of macrophages, lymphocytes, and plasma cells, rather than by the plasma exudative and neutrophilic infiltrate response of acute inflammation. In chronic inflammation, fibroblasts and abnormal vascular permeability are prominent characteristics of the process. ^{67}Ga, since it is not dependent on migration of neutrophilic leukocytes (as are ^{111}In leukocytes), accumulates relatively well at sites of chronic inflammation. In a rabbit abscess model, Bitar and others demonstrated the difference in biokinetic behavior of gallium and indium leukocytes over 7 days. Although gallium uptake in the abscess was not affected by abscess age, ^{111}In leukocyte uptake progressively decreased with time. Furthermore, early images of ^{111}In leukocytes were clearly superior to ^{67}Ga images, at 7 days the two agents showed similar quantitative uptake in the abscesses.

LABORATORY APPLICATION

81

GALLIUM-67 IMAGING FOR INFECTION AND INFLAMMATION

Purpose and indications

The clinical indications for ^{67}Ga imaging of infection and inflammation span a wide variety of disease states, including the following:

1. Fever of unknown origin
2. Pulmonary disorders
3. Acquired immunodeficiency syndrome (AIDS)
4. Osteomyelitis
5. Myocardial or pericardial inflammatory processes

Procedure

Materials

1. Scintillation gamma camera with medium energy collimator for the 184- and 296-keV energy emissions of gallium-67.
2. ^{67}Ga citrate, 5 to 10 mCi (185 to 370 MBq).

Patient preparation

1. Intravenously inject 5 to 10 mCi (185 to 370 MBq) of ^{67}Ga. Imaging times are as follows:
   a. 6 hours postinjection if an early image evaluation for infection is required.
   b. Ideally imaging is performed later, although a 24-hour image followed by a 48-hour or 72-hour examination is generally performed.
2. Explain the entire procedure to the patient.

Technique

1. Whole-body planar imaging is routine unless a limited examination is requested.
2. Note that SPECT capability is desirable and frequently performed for better localization or identification of a region of abnormal uptake. (If SPECT is anticipated, a higher dose of gallium is desirable.)
3. Perform images using medium-energy collimation for the 184- and 296-keV energy emissions of gallium-67.
4. Set windows of 25% around those peaks.
5. Acquire images for 1000K counts, anteriorly and posteriorly to include the head, chest, abdomen, pelvis, and extremities, as warranted.
6. If multihead detector equipment or scanning whole-body table detector arrangements are available, the study time can be reduced.

Continued.

Image diagnosis

Fever of unknown origin

Petersdorf and Beeson defined fever of unknown origin (FUO) as elevated body temperature in a cyclical pattern that has persisted for at least 3 weeks. Typically, localizing signs to direct the search for the source of the fever are lacking. About 20% of such patients have occult tumor, such as lymphoma, not infection. Thus, a whole-body image of ^{67}Ga distribution, an agent that localizes in either infection or occult tumor sites, is probably the preferred radionuclide screening test for FUO. An alternative to whole-body gallium imaging might be ^{111}In leukocytes. Certainly for imaging in the abdomen, the ^{111}In-leukocyte study has an advantage over gallium because of the normal bowel excretion of gallium that often obscures identification of pathologic conditions in the abdomen. However, since FUO is a process of at least 3 weeks duration, gallium is again preferred because of its possible superiority in chronic conditions. Published studies that have evaluated ^{67}Ga imaging in patients with fever of unknown origin have shown high yield for gallium images: 17 of 22 patients had abnormal studies, and 50 of 67 studies were abnormal in the second report. In a study of CT images, patients with fever of unknown origin yielded a much smaller percentage of abnormal findings: 23 of 78 images were abnormal. Since FUO typically has no focus to identify a regional site for CT imaging, the whole-body gallium image provides a much more comprehensive and rational screening modality.

Tumor and fever

A special problem is presented by patients with a known tumor who have fever, because the fever may be related to the tumor, chemotherapy, or an infection or inflammatory lesion. If localizing signs exist, CT or sonography to evaluate the focus of suspicion is warranted. In the absence of localizing signs, however, a whole-body indium-111 leukocyte scan or gallium scan is preferable to search for an asymptomatic (except for fever) focus. But which of these two whole-body studies would be superior in resolving this problem? Palestro and others reported on 10 febrile patients with known tumors who had both gallium and indium-labeled leukocyte scans. Fever was chemotherapy-and/or tumor-related in nine, and abscess-related in one. Only 1 of 14 known tumor sites was seen on indium-leukocyte images; 7 of 14 tumor sites were positive on gallium scans. The conclusions were that normal findings on gallium and indium-leukocyte scans indicate that the fever is chemotherapy-tumor-related, whereas indium-leukocytes positivity shows infection foci and is unlikely to show uptake by tumor, regardless of the tumor's affinity for gallium. The message is that indium-leukocyte scanning is preferable for patients with known tumor and fever who are thought to have infection or abscess but no localizing signs.

Lung inflammatory lesions

Siemsen and others reported a large patient study of gallium imaging in pulmonary disorders. In that report, 100 normal patients had no abnormal gallium chest images; 264 patients with lung cancer showed gallium image abnormalities in 90% of their images; 149 patients with lymphoma showed abnormal tumor uptake in 80% of their images; 197 patients with active tuberculosis showed abnormalities in the area of tuberculosis in 97% of their images; 32 cases of inactive tuberculosis showed no abnormalities; 98 cases of silicosis showed abnormalities in 100% of their images; 18 cases of pulmonary abscess showed abnormalities in 100% of their images; 12 cases of asbestosis showed abnormalities in 100% of their images.

Gallium-67 imaging has been evaluated in idiopathic pulmonary fibrosis and correlated with bronchoalveolar lavage results. Studies have shown good correlation of quantitative computer analysis of gallium lung images and presence of neutrophils in lavage samples. A general conclusion is that the degree of gallium lung uptake correlates with the degree of activity of the inflammatory state. Thus, the gallium lung study is a useful quantitative index of staging activity of disease and following the response to therapy over extended periods of time. Figure 28-1 demonstrates varying degrees of active inflammation in five patients with interstitial fibrotic disease.

Gallium lung imaging is used for staging pulmonary sarcoidosis and quantitating activity of disease. In sarcoid, comparisons of quantitative gallium lung images with numbers of lymphocytes in

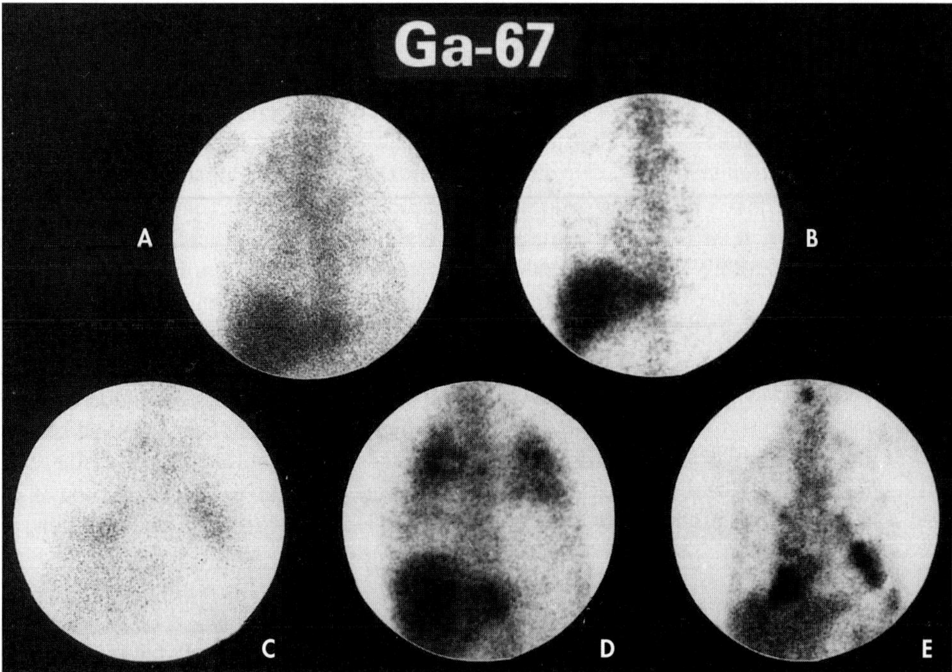

Fig. 28-1. Anterior chest views of gallium-67–citrate images taken in five patients with interstitial pulmonary fibrosis. Images show varying degrees of active inflammation. **A,** gallium image shows very mild increased gallium uptake in the perihilar lung regions. **B,** Image shows a slightly higher degree of increased gallium uptake in the inferior medial right lung region. **C,** Image shows slightly higher increased gallium uptake in both inferohilar lung regions, and mild increased uptake in hilar and mediastinal nodes. Note the comparative uptake in abnormal regions of lung relative to the liver and the bone marrow. **D,** Image shows a high degree of abnormal gallium uptake in the upper lung fields. The activity far exceeds the normal activity in the sternum and in this case is similar to the degree of activity in the liver. **E,** Image shows the highest degree of abnormal uptake in the perihilar inferior lungs. In this patient the degree of activity far exceeds the activity in the liver or bone marrow, indicating very active inflammatory disease.

bronchoalveolar lavage fluid showed excellent correlations in inactive disease (<25% of lavage lymphocyte count and low gallium computer-derived index of uptake). In the active disease category, in 4 of 14 cases there was disagreement between lymphocyte counts and gallium uptake. In addition to lung evaluation in sarcoidosis, the gallium image indicates extent of nodal involvement.

Abdominal inflammatory lesions

Because of the difficulty of discriminating between normal bowel excretion of gallium and abnormal uptake, ^{111}In leukocytes are widely used in abdominal inflammatory problems in preference to gallium. For gallium, various approaches to bowel preparation including enemas, laxatives, or no preparation, have been evaluated with clinically varying results. Results are variable, gallium excretion through the colonic wall is continuous, and GI transport of excreted gallium is unpredictable; because of these factors, many nuclear medicine physicians prefer not to subject the patient to any bowel preparation. Rather, laxatives and/or enemas are reserved to determine if a suspected abnormal focus of gallium uptake on routine images moves on images made after enema 24 hours later. Movement implies intraluminal normal excretion, while no movement after enema or laxative implies greater likelihood of a fixed pathologic focus of uptake.

Published reports have indicated a variety of clinical results of sensitivity for gallium imaging in abdominal infections. These have ranged from 59% to 91%, with specificities ranging from 57% to 93%. Indium-111 leukocytes, on the other hand, have shown much more consistent high sensitivity and specificity results for identifying abdominal abscesses (85% to 95% sensitivities and specificities).

Continued.

Posterior abdominal images at 72 hours normally show no uptake in the kidneys. Renal or perirenal infection is the most obvious cause of abnormal gallium renal uptake. However, abnormal gallium kidney uptake has also been described in noninfectious interstitial nephritis, Wegener's granulomatosis, polyarteritis nodosa, the primary glomerulopathies, allograft rejection, amyloidosis, and lupus nephritis. In a study of gallium imaging in lupus nephritis, a high correlation was found between delayed gallium visualization of the kidneys and active lupus nephritis. Sixteen of the 18 cases of active renal disease showed abnormal gallium uptake (89%), and no gallium kidney uptake predicted absent, resolved, or minimal renal disease in 93% of cases. Others have used gallium to distinguish between upper tract and lower tract urinary infections. Experimental studies in rats have shown that short-term use of nephrotoxic agents such as aminoglycosides or amphotericin is unlikely to cause increased renal gallium uptake.

Patients without renal disease have been reported to show abnormal delayed gallium kidney uptake in association with severe hepatocellular disease. The abnormal uptake in these cases was bilateral and symmetrical. A possible explanation for this phenomenon is that patients with advanced liver disease may accumulate less gallium in their livers (normally 20% of the injected dose), leaving more available for renal excretion. Also, these patients may have less circulating transferrin (protein produced by the liver) to bind gallium in blood, leaving even more gallium available for renal excretion.

Acquired immunodeficiency syndrome (AIDS)

AIDS patients present with a variety of infections, the most common of which is *Pneumocystis carinii* pneumonia (PCP). Other infections seen in AIDS patients include candida esophagitis, cytomegalovirus, cryptococcus, herpes simplex, toxoplasmosis, and *Myciobacterium avium-intracellulare* (MAI). Kaposi's sarcoma, lymphoma, and other neoplasms are also commonly seen in these patients. Several recent reports of the experience with ^{67}Ga images in patients with AIDS have indicated a high degree of clinical utility. In a report of gallium chest images performed in 71 patients with AIDS, 45 of whom also had Kaposi's sarcoma, 29 of 57 abnormal images were correlated with abnormal chest x-ray studies while 27 positive gallium images had accompanying normal chest x-ray studies. The gallium image abnormalities included diffuse increased lung uptake, most commonly seen with PCP. Focal uptake corresponding to lymph nodes was frequently seen with *Mycobacterium avium-intracellulare* and with lymphoma, while localized intrapulmonary uptake was seen with bacterial pneumonias. When chest x-ray examinations were abnormal and gallium images were normal, the most common diagnosis was pulmonary Kaposi's sarcoma, a tumor which does not concentrate gallium. In another study, of 32 patients with AIDS, gallium images showed the same three patterns of abnormal uptake described by others including lymph node uptake alone, diffuse pulmonary uptake, and normal image. The gallium images were useful in identifying clinically occult *Pneumocystis carinii* pneumonia in 7 of 15 patients with AIDS-related complex who were asymptomatic and had normal chest x-ray studies. Woolfenden reported on 164 gallium images in 95 patients. Nineteen of 20 patients with PCP had positive gallium lung images for a sensitivity of 95%. Gallium uptake was less intense in patients receiving therapy for PCP and more intense in untreated PCP patients. Figure 28-2 shows a gallium image in an AIDS patient with *Mycobacterium avium-intracellulare*.

Although technically demanding, immunofluorescent examination of liquefied, induced sputum correctly diagnoses 80% of PCP cases, and if reliably available, may diminish the need for gallium scans in some patients. But, investigators have shown that gallium is positive in the lungs in 100% of patients with AIDS and PCP, even if infection is subclinical. Fiberoptic bronchoscopy also showed *P. carinii* in the bronchial washings of all patients with PCP and abnormal gallium scan, but only 81% of transbronchial biopsy tissue results in those patients showed *P. carinii*. The important message of these studies is that despite pulmonary symptoms, a gallium scan in AIDS patients with normal chest x-ray studies shows objective evidence of PCP and indicates extent, severity, and localization of the infection, all of which may be useful for guiding further diagnostic interventions.

Febrile AIDS patients who present without localizing signs are another special problem. Fineman and others conducted a comparative study of gallium and indium-labeled leukocytes in a group of these patients to determine which is the most effective imaging agent to identify the cause of the fever. Of 27 sites confirmed by biopsy, 15 appeared abnormal only on indium-leukocyte scans (co-

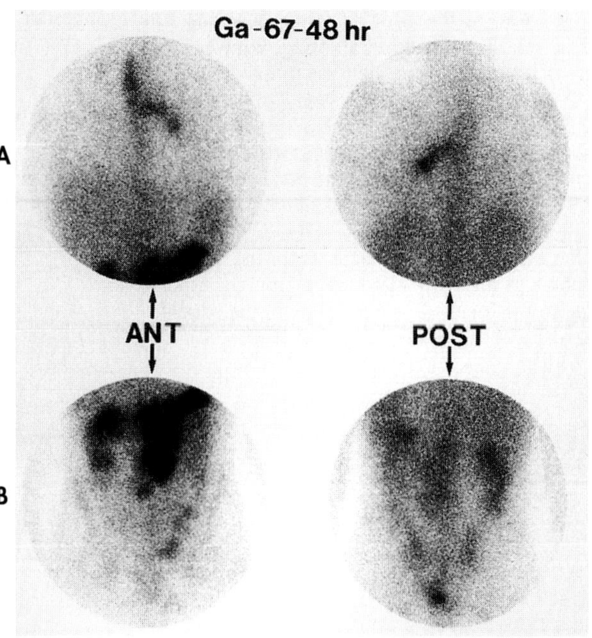

Fig. 28-2. **A,** Anterior and posterior chest images of gallium-67–citrate scans done at 48 hours postinjection in a patient with AIDS and mycobacterium avium intracellulare. Image shows abnormal increased uptake in right paratracheal nodes and hilar-, mediastinal-, and broncho-pulmonary lobes. **B,** Shows anterior and posterior abdomen-pelvis images. There is significant increased uptake, probably in inflamed lymph nodes.

litis, sinusitis, focal bacterial pneumonia), six sites were seen only on gallium scans (PCP and lymphadenopathy), and six were seen on both gallium and indium-leukocyte scans (pulmonary lesions).

Thus, indium leukocytes showed 78% of abnormalities, while gallium showed 44%. The key message is that febrile patients with AIDS who lack localizing signs and are not suspected of having lung infection should be examined with indium leukocytes to image an infection site. If lung infection is suspected, gallium would be preferred, since gallium is clearly superior as an indicator of PCP than is the indium-leukocyte scan, which may be completely normal in the presence of PCP.

Osteomyelitis

Most nuclear-medicine physicians would probably agree that ^{99m}Tc phosphonate three- or four-phase bone imaging should be the first nuclear imaging test for evaluation of osteomyelitis. Gallium-67 citrate and indium-111–labeled leukocyte images are also used to complement the three- or four-phase ^{99m}Tc phosphonate bone scan, primarily to increase specificity in diagnosing osteomyelitis and in monitoring the response to therapy. The gallium image has been particularly useful in small children because of the reported high false-negative rate for ^{99m}Tc phosphonate bone images in young children. False-negative results are minimized when pinhole magnification and high-resolution techniques are used. If, however, a normal bone image is obtained in a young child suspected of having bone infection, a gallium image should be performed. The false-negative rate for ^{99m}Tc phosphonate bone images in neonates and young children has varied from reports of 5% to 60%. Those reports, however, were based on single static images of bone at about 2 hours following administration of the radiopharmaceutical, rather than the three- or four-phase bone images. In adults, sensitivity for the three-phase bone image to detect osteomyelitis has been reported as 92%, and specificity as 89%. In adults with peripheral vascular disease and suspected osteomyelitis, the four-phase bone image showed sensitivity of 80% and specificity of 87%, which was slightly better than the three-phase study in the same patient group.

Cases of osteomyelitis missed on ^{99m}Tc phosphonate bone images that are detected on gallium- or indium-leukocyte studies often involve bony regions that have high metabolic activity and therefore normally exhibit high levels of uptake on ^{99m}Tc phosphonate images. Figure 28-3, *A* and *B* shows a case of sacroiliac osteomyelitis with an apparently normal bone scan and a positive gallium image in a 21-year-old drug abuser. The mechanisms of bone-scan positivity depend on changes in bone-blood flow and increased osteoblastic activity. In early osteomyelitis, blood flow may be decreased by vascular thrombosis or compression from surrounding edema in the marrow space where hematogenously spread osteomyelitis starts. Thus, the ^{99m}Tc phosphonate bone image may be normal or even photo-

Continued.

Fig. 28-3. A, Posterior view from a technetium-99m–MDP bone scan showing equivocal increased uptake in the right sacroiliac region. **B,** Posterior view of the whole-body gallium scan in the same patient, a 21-year-old drug addict who appeared in the emergency room with a complaint of right hip pain. Initially the bone scan *(above)* was performed, but because of inconclusive results, a gallium injection was done. The gallium scan clearly shows notable abnormal increased uptake in the right sacroiliac region corresponding to the focus of osteomyelitis in the patient.

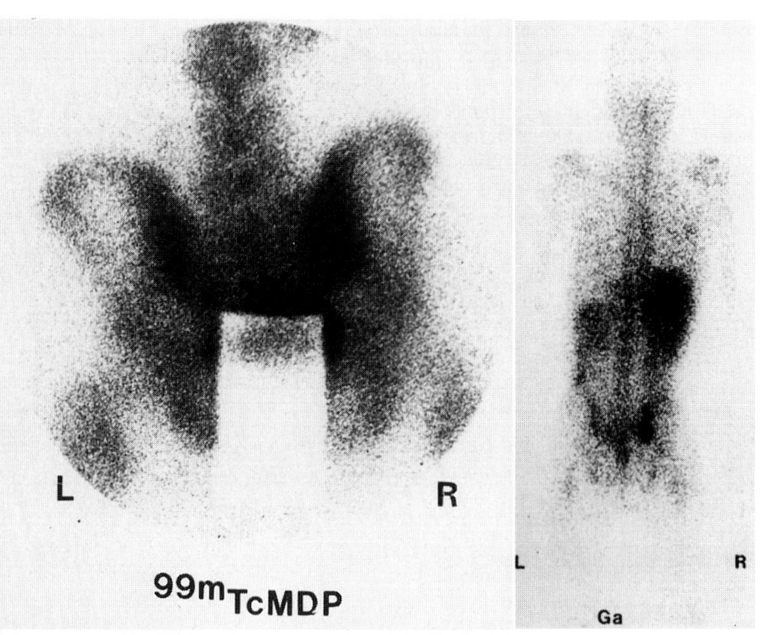

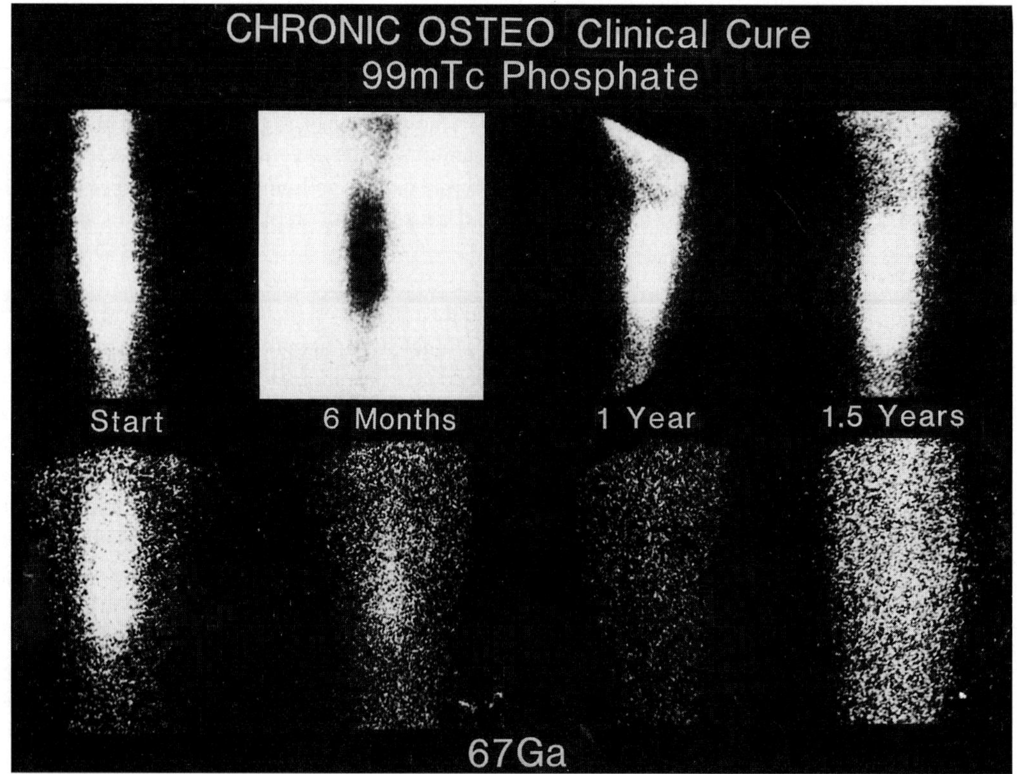

Fig. 28-4. Technetium-99m–phosphonate bone scans *(above),* and gallium-67–citrate scans *(below)* performed at 6-month intervals over a period of 1½ years in a patient with known chronic osteomyelitis. At the start of intensive antibiotic therapy, both the bone scan and the gallium scan show abnormal uptake in the tibia. Following 6 months on the antibiotics, both the bone scan and the gallium scan show considerable improvement. Antibiotic therapy was discontinued soon after the 6-month image, after which the gallium scan reverted to normal while the bone scan remained abnormal (see 1-year images). A follow-up gallium scan at 18 months following the start of therapy and about 1 year following cessation of antibiotic therapy remains normal while the bone scan remains abnormal. Clinically, the patient responded to antibiotic therapy. Radiographs showed old trauma and changes of chronic osteomyelitis.

penic early in osteomyelitis. But exudation of serum proteins and neutrophils occurs very early in infection, facilitating early localization of gallium citrate and/or indium leukocytes.

Animal studies that compare ^{99m}Tc methylene diphosphonate and ^{67}Ga citrate for detecting acute osteomyelitis have indicated that gallium is positive earlier than is ^{99m}Tc phosphonate in the course of infection. In one study, on day 2 after inoculation of bone with microorganisms, gallium images were positive, while no ^{99m}Tc MDP images showed abnormality until day 3. Thereafter, however, there was close correlation between the ^{67}Ga and the ^{99m}Tc MDP images.

As a predictor of cure of osteomyelitis being treated, ^{67}Ga serial images showed a progression towards normal. This correlated with negative bacteriologic cultures of previously infected bone. Persistently positive gallium images correlated with positive bacteriologic cultures in 11 of 18 animals, and negative cultures in 7 of 18 animals. Thus, both animal and patient studies indicate that sequential ^{67}Ga images may be useful in predicting the cure of osteomyelitis during treatment. Comparisons with ^{99m}Tc MDP images showed that the conversion of the ^{99m}Tc study to normal was significantly delayed, and in fact not identified in any of the animal studies performed. Figure 28-4 illustrates a chronic osteomyelitis case that responded to antibiotic therapy given over many months. The ^{67}Ga image reverted to normal, while the bone image remained abnormal.

Postoperative sternal osteomyelitis occurs as a complication of median sternotomy for cardiovascular surgery in less than 1% of cases. Prognosis for patients with sternal-wound infections has been related to the length of time required for institution of treatment and adequacy of initial therapy. In a study of gallium imaging in postcoronary artery bypass grafting surgery patients suspected of having sternal osteomyelitis, results indicated a sensitivity of 83% and specificity of 96% for gallium imaging. Thus, despite the increased gallium uptake that is expected following recent surgical trauma, using degree of increased uptake and the pattern of increased uptake (uniform vs. nonuniform), the gallium image was interpreted successfully to indicate presence or absence of sternal osteomyelitis in most of the cases evaluated. In addition, the use of SPECT imaging in such cases is particularly helpful to identify the presence or confirm the absence of mediastinitis. From planar gallium imaging it may be difficult to determine posterior extent of abnormal uptake behind the sternum. SPECT images more clearly indicate the presence or absence of abnormal gallium uptake in the mediastinum posterior to the sternum (Fig. 28-5, *A* and *B*). The importance of this capability is highlighted by a report of 39 patients who had sternal wound complications after cardiac surgery. Nineteen of those patients died; all 19 had septicemia and mediastinal abscess.

Many of the patients prone to osteomyelitis are individuals who have had previous bone trauma or other bone diseases. This is a particularly difficult group of patients for diagnosing osteomyelitis. The bone image will often be abnormal at the sites of old trauma, particularly when healing has been incomplete or there is a bony deformity and/or degenerative disease that may not be differentiable from acute bone infection on the Tc phosphonate bone image. Likewise, the gallium image may show abnormal increased uptake on the basis of gallium's behavior as a bone imaging agent in a bony proliferative process such as degenerative change or trauma. Several studies have examined the patterns of abnormal uptake that can be identified and used to distinguish between other bony abnormalities and osteomyelitis. These studies have shown that if ^{67}Ga uptake exceeds the ^{99m}Tc bone image at a given location, active osteomyelitis can be diagnosed. Also when ^{67}Ga and ^{99m}Tc bone uptake localize discordantly, bone infection is likely. These criteria for image diagnosis of osteomyelitis, however, are satisfied in only one fourth of cases of bone infection imaged with ^{67}Ga and ^{99m}Tc MDP. A normal gallium image accurately excludes osteomyelitis, but an abnormal image is only a nonspecific indicator of osteomyelitis. Figure 28-6 illustrates gallium and technetium bone images in a patient with cellulitis and osteomyelitis.

In a comparative study of ^{67}Ga and ^{99m}Tc methylene diphosphonate in early rabbit osteomyelitis and fracture repair, Hartshorne, et al showed preferential accumulation of gallium over ^{99m}Tc MDP within the first 48 hours, in both infection and fracture, while images at 5 to 7 days showed predominance of the ^{99m}Tc MDP over the ^{67}Ga. This was demonstrated by a simultaneous digital acquisition of the gallium and the technetium images and subsequent division of the gallium image by the technetium image on a pixel-by-pixel basis, to produce a parametric ratio image to characterize the relative localization of the two radiopharmaceuticals. Through this approach, the dual-image study characterizes the amount of inflammation relative to the amount of bone repair.

Continued.

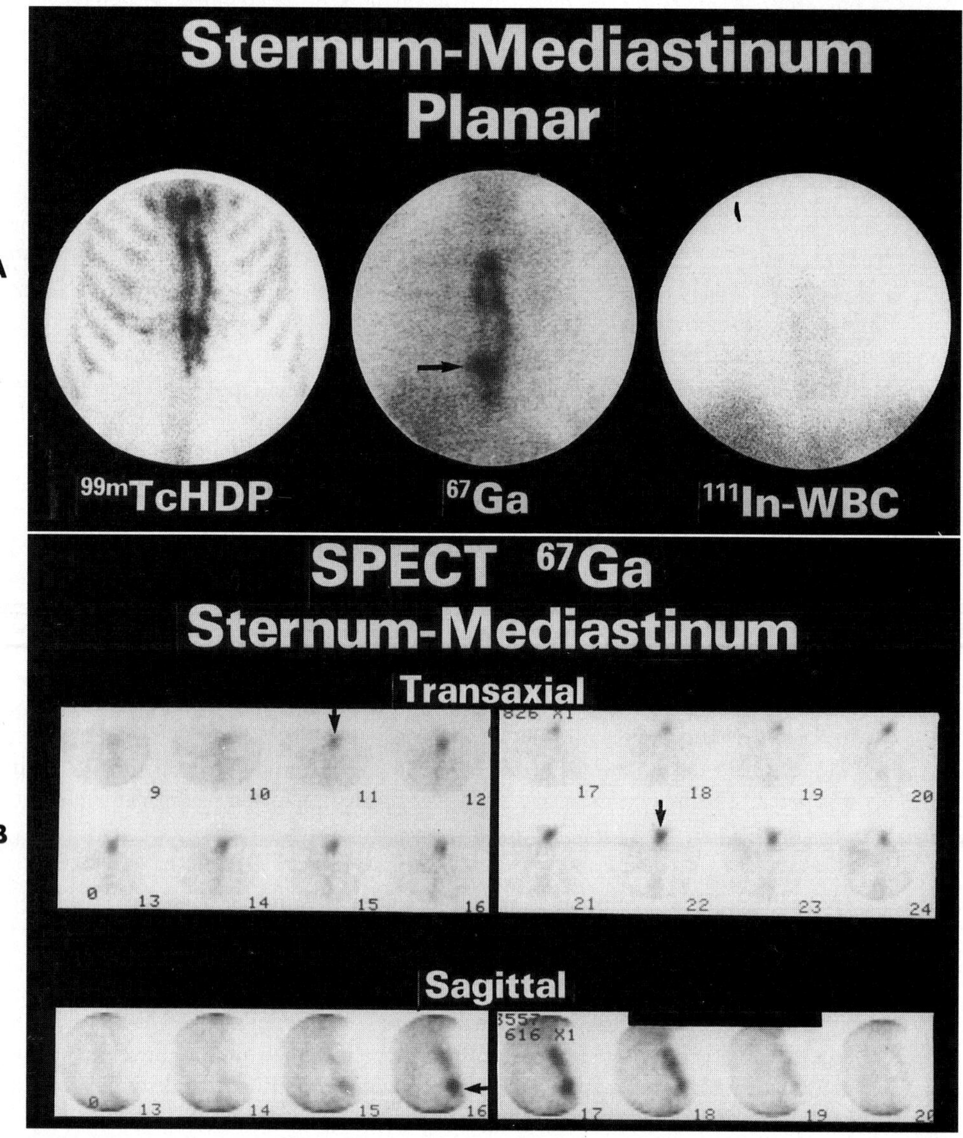

Fig. 28-5. **A,** Two weeks after coronary artery bypass and median sternotomy, this patient was studied with technetium-99m–HDP bone scan, gallium-67–citrate scan, and indium-111–leukocyte scans of the sternum to assess the possibility of osteomyelitis. Abnormalities secondary to surgical trauma are seen on the bone scan, the gallium scan, and very faintly on the indium-leukocyte scan. However, the gallium scan clearly shows discordant abnormal uptake in the sternum inferiorly, indicated by the arrow. The abnormality is not well defined on the indium leukocyte scan in this case. **B,** In addition to osteomyelitis, there is clinical concern about posterior extent of infection into the mediastinum. SPECT imaging of the gallium-67 distribution was performed. Transaxial slices *(above)* and sagittal slices *(below)* are shown in this figure. Arrows indicate the abnormal increased inferior sternal uptake (slice 22 in the transaxial views and number 16 in the sagittal views). It is clear that there is no abnormal increased gallium uptake posterior to the sternum. Thus the gallium was useful in excluding mediastinitis.

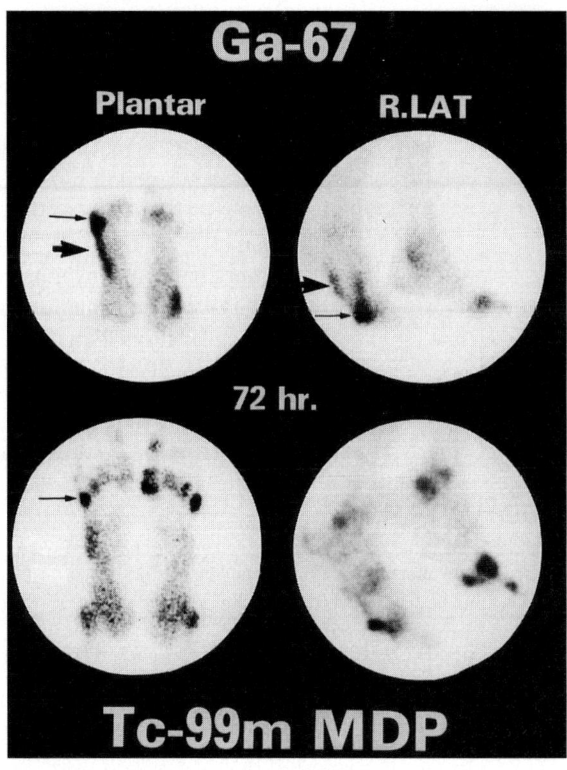

Fig. 28-6. Gallium-67 and technetium-99m–MDP bone scans in a patient with a nonhealing ulcer at the lateral margin of the distal fifth metatarsal bone. This patient had degenerative bony changes in the foot and toes, with multiple abnormal foci of increased uptake on the technetium-99m–MDP bone scan. The gallium scan, however, shows discordant increased gallium uptake in the region of the distal fifth metatarsal, with extent of the abnormal gallium uptake into the soft tissues (*large black arrow* on plantar image). Significantly abnormal gallium uptake is not seen in any of the other abnormal foci of technetium-99m–MDP uptake; these foci are therefore probably related to the degenerative changes in the bones, rather than to infection.

Sensitivity, specificity

The three-phase bone scan has been reported to have sensitivity of 90% to 100% and specificity of 73% to 81%. Addition of the fourth phase increases the specificity slightly to a maximum reported 87%. Reports of sensitivity and specificity are always greatly influenced by the character of the patients selected for the particular study. Some investigators have indicated that presence of soft-tissue ulcers of cellulitis, and not peripheral vascular disease or antibiotic therapy, substantially affects the radionuclide results. Others claim decreased sensitivity (70%) and specificity (43%) of three-phase bone scanning for detecting pedal osteomyelitis in patients with diabetes, peripheral vascular disease, and complicating soft-tissue ulcerations and/or necrosis.

Comparative studies in patients with a mixture of acute and chronic complicated orthopedic bone problems have reported for gallium/^{99m}Tc MDP sensitivities of 38% to 80% and specificities of 67% to 86% for detecting osteomyelitis. For indium-111 leukocytes, reports indicate sensitivities of 80% to 83% and specificities of 83% to 86% for infection. An important article by Schauwecker noted that the sensitivity for indium leukocytes varied for different bone locations, as well as for chronic versus acute osteomyelitis. Specifically, he retrospectively reviewed 485 cases and reported sensitivity of 90% to 95% in acute osteomyelitis for indium-111 for leukocytes for all bones, but for chronic osteomyelitis, sensitivity was 94% for peripheral bones, 80% for middle bones, and 53% for central skeletal locations. Thus, particularly for bones in which there exist other complicating conditions such as trauma and degenerative disease, indium-leukocyte imaging is the superior radionuclide imaging approach for diagnosis of osteomyelitis, unless the condition is chronic and in the central skeletal bones. In those cases, the gallium-technetium combination can be considered. In bones without old trauma or degenerative changes, as in children, gallium offers an excellent alternative. Gallium is in fact preferred in children because of its more favorable radiation exposure, particularly for young children who receive higher organ-absorbed exposures in rad per dose administered than do adults because of their larger organ sizes relative to whole-body size. For indium leukocytes, the critical organ is the spleen, which for children has been calculated to receive 13.7 ± 10.6 rad per dose administered. In the case of gallium, calculated dosimetry is more favorable.

Continued.

Magnetic resonance imaging

Magnetic resonance imaging (MRI) in osteomyelitis is reported to be quite sensitive but not as highly specific. For example, although most bone-infection lesions show increased signal on T1- and T2-weighted images, some culture-proven cases of osteomyelitis show low signal on T1- and T2-weighted images, precluding differentiation from fibrous dysplasia, bone infarct, or benign sclerosis. The pattern seen in most osteomyelitis cases of increased signal on T2-weighted images may mimic neoplasm and trauma. Nonetheless, MR studies show sequestra, sinus tracts, and soft-tissue abscesses in chronic osteomyelitis; this gives it advantages over CT and radionuclide imaging. In a report of vertebral osteomyelitis comparing gallium-bone scans with the MRI, sensitivity was 96% for MRI, 90% for bone-gallium scans; specificity was 92% for MRI and 100% for bone-gallium. Since MRI is an exquisitely high resolution tomographic technology, meaningful comparisons can only be made to SPECT gallium-bone images, preferably using multiheaded equipment for high-count imaging.

BIBLIOGRAPHY

Al-Sheikh, W., Sfakianakis, G.N., Mnaymneh, W., and others: Subacute and chronic bone infections: diagnosis using In-111, Ga-67 and Tc-99m MDP bone scintigraphy and radiography, Radiology 155:501-506, 1985.

Alazraki, N., Dries, D., Datz, F., Lawrence, P., Greenberg, E., and Taylor, A.: The value of a 24-hour image (four phase bone scan) in assessing osteomyelitis in patients with peripheral vascular disease, J. Nucl. Med. 26:711-717, 1985.

Alazraki, N.: Usefulness of gallium imaging in the evaluation of lung cancer, CRC Crit. Rev. Diag. Imaging 249-247, 1980.

Alazraki, N., Sterkel, B., and Taylor, A.: Renal gallium accumulation in the absence of renal pathology in patients with severe hepatocellular disease, Clin. Nucl. Med. 85:200-204, 1983.

Ash, J.M., and Gilday, D.L.: The futility of bone scanning in neonatal osteomyelitis: concise communication, J. Nucl. Med. 21:417-420, 1980.

Aulbert, E., Gebhardt, A., Schulz, E., and Haubold, U.: Mechanism of Ga-67 accumulation in normal rat liver lysosomes, Nuklearmedizin 15:185, 1976.

Bakir, A.A., Lopez-Majano, V., Hryhorczuk, D.O., Rhee, H.L., and Dunea, G.: Appraisal of lupus nephritis by renal imaging with gallium-67, Am. J. Med. 79:175-182, 1985.

Biello, D.R., Levitt, R.G., and Melson, G.L.: The roles of gallium-67 scintigraphy, ultrasonography, and computed tomography in the detection of abdominal abscesses, Semin. Nucl. Med. 9:58-65, 1979.

Bitar, R.A., Scheffel, U., Murphy, P.A., and Bartlett, J.G.: Accumulation of In-111 labeled neutrophils and gallium-67 citrate in rabbit abscesses, J. Nucl. Med. 27:1883-1889, 1986.

Bitran, J., Bekerman, C., Weinstein, R., Bennett, C., and Ryo, U.: Patterns of gallium 67 scintigraphy in patients with acquired immune deficiency syndrome, J. Nucl. Med. 28:1103-1106, 1987.

Fineman, D.S., Palestro, C.J., Kim, C.K., and others: Detection of abnormalities in febrile AIDS patients with In-111 labeled leukocyte and Ga-67 scintigraphy, Radiology 170:677-680, 1989.

Fortun, J., Vavas, E., Marti-Belda, P., and others: *Pneumocystis carinii* pneumonia in HIV-infected patients: diagnostic yield of induced sputum and immunofluorescent stains with monoclonal antibodies, Eur. Respir. J. 5:655-659, 1992.

Gainey, M.A., Siegel, J.A., Smergel, E.M., and others: Indium-111 labeled white blood cells: dosimetry in children, J. Nucl. Med. 29:689-694, 1988.

Graham, G.D., Lundy, M.M., Frederick, R.J., Berger, D.E., O'Brien, A.W., and Brown, T.J.: Predicting the cure of osteomyelitis under treatment: concise communication, J. Nucl. Med. 24:110-113, 1983.

Habibian, M.R., Stabb, E.V., and Matthews, H.A.: Gallium citrate Ga-67 scans in febrile patients, JAMA 233(10):1073-1076, 1975.

Handmaker, H.: Acute hematogenous osteomyelitis: has the bone scan betrayed us? Radiology 135:787-789, 1980.

Hartshorne, M.F., Graham, G., Lancaster, J., and Berger, D.: Gallium-67 technetium-99m methylene diphosphonate radio imaging: early rabbit osteomyelitis and fracture, J. Nucl. Med. 26:272-277, 1985.

Hayes, R.L.: The tissue distribution of gallium radionuclides, J. Nucl. Med. 18:740, 1977.

Hoffer, P.B., Huberty, J., and Khayam-Bushi, H.: The association of Ga-67 and lactoferrin, J. Nucl. Med. 18:713, 1977.

Hoffer, P.B.: Mechanisms of localization: In Hoffer, P.B., Bekerman, C., and Henkin, R.E., editors: Gallium-67 imaging, New York, 1978, John Wiley & Sons, pp. 3-8.

Hurwitz, S.R., Kessler, W.O., Alazraki, N.P., and others: Gallium-67 imaging to localize urinary tract infections, Br. J. Radiol. 49:156, 1976.

Johnson, D.G., Johnson, S.M., Harris, C.C., Piantadosi, C.A., Blinder, R.A., and Coleman, R.E.: Ga-67 uptake in the lung in sarcoidosis, Radiology 150:551-555, 1984.

Kissin, M.W., and Williamson, R.C.N.: Gallium-67 scanning in pyrexia of unknown origin, BMJ 2:1330-1331, 1979.

Kolyvas, E., Rosenthall, L., Ahronheim, G.A., Lisbona, R., and Marks, M.I.: Serial Ga-67 citrate imaging during treatment of acute osteomyelitis in childhood, Clin. Nucl. Med. 3(12):461-466, 1978.

Kramer, E.L., Sanger, J.J., Garay, S.M., Greene, J.B., Tiu, S., Banner, H., and McCauley, D.I.: Gallium 67 scans of the chest in patients with acquired immune deficiency syndrome, J. Nucl. Med. 28:1107-1114, 1987.

Larson, S.M., Rasey, J.S., Allen, D.R., and Grunbaum, Z.: A transferrin mediated uptake of gallium-67 by EMT-6 sarcoma: II, Studies in vivo (Balb/c Mice), J. Nucl. Med. 20(8):843, 1979.

Lavendar, J.P., Lowe, J., Baker, J.R., and others: Gallium-67 citrate scanning in neoplastic and inflammatory lesions, Br. J. Radiol. 44:361-366, 1971.

Line, B.R., Fulmer, J.D., Reynolds, H.Y, and others: Gallium scanning in the staging of idiopathic pulmonary fibrosis: correlation with physiologic and morphologic features and broncho-alveolar lavage, Am. Rev. Respir. Dis. 118:355, 1978.

Lisbona, R., and Rosenthall, L.: Observations on the sequential use of ^{99m}Tc phosphate complex and Ga-67 imaging in osteomyelitis, cellulitis and septic arthritis, Radiology 123:123-129, 1977.

Maurer, A.H., Chan, D.P.C., Camargo, E.E., Wong, D.F., Wagner, A.N., and Alderson, P.O.: Utility of three-phase skeletal scintigraphy in suspected osteomyelitis: concise communication, J. Nucl. Med. 22:941-949, 1981.

McNeil, B.J., Sanders, R., Alderson, P.O., and others: A prospective study of computed tomography, ultrasound, and gallium imaging in patients with fever, Radiology 139:647-653, 1981.

Medical Internal Radiation Dose (MIRD) Committee, Society of Nuclear Medicine, Dose estimate report no. 2, J. Nucl. Med. 11(10):755, 1973.

Merkel, K.D., Brown, M.L., Dewanjee, M.K., and Fitzgerald, R.H.: Comparison of indium labeled leukocyte imaging with sequential technetium gallium scanning in the diagnosis of low grade musculoskeletal sepsis, J. Bone and Joint Surg. 67:465-476, 1985.

Palestro, C.J., Fineman, D.S., Needle, L.B., and others: Utility of In-111 labeled autologous leukocytes and Ga-67 citrate imaging in patients with tumor, Radiology 165:173, 1987 (abstract).

Petersdorf, R.G., and Beeson, P.B.: Fever of unexplained origin: report on 100 cases, Medicine 40:1-30, 1961.

Pope, T.L., Teague, W.G., Kossack, R., Bray, S.T., and Slannery, D.B.: Pseudomonas sacroiliac osteomyelitis: diagnosis by gallium citrate Ga-67 scan, Am. J. Dis. Child 136:649-650, 1982.

Quinn, M.J.U., Sheedy, P.F., Stephens, D.H., and Hattery, R.R.: Computed tomography of the abdomen in evaluation of patients with fever of unknown origin, Radiol 136:407-411, 1980.

Salit, I.E., Detsky, A.S., Simor, A.E., Weisel, R.D., and Feiglin, D.: Gallium-67 scanning in the diagnosis of postoperative sternal osteomyelitis: concise communication, J. Nucl. Med. 24:1001-1004, 1983.

Schauwecker, D.S., Park, H.M., Mock, B.H., Burt, R.W., Kernick, C.B., Ruoff, A.C., Sinn, H.J., and Wellman, H.N.: Evaluation of complicating osteomyelitis with Tc-99m MDP, In-111 granulocytes and Ga-67 citrate, J. Nucl. Med. 25:849-853, 1984.

Seldin, D.W., Heiken, J.P., Feldman, F., and others: Effect of soft-tissue pathology on detection of pedal osteomyelitis in diabetes, J. Nucl. Med. 26:988-993, 1985.

Serry, C., Bleck, P.C., Javid, H., Hunter, J.A., Goldin, M.D., DeLaria, G.A., and Najafi, H.: Sternal wound complications: management and results, J. Thorac. Cardiovasc. Surg. 80:861-867, 1980.

Sfakianakis, G.N., Al-Sheikh, W., Heal, A., and others: Comparison of scintigraphy with In-111 leukocytes and Ga-67 in the diagnosis of occult sepsis,

Siemsen, J.K., Siegfried, G.F., and Wazman, A.D.: The use of Ga-67 in pulmonary disorders, Semin. Nucl. Med. 3:235-249, 1978.

Swartzerndruber, D.C., Nelson, B., and Hayes, R.L.: 67 gallium localization in lysosomallike granules of leukemic and nonleukemic murine tumors, J. Natl. Cancer Inst. 46:942, 1971.

Taylor, A., Nelson, H., Vasquez, M., and Hollenbeck, J.: Renal gallium accumulation in rats with antibiotic-induced nephritis: clinical implications, J. Nucl. Med. 21:646-649, 1980.

Thakur, M.: Cell labeling: achievements, challenges and prospects, J. Nucl. Med. 22:1011-1014, 1981.

Tsan, M.F.: Mechanism of gallium-67 accumulation in inflammatory lesions, J. Nucl. Med. 26:88-92, 1985.

Tuazon, C.U., Delaney, M.D., Simon, G.L., and others: Utility of ^{67}Ga-scintigraphy and bronchial washings in the diagnosis and treatment of *pneumocystis carinii* pneumonia in patients with acquired immune deficiency syndrome, Am. Rev. Respir. Dis. 132:1087-1092, 1985.

Tumeh, S., Rosenthal, D.S., Kaplan, W.D., English, R.J., and Halman, B.L.: Lymphoma: evaluation with Ga-67 SPECT, Radiology 164:111-114, 1987.

Woolfenden, J.M., Carrasquillo, J.A., Larson, S.M., Simmons, J.T., Masur, H., Smith, P.D., Shelhamer, J.H., Ognibene, F.P.: Acquired immunodeficiency syndrome: Ga-67 citrate imaging, Radiology 162: 383-387, 1987.

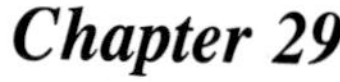

Chapter 29

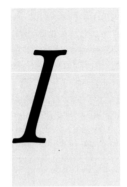

INDIUM-111 LABEL IN INFLAMMATION AND NEOPLASM IMAGING

DAVID F. PRESTON

■ ANATOMY AND PHYSIOLOGY

Inflammation, infection, and abscess may be found in any organ and at any location. The terms are not synonymous. Inflammation is a fundamental response of most tissues to a noxious stimulus. Mechanical trauma and allergic stimuli, as well as thermal, chemical, electrical, electromagnetic injury initiate a sequence of similar events in tissue that results in inflammation. These stimuli cause release of vasoactive chemicals, histamine, bradykinin, serotonin, and other substances that cause increased blood flow, increased capillary permeability, and leakage of plasma into the tissue. White blood cells are attracted to the region. The external manifestations of this sequence are redness, warmth, swelling, and pain—all consequences of inflammation.

There are two groups of white cells, *granulocytes* and *lymphocytes*. Granulocytes are produced by the bone marrow and contain stainable granules. Granulocytes may be divided into neutrophils, eosinophils, basophils, and monocytes. Their names are derived from the color their granules stain. The individual functions of each type of granulocyte is given in Table 29-1.

Lymphocytes are the second group of white cells. There are two subgroups of lymphocytes, B-lymphocytes and T-lymphocytes. B-lymphocytes become plasma cells and produce antibodies, while T-lymphocytes control many diverse activities of the immune system including the production of granulocyte-colony–stimulating factor. These complex factors stimulate specific cell groups. Up to this time, isolated populations of lymphocytes have not been tagged with a radiotracer.

Infection is the active growth of bacteria, fungi, or viruses in a tissue. Infection almost always results in local inflammation. As the infection and the resultant inflammation progress, white blood cells, especially neutrophils, are attracted to the area. For the neutrophil to locate and ingest an invading organism, it needs an intact cell surface with appropriate numbers and types of cell surface receptors. The cell surface receptors are stimulated and maintained by monocyte-macrophage–colony stimulating factors and granulocyte-colony–stimulating factors released by subsets of T-lymphocytes. When neutrophils ingest or phagocytize a bacterium, potent intracellular enzymes are activated. These enzymes have the power to digest bacteria. Enzyme activation results in the death of the white cell. The dead neutrophils and bacteria and associated tissue fluid are pus. The body also lays down a layer of fibrin to surround and localize the active infection. This is the *pyogenic membrane*. The local inflammation or cellulitis has developed into an abscess. Abscess formation is important to identify because surgical drainage is usually necessary. Modern antibiotic therapy may not be effective in the treatment of an undrained abscess. Pus under pressure is dangerous; the living bacteria in the pus can enter the blood stream, causing septicemia or blood poisoning. If bacteria colonize and grow on a heart valve, the term is *bacterial endocarditis*. If bacteria infect bone, the result is *osteomyelitis*. Osteomyelitis can occur from direct extension from surrounding soft-tissue infection or from hematogenous spread from bloodborne bacteria.

Monocytes are also involved in host defense and are precursors of tissue macrophages. Their life span is about 3 days. Monocytes and macrophages are seen in the more chronic stages of infection, perhaps 2 weeks or more after the onset, while the neutrophil is seen within hours after the onset of the infection. The eosinophil response is di-

Table 29-1. Function of granulocytes

	Life span	Defense against
Neutrophil	7 hours in blood 2-3 days in tissue	Bacteria
Eosinophil	Unknown	Parasites, allergies
Basophil	Unknown	Inflammation, allergies
Monocyte	3 days	Immune surveillance

rected primarily against parasites and allergies; its life span is unknown. The basophil is involved in responses to inflammation and allergy; its life span in the blood is also unknown.

■ WHAT IS CANCER?

Cancer is defined as the uncontrolled overgrowth of cells. The natural course of cancer leads to a fatal outcome. The tissue where the cancer originates defines the type of cancer. For instance, breast cancer originates in the female or less often in the male breast. The usual progress of breast cancer is different from that expected from prostate, thyroid, or lung cancer. The ability of a cancer to disseminate to remote parts of the body, to metastasize, is a characteristic of most malignant cancers. Typically, a cancer of the breast located in the lateral aspect of the breast will initially spread by lymphatic drainage into the adjacent axilla. Later there may be spread to the lung. Still later, the bone may become the site of breast-cancer metastases. This situation is often incorrectly called *bone cancer* when in reality it is breast cancer that has metastasized to bone. The term *bone cancer* should be reserved for cancer that has originated in bone, such as osteosarcoma or Ewing's tumor.

The term *tumor* means the presence of a swelling or enlargement of a tissue. Neoplasm is defined as the development of new tissue. There are benign neoplasms, which are localized tumors that do not metastasize, and there are malignant tumors that do metastasize. In general, a cancer must metastasize to vital organs before the cancer can kill a patient.

No one knows the cause or time of origin of a cancer. For the last century, cancers have been thought of as abnormal masses of cells, and surgeons have been called on to remove these masses. In reality, cancer begins as a biochemical intracellular change that may precede the presence of a mass by years or decades. For example, one of the first known changes of breast cancer may be the loss of the breast cell to control the amount of estrogen receptors in the breast cell. The excess of estrogen receptor may allow normal estrogen concentrations to stimulate intracellular protein growth within the breast cell. The histology, if examined at this stage, may remain normal for years. Eventually, after prolonged excess estrogen stimulation, there may be a change in a breast cell surface antigen such as CA 15.3. This antigen can be detected by radioimmunoassay. Imaging of metastatic breast cancer using an ^{111}In-labeled MAb has been reported. During the cellular changes associated with early cancer, there are increases in regional metabolism and blood flow. F-18 fluoro-d-oxyglucose (FDG) and Tl-201 breast imaging will become abnormal. After more time, increased density of tissue may be recognized as an abnormality by mammogram. Much later, a mass may develop that is eventually palpated by the patient. If a radiotracer could demonstrate estrogen receptor excess in the intact breast, nuclear medicine would have an opportunity to identify breast cancer months to years before anatomic changes.

■ WHAT IS AN ANTIGEN?

An antigen is any substance able to trigger an immune response with subsequent antibody formation. The probability and degree of the immune response is dependent on molecular weight, shape, and duration of contact. Below a certain molecular size, no antigenic response occurs.

The immune response is quite specific for a given antigen and is elicited by a very small region of the antigen called the *epitope*. Unfortunately, the same antigen may be found on various tissues, thereby causing nonspecific localization. Some tumors "shed" or lose significant amount of their antigen to the interstitial fluid and vascular compartment. If the circulating antigen binds to a radiolabeled antibody, the background will be increased. An antigen may exist at perhaps a million sites on the surface of an intact tumor cell. In some tumors, when an antibody reacts with an antigen at the tumor surface, many of the surrounding antigenic sites become inactive and therefore unavailable to be detected by a labeled antibody. Several good introductory texts exist.

■ ANTIBODY PRODUCTION

Initially, a B-lymphocyte is sensitized to a single antigen. A structure, really a biologic factory, is created in the now-sensitized B-lymphocyte to produce a great many copies of the antibody specific to the exact antigen to which it was sensitized. The sensitized B-lymphocyte may wait years or decades before again encountering the precise antigen. Antibody production in animals is initiated by the presentation of the antigen to a macrophage that modifies the antigen to a more antigenic form. T-helper lymphocytes are involved in recognizing the "foreignness" of the antigen. The B-lymphocyte, previously sensitized to the one specific antigen, is transformed into a plasma cell that then makes many copies of the single antibody to the single antigen. In a clinical situation, a single virus or bacterium will contain several distinct antigens, resulting in a distinct antibody for each antigen.

■ TYPE OF ANTIBODIES

Antibodies are immunoglobulins (Ig). There are five types of immunoglobulins: IgA, IgD, IgE, IgG, and IgM.

IgG is found in the greatest concentrations and is the type used for tumor imaging. IgG has a molecular weight of 150,000 daltons (150 kd). The various types of immunoglobulins can be separated from each other, but it is very difficult to separate various IgG from each other. Even purified mixtures of radiolabeled IgG will contain antibodies to a mixture of antigens, a polyclonal mixture, which may cause nonspecific localization.

■ THE HYBRIDOMA

In 1975, Kohler and Milstein developed the hybridoma technique. They developed a method in which a previously sensitized B-lymphocyte was fused to a mouse myeloma cell. The myeloma cell is a hardy cell, able to survive and reproduce under proper in vitro laboratory conditions. The sensitized B-lymphocyte contains the logic and structure for making multiple copies of a single antibody specific for the single antigen to which it has been sensitized. This resultant combined cell, part mouse myeloma and part sensitized human B-lymphocyte, is the hybridoma cell. After fusion, a single fused cell is placed in a separate container where it multiplies into a homogenous clone containing many identical cells, all making the same identical antibody. The antibody output of clones is tested to identify those clones making the desired antibody. The antibodies produced by a single clone are identical in structure and antigenic function. This is the monoclonal antibody.

■ ANTIBODY ANATOMY

IgG is the antibody type currently used for tumor imaging. The general shape is that of the letter "Y." The tips of the two arms of the Y are the sites of the antigen-antibody reaction. The IgG molecule is composed of four linear structures. There are two short or "light" chains and two longer or "heavy" chains. A combination of one light and one heavy chain joined by disulfide bonds makes up each of the upper limbs of the Y. Two identical light and heavy chain combinations, joined together by more disulfide bonds, make the complete IgG molecule (Fig. 29-1). The IgG is large, with a molecular weight of 150,000 or 150 kilodaltons (150 kd). It is a large structure and must pass out of the intravascular space into the interstitial fluid before it can encounter the specific antigen on a tumor cell.

Only the tips of the arms of the Y are the site of the antigen-antibody–binding reactions. This is called the *variable region* and it is different from one antibody to another. The lower part of the Y contains a region that is similar from one antibody to another and appears to be species-specific. Attempts have been made to remove the constant region (Fc) and to split the antibody apart, still maintaining the antibody function at the tips of the Y. This can be accomplished through the use of the enzymes pepsin and papain.

Fragments of the antibody are called Fab or fractional antibody. Pepsin removes the distal end of the Y (the Fc region), producing a Y with two antigenic-binding sites but

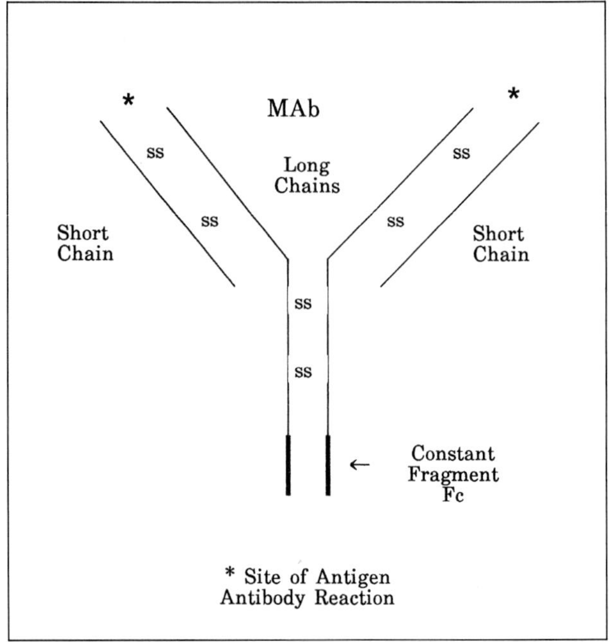

Fig. 29-1. Schematic representation of an intact monoclonal antibody (MAb). Labeling must not block the site of antigen antibody reaction.

a much shorter stem. This smaller molecule is called an F(ab')2 (Fig. 29-2). Papain cleaves the Y into two identical pieces, each with an individual binding site, and removes the Fc component (Fig. 29-3). An added benefit to this structural change is that the smaller fragments are less antigenic and leave the vascular space more quickly than does the large intact IgG. Even smaller immunoreactive structures constructed of peptides have been created. These immunoreactive units clear the vascular pool even more quickly and are less antigenic than the intact antibody or its fragments. IgG clears very slowly from the vascular space with a half-time clearance of perhaps 40 hours. F(ab')2 clears with a half-time of 20 hours and the smallest fragments, Fab, appear to have a half-time clearance of about 1 hour. An excellent editorial discussing the pharmacokinetics of antibodies is presented by Goodwin.

■ THE HAMA REACTION

Since most current monoclonal antibodies are produced from mice, the injection of a mouse antigen into a human may be accompanied by the production of antimouse antibodies by the human. If a second injection of mouse-derived antibody is made, the *H*uman *A*nti*M*ouse *A*ntibodies (HAMA) recognize the mouse origin of the antibody and bind to the newly injected mouse antibody, which is then cleared more rapidly from the vascular space. The murine tracer-human antibody complex is cleared by the reticuloendothelial system, which of course is predominantly in the liver. There is less labeled antibody available to bind with the desired tumor antigen, and liver activity is increased.

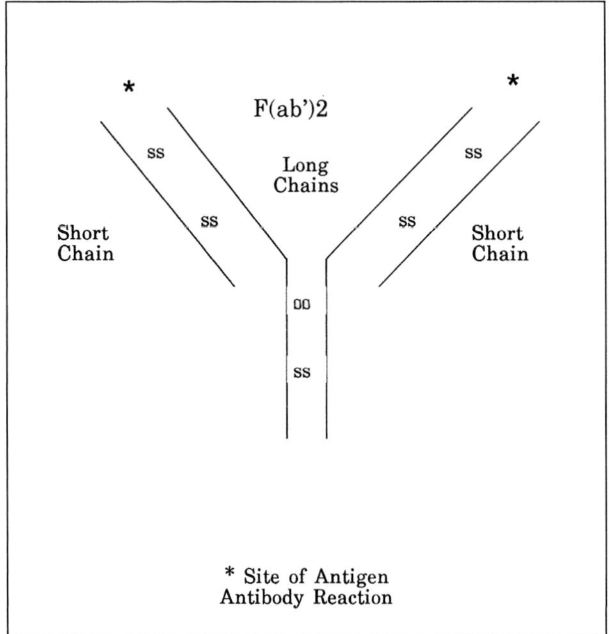

Fig. 29-2. The constant fragment (Fc) has been removed. F(ab′)2 maintains the divalent character of the MAb, but it is about 100,000 in molecular weight.

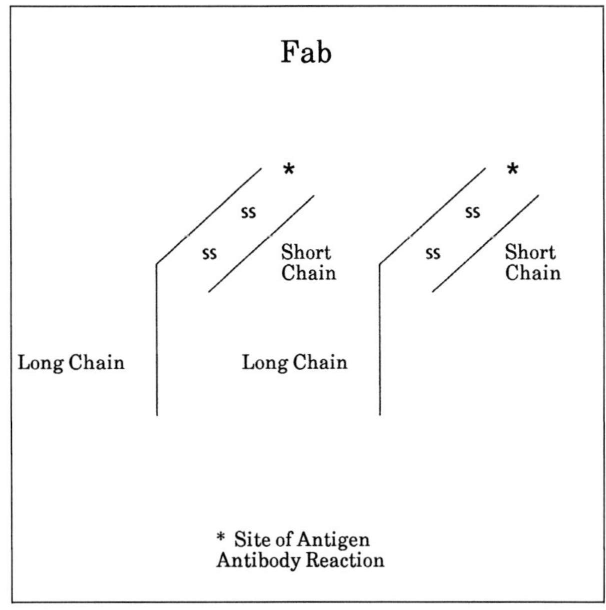

Fig. 29-3. Fab is monovalent. Molecular weight is about 50,000.

Removal of the Fc fragment decreases the human anti-mouse response.

■ THE RADIOACTIVE LABEL

The radionuclides most used in labeled antibody tumor imaging are listed in Table 29-2. Each radionuclide has unique advantages and disadvantages. ^{131}I and ^{123}I can easily tag exposed tyrosine molecules. Unfortunately the iodine tyrosine bond is attacked by circulating iodinases in the blood stream. This results in an unwanted increase in background activity. ^{131}I has an energetic beta particle that causes increased radiation exposure to the patient as well as to the monoclonal antibody. ^{123}I is more expensive and its 159 keV photon is better matched with current-day gamma cameras, but its 13-hour half-life is somewhat limiting because most monoclonal-antibody-tumor imaging is performed several days after tracer injection.

^{111}In has an excellent half-life of 67.4 hours and is quite appropriate for the usual scanning delay. The tagging process is more complex than that with iodine. ^{111}In must first be chelated with DTPA; the complex is attached to the antibody through an amide linkage.

Technetium-99m DTPA has been used as a label but with less satisfactory results. When coupled with an intact MAb that clears slowly from the blood, the 6-hour physical half-life is too short to be optimal. There is partial compensation for the slow clearance by administering multi millicurie doses. Adequate ^{99m}Tc may still be present at 1 to 2 days to obtain an adequate scan.

Table 29-2. Radionuclides most used in labeled antibody tumor imaging

Nuclide	Half-life	Gamma emission (keV)
^{131}I	8 days	364*
^{123}I	13 hours	159
^{111}In	67.4 hours	173,247
^{99m}Tc	6 hours	140

*Beta emission

■ PRODUCTION OF ^{111}In

Indium-111 (^{111}In) currently is the radioactive tag of choice for labeling white cells, platelets and several monoclonal antibodies of great potential to the future of nuclear medicine, and progress in nuclear medicine is directly related to radiotracer development. The ability to tag the formed elements of the blood and to have those structures retain a major portion of their function is a major event in the progress of nuclear medicine.

^{111}In is a cyclotron product, produced by bombardment of a cadmium-112 target by 12 to 22 MeV protons. Indium is an active metal. A one-half to one-millicurie dose (18.5 to 37 MBq) is currently administered for white-cell imaging. Five millicuries of ^{111}In is administered for antibody

Table 29-3. Indium-111 summary

Production cadmium-112 (p, 2n) indium-111
Physical half-life 67.4 hours
Decay electron capture
173 keV (85%)
247 keV (94%)
Decay is to stable cadmium-111

imaging. Five millicuries delivers only 120 pg of indium to the human patient, an amount far below that associated with chemical toxicity. ^{111}In has a physical half-life of 67.4 hours. Decay is by electron capture. Two photons with energies of 173 keV (85%) and 247 keV (94%) are produced. Both energies are excellent for imaging with current gamma cameras. The combined frequencies of useful emissions of 85% and 94% yield 1.8 photons per disintegration, a figure well above any other radionuclide currently used in clinical nuclear medicine (see Table 29-3). ^{111}In decays to stable cadmium-111, also a chemical toxin in milligram amounts but of no known hazard in picogram quantities resulting from diagnostic doses of ^{111}In.

■ INDIUM-111 CHLORIDE

^{111}In first appeared in clinical nuclear medicine in the early 1970s. As ^{111}In chloride, it was considered an alternative to gallium-67 (^{67}Ga) in the detection of tumors and abscesses. The advantage of indium-111 as compared with ^{67}Ga was its lack of concentration in the GI tract—a distinct advantage when examining the abdomen. Clinical results were no better than those obtained with ^{67}Ga, and the cost was greater. ^{111}In chloride therefore disappeared from the mainstream of tumor and abscess imaging. ^{111}In chloride is again available as the radiolabel for a recently released antibody tracer for colon and ovarian cancer. ^{111}In chloride has equal sensitivity to ^{111}In-labeled white cells in the detection of osteomyelitis abscess formation, tumor detection, and visualization of the distribution of red marrow.

^{111}In chloride is administered intravenously in doses of 1 to 2 mCi (37 to 74 MBq); imaging is carried out at 24 hours. Both 173 keV and 247 keV photopeaks can be summed if a dual-energy pulse-height analyzer is available. A 15% to 20% window is used. The collimator should be a medium-energy collimator, or, depending on the energy rating of the medium-energy collimator, a high-energy collimator (though this is a less optimal choice). A low-energy, all-purpose collimator is not adequate. Five-hundred-thousand counts can be acquired in about 5 minutes. ^{111}In chloride has the advantage of no normal gastrointestinal activity, but there is the disadvantage of physiologic renal activity normally being seen. Despite the renal activity, the abdomen is easier to evaluate with ^{111}In chloride than with ^{67}Ga.

■ LABELED NEUTROPHIL AS A RADIOTRACER

In one cubic microliter of blood there are about 5,000,000 red cells and 5000 to 10,000 white cells, a ratio of about 1000 red cells for each white cell. Currently, tagging methods require the red cells to be separated from the white cells. Even methods that remove 99% of red cells are not adequate because there would be equal numbers of red and white cells under those conditions. Since about 60% of white cells are neutrophils, 3% are eosinophils, 1% are basophils, 5% are monocytes, and 30% are lymphocytes, most of the white cells tagged will be neutrophils.

The tagging method must not significantly damage the surface sensors responsible for migration of the neutrophil to the site of infection. There are several methods for the tagging of white cells, but the indium-oxime method has had the greatest use. Indium oxime is a neutral lipid soluble complex that penetrates the lipid membrane of the white cell. Once in the cell, the ^{111}In dissociates from the oxine and attaches to intracellular components. Little ^{111}In leaves the cell. The greatest amount of ^{111}In can be placed on a neutrophil in a media free of plasma, but this results in damage to the neutrophil. Labeling in plasma preserves neutrophil function but results in decreased labeling. The current oxime method attempts to tag the neutrophil in a reduced amount of plasma.

A method using tropolone has also been used successfully. The oxime method, however, is readily available from local commercial radiopharmacies.

■ ^{111}In OXINE METHOD FOR LEUKOCYTE SEPARATION AND WHITE CELL TAGGING

1. 50 ml of venous blood is collected in a 60-ml syringe predosed with 1 ml of 1000 U/ml preservative-free heparin. An 18- or 19-gauge needle should be used, to prevent cell trauma.
2. Add 5 ml of 6% hetastarch to increase the settling rate of red cells. Suspend the syringe for 60 minutes with the needle up.
3. After settling of the red cells, the leukocyte-rich plasma contains 50% to 70% of the leukocyte content of the whole blood. Through a large-gauge butterfly, the leukocyte-rich plasma is slowly ejected into sterile plastic tubes.
4. Centrifuge the leukocyte-rich plasma at 300 *g* for 5 minutes to deposit the leukocytes in a pellet at the bottom of the centrifuged tube.
5. Remove the leukocyte-poor plasma and transfer to fresh plastic tubes. Centrifuge at 100 *g* for 15 minutes to separate the platelets. Remove the platelet-poor plasma and save for a later step.
6. Add 5 ml of normal saline, mix gently, and resuspend the leukocyte button.
7. Drop by drop, add 0.5 to 1.0 mCi (18.5 to 37 MBq) ^{111}In oxine to the leukocyte suspension. Gently mix

and incubate at room temperature for 20 minutes.

8. Add 5 ml of platelet-poor plasma from the previous step to bind any indium not labeled to the leukocytes.
9. Centrifuge at 300 *g* for 5 minutes to deposit the tagged leukocytes at the bottom of the centrifuge tube. Remove the supernatant and place into a test tube.
10. Add 2 ml of platelet-poor plasma to the labeled white cells without resuspending the white cells. Remove the platelet-poor plasma.
11. Resuspend the labeled white cells in 5 ml of platelet-poor plasma.
12. Inject slowly into the patient through a large bore needle.

About 200 to 500 μCi of ^{111}In-labeled white cells may be injected into the patient. The labeled white cells should be injected slowly through a large bore needle to avoid mechanical trauma. Injection through plastic tubing should be avoided if possible. Following intravenous injection, there is immediate transit accumulation in the lungs. The half-time in the lung is about 15 minutes, and by 3 hours the lungs should be clear of indium-labeled white cells. Twenty percent to 50% of activity is seen in the spleen, the liver, and the bone marrow. The relative distribution of activity does not change after the first 4 hours. Unlike ^{67}Ga imaging, there is no merit in images delayed beyond 24 hours.

Localization at inflammatory sites has been reported at 4 hours, but most clinical images are performed at 24 hours (Fig. 29-4). Bowel and renal activity will not confuse evaluation of the abdomen. Normal uptake in normal marrow can be a problem, and it can be solved only by consistent technique and physician experience. Recent fractures, metastases, and tumors have been reported to occasionally retain ^{111}In white cells.

The diagnosis of osteomyelitis has been aided by the ^{111}In white cell scan and the ^{99m}Tc MDP bone scan. The combined study has demonstrated good overall sensitivity and specificity for the diagnosis of osteomyelitis. It is difficult to make the diagnosis of osteomyelitis in the periarticular areas if there has been prior trauma. In this situation, a normal ^{111}In WBC scan was reliable in predicting the absence of osteomyelitis. Using the visual criteria of the authors, there was an increase of ^{111}In-labeled WBC in the periarticular regions when there had been prior periarticular trauma. The periarticular accumulations of ^{111}In WBC were falsely identified as sites of osteomyelitis. Since all healing is accompanied with some degree of inflammation and white-cell accumulation, this result is not surprising and indicates that consistency in imaging technique is very important in allowing a proper diagnosis to be made.

^{111}In WBC is a sensitive diagnostic test for the presence of inflammatory bowel disease. Many general internists, family practice physicians, gastroenterologists, and surgeons have no idea this is a practical diagnostic test. There are even physicians responsible for nuclear medicine who are uninformed regarding the potential for ^{111}In WBC to make the diagnosis. Only by informing the referring physician about such advances will this excellent application be used.

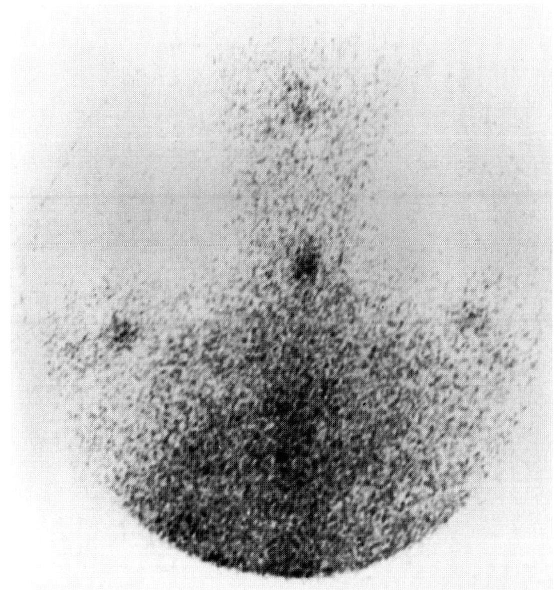

Fig. 29-4. Twenty-four–hour anterior image of ^{111}In WBC accumulation in abscess from esophageal perforation.

Adult imaging is best accomplished using a large field of view camera and a medium- or high-energy collimator. If a dual-energy pulse-height analyzer is available, both the 173 and 247 keV energies may be summed together. A 20% window is appropriate. If the patient has received a ^{99m}Tc-radiotracer in the previous 2 days, a background image at the 173 keV window may discover significant technetium counts. ^{99m}Tc sulfur colloid in the liver, bone scanning agents in fractures, or free pertechnetate in the stomach, thyroid, or bowel may cause clinical concern that may be recognized by the background image. A previous ^{67}Ga injection within the prior week may cause clinical confusion.

Anterior and posterior views of the head, chest, abdomen, and pelvis should be performed. The extremities should be imaged if there is clinical suspicion of infection in shunts or prostheses. The indium image is a low-count image. Acquisition times of 10 minutes per image are appropriate. Special care should be used in the upper abdomen because the liver and spleen will contain intense activity, and often the abscess activity will be suppressed into the background. Recording on a computer and photographing two images, one satisfactory for the dynamic range of the liver and spleen and the other contrasted in such a way as to overexpose the liver and spleen, bring out the background that may harbor the abscess in a method to overcome the dynamic range problem (Fig. 29-5).

In the past 5 years, whole-body imaging devices have

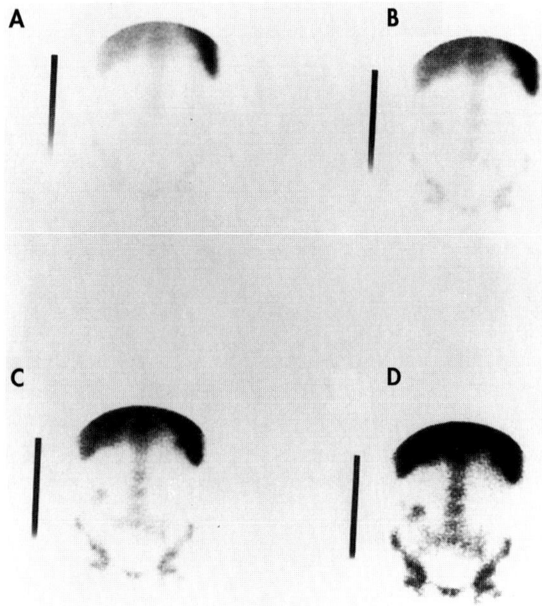

Fig. 29-5. Images of abdominal abscess presented at four successive levels of contrast. **A,** Image scaled to maximum count in liver. There is no contrast enhancement. Image presented at 100% of full scale. **B,** 50% of full scale. **C,** 25% of full scale. **D,** 12% of full scale. Increasing contrast allows the abscess to be seen.

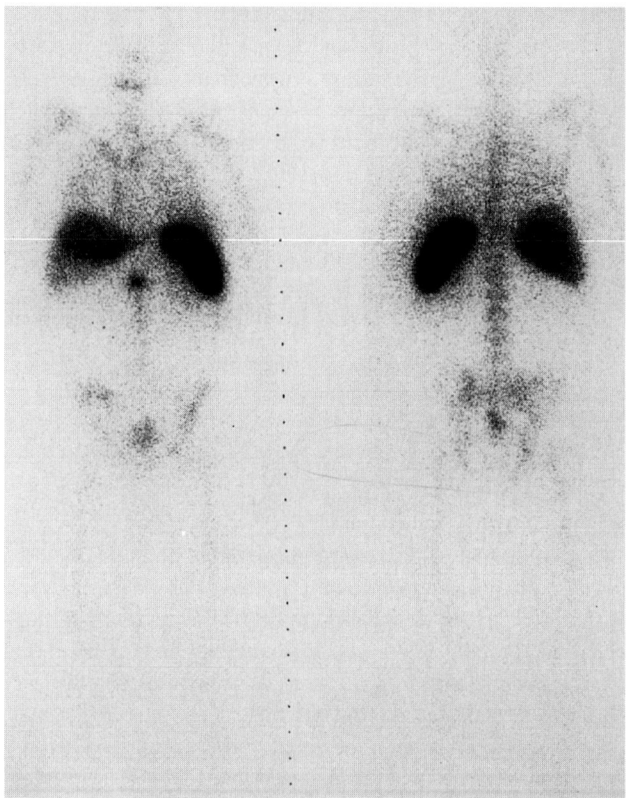

Fig. 29-6. Whole body ^{111}In white blood cell scan obtained 18 hours after injection. The anterior image is to the left and the posterior image to the right. The patient had a known osteomyelitis of the mandible that had been adequately treated. There had been severe maxillofacial and neck injuries. Unexplained fever developed. CT and sonography demonstrated no evidence of focal infection. The increased focal activity in the epigastrium is due to a gastrostomy, not abscess, and is commonly seen with a gastrostomy. This may be a normal finding and must be properly identified by the physician or the technologist. The diffuse increase ^{111}In WBC activity in the lungs is due to a pneumonia that became radiographically apparent the next day. Asymmetrical increased left sacro-illac uptake is due to partially treated osteomyelitis, which was identified by this scan. The pneumonia was probably due to multiple septic pulmonary emboli. Note the uptake in the marrow and the intense uptake in the liver and spleen, which are normal findings.

become available. They permit imaging from head to foot, a significant and unique nuclear medicine capability (Fig. 29-6). Computed tomography (CT), magnetic resonance imaging (MRI), and ultrasound (US) are limited to looking at small regions of the body. These anatomic modalities require either a change in electron density, as with CT; proton density, as with MRI; or a local change in acoustic impedance characteristics, as in US. Usually the presence of a localized abscess is required for diagnosis. Labeled white-cell imaging requires only the presence of inflammation and may be positive when US, CT, or MRI are negative. A whole-body image taking 45 minutes is often adequate. It is a self-defeating attitude to conclude that nuclear medicine has nothing to offer diagnostically just because CT and MRI cannot find the cause of symptoms.

■ ^{99m}Tc-LABELED WHITE CELLS

From the imaging standpoint, ^{99m}Tc is superior to ^{111}In in terms of cost, availability, and compatibility with current cameras. In 1986 a method using ^{99m}Tc-labeled HMPAO was developed; it was modified in 1988. There have been numerous clinical studies attesting to the clinical equality if not superiority of the ^{99m}Tc HMPAO method. ^{99m}Tc WBC scans have been especially satisfactory for the detection of osteomyelitis in the extremities (Fig. 29-7). The superior count rate, when compared with ^{111}In WBC in the hands and feet (especially of diabetics or other patients with poor peripheral circulation) allows individual fingers and toes to be seen (Figs. 29-8, 29-9). Images utilizing a low-energy, all-purpose collimator or high-resolution, low-energy collimator or pinhole collimator can be obtained within less than 5 minutes. With ^{111}In WBC, the hands and feet are difficult to visualize even with views of 5- to 10-minute duration. SPECT imaging of the thorax, abdomen, pelvis, or head make a significant contribution to our diagnostic ability.

■ TUMOR IMAGING WITH ^{111}In-LABELED MONOCLONAL ANTIBODIES

With proper use, nuclear medicine imaging has always been a sensitive but not always specific modality. In the

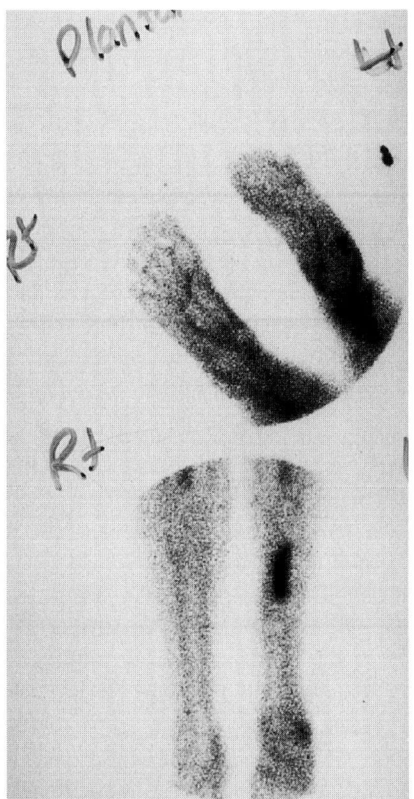

Fig. 29-7. Five years previously, this 30-year-old male had suffered a fracture and dislocation and subsequent osteomyelitis of the left ankle and closed fractrue of the left mid-tibia. Due to unexplained fever, the cutaneous inflammation remaining over the left lateral malleolus was the site of clinical concern for residual osteomyelitis. There was minor increased ^{99m}Tc WBC activity over the left lateral malleolus but major intense linear activity within the mid-shaft of the left tibia seen 2 hours after the injection of ^{99m}Tc WBC. The mid-tibial region proved to be active osteomyelitis, the cause of the fever. The region of the left lateral malleolus was within normal limits on bone scan, which is not shown. ^{99m}Tc WBC imaging provides adequate photons to demonstrate the distal foot, which is usually poorly seen with ^{111}In WBC.

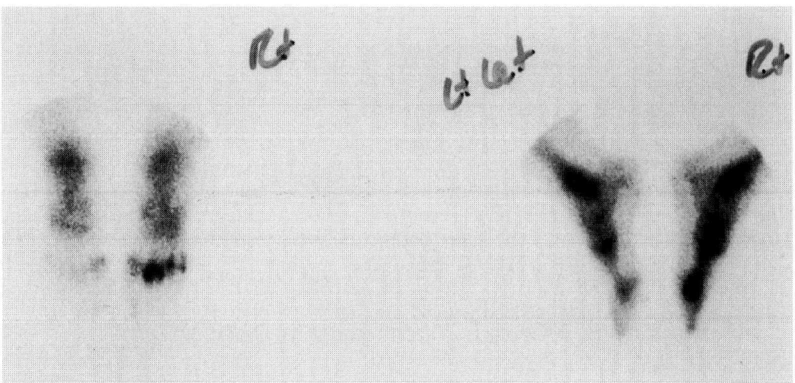

Fig. 29-8. MDP bone scan of feet in 45-year-old diabetic male with pain, redness, and swellling of distal right foot. From the bone scan, this active reparative process involving the right distal second and third metatarsal could be either osteomyelitis or fracture.

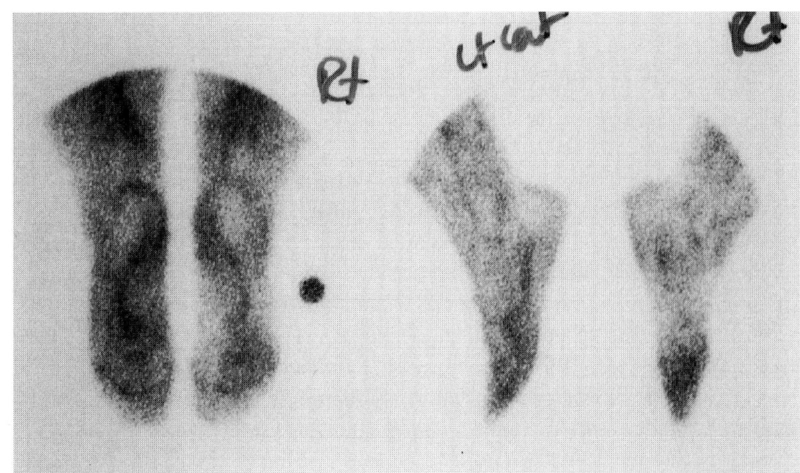

Fig.29-9. The ^{99m}Tc WBC plantar image of the feet demonstrates no abnormal focal activity to suggest active infection. Fracture without osteomyelitis was the eventual diagnosis.

last 10 years, however, enormous progress has been made in the production of radiolabeled monoclonal antibodies specific to individual tumor antigens. ^{111}In has frequently been the radiolabel for these antibodies. Carcinoembryonic antigen and alphafetoprotein are two antigens found in fetal development. Antibodies to these substances have been used for tumor imaging in the specific situations in which tumors express those antigens. There has been no FDA-approved radiotracer to exploit the unique capabilities of CEA or AFP.

The greatest experience with human tumors have been with neuroblastoma, melanoma, and colon cancer. The literature is complex because there may be three different forms of the antibody: the intact antibody, the divalent antibody, and the monovalent fraction. There are hundreds of antigens expressed on the surface of a tumor cell, and none may be unique to the specific tumor. For each chosen antibody and its fragments, iodine or indium or technetium may be used as the radiolabel.

Miraldi in 1986 demonstrated metastatic neuroblastoma in humans using the intact IgG MAb 3F8 tagged with ^{131}I. Images were obtained from 10 to 72 hours postinjection with optimal visualization occurring at about 48 hours postinjection. The imaging technique would be similar to the white-cell technique mentioned earlier in this chapter. In addition, the imaging technique must permit background activity to be seen.

Melanoma may occur on the skin or in the eye; in both

areas it has been detected by imaging techniques. SPECT imaging of a ^{99m}Tc-labeled monoclonal antibody 225.28S, F(ab')2, has been successfully used.

In a wide-ranging study, Halpern has compared intact ^{111}In MAb with the F(ab')2 and found superior lesion detectability using the F(ab')2 fragment in comparison with the intact monoclonal antibody.

An excellent review of the basic science and current clinical applications is presented in a concise monograph by Grossman.

In early 1993, the first commercially available monoclonal tracer was released for routine diagnostic human use. The tracer, tagged with ^{111}In, is a murine product with the ability to localize the presence and extent of colorectal and ovarian cancers. Most colorectal and ovarian cancers express a high-molecular-weight antigen, a tumor-associated glycoprotein identified as TAG-72. A murine monoclonal antibody (MAb B72.3) localizes to TAG-72 of colorectal and ovarian cancers and is the basis for the commercial product. Eighty-three percent of colorectal adenocarcinomas and 97% of common epithelial ovarian cancers are found to react with B72.3, which is generally not reactive with most adult tissues. There is some cross reactivity with salivary duct glands, postovulatory endometria, benign ovarian tumors, and fetal intestinal tissue.

The B72.3 antibody is labeled with a unique "linking" process. To a carbohydrate on the B72.3 antibody, DTPA is attached. The DTPA is then labeled with ^{111}In. This method provides a high specific activity product. The method is described in more detail in Rodwell et al (1986).

Colorectal cancer is the third most common noncutaneous malignancy. In 1992 there were 111,000 new colon cancer cases and 45,000 new rectal cancer cases. Fifty-one thousand humans died of colon cancer and 7300 died of rectal cancer, making colorectal cancer a significant health problem. Identifying colon cancer before spread beyond the submucosa is associated with a 5-year survival of greater than 90%. When there is transmural penetration, 5-year survival is 60% to 80%. If less than four lymph nodes are involved, 5-year survival approximates 56%. If more than four nodes are involved, there is 33% survival. Five-year survivals are slightly less for rectal cancer. For both colon and rectal cancers there is frequent recurrence.

The methods to detect recurrence of colorectal cancer include all the modern imaging technologies. Since these methods use such physical attributes as electron density, acoustic impedance mismatch, and proton density, they are unable to detect disease before the presence of a mass. Barium enema and colonoscopy are limited to mucosal disease. Computed tomography, although excellent in detecting metastases in the liver, has a difficult time detecting lymph node metastases and in differentiating postoperative scar from recurrent tumor in the abdomen and pelvis. Magnetic resonance imaging of the liver may detect even smaller metastases than can be seen by CT, but MRI also has diagnostic difficulty in the postoperative and postradiation-therapy pelvis. There is a need for earlier detection of recurrent disease. The early trials indicate the immunoscintigraphy method aids in clinical management. The immunoscintigraphy method has proved useful in identifying the following:

1. The location of recurrent cancer in patients with an increasing CEA and otherwise normal evaluation
2. The presence of extrahepatic abdominal and pelvic involvement in patients thought to have isolated and resectable recurrence
3. Active disease, and differentiating it from postsurgical and postradiation changes

Immunoscintigraphy using labeled B72.3 has not been as sensitive as CT or MRI in looking for metastases in the liver. On average, the immunoscintigraphy method is superior to CT and MRI in the pelvis and extrahepatic abdomen. The method detects about 70% of surgically confirmed colorectal cancer. The tracer correctly identified 76% of patients found to be free of disease. In 50% of patients, the first recurrence was in the extrahepatic abdomen and pelvis, exactly the area where the method can provide the most help.

Pregnant or lactating women or children have not been examined at this time, and caution is advised in examining these groups. Fetal gastrointestinal tissue has been shown to concentrate the tracer, which in theory could produce a false-positive examination. At this time, repeat injections are discouraged. After a single injection, 40% of patients developed detectable antimouse antibodies. The antimouse antibodies became undetectable after 4 to 12 months in half of those patients. There is a clinical caution, however. The induction of antimouse antibodies will produce false elevations of both CEA and CA-125 laboratory values. This may cause clinical concern because the CEA is commonly used in evaluation of colorectal cancer and the CA-125 is used in ovarian cancer. There is a standard technique available to correct for the antimouse antibody elevation, but it must be specifically requested. The Knoll/Cytogen representative can be helpful in providing support for this problem.

In preparation of the labeled antibody, there are times when the ideal total 5 mCi cannot be injected. This is not a serious problem with planar imaging because each view may be acquired for longer duration. One milligram of antibody protein labeled with 3 to 5 mCi of ^{111}In is injected into a peripheral vein over 5 minutes. Following injection of the tracer, chills, fever, hypotension and hypertension, rash, itching, and sweating have been recorded in 5% of patients. One should be prepared to treat anaphylaxis or lesser allergic reactions. Imaging is usually delayed for at least 48 to 72 hours. Five-day delayed imaging is possible and allows a reasonable trade-off between blood clearance and remaining signal for planar imaging. An excellent monograph has been produced summarizing experience with the B72.3 ^{111}In-labeled tracer. Another more general discussion is found in a book by Chatal.

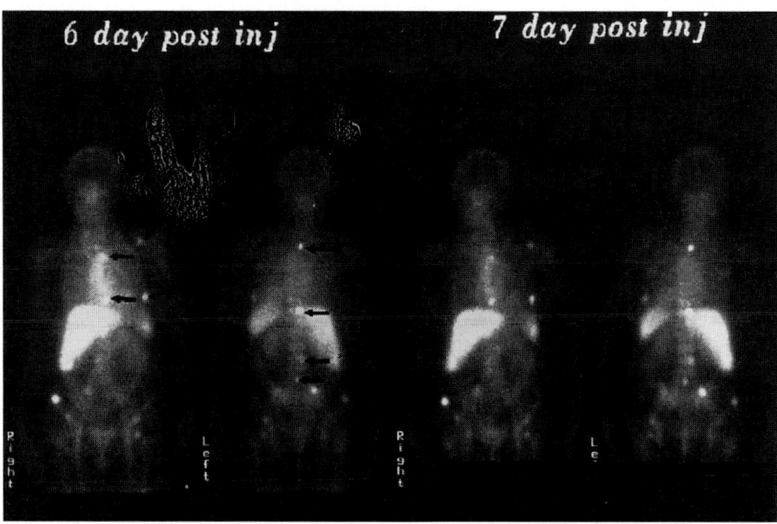

Fig. 29-10. A 46-year-old female, 4 months post-operative who had "total" removal of ovarian carcinoma with rising serum levels of CA-125. Six and seven day anterior and posterior whole body images following the adminstration of 5 mCi ^{111}In Oncoscint reveal multiple foci of metastatic disease *(arrows)*. The focus in the right pelvis is in a mesenteric lymph node (surgically confirmed), and all other sites are in the bone marrow (^{99m}Tc MDP bone images were negative).

Planar imaging and SPECT imaging are both appropriate. A medium-energy collimator, 128 × 128 or 64 × 64 acquisition matrix are acceptable. Both the 171 and 247 keV energies, a 20% symmetric window and a 10-minute acquisition time per image will provide adequate imaging statistics for planar imaging.

The full 5 mCi (185 MBq) is much preferred for a standard adult as a lesser dose may require a longer duration of acquisition. With a full 5-mCi dose and a single-head camera, acquisition times of 40 seconds for 64 stops produce adequate statistics at 4 to 5 days postinjection. Total acquisition time is about 50 minutes. Multihead cameras for the same duration of acquisition will produce a significant improvement in statistics of the projection data.

A low-pass filter such as a Butterworth with 0.4 Nyquist cutoff and perhaps order 7 has produced good images. Of course the poorer the statistics of the projection data, the greater the need to limit high frequencies to produce an adequate reconstruction. The more high frequencies are limited, the less spatial resolution there is and the larger the tumor must be before it can be seen. The major problem when starting antibody imaging is false positive sites caused by a filter that permits too much noise in the reconstruction and the lack of experience in interpreting such noisy images. It is better to start with images that limit noise and allow the large lesions to be seen. Experience gained from other low-count SPECT studies such as ^{67}Ga will help. There is no substitute for using a low-pass, intermediate-pass, and high-pass filter on the same data and seeing first-hand the effects in the final image.

Another complicating factor is the difference between vendors' SPECT systems. Some experimentation with filters is needed to produce an adequate reconstruction because the optimal filter will vary depending on the statistical validity of the projection data. There is an almost infinite variety of Butterworth filters. To say an image was reconstructed with a Butterworth filter is almost meaningless, unless the cutoff, the order and the computer are specified.

With an administered dose of 3 mCi (111 MBq) of radiotracer, SPECT imaging can still be performed. Despite statistical difficulties, antibody imaging is clinically useful and unique. Diagnostic information that will change the management of 26% of patients with colon and ovarian cancer can be obtained (Fig. 29-10).

BIBLIOGRAPHY

Barrett, J.T.: Basic immunology and its medical applications, ed. 2, St. Louis, Mo., The C.V. Mosby Co.

Becker, W., Schoman, E., Fischbach, W., and others: Comparison of ^{99m}Tc-HMPAO and ^{111}In-oxine labelled granulocytes in man: first clinical results, Nucl. Med. Commun. 9:435-447, 1988.

Bomanji, J., Nimmon, C.C., Hungerford, J.L., and others: Ocular radioimmunoscintigraphy: sensitivity and practical considerations, J. Nucl. Med. 29:1038-1044, 1988.

Callcott, F., Gordon, L., Schabel, S.I., and others: Indium-111 WBC imaging—false positive in a simple fracture, J. Nucl. Med. 29:571-572, 1988.

Cancer Facts and Figures, 1992: American Cancer Society, Inc.: Atlanta

Carrasquillo, J.A., Abrams, P.G., Schroff, R.W., and others: Effect of antibody dose on the imaging and biodistribution of indium-111 9.2.27 antimelanoma monoclonal antibody, J. Nucl. Med. 29:39-47, 1988.

Cohen, A.M., Shrank, B., and Friedman, M.A.: Colorectal cancer. In DeVita, V.T., Jr., Hellman, S., and Rosenberg, S.A., editors: Cancer: principles and practice of oncology, ed. 3, Philadelphia, 1989, J.B. Lippincott Co., pp. 895-964.

Collier, B.D., Abdel-Nabi, H., Doerr, R.J., and others: Immunoscintigraphy performed with In-111 labeled CYT-103 in the management of colorectal cancer: comparison with CT, Radiology 185:179-186, 1992.

Danpure, H.M., Osman, S., and Brady, F.: The labeling of blood cells in plasma with In-111 Tropolonate, Br. J. Radiol. 55:247-249, 1982.

Danpure, H.J., Osman, S., and Caroll, M.J.: The development of a clinical protocol for the radiolabeling of mixed leukocytes with ^{99m}Tc-hexamethylpropyleneamine oxime, Nucl. Med. Commun. 9:465-475, 1988.

Doerr, R.J., Abdel-Nabi, H., Krag, D., and others: Radiolabeled antibody imaging in the management of colorectal cancer: results of a multicenter clinical study, Ann. Surg. 214:118-124, 1991.

Farrer, P.A., Saha, G.B., and Shibata, H.N.: Evaluation of 111-In transferrin as a tumor scanning agent in humans, J. Nucl. Med. 13:429, 1972.

Galandiuk, S., Wieand, H.S., Moertel, C.G., and others: Patterns of recurrence after curative resection of carcinoma of the colon and rectum, Surg. Gynecol. Obstet. 174:27-32, 1992.

Gilbert, E.H., Earle, J.D., Goris, M.L., and others: The accuracy of 111-In Cl as a bone marrow scanning agent, Radiology 117:167-168, 1976.

Golde, D.W., and Gasson, J.C.: Hormones that stimulate the growth of blood cells, Scientific American, July 1988, pp. 62-79.

Goodwin, D.A.: Pharmacokinetics and antibodies, J. Nucl. Med. 28:1358-1362, 1987.

Grossman, Z.D., and Rosebrough, S.F.: Clinical radioimmuno imaging, Orlando, Fla., 1988, Grune & Stratton, Inc.

Halpern, S.E., Dillman, R.O., Witzum, K.F., and others: Radioimmunodetection of melanoma utilizing In-111 96.5 monoclonal antibody: a preliminary report, Radiology 155:493-499, 1985.

Halpern, S.E., Haindl, W., Beauregard, J., and others: Scintigraphy with In-111 labeled monoclonal antitumor antibodies: kinetics, biodistribution and tumor detection, Radiology 168:529-536, 1988.

Hawker, R.J., Hall, C.E., and Gunson, B.K.: Re: Indium-111 tropolone vs. oxine, J. Nucl. Med. 24:367, 1983.

Hunter, W.W., and Riccobono, X.J.: Clinical evaluation of ^{111}In for localization of recognized neoplastic disease, J. Nucl. Med. 11:328-329, 1970.

Iles, S.E., Ehrlich, I.E., Saliken, J.C., and Martin, R.H.: Indium-111 chloride scintigraphy in adult osteomyelitis, J. Nucl. Med. 28:1540-1545, 1987.

Johnson, J.A., Christie, M.J., Sandler, M.P., Parks, P.F., Jr., Homra, L., and Kaye, J.J.: Detection of occult infection following total joint arthroplasty using sequential technetium-99m HPD bone scintigraphy and indium-111 WBC imaging, J. Nucl. Med. 29:1347-1353, 1988.

Kohler, G., and Milstein, C.: Continuous culture of fused cells secreting antibody of predefined specificity, Nature 256(5517):495-497, 1975.

Kramer, E.L., DeNardo, S.J., Liebes, L., and others: Radioimmunolocalization of metastatic breast cancer using indium-111-methyl benzyl DTPA BrE3 monoclonal antibody: phase I study, J. Nucl. Med. 34:1067-1074, 1993.

Lamb, J.F.: Commercial production of radioisotopes for nuclear medicine, 1970-1980, IEEE Transactions on Nuclear Science, vol. NS-28, no. 2, 1982, pp. 1916-1920.

Larsen, S.M., Carrasquillo, J.A., McGriffin, R.W., and others: Use of I-131 labeled murine Fab against high molecular weight antigen of human melanoma: preliminary experience, Radiology 155:487-492, 1985.

Magnuson, J.E., Brown, M.L., Hauser, M.F., Berquist, T.H., Fitzgerald, R.H., Jr., and Klee, G.G.: In-111-labeled leukocyte scintigraphy in suspected orthopedic prosthesis infection: comparison with other imaging modalities, Radiology 168:235-239, 1988.

Maguire, R.T., and Van Nostrand, D.: Diagnosis of colorectal and ovarian carcinoma: application of immunoscintigraphic technology, New York, Basel, Hong Kong, Marcel Dekker, Inc.

McCarthy, K., Velchik, M.G., Mandell, G.A., Esterhai, J.L., and Goll, S.: Indium-111-labeled white blood cells in the detection of osteomyelitis complicating a pre-existing condition, J. Nucl. Med. 29:1015-1021, 1988.

Merkel, K.D., Brown, M.L., Dewanjee, M.K., and Fitzgerald, R.H., Jr.: Comparison of indium-labeled-leucocyte imaging with sequential technetium-gallium scanning in the diagnosis of low-grade musculoskeletal sepsis, J. Bone Joint Surg. [Am.] 67:465-476, 1985.

Metcalf, D.: The granulocyte-macrophage colony stimulating factors, Science 224:(4708), 1985, pp. 18-22.

Milstein, C.: Monoclonal antibodies, Scientific American, Oct. 1980, pp. 66-75.

Miraldi, F.D., Nelson, A.D., Kraly, C., and others: Diagnostic imaging of human neuroblastoma with radiolabeled antitumor antibody, Radiology 161:413-418, 1986.

Mountford, P.J., Kettle, A.G., O'Doherty, M.J., and Coackly, A.J.: Comparison of technetium-99m-HMPAO leukocytes with indium-111-oxime leukocytes for localizing intra-abdominal sepsis, J. Nucl. Med. 31:311-315, 1990.

Murray, J.L., Rosenblum, M.G., Lamki, L., and others: Clinical parameters related to optimal tumor localization of indium-111 labeled mouse antimelanoma monoclonal antibody ZME-018, J. Nucl. Med. 28:25-33, 1988.

Nabi, H.A., and Doerr, R.J.: Radiolabeled monoclonal antibody imaging (immunoscintigraphy) of colorectal cancers: current status and future perspectives, Am J. Surg. 163:448-456, 1992.

Peters, A.M., Danpure, H.J., Osman, S., and others: Clinical experience with ^{99m}Tc-hexamethylpropyleneamine for labeling and imaging inflammation, Lancet i:946-949, 1986.

Reynolds, J.H., Graham, D., and Smith, F.W.: Imaging inflammation with ^{99m}Tc HMPAO labelled leukocytes, Clin. Radiol. 42:195-198, 1990.

Roddie, M.E., Peters, A.M., Danpure, H.J., and others: Inflammation: imaging with Tc-99m HMPAO-labeled leukocytes, Radiology 166:767-772, 1988.

Rodwell, J.D., Alvarez, V.L., Lee, C., and others: Site specific covalent modification of monoclonal antibodies: in vitro and in vivo evaluations, Proc. Natl. Acad. Sci. USA 83:2632-2636, 1986.

Rodwell, J.D.: Engineering monoclonal antibodies: a perspective of the future, Nature 342:99-100, 1989.

Sayle, B.A., Balachandron, S., and Rogers, C.A.: Indium-111 chloride imaging in patients with suspected abscesses, J. Nucl. Med. 24:114, 1983.

Seabold, J.E., Nepola, J.V., Conrad, G.R., and others: Detection of osteomyelitis at fracture non-union sites: a comparison of two scintigraphic methods, AJR 152:1021-1027, 1989.

Schauweeker, D.S., Park, H.M., Mock, B.H., and others: Evaluation of complicating osteomyelitis with Tc-99m, In-111 granulocytes, and Ga-67 citrate, J. Nucl. Med. 25:849-853, 1984.

Schmidt, K.G., Rasmussen, J.W., Wedebye, I.M., and others: Accumulation of indium-111 labeled granulocytes in malignant tumors, J. Nucl. Med. 29:479-484, 1988.

Sfakianakis, G.N., Mnaymneh, W., Ghandur-Mnaymneh, L., and others: Positive indium-111 leukocyte scintigraphy in a skeletal metastasis, Am. J. Roentegenol. 139:601-603, 1982.

Stramignoni, D., Bowen, R., Atkinson, B.F., and Schlom, J.: Differential reactivity of monoclonal antibodies with human colon adenocarcinomas and adenomas, Int. J. Cancer 31:543-552, 1983.

Taylor, A., Milton, W., Eyre, H., and others: Radioimmunodetections of human melanoma with indium-111 monoclonal antibody, J. Nucl. Med. 29:329-337, 1988.

Van Nostrand, D., Abreu, S.H., Callaghan, J.J., and others: In-111 labeled white cell uptake in noninfected closed fracture in humans: prospective study, Radiology 167:495-498, 1988.

Zakhireh, B., Thakur, M.L., Malech, H.L., and others: Indium-111 labeled human polymorpholnclear leukocytes: viability, random migration, chemotaxis, bacterial capacity and ultrastructure, J. Nucl. Med. 29:741, 1979.

Chapter 30

SPECIAL IN VITRO PROCEDURES

D. BRUCE SODEE

■ BLOOD: GENERAL CONCEPTS

Circulating blood contains extracellular fluid and the intracellular fluid that is found in red blood cells. The average blood volume of a normal adult is 5000 ml—3000 ml of plasma and 2000 ml of red blood cells. Of the total of 40 liters of fluid in the body, 25 liters comprise the intracellular fluid found in the 75 trillion cells of the body. The plasma is the portion of the blood that is noncellular and makes up a large portion of the extracellular fluid volume; it is constantly being exchanged with the interstitial fluid through the capillaries. The plasma proteins contained by colloid and osmotic pressure decrease the amount of fluid lost through the capillary pores. Serum is that portion of blood remaining after clot formation has removed the cells and proteins consumed in the clotting process.

■ Plasma

Plasma is a watery fluid with various ions and inorganic and organic molecules. Its solid portion is made up of plasma proteins, which are composed of albumin, globulin, and fibrinogen. These proteins exert an osmotic force, which tends to hold water in the capillaries. The globulin fraction has varied functions, including blood clotting, the transporting of hormones, and transporting the immune mechanism of the body. Albumin and blood-clotting proteins are produced by the liver. Globulins and fibrinogen are formed by the plasma cells, lymphoid tissue, and the reticuloendothelial system.

■ Red blood cells

Red blood cells primarily transport hemoglobin, which carries oxygen from the lungs to the tissues. They also contain carbonic anhydrase, which catalyzes the reaction between water and carbon dioxide and makes it possible for the blood to transport carbon dioxide from the tissues to the lungs. Red blood cells are biconcave disks with an average volume of 83 cubic microns. A red blood cell can take any shape as it passes through capillaries. The average adult has approximately 5 million red blood cells per cubic millimeter of whole blood. Whole blood contains approximately 16 gm of hemoglobin per 100 ml. When a sample of blood is centrifuged or allowed to settle, the sediment, which is primarily made up of red cells, is approximately 45%, with the supernatant plasmacrit being 55%. White cells and platelets make up a small part of the formed sediment.

During the midtrimester of gestation, in the fetus the liver is the main organ for production of red cells, as well as the spleen and lymph nodes. During the third trimester and after birth, red blood cells are primarily formed in bone marrow. Until approximately 5 years of age the bone marrow of all bones produces red blood cells. The shaft of the femur and tibia continue to produce some red cells through the early 20s. Thereafter the primary red blood cell production is in the vertebra, the sternum, and the ribs.

Red cells are produced by a unipotential stem cell. It is first identified as a basophilic erythroblast, which has the ability to synthesize hemoglobin. As the cell matures, the nucleus shrinks, and the cell becomes a normoblast. Before the red cell leaves the bone marrow, the nucleus is extruded and the cell is called a *reticulocyte* because it still contains a slight amount of basophilic endoplasmic reticulum in the cytoplasm. While in this stage the cells squeeze through the pores of the blood capillaries. In normal blood the total number of reticulocytes among all red blood cells is less than 1%. The basic regulator of red blood cell production is tissue oxygenation; thus high altitudes, cardiac failure, or severe lung diseases cause tissue hypoxia, which results in an increase in the rate of red cell production. The primary stimulator of red cell production in response to hypoxia is erythropoietin, which is a specific glycoprotein that appears in the blood in response to hypoxia. Erythropoietin production is also primarily dependent on the kidneys, which in response to hypoxia release renal erythropoietic factor. The rate of red cell production in a human can be stimulated 6 to 8 times normal production. Red blood cells have an average life span of between 100 and 120 days. Senescent red blood cells are primarily destroyed in the spleen.

■ SPECIAL IN VITRO PROCEDURES

LABORATORY APPLICATION

82

BLOOD VOLUME DETERMINATION

Purpose

Blood volume is tightly controlled and kept constant by the following mechanisms. If blood volume is decreased, cardiac output and arterial pressure decrease. The kidneys in turn retain fluid, and progressive accumulation of fluid brings the blood volume back within normal limits. If blood volume is increased, cardiac output and arterial pressure increase, which causes loss of fluid from the kidney and which in turn brings the blood volume back within normal limits. Many drugs and diseases, however, have a great influence on these control mechanisms. In bleeding, the above mechanisms bring the blood volume back to normal by increasing the plasma volume. The red cell mass remains low.

A simple hematocrit reading can be misleading in estimating blood volume or the true number of red cells circulating in the body; for example, if the patient has a low plasma volume the hematocrit will be falsely elevated, or if the patient has an increased plasma volume the hematocrit will be falsely low.

Thus radioactive tracers were introduced into the measurement of blood volume. They have proved extremely accurate, particularly when combined with a labeled protein tracer such as ^{125}I RISA, which measures the plasma compartment, and the ^{51}Cr-labeled red cell procedure that accurately measures the red cell mass.

Indications

1. For evaluation of blood loss and blood-replacement therapy
2. For evaluation of extensive trauma and burns
3. For preoperative evaluation of the elderly patient
4. For evaluation of a patient with anemia
5. For evaluation of a patient with possible polycythemia

Procedure: plasma volume determination

Materials

1. ^{125}I RISA, 10 to 20 μCi, (0.37 to 0.74 MBq) contained in a 1.5-ml volume
2. Uncontaminated 22-gauge needle
3. Well adaptor

Patient preparation

1. No preparation of the patient is required.
2. Explain the entire procedure to the patient.

Technique

1. Place the syringe (^{125}I RISA) in the well adaptor; collect and record counts.
2. Inject the RISA dose intravenously in the arm contralateral to the arm to be used for obtaining postinjection blood samples. Rinse the syringe three times with the patient's blood. Record the time of injection.
3. Draw 1.5 ml of tap water into the syringe through the needle used for injection.
4. Replace needle with a new uncontaminated 22-gauge needle and again obtain counts of the syringe above the well in the well adaptor. Record count rate.

5. Withdraw three 15-ml blood samples at 15, 25, and 35 minutes after injection. Record times of blood samples withdrawn.
6. Patient blood samples are centrifuged and divided into 5-ml aliquots.

Calculations

1. Count each 5-ml sample for 1 minute, or for 10,000 counts. Reduce the result of cpm/ml and record values.
2. If extrapolation is not necessary, select the highest value of the three 15-, 25-, and 35-minute plasma count rates and use this value for the patient sample.
3. The circulating plasma volume is derived by the following formula:

$$\text{PL volume} = \frac{(\text{Full syringe} - \text{empty syringe}) \times \text{CF}}{\text{Patient sample}}$$

Key points

1. If the concentration of RISA is high, it may be diluted with saline to obtain the 10 to 20 μCi (0.37 to 0.74 MBq)/1.5 ml dose needed.
2. The RISA syringe must be counted above the well, since it is too "hot" to count in the well. Counting the syringe in the well produces an inaccurately low count rate that is not representative of the true activity.
3. The same-gauge needle is necessary during syringe counting in the well adaptor. Different size needles for the "full syringe" and "empty syringe" counts may increase or decrease activity detected by the crystal. Remember, ^{125}I emits a low-energy gamma and is easily absorbed.
4. The correction factor for an individual well can be determined by the following steps:
   a. Count 10 to 20 μCi (0.37 to 0.74 MBq) of ^{125}I RISA in a 2.5 ml syringe in a well adaptor above the well. The volume of the activity should be 1.5 ml. Record the counts.
   b. Dispense syringe contents into a 2000-ml volume of water containing 5 to 15 ml of patient plasma. (This reduces the tendency of iodine to adhere to the walls of the glass or plastic container.) Mix well.
   c. Accurately pipette 5 ml into a large-well vial and count in the well.
   d. Record the counts and reduce the result to counts per minute per milliliters.
   e. Derive the correction factor by the following formula:

$$\text{CF} = \frac{\text{cpm/ml from 5-ml volume} \times 2000}{\text{cpm from syringe above well}}$$

   f. Repeat procedure to ensure accuracy of the derived CF.
5. Protein-bound tracers such as ^{125}I albumin (RISA) transfer in and out of vascular/extravascular beds in the same manner as untagged proteins. Therefore the RISA injection may not remain in the vascular space during the mixing time. The amount of ^{125}I albumin that diffuses or "leaks" out during the mixing and withdrawal time of the plasma volume determination can be estimated by establishing a disappearance curve. This is accomplished by plotting the dilution count (15-minute, 25-minute, and 35-minute patient samples corrected for background) versus time

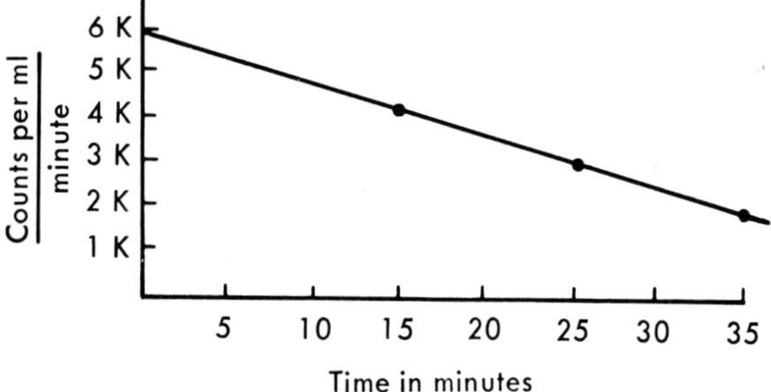

Fig. 30-1. Extrapolated to zero time, there were 6000 counts before diffusion occurred.

Continued.

(Fig. 30-1). The correct dilution count before diffusion can be derived by extrapolating the curve back to zero time. If there is less than 5% difference between any of the three RISA withdrawals, extrapolation is not necessary.

6. Iodine has a tendency to adhere to glass, metal, plastic, and tissue such as the vascular wall at the site of injection.
7. A contaminated syringe cap on the "full" or "empty" syringe results in an inaccurate, high determination.
8. If a single determination is done with RISA, be sure to take a background blood sample before starting the procedure.
9. If needed or desired, total blood volume or red cell mass can be calculated from the plasma volume determination using the following formula:

$$\text{TBV} = \frac{\text{PL volume}}{\text{Corrected PL crit}} = \frac{\text{PL volume}}{1 - (\text{Hct} \times 0.97 \times 0.91)}$$

Hct = Patient hematocrit, determined from one of the patient's blood samples

$$\text{RCM} = \text{TBV} - \text{PL volume}$$

10. Microhematocrit readings are given in Table 30-1. Normal values can be found in Tables 30-2 and 30-3. The box on page 732 lists pitfalls in blood volume measurement.

Procedure: labeling red blood cells

Materials

1. ^{51}Cr, 100 μCi (3.7 MBq)
2. ACD solution and standard tagging vial
3. Ascorbic acid, 50 mg
4. Heparin solution, 2.5 ml (1000 units/ml)
5. Counting vials, 10 and 15 ml
6. Pipettes, 1 and 5 ml
7. Microhematocrit tubes and centrifuge
8. Syringes
9. Butterfly infusion set, 19-gauge
10. Scintillation counting system

Patient preparation

1. No preparation of the patient is required.
2. Explain the entire procedure to the patient.

Technique

1. Draw up 7 ml of ACD solution into a 50-ml syringe. Dispose of 2 ml of the solution so that 5 ml remains in the syringe
2. Perform a venipuncture with the infusion set.
3. Using the 50-ml syringe with the 5 ml of ACD solution, withdraw 40 ml of whole blood from the patient (the ACD solution acts as an anticoagulant).
   a. Pinch the butterfly tubing, disconnect the 50-ml syringe, and connect the 2.5-ml syringe filled with heparin solution
   b. Inject 0.5 ml of heparin to keep the infusion set patent
4. Cap the 50-ml syringe and gently mix ACD solution and blood to prevent clotting.
5. Inject 30 ml of the total 45 ml into the ACD bottle.
6. Place the remaining 15 ml in a counting vial and label background. Place this vial in the well and check for background activity using the ^{51}Cr window. (If plasma volume determination is being performed in conjunction with red cell labeling, background activity should be checked in the ^{125}I window also.)

   If background activity exceeds 20% of expected count rate of either fraction of the blood samples, the dose must be doubled.
7. Inject 100 μCi (3.7 MBq) of ^{51}Cr into the ACD bottle and incubate for 20 minutes at room temperature.

Table 30-1. Microhematocrit readings centrifuged 4 minutes, corrected for trapped plasma with corresponding D_f factors*

	1 LVH				1 LVH				1 LVHd		
LVH†	Corr.	Corr.	D_f	LVH	Corr.	Corr.	D_f	LVH	Corr.	Corr.	D_f
				30	28.9	71.1	0.965	50	47.0	53.0	0.930
				30.5	29.4	70.6	0.965	50.5	47.5	52.5	0.930
				31	29.9	70.1	0.965	51	47.9	52.1	0.930
				31.5	30.3	69.7	0.965	51.5	48.4	51.6	0.930
				32	30.8	69.2	0.965	52	48.8	51.2	0.925
				32.5	31.2	68.8	0.965	52.5	49.2	50.8	0.925
13	12.8	87.2	0.985	33	31.7	68.3	0.960	53	49.7	50.3	0.925
13.5	13.3	86.7	0.985	33.5	32.2	67.8	0.960	53.5	50.1	49.9	0.925
14	13.8	86.2	0.985	34	32.6	67.4	0.960	54	50.5	49.5	0.920
14.5	14.2	85.8	0.985	34.5	33.1	66.9	0.960	54.5	51.0	49.0	0.920
15	14.7	85.3	0.985	35	33.5	66.5	0.960	55	51.4	48.6	0.920
15.5	15.2	84.8	0.985	35.5	34.0	66.0	0.960	55.5	51.8	48.2	0.920
16	15.7	84.3	0.985	36	34.5	65.5	0.960	56	52.3	47.7	0.915
16.5	16.2	83.8	0.985	36.5	35.0	65.0	0.960	56.5	52.7	47.3	0.915
17	16.7	83.3	0.985	37	35.4	64.6	0.955	57	53.1	46.9	0.915
17.5	17.1	82.9	0.985	37.5	35.8	64.2	0.955	57.5	53.6	46.4	0.910
18	17.6	82.4	0.985	38	36.3	63.7	0.955	58	54.0	46.0	0.910
18.5	18.1	81.9	0.985	38.5	36.7	63.3	0.955	58.5	54.4	45.6	0.910
19	18.6	81.4	0.980	39	37.2	62.8	0.955	59	54.9	45.1	0.905
19.5	19.0	81.0	0.980	39.5	37.6	62.4	0.955	59.5	55.2	44.8	0.905
20	19.5	80.5	0.980	40	38.1	61.9	0.950	60	55.7	44.3	0.905
20.5	20.0	80.0	0.980	40.5	38.6	61.4	0.950	60.5	56.2	43.8	0.905
21	20.5	79.5	0.980	41	39.0	61.0	0.950	61	56.6	43.4	0.905
21.5	20.9	79.1	0.980	41.5	39.5	60.5	0.950	61.5	57.0	43.0	0.900
22	21.4	78.6	0.980	42	39.9	60.1	0.950	62	57.4	42.6	0.900
22.5	21.9	78.1	0.980	42.5	40.4	59.6	0.950	62.5	57.9	42.1	0.900
23	22.4	77.6	0.980	43	40.8	59.2	0.950	63	58.3	41.7	0.895
23.5	22.8	77.2	0.975	43.5	41.3	58.7	0.945	63.5	58.7	41.3	0.895
24	23.3	76.7	0.975	44	41.7	58.3	0.945	64	59.1	40.9	0.895
24.5	23.8	76.2	0.975	44.5	42.1	57.9	0.945	64.5	59.6	40.4	0.890
25	24.3	75.7	0.975	45	42.6	57.4	0.940	65	60.0	40.0	0.890
25.5	24.7	75.3	0.975	45.5	43.0	57.0	0.940	65.5	60.4	39.6	0.890
26	25.2	74.8	0.975	46	43.5	56.5	0.940	66	60.8	39.2	0.885
26.5	25.7	74.3	0.975	46.5	43.9	56.1	0.940	66.5	61.3	38.7	0.885
27	26.1	73.9	0.970	47	44.4	55.6	0.940	67	61.7	38.3	0.880
27.5	26.6	73.4	0.970	47.5	44.8	55.2	0.935	67.5	62.1	37.9	0.880
28	27.1	72.9	0.970	48	45.3	54.7	0.935	68	62.5	37.5	0.875
28.5	27.5	72.5	0.970	48.5	45.7	54.3	0.935	68.5	62.9	37.1	0.875
29	28.0	72.0	0.970	49	46.1	53.9	0.935	69	63.3	36.7	0.870
29.5	28.5	71.5	0.970	49.5	46.6	53.4	0.930	69.5	63.8	36.2	0.865

*Dilution volume (obtained with plasma tracer) × D_f = Corrected total blood volume.
†Large-vessel hematocrit.

Continued.

Table 30-2. Normal blood volume values in milliliters for men

	Height in inches									
Wt (lb)	**60**	**62**	**64**	**66**	**68**	**70**	**72**	**74**	**76**	**Wt (kg)**
90	3,150	3,250	3,350	3,450	3,550	3,650	3,750	3,850	3,950	40.8
95	3,250	3,350	3,450	3,550	3,650	3,750	3,850	4,000	4,100	43.1
100	3,350	3,450	3,550	3,650	3,800	3,900	4,000	4,100	4,200	45.4
105	3,450	3,550	3,650	3,750	3,900	4,000	4,100	4,200	4,300	47.6
110	3,500	3,650	3,750	3,850	4,000	4,100	4,200	4,300	4,400	49.9
115	3,600	3,750	3,850	3,950	4,100	4,200	4,300	4,400	4,500	52.2
120	3,700	3,850	3,950	4,050	4,200	4,300	4,400	4,500	4,650	54.4
125	3,800	3,900	4,050	4,150	4,250	4,400	4,500	4,600	4,750	56.7
130	3,900	4,000	4,150	4,250	4,350	4,500	4,600	4,700	4,850	59.9
135	3,950	4,100	4,200	4,350	4,450	4,600	4,700	4,800	4,950	61.2
140	4,050	4,150	4,300	4,400	4,550	4,650	4,800	4,900	5,050	63.5
145	4,100	4,250	4,400	4,500	4,650	4,750	4,900	5,000	5,150	65.8
150	4,200	4,350	4,450	4,600	4,700	4,850	4,950	5,100	5,200	68.0
155	4,300	4,400	4,550	4,650	4,800	4,950	5,050	5,200	5,300	70.3
160	4,350	4,500	4,600	4,750	4,900	5,000	5,150	5,250	5,400	72.6
165	4,450	4,550	4,700	4,850	4,950	5,100	5,200	5,350	5,500	74.8
170	4,500	4,650	4,750	4,900	5,050	5,150	5,300	5,450	5,550	77.1
175	4,550	4,700	4,850	5,000	5,100	5,250	5,400	5,500	5,650	79.4
180	4,650	4,800	4,900	5,050	5,200	5,350	5,450	5,600	5,750	81.6
185	4,700	4,850	5,000	5,150	5,250	5,400	5,550	5,700	5,800	83.9
190	4,800	4,900	5,050	5,200	5,350	5,500	5,600	5,750	5,900	86.2
195	4,850	5,000	5,150	5,300	5,400	5,600	5,700	5,850	6,000	88.5
200	4,900	5,050	5,200	5,350	5,500	5,650	5,750	5,900	6,050	90.7
205	4,950	5,100	5,250	5,400	5,550	5,700	5,850	6,000	6,150	93.0
210	5,050	5,200	5,350	5,500	5,650	5,800	5,900	6,050	6,200	95.3
215	5,100	5,250	5,400	5,550	5,700	5,850	6,000	6,150	6,300	97.5
220	5,150	5,300	5,450	5,600	5,750	5,900	6,050	6,200	6,350	99.8
225	5,200	5,400	5,550	5,700	5,850	6,000	6,150	6,300	6,450	102.1
230	5,300	5,450	5,600	5,750	5,900	6,050	6,200	6,350	6,500	104.3
235	5,350	5,500	5,650	5,800	5,950	6,100	6,250	6,400	6,550	106.6
240	5,400	5,550	5,700	5,900	6,050	6,200	6,350	6,500	6,650	108.9
245	5,450	5,600	5,800	5,950	6,100	6,250	6,400	6,550	6,700	111.1
250	5,500	5,700	5,850	6,000	6,150	6,300	6,450	6,650	6,800	113.4
255	5,600	5,750	5,900	6,050	6,200	6,400	6,550	6,700	6,850	115.7
260	5,650	5,800	5,950	6,100	6,300	6,450	6,600	6,750	6,900	117.9
265	5,700	5,850	6,000	6,200	6,350	6,500	6,650	6,800	7,000	120.2
270	5,750	5,900	6,100	6,250	6,400	6,550	6,750	6,900	7,050	122.5
275	5,800	5,950	6,150	6,300	6,450	6,650	6,800	6,950	7,100	124.7
280	5,850	6,000	6,200	6,350	6,500	6,700	6,850	7,000	7,150	127.0
285	5,900	6,100	6,250	6,400	6,600	6,750	6,900	7,100	7,250	129.3
290	5,950	6,150	6,300	6,450	6,650	6,800	6,950	7,150	7,300	131.5
295	6,000	6,200	6,350	6,550	6,700	6,850	7,050	7,200	7,350	133.8
300	6,050	6,250	6,400	6,600	6,750	6,900	7,100	7,250	7,450	136.1
305	6,100	6,300	6,450	6,650	6,800	7,000	7,150	7,300	7,500	138.3
310	6,150	6,350	6,500	6,700	6,850	7,050	7,200	7,400	7,550	140.6
315	6,200	6,400	6,550	6,750	6,900	7,100	7,250	7,450	7,600	142.9
	1.52	1.57	1.63	1.68	1.73	1.78	1.83	1.88	1.93	
	Height in meters									

From Hidalgo, J.U., Nadler, S.B., and Bloch, T.: J. Nucl. Med. 3:94, 1962.

Table 30-3. Normal blood volume values in milliliters for women

Wt (lb)	Height in inches 58	60	62	64	66	68	70	72	74	Wt (kg)
80	2,300	2,400	2,500	2,600	2,750	2,850	2,950	3,050	3,150	36.3
85	2,400	2,550	2,650	2,750	2,850	2,950	3,050	3,150	3,250	38.6
90	2,550	2,650	2,750	2,850	2,950	3,050	3,200	3,300	3,400	40.8
95	2,650	2,750	2,850	2,950	3,100	3,200	3,300	3,400	3,500	43.1
100	2,750	2,850	2,950	3,100	3,200	3,300	3,400	3,500	3,650	45.4
105	2,850	2,950	3,050	3,200	3,300	3,400	3,500	3,650	3,750	47.6
110	2,950	3,050	3,150	3,300	3,400	3,500	3,650	3,750	3,850	49.9
115	3,000	3,150	3,250	3,350	3,500	3,650	3,750	3,850	4,000	52.2
120	3,100	3,250	3,350	3,500	3,600	3,750	3,850	3,950	4,100	54.4
125	3,200	3,350	3,450	3,600	3,700	3,850	3,950	4,050	4,200	56.7
130	3,300	3,400	3,550	3,650	3,800	3,950	4,050	4,200	4,300	59.0
135	3,350	3,500	3,650	3,750	3,900	4,000	4,150	4,250	4,400	61.2
140	3,450	3,600	3,700	3,850	4,000	4,100	4,250	4,350	4,500	63.5
145	3,550	3,650	3,800	3,950	4,050	4,200	4,350	4,450	4,600	65.8
150	3,600	3,750	3,900	4,050	4,150	4,300	4,450	4,550	4,700	68.0
155	3,700	3,850	3,950	4,100	4,250	4,400	4,500	4,650	4,800	70.3
160	3,750	3,900	4,050	4,200	4,350	4,450	4,600	4,750	4,900	72.5
165	3,850	4,000	4,150	4,250	4,400	4,550	4,700	4,850	4,950	74.8
170	3,900	4,050	4,200	4,350	4,500	4,650	4,800	4,900	5,050	77.1
175	4,000	4,150	4,300	4,450	4,600	4,700	4,850	5,000	5,150	79.4
180	4,050	4,200	4,350	4,500	4,650	4,800	4,950	5,100	5,250	81.6
185	4,150	4,300	4,450	4,600	4,750	4,900	5,000	5,150	5,300	83.9
190	4,200	4,350	4,500	4,650	4,800	5,000	5,100	5,250	5,400	86.2
195	4,250	4,450	4,600	4,750	4,900	5,050	5,200	5,350	5,450	88.5
200	4,350	4,500	4,650	4,800	4,950	5,100	5,250	5,400	5,500	90.7
205	4,400	4,550	4,700	4,900	5,000	5,200	5,350	5,500	5,560	93.0
210	4,450	4,650	4,800	4,950	5,100	5,250	5,400	5,550	5,700	95.3
215	4,550	4,700	4,850	5,000	5,150	5,350	5,500	5,650	5,800	97.5
220	4,600	4,750	4,900	5,100	5,250	5,400	5,550	5,700	5,850	99.8
225	4,650	4,850	5,000	5,150	5,300	5,450	5,650	5,800	5,950	102.1
230	4,700	4,900	5,050	5,200	5,400	5,550	5,700	5,850	6,000	104.3
235	4,800	4,950	5,100	5,300	5,450	5,600	5,750	5,950	6,100	106.6
240	4,850	5,000	5,200	5,350	5,500	5,700	5,850	6,000	6,150	108.9
245	4,900	5,100	5,250	5,400	5,600	5,750	5,900	6,050	6,250	111.1
250	4,950	5,150	5,300	5,500	5,650	5,800	6,000	6,150	6,300	114.4
255	5,000	5,200	5,350	5,550	5,700	5,900	6,050	6,200	6,350	115.7
260	5,100	5,250	5,450	5,600	5,750	5,950	6,100	6,300	6,450	117.9
265	5,150	5,300	5,500	5,650	5,850	6,000	6,150	6,350	6,500	120.2
270	5,200	5,350	5,550	5,700	5,900	6,050	6,250	6,400	6,600	122.5
275	5,250	5,450	5,600	5,800	5,950	6,150	6,300	6,450	6,650	124.7
280	5,300	5,500	5,650	5,850	6,000	6,200	6,350	6,500	6,700	127.0
285	5,350	5,550	5,700	5,900	6,100	6,250	6,450	6,600	6,750	129.3
290	5,400	5,600	5,800	5,950	6,150	6,300	6,500	6,650	6,850	131.5
295	5,450	5,650	5,850	6,000	6,200	6,400	6,550	6,750	6,900	133.8
300	5,500	5,700	5,900	6,100	6,250	6,450	6,600	6,800	6,950	136.1
305	5,600	5,750	5,950	6,150	6,300	6,500	6,650	6,850	7,050	138.3
310	5,650	5,800	6,000	6,200	6,350	6,550	6,750	6,900	7,100	140.6
315	5,700	5,850	6,050	6,250	6,450	6,600	6,800	6,950	7,150	142.9
	1.47	1.52	1.57	1.63	1.68	1.73	1.78	1.83	1.88	
	Height in meters									

From Hidalgo, J.U., Nadler, S.B., and Bloch, T.: J. Nucl. Med. 3:94, 1962.

Continued.

Pitfalls in blood volume measurement

General errors

1. There may be errors in the techniques of administering tracer and blood sampling.
2. Errors may result from improper equilibration of tracer in the bloodstream.

Inherent errors caused by the characteristics and distribution of tracers

1. Dilution ratio does not signify blood volume.
2. Large-vessel hematocrit (LVH) differs from whole-body hematocrit (WBH).
3. The F_{cell} ratio figures in calculations.

Labeled red cells as tracers

1. There may be clots and aggregation of cells in the tracer dose administered.
2. There may be an excessive amount of free chromium ions.
3. The calculated plasma and blood volume are approximated.

Labeled albumin as tracers

1. There is a high rate of loss from the intravascular bed.
2. There is an excessive amount of free iodine in the preparation.
3. The calculated red cell and blood volume are approximated.

Errors in repeat measurement

1. There is a fluctuating background.
2. There are differences in the hematocrit values between samples.

8. At 20 minutes inject 50 mg of ascorbic acid into ACD bottle and incubate for 10 minutes; this reduces the ^{51}Cr from a +6 valence to a +3 valence state. In a +3 state ^{51}Cr cannot penetrate the red cell membrane and will not tag red cells in vivo after reinjection.
9. Withdraw 20 ml of the patient's whole blood from the ACD bottle and inject into the patient's opposite arm with the infusion set.
10. Allow a circulation time of 20 minutes before withdrawing a 20-ml sample.
11. Remove the butterfly infusion set after the 20-minute sample is obtained.
12. Divide the patient's blood sample into various aliquots and place in vials for counting purposes. It is suggested that blood be identified in the following manner:
    a. Standard whole-blood sample taken from the ACD bottle (Std WB)
    b. Standard plasma taken from the ACD bottle (Std PL)
    c. The 20-minute blood (20 min WB)
    d. The 20-minute plasma (20 min PL)
    e. The background activity sample (Bkg)
13. Hematocrit determination and blood sample volumes needed for the calculation are made up of the following:
    a. Hematocrit of Std WB
    b. Hematocrit of 20 min WB (Both hematocrits are performed in duplicate)
    c. 0.5 ml of Std WB should be placed in 4.5 ml of water or distilled water

d. 5 ml of Std PL may be obtained by spinning the remaining Std WB after the hematocrit and 0.5-ml samples are removed
e. 5 ml of 20 min WB
f. 5 ml of 20 min PL

Calculations

1. Count all samples (5-ml Std WB, 5-ml Std PL, 5 ml of 20-min WB, 5 ml of 20-min PL) for at least 10,000 counts and reduce results to counts per minute per ml (cpm/ml).
2. Derive the circulating red cell mass by the following formula:

$$\text{RCM} = \frac{([\text{Std WB cpm/ml}] - [\text{Std PL cpm/ml} \times \text{Std PL crit}]) \times \text{volume injected} \times \text{20-minute Hct}}{(\text{20-minute WB cpm/ml}) - (\text{20-minute PL cpm/ml} \times \text{20-minute PL crit})}$$

Key points

1. Uniformity of cell distribution in a sample may be offset by clots, agglutinations, or aggregation of cells and may cause erroneous results. This is why all blood samples are heparinized and mixed well. All samples containing red cells should be remixed just before counting.
2. ^{51}Cr should not be added to the ACD solution before the patient's blood is placed in the vial for tagging. Dextrose contained in the ACD solution acts as as reducing agent.
3. ^{51}Cr will not properly label the red cells from patients receiving antibiotics or polyvitamins. These act as a reducing agent and reduce the hexavalent C to a trivalent state before it can tag the red cells in the standard whole blood (ACD vial).
4. Hemolysis of the standard whole blood red cells or hemolysis of these cells during or after injection results in an inaccurate larger red cell mass.
5. If needed or desired, the total blood volume or plasma volume can be calculated from the red cell mass determination using the formula:

$$\text{TBV} = \frac{\text{Red cell mass}}{\text{Corrected patient hematocrit}} = \frac{\text{Red cell mass}}{\text{Patient Hct} \times 0.91 \times 0.97}$$

PL volume = TBV − Red cell mass. However, this method is not recommended.

6. Plasmacrits as well as hematocrits are often expressed in percent. Plasmacrits can be determined by knowing the hematocrit and subtracting the decimal equivalent from 1.00, as in the following:

Hematocrit = 42%
Decimal equivalent = 0.42
Plasmacrit = 1.00 − 0.42 = 0.58 or 58%

The formula in step 13 is designed to use the decimal equivalent whenever a hematocrit or plasmacrit is required. For example:

If 20-minute plasmacrit = 58%, use 0.58 in formula

Procedure: combined ^{125}I RISA plasma volume and ^{51}Cr red cell mass

Materials

See plasma volume and red cell mass procedures, pp. 726-728 and 728-733.

Patient preparation

1. No preparation of the patient is required.
2. Explain the entire procedure to the patient.

Technique

Time sequence chart—plasma volume and red cell mass

Single determination (plasma volume)	Lapsed time (minutes)	Single determination (^{51}Cr red cell mass)
	0	Insert infusion set in patient's arm. Withdraw 40 ml of whole blood.
Inject RISA "full syringe," mark time.	1	
	2	Place 30 ml of WB in ACD vial. Inject ^{51}Cr, mix, incubate.
Withdraw 15 ml of 15-min WB.	16	
	22	Add ascorbic acid, mix, incubate.
Withdraw 15 ml of 25-min WB.	26	
	32	Prepare 20 ml of Std WB from ACD vial for injection
Withdraw 15 ml of 35-min WB. Patient may leave if only RISA procedure is being performed. Determine Hct (if this is a single study), spin blood.	36	
	37	Inject Std WB.
Complete procedure for single determination.	Approx. 55	
	57	Withdraw 20 ml of 20-min WB. Patient may leave. Determine Hct, spin blood.
	Approx. 120	Complete dual-determination procedure.

LABORATORY APPLICATION

83

RED CELL SURVIVAL

Purpose

The red cell survival test determines the functional half-clearance time of ^{51}Cr-labeled isologous red cells. The study is used primarily to study the life-span of red cells in patients with suspected hemolytic anemia.

Indications

1. To determine survival of isologous red cells in hemolytic anemia
2. To determine the life span of hemologous red cells in the study or therapy of hemolytic anemia
3. To study the effect of therapy on patients with hemolytic anemia

Procedure

Materials

1. Scintillation detector and readout system
2. Hematocrit tubes
3. Red cell survival data sheet
4. Semilogarithmic graph paper

Patient preparation

1. Patient is to have ^{51}Cr blood volume procedure.
2. Explain the procedure to the patient. Blood samples are taken three times a week for approximately 2 weeks. (Try to arrange test to be done on Monday, Wednesday, and Friday.)

Technique

1. On Day 1 withdraw 20 ml of patient's heparinized whole blood and record hematocrit.
2. Pipette 5 ml of whole blood into test tubes and label appropriately.
3. Centrifuge remaining blood.
4. Pipette 5 ml of plasma into sample test tubes and label appropriately.

5. Repeat three times a week for 2 weeks.
6. All patient samples should be refrigerated during this time.

Calculations

1. After all samples have been obtained, count all whole-blood and plasma samples for minimum of 10,000 counts, or 5 minutes each. Whole-blood samples should be mixed well before counting to maintain geometry.
2. Determine 5-minute counts for each sample.
3. Determine net red cell counts for each sample.

   Net red cell counts in 5 ml of whole blood = Whole blood counts/5 ml − Plasma counts/5 ml

4. Determine 5-minute counts for red cells.

$$\text{Net counts of red cells} = \frac{\text{Net red cell counts of whole blood}}{\text{Sample hematocrit}}$$

5. Express counts of red cells for each sample as a percent of Day 1 red cell counts.

$$\text{\% tagged red blood cells} = \frac{\text{Sample net counts of red cells} \times 100}{\text{Day 1 net counts of red cells}}$$

6. Using semilogarithmic graph paper, determine red cell survival half-time by plotting percent on the log scale and the time lapse in days on the linear scale. Draw a line through 50% and determine number of days elapsed.

Diagnosis

The red cell survival procedure, if carefully performed, is an accurate index of the life span of injected ^{51}Cr-labeled red cells. This study has to be carefully monitored because the results may be invalidated by therapy (for example, blood transfusions). The study is an accurate index of low-grade red blood cell destruction, which may be missed by standard hematologic examination and may be used to determine if increased red blood cell destruction results from red blood cell defects or from an intravascular cause. Cause and relationship may be established by using isologous or homologous chromium-labeled red cells in the study. Normal half-time ^{51}Cr red blood cell survival is approximately 28 days. Each laboratory should determine normal values.

LABORATORY APPLICATION

84

VITAMIN B_{12} ABSORPTION (SCHILLING TEST)

Purpose

This study helps to determine whether a patient is able to absorb orally administered vitamin B_{12}.

Vitamin B_{12} is necessary for the maturation of all tissues in the body. The organ systems most profoundly affected by vitamin B_{12} deficiency are the bone marrow and GI and neurologic systems. Systemic symptoms are primarily related to anemia. Bone marrow is hyperplastic, with many red cell precursors. Peripheral blood reveals a macrocytic anemia with many bizarre red cell forms. Leukocytes are large and multisegmented and reduced in number. Platelets are bizarre and also reduced in number. GI symptoms are related to mucosal atrophy and appear as a sore tongue, abdominal pain, and diarrhea. Neurologic symptoms result from degeneration of the posterolateral columns of the spinal cord and peripheral nerves. The classic vitamin B_{12} deficiency syndrome is pernicious anemia, which results from a deficiency in the gastric secretion of intrinsic factor necessary for absorption of vitamin B_{12}.

The Schilling test entails the collection of urine for 48 hours after the oral administration of radioactive cobalt-labeled vitamin B_{12}. If the initial collection has a reduced amount of excreted vitamin, the test is repeated with a second sample of radioactive cobalt-labeled vitamin B_{12} and intrinsic factor.

The following are possible causes of a vitamin B_{12} deficiency:

1. Failure of the stomach to secrete intrinsic factor. This could be a result of gastrectomy or of

Continued.

gastric atrophy, possibly caused by the immune mechanism. Antibodies to various components of gastric secretion have been isolated in patients with pernicious anemia.
2. Absorption deficiency. Malabsorption syndrome may be caused by regional enteritis.
3. Intraintestinal destruction of vitamin B_{12} by intestinal bacterial overgrowth, for example, in the "blind loop" syndrome.

These studies should be preceded by a plasma vitamin B_{12} assay (RIA). However, the Schilling test has been found to be more accurate in the diagnosis of pernicious anemia, since many patients have had vitamin B_{12} administered before a complete evaluation.

Indications

1. Evidence of anemia suggestive of pernicious anemia.
2. Neurologic signs that suggest vitamin B_{12} deficiency.

Procedure

Materials

1. Scintillation detector and readout system
2. Urine specimen collection containers
   a. 1 quart urine bottle
   b. 1 small urine cup
3. Radioactive B_{12}
   a. 1 capsule 0.5 μCi (.0185 MBq) ^{57}Co
   b. ^{57}Co reference standard
   c. 1 capsule intrinsic factor (where applicable)
4. Disposable counting tubes, 10 ml vacutainer tubes
5. A 5- or 10-ml pipette

Patient preparation

1. The patient should not be allowed anything orally from midnight the evening before the test is to begin.
2. Preferably the patient should not have had recent administration of radionuclides that were eliminated by the urinary system.
3. Explain the entire procedure to the patient, giving special instructions concerning collection of urine.

Technique

1. Obtain a background urine sample from the patient.
2. Administer ^{57}Co orally.
3. Instruct the patient not to eat for the next 3 hours.
4. Instruct the patient to save all urine for the next 48 hours.
5. The patient is to receive 2 injections of vitamin B_{12} intramuscularly (1000 μgm each) 2 to 6 hours after dose administration.
6. Collect urine container after 48 hours.

Calculations

1. Total urine volume can be read from calibrated urine containers.
2. Mix containers thoroughly. Pipette 4 ml of urine into a vial and label appropriately. Pipette 4 ml of background urine into another vial and label.
3. Count each vial in the ^{57}Co window for statistical counts and record on work sheet.
4. Count ^{57}Co reference standard and reduce to cpm.
5. Calculate results using following formula:

$$\frac{^{57}\text{Co urine cpm} - \text{bkg urine cpm} \times \text{urine vol} \times 100}{^{57}\text{Co standard cpm} \times \text{Dilution factor}} = \text{Percent excretion}$$

6. Record all results.

Results

Borderline abnormal range for Schilling's I is 8% to 10%; below 8% is abnormal. For Schilling's II, an improved percentage is compatible with pernicious anemia, while no change in the percentage is compatible with malabsorption.

Key points

1. Previous studies with high-energy radionuclides may interfere.
2. The urine collection is usually the problem area. Any lost urine should be noted and taken into consideration in the diagnosis of results. Should an inaccurate collection be suspected, do not discard urine. A determination on the partial specimen may yield normal results.
3. A normal creatinine determination can be used to confirm a 100% collection. An abnormal creatinine can result from an incomplete urine collection or kidney damage. Normal kidneys are expected to excrete 1000 ml/24 hours. The excretion of vitamin B_{12} is both delayed and decreased with renal disease, even when the urine volume is normal.
4. To prevent contamination of the samples, it is important for the technologist to wear gloves and check pipettes for contamination before handling the urine samples.
5. After the results have been interpreted by the physician, all urine samples may be discarded via the commode with one additional flushing.
6. The dilution factor in the formulas is necessary to bring standard counts to the activity given the patient.
7. Check standards to calculate correct dilution factor.
8. Correct dilution factor. (The dilution factor is equal to 50 when 1 ml of the standard is 2% of the administered dose.)

Diagnosis

Unless the flushing dose (1000 μ of nonradioactive vitamin B_{12}) is parenterally administered 1 to 3 hours after the oral radioactive vitamin B_{12} is given, no radioactivity will be found in the urine in normal or vitamin B_{12}-deficient patients in the Schilling test.

Normal subjects excrete 11% to 26% of the orally administered vitamin B_{12} in a 48-hour urine sample. Patients with renal disease, even with normal urine volume, have diminished and delayed excretion of vitamin B_{12}. If the results are abnormal, the Schilling test should be repeated with intrinsic factor. This test is referred to as *Schilling test II*.

Malabsorption

There will be defective absorption of vitamin B_{12} on the initial study as well as in the repeat vitamin B_{12}–intrinsic factor study in the intestinal malabsorption syndromes (vitamin B_{12} is absorbed at the level of the ilium). This can be seen in sprue or regional enteritis. In the "blind-loop" syndrome, vitamin B_{12} absorption returns to normal after the bacterial overgrowth has been eliminated by specific antibiotic therapy.

Pernicious anemia

In pernicious anemia patients, less than 7% of the administered dose is excreted in the initial study; in the repeat study done with simultaneous administration of intrinsic factor, 3% to 30% of the dose is excreted. In those patients who have diminished excretion of vitamin B_{12} with the addition of intrinsic factor, pernicious anemia may still exist, since there may be intestinal malabsorption with this disease. If the clinical picture suggests pernicious anemia, a therapeutic trial of parenteral vitamin B_{12} should be carried out for 3 to 6 weeks. During this time period the malabsorption defect will have cleared, and a repeat Schilling test with intrinsic factor will be compatible with the syndrome of pernicious anemia. Results of these studies are usually correlated with a plasma level of vitamin B_{12} (RIA) drawn before vitamin B_{12} is administered to the patient.

BIBLIOGRAPHY

General

Bernier, D.R., Langan, J.K., and Wells, L.D.: Nuclear medicine technology and techniques, ed. 2, St. Louis, 1989, The C.V. Mosby Co.

Guyton, A.C.: Textbook of medical physiology, ed. 7, Philadelphia, 1986, W.B. Saunders Co.

Wyngaarden, J.B., and Smith, L.H., Jr., editors: Textbook of medicine, ed. 18, Philadelphia, 1988, W.B. Saunders Co.

Blood volume

Albert, S.N.: Blood volume, Springfield, Ill., 1963, Charles C. Thomas, Publisher.

Albert, S.N.: Blood volume and extracellular fluid volume, ed. 2, Springfield, Ill., 1971, Charles C. Thomas, Publisher.

Albert, S.N.: Blood volume measurement. In Rothfeld, B., editor: Nuclear medicine in vitro, ed. 2, Philadelphia, 1983, J.B. Lippincott Co.

Belcher, E.H., and others: Recommended methods for measurement of red cell and plasma volume, J. Nucl. Med. 21:793, 1980.

Davidson, I., and others: Intravascular volumes and colloid dynamics in relation to fluid management in living related kidney donors and recipients, Crit. Care Med. 15(7):631-636, July 1987.

Grable, E., and Williams, J.A.: Simplified method for simultaneous determinations of plasma volume and red cell mass with ^{125}I-labeled albumin and ^{51}Cr-tagged red cells, J. Nucl. Med. 9:219, 1968.

Hidalgo, J.U., Nadler, S.B., and Bloch, T.: The use of electronic digital computer to determine best fit of blood volume formulas, J. Nucl. Med. 3:94, 1962.

Kirsch, K.A., Johnson, R.F., and Goiten, R.J.: Significance of total-body hematocrit in measurement of blood compartments, J. Nucl. Med. 12:17, 1971.

Kirschbaum, B.: Comparison of indirect methods to estimate plasma volume changes during hemodialysis, Int. J. Artif. Organs 12(5):307-313, 1989.

Nusynowitz, M.L., Strader, W.J., III, and Waliszewski, J.A.: Predictability of red cell volume from RISA blood volume, Am. J. Roentgenol. 109:820, 1970.

Pinto, P.C., Amerian, J., and Reynolds, T.B.: Large-volume paracentesis in nonedematous patients with tense ascites: its effect on intravascular volume, Hepatology, 8(2):207-210, March-April 1988.

Pivarnik, J.M., Goetting, M.P., and Senay, L.C., Jr.: The effects of body position and exercise on plasma volume dynamics, Eur. J. Appl. Physiol. 55(4):450-456, 1986.

Red cell survival

Belcher, E.H., and others: Recommended methods for radioisotope red-cell survival studies, Br. J. Haematol. 21:241, 1971.

Levy, G.J., and others: Clinical significance of anti-Yt (b). Report of a case using a 51 chromium red cell survival study, Transfusion 28(3):265-267, May-June 1988.

Marcus, C.S., and others: Radiolabeled red cell viability: I. Comparison of ^{51}Cr, ^{99m}Tc, and ^{111}In for measuring the viability of autologous stored red cells, Transfusion 27(5):415-419, Sept.-Oct. 1987.

Ottenwaelder, H., and others: Uptake of ^{51}Cr (VI) by human erythrocytes: evidence for a carrier-mediated transport mechanism, Sci. Total Environ. 71(3):561-566, June 1, 1988.

Panzer, S., and others: Haemolytic transfusion reactions due to HLA antibodies: a prospective study combining red-cell serology with investigations of chromium-51-labeled red-cell kinetics, Lancet 1(8531):474-478, Feb. 18, 1987.

Peters, A.M., and others: Erythrocyte radiolabelling: in vitro comparison of chromium, technetium, and indium in undamaged and heat damaged cells, J. Clin. Pathol. 39(7):717-721, July 1986.

Schilling test

Bergesen, O., and others: Is vitamin B-12 malabsorption in bile fistula rats due to bacterial overgrowth? A study of bacterial metabolic activity in the small bowel, Scand. J. Gastroenterol. 23(4):471-476, May 1988.

Briedis, D., and others: An evaluation of a dual isotope method for the measurement of vitamin B-12 absorption, J. Nucl. Med. 14:135, 1973.

Carethers, M.: Diagnosing vitamin B-12 deficiency, a common geriatric disorder, Geriatrics 43(3):89-94, 111-112, 1988.

Carmel, R., and others: Atypical cobalamin deficiency: subtle biochemical evidence of deficiency is commonly demonstrable in patients without megaloblastic anemia and is often associated with protein-bound cobalamin malabsorption, J. Lab. Clin. Med. 109(4):454-463, 1987.

Carmel, R., and others: Food cobalamin malabsorption occurs frequently in patients with unexplained low serum cobalamin levels, Arch. Intern. Med. 148(8):1715-1719, 1988.

Gross, J.S., and others: Pernicious anemia in the demented patient without anemia or macrocytosis: a case for early recognition, J. Am. Geriatric Soc. 34(8):612-614, 1986.

Herbert, V.: Detection of malabsorption of vitamin B-12 due to gastric or intestinal dysfunction, Semin. Nucl. Med. 2:220, 1972.

Herbert, V.: Folic acid and vitamin B-12. In Rothfeld, B., editor: Nuclear medicine in vitro, ed. 2, Philadelphia, 1983, J.B. Lippincott Co.

Henze, E., and others: The Schilling test cannot be replaced by an absorption test with unlabeled vitamin B-12, Klin. Wochenschr. 66(8):332-336, 1988.

Jones, B.P., and others: Incidence and clinical significance of protein-bound vitamin B-12 malabsorption, Eur. J. Haematol. 38(2):131-136, 1987.

Karnaze, D.S., and Carmel, R.: Low serum cobalamin levels in primary degenerative dementia: do some patients harbor atypical cobalamin deficiency states? Arch. Intern. Med. 147(3):429-431, 1987.

Marcuard, S.P., and others: Absence of luminal intrinsic factor after gastric bypass surgery for morbid obesity, Dig. Dis. Sci. 34(8):1238-1242, 1989.

Nilsson-Ehle, H., and others: Cyanocobalamin absorption in the elderly: results for healthy subjects and for subjects with low serum cobalamin concentration, Clin. Chem. 32(7):1368-1371, 1986.

Nilsson-Ehle, H., and others: Low serum cobalamin levels in a population study of 70- and 75-year-old subjects: gastrointestinal causes and hematological effects, Dig. Dis. Sci. 34(5):716-723, 1989.

Schilling, R.F.: Intrinsic factor studies. II. The effect of gastric juice on the urinary excretion of radioactivity after the oral administration of radioactive vitamin B-12, J. Lab. Clin. Med. 42:860, 1953.

Shaw, S., and others: The ileum is the major site of absorption of vitamin B-12 analogues, Am. J. Gastroenterol. 84(1):22-26, 1989.

Shermann, A.A., and others: Plasma level of 57 Co-vitamin B-12 as an adequate substitute for the Schilling test. Presented at the Seventeenth Annual Meeting of the Society of Nuclear Medicine, July 12, 1970, Washington, D.C.

Silberstein, E.B.: Value of 48 or 72 hour urine collections in performing the Schilling test, J. Nucl. Med. 24:692, 1973.

Smith, J.P., and Graham, M.M.: Schilling evaluation of pernicious anemia (letter), J. Nucl. Med. 26(9):1099-1100, 1985.

Solanki, D.L., and Garcia, R.: Serum only Schilling's test in patients with subtotal gastrectomy (letter), JAMA Dec. 23-30; 250(24):3283, 1983.

Sriram, K., and others: Absorption of cobalamin (vitamin B-12) administered via jejunostomy. J. Am. Coll. Nutr. 8(1):75-81, 1989.

Thompson, W.B., and others: Evaluation of current criteria used to measure vitamin B-12 levels. Am. J. Med. 82(2):291-294, 1987.

Zuckier, L.S., and Chervu, L.R.: Schilling evaluation of pernicious anemia: current status, J. Nucl. Med. 25(9):1032-1039, 1984.

Chapter 31

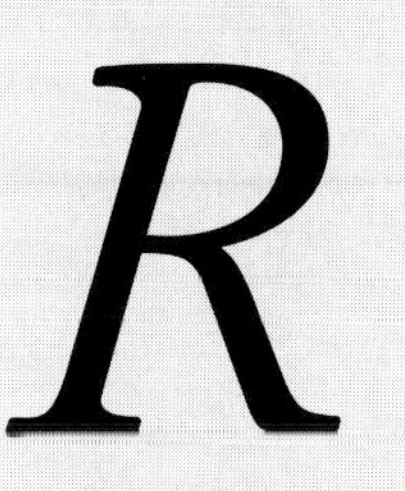

ADIOPHARMACEUTICALS FOR POSITRON EMISSION TOMOGRAPHY (PET)

MARK A. GREEN
MICHAEL J. WELCH

Positron emission tomography (PET) allows the physician to obtain a patient image that is essentially a low-resolution "autoradiograph" showing the regional concentration of a positron-emitting nuclide inside the *living* body. By application of appropriate tracer kinetic models, it is possible to extract from the PET image information about a variety of physiologic and biochemical processes, information that is not accessible with other diagnostic imaging modalities. Imaging applications in which PET has shown great use include mapping of regional blood flow (perfusion), mapping of regional blood volume, mapping the rates of use of metabolic substrates, and mapping receptor-specific tracer binding (Table 31-1). Historically, PET imaging has evolved with its main focus on studies of the brain and heart; it is here that PET should have its greatest clinical impact. However, it should be recognized that applications of PET measurements in the study of other organ systems and tumors could expand the use of this technology in the future.

When a radionuclide inside the body decays by emission of a positron (a positively charged electron), that particle travels only a short distance before expending its kinetic energy and combining with an electron. The positron path length in body tissues or water is in the range of 1 to 4 mm, with the mean path length increasing with increasing positron energy (Table 31-2). The positron-electron transmutation usually produces two 511-keV gamma photons that must be emitted in opposite directions, their angle of nearly 180° a requirement for conservation of momentum. It is the angular relationship between the emitted photon pair that is exploited in PET imaging to allow electronic collimation of the radiation and determination of the spatial location of the decay source.

The PET camera consists of multiple rings of gamma detectors, generally bismuth germanate or barium fluoride crystals coupled to photomultiplier tubes that surround the body of the patient (Fig. 31-1). Each of the detectors in this ring operates in a "coincidence circuit" with an array of detectors on the opposite side of the ring, allowing pairwise detection of the gamma photons produced by individual positron decays inside the patient's body. Tomographic image reconstruction from the resulting data is achieved by application of algorithms analogous to those used in reconstruction of computed tomography (CT) images. In the "time-of-flight" PET camera, the statistical significance of the image is improved through further localization of the transmutation event by use of timing circuits that measure the time differential for arrival of the photon pair at their respective detectors. Using electronic timing circuits capable of resolving events at nanosecond time intervals, it is possible to collect data at activity levels of up to 10 mCi within the camera field of view. Tomographic images obtained in this manner can have an axial resolution or slice thickness of 5 to 8 mm and an in-plane resolution in the range of 5 mm. The fundamental limit to resolution in a PET image is determined by the positron path length; however, in the current commercial PET imaging devices the limits of resolution are instead determined by instrumental factors.

The nature of the tracers that can be used in PET imaging—natural biochemicals labeled with radionuclides of carbon, nitrogen, oxygen, and fluorine—allows image analysis in terms of physiology and biochemistry at a level of sophistication beyond that encountered in the traditional nuclear medicine procedures that rely predominantly on ^{99m}Tc-labeled tracers. PET image processing generally goes beyond simple reconstruction of the spatial distribution of the radionuclide. Quantitative mapping of regional rates of

Table 31-1. Positron-emitting radiopharmaceuticals used in common PET imaging procedures

Radiopharmaceutical	Application	Typical dose/procedure*
[^{15}O]-O_2	Cerebral oxygen extraction and metabolism	100 mCi
[^{15}O]-CO	Cerebral blood volume	100 mCi
	Myocardial blood volume	100 mCi
[^{15}O]-H_2O	Cerebral blood flow	80 mCi
	Myocardial blood flow	150 mCi
[^{13}N]-ammonia (NH_3)	Myocardial blood flow	15-25 mCi
[^{11}C]-*n*-butanol	Cerebral blood flow	50 mCi
[^{11}C]-palmitate	Myocardial metabolism	30 mCi
[^{11}C]-acetate	Myocardial metabolism	30 mCi
[^{11}C]-glucose	Cerebral glucose metabolism	40 mCi
[^{11}C]-*N*-methylspiperone	Dopamine receptor binding	20 mCi
[^{18}F]-fluorodeoxyglucose	Cerebral glucose metabolism	5-10 mCi
	Myocardial glucose metabolism	5-10 mCi
	Tumor glucose metabolism	5-10 mCi
[^{18}F]-spiperone	Dopamine receptor binding	6 mCi
[^{18}F]-16α-fluoro-17β-estradiol	Estrogen receptor binding	6 mCi
[^{82}Rb]-Rb^+	Myocardial blood flow	4-10 mCi
[^{68}Ga]-citrate/transferrin	Plasma volume	4-8 mCi

*Note that many PET studies combine multiple PET imaging procedures (e.g., measurements of both blood flow and metabolism); the doses given here are typical of those actually used in each procedure of the study. For a single imaging procedure, an allowable dose (i.e., a dose that does not lead to excessive radiation exposure) may be significantly higher than these values.

Table 31-2. Selected positron-emitting radionuclides

Radionuclide	Half-life (minutes)	Positron yield	Positron energy (MeV)
Cyclotron-produced			
^{15}O	2.04	99+%	1.72
^{13}N	9.96	99+%	1.19
^{11}C	20.40	99+%	0.96
^{18}F	110.00	96.9%	0.64
Generator-produced			
^{82}Rb	1.27	96%	3.35
^{62}Cu	9.80	98%	2.93
^{68}Ga	68.10	90%	1.90

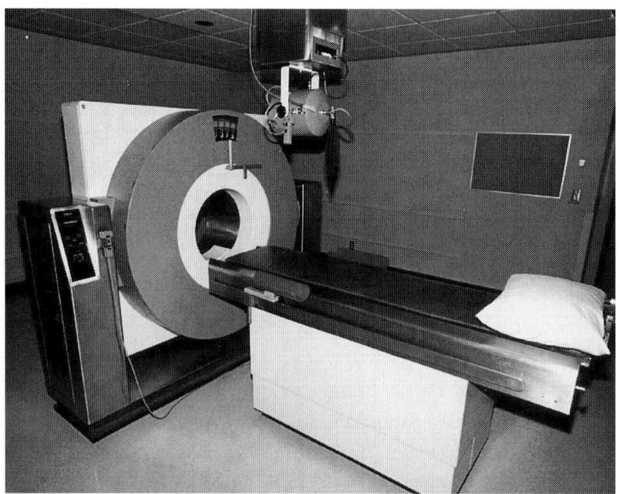

Fig. 31-1. Photograph of modern time-of-flight PET camera with barium-fluoride detectors installed at Mallinckrodt Institute of Radiology, Washington University School of Medicine, St. Louis, Missouri. (Courtesy of Dr. M.M. Ter-Pogossian, Division of Radiation Sciences, Washington University School of Medicine, St. Louis, MO.)

various physiologic and biochemical processes is achieved by application of appropriate mathematic models describing tracer distribution and kinetics. Obviously the accuracy of the biochemical information that can be extracted depends on the use of suitable tracers along with tracer kinetic models that accurately correlate the measured tissue radioactivity with the process of interest. In some cases, accurate modeling requires, in addition to the PET data describing tissue concentrations of tracer, knowledge of the arterial blood concentration of tracer integrated over the time frame of the study. This allows the model to include the input function describing the rate of tracer delivery to tissue. If a tracer undergoes metabolism during the PET study, the model must also account for the presence and behavior of labeled metabolites in the blood and tissues of interest. Whenever possible, it is desirable to select labeled tracers that are amenable to study over a time frame in which tracer metabolism does not complicate image interpretation.

■ POSITRON-EMITTING RADIOPHARMACEUTICALS

■ General concepts

Radionuclides that decay by positron emission (see Table 31-2) offer several features that make them attractive labels for radiopharmaceuticals to be used in diagnostic nuclear medicine. For example:

- They allow quantitative tomographic imaging of tracer distribution by positron emission tomography.
- They generally have very short half-lives, permitting administration of large doses of activity without subjecting the patient to excessive radiation exposure (see Table 31-1). The resulting high count rates allow collection of statistically significant images in very short time intervals, facilitating dynamic studies of physiologic processes that produce rapid fluctuation in tissue concentrations of tracer. These short half-lives also facilitate repeat imaging studies at reasonably brief time intervals without interfering background activity from previous injections.
- Radionuclides such as carbon-11, oxygen-15, nitrogen-13, and fluorine-18 allow tracer studies of natural biochemicals and therapeutic drugs that have been labeled by isotopic substitution at an appropriate site in the molecule.

It is desirable to label radiopharmaceuticals using radionuclides with the shortest half-life that is compatible with the time-scale of the physiologic process to be studied. However, a practical consequence of using short-lived ($t_{1/2}$ < 1 hr) radionuclides in diagnostic medicine is the necessity for radionuclide production and radiotracer synthesis to occur within the hospital where the imaging procedure will be performed. The radionuclides around which PET imaging has developed, ^{11}C, ^{13}N, ^{15}O, and ^{18}F are generally produced using a biomedical cyclotron located in the hospital. Despite their short half-lives, these radionuclides have been incorporated into a diverse spectrum of radiopharmaceuticals. For those tracers that have exhibited the greatest utility in PET imaging studies, robotic techniques and automated systems have been developed for performance of radiopharmaceutical synthesis on a routine basis. Although these systems can not substantially reduce the personnel needed to supply positron-emitting radiopharmaceuticals, the automatic systems allow frequent syntheses using large amounts of activity to be performed without subjecting the chemistry staff to excessive or unnecessary radiation exposure. The following section surveys some of the most common synthetic methods that have been applied in the preparation of positron-emitting radiopharmaceuticals and should serve as a guide to the types of tracers that can be obtained. The reader is referred to a number of comprehensive reviews of this subject that have appeared in the recent literature.

■ Oxygen-15 radiopharmaceuticals

With a half-life of 2.04 minutes, oxygen-15 is the longest-lived radionuclide of oxygen. PET imaging studies employing oxygen-15 are restricted to the use of a few relatively simple molecules because very little time is available for tracer synthesis, purification, and delivery. However, the four oxygen-15 radiopharmaceuticals that are available—^{15}O-oxygen gas (^{15}OO), ^{15}O-carbon monoxide ($C^{15}O$), ^{15}O-carbon dioxide ($CO^{15}O$), and ^{15}O-water ($H_2{}^{15}O$)—have been used to great advantage in hemodynamic studies that exploit the short half-life to allow administration of large doses of activity (up to 100 mCi) in imaging procedures that can be repeated at 8- to 10-minute intervals.

Oxygen-15 is most conveniently produced for medical use by the $^{14}N(d,n)^{15}O$ nuclear reaction. Using a nitrogen gas (N_2) target containing 1% O_2, oxygen-15 is obtained as labeled oxygen gas, ^{15}O-^{16}O. If a deuteron beam is not available, oxygen-15 can be produced by the $^{15}N(p,n)^{15}O$ reaction; however, this requires the expense of a target enriched in nitrogen-15 (natural abundance 0.37%).

Labeled oxygen gas can be used directly in studies of O_2 metabolism or can be converted to CO, CO_2, or H_2O (Fig. 31-2). Production of ^{15}O-labeled carbon oxides is accomplished by passing the ^{15}O-O through an activated carbon furnace, with the selectivity for $C^{15}O$ or ^{15}OCO production determined by the furnace temperature. Since oxygen-15 can be prepared in high specific activity, ^{15}O-carbon monoxide can be safely administered to patients via inhalation to serve as a tracer for red blood cell volume upon binding of the $C^{15}O$ to hemoglobin.

Oxygen-15–labeled water can be used in equilibrium measurements of tissue water content; it finds its greatest use, however, as a tracer for regional blood flow. Oxygen-15 water is the most commonly used tracer in PET

^{15}O-Oxygen (O_2; ^{15}O-O):

$^{14}N(d,n)^{15}O$ on N_2 gas/1% O_2

^{15}O-Carbon Monoxide (CO):

$$^{15}O\text{-}O \xrightarrow[900^\circ\ C]{\text{carbon}} C^{15}O + CO$$

^{15}O-Carbon Dioxide (CO_2):

$$^{15}O\text{-}O \xrightarrow[400^\circ\ C]{\text{carbon}} CO^{15}O$$

$^{14}N(d,n)^{15}O$ on N_2 gas/2.5% CO_2

^{15}O-Water (H_2O):

$$CO^{15}O + H_2O \rightleftharpoons H_2CO_2{}^{15}O \rightleftharpoons CO_2 + H_2{}^{15}O$$

$$^{15}O\text{-}O + H_2 \xrightarrow[150^\circ\ C]{\text{Pd}} H_2{}^{15}O$$

Fig. 31-2. Synthesis of oxygen-15 radiotracers and synthetic precursors.

evaluations of cerebral and myocardial perfusion, with the advantages of its 2-minute half-life outweighing limitations in its ability to freely diffuse across the blood-brain barrier at high flow rates. Labeled water can be produced from ^{15}O-carbon dioxide via the carbonic acid mediated exchange reaction (Fig. 31-2) that occurs when CO_2 is placed in aqueous solution. Bubbling of $CO^{15}O$ through normal saline produces ^{15}O-water in a form suitable for I.V. injection. Alternatively, the gaseous $CO^{15}O$ can be administered to a patient via inhalation, leading to formation of ^{15}O-water in the lungs and blood. Blood-flow measurements can be made following either mode of administration by application of appropriate kinetic models. The I.V. infusion of ^{15}O-water may be the preferred technique because of a greater linearity in the correlation between tissue counts and blood flow; however, for a detailed comparison of the relative merits of these tracer techniques, the reader is referred to a 1985 review of this subject by Ter-Pogossian and Herscovitch. As an alternative method of production, $[^{15}O]$-H_2O can be obtained directly from reaction of $O^{15}O$ with H_2 over a palladium catalyst.

PET images generated using oxygen-15 tracers are shown in Figs. 31-3 to 31-5. Figure 31-3 shows an image of myocardial blood flow in a normal subject. This image has been generated following the consecutive administration of water labeled with oxygen-15 and carbon monoxide labeled with oxygen-15. The water image was taken over a period of 1 minute and the blood pool subtracted to afford the image showing regional perfusion. Homogeneous uptake of the tracer in this normal subject is observed. Figure 31-4 shows cerebral blood flow (upper left), blood volume (upper right) and oxygen metabolic rate (lower left) in a subject with left common carotid artery occlusion. Although the blood flow in the occluded area is severely reduced, the oxygen metabolic rate is almost normal in this area of the brain. Figure 31-5 shows a subtracted image of blood flow in a normal human. One image was obtained during visual stimulation and the other during a control state. The subtracted image is shown as a sagittal reconstruction where the increase in blood flow in the visual cortex is clearly observed. For anatomic positioning, the magnetic resonance imaging (MRI) of the patient is shown on the left.

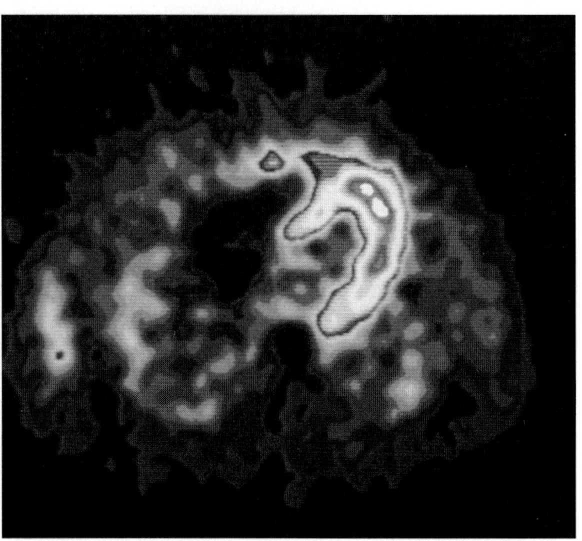

Fig. 31-3. Myocardial blood flow measured utilizing oxygen-15-labeled water in a normal subject. (Courtesy Dr. E. Geltman, Division of Cardiology, Department of Internal Medicine, Washington University School of Medicine, St. Louis, MO.)

■ Nitrogen-13 radiopharmaceuticals

Nitrogen-13 is best produced with a biomedical cyclotron using the $^{16}O(p,\alpha)^{13}N$ nuclear reaction. With oxygen-16 being the naturally abundant isotope of oxygen, this nuclear reaction can be conveniently performed using a water target to yield nitrogen-13 in the form of the aqueous nitrate ion, $^{13}NO_3{}^-$. The labeled nitrate can be converted to ^{13}N-ammonia by reaction with titanium (III) chloride:

$$^{13}NO_3{}^- + H_2O \xrightarrow{TiCl_3} {}^{13}NH_3(aq)$$

Alternatively, ^{13}N-ammonia can be obtained directly from the cyclotron target, if a trace of ethanol is added to the

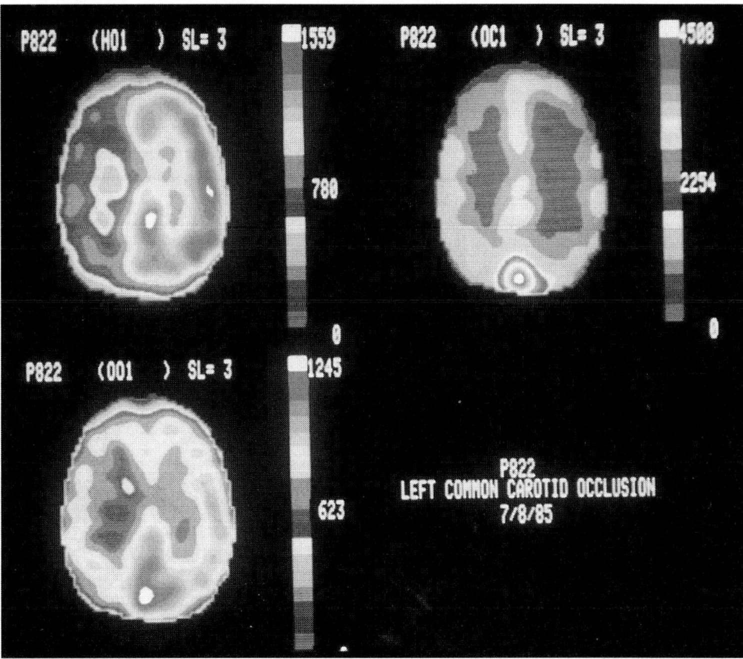

Fig. 31-4. Blood flow, blood volume, and oxygen metabolic images in a subject with left common carotid artery occlusion. (Courtesy Dr. M.E. Raichle, Departments of Neurology, Radiology and Neurobiology, Washington University School of Medicine, St. Louis, MO.)

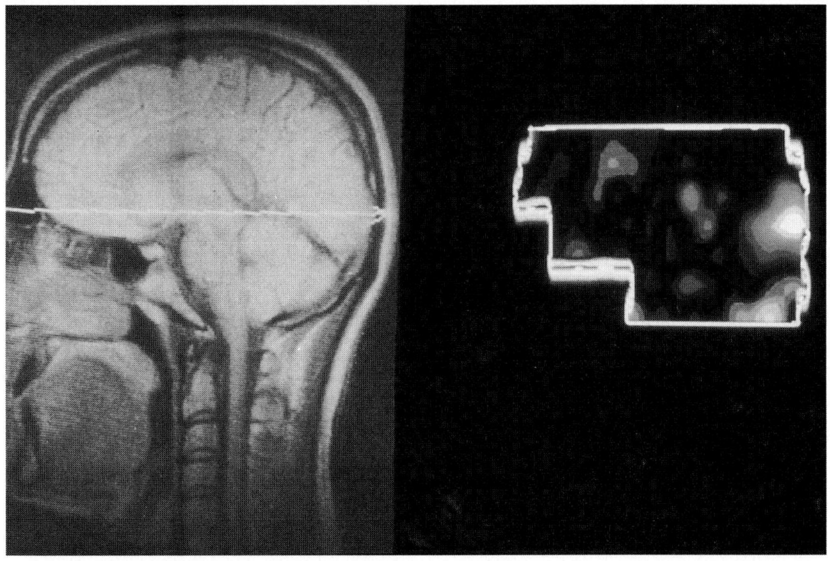

Fig. 31-5. Increase in blood flow following visual stimulation in a normal human subject. (Courtesy Dr. M.E. Raichle, Departments of Neurology, Radiology, and Neurobiology, Washington University School of Medicine, St. Louis, MO.)

target water prior to irradiation. Nitrogen-13 ammonia has been used as a tracer for cerebral and myocardial blood flow, undergoing relatively high extraction into these organs and exhibiting prolonged retention as a major fraction of extracted tracer is metabolically incorporated into amino acids.

Numerous nitrogen-13–labeled amino acids have been synthesized for use in the study of amino acid metabolism by PET. A number of enzymatic methods have been reported that allow the stereospecific synthesis of L-^{13}N-amino acids from ^{13}N-ammonia (for a review see Fowler and Wolf, 1982). For example, glutamic acid dehydrogenase is sufficiently nonselective that it can be used to prepare ^{13}N-valine, ^{13}N-alanine, ^{13}N-leucine, and ^{13}N-methionine, as well as ^{13}N-glutamate, from $^{13}NH_3$ and the appropriate α-ketoacids:

$$NH_3 + R\text{-}\overset{\overset{O}{\|}}{C}\text{-}\overset{\overset{O}{\|}}{C}\text{-}OH \xrightarrow{\text{glutamic acid dehydrogenase}} R\text{-}\overset{\overset{^{13}NH_2}{|}}{CH}\text{-}COOH \quad \text{L-form}$$

Nitrogen-13–labeled nitrogen gas, $N^{13}N$, is obtained by proton or deuteron bombardment of carbon dioxide containing a trace of N_2 via the $^{16}O(p,\alpha)^{13}N$ or $^{12}C(d,n)^{13}N$ nuclear reactions. For studies of pulmonary ventilation, $N^{13}N$ gas is superior to the radioactive noble gases (e.g., ^{127}Xe, ^{133}Xe, ^{81m}Kr) because of its lower solubility in blood. However, the chemical stability of $N^{13}N$ makes it a poor precursor for the synthesis of other nitrogen-13–labeled tracers.

■ Carbon-11 radiopharmaceuticals

Carbon-11 is prepared as $^{11}CO_2$ by proton bombardment of a nitrogen gas target containing a trace of O_2 ($^{14}N(p,\alpha)^{11}C$). Despite the limitations imposed by a 20-minute half-life, carbon-11 has been incorporated into a variety of organic molecules for use in diagnostic imaging. The literature on the synthesis of carbon-11 radiopharmaceuticals is extensive and the reader is referred to the reviews on this subject for a comprehensive survey of the methods that have been developed. The majority of carbon-11 tracers have been synthesized directly from $^{11}CO_2$ or a few other relatively simple building blocks, with ^{11}CO, $^{11}CH_3I$, and $H^{11}CN$ being the most common.

These ^{11}C-synthetic precursors are readily prepared (Fig. 31-6) from $^{11}CO_2$ using automated systems that are provided by the current biomedical cyclotron manufacturers. Carbon-11–labeled carbon monoxide is prepared by reduction of $^{11}CO_2$ in a zinc furnace and can serve as a red blood cell volume tracer with a half-life significantly longer than that of oxygen-15 carbon monoxide. Labeled cyanide can be prepared from $^{11}CO_2$ in a two-step process in which carbon dioxide is first converted to [^{11}C]-methane that is then reacted with ammonia over a platinum catalyst to yield $H^{11}C{\equiv}N$. The preparation of methyl iodide also requires a two-step process. Initially $^{11}CO_2$ is reacted with lithium aluminum hydride and on hydrolysis provides labeled methanol, which can be converted to methyl iodide by reaction with HI.

Labeled carboxylic acids and alcohols. The synthesis of carbon-11–labeled carboxylic acids, such as acetate and palmitate, is facilitated by the facile insertion of CO_2 into the metal-carbon bonds of Grignard reagents and organo lithium salts. The resulting metal carboxylate is then hydrolyzed to yield the free acid labeled at the C-1 position:

$$^{11}CO_2 + R\text{-}M \longrightarrow R\text{-}^{11}\underset{\underset{O}{\|}}{C}\text{-}O\text{-}M \xrightarrow{H_2O} R\text{-}^{11}\underset{\underset{O}{\|}}{C}\text{-}OH + HO\text{-}M$$

where M = Li, MgCl, MgBr.

^{11}C-Carbon Dioxide (CO_2)

$^{14}N(p,\alpha)^{11}C$ on N_2 gas/trace O_2

^{11}C-Carbon Monoxide (CO)

$$^{11}CO_2 \xrightarrow[400^\circ\ C]{Zinc} {}^{11}CO$$

^{11}C-Hydrogen Cyanide (HCN)

$$^{11}CO_2 + H_2 \xrightarrow[350^\circ\ C]{Ni} {}^{11}CH_4 + H_2O$$

$$^{11}CH_4 + NH_3 \xrightarrow[1000^\circ\ C]{Pt} H^{11}CN$$

^{11}C-Methanol (CH_3OH)

$$^{11}CO_2 + LiAlH_4 \longrightarrow \xrightarrow[H_2O]{H^+} {}^{11}CH_3OH$$

^{11}C-Methyl Iodide (CH_3I)

$$^{11}CH_3OH + HI \longrightarrow {}^{11}CH_3I + H_2O$$

Fig. 31-6. Preparation of carbon-11 radiotracers and synthetic precursors.

One of the carboxylic acids that has had the most use to date in positron emission tomography is palmitic acid. This tracer has been used for the study of myocardial metabolism. Figs. 31-7 and 31-8 show the distribution of carbon-11–labeled palmitic acid in a normal subject (Fig. 31-7) and in a patient with an anterior myocardial infarct (Fig. 31-8). The normal subject is the same subject in whom blood-flow distribution is shown in Fig. 31-3.

If the metal carboxylate is reacted with lithium aluminum hydride before hydrolysis, carbon-11 alcohols are obtained with the label in the C-1 position:

$$R\text{-}^{11}\underset{\underset{O}{\|}}{C}\text{-}O\text{-}M \xrightarrow{LiAlH_4} \xrightarrow{H_2O} R\text{-}^{11}CH_2OH$$

Carbon-11–labeled n-butanol prepared in this manner has been shown to behave as a freely diffusible tracer over a broad range of blood flows and is a suitable radiopharmaceutical for evaluation of cerebral and myocardial perfusion.

Labeled amines and amino acids. Primary amines labeled with carbon-11 can be prepared by $LiAlH_4$ reduction

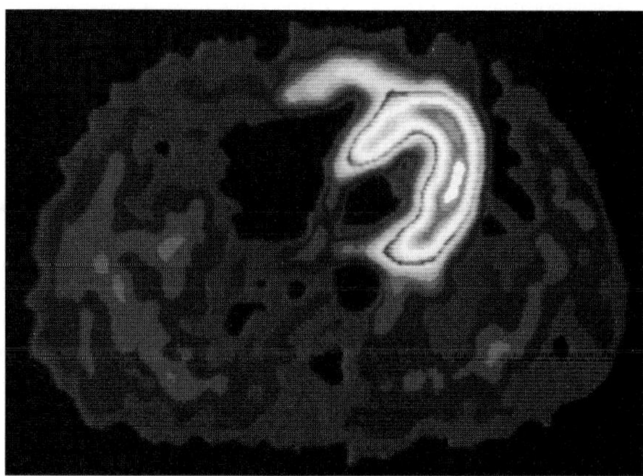

Fig. 31-7. ^{11}C-palmitic acid distribution in a normal volunteer. (Courtesy Dr. E. Geltman, Division of Cardiology, Department of Internal Medicine, Washington University School of Medicine, St. Louis, MO.)

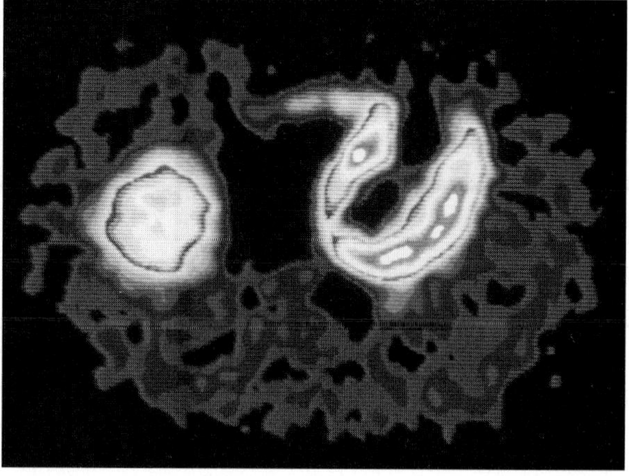

Fig. 31-8. ^{11}C-palmitate distribution in a patient with an anterior myocardial infarct; lack of uptake in the tracer in the myocardial wall is clearly observed. Liver uptake of palmitic acid is also apparent on the left side of this transaxial slice. (Courtesy Dr. E. Geltman, Division of Cardiology, Department of Internal Medicine, Washington University School of Medicine, St. Louis, MO.)

of the nitrile formed on the reaction of an alkyl halide with [^{11}C]-cyanide:

$$H^{11}CN + R\text{-}Cl \longrightarrow R\text{-}^{11}CN \xrightarrow{LiAlH_4} R\text{-}^{11}CH_2NH_2$$

Carbon-11–labeled methyl amines are readily obtained by reaction of ^{11}C-methyliodide with an amine:

$$^{11}CH_3I + H\text{-}N \longrightarrow {}^{11}CH_3\text{-}N$$

Methyl iodide undergoes similar reactions with RO-H and RS-H bonds to form labeled methyl ethers and mercaptans. This method has been used in the conversion of spiperone into [^{11}C]-methylspiperone for the study of brain dopamine receptors.

F-C$_6$H$_4$-C(=O)-(CH$_2$)$_3$-N (spiperone, N-H) $\xrightarrow{^{11}CH_3I}$ F-C$_6$H$_4$-C(=O)-(CH$_2$)$_3$-N (N-^{11}CH$_3$)

Amino acids labeled with carbon-11 are prepared from ^{11}C-cyanide and appropriate aldehydes using a modified Bucherer-Strecker synthesis (Washburn and others, 1979):

R-C(=O)-H + Na^{11}CN → hydantoin (H, R, ^{11}C=O, NH, HN, C=O) $\xrightarrow{NaOH}$ $\xrightarrow{H^+}$ R-C(H)(NH$_2$)-^{11}COOH

The resulting mixture of D- and L-amino acids can be resolved by liquid chromatography using a chiral column matrix to provide the purified natural L-amino acid.

Labeled sugars. Randomly ^{11}C-labeled glucose has been produced photosynthetically for use in studies of cerebral glucose metabolism. A variety of plant materials have been used to effect this conversion of $^{11}CO_2$ into labeled sugars (see Fowler and Wolf, 1982). In a typical procedure, a light-starved Swiss chard leaf is exposed to $^{11}CO_2$ and illuminated. After about 20 minutes, the labeled sugars are extracted into alcohol, hydrolyzed, and the ^{11}C-glucose separated by high-pressure liquid chromatography (HPLC) (see below). A product suitable for I.V. injection can be obtained in less than 60 minutes using automated systems that have been developed. Production of 50 mCi ^{11}C-glucose requires approximately 1 Ci of $^{11}CO_2$ at the beginning of the synthetic procedure.

The use of ^{11}C-glucose for measurement of cerebral glucose metabolism requires an imaging procedure of less than

$^{11}CO_2$ + Starved Swiss Chard Leaves

1. Photosynthesis
2. Alcohol extraction

→ ^{11}C-Glucose, ^{11}C-Fructose, ^{11}C-Sucrose + Phosphates

1. H$^+$
2. Neutralize

→ ^{11}C-Glucose, ^{11}C-Fructose $\xrightarrow{HPLC}$ ^{11}C-Glucose

5 minutes' duration following injection. At longer time intervals, the presence of substantial quantities of the metabolic product $^{11}CO_2$ interferes with the tracer kinetic models needed to correlate tissue counts and metabolism.

2-Deoxy-D-glucose labeled with carbon-11 exclusively at the C-1 position has been prepared from $H^{11}CN$ using a modification of the Kiliani-Fischer cyanohydrin synthesis.

■ Fluorine-18 radiopharmaceuticals

The 110-minute half-life of fluorine-18 allows a relatively long time for radiopharmaceutical synthesis and opens the possibility for delivery of this radionuclide to imaging centers located some distance from cyclotron-production facilities. In fact, at one time a U.S. radiopharmaceutical manufacturer had a nationwide distribution network for ^{18}F-fluoride.

The half-life of ^{18}F coupled with its availability in high specific activity make it an attractive label for radiopharmaceuticals used in the study of receptor-specific tracer binding, an application in which ^{18}F is finding increasing use. However, the major use of ^{18}F in PET imaging remains in the study of cerebral, myocardial, and tumor metabolism with ^{18}F-2-fluorodeoxyglucose (FDG). Fluorodeoxyglucose undergoes carrier-mediated uptake into the brain as a glucose analog and serves as a substrate for hexakinase. The ^{18}F-radiolabel is metabolically trapped in the cell because phosphorylation cannot proceed past the C-1 carbon. In brain-imaging studies, FDG maps normal brain metabolic activity, while in cardiac studies FDG is used to delineate ischemic regions in which glucose metabolism increases as a consequence of diminished fatty acid metabolism. Glucose metabolism is increased in malignant tissues. Therefore FDG localization has become a major part of oncologic PET imaging research.

Fluorine-18 is produced by either the $^{20}N(d,\alpha)^{18}F$ or the $^{18}O(p,n)^{18}F$ nuclear reaction. Use of a neon gas target containing 1% F_2 provides labeled fluorine gas, $^{18}F\text{-}^{19}F$. While the high reactivity of $[^{18}F]\text{-}F_2$ facilitates its incorporation into organic compounds—for example, in the preparation of fluorodeoxyglucose—it is unfortunately an agent with little selectivity:

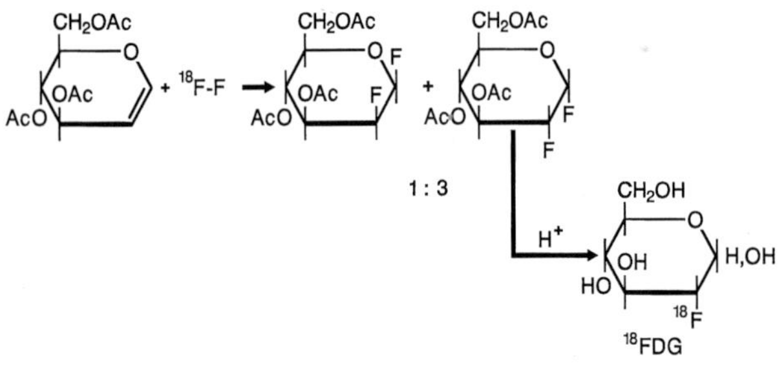

1 : 3

^{18}FDG

The selectivity of the electrophilic addition to a C=C double bond can be improved by first preparing acetyl hypofluorite, which adds as desired to the least hindered side of the molecule:

$$^{18}F\text{—}F + NH_4OAc \rightarrow {}^{18}FOAc$$

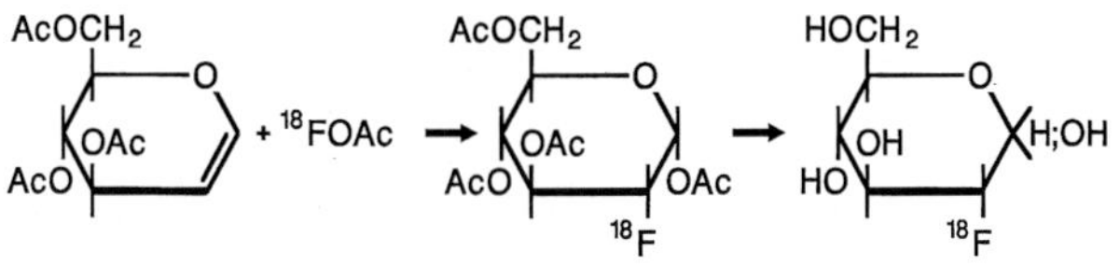

In recent years techniques have been developed that allow organic syntheses using the aqueous ^{18}F-fluoride ion produced by proton bombardment of water enriched in oxygen-18, making the $^{18}O(p,n)^{18}F$ nuclear reaction the preferred method for ^{18}F production. Formation of carbon-fluorine bonds with $^{18}F^-$ can be achieved either by nucleophilic displacement of a good leaving group (e.g., trifluoromethanesulfonate, $CF_3SO_3^-$ or OTf) from an alkyl carbon

$$\underset{\text{(anhydrous)}}{^{18}F^-} + R_2CH\text{-}\overset{\overset{\text{OTf}}{|}}{C}R_2 \longrightarrow R_2CH\text{-}\underset{\underset{^{18}F}{|}}{C}R_2 + {}^-OTf$$

or by an olefin halofluorination reaction

$$\underset{\text{(anhydrous)}}{^{18}F^-} + RCH = CH_2 \xrightarrow[\text{NIS} \; CH_2Cl_2]{H_2SO_4} R\text{-}\underset{^{18}F}{CH}\text{-}\underset{I}{CH_2}$$

The latter method provides a labeled alkane containing a reactive carbon-iodine bond that can be the site for further functionalization.

The triflate displacement reaction has been exploited in the stereospecific synthesis of $[^{18}F]$-2-fluorodeoxyglucose as described by Hamacher and others in 1986,

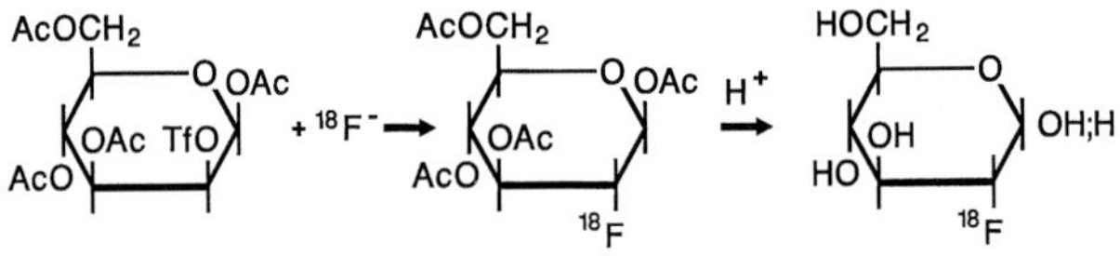

and in the synthesis of ^{18}F-labeled estrogens for study of receptor-positive breast tumors (Mintum, 1988):

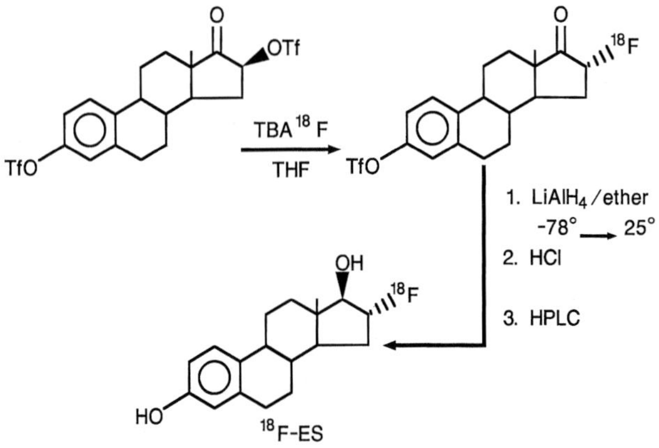

TBA ^{18}F / THF

1. $LiAlH_4$/ether $-78° \rightarrow 25°$
2. HCl
3. HPLC

^{18}F-ES

It was noted above that *N*-methyl spiperone labeled with carbon-11 can be used to study tracer uptake by brain dopamine receptors. Spiperone is also an attractive molecule for ^{18}F labeling because it naturally contains a fluorine atom. In addition, a 2-hour half-lived tracer permits study of tracer uptake and egress over a substantially longer time frame than possible with ^{11}C. Unfortunately, formation of the bond between fluorine and an aromatic carbon atom poses a difficult synthetic challenge. ^{18}F-spiperone has been prepared by fluoride displacement of a nitrogroup.

$$O_2N\text{-}C_6H_4\text{-}C(=O)(CH_2)_3N\text{(spiro)} \xrightarrow[\text{DMSO, }150°C]{^{18}F^-} {}^{18}F\text{-}C_6H_4\text{-}C(=O)(CH_2)_3N\text{(spiro)}$$

However, this reaction provides only a very low yield of the desired product. To circumvent this synthetic difficulty, a number of research groups have prepared spiperone derivatives containing an *N*-fluoroalkyl group.

$$F\text{-}C_6H_4\text{-}C(=O)(CH_2)_3N\text{(spiro, NH)} + Br\text{-}(CH_2)_n\text{-}^{18}F \rightarrow F\text{-}C_6H_4\text{-}C(=O)(CH_2)_3N\text{(spiro, N-}(CH_2)_n\text{-}^{18}F)$$

Welch and Katzenellenbogen reported the fluoropropyl compound (n = 3) to be the "ideal" ^{18}F-labeled spiperone derivative for use in PET studies of dopamine receptor binding, since it retains the receptor specificity of spiperone. Equally important is the observation that the labeled products produced by metabolism of [^{18}F]-fluoropropylspiperone do not penetrate the blood-brain barrier thus avoiding a complication in the correlation of brain activity with receptor binding.

Spiperone labeled in the various positions has been used to study dopaminergic receptors in both normal and diseased subjects. Figure 31-9 shows the uptake 2 hours after administration of ^{18}F-spiperone in an untreated symptomatic subject with MPTP-induced Parkinsonism and an age-matched normal volunteer. Although Fig. 31-9 shows similar distribution, computer modeling of the data shows that the product of the maximum number of available specific binding sites multiplied by the association rate constants is many times elevated in the MPTP-induced Parkinson's patient. This observation provides potential new insights, not only in the pathophysiology of the disease but in the clinical importance of dopamine receptor function.

■ Generator-produced positron-emitting radiopharmaceuticals

Parent/daughter generator systems are attractive sources for positron-emitting radiopharmaceuticals, since they

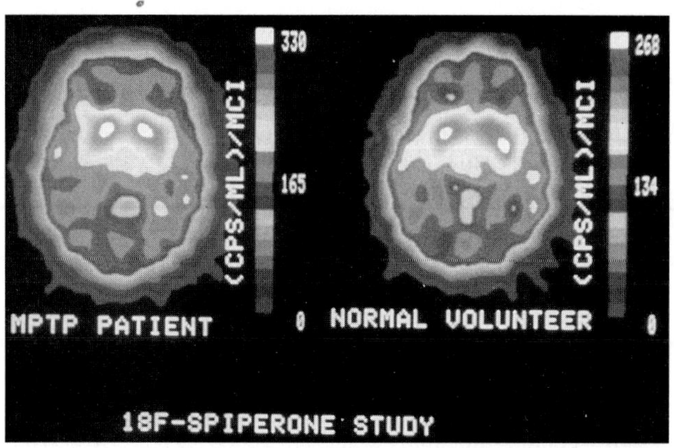

Fig. 31-9. Distribution of fluorine-18-labeled spiperone in MPTP induced Parkinson patient and a normal volunteer. (Courtesy Dr. Joel S. Perlmutter, Departments of Neurology and Neurological Surgery and Radiology, Washington University School of Medicine, St. Louis, MO.)

could free PET imaging from its dependence on radionuclides that require cyclotron production within the hospital. The availability of positron-emitting radiopharmaceuticals labeled with generator-produced radionuclides could thus have a significant impact on the economic viability of PET as a routine tool in clinical diagnosis. Unfortunately, the number of positron emitters that can be delivered by parent/daughter generator systems is relatively small (Table 31-3). Only two of these radionuclides, rubidium-82 and gallium-68, have received a great deal of attention in the nuclear medicine literature. A $^{82}Sr/^{82}Rb$ generator system consisting of a tin dioxide-adsorbent column from which the ^{82}Rb can be selectively eluted in normal saline has been approved by the U.S. Food and Drug Administration and is marketed by Squibb Diagnostics. The ^{82}Sr parent is produced at Los Alamos National Laboratory by spallation of a molybdenum target and is contaminated with ^{85}Sr in a ratio of at least 1:1. Because of its 65-day half-life, the ^{85}Sr can account for a major portion of the patient radiation dose following administration of ^{82}Rb, unless the strontium breakthrough is kept very low. The 75-second half-life of ^{82}Rb is desirably short, allowing rapid repeat imaging studies. However, this short half-life, along with the limited chemistry of the alkali metal ion, severely restricts its potential applications in nuclear medicine.

The short half-life of ^{82}Rb also poses practical problems associated with generator elution, dosage measurement, and administration. To deal with these problems, a calibrated continuous infusion system has been developed (Fig. 31-10) that allows elution of the generator directly into an intravenous catheter. Using this infusion system, the dosage of ^{82}Rb to be administered (typically 20 to 40 mCi [740 MBq, 1.4 GBq]), the total volume of the $^{82}Rb^+$/saline infusion, and the infusion rate are preselected by push buttons on the control panel. Infusion begins with the depression of an "inject button" and automatically continues until the preset dose has been delivered. The 25-day half-life of the ^{82}Sr parent allows a single generator to remain clinically useful for a period of 4 to 6 weeks.

The principal use of ^{82}Rb will be in the evaluation of myocardial blood flow because the Rb^+ cation exhibits myocardial uptake as a potassium analog, similar to $^{201}Tl^+$ (for comparison, the Pauling ionic radii for the K^+, Tl^+, and Rb^+ cations are 1.33 Å, 1.40 Å, and 1.48 Å, respectively). In general clinical practice, $^{82}Rb^+$ will be used only to provide a qualitative map of myocardial perfusion, since myocardial $^{82}Rb^+$ uptake shows a nonlinear dependence on blood flow and is significantly influenced by the presence of ischemia. Drug-induced coronary vasodilation before ^{82}Rb infusion may enhance the ability of this tracer to detect the presence and severity of coronary artery disease. A method for quantification of myocardial blood flow with ^{82}Rb using beta probes to measure both ^{82}Rb uptake and extraction fraction has been reported in experiments with open-chested dogs; however, the suitability of this technique for human studies with fast time-of-flight positron cameras remains to be demonstrated.

Aside from myocardial imaging, $^{82}Rb^+$ has been reported to have potential for study of defects in the blood-brain barrier and for study of some brain tumors as well. Extravasation of $^{82}Rb^+$ into the brain is indicative of blood-brain–barrier disruption and may provide information about the size and vascularity of a lesion.

The germanium-68/gallium-68 generator is possibly the "best" generator system for providing positron-emitting radiopharmaceuticals for clinical practice. The long half-life of the ^{68}Ge parent affords this generator an attractively long useful shelf-life, while the 68-minute half-life of the daughter gallium-68, which though reasonably short might allow the synthesis of a diverse array of radiopharmaceuticals. A number of methods have been described for efficient sepa-

Table 31-3. Parent→daughter generator systems for positron-emitting nuclides

Parent isotope	Parent half-life	Daughter isotope	Daughter half-life	Daughter positron yield (%)	Daughter positron energy (MeV)	Daughter decay product (stable)
^{68}Ge	288 days	^{68}Ga	68.1 min	90	1.899	^{68}Zn
^{82}Sr	25.0 days	^{82}Rb	75 sec	96	3.15	^{82}Kr
^{62}Zn	9.2 hrs	^{62}Cu	9.73 min	98	2.93	^{62}Ni
^{52}Fe	8.27 hrs	^{52m}Mn	21.1 min	98	2.63	^{52}Cr
^{122}Xe	20.1 hrs	^{122}I	3.6 min	77	3.12	^{122}Te
^{118}Te	6.0 days	^{118}Sb	3.5 min	—	2.70	^{118}Sn
^{128}Ba	2.43 days	^{128}Cs	3.6 min	61	2.88	^{128}Xe
^{72}Se	8.4 days	^{72}As	26 hrs	77	3.32	^{72}Ge
^{44}Ti	47 yrs	^{44}Sc	3.9 hrs	95	1.47	^{44}Ca

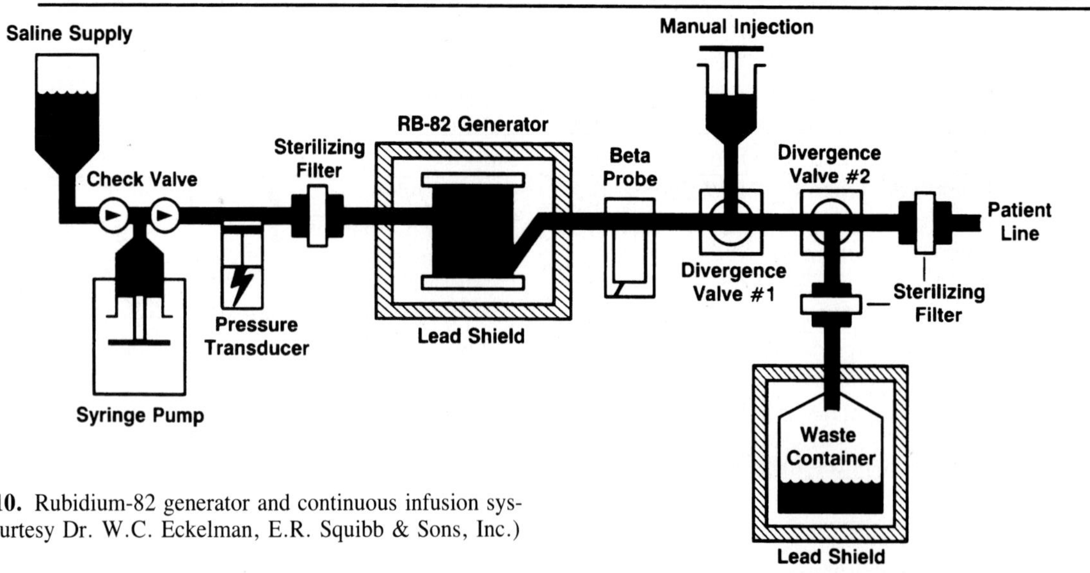

Fig. 31-10. Rubidium-82 generator and continuous infusion system. (Courtesy Dr. W.C. Eckelman, E.R. Squibb & Sons, Inc.)

ration of gallium-68 from its parent. The generator system that offers the most versatility for chemical synthesis following elution contains ^{68}Ge adsorbed to a tin dioxide column from which the gallium-68 daughter can be eluted in high yield with 1N hydrochloric acid. The hydrated $^{68}Ga^{3+}$ ion obtained in this manner is suitable for preparation of a variety of radiotracers; only a few of these have found use in human studies, however (see Table 31-4). Gallium-68 labeling of albumin microspheres is effected either by hydrolysis and precipitation of gallium-68 in the presence of these albumin particles or by using a "bifunctional chelate"

Table 31-4. Gallium-68 radiopharmaceuticals used in human studies

Tracer	Application
^{68}Ga-Albumin microspheres	Blood flow
^{68}Ga-citrate/^{68}Ga-transferrin	Plasma volume
^{68}Ga-EDTA	Blood-brain–barrier integrity

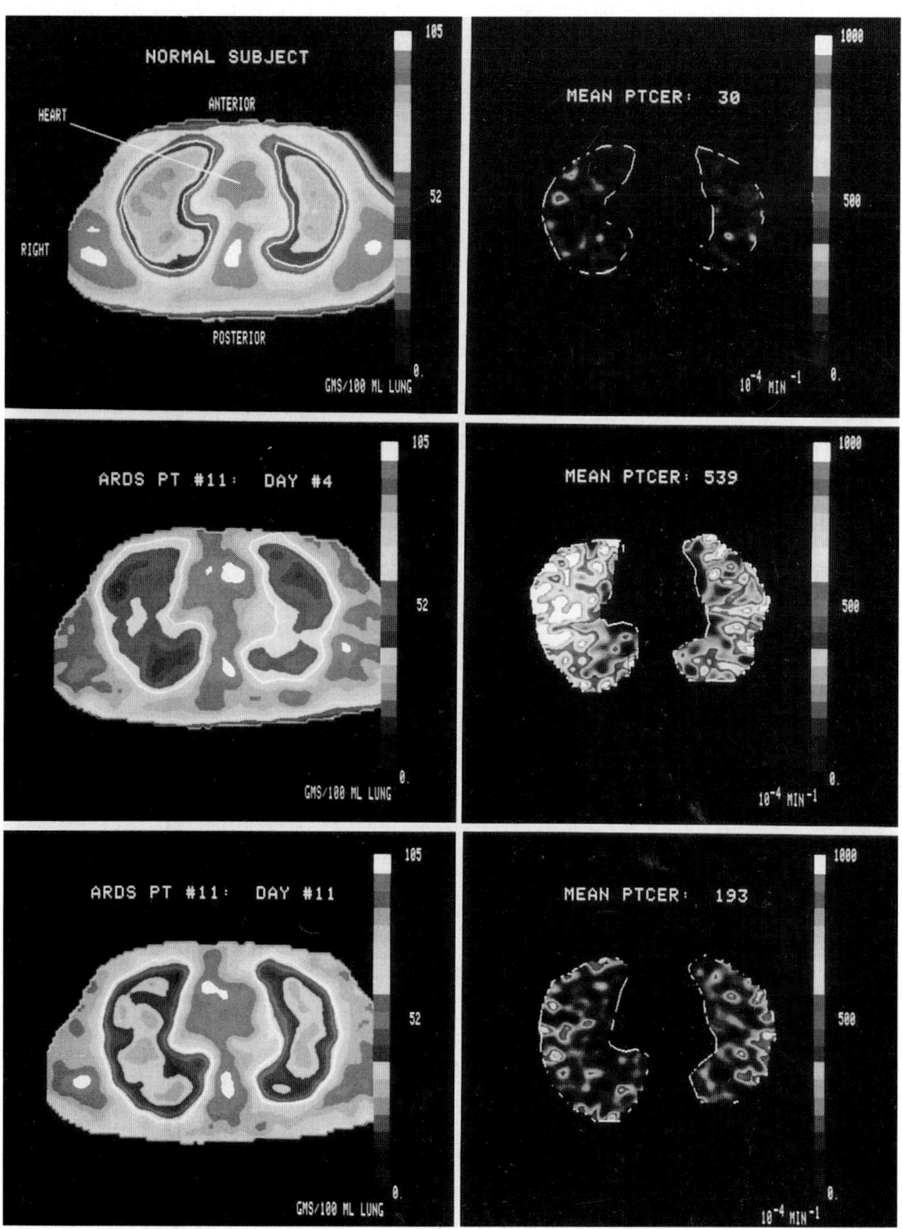

Fig. 31-11. Transmission scans and functional images of pulmonary transcapillary exchange rate in a normal subject and an ARDS patient 4 and 11 days after onset of disease. (Courtesy Dr. Daniel Schuster, Pulmonary Division, Department of Internal Medicine, Washington University School of Medicine, St. Louis, MO.)

approach that involves covalent attachment of a gallium-chelating ligand to the microsphere surface. While the latter method should provide the more stable product, the hydrolysis method is far more convenient and yields a product with acceptable radiochemical purity and stability. The major use of ^{68}Ga-albumin microspheres has been as a reference flow marker in imaging studies that validate the kinetic models employed for PET measurement of myocardial and pulmonary blood flow with PET and freely diffusible tracers (e.g., ^{11}C-n-butanol and ^{15}O-water).

Gallium-68 is rapidly bound by the iron-binding sites of transferrin following intravenous injection of ^{68}Ga-citrate, making this simple chelate complex a convenient radiopharmaceutical for use in studies of regional plasma volume. When combined with an [^{15}O]-carbon monoxide measurement of regional red blood cell volume, the ^{68}Ga-transferrin PET study allows calculation of regional hematocrit. ^{68}Ga-transferrin has also been used in pulmonary studies of vascular permeability. Gallium-68 transferrin has received the most interest in the study of the pulmonary transcapillary exchange rate in patients suffering from acute respiratory distress syndrome. Figure 31-11 shows the transmission images in a normal subject and an ARDS patient 4 days and 11 days after diagnosis, along with metabolically generated images of the pulmonary transcapillary exchange rate. It is seen that in the 4 days after disease onset, the pulmonary transcapillary exchange rate is some 18 times that of a control, while at day 11, the rate has dropped by approximately a factor of 3.

Ethylenediaminetetracetic acid (EDTA) forms an ionic chelate complex with gallium-68 that is normally excluded from the brain by the blood-brain barrier following IV injection. This tracer, therefore, has been used in brain-imaging studies to assess the size and extent of blood-brain barrier–disruption in patients with brain tumors.

BIBLIOGRAPHY

ACNP/SNM Task Force on Clinical PET: Positron emission tomography clinical status in the United States in 1987, J. Nucl. Med. 29:1136, 1988.

Bergmann, S.R. and Sobel, B.E., editors: Positron emission tomography of the heart, Mount Kisco, NY, 1992, Futura Publishing Co.

Bergmann, S.R., Fox, K.A.A., Rand, A.L., McElvany, K.D., Welch, M.J., Markham, J., and Sobel, B.E.: Quantification of regional myocardial blood flow in vivo with $H_2{}^{15}O$, Circulation 70:724, 1984.

Brandes, S.J., and Katzenellenbogen, J.A.: Fundamental considerations in the design of fluorine-18 labeled progestins and androgens as imaging agents for receptor-positive tumors of the breast and prostate, Nucl. Med. Biol. 15:53, 1988.

Daghighian, F., Sumida, R., and Phelps, M.E.: PET imaging an overview and instrumentation, J. Nucl. Med. Tech. 18:1, 1990.

Dence, C.S., Lechner, K.A., Welch, M.J., and Kilbourn, M.R.: Remote system for production of carbon-11 labeled glucose via photosynthesis, J. Labeled Cmpds. Radiopharm. 21:743, 1984.

Fowler, J.S., and Wolf, A.P.: The synthesis of carbon-11, fluorine-18, and nitrogen-13 labeled radiotracers for biomedical applications, Springfield, Va., 1982, Technical Information Center, U.S. Dept of Energy, NAS-NS-3201.

Fujiwara, T., and others: Relationship between histologic type of primary lung cancer and carbon-11-L-methionine uptake with positron emission tomography, J. Nucl. Med. 30(1):33-37, 1989.

Gennaro, G.P., Neirinckx, R.D., Bergner, B., Muller, W.R., Waranis, A., Haney, T.A., Barker, S.I., Loberg, M.D., and Yarnais, A.: A radionuclide generator and infusion system for pharmaceutical quality Rb-82. In Knapp, F.F., Butler, T.A., editors: ACS Symposium Series 241, Radionuclide generators, Washington, D.C., 1984, American Chemical Society, pp. 135.

Goldstein, R.A., Mullani, N.A., Marani, S.K., Fisher, D.J., Gould, K.L., and O'Brien, H.A.: Myocardial perfusion with rubidium-82. II. Effects of metabolic and pharmacologic interventions, J. Nucl. Med. 24:907, 1983.

Green, M.A., and Welch, M.J.: Gallium radiopharmaceutical chemistry, Nuclear Med. and Biol. 16:435, 1989.

Hamacher, K., Coenen, H.H., and Stocklin, G.: Efficient stereospecific synthesis of no-carrier-added 2-[^{18}F]-fluorodeoxy-D-glucose using aminopolyether supported nucleophilic substitution, J. Nucl. Med. 27:235, 1986.

Hawkins, R.A., Pheps, M.E., Huang, S.C., Wapenski, J.A., Grimm, P.D., Parker, R.G., Juillard, G., and Greenberg, P.: A kinetic evaluation of blood-brain permeability in human brain tumors with Ga-68 EDTA and PET, J. Cereb. Blood Flow Metab. 4:507, 1984.

Hubner, K.F.: Clinical positron emission tomography, St. Louis, 1992, Mosby-Year Book, Inc.

Hubner, K.F., Collmann, J., Buonocore, E., and Kabalka, G.W.: Clinical positron emission tomography, St. Louis, 1992, Mosby.

Hubner, K.F.: PET imaging in neurology, J. Nucl. Med. Tech. 18:229, 1990.

Ito, K., and others: Recurrent rectal cancer and scar: differentiation with PET and MR imaging, Radiology 182(2):549-552, 1992.

Jacobson, H.G., editor: Cyclotrons and radiopharmaceuticals in positron emission tomography, J. Am. Med. Assoc. 259:1854, 1988.

Kameyama, M., and others: The accumulation of ^{11}C-methionine in cerebral glioma patients studied with PET, Acta Neurochirurgica 104(1-2):8-12, 1990.

Kessler, R.M., Goble, J.C., Bird, J.H., Girton, M.E., Doppman, J.L., Rapoport, S.I., and Barranger, J.A.: Measurement of blood-brain barrier permeability with positron emission tomography and Ga-68 EDTA, J. Cereb. Blood Flow Metab. 4:323, 1984.

Leskinen-Hallio, S., and others: Carbon-11-methionine and PET is an effective method to image head and neck cancer, J. Nucl. Med. 33(5):691-695, 1992.

Lilja, A., and others: Positron emission tomography and computed tomography in differential diagnosis between recurrent or residual glioma and treatment-induced brain lesions, Acta Radiologica 30(2):121-128, 1989.

MacGregor, R.R., Fowler, J.S., Wolf, A.P., Shiue, C.Y., Lade, R.E., and Wan, C.N.: A synthesis of 2-deoxy-D-[^{11}C]-glucose for regional metabolic studies, J. Nucl. Med. 22:800, 1981.

Mankoff, D., Nader, R.G., and Elsen, H.J.: Cardiac application of positron emission tomography, J. Nucl. Med. Tech. 18:69, 1990.

Mintun, M.A., Ter-Pogossian, M.M., Green, M.A., Lich, L.L., and Schuster, D.P.: Quantitative measurement of regional pulmonary blood flow with positron emission tomography, J. Appl. Physiol. 60:317, 1986.

Mintun, M.A., Dennis, D.R., Welch, M.J., Mathias, C.J., and Schuster, D.P.: Measurements of pulmonary vascular permeability with PET and gallium-68 transferrin, J. Nucl. Med. 28:1704, 1987.

Muehllehner, G., and Karp, J.S.: Positron emission tomography—technical considerations, Semin. Nucl. Med. 16:35, 1986.

Mullani, N.A., Goldstein, R.A., Gould, K.L., Marani, S.K., Fisher, D.J., O'Brien, H.A., and Loberg, M.D.: Myocardial perfusion with Rb-82. I. Measurement of extraction fraction and flow with external detectors, J. Nucl. Med. 24:898, 1983.

Ogawa, T., and others: Clinical value of PET with ^{18}F-fluorodeoxyglucose and L-methyl-^{11}C-methionine for diagnosis of recurrent brain tumor and radiation injury, Acta Radiologica 32(3):197-202, 1991.

Okazumi, S., and others: Evaluation of liver tumors using fluorine-18-fluorodeoxyglucose PET: characterization of tumor and assessment of effect of treatment, J. Nucl. Med. 33(3):333-339, 1992.

Perlmutter, J.S., Kilbourn, M.R., Raichle, M.E., and Welch, M.J.: MPTP induced up-regulation of in vivo dopaminergic radioligand-receptor binding in man, Neurology 37:1575, 1987.

Phelps, M.E., Mazziotta, J.C., and Schelbert, H.R., editors: Positron emission tomography and autoradiography, New York, 1986, Raven Press.

Reivich, M., and Alavi, A.: Positron emission tomography, New York, 1985, A.R. Liss, Inc.

Robison, G.D.: Generator systems for positron emitters. In Positron emission tomography, New York, 1985, A.R. Liss, Inc., pp. 81.

Schuster, D.P., Mintun, M.A., Green, M.A., Ter-Pogossian, M.M.: Regional lung water and hematocrit determined by positron emission tomography, J. Appl. Physiol. 59:860, 1985.

Selwyn, A.P., Allan, R.M., L'Abbate, A., Horlock, P., Camili, P., Clark, J., O'Brien, H., and Grant, P.M.: Relation between regional myocardial uptake of Rb-82 and perfusion: absolute reduction of cation uptake in ischemia, Am. J. Cardiol. 50:112, 1982.

Ter-Pogossian, M.M., Raichle, M.E., and Sobel, B.E.: Positron emission tomography, Sci. Am. 243:170, 1980.

Ter-Pogossian, M.M.: Positron emission tomography instrumentation. In Reivich, M., and Alavi, A., editors: Positron emission tomography, New York, 1985, A.R. Liss, Inc., pp. 43.

Ter-Pogossian, M.M., and Herscovitch, P.: Radioactive oxygen-15 in the study of cerebral blood flow, blood volume, and oxygen metabolism, Semin. Nucl. Med. 15:377, 1985.

van der Wall, E.E., Sochor, H., Righetti, A., and Niemeyer, M.G., editors: What's new in cardiac imaging? Dordrecht, 1992, Kluwer Academic Publishers.

Washburn, L.C., Sun, T.T., Byrd, B.L., Hayes, R.L., Butler, T.A., and Callahan, A.P.: High level production of C-11-carboxyl-labeled amino acids, In Radiopharmaceutical II, New York, 1979, Society of Nuclear Medicine, pp. 767.

Waters, S.L., and Coursey, B.M., editors: The strontium-82/rubidium-82 generator. Applied radiation and isotopes, Int. J. Rad. Appl. Instrum., A, vol. 38, no. 3, 1987.

Welch, M.J., Kilbourn, M.R., and Green, M.A.: Radiopharmaceuticals labeled with short-lived positron-emitting radionuclides, Radioisotopes (Japan) 34:170-179, 1985.

Welch, M.J., and Kilbourn, M.R.: Clinical potential of positron-emitting radiopharmaceuticals. In Fritzberg, A.R., editor: Radiopharmaceuticals: progress and clinical perspectives, vol. 2, Boca Raton, Fla., 1986, CRC Press, p. 115.

Welch, M.J., Katzenellenbogen, J.A., Mathias, C.J., Brodack, J.W., Carlson, K.E., Chi, D.Y., Dence, C.S., Kilbourn, M.R., Perlmutter, J.S., Raichle, M.E., and Ter-Pogossian, M.M.: N-(3-[^{18}F]-fluoropropyl)-spiperone: the preferred ^{18}F-labeled spiperone analog for positron emission tomographic studies of the dopamine receptor, Nucl. Med. Biol. 15:83, 1988.

Wolf, A.P., and Fowler, J.S.: Positron emitter-labeled radiotracers, chemical considerations. In Reivich, M., and Alavi, A., editors: Positron emission tomography, New York, 1985, A.R. Liss, Inc., p. 63.

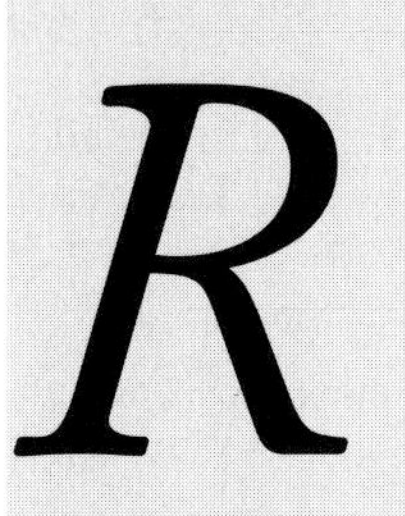

Chapter 32

RADIONUCLIDE THERAPY

JAMES H. LAROSE

■ TREATMENT OF HYPERTHYROIDISM

■ Graves' disease

Graves' disease is usually suspected on the basis of clinical evidence of hypermetabolism such as weight loss despite good appetite, heat intolerance, tachycardia, anxiety, tremor, palpitations, goiter, lid lag, extraocular muscle weakness, and brittle hair. Medical therapy is designed to temporarily suppress secretion of thyroid hormone into the plasma. If successful the derangement driving the thyroid into uncontrolled secretory activity seems to abate, and in months or years the gland is able to reestablish a normal homeostatic relationship with the pituitary gland and to supply the body with the proper physiologic amounts of thyroid hormone.

Nonradioactive iodine immediately inhibits the release of thyroid hormone from the gland. Unfortunately, its effectiveness in controlling thyrotoxicosis is only partial and frequently not sustained. It is also used preoperatively to decrease the vascularity of the thyroid gland. Propylthiouracil (PTU) inhibits the synthesis of thyroid hormone but does not affect the storage or release of preformed thyroid hormone. This explains the delayed onset of clinical change in many cases. Prolonged remission has been reported in 45% to 72% of patients who received long-term therapy (follow-up period of 4 years or more). Methimazole (Tapazole™) is at least 10 times more potent than PTU and therefore is given in proportionately lower doses. Neither drug has an overwhelming advantage over the other. Propranolol (Inderal™), by virtue of its ability to block beta-adrenergic receptors, is used as an adjunct in the treatment of thyrotoxicosis. One advantage of this regimen is prompt protection of the heart.

Use of $Na^{131}I$ is an acceptable method of treatment in practically all adults with Graves' disease except those who are pregnant or lactating. Since the average range of beta particles in tissue is 0.5 mm, there is no significant extrathyroidal radiation. There are only two reports of possible injury to parathyroid glands or other perithyroidal tissues. Salivary gland amylase has been noted to be depressed temporarily after radioiodine therapy. This can be substantially reduced by administering 0.4 mg atropine along with the radioiodine dosage to decrease iodine accumulation in the salivary glands. It is probably safe to treat females during or shortly after their menstrual periods.

Treatment includes a single dosage designed to deliver 80 μCi (2.96 MBq) $Na^{131}I$/gm of thyroid tissue to the gland at 24 hours:

$$D(\mu Ci) = \frac{80\ \mu Ci\ (2.96\ MBq)/g \times (\text{Gram weight of gland})}{\text{24-hr radioiodine uptake (fraction)}}$$

For example, a patient with a 45-g gland and an RAIU of 45% would be calculated as follows:

$$D(\mu Ci) = \frac{80\ \mu Ci\ (2.96\ MBq)/g \times 45\ g\ (\text{estimated weight of gland})}{0.45\ (\text{radioiodine uptake})}$$

$$\text{Dose} = 8000\ \mu Ci\ (2.96\ MBq)\ Na^{131}I$$

If the gland is greater than 50 g, then the dose for that part of the gland over 50 g should be reduced to 40 μCi (1.48 MBq) $Na^{131}I$/g. Some practitioners prefer to deliver 3.2 mCi (118.4 MBq) $Na^{131}I$ to the gland, which is essentially the same technique just mentioned except that all glands are assumed to be approximately 40 g. Reevaluation should take place in 2 to 3 months after the first dose, and the decision to retreat should be both a clinical and laboratory decision.

Nordyke places too much emphasis on size, gland weight, and radioiodine uptake. He notes that hypothyroidism is common after radioiodine therapy and stresses that the goal should be cure of hyperthyroidism rather than avoidance of hypothyroidism. He uses a base dose of 10 mCi (370 MBq) $Na^{131}I$, increasing it for unusually large glands or for special patient circumstances.

Culver and Dworkin have established guidelines in conformity with the NCRP. They showed that all of their patients treated with <12 mCi (444 MBq) of $Na^{131}I$ had radiation levels <2.0 mR/hr at 1 meter on Day 0 and therefore no restrictions. This level was reached in 25 of 29 patients at 0.6 meter in 2 to 4 days.

■ Toxic nodular goiter

There is no uniform agreement about the role of radioiodine therapy in toxic nodular goiter. Dose calculations are less accurate here than for Graves' disease because (1) the iodine uptake is irregularly distributed, and many of the nodules receive little or no radiation because of a low uptake, (2) there is difficulty in estimating the gland size because of the irregularity and frequent retrotracheal and substernal extensions, and (3) relapses are more likely to occur in this disease. Hamburger and co-workers suggest treating "small gland" with 8 mCi retained in the gland, and the largest glands with up to 20 mCi (740 MBq) $Na^{131}I$ retention, with administered doses of 20 to 50 mCi (740 to MBq) $Na^{131}I$.

Thyrocardiac symptoms are particularly troublesome in Plummer's disease, true autonomous toxic nodular goiter. An initial retained dose of 20 mCi (740 MBq) $Na^{131}I$ has been suggested by Skillern and co-workers. Myxedema is seldom seen after radioiodine therapy because the normal suppressed gland receives little radiation.

The Cooperative Thyrotoxicosis Therapy Follow-up Study of over 36,000 treated hyperthyroid patients showed an age-adjusted leukemia incidence of 11 per 100,000 patient years for radioiodine-treated patients and 14 per 100,000 patient years in patients treated with surgical thyroidectomy. Radioiodine therapy delivered about 13 to 14 cGy (rad) to the total body in these cases. This finding is consistent with the two other existing dose-effect studies of radiation leukemogenesis in human adults (that is, atomic bomb survivors and ankylosing spondylitis studies). All three studies fail to demonstrate induction of leukemia at low total-body doses of irradiation.

■ THYROID CARCINOMA

Thyroid carcinoma is a relatively rare disease, with an incidence rate of 3.9 cases per 100,000 population per year in the United States. This is an increase in the incidence reported by the Second National Cancer Survey in 1947, when the occurrence rate was 2.4 per 100,000 population.

For several decades, beginning in the 1920s, radiation therapy was considered good medical practice and very effective treatment for patients with such conditions as enlargement of the thymus gland, hypertrophy of tonsils and adenoids, deafness caused by hypertrophied lymphoid tissue around the eustachian tubes, cervical adenitis, hemangiomas of the head and neck, tinea capitus, and acne.

A linkage of thyroid tumors with prior irradiation was not recognized until these tumors began to be diagnosed with increasing frequency in individuals more than 5 years after their initial treatments. It is now recognized that the effect of these treatments continues into adult life, and intervals of more than 35 years between irradiation and carcinoma have now been recorded.

The majority of thyroid carcinomas are likely to be fully removable by surgery, which further reduces the frequency with which they are seen by the nuclear medicine physician. They are also frequently well differentiated, which has led to confusion and the introduction of inherently contradictory terms such as "benign metastasizing thyroid" and "lateral aberrant thyroid." The thyroid is an embryologically midline organ, and it is the general consensus that any lateral tissue is a metastasis. Fortunately radioiodine has been found to concentrate in about 80% of all differentiated adenocarcinomas of the thyroid, provided that tests are performed after total ablation of all normal thyroid tissue. Not just the follicular but also occasionally papillary carcinomas have been shown to accumulate radioiodine. Undifferentiated, medullary, and Hürthle cell carcinomas rarely concentrate efficiently, nor do they respond to radioiodine therapy. A few adenocarcinomas have been shown to be autonomous, that is, to concentrate radioiodine in the presence of normal functioning thyroid tissue. Usually, uptake develops only after removal or ablation of all normal thyroid tissue so that the TSH rises. Radioiodine therapy should be attempted no matter what the uptake or histopathology shows, since radiosensitivity does not correlate with iodine uptake; a biopsy showing an undifferentiated carcinoma may be incomplete, and a treatable adenocarcinoma may also be present.

When a histologically differentiated tumor is found by biopsy or at surgery, it is now common surgical practice to attempt a total thyroidectomy as well as total removal of recognizable thyroid tissue, since any intrathyroidal or multicentric tumor development is thereby dealt with and since radioiodine concentration is maximized in any tumor tissue that remains. Some clinics prefer hemithyroidectomy followed by radioiodine ablation with 80 to 100 mCi (2960 to 3700 MBq) $Na^{131}I$ of the remaining normal functioning thyroid tissue. This is done to reduce the incidence of surgical hypoparathyroidism.

After removal of the normal thyroid tissue, Pochin prefers to treat differentiated thyroid adenocarcinomas with repeated dosages of 150 mCi (5550 MBq) $Na^{131}I$. Pretreatment serum TSH values should be greater than 50 μIU/ml. He typically uses three to seven therapeutic dosages given over a course of 2 to 5 years until all clinical and serum evidence of remaining tumor tissue is abolished. After ablation of normally functioning thyroid tissue, a recurrent tumor can best be predicted by a rise in serum thyroglobulin. Blahd's group believes that serum thyroglobulin levels below 20 indicate the absence of thyroid carcinoma. This is more sensitive than radioiodine imaging and is the recommended follow-up procedure.

Marrow depression is found to be uncommon on normal

dosage regimens except when bone metastases are present. In these cases longer intervals between dosages, at least after the first few dosages, are desirable.

Patients are treated with replacement/suppressive dosages of thyroxine during the months between radioiodine dosages. In the past, TSH was used to enhance uptake, but this hormone is of bovine origin and has occasionally been known to cause sloughing at the injection site and is not currently recommended.

Culver and Dworkin note that there is no evidence suggesting that the residual radiation present in ^{131}I thyroid cancer therapy patients (following release from the hospital) causes health problems in others. However, the NCRP recommends that family members of a radioactive patient receive less than 500 mrem in any one year. Therefore the criterion for removing restrictions is when the average exposure rate measures 2 mR/hr at 1 m from the patient.

Beierwaltes notes that in their retrospective study of 33 children and adolescents treated with large doses of ^{131}I for thyroid cancer, there was no subsequent detrimental effect on their fertility or birth histories. He finds that suggestions that the mother of young children hire a babysitter for 2 or 3 weeks to avoid radiation hazard to the children usually alarms the mother who is already frightened by her "cancer."

■ POLYCYTHEMIA VERA

Polycythemia vera is a chronic hematologic disorder characterized by increased proliferative activity of erythroid, myeloid, megakaryocytic, and fibroblastic cell lines. The early erythrocytotic phase often progresses to a phase of myelofibrosis with myeloid metaplasia (MMM), also called the spent phase. It is marked by anemia, a leukoerythroblastic blood picture, and hepatosplenomegaly. This eventually progresses to an accelerated malignant phase indistinguishable from acute myeloblastic leukemia (AML).

Elevated hematocrit and hemoglobin levels or RBC counts do not suffice for a diagnosis of polycythemia vera. An absolute increase in the red cell mass must be determined by direct measurement using ^{51}Cr (or ^{32}P) labeled autologous erythrocytes. Compensatory erythrocytosis resulting from tissue hypoxia must be ruled out by the demonstration of normal arterial O_2 concentration and the absence of an abnormal hemoglobin with increased O_2 affinity or diminished O_2 carrying capacity. Erythropoietin-secreting tumors must be ruled out. Once these possibilities have been eliminated, confirmatory evidence of panmyelosis must be obtained, including the finding of splenomegaly or two or more of the following: leukocytosis greater than 12,000, thrombocytosis greater than 400,000, elevated leukocyte alkaline phosphatase, or elevated serum unsaturated B_{12} binding capacity.

After confirmation of the disease process, therapy can include phosphorous-32. Three to 5 mCi (111 to 185 MBq) sodium phosphate ^{32}P solution is injected intravenously. It is important to confirm before injection that the dose is in a clear liquid, because ^{32}P chromic phosphate suspension is cloudy and should not be injected. Patients are reevaluated at 10 to 12 weeks, and this dose is repeated if the patient's clinical status and laboratory data so indicate. At least this much time is necessary because the circulating red cells normally disappear from circulation so slowly that a significant change could not be expected any earlier. A single course of therapy may induce a remission lasting several years. The ^{32}P dosage probably should not exceed 6 mCi (222 MBq) during any 6-month period. Treatment with ^{32}P should preferably not be used if the platelet count is less than 15,000, or the reticulocyte count is less than 0.2%, or the white blood cell count is less than 3000. Phosphorus-32 therapy is generally reserved for patients who cannot be relied on to take hydroxylurea according to instructions, and for the elderly, so that there is minimal concern about subsequent development of acute leukemia.

In 1969 Lawrence's group observed 181 patients treated with ^{32}P to termination. Fourteen percent developed an acute myelogenous leukemia-like state, and 25% developed significant splenic myeloid metaplasia. These investigators believe that the increased incidence of both acute leukemia and splenic myeloid metaplasia was a result of prolonged survival, since these patients were younger at the time of diagnosis and survived longer than those ^{32}P-treated patients who died of causes other than myeloid metaplasia or acute leukemia. The massive retrospective survey of Modan and Lilienfeld showed an 11% incidence of acute leukemia in ^{32}P-treated patients and an 8.9% incidence in irradiated subjects. The significance of the less than 1% incidence of acute leukemia in the nonirradiated group is subject to the limitations the researchers so ably discuss—improper diagnostic criteria, lack of selection of comparable cases, differences in quality of medical care, and inadequate follow-up visits.

A Polycythemia Vera Cooperative Study has been in progress for 25 years under the sponsorship of the National Cancer Institute. A total of 432 patients with proven polycythemia vera were randomized into this three-arm study in the late 1960s. One third of the patients were treated with phlebotomy, another third with chlorambucil, and the rest with sodium phosphate ^{32}P solution. Acute leukemia has been found in only 8.6% of the patients: 3 who were treated with phlebotomy, 15 who were treated with phosphorus-32, and 19 who were treated with chlorambucil. In addition to the increased incidence of leukemia, the patients receiving chlorambucil also had an increase in carcinomas of the skin and GI tract. This chlorambucil portion of the study was discontinued because "the risk of neoplasia increased with time . . . and there was no benefit in morbidity or mortality compared to ^{32}P."

■ INTRACAVITARY USE OF RADIOACTIVE COLLOIDS

The control of recurrent effusions in the pleural and peritoneal cavities resulting from a malignant disease presents a serious and difficult problem. Not only is the repeated drainage of these cavities an uncomfortable procedure for the patient, but also it usually has to be repeated at frequent intervals with a resulting loss of vital body proteins. Solutions are not suitable because they are absorbed into the bloodstream, thus subjecting the patient to significant total body radiation. Colloids introduced into the cavity are first engulfed by the floating macrophages and then fixed by the tissue macrophages lining the wall of the serous cavity. Some of the material reaches the local lymph nodes and are deposited there.

Patients with Stage I or II ovarian carcinoma are often treated with 15 mCi (555 MBq) of colloidal chromic phosphate ^{32}P premixed with 250 ml of normal saline. It is important to make sure that the preparation is a cloudy, brownish-green colloidal suspension and not the clear ^{32}P solution used for IV injection (as for polycythemia vera). Confirmation that fluid will disperse can be done by a ^{99m}Tc sulfur colloid technique or by injecting a water-soluble radiopaque and taking a KUB. After instillation, the patient is turned frequently. Gamma cameras can be used to image the Bremsstrahling radiation with a high-energy collimator and an energy window of 150 to 450 keV. Spanos prefers to deliver the ^{32}P in the immediate postoperative period, finding that this results in significantly fewer GI complications.

Intrapleural use of colloidal chromic phosphate ^{32}P requires a lesser dosage of about 10 mCi (370 MBq).

Sprengelmeyer suggests that pericardial administration of phosphorus-32 colloidal chromic phosphate is the treatment of choice for malignant pericardial effusion.

■ METASTATIC BONE DISEASE

In clinical practice, breast, prostate, bronchial, renal, and thyroid carcinomas account for most of the metastatic bone disease seen. Thyroid carcinoma has been discussed previously. Control of bone pain has always been the objective of radionuclide therapy because it was immediately apparent that the soft tissue component was unreachable.

The Maxfields stimulated humeral-dependent prostate metastases with aqueous testosterone and showed by means of autoradiography that a 20:1 tumor-to-nontumor ratio could be achieved with sodium phosphate ^{32}P solution. This technique showed that sodium phosphate ^{32}P solution was taken up in new bone rather than in the adjacent tumor tissue. Most series indicate success in relieving bone pain, but this relief has been accompanied by an unacceptable incidence of bone-marrow depression.

Robinson's group investigated strontium-89 chloride, which interestingly was the first radionuclide employed for therapy of metastatic bone disease. They note that not only is there significant uptake of strontium at sites of osteoblastic skeletal metastases, but that unlike adjacent normal bone, the radiostrontium remained essentially in the same concentration at the tumor sites for 100 days following injection. In almost 500 patients, the overall response rate in terms of decrease in pain and improved quality of life is now 79% for prostate metastases and 83% for breast metastases. Strontium-89 decays by beta emission with a physical half-life of 50.5 days. The maximum beta energy is 1.463 MeV (100%). The maximum range of the beta particle in tissue is approximately 8 mm. This radiopharmaceutical (Metastron-Amersham) was approved by the FDA in June 1993. Candidates for strontium-89 therapy should have multiple bone metastases, bone pain, a platelet count over 60,000, and a white blood cell count over 2400. All patients who have failed hormonal therapy management of prostate cancer metastases to bone are candidates for strontium-89 therapy. The minimal effective dose is 40 μCi/kg (1.48 MBq/kg) ^{89}SrCl. Doses up to 60 μCi/kg (2.22 MBq/kg) ^{89}SrCl are probably ideal. Average body weight patients are generally dosed with 4 mCi (148 MBq). Patients should be retreated as early as 10 weeks if symptoms begin to recur. Concurrent use of multiple site or hemibody external radiation with strontium-89 therapy should be carefully evaluated for toxicity implications. Platelet counts are the most sensitive indicator of hematologic toxicity.

A New Drug Application has been filed with the FDA for another pair of therapeutic agents. Both rhenium-186 HEDP and samarium-153 EDTMP are chelates that show excellent biolocalization characteristics similar to technetium-99m diphosphonates, including rapid blood clearance, selective skeletal uptake, and high lesion affinity. The efficacy of the samarium chelate has been demonstrated in dogs with spontaneous bone cancer. The beta particles of the radionuclides make them capable of delivering highly localized radiation doses, while confirmation of localization in each patient is easily accomplished by imaging using the gamma photon emissions of these radionuclides.

■ RHEUMATOID ARTHRITIS

Rheumatoid arthritis (RA) causes chronic synovial inflammation that can lead to pannus formation and eventual destruction of the articular cartilage. Medical therapy includes aspirin, nonsteroidal antiinflammatory agents, steroids, remission-inducing agents (gold, D-penicillamine) and intraarticular corticosteroid injections. Chemical synovectomy using osmic acid or alkylating agents like Thiotepa-T have achieved only limited acceptance. Surgical synovectomy can be expected to give 2 to 3 years of relief. This procedure is technically difficult, and complete removal of the synovium is usually not achieved.

Patients with Stage I or Stage II RA are candidates for radiation synovectomy if they have failed the medical regimen and have not had knee surgery. Zuckerman's group uses dysprosium-165 ferric hydroxide macroaggregates (^{165}Dy-FHMA) obtained from a local nuclear reactor. The ^{165}Dy has a half-life of 2.3 hours, which is 25 times shorter than previously used ^{90}Y or ^{198}Au. The shortened half-life limits the leakage dose and also allows the patients to be discharged in 8 hours instead of 3 days. The extraarticular leakage to the liver was measured at 0.64% of the injected dosage and gave a mean radiation liver dose of 3.2 rad. In Stage I knees 94% of patients showed good or fair results and in Stage II 78% had similar results.

Davis and Chinol prefer yttrium-90 particulate agents for the 2.3 MeV maximum energy of this pure beta particle emitter. It deposits 80% of its energy in the first 4 to 5 mm of tissue and has a short 237-day half-life. Both calcium oxalate and ferric hydroxide macroaggregates are acceptable particulate agents. Leakage is reduced by using proper-sized aggregates, by immobilizing the joint, and by using this short half-life radionuclide.

■ POSTOPERATIVE IRRADIATION OF PTERYGIUM

Surgical ablation is essential in the treatment of pterygium (a triangular patch of hypertrophied bulbar subconjunctional tissue), regardless of whether the lesion is primary or recurrent after previous treatment. However, an overall 20% to 30% recurrence rate follows surgery alone. To reduce this rate of recurrence, prophylactic postoperative irradiation has been advocated and has proved successful in many centers. If beta radiation of low tissue penetration is used, the dose to the lens is very low and the incidence of radiation cataract is correspondingly reduced to negligible proportions. A series of 1300 pterygia were reported by van den Brenk, who used a flat, circular ^{90}Sr applicator to the limbus over the bare area produced at surgery. The pterygium received either an 800- or 1000-rad surface dose of beta radiation, respectively, on postoperative days 0, 7, and 14. The recurrence rate was reduced to less than 2%, as compared with the 25% recurrence rate with two doses of 900 rad. Three doses of 1000 rad often caused a diffuse erythematous reaction at the site of irradiation with some edema and formation of a fibrinous exudate, but this reaction invariably resolved within 1 to 2 weeks of the first dose. Scleral or corneal damage or both occurred in only five cases. No cases of cataract formation were seen.

BIBLIOGRAPHY

Blahd, W.H., and others: Serum thyroglobulin, a monitor of differentiated thyroid carcinoma in patients receiving thyroid hormone suppression therapy: concise communication, J. Nucl. Med. 25:673-676, 1984.

Beierwaltes, W.H., and Widman, J.: How harmful to others are iodine-131 treated patients, J. Nucl. Med. 33:2116-2117, 1992 (editorial).

Culver, C.M., and Dworkin, H.J.: Radiation safety considerations for post-iodine-131 hyperthyroid therapy, J. Nucl. Med. 32:169-173, 1991.

Culver, C.M., and Dworkin, H.J.: Radiation safety considerations for post-iodine-131 thyroid cancer therapy, J. Nucl. Med. 33:1402-1405, 1992.

Davis, M.A., and Chinol, M.: Radiopharmaceuticals for radiation synovectomy: evaluation of two yttrium-90 particulate agents, J. Nucl. Med. 30:1047-1055, 1989.

Ketring, A.R.: ^{153}Sm-EDTMP and ^{186}Re-HEDP as bone therapeutic radiopharmaceuticals, Nucl. Med. Biol. 14:223-232, 1987.

Lawrence, J.H., Winchell, H.S., and Donald, W.G.: Leukemia in polycythemia vera: relationship to splenic myeloid metaplasia and therapeutic radiation dose, Ann. Intern. Med. 70:763, 1969.

Maxfield, J.R., Jr., Maxfield, J.J.G., and Maxfield, W.S.: Use of radioactive phosphorus and testosterone in metastatic bone lesions from breast and prostate, South. Med. J. 51:320, 1958.

Modan, B., and Lilienfeld, A.M.: Polycythemia vera and leukemia: the role of radiation treatment: a study of 122 patients, Medicine 44:305, 1965.

Muller, W., Pavelka, K., and Fridrich, R.: Treatment of chronic arterial effusions with 90-yttrium (^{90}Y), Scand. J. Rheumatol. 4:216, 1975.

Murphy, S.: Polycythemia vera, Dis. Mon. 38:158-212, 1992.

Nordyke, R.A., and Gilbert, F.J.: Optimal iodine-131 dose for eliminating hypothyroidism in Graves' disease, J. Nucl. Med. 32:411-416, 1991.

Pochin, E.E.: Radioiodine therapy of thyroid cancer, Semin. Nucl. Med. 1:503, 1971.

Robinson, R.G., and others: Radionuclide therapy of intractable bone pain: emphasis on strontium-89, Semin. Nucl. Med. 22:28-32, 1992.

Sarkar, S., and others: Subsequent fertility and birth histories of children and adolescents treated with ^{131}I for thyroid cancer, J. Nucl. Med. 17:460, 1976.

Skillern, P.G., McCullagh, E.P., and Clamen, M.: Radioiodine in diagnosis and therapy of hyperthyroidism, Arch. Intern. Med. 110:888, 1962.

Spanos, W.J., Jr., and others: Complications in the use of intraabdominal ^{32}P for ovarian carcinoma, Gynecol. Oncol. 45:243-247, 1992.

Sprengelmeyer, J.T., and McDermott, R.L.: Phosphorus-32 colloidal chromic phosphate: treatment of choice for malignant pericardial effusion, J. Nucl. Med. 31:2034-2036, 1990.

U.S. Department of Health, Education, and Welfare: Information for physicians—irradiation related thyroid cancer, DHEW Pub No. (NIH) 77-1120, Washington, D.C., 1977.

van den Brenk, H.A.S.: Results of prophylactic postoperative irradiation in 1,300 cases of pterygium, Am. J. Roentgenol. 103:723, 1968.

Zuckerman, J.D., and others: Treatment of rheumatoid arthritis using radiopharmaceuticals, Nucl. Med. Biol. 14:211-218, 1987.

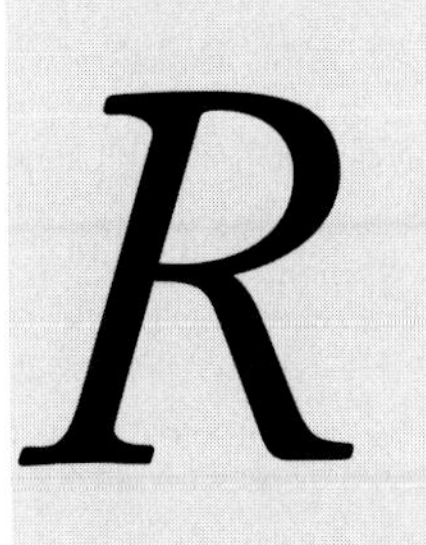

Chapter 33

RADIOASSAY

ALBERT V. HEAL

Before proceeding into this chapter, a few terms used to describe different methodologies must be clarified. In the early development of this technique only two very similar methodologies existed and the interchange of terminology was of little consequence. In recent years, however, new and varied techniques have evolved that make the proper use of terminology extremely important. Figure 33-1 illustrates the various terms that have evolved and their relationship to each other.

In the late 1950s and early 1960s only the competitive protein binding assay (CPB) and radioimmunoassay (RIA) procedures were being used clinically; these terms were used interchangeably, since all RIAs are CPBs. However, the reverse is not true. With the development of new methodologies, more descriptive and general terminology was needed to properly separate them. This chapter deals with *radioassay,* a very general term. The actual subject covered in this chapter is only a portion of radioassay, since any assay, test, or determination involving radionuclidic material can be considered a radioassay. The portion of radioassay discussed here can be considered as *binding assay,* which includes all the techniques discussed here plus those assays that use a nonisotopic label. Most of these techniques can be further classified according to their procedure and are described by other terminology. Also, those assays using an antibody as the binder can be further classified as *immunoassays*. All of these methodologies, including other terminology used, are discussed.

■ GENERAL CONCEPTS

RIA was the first binding assay method developed and came out of the early works of Berson and Yalow in the early 1950s. At the 1955 annual meeting of the Society of Nuclear Medicine, Berson and Yalow reported on an insulin-binding protein using ^{131}I-labeled insulin in the blood of insulin-treated diabetics. Berson and Yalow, however, originally reported this protein as insulin antibody but were refused publication unless it was changed to insulin-binding protein. The scientific community at that time was not ready to believe that an antibody to insulin could be produced in humans. This, however, was the beginning of what eventually led to the development of an RIA insulin test. In 1959 Berson and Yalow reported on the first RIA for insulin in human blood using guinea pig antibody, for which Dr. Yalow won the 1977 Nobel Prize.

At the same time Berson and Yalow were developing RIA in the United States, Ekins in England and later Murphy in Canada were looking at naturally occurring serum-binding assays. Ekins' early work was first reported in 1960, and some, therefore, feel he should have shared the Nobel Prize. Both of these investigators made important and significant contributions to the development of binding assays, but it was the development of RIA that had the greatest impact on the subsequent proliferation of immunoassays.

The early development of binding assays for clinical use was slow, but as better techniques were developed for producing antibody and radiolabeling, such as the chloramine-T iodination procedure by Greenwood and others in 1963, binding assays began to proliferate both for the various substances assayed and for the number of laboratories performing these assays. The 1970s showed the greatest advance in binding assays with (1) the production of more and better antibodies; (2) different labeling techniques; (3) solid phase techniques; (4) new methodologies; (5) new instrumentation for performing binding assays; and (6) more accurate data reduction techniques, primarily formulated by Rodbard. However, the most significant advance was the technique, equivalent only to the discovery of RIA itself, to produce an unlimited supply of antibodies to a single antigenic determinant (monoclonal antibodies). Kohler and Milstein described this technique in 1975, but it was not until the 1980s that the full impact of this discovery was felt in the immunoassay area. Since then immunoassay has undergone tremendous changes, which will be discussed later in this chapter.

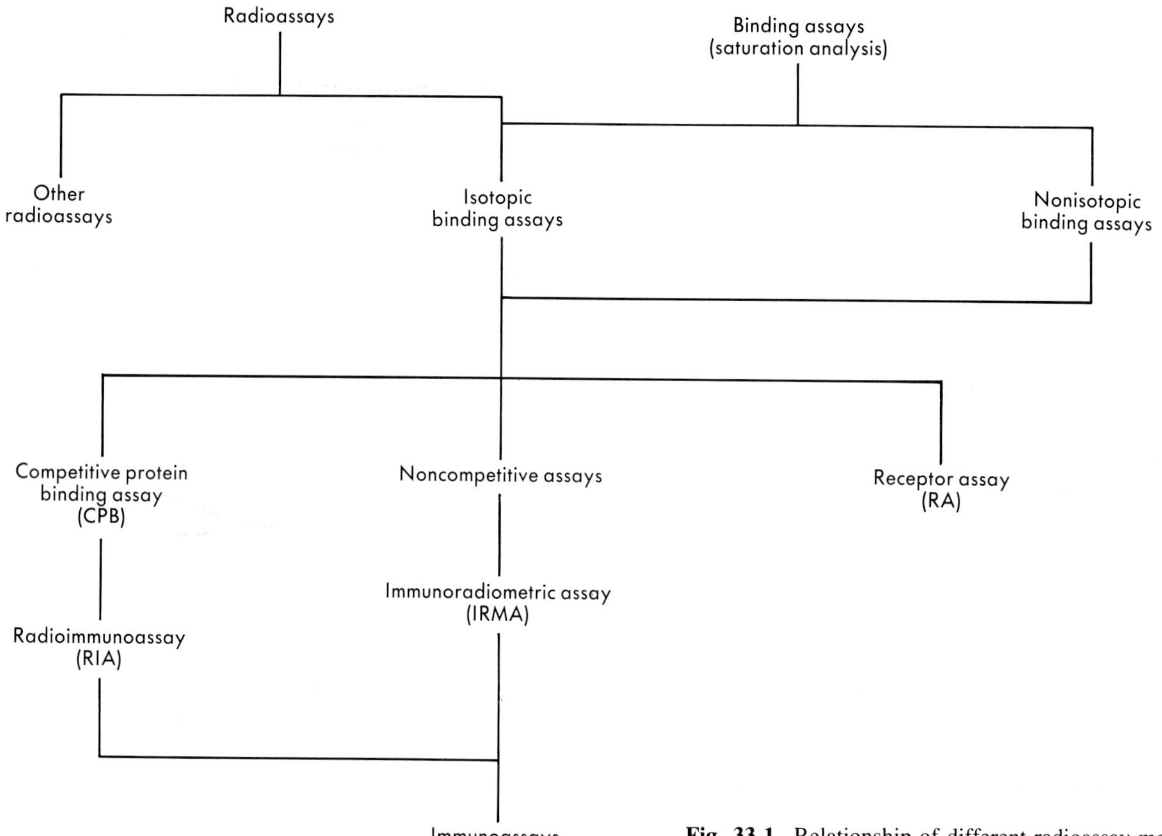

Fig. 33-1. Relationship of different radioassay methods.

Before the development of RIA, substances in biologic fluids were measured by chemical analysis or bioassay. These methods, however, lacked sensitivity, specificity, and accuracy and were usually laborious, expensive, and time-consuming. RIA is rapid, sensitive, specific, and inexpensive, but the one objection to RIA is that it measures immunologic activity and not biologic activity. Fortunately, direct correlation between immunologic activity and biologic activity has been demonstrated for most substances measured.

■ BASIC ANTIGEN-ANTIBODY REACTION

The basic principles of antigen-antibody reactions are quite simple and apply to all binding assays, not just immunoassays. The reaction between antigen and antibody to form the antigen-antibody complex is a reversible reaction described thus:

$$Ag + Ab \underset{K_2}{\overset{K_1}{\rightleftarrows}} Ag\ Ab$$

In this equation K_1 represents the rate constant or association constant for the formation of the complex and K_2 represents the rate constant or dissociation constant for the breakdown of the Ag-Ab complex. The rate constants represent that fraction of available molecules reacting within a unit of time in each direction, and the absolute rate, which is the number of molecules reacting within a unit of time, is dependent on concentration. Therefore at the start of the reaction the concentration of free Ag and Ab is high and the absolute rate in the direction of the complex will be greatest. As more and more complex is formed, the absolute rate to the right decreases (association) and the absolute rate to the left increases (dissociation) until the absolute rates in both directions are equal. At this point equilibrium is reached and no further changes in concentrations of the molecules on either side of the equation will result.

This reaction is described by the law of mass action, which states that the ratio of the products of the concentration on the two sides of the equation are a constant, K:

$$\frac{[Ag\ Ab]}{[Ag]\ [Ab]} = K$$

[Ag Ab], [Ag], and [Ab] are the concentrations of the antigen-antibody complex, free antigen, and free antibody, respectively, and K is the equilibrium or affinity constant. The exact concentrations are determined by the rate constants of the forward and reverse reactions and therefore:

$$K_a = \frac{K_1}{K_2}$$

The affinity constant is a measure of the energy of reaction between Ag and Ab. The concentration of complex formed [Ag Ab] is directly related to the affinity constant K_a. The higher the K_a, the greater the concentration of complex formed.

All binding assays, whether antigen-antibody, ligand–specific protein, or ligand-receptor–type assays, follow the basic immune reaction and the law of mass action. Radiobinding assays differ from this basic reaction by the addition of a radiolabeled antigen, ligand, or binder; the use of binders other than antibody; and the reaction methodology, an example of which is as follows:

$$\begin{matrix} L & & & K_1 & LB \\ & + & B & \rightleftarrows & + \\ L^* & & & K_2 & L^*B \end{matrix}$$

where L and L* represent ligand, antigen, or analyte, unlabeled and radiolabeled, respectively, and B represents specific binder, protein, or antibody. Before discussing binding assay reactions, a discussion of the reactants must precede.

■ LIGANDS

A ligand is defined as any substance that will bind to an appropriate binder and refers to both unlabeled and labeled reagent. This is a very general term and refers basically to any substance for which there is a binding assay. An antigen is a specific type of ligand, but not all ligands are antigens.

The development and routine use of a binding assay depends on an ample supply of highly purified ligand. This is necessary for several reasons:

1. Standardization of the assay
2. Preparation of tracer
3. Monitoring recovery
4. In the case of immunoassays, for immunization

The availability of pure ligand varies, depending on the kind of ligand needed. Ligands may be purified from natural or synthetic material. Those purified from natural material usually present the most problems, such as large-protein hormones and tumor-associated ligands. This is not as much of a problem today as it was in the past, since many ligands that were only available from natural sources are now synthesized. However, there are still many ligands that are difficult to purify completely or that are in short supply. To overcome these difficulties the World Health Organization (WHO) has established standards for most ligands designated the first international reference preparation (IRP) and the second international standard (IS). All assays can be standardized against these values for greater consistency of results. It many cases the international standards are not as pure as can be prepared today; they cannot be quantitated in absolute units, only international units (IU), but they are still useful for standardization of results.

Steroid hormones, small peptide hormones, and drugs are mostly prepared chemically; therefore virtually 100% purity is usually available. Although these ligands are synthetically produced, it should not be assumed that they are 100% pure. Occasionally purity must be checked by various methods, such as thin-layer chromatography. These and the naturally occurring ligands may also break down when stored, changing their purity. Therefore stability studies must be performed to determine at what storage condition they are most stable. Generally, most ligands should be stored at −20° C for greatest stability.

One of the most important qualities of a ligand is that it be identical with the endogenous ligand being measured. Dissimilarities can affect the assay's specificity, sensitivity, and accuracy; therefore a ligand as identical as possible to endogenous ligand should be sought. Among the many things that can affect ligand similarity are the following:

1. Species differences caused by use of animal ligands for the detection of human ligands.
2. Tissue differences of origin of the ligand. The same ligand may be very different when extracted from different tissues, for example, adrenocorticotropic hormone (ACTH) from the pituitary gland differs from that of ACTH-secreting tumors.
3. Various forms of the ligand with endogenous material may exist. These include large and small gastrin, insulin, and proinsulin.

■ Antigens

Since most of the binding assays to be considered will be immunoassays, the ligand is called an *antigen*. An antigen is defined as any substance capable of stimulating an antibody response. For a substance to be antigenic, it must be foreign to the host animal and have a molecular weight greater than 5000; typically molecular weights greater than 10,000 are necessary for antibody stimulation. The antigen used to stimulate antibody production is also termed an *immunogen*, and the antigen being measured in the patient sample is often termed an *analyte*. As mentioned previously, to develop a clinically useful immunoassay the antigen must be pure for use as a standard, labeled antigen and for the production of highly specific antibody. It must also be identical to endogenous analyte as far as immunoreactivity is concerned.

■ Haptens

Haptens are substances that cannot stimulate an antibody response when injected into a host but can be rendered antigenic when coupled to a high molecular weight substance such as a protein. The molecular weight of haptens is typically less than 5000 (drugs, antibiotics, etc.) and the most common protein used for conjugation to haptens is bovine serum albumin (BSA) or bovine thyroglobulin.

To couple a hapten to BSA, it is usually necessary to form a hapten "bridge" (Figs. 33-2 and 33-3). A hapten bridge is simply a small molecule that is capable of linking the hapten with BSA by binding them on two different sites of the hapten bridge molecule. The choice of bridge depends on site of attachment, bridge length, steroid nucleus orientation, and desired immunogenicity. The two most

O-CARBOXYMETHYL OXIMES

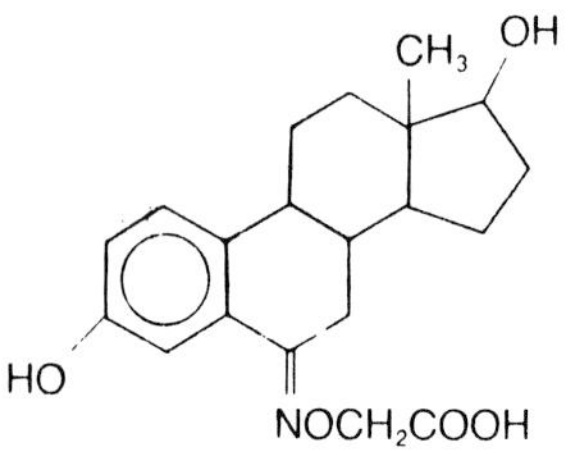

$NOCH_2COOH$

Estradiol-6-O(carboxymethyl) oxime

CARBOXYMETHYL STEROIDS

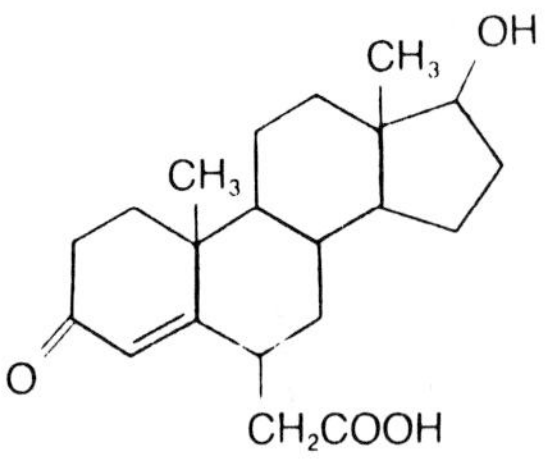

CH_2COOH

6-β carboxymethyl testosterone

HEMISUCCINATES

$COOHCH_2CH_2CO$

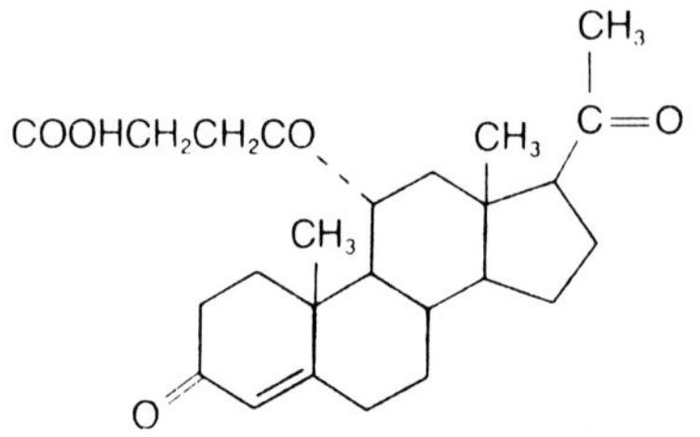

Progesterone-11 α hemisuccinate

GLUCURONIDE

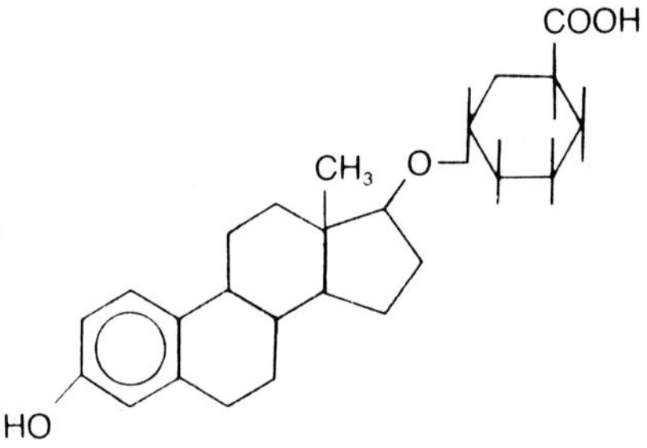

Estradiol-17 β glucuronide

MERCAPTOACETATES

$S—(CH_2)_N—COOH$

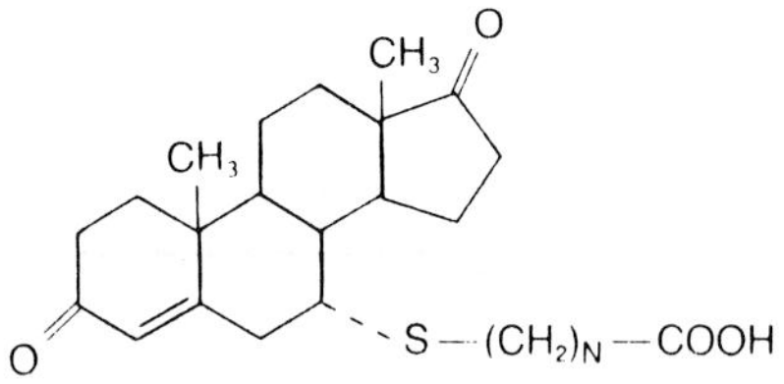

Androstenedione-7 α carboxymethyl thioether

Fig. 33-2. Molecules used for the formation of a hapten bridge. (From Bio-Educational Publications Slide/Seminar Education Programs: Radioimmunoassay, vol. 2, Rochester, N.Y., 1982, Bio-Educational Publications.)

SULFATES

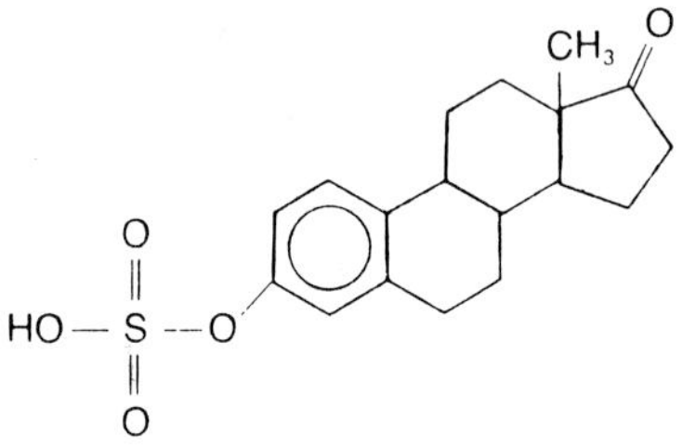

Estrone-3-sulfate

Fig. 33-3. Molecules used for the formation of a hapten bridge. (From Bio-Educational Publications Slide/Seminar Education Programs: Radioimmunoassay, vol. 2, Rochester, N.Y., 1982, Bio-Educational Publications.)

common methods of hapten-BSA coupling are (1) mixed anhydride reaction and (2) the carbodiimide reaction (Figs. 33-4 and 33-5).

■ Standards

The various reactants in binding assays are highly variable from laboratory to laboratory for the detection of the same analyte; if not adjusted this variance would result in highly variable analyte values. To overcome this situation, ligand used as standard should be standardized against a known universal reference material for that ligand supplied by the World Health Organization (WHO). This permits different laboratories to express their results in relation to a common reference material. For the most part this system of standardization works well, but there are some problems with the system:

1. Some standards are not fully characterized and as such are quantitated in international units. Various laboratories will convert international units into an absolute estimate of weight by use of a conversion factor based on biologic activity per unit weight. This may not be correct and will give a false sense of accuracy.
2. In some cases two international standards are available for the same ligand; there is some controversy over which one is correct. This creates some confusion when different laboratories standardize against different international standards.

Material intended to be used as a standard should conform to certain characteristics:

1. There should be ample quantities available to supply many laboratories for many years.
2. Storage effects should be known, and the material should be stable for several months.
3. It should not contain any interfering substances but

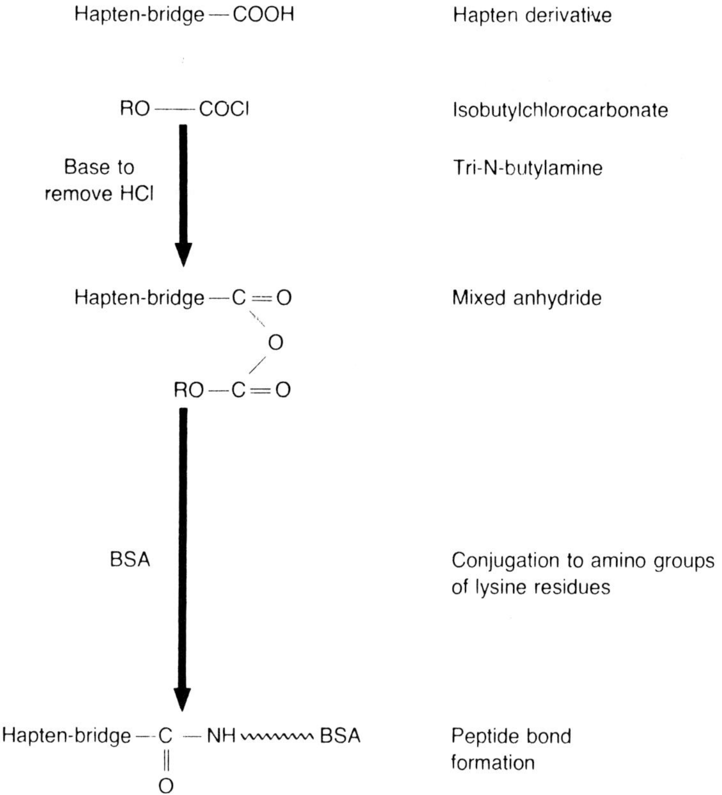

Fig. 33-4. Method of hapten coupling or conjugation using the mixed anhydride reaction. (From Bio-Educational Publications Slide/Seminar Education Programs: Radioimmunoassay, vol. 2, Rochester, N.Y., 1982, Bio-Educational Publications.)

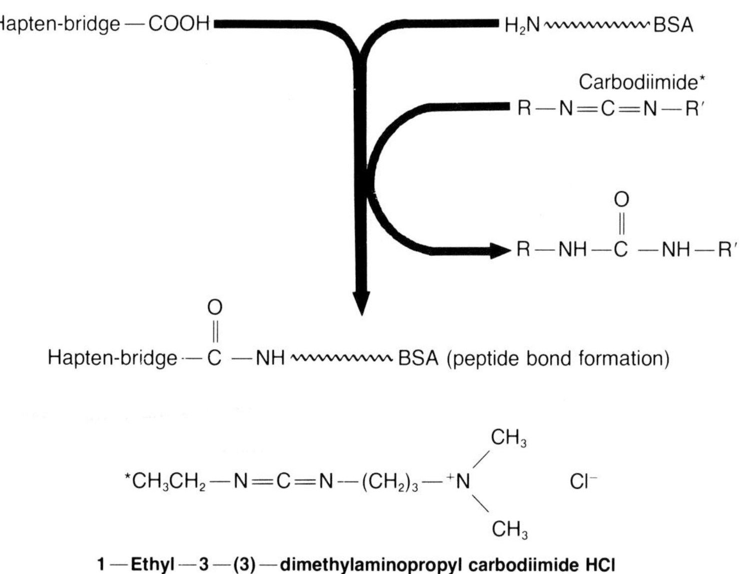

Fig. 33-5. Method of hapten coupling or conjugation using the carbodiimide reaction. (From Bio-Educational Publications Slide/Seminar Education Programs: Radioimmunoassay, vol. 2, Rochester, N.Y., 1982, Bio-Educational Publications.)

Table 33-1. List of radionuclides

Status	Nuclide	Type of decay	Energy of radiation	Half-life	Counting efficiency (%)
Currently used	^{125}I	γ and x rays	35,69 keV	60 days	80
		e^-	30 keV		
	^{57}Co	α and x rays	14,122,126,692 keV	270 days	90
		e^-	7,13,115,129 keV		
	^{75}Se	γ	66,97,121,136,265,280,401 keV	120 days	
		β^-	85,95,109,124,253 keV		
	^{59}Fe	β^-	1.57 maximum and 0.475 maximum MeV	45.6 days	
		γ	0.143,0.192,1.095,1.292 MeV		
	^{3}H	β^-	average 5.7 keV, maximum 18.6 keV	12.6 yrs	55
No longer in general use	^{131}I	β^-	Maximum 806,606 keV	8 days	35
		e^-	46,330 keV		
		γ	80,284,364,637,723 keV		
	^{14}C	β^-	average 45 keV, maximum 156 keV	5.730 yrs	85

should be as identical as possible to the patient sample in the final reaction mixture.

4. Ideally it should be highly purified, but actually this is not always necessary, possible, or desirable.

Standards for an immunoassay procedure are usually produced by using a standard with a value above the clinical range with a number of serial dilutions to be below the clinical range adequate to reproduce an accurate standard curve. These dilutions may be freeze-dried and stored until used and then reconstituted; or frozen and stored until used, or used directly without further preparation. Care should be taken when freeze-drying, since some molecules may undergo alteration.

■ RADIOLABELING ANTIGEN

Radiolabeled antigen is simply highly purified antigen containing 1 or more atoms of a radionuclide. The labeled antigen may be identical to the standard or analyte being measured, but this is not absolutely necessary. The only requirement is that the labeled antigen possess the same immunoreactivity as the standard and analyte in the unknown sample. Antigen may be labeled directly or by conjugation with a prelabeled molecule.

Several radionuclides have been used as labels for antigens in immunoassays since Berson and Yalow first used ^{131}I; some of these are ^{14}C, ^{3}H, ^{131}I, ^{32}P, ^{75}Se, ^{59}Fe, and ^{57}Co. At present, however, primarily ^{125}I, ^{57}Co, ^{59}Fe, and ^{3}H are used (Table 33-1). ^{125}I is the principal radionuclide used today (in better than 90% of the assays). ^{57}Co is used primarily for the B_{12} assay, and ^{59}Fe for the serum iron assay. ^{3}H is used for those ligands that are difficult to label with ^{125}I or for which a longer shelf life is needed because of low assay volume.

The ideal radionuclide is one that (1) has a high isotopic abundance, (2) has a high counting efficiency, (3) has a moderately long half-life, (4) can be bound to antigen easily, and (5) has a low or negligible radiation risk (Table 33-1).

Although assay sensitivity ultimately depends on the affinity of the antibody, the half-life and specific activity also have an effect on sensitivity. The shorter the half-life and the greater the specific activity, the greater the sensitivity. The greater the number of radioactive decays in a shorter period of time, the fewer molecules that can be detected and thus the greater the sensitivity. However, the half-life is limited by the fact that too short a half-life limits the useful life of the assay, and the increase in specific activity appears to be limited by the fact that there is a minimum radioisotope level below which no further increase in sensitivity occurs and the stability of the antigen or ligand is affected.

Many methods have been developed for labeling antigen with radionuclides, but it was the chloramine-T method of iodination that accelerated the advance of radiobinding assays. The method used for labeling an antigen will depend on the molecule to be labeled and the nuclide to be used.

^{3}H requires a liquid scintillation counter for detection and ^{125}I requires a sodium iodide gamma scintillation counter, although it may be counted efficiently by liquid scintillation if necessary; each requires a different labeling method.

Antigens are labeled with ^{3}H by various methods, such as the following:

1. Exchange reactions by such methods as the Wilzbach technique, which works by exchange of ^{3}H for stable hydrogen on the molecule. The method, however, does not provide uniform labeling or specific labeling sites on the molecule.
2. Chemical synthesis using simple molecules already labeled with ^{3}H.
3. Biologic synthesis, which is the production of mole-

cules by biologic systems in vivo or in vitro using ^{3}H-labeled precursors.

4. Neutron activation, which is seldom used because it is nonselective and can disrupt the molecule.

Iodination of antigen or ligands is accomplished either directly or indirectly by conjugation of a prelabeled tyrosine molecule to the antigen. ^{125}I is substituted for hydrogen into the aromatic side chain of tyrosine residues by conversion of the relatively unreactive (I^-) to the highly reactive (I^+) state. Iodine may also substitute into other amino acids, including histidine, but not as efficiently. For large protein molecules, direct labeling is usually not a problem, since they will usually contain tyrosine residues. The amount of labeling that occurs will depend on the specific activity of the iodine used and the number and location of the tyrosine residues. For molecules that do not contain a tyrosine residue, that are too small to incorporate a large iodine atom, or where direct incorporation may affect immunoreactivity, iodination may be accomplished by conjugation with a preiodinated molecule.

The following methods of iodination have been used extensively and are thoroughly described in the literature:

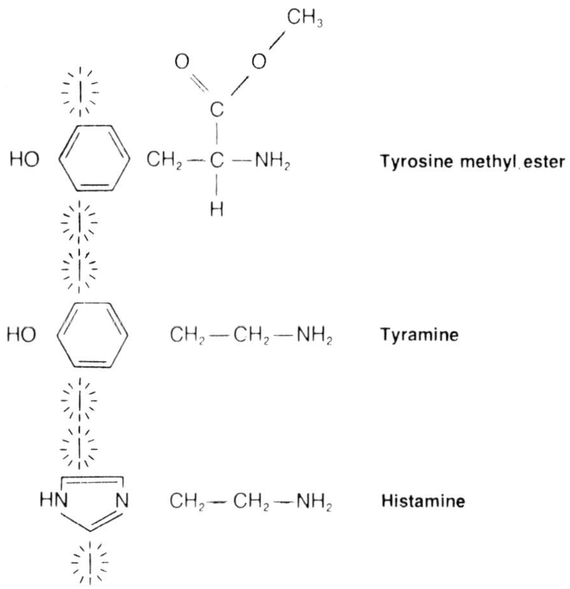

1. *Chloramine-T method.* Originally marketed as a disinfectant, chloramine-T was found to oxidize ^{125}I-labeled sodium iodide for reaction with tyrosine residues. This method is useful for iodinating peptides and proteins. The chloramine-T method is inexpensive and simple, uses commonly available reagents, is quick, avoids pH extremes, and produces minimal radiation exposure. Sometimes, however, loss of immunologic or biologic activity of the iodinated antigen may result; therefore less harsh methods may be used.
2. *Lactoperoxidase method.* This method was first reported in the literature by Marchalonis in 1969 and was developed as a less harsh alternative to the chloramine-T method. Lactoperoxidase is a high–molecular-weight protein obtained from unpasteurized bovine milk; in the presence of hydrogen peroxide it allows the iodination of proteins and peptides without loss of immunologic or biologic activity. This method produces primarily external tyrosine labeling, leaving internal tyrosine molecules free for maintenance of structural integrity.
3. *Conjugation labeling.* This procedure was developed by Bolton and Hunter in 1973 for indirect labeling by first coupling iodine to a carrier molecule and conjugating it to an antigen or hapten by a bridge (Fig. 33-6). This technique has been found to be very useful for several reasons: (a) It does not expose ligand to chemical damage; (b) it can be applied to ligands without tyrosine residues; and (c) it is a simple procedure.

   There are certain disadvantages such as the size of the labeled molecule may alter immunoreactivity and the bridge may be common to both labeling and antibody production, leading to nonspecific binding to the bridge, which cannot be displaced by unlabeled ligand.
4. Iodogen method. This method is becoming one of the most popular methods of labeling because it is simple, rapid, effective and not damaging to most molecules. The method, which has undergone some modifications since it was first described by Fraker and Spect in 1978, uses a water-insoluble compound 1,3,4,6-tetrachloro-3 alpha, 6 alpha-diphenyl glycoluril (Iodogen). The Iodogen is simply coated to the side of a glass or polyethyline tube, and protein and radioactive iodine added. After the reaction is complete, which usually takes 5 to 10 minutes, the reaction is terminated simply by removing the contents from the tube. Protein damage is minimal since it is not exposed to soluble oxidizing agents and labeling efficiency is high, usually greater than 90%. The primary amino acid to be labeled is tyrosine.

Tyrosine methyl ester: HO–(benzene ring)–CH_2–C(H)(NH_2)–C(=O)–O–CH_3

Tyramine: HO–(benzene ring)–CH_2–CH_2–NH_2

Histamine: (imidazole ring, HN, N)–CH_2–CH_2–NH_2

Fig. 33-6. Carrier molecules used for radioactive iodine coupling. (From Chard, T.: An introduction to radioimmunoassay and related techniques, New York, 1981, North Holland Publishing Co.)

■ Haptens

Haptens can be labeled by any of these methods also but usually must be labeled indirectly by conjugation of a labeled molecule. As mentioned previously, there are certain disadvantages:

1. The size of the conjugated molecule may be large compared to the hapten and thus affect immunoreactivity.
2. Because of a common bridge for labeling and antibody production, antibody may be produced that is directed to the bridge rather than to the hapten. This can be overcome by using a different bridge for each procedure (Fig. 33-7).

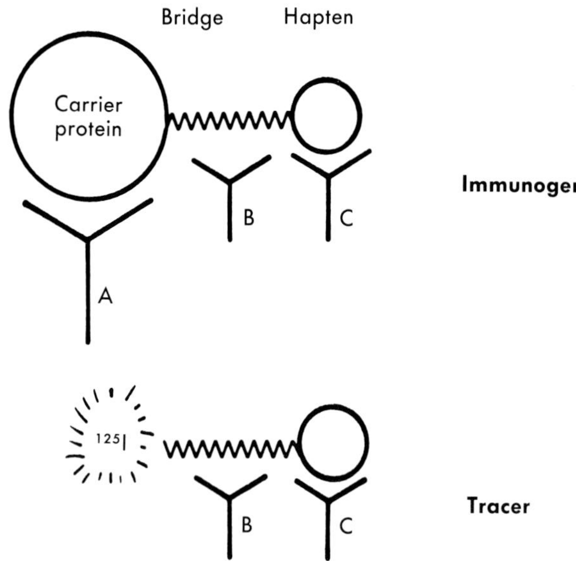

Fig. 33-7. Antibody to common bridge used for both carrier protein and radioactive iodine coupling. (From Chard, T.: An introduction to radioimmunoassay and related techniques, New York, 1981, North Holland Publishing Co.)

■ Other ligands and antibodies

Some types of assays may require other ligands such as receptors or antibodies to be labeled. However, the same labeling methods as described previously may be employed to label their substances as long as the appropriate binding sites are available on the molecule, or they may be labeled as haptens.

■ Other labeling procedures

In addition to those procedures already mentioned, there are other, less commonly used methods:

1. Iodine monochloride
2. Chlorine and hypochlorite
3. Electrolysis
4. Iodine vaporization

■ Quality assurance of labeled ligand

1. Radiochemical purity. This is performed by use of column chromatography and later by checking maximum binding and nonspecific binding (NSB).
2. Immunoreactivity. This is checked by use of excess antibody and a small amount of labeled ligand. If a significant portion of the label does not bind, it denotes nonimmunoreactivity.
3. Specific activity. This is simply a measure of the curies of radioactive isotope per unit weight of both labeled and unlabeled ligand. The degree of specific activity can affect the assay sensitivity.
4. Stability. This includes half-life, storage, chemical breakdown resulting from radioactive decay, radiation damage, and loss of immunoreactivity.

■ BINDERS

In binding assays there are three basic types of binders: antibodies, circulating binding proteins, and cell receptors. The three most important characteristics of a binder are affinity, specificity, and availability.

■ Antibodies

Antibodies are immunoglobulins produced in response to an antigen or immunogen and combine specifically with it. Serum proteins can be separated in terms of their mobility, from greatest to least, into albumin and alpha, beta, and gamma globulin. Antibodies or immunoglobulins are found among the beta and gamma globulins. The immunoglobulins consist of five distinct classes; IgG, IgM, IgA, IgD, and IgE. All the immunoglobulins have a common basic structure, but each class has its own characteristic function. For example, IgE is responsible for allergic reactions, and IgM is a primitive immunoglobulin that is the earliest of the immune responses and eventually disappears. The immunoglobulin class of greatest importance to immunoassays and the class that includes the vast majority of antibodies to bacterial and viral antigens responsible for the body's defense mechanisms is IgG. Although the immunoglobulins' basic structures are very similar, their physicochemical properties and biologic activity are quite diverse. Antibodies react with foreign substances by (1) neutralization, (2) formation of antigen-antibody complexes, (3) agglutination, (4) bacteriolysis, and (5) opsonization.

The IgG molecule is a Y-shaped structure consisting of four peptide chains linked by disulfide bonds (Fig. 33-8), two "heavy" (H) chains with a molecular weight of 55,000 to 90,000, and two "light" (L) chains with a molecular weight of 25,000. Different portions of the IgG molecule exhibit different functional activity and were originally defined on the basis of the fragments produced by enzyme digestion. Papain splits IgG into three fragments, two of which are composed of the light chains and the adjacent portion of the heavy chains, called the Fab fragments because they retain specific antigen-binding ability, and a third fragment consisting of the remaining portion of the heavy chains, called the Fc fragment because it can be crystallized. IgG may also be fragmented by pepsin, an enzyme that produces an Fc fragment and a large fragment called $F(ab)_2$, which has divalent specific antigen-binding abilities. An IgG molecule is capable of binding two antigen molecules.

Two distinct functional regions exist for each heavy and light chain: an amino (N) terminal portion called the *variable region* and the carboxy (C) terminal portion or *constant region*. The amino acid sequence heterogeneity of the variable region provides the diversity necessary for the production of highly specific antibodies. This region can virtually produce 100 million unique antibody specificities, which, in addition to binding to hydrogen bonds, hydrophobic bonds, coulombic forces, and van der Wall's forces, form three-dimensional structures that complement a spe-

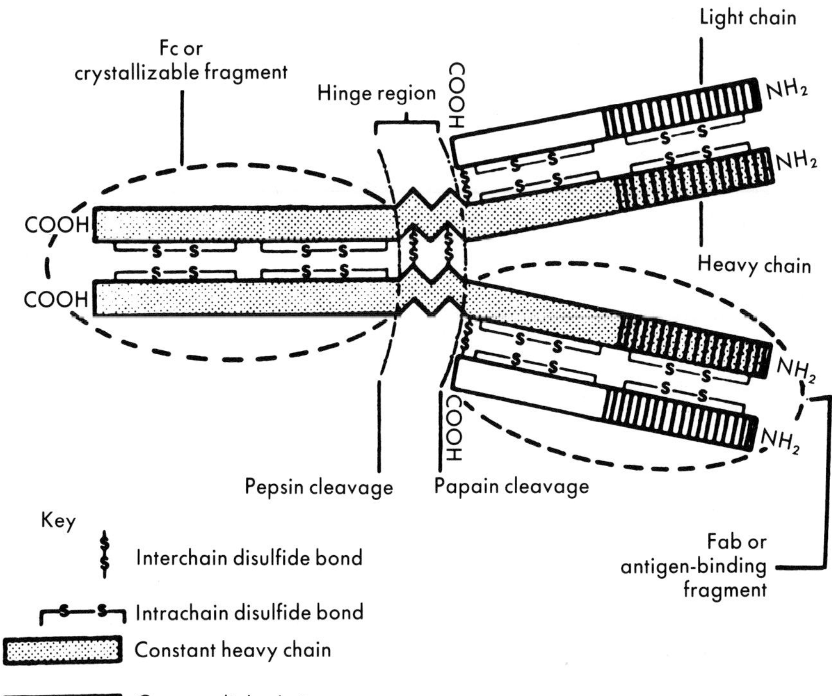

Fig. 33-8. Diagrammatic structure of an IgG molecule showing heavy and light chains and Fab and Fc fragments. (From Bowry, T.R.: Immunology simplified, New York, 1978, Oxford University Press.)

cific antigenic determinant on a vast number of antigens, much like a lock and key fit together. The carboxy or constant region of the heavy and light chains has the same amino acid sequence for all immunoglobulins in a given subclass. The constant region is responsible for complement fixation, macrophage binding, antigen aggregation, and precipitation.

Antibody production in humans is brought about by the lymphocyte population. Lymphocytes can be divided into B lymphocytes and T lymphocytes. On entering the body, antigen interacts with a macrophage and is carried to a lymph node. The antigen interacts with T lymphocytes, which differentiate into memory cells and control celis (helpers and suppressors) and regulate antibody production. T lymphocytes are long-lived and are responsible for future antibody production. B lymphocytes are found in the peripheral blood and lymph nodes and in the presence of a macrophage-antigen complex differentiate and proliferate into plasma cell clones that produce specific antibody. Antigens contain many antigenic determinants that stimulate antibody-producing clones, giving rise to a variety of antibodies with varying specificities and affinities.

■ Polyclonal antibody production

Polyclonal antibodies are produced in response to a variety of antigenic determinants on a immunogen injected into an animal. Each antigenic determinant produces an antibody with its own affinity and specificity that forms a mixture of antibodies to the same antigen, also called *antiserum*. Useful antisera are generally achieved by injection of an immunogen into a host animal with subsequent purification of specific immunoglobulins from blood. To produce specific antisera certain details must be followed as closely as possible (Fig. 33-9):

1. The immunogen must be as pure as possible for the production of highly specific antisera. If the immunogen is a hapten, care must be taken that the antibody is not produced to the bridge between the hapten and protein conjugate, especially if the same bridge is also used for labeling.
2. Small amounts (micrograms to milligrams) of immunogen, with regular intervals of booster shots, should be used.
3. Immunogen should be injected in complete Freund's adjuvant, a mixture of mycobacteria, mineral, and emulsifier that enhances the immune response and allows for slow absorption into the system.
4. A variety of routes of administration have been used, but one of the most satisfactory has been multisite intradermal injections; however, subcutaneous injections are generally used.
5. A variety of host animals, such as rabbits, sheep, goats, and guinea pigs, have also been used. The selection of host animals depends on three things:
   a. Volume of antisera needed
   b. Foreignness of immunogen to host animals
   c. Available animal facilities
6. Booster injections are given every 6 to 8 weeks with testing of blood 1 to 2 weeks after the booster shots

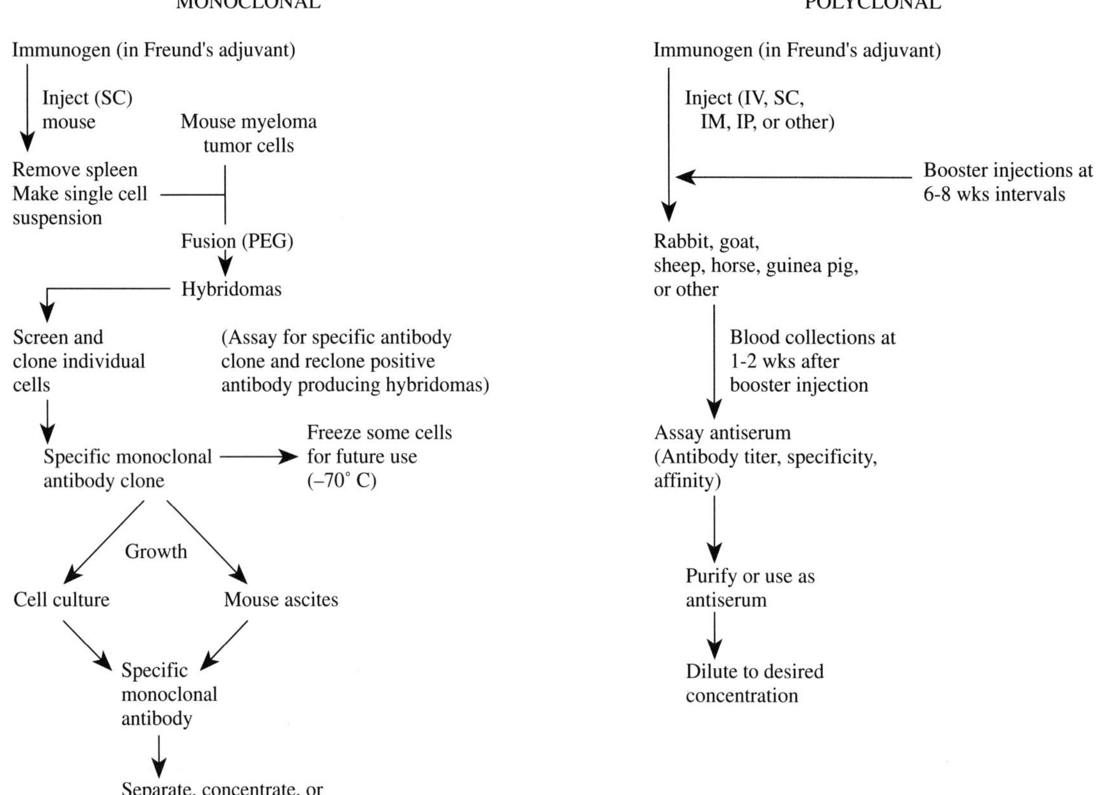

Fig. 33-9. Flow chart for production of monoclonal and polyclonal antibody.

for titer, specificity, and affinity. Maximum specificity and general affinity will be reached at 6 to 8 months.

7. Many animals must be injected, since each animal will respond differently. It may take several animals to get one animal producing useful antibody.
8. Antisera must be purified by absorption with BSA to remove carrier protein antibody and affinity chromatography for specific separation of antigen-specific antibody.

■ Monoclonal antibody production

Monoclonal antibody production, also known as the *hybridoma technique,* was developed by Kohler and Milstein in 1975. Using this technique clones can be grown producing a single antibody that is specific for only one antigenic determinant.

Monoclonal antibodies are produced as follows (Fig. 33-9):

1. A mouse is injected with the immunogen.
2. After a period of time B lymphocytes are isolated from the mouse spleen and fused with myeloma cells by use of an appropriate medium.
3. The secretions from different cell fusions are tested for specificity and affinity.
4. The cell fusion or hybridoma secreting the best antibody is then grown or cloned in a growth medium or as ascites in mice.
5. Antibody is extracted from the fluid in which the hybridoma is growing.
6. Using this technique a continuous, adequate supply of a single antibody is assured for a long time.

■ Antibody assessment

Titer. Titer is the dilution of antiserum binding a predetermined percentage of tracer, usually equal to the concentration to be used in the assay, and usually that which will bind 50% (30% to 70%) of it. This is most conveniently done by incubating serial dilution of antibody or antiserum with a fixed amount of tracer and plotting percent bound against dilution. That dilution giving 50% bound is the antibody titer. The higher the titer, the greater the number of assays that can be performed. Titer is proportional to the product of antibody concentration and the affinity constant of the antiserum.

Affinity. Affinity is a measure of the force of attraction of antigen to antibody or a measure of antigen-antibody binding energy. Sensitivity is closely related to affinity, or K_a value, of the antibody. The higher the K_a value, the greater the sensitivity of the antibody and the more rapid the attainment of equilibrium, since it is also related to a fast association constant, as described earlier. The equation is:

$$\text{Ag} + \text{Ab} \underset{K_2}{\overset{K_1}{\rightleftarrows}} \text{AgAb}$$

where:

K_1 = Association constant
K_2 = Dissociation constant

and

$$\frac{K_1}{K_2} = K_a$$

where:

K_a = Affinity or equilibrium constant

Related to this is *avidity,* which is a measure of the strength of the bound antigen-antibody. The greater the avidity, the greater the concentration of the antigen-antibody complex formed and the smaller the dissociation constant.

Affinity, or K value, can be determined by the use of a Scatchard plot, which will also give a determination of concentration of binding sites and antibody as well as heterogeneity of antiserum. This type of plot will be discussed in another section in greater detail.

Specificity. Specificity is the primary criterion for the selection of an antibody. Without a highly specific antiserum or antibody a high titer or affinity is of no value. Specificity is defined as the degree to which an antiserum or antibody will react with the substance to be assayed and only that substance. Inversely, it can be defined as the degree of interaction or cross-reactivity with other substances that are closely related or structurally similar to the substance in question. Usually the interaction energies with cross-reacting substances are much lower than the original antigen and thus, although there is some interaction, may be insignificant. Occasionally molecules of different substances may have portions in common that would give rise to a common antibody—thus 100% cross-reactivity for all related substances, such as the alpha chains of luteinizing hormone (LH), follicle-stimulating hormone (FSH), thyroid-stimulating hormone (TSH), and human chorionic gonadotropin (HCG). Antibody directed to the alpha chain of one of these hormones would be useless for its detection when used in the presence of any of the other hormones. Therefore to develop a highly specific assay, specific antibody must be produced to a portion of the molecule that is unique for that substance, such as the beta chain of HCG.

Specificity testing is usually performed comparing serial dilutions of the original antigen to related substances using the same antibody and plotted on a dose-response curve. All substances are usually compared at 50% displacement, and a ratio or percentage of the concentration of the original substance to the concentration of related substances is calculated. This then would give the percent cross-reactivity for each related substance:

$$\frac{\text{Concentration of antigen at 50\% displacement}}{\text{Concentration of cross-reacting substance at 50\% displacement of antigen}} \times 100 = \%\ \text{cross-reactivity}$$

■ Circulating binding proteins

Steroid and thyroid hormones are associated with specific binding proteins in the circulation. Ekins and Murphy both took advantage of this fact and the availability of proteins for use in assays for thyroid hormones, cortisol, estrogens, androgens, progesterone, etc. These CPBs were more widely used for many years but have now mostly been replaced by RIAs because of certain disadvantages with binding proteins such as (1) low affinity constants, thus less sensitivity; (2) poor specificity; (3) temperature dependency; and (4) a high concentration of binder needed because of low affinity constant.

■ Cell receptors

The effects of many protein hormones are exerted by first coupling to specific receptor sites on cell membranes. This fact has been taken advantage of in the development of an assay method using isolated cell membrane receptor sites as the specific binder. These assays are called radioreceptor assays (RRA), and their principal advantage is that the receptor actually measures biologic activity, whereas immunoassays measure immunologic activity. Cell receptors usually have high affinity constants and therefore give rise to very sensitive assays. However, there are certain technical problems associated with receptors:

1. They are derived from diverse tissue and not completely solubilized.
2. They are present in low concentrations.
3. They are unstable.
4. They are easily damaged.

■ BINDING ASSAY METHODS

As described earlier, the basic reaction of all binding assays is similar, but by applying small modifications to this, several different types of binding assays can be achieved, leading to improved speed, efficiency, precision, sensitivity, accuracy, specificity, etc. The reactants needed in binding assays are binder, standard or unknown ligand and a labeled material, in most cases labeled ligand, but possibly also labeled antibody. In addition to this, there must be some method of separating bound ligand from free ligand. Although not mentioned previously, the separating method is a very important part of the binding assay and may actually have an effect on the final result. In addition, some method of data reduction and quality control must be employed. The general method of CPBs or RIAs will be dis-

Table 33-2. Typical RIA procedure

			Standard dilution							**Controls**			**Unknown patient samples**					
	Total	**NSB**	**A**	**B1**	**C2**	**D4**	**E8**	**F16**	**G32**	**I**	**II**	**III**	**1**	**2**	**3**	**4**	**5**	**6**
Tube no.	1	3	5	7	9	11	13	15	17	19	21	23	25	27	29	31	33	35
	2	4	6	8	10	12	14	16	18	20	22	24	26	28	30	32	34	36
Buffer (μl)	—	200	100	—	—	—	—	—	—	—	—	—	—	—	—	—	—	—
Standard (μl)	—	—	—	100	100	100	100	100	100	—	—	—	—	—	—	—	—	—
Controls (μl)	—	—	—	—	—	—	—	—	—	100	100	100	—	—	—	—	—	—
Unknown (μl)	—	—	—	—	—	—	—	—	—	—	—	—	100	100	100	100	100	100
Labeled Ag (μl)	100	100	100	100	100	100	100	100	100	100	100	100	100	100	100	100	100	100
Antibody (μl)*	—	—	100	100	100	100	100	100	100	100	100	100	100	100	100	100	100	100
Vortex and incubate																		
Separating reagents (μl)	—	500	500	500	500	500	500	500	500	500	500	500	500	500	500	500	500	500
†Vortex, centrifuge, decant supernate, and count																		

*For antibody-coated tube assay, skip to last step after appropriate incubation and no centrifuging.
†Some assays may require a second incubation before centrifuging.

cussed through data reduction before considering other modified methods, since this is the basic method from which the others were derived.

■ Competitive protein-binding assays and radioimmunoassays

CPBs and RIAs are being considered together because of their similarity. CPB reagents are a ligand or analyte, labeled ligand, and specific binding protein. RIA reagents are an antigen or analyte, labeled antigen, and a specific antibody, which is usually more specific and sensitive than binding proteins. These assays are based on two general reactions.

$$L + B \overset{K_a}{\rightleftarrows} L\,B$$

$$L^* + B \overset{K_a^*}{\rightleftarrows} L^*\,B$$

where:

L = Ligand or analyte or antigen
L* = Labeled ligand or antigen
B = Specific protein binder or antibody
LB and L*B = Bound forms of reactants

Combining these reactions to form the competitive assay reaction:

CPB:

$$\begin{matrix} L \\ \\ L^* \end{matrix} + B \overset{K_a}{\rightleftarrows} \begin{matrix} L\,B \\ + \\ L^*\,B \end{matrix}$$

RIA:

$$\begin{matrix} Ag \\ \\ Ag^* \end{matrix} + Ab \overset{K_a}{\rightleftarrows} \begin{matrix} Ag\,Ab \\ + \\ Ag^*\,Ab \end{matrix}$$

Based on these reactions the ideal competitive radioassay (CPB) and RIA) should have the following criteria:

1. Both nonradioactive and radioactive ligands or antigens should be chemically and immunologically indistinguishable.
2. Both reactions go to completion: $K_a = K_a^* = \infty$
3. Antigen and antibody binding sites react in a one-to-one ratio.
4. The antibody is specific for a single antigen. Only the preceding reactions occur.
5. There is an excess of antigen over antibody (L + L* or Ag + Ag*).
6. The antibody binding sites are independent of one another.

The purpose of binding assays is to determine the concentration of antigen or analyte in patient's serum or plasma or other body fluids. To perform this function a dose-response curve must be constructed using serial dilutions of known concentrations of ligand or antigen, called *standard*. This then is known as a standard curve and is used to determine patient analyte concentration. The performance of RIA or CPB procedures involves the addition of the three reactants in a single tube for each standard and unknown (Table 33-2). The labeled ligand or antigen and antibody volumes remain constant in all tubes, and the only variable is the standard or unknown (Fig. 33-10). In the

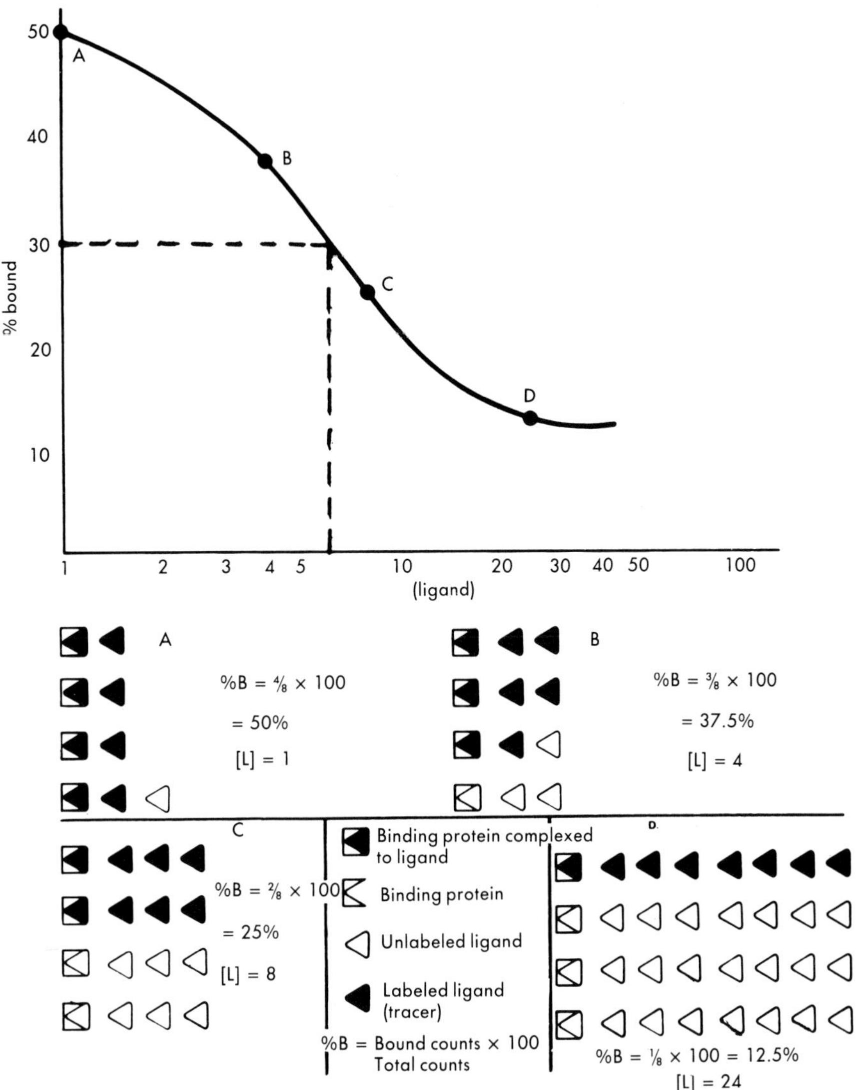

Fig. 33-10. Representation of the generation of a typical standard curve showing serial dilution of standards and relationships of bound to free fractions. Dotted line demonstrates how a patient result is determined from a standard curve. The patient response is found on the Y-axis and the result read on the X-axis. (From Travis, J.C.: Fundamentals of RIA and other ligand assays, Anaheim, Calif., 1979, Sci. Newsletter, Inc.)

general RIA or CPB procedure the unlabeled ligand (standard and analyte in patient sample) competes for binding sites on the antibody or binding protein with the labeled ligand or antigen. The reaction proceeds until equilibrium is reached, that is, until the number of antigen-antibody complexes being formed is equal to the number of complexes being dissociated. The time for equilibrium to be reached depends on the *affinity constant,* also called the *equilibrium constant*. The affinity constants for binding assays, especially for antibody-antigen complexes are extremely high (ranging from 10^7 to 10^8 and 10^9 to 10^{12} liters/mole for CPB and RIA, respectively); thus the antigen-antibody complex formation is favored even though the reaction is reversible.

The antibody in the RIA (or CPB) reaction is unable to distinguish between labeled and unlabeled antigen, both having the same binding affinity. According to the law of mass action, the greater the concentration of antigen (labeled and unlabeled) present, the more antibody binding sites that will be occupied. Since the only variable is the concentration of unlabeled antigen or analyte, the amount of labeled antigen complexed with antibody will depend on the increasing concentrations of unlabeled antigen. Simply put, in the absence of unlabeled antigen, there will be a specific and maximum amount of labeled antigen complexed to antibody. As the concentration of unlabeled antigen is increased, more and more labeled antigen complexed to antibody is displaced. Since the antibody-antigen complex on the right-hand side of the equation, called the *bound fraction,* is usually counted and as the unlabeled antigen increases, the labeled antigen-antibody complex decreases, the radioactivity counts in the bound fraction are inversely related to the unlabeled antigen concentration (Fig. 33-10). To count the bound fraction it must be separated from the unbound or free fraction (labeled and unlabeled antigen) or the left-hand side of the equation. There are various methods for performing this separation, but the two basic means of separation are either by adding a substance that will separate bound from free fractions (called *liquid phase*) or by having the antibody already complexed to a separating system, therefore not requiring the addition of the separating substance *(solid phase).*

By plotting counts (or percent bound or one of several other calculations based on counts) versus increasing concentrations of known antigen, a standard curve can be constructed so that when comparing the unknown counts to the curve, the concentration of antigen or analyte in the unknown sample can be calculated (Fig. 33-10).

In addition to the standard and unknown sample tubes, other samples must be included in the performance of an RIA:

total activity tubes Tubes containing only the total activity representative of the total activity used in each assay tube.

nonspecific binding (NSB) tubes Tubes containing all reagents present in sample tubes except antibody and used to determine binding not resulting from specific antigen-antibody reaction. Also called *assay blank tubes* or *background,* if no NSB.

maximum binding (Bo) tubes Tubes containing all reagents present in standard tubes except standard. Also called *zero standard concentration tubes.*

controls Tubes containing known amounts of antigen and handled as an unknown in the assay. Used to determine precision and/or accuracy of the assay.

So far one general RIA type has been considered using two different separating methods, which will be considered in greater detail in the next section. However, there are three general RIA types that should be mentioned before continuing. These methods are also referred to as *limited-reagent methods* because the binder is present in limited quantity.

1. Equilibrium assays. This is the type of assay previously discussed and is the most common type of RIA. It is the simultaneous incubation of unlabeled and labeled antigen and antibody.
   a. Indirect liquid phase, so named because of the inverse relationship of unlabeled antigen to labeled antibody-antigen complex and the separate addition of the separating substance. Applies to other types of RIAs also.
   b. Indirect solid phase, which is similar to the previous method except antibody is prelinked to a solid separating system, not requiring the separate addition of a separating substance. Also applies to other types of RIAs.
2. Displacement assays. Labeled antigen is allowed to first complex with antibody. Unlabeled antigen is then added to the complex, displacing the labeled antigen.
3. Sequential assay. Unlabeled antigen or analyte is allowed to react with an excess of antibody, after which labeled antigen is added, binding to the remaining antibody binding sites. This method allows for increased sensitivity in some assays, especially those with low-affinity constants, but reduces the effective concentration range.

■ Immunoradiometric assays (IRMA)

The conventional IRMA can be represented by the following reaction:

$$\text{(Free) Ag} + \text{Ab}^* \underset{K_2}{\overset{K_1}{\rightleftarrows}} \text{Ag Ab}^* \text{ (Bound)}$$

As can be seen, this reaction is similar to the RIA reaction but differs in several aspects: (1) antibody is labeled instead of antigen, (2) antibody is used in excess, (3) there is no competition for binding sites, (4) free antibody is separated from bound antibody (not antigen), and (5) counts are directly related to antigen concentration. Bound complex is separated from free labeled antibody by binding free antibody to an excess of immobilized antigen (antigen bound to a solid support system). For this reason this method is also referred to as the *excess reagent method;* it is performed as follows:

1. Add excess labeled specific antibody to microliter amounts of antigen (unknown sample or standard).
2. Incubate to equilibrium.
3. Separate free labeled antibody from bound complex by adding excess antigen linked to solid phase support.
4. Determine radioactivity counts in the supernate that contains the bound complex and relates directly to antigen concentration.

The technique significantly shortens the incubation or equilibrium time because of the addition of excess antibody, allows for less precision of pipetting antibody, and is potentially more sensitive. Whereas in the RIA methodology sensitivity is ultimately dependent on the antibody affinity constant, in the IRMA methodology sensitivity is only limited by the specific activity of the label. This potentially makes IRMA procedures more sensitive than RIA, but at present in most cases this has not been realized because of limitations on labeling, precision, NSB, etc.

A modification of this method is the two-site and three-site sandwich IRMA. These techniques are becoming more and more popular primarily because of their increased specificity, sensitivity, speed, and simplicity. In the two-site

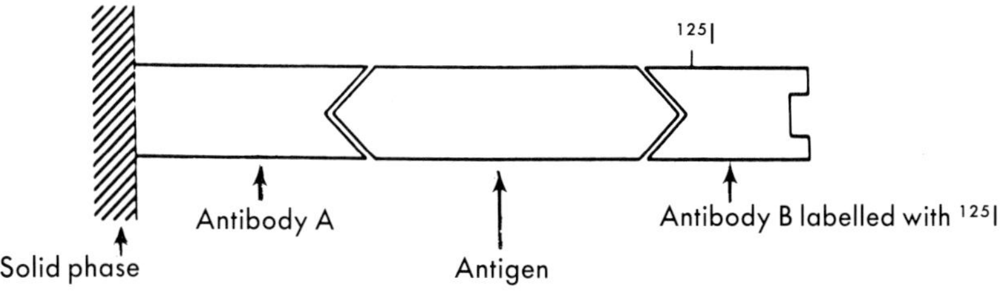

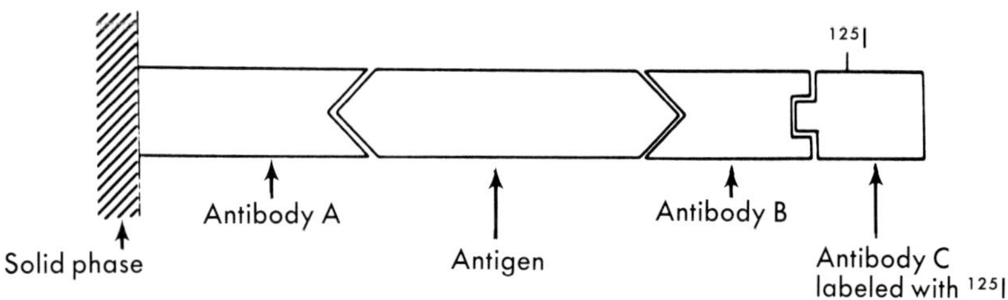

Fig. 33-11. Diagrammatic representation of a two- and three-site immunoradiometric assay (IRMA). (From Al-Shawi, A., and others: Ligand Q. 4(4):43-51, 1981.)

IRMA excess, solid phase specific antibody and free labeled antibody are incubated with antigen. After equilibrium is attained, the free labeled antibody is separated and the bound complex is counted (Ab-Ag-Ab*) (Fig. 33-11). Many antigens have several binding sites for the same antibody, and therefore the two antibodies used in this method may be the same or two different populations of antibody with different specific binding sites. This provides increased specificity, since two specific antibodies are bound to the same antigen instead of one, as in the RIA method. If the two antibodies used are the same, separate antibody incubations are necessary, with separation of the free antigen before the second antibody addition. This is finding increased use for antigens with two chains or monomers that by themselves are not specific, but when combined as the dimer become a specific molecule. These molecules are difficult to produce antibody to, since both chains or monomers must be detected to attain a specific assay. An example of this is the enzyme CK-MB, where the M monomer and/or the B monomer are common to CK-MM and CK-BB; therefore antibody to the M or the B monomer would still be nonspecific. However, by producing specific antibody to the M and B monomer and using a two-site IRMA with one antibody linked to a solid phase and the other labeled, a highly specific assay can be produced.

The advantages of the two-site IRMA over the conventional IRMA are that large amounts of antigen are not required and specificity is improved. The three-site IRMA is essentially similar to the two-site method except that the third antibody is labeled instead of the second. This allows the use of a nonspecific anti-IgG molecule for the third antibody, which can be universally applied to almost all IRMAs (Fig. 33-11). The advantages of the three-site IRMA are the same as for the two-site assay.

■ Receptor assays

In addition to specific antibody and circulating binding proteins, specific cellular receptor sites may be used as the sources of binding material. The interest in this type of assay is based on the belief that the biologic interaction is more specific than the immunologic interaction and that interaction of receptor and hormone is more relevant to clinical problems. However, receptor assays are slow, more technically demanding, and less specific and the binders are unstable. In spite of these shortcomings, estrogen and progesterone receptor assays have gained great popularity in the detection of breast cancers.

A comparison of the various binding assay techniques can be seen in Table 33-3.

■ SEPARATION METHODS

The purpose of a separation method is to isolate the bound fraction from the free fraction in an RIA procedure so that one or each fraction can be counted without interference from the other. The ideal separation procedure should be (1) clean (complete separation of bound and free fractions), (2) uninfluenced by serum or other nonspecific substances, (3) reproducible, (4) technically simple, (5) rapid, (6) inexpensive, and (7) not interfering with the antigen-antibody reaction.

None of the separation methods available today are entirely satisfactory, but each has its advantages and disad-

Table 33-3. Comparison of CPBs, radioreceptor assays, and RIAs*

			RIA	
Property	**CPB binding protein**	**RRA tissue receptor**	**Polyclonal antibody**	**Monoclonal antibody**
Specificity	High	Very high	Very high	Potentially highest
Relationship to biologic activity	High	Very high	Variable	
Reproducible source of binder	High	High	Variable	Very high
Stability on storage	Stable	Variable	Very stable	
Titer	Low	Low	Very high	
Preparation	Simple dilution of plasma	Cell fractionation	Immunization	Hybridoma production

*Using both polyclonal and monoclonal antibodies. (From Bio-Educational Publications Slide/Seminar Education Programs: Radioimmunoassay, vol. 2, Rochester, N.Y., 1982, Bio-Educational Publications.)

vantages. The resultant components of a separation method can be divided into three parts: free fraction, bound fraction, and NSB fraction. In all separation methods some part of the free fraction will be separated with the NSB fraction. This can be a problem in some assay systems and data-reduction methods, especially if there are inconsistent NSB fractions between standards and patient samples. Therefore NSB must be calculated and corrected for in many assays. NSB can be caused by various situations:

1. Entrapment of free fraction in precipitate
2. Labeled contaminants precipitated
3. Adsorption of tracer on tube surface
4. Poor separating technique
5. Incomplete separation of bound from free fractions

There are large numbers of separation methods in use today because of these problems. The earliest methods included electrophoresis and chromatography, which are not generally used today because they are so labor intensive. The following are the most popular methods in use today.

■ Nonspecific adsorption of antigen

The primary substance used in nonspecific adsorption of antigen is charcoal and dextran-coated charcoal. This method was very popular in the early development of RIA and is still popular for certain assays. Separation is achieved by adsorption of the free fraction and, after centrifugation of the charcoal-free fraction (pellet), the decanting and counting of the bound fraction (supernate). This method is useful for small antigen molecules where there is a large charge difference.

Several other adsorbents have been used successfully by this method, for example, resins, talcs, silicas, hydroxyapatite, and fluorouracil.

The advantages are that this method is (1) reproducible, (2) rapid, and (3) inexpensive. The disadvantages are that (1) it is affected by varying protein concentrations, (2) it may cause "stripping" of bound antigen from antibody, (3) it is time-dependent, (4) it is temperature-dependent, and (5) it is pH- and ionic-strength–dependent.

■ Nonspecific precipitation of antigen-antibody complexes

Neutral salts and organic solvents have been useful in a few RIA procedures for separation of free from bound fractions. Some common substances used are ethanol, polyethylene glycol (PEG), and ammonium sulfate. These substances function by causing precipitation of the antigen-antibody complex; ethanol precipitates large molecular weight proteins (Ab); PEG and ammonium sulfate precipitate by binding the water making the bound complex insoluble.

The advantages are that this method is (1) simple, (2) inexpensive, (3) rapid, and (4) reproducible. The disadvantages are that (1) it is nonspecific (coprecipitation of free fraction), (2) it gives incomplete removal of bound fraction, (3) it is pH-dependent, (4) it is time-dependent, (5) it is temperature-dependent, (6) it is protein-concentration–dependent, (7) it is salt- or solvent-concentration–dependent, and (8) it gives a high NSB.

■ Immunoprecipitation of antigen-antibody complex (double antibody)

Immunoprecipitation has proved to be the most useful and sensitive method. In this method a second antibody to the primary antibody is produced by immunizing a different host animal with the primary antibody and purifying the second antibody. The binding of the second antibody to the first antibody forms an insoluble immune complex of the bound fraction:

$$\begin{matrix} Ag\ Ab_1 \\ Ag^*\ Ab_1 \end{matrix} + Ab_2 \rightarrow \begin{matrix} Ag\ Ab_1\ Ab_2 \\ + \\ Ag^*\ Ab_1\ Ab_2 \end{matrix}$$

The advantages of this method are that it is (1) specific, (2) clean, (3) not interfering with the primary reaction, and

Table 33-4. Various parameters used to graph radioassay standard curves

X-axis (dose)	Y-axis (response)						
P	B/F		F/B		1/F		F
Log P	B/T		T/B		B		1/B
Log P	T/F		F/T		log 1/F		log F
1/P	log B/F	or	log F/B	or	log B	or	log 1/B
P_n	log B/T		log T/B		log %B		%F
	log T/F, counts		log F/T, 1/counts		$\%B/B_0$		

KEY: P, Ligand or antigen concentration; B, bound counts; F, free counts; T, total counts; % B = B/T × 100; B_0 = zero standard counts or maximum binding.

(4) time- and temperature-independent. The disadvantages are (1) the second long incubation and (2) the fact that it may be protein-dependent.

This method can be made more rapid by combining with PEG; this solves two problems—shortening the second incubation time to a few minutes and eliminating the high-NSB problem with PEG alone.

■ Solid-phase adsorption of antigen

In solid-phase adsorption, antibody is previously bound to a solid surface such as plastic or glass (coated tubes and beads are examples of this). The assay is performed simply by adding labeled and unlabeled antigen to the antibody-coated surface, incubating, decanting or washing, and counting for bound complex. The important consideration is to bind the antibody to the surface so that it does not interfere with the reaction.

The advantages are that this is (1) simple, (2) rapid, (3) irreversible, (4) less technically difficult, and (5) associated with minimal NSB. The disadvantages are (1) the large amounts of antibody necessary, (2) the complex preparation of tubes, and (3) the slower reaction rates (and lessened sensitivity). Modifications of this method have given rise to such methods as double antibody solid phase (DASP) and magnetizable antibody-coated particles.

■ Protein A

A method that has not gained much popularity but is useful for RIAs is protein A. This is a cell wall constituent of *Staphylococcus aureus,* which binds IgG specifically. Protein A is as sensitive as DASP, is rapid, and only requires centrifugation.

■ DATA REDUCTION

This section deals with the most common methods of data reduction. The reader is encouraged to read more on the subject, since with the increased use and capacities of the computer it is becoming more important to know what method to use.

After the binding assay has reached equilibrium and bound and free fractions are separated by an appropriate method, the next step is to decide whether one fraction or both should be counted and how the results should be plotted to arrive at the correct result. The response (counts or various calculations from the counts) is usually plotted on the Y-axis, and the ligand dose for each standard is usually plotted on the X-axis. Some examples of how each parameter may be plotted are shown in Table 33-4. If the dose on the X-axis is plotted against the response on the Y-axis from columns 1 and 3 in Table 33-4, an inverse curve will result. If columns 2 and 4 are plotted, a direct relationship or curve will result. Each curve has its own characteristics, and no one curve may be entirely useful for all binding assay data. A few examples of the various curves possible are shown in Fig. 33-12.

Some data-reduction methods can be performed easily by manual means, but others are impossible without the aid of a computer. The use of the computer in data reduction has many advantages, such as speed, improved accuracy and precision, elimination of calculation and transcription errors, additional quality-control data, less technologist time, and elimination of curve variation in manual plotting. The only possible disadvantages of the computer might be the hardware expense and required programming. However, the computer can provide information on the standard curve and unknowns that was previously almost impossible to acquire manually, such as the following:

Standard curve:

1. Curve statistics such as slope, intercepts, and correlation coefficients
2. Precision of replicates and 95% confidence limits
3. Rejection of erroneous data points during curve fitting
4. Storage and comparison with previous curves of quality control data such as slope, intercepts, and correlation coefficients

Unknowns:

1. The result
2. Precision of replicates and 95% confidence limits
3. Interassay and intrassay coefficients of variations
4. Tests for parallelism
5. Miscellaneous calculations

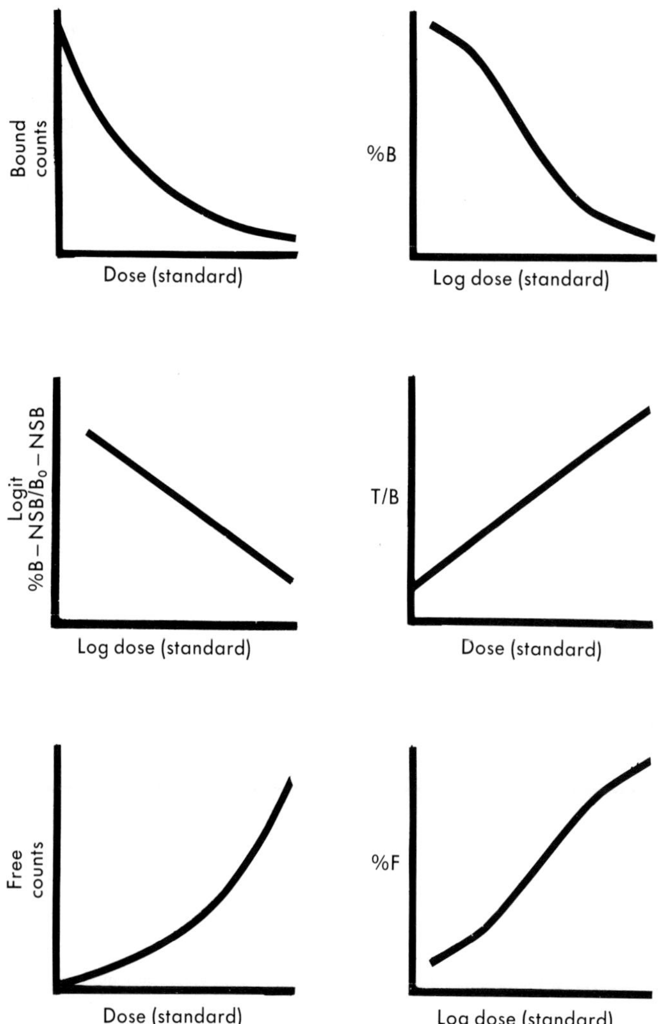

Fig. 33-12. Representation of several possible standard curves using different dose and response variables.

■ Hyperbolic curve fit

Data reduction via hyperbolic curve fit is the simplest procedure and can be plotted manually or by computer. For this type of curve the dose (standard concentrations) is plotted on a linear scale (X-axis) versus the response (counts, %B/T, %B/B_0, etc.) plotted on a linear scale (Y-axis) (Fig. 33-12). The response may be calculated as follows:

$$\%B/T = \frac{\text{Bound counts} - \text{NSB counts}}{\text{Total counts}} \times 100$$

$$\%B/B_0 = \frac{\text{Bound counts} - \text{NSB counts}}{\text{Zero standard counts} - \text{NSB counts}} \times 100$$

where:

NSB = Nonspecific binding (this may or may not be subtracted in the calculation)

This curve may be drawn in two ways: a linear interpolation, which is a point-to-point linear plot, or a polygonal interpolation, which is a best fit curve through all points.

The main advantages of this method are that it is simple, and rapid and does not require a computer. The disadvantages of this plot are that it is easy to make calculations and/or transcription errors and very little quality control data are available on the curve. There is greater error when using the linear interpolation, since the linearization of the curve between points further increases the error from the true curve between points.

■ Sigmoidal curve fit

Sigmoidal curve fit plots the response (counts, B/T, B/B_0, etc.) on the Y-axis versus the logarithm of the dose (standard antigen concentration) on the X-axis and results in a straightening of the hyperbolic curve. The resulting curve is sigmoidal or S-shaped (Fig. 33-12).

The advantages of this method are similar to those of the previous curve except that it is easier to draw a best fit curve, since the central portion of the curve is nearly linear, and the interpretation of results is more accurately determined. The disadvantage for manual plotting are calculation and transcription errors. In addition, the log scale does not begin at zero antigen concentration, and therefore zero binding information is not available on the curve.

The reciprocal of the response variable used in the hyperbolic or sigmoidal curve fit plotted on the X-axis versus the linear dose (antigen concentration) on the Y-axis will yield a direct, straight-line relationship between the dose concentration and the inverse response (T/B, B_0/B, etc.) (Fig. 33-12).

This method is simple, rapid, and nearly linear but should only be used for certain RIA procedures. It has a limited range of linearity, and small changes in the response variable may have large effects on the reciprocal.

■ Logit-log curve fit

The logit-log curve fit method of data reduction is probably the most popular curve-fitting model in use today, both manually and by computer. First introduced by Rodbard in 1970, it has since been widely applied because of the ability to linearize the hyperbolic and sigmoidal standard curves and thereby eliminate the subjectivity of drawing a standard curve. In this model the response is plotted as the logit of B/B_0 on the Y-axis, but NSB must be corrected for as follows:

$$\text{Logit } B/B_0 = \text{Log}_e \left[\frac{\left(\dfrac{B - NSB}{B_0 - NSB}\right)}{\left(1 - \dfrac{B - NSB}{B_0 - NSB}\right)} \right]$$

versus the log of the dose or antigen concentration on the X-axis. The resulting dose-response curve is a straight line fitted by linear regression analysis. This calculation is too difficult to be handled manually and is computerized. Logit-log plots are performed quite frequently, however, by the use of logit-log graph paper and a simple calculation for the logit scale as a percent B/B_0 (Fig. 33-12).

$$\% \text{ Response} = \frac{B - NSB}{B_0 - NSB} \times 100$$

This method has several advantages, such as the facts that it is linear and simple, it can be plotted both manually and by computer, it can be applied to a large number of binding assays, and it provides good quality control data (slope, intercept, correlation coefficient, etc). Although at first this seems like the perfect solution to the data reduction problems, there are certain serious disadvantages that are often overlooked:

1. All response values must be corrected for the assay blank value (NSB) before the logit is calculated; otherwise it will yield a nonlinear response.
2. The upper and lower 10% of a standard curve should be eliminated, since this portion of the curve is frequently nonlinear in logit transformation and should not be used for the calculation of results.
3. In some RIA systems the logit transformation does not yield a straight line, probably because of the heterogeneity of the antiserum. Actually most RIA data are not linear on logit-log plots but slightly S curved, and the assumption of linearity can introduce increased errors in parts of the curve.
4. At different parts of the response, variable precision occurs, referred to as heteroscedasticity, and best-fit linearization can occur only after weighting. This requires the calculation of the standard deviation (SD) for each response; if this indicates a large scatter, the reciprocal of SD^2 (the variance) is used as the weighting factor in the linear regression. The technique requires the use of a computer.
5. It does not linearize some sequential RIAs.

■ Spline function curve fit

The spline function or cubic spline function curve fit is a computerized version of the French curve that describes any given point on the curve by a cubic polynomial. By dividing the curve into sections and performing computation, a smooth curve is constructed that is not forced through the standard points. This method provides a good fit for irregular curves without transformation of the response and good uniformity of variance throughout the curve. Although not very popular in this country, it is used extensively in Europe. This method has some disadvantages, however, one of which is uncertainty as to how many points are necessary and where they should be to arrive at a best-fit curve. Other disadvantages include lack of some quality-control data and the effect of outlying points on the spline function between standard points.

■ Four-parameter logistic curve fit

The four-parameter logistic curve fit method of data reduction is more versatile than the two-parameter logit-log method. To describe the dose response curve by this model, four curve parameters are necessary:

$$y = \frac{a - d}{1 + (x/c)^b} - d$$

where:

y = Response
x = Dose or antigen concentration
a = Response when $\times = 0$
b = Slope (-1 times slope of logit-log plot)
c = 50% intercept
d = Predicted response at infinit of labeled antigen concentration ($\approx$NSB)

To achieve the best possible fit the B_0 and NSB are computer adjusted throughout the standard curve. The advantages of this method are a more natural curve fit, wide applicability to most binding assays, and calculation of a 50%

intercept, which is useful for quality control and calculating cross-reactivity. The four-parameter logistic model, however, requires the curve to be symmetric about the midpoint, which may fail for certain curves, usually requires weighting, and requires more computer memory.

• • •

There are other methods of data reduction that may be applied to binding assays; however, the methods described here are those most widely used. These methods can be applied to most binding assays.

■ PATIENT SAMPLES

Patient samples are handled and calculated similarly to the standard in the binding assay procedures (occasionally patient samples require preextractions). The dose of the patient sample is determined by comparing the patient response to the standard curve (Fig. 33-10). Patient samples may be serum, plasma, urine, cerebral spinal fluid, etc. The exact nature of the sample and whether a preextraction is needed depend on the requirements of the binding assay.

Care must be taken in accepting the proper specimens for testing, since certain problems may affect the binding assay. The following are the criteria that should be followed for rejecting specimens:

1. If specimens are from unidentified patients, are improperly labeled or do not come from the correct patient. The data on the tube label and the data on the voucher must match.
2. If specimen was not drawn or transported under the right temperature specifications or if specimen was collected in the wrong type of tube.
3. If amount of specimen is not sufficient for the test required.
4. If specimen is grossly lipemic.
5. If specimen is grossly hemolyzed. Some specimens for testing, for example, folate or plasma renin activity, cannot be accepted even if they are slightly hemolyzed, since it will affect the results.
6. Nonfasting specimens, if fasting is a requirement.
7. Contaminated specimens.
8. Specimens that are radioactive, if the test requested is affected by the radioisotope used. This type of specimen should be handled as follows:
   a. All specimens received in the laboratory must be counted before centrifugation using a ^{125}I window or setting for whatever radionuclide will be counted in the assay. If the specimen is radioactive, a red tape, or some other indicator must be attached to the specimen's tube and to the specimen's aliquots after centrifugation.
   b. If specimen is radioactive (red tape), before running an assay check for radioactivity by counting the same amount of sample that is required for the assay. If significant counts are obtained, the test may not be able to be run. Some tests are not affected, others should include a blank, and still others should not be run (for example, HCG, B_{12}, folate).
   c. In general the interference of various radioisotopes in RIA is largely determined by the separation procedure of the particular assay. However, the problem is more complex than first realized because the degree of contamination of the patient sample is also dependent on a number of other factors, including (1) which radioisotope the patient received and how much of it was given, (2) the rate of clearance of this radioisotope from the patient's serum, (3) when the blood sample was drawn in relation to when the radioisotope was administered, (4) when the laboratory runs the blood sample (since further radioactive decay will occur in vitro), and (5) sample size used in the assay.
   d. If a specimen cannot be used because of radioactive contamination, inform the nursing station or physician requesting the test that a new specimen should be submitted after enough time has been allowed for the radioisotope to decay or be excreted to a level where it will not interfere with the assay.

■ INSTRUMENTATION

Various types of instruments are used in the binding assay laboratory, most of which are also common to the other clinical laboratories. However, the progress of binding assays has increased the development of certain tools unique to the binding assay laboratory, but some are also used in other laboratories. Attempts have been made to automate these techniques, but because of difficulties in the procedures, full automation has only partially been possible, with many tests still being performed manually. This section will briefly discuss many of the unique instruments and system used in the binding assay laboratory, as well as their use in assay procedures or systems.

■ Manual and semiautomated instruments/systems

Pipettes and dilutor dispensers. Over the last 10 years pipettes have evolved from simple glass and capillary pipettes to complex pipetting stations capable of pipetting the sample and three or more reagents at the same time with dilutions mixing. This has not necessarily improved the accuracy of pipetting, but it has improved reproducibility and speed. There are several types of pipetting equipment that will be discussed: the capillary type, first used to perform radioassay; air displacement and positive displacement pipettes; repeating pipettes; dispensers; automatic pipettes; dilutor/dispensers; and automatic pipetting stations.

Capillary-type pipettes were used in the 1960s and early 1970s when radioassay was in its infancy. These pipettes filled by capillary action but had to be blown out and rinsed. They were very accurate but difficult to use, so that reproducibility was poor and pipetting was slow. These were replaced in the early 1970s by manually operated sampler pipettes. The first of these was the air displacement pipettes such as Eppendorf, Oxford, and Versapetter. These pipettes require a replaceable plastic tip that should be changed after pipetting each different reagent to prevent cross-contamination. This type of pipette is still used and has been found to be quite accurate and reproducible as long as the tip is changed, rinsed in the sample first, watched for bubbles and improper filling, and used slowly. The volumes of these pipettes range from 5 μl to 1 ml and have accuracy errors of <2% and coefficients of variation (CVs) of <1%, depending on the volume. The use of these pipettes increased the speed at which radioassay procedures could be performed by a factor of 5.

The next type of pipette on the market was the *positive displacement pipette* such as the S.M.I., which used a glass or plastic tip with an internal Teflon plunger. These pipette tips do not have to be changed, but the tips must be wiped off carefully with the plunger out after each pipetting to avoid any contamination. If care is taken to watch for bubbles and incomplete filling, the speed of the pipette could be increased even more; <1% carryover with volumes from 10 μl to 1 ml and <2% with the 5 μl volume; an error of <2% depending on volume; and CVs of <1%.

There are two basic types of *repeating pipettes*. One type uses a self-filling pipette or syringe similar to a Cornwall pipette that is attached to a two-way valve and tubing, which is submerged into the reagent to be pipetted. This type of pipette is generally used for the continuous pipetting of a single reagent at volumes from 0.2 to 10 ml. The percent error and CVs for these pipettes is less than 3% and 2%, respectively, depending on the kind of pipette and volume used. The other type of repeating pipette is also a syringe-type pipette that is attached to a push-button, hand-held mechanism. With this type of pipette the syringe is filled to the necessary volume, and by using the push button a volume equal to a set fraction of the total volume of the pipette is dispensed. By changing to different-sized syringes, different volumes can be dispensed. These pipettes are very accurate, with an error of <1% and CVs of <1%. Although they may be used in volumes up to 1000 μl, they are generally used for smaller volumes, from 5 to 200 μl, and are very rapid. Both of these types of repeating pipettes are usually used for rapid pipetting of a single reagent to many tubes.

Dispensers are similar to a small pump attached to a reservoir, which is the reagent, either directly or by tubing. They are available both at a set volume or at adjustable volumes. Some repeating pipettes may be considered dispensers and vice versa. These may be considered an intermediate step from manual pipetting to automatic pipettes, dilutor/dispensers, and pipetting stations. They are available as manual or automatic dispensers, usually for volumes greater than 1 ml. The error and CVs on these dispensers can be as high as 3% to 5% or as low as <1%, depending on the type used.

Automatic pipettes, dilutor/dispensers, and automatic pipetting stations are all similar, except for their uses. Most use a syringe-type pump with a two-way valve and may have an adjustable or a set volume. Others use a peristaltic pump that may or may not be adjustable, usually simply by changing the size of the tubing used. All are easy to operate and very rapid; they usually can be operated by a push button or foot switch, or they may be continuous, stopping only after there are no more tubes to pipette or when stopped. Many automatic pipettes usually require a large priming volume and therefore make it undesirable for pipetting reagents that are in short supply. Dilutor/dispensors, on the other hand, allow picking up and pipetting only the volume of a scarce reagent needed along with the dispensing of another reagent, usually a buffer. With this system two reagents can be pipetted at the same time, and if two systems are used together, four reagents can be pipetted. Both of these systems, although very rapid and accurate, still require the operator to transfer the pipette tip from tube to tube. The pipetting station can do all of this plus more. Besides withdrawing the sample or standard and pipetting it along with the radiolabel, binder, and buffer, the pipetting station will pipette singly, in duplicate, or in triplicate; it will mix, and start and stop automatically when all the tubes are completed. This system is usually set up with its own test tube rack that can be centrifuged and counted without ever touching the tubes. The pipetting station is rapid, highly accurate, and precise, and once started it allows the operator to do other things until all pipetting is complete.

Gamma scintillation counters. Most radioassay procedures currently use either ^{125}I or ^{57}Co as the radiolabel. Most laboratories, therefore, only require a gamma scintillation counter to count these isotopes. In the early 1970s many radioassay procedures used other isotopes (^{3}H and ^{14}C) that required liquid scintillation counters. Because liquid scintillation is generally no longer used except for very esoteric assays, discussion will concentrate on gamma scintillation counters.

Ten years ago the radioassay test volume was small; therefore gamma counting of the tubes required no more than a tabletop counter that manually counted one tube at a time and required each count to be recorded by hand. As radioassay volumes increased, more efficient automatic counters were needed. Gamma counters then were developed that would allow 100 or more samples to be placed on the machine and counted. They had two or three channels for counting more than one isotope at a time, they automatically started and stopped, and they gave an automatic printout of counting time, tube number, and total count, counts per minute, or both. These counters still presented problems to the increasing radioassay volumes. For example, they were generally too slow because of the time it took to go from one tube to the next, and they were not very efficient. Also, each isotope had to be set manually and the instrument had to be constantly calibrated.

The next generation of gamma counters offered much more automation. The following features were added to decrease counting and technologist time:

1. Automatic counting of up to 300 samples
2. Rapid sample changing, less than 2 seconds per sample
3. Automatic calibration
4. Automatic nuclide setting
5. Ability to count various size tubes
6. On-line capabilities with data reduction systems such as programmable calculators or computers

These new counters gave the laboratory more free time for other work and more flexibility, but this was still not enough. What was wanted was faster, completely self-contained systems with data reduction. As a consequence, the next generation of gamma counters gave some or all of the following features:

1. Two, 4, 10, 16, 20, up to 48 counting wells, allowing 2 to 48 tubes or whole assays to be counted at the same time with automatic or manual sample changing
2. Built-in data reduction, either by programmable calculator or computer

Other gamma counters are also available that are modifications of those already discussed. For instance, gamma counters are available with rack systems that allow the performance of a complete radioassay procedure without ever touching a tube; other counters are very compact and count 16 samples at one time but must be performed manually. Some counters only count two isotopes, ^{125}I and ^{57}Co, but are multiwell counters capable of very large volumes of tubes (up to 1000).

Data-reduction systems. This section will not discuss data-reduction systems in any great detail (this is the subject of another section) but will simply give some information on what is currently available.

Data reduction systems can be programmable calculators or computers. They may be on-line, built in to a gamma counter, or off-line. It has only been within the last 5 years that data-reduction systems have been small, simple, and inexpensive enough for general use in the radioassay laboratory. Since then, they have progressed at a fantastic rate.

Programmable calculators are limited in their capabilities, but for many applications they are adequate. They are usually on-line to a gamma counter so that results are calculated as soon as they are counted. These systems usually use a cartridge tape that contains the programs for each assay and stores memory. Generally they have the following capabilities:

1. Simple calculations and curve fittings, usually a simple logit-log plot or modified logit-log plot
2. Preprogrammable for several assays in succession
3. Printout of curve data and quality-control information, sample counts or percents, and results with percent error or standard deviation
4. Limited memory storage, usually only quality-control information such as curve data or quality-control sample results
5. Preprogrammed tapes or manually programmable

The problem with programmable calculators is their limitations. There is not enough memory storage, the curves or results cannot be saved and retrieved later, and many assays do not fit the logit-log curve available in most programmable calculators.

Computers gave the laboratory much more capability and flexibility in performing radioassay procedures. They should more correctly be called minicomputers, since they are designed to perform a specific task. They may be on-line or built into the counter, and they can perform all of the same functions as the programmable calculators plus:

1. Complex calculations, usually six to eight different data-handling calculations and six to eight curve fits, making it possible to fit the assay to a curve, including difficult nonequilibrium assays
2. Printouts of all curve and sample information, including curve and sample calculations
3. More storage and retrieval capability, including curve data, quality control, and sample results; some systems can even store, on permanent disk or tape, patient information such as name, hospital number, and result, with hard copy capability
4. Full programmability for any assay or even other uses for the laboratory

Combination of systems for radioassay testing. The right combinations of instruments depend on many things, such as number of different assays being performed, sample volume, economics, other uses for the equipment, and technical staff. Based strictly on work load, I will demonstrate how any laboratory can have some degree of semiautomation.

Laboratories performing only a few assays, but with a moderate to high sample volume, do not need technical help, but with large sample volumes it is necessary to rapidly pipette. This laboratory might function more efficiently and economically using repeating pipettes and manually operated sampler pipettes in conjunction with a simple single-channel automatic gamma counter with a programmable calculator. The incubation and separation steps cannot be automated, but, after vortexing, the incubation is usually carried out at room temperature or in a 37° C agitating water bath and separation is simply by centrifugation and decanting, or only decanting in the case of some solid-phase assays. Since there is adequate technologist time and not many assays to tie up the instruments, this combination would meet the needs of this laboratory quite adequately.

In the laboratory with a great number of different assays but with low to moderate sample volumes, although the workload is low, the performance of many different assays actually takes much more technologist time. This means that there is a need to reduce the number of pipetting steps and increase the data reduction capabilities to handle the different assays. In this case an automatic diluter/dispenser would be valuable to reduce the pipetting steps; however, the sample volume does not justify a pipetting station. A dual channel single-well or multiwell gamma counter with an on-line or built-in computer should be used for rapid throughput with maximum capabilities. The incubation and separation steps are the same as those described previously.

The last type of laboratory to be considered is the one with many different assays and a high sample volume. In this case maximum capabilities are needed in pipetting, counting, and data reduction. A possible combination for this laboratory might be a rack system, a pipetting station using racks in which the tubes can be incubated and centrifuged with a special centrifuge head. The racks would then be put directly on a gamma counter designed to accept the racks, with an on-line computer for maximum capability.

There are many other combinations that can be used, but any combination depends on the requirements of the particular laboratory.

■ Automated systems

Although automation has been commonplace in the clinical laboratory for many years, it has only become available for radioassay procedures for a few years. You may now be saying to yourself, "But I have been using automation to perform radioassay procedures for at least 10 years." This is true, if you consider automation as the mechanization of any one of the separate steps in the radioassay procedure. But relative to radioassay, this is considered semiautomation, since only a portion of the whole procedure is automated. True, total, or full automation—whichever adjective is used—is a self-containing system that, once started, will proceed without technologist intervention through the printout of the final result.

In the late 1970s, radioassay evolved to the point where the volume and diversity of tests were overwhelming the laboratory. Full automation was now needed to free the technologist from the high-volume routine tests in order to perform the more esoteric and difficult low-volume test, but unfortunately progress has been slow. This delay in the application of automation to radioassay has been the result of the unique characteristics associated with this type of assay.

First, radioassay procedures consist of separate unique steps, in particular the method of separation of free from bound radiolabel, which makes them difficult to automate. This same problem also applies to dissimilarities of the methods from assay to assay, which has been probably the major cause of the delays in the progress of fully automated systems. Portions of the radioassay methodology can easily be automated, such as pipetting and counting with data reduction, even between highly diverse assays. Other portions of the assay, such as the incubation and separation steps, have been consistently difficult to adapt to automation. For this reason few assays have thus far been fully automated, but instead many have been semiautomated by separately automating each step in the procedure.

A second situation that has made full automation prohibitive is the radioassay work load. Most radioassays are low-volume tests compared with other clinical chemistry tests, and each requires a unique methodology. Automation is usually applied to high-volume tests performed daily, but few tests in radioassay qualify as high-volume tests.

It appears that there are four basic problems an automated system must deal with if it is to be widely accepted:

1. The uniqueness of the radioassay methodology
2. The diversity of the methodology from assay to assay
3. The limited number of high-volume tests and lack of screening tests or profiles
4. The necessity to be locked in to a single supplier for reagents

There have been several automated systems on the market in the past few years, but at present only three are enjoying any significant use. One system, the Centria 2 system, although considered an automated system is actually semiautomated because tests are performed on three separate modular sections with technologist intervention between each section. This system consists of a pipetter, incubator/separator, and counter/data-reduction module, and the assays are performed by a double antibody solid phase procedure.

The other two automated systems in use are fully automated. One system, Micromedic's Concept IV, performs assays by the use of antibody-coated tubes; the other, B-D Immunodiagnostic's ARIA-HT and ARIA II, performs assays by the use of antibody-coated, reusable chambers. The only difficulty with these two systems is that you are completely dependent on the manufacturer for all your assay needs.

■ QUALITY CONTROL

The most important part of any laboratory is its quality-control program. Without a good quality-control program, not only are the results reported by the laboratory questionable, but the laboratory is vulnerable for a medical malpractice suit. Most states require that certain quality-control procedures be followed and that all quality-control information be kept available for a specified number of years. There has been talk of federal government control of laboratory licensing, which would put more emphasis on quality control. Hospital accreditation is contingent on a good quality-control program.

Aside from the legal applications, the competence of the laboratory is dependent on its quality-control program. Although the director is responsible for the quality of the laboratory, everyone in the laboratory, from the person who washes the glassware to the person who types the results, must participate in the program for the laboratory to work effectively. A well-run laboratory increases the morale and pride of the personnel. The precision of the laboratory is improved when the technologists are constantly aware of the quality of their work, and they will try harder to improve.

Every instrument in the laboratory, binding assay reagents or kits, and procedures must be quality-controlled. Quality control can be divided into three sections: (1) instrument quality control, (2) initial assay quality control and (3) daily assay quality control.

■ Instrument quality control

Besides the obvious quality control necessary on the methods for the different assays involved, some quality control should be instituted on all instruments used in the laboratory. For example:

1. Automatic pipetting equipment should be calibrated and checked for accuracy at various times. This can be checked by pipetting a radioactively labeled sample 10 times and comparing the counts with the counts pipetted using a certified capillary pipette. An accurate pipette should have a less than 1% error and should be reproducible. The following are general quality-control procedures for pipetting equipment. The methods for performing these quality-control procedures may differ from laboratory to laboratory or with different types of pipettes, but the quality-control information sought is the same.
   a. *Service and maintenance.* The instruments must be cleaned every month or whenever less than optimum operation is noted by the technologist. This should include cleaning the cylinder wall, the O-ring seat, and the piston of all deposits and old lubricant. The O-ring is relubricated by working a small amount of lubricant well into the mounting groove. If fluid is accidentally drawn inside the instrument, it should be disassembled and the piston, O-ring, and small-bore tubing connecting the piston area to the outlet should be cleaned and dried, preferably by blowing out with air. If any fluid has dried in the connecting tubing's bore, it may be cleaned by inserting the cleaning wire through its length. The O-ring must be replaced every 3 to 6 months or whenever necessary, according to the use of the pipette.
   b. *Accuracy.* Pipettes should be checked for accuracy before initial use and once a month thereafter. To check for accuracy, a radioactive solution (^{125}I) is used with at least 10,000 counts for the volume being tested. Pipetting is done repetitively into 10 plastic tubes, dispensing sufficient distilled water into each tube to bring the total volume to approximately 1.0 ml. This ensures standard counting geometry. Calculation is made of the mean counts of the 10 samples, the standard deviation (SD), and the coefficient of variation. The counts are compared with the counts pipetted using a certified capillary pipette. The accuracy should be less than $\pm 5\%$ of the stated value of pipette.
   c. *Precision.* All pipettes should be checked for precision before initial use and once a month thereafter. To check for precision, a radioactive solution (^{125}I) is pipetted repetitively into 10 plastic tubes, dispensing sufficient distilled water into each tube to bring the total volume to approximately 1.0 ml. This ensures standard counting geometry. Radioactivity is counted (at least 10,000 counts). Calculation is made of the mean, SD, and CV. The CV should be 3% or less, based on the number of counts per measurement. Pipettes found to be outside the limits specified for accuracy, or precision, or both should not be used. They are defective, probably because of wear of the spring, and must be replaced. For multiple-volume pipettes, these procedures should be done at the low-, medium- and high-volume settings.
2. The centrifuges should be checked for correct revolutions per minute (rpms), G forces, and temperature for refrigerated centrifuges. The rpm checks and routine maintenance should be performed at regular intervals and records kept of everything done, including breakdowns and repairs. Temperature readings should be taken daily and a record kept.
3. Refrigerators, freezers, and water baths should have daily records kept of temperature, maintenance, and repair. Frost-free refrigerator and freezers should not be used because of large temperature changes in the defrost cycle.
4. Gamma and liquid scintillation counters should be checked for efficiency and daily reliability. By making up a standard of the radionuclide used in the laboratory (for example, ^{125}I, ^{57}Co, and ^{51}Cr), counting every day, and plotting either as counts per minute or percent of initial count on a decay graph (Fig. 33-13), daily fluctuations in the instrument can be detected and would indicate whether the instrument should be recalibrated. By using this method, it may only be necessary to calibrate the instrument once a month. All counts and graphs should be recorded and saved. Radioactivity counters should be checked daily for background and less than a certain maximum background maintained (<50 cpm or whatever is appropriate for your counter and environmental conditions). High background counts indicate contamination; the instrument should be shut down and decontaminated. Precision or replicate counting should

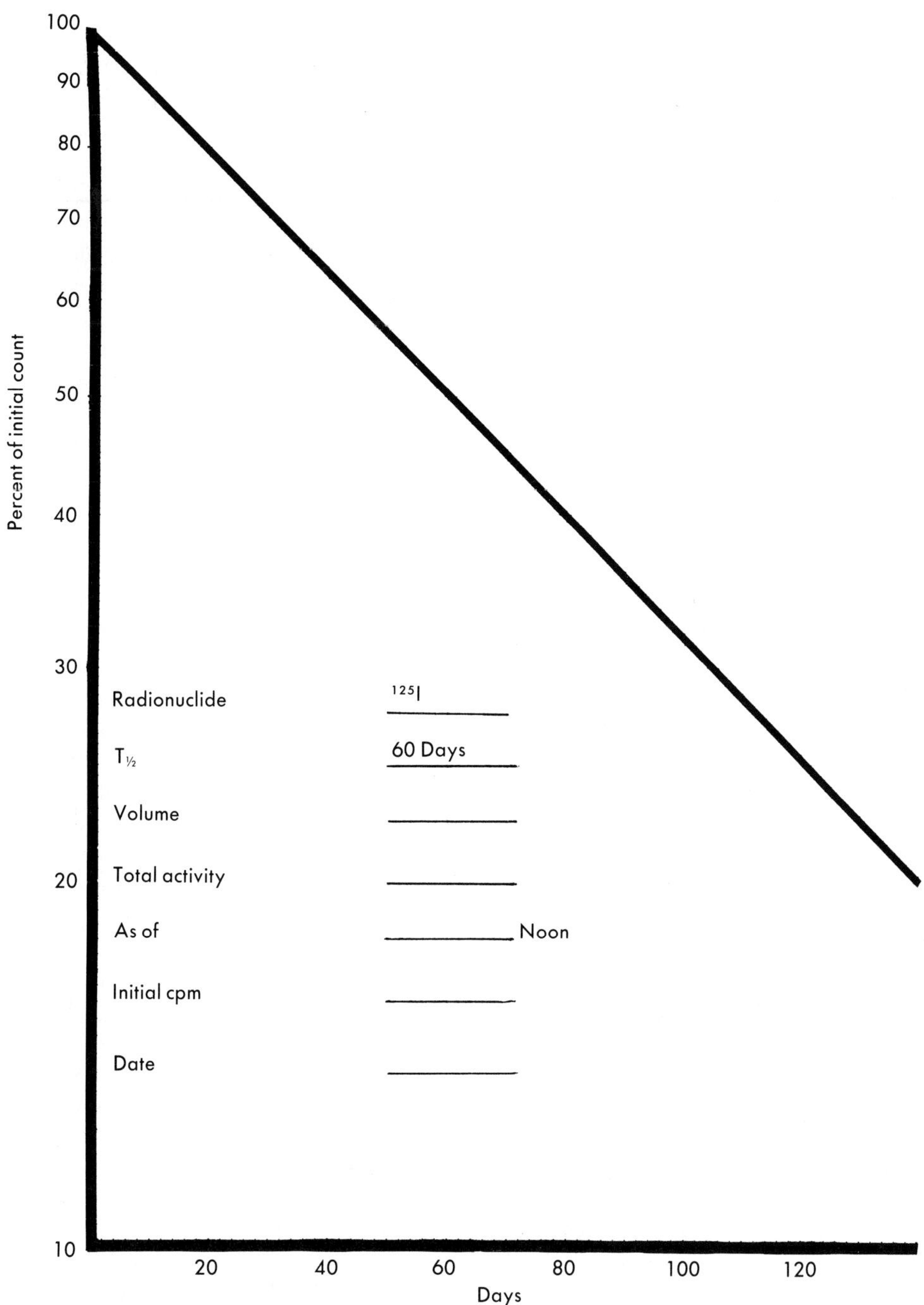

Fig. 33-13. Decay curve of ^{125}I for the quality control of gamma scintillation counters.

also be determined by counting a sample at least 20 times and an SD and CV calculated. The CV should be less than 1%. Efficiency for counting each isotope used in the laboratory should be calculated. This is performed by a radioactive source with known disintegrations per minute (dpm) and compared to counts per minute (cpm) obtained on the counter (cpm/dpm × 100 = %). Efficiencies for ^{125}I range from 75% to 85% and for ^{3}H, 35% to 45%. The higher the efficiency, the shorter the counting time.

NOTE—Even though the daily quality control may be correct, there may still be problems in counting your samples, which may result from other sources of error. Some sources of error in the radioactivity counting are as follows:

a. The accumulation of sufficient counts will reduce the statistical variation to within acceptable limits, for example, the SD on 10,000 counts is 1%.
b. Patient samples must be counted before centrifugation to check for radioactivity from in vivo proce-

PERSONNEL QUALITY CONTROL

Technologist's name:

Date started:

Instrument:

1. Theory does the technologist have a knowledge of the basic principles of how the instrument works?
2. Knowledge of instrument control knobs and how to use them.
3. Knowledge of how to set up and process samples.
4. Knowledge of instrument programming for sample handling.
5. Quality control performance on instrument.
6. Troubleshooting knowledge of what to do when certain problems arise and how to correct them.
7. Knowledge of what should be done in the event of instrument breakdown.

Completion date:

Technologist's signature:

Supervisor's signature:

Fig. 33-14. Record of training and knowledge of the instruments used in the laboratory for each technologist.

dures. If the sample is *hot* (containing radioactivity), a red tape or some other indicator should be attached to the sample tube. After centrifugation and separation of the serum, red tapes should be attached to the serum tubes. Before assaying, the specimen must be counted, and if it is hot, a sample blank must be run (this is necessary only if sample counts are significantly high enough to effect the assay). This blank will contain the sample and all reagents, except the tracer. The counts per minute from this tube should be subtracted from the counts per minute of the test sample. If the sample cannot be handled in this way, the requesting physician should be notified, so that a new sample can be drawn or other appropriate measures taken.

c. The use of glass containers for secondary containment in the gamma counter should be avoided, since the attenuation of glass for the low-energy ^{125}I radiation is relatively high. Not only is the count rate significantly reduced, but serious errors may arise from variations in the wall thickness of the glass container. Where secondary containment is required, molded plastic tubes or vials are recommended.

d. Possible variations in count rates caused by positioning of the assay tubes in the gamma counter should also be checked. This is referred to as counting geometry, and although it may seem insignificant, it can have a tremendous effect on counting precision.

5. Although not thought of as an instrument, technologists are one of the most variable instruments in the laboratory and therefore must have some control or checks on their abilities. Personnel quality control is often taken for granted, but it also requires monitoring. Technologists should be monitored for knowledge of operation, quality control, maintenance, and trouble shooting of all instruments. A record of all training and abilities should be maintained, as shown in Fig. 33-14.

■ Initial assay quality control

Assessing the quality of RIA tests is extremely important, regardless of whether you are using a kit or components, since incorrect results can lead to disasterous effects for the patient. Although the manufacturers of kits and components must report certain quality-control data for each lot of material, it is still a good idea to check these, since most manufacturers do not change their data with different lots of reagents, or the quality control data may be different under your laboratory conditions. WHO recommends that manufacturers supply certain information with an RIA kit, such as the following:

1. Basic statistics—SD, detection range, slope, and intercepts for the standard curve
2. Cross reactivity—specificity
3. Parallelism of standard and unknown
4. Recovery
5. Intraassay and interassay CVs at three dose levels
6. Sensitivity—lowest detectable dose
7. Antibody dilution curve
8. Clinical correlation studies
9. Normal-range study
10. Effects of different variables such as time, temperature, pH, and serum proteins
11. Comparison with other methods
12. Scatchard plots and equilibrium constants

Most of these data, but not all, are supplied by the manufacturer to varying degrees; however, because of the variations between kits, components, or even "homemade" reagents from lot to lot and manufacturer to manufacturer, it is a good idea for each laboratory to perform its own evaluation. Because of the expense and time involved in doing a complete evaluation, only certain key parameters are usually checked: specificity, sensitivity, precision, accuracy, clinical correlation, and normal range.

Specificity. The ability of the binder to react with one and only one ligand is termed specificity. Because of the nonspecificity of some protein binders, heterogeneity of polyclonal antibody, and similarities in binding sites for ligands other than the one being measured, binding to substances other than the one being measured will occur to varying degrees, which is termed cross reactivity. Binders may react with precursors or prohormones and metabolites or fragments of the ligand of interest or may react with portions of the molecule that are common to other molecules. Cross-reaction or nonspecificity may be reduced by several means.

1. Producing antibody to those sites on the molecule that are unique for that ligand
2. Absorption of the cross-reacting antibodies by the addition of the cross-reacting substance to the antiserum, thus blocking those binding sites
3. Extraction of ligand from cross-reacting substances
4. Production of monoclonal antibodies to unique binding sites on the molecule

By far the greatest development toward the improvement of specificity has been the use of monoclonal antibodies by the hybridoma technique.

The classic example of improved specificity is the assay for HCG. HCG is composed of two different chains, alpha and beta. The alpha chain is similar to the alpha chain of LH, FSH, and TSH. Therefore an antibody directed against the alpha chain would cross-react with all four. The beta chain, however, is unique for each of these hormones; thus a beta-specific HCG antibody can be produced that will not cross-react with LH, FSH, or TSH. But because of the heterogeneity of polyclonal antibody, some cross-reactivity may still occur. If it is significant, the cross-reacting antibody can be absorbed by addition of the cross-reacting substance, thus significantly increasing the specificity. However, the use of monoclonal antibodies has solved these problems, since virtually limitless amounts of a single antibody specific to a unique binding site on the HCG beta chain can be produced with no cross-reactivity to LH, FSH, or TSH.

The specificity of the binders in most commercial kits is usually adequate for their intended use; however, it is a good idea to check specificity. This is not always possible, since the suspected cross-reacting substances may be difficult or expensive to acquire in a pure or even impure form. Therefore it may only be possible to check for a few of the suspected cross-reacting substances, but this is still better than not checking at all. Cross-reactivity is checked by performing the standard assay (Fig. 33-15, curve A) and then performing the assay using the same antibody but substituting serial dilutions of the suspected cross-reacting ligand for the standard in the original assay (Fig. 33-15, curves B and C). The percent of cross reactivity is then expressed as the ratio of the dose of the ligand of interest to the dose of the cross-reacting substance at 50% displacement multiplied by 100. As can be seen in Fig. 33-15, substance B has a 25% cross-reactivity, but substance "C" has no significant cross-reactivity. What this simply means is that 24 units of substance B at 50% binding will give a value of 6 units of ligand A, which may not be present at all. One word of caution when using cross-reactivity values from curves. Sometimes there may be a high cross-reactivity for a substance other than the one being measured, but the cross-reacting substance may be present in such minute amounts as to make it insignificant to the final result of the ligand of interest.

Sensitivity. Sensitivity is usually defined as the smallest amount of unlabeled ligand that can be distinguished for no ligand. This is the minimum detection limit of the assay and may be less than the first standard used on the assay curve other than the zero standard. This value is usually determined by performing the assay and including at least 10 zero standard samples as unknowns. The mean and a 2-SD value are calculated for the 10 zero sample counts, and the 2-SD value from the zero mean counts is taken as the least detectable value (95% confidence level).

The sensitivity of an assay is basically determined by two things, the labeled ligand and the antibody or binder. Generally the greater the specific activity of the labeled ligand, the more sensitive the assay; if 1 molecule out of 10^6 molecules is radioactive, then the assay can detect no less

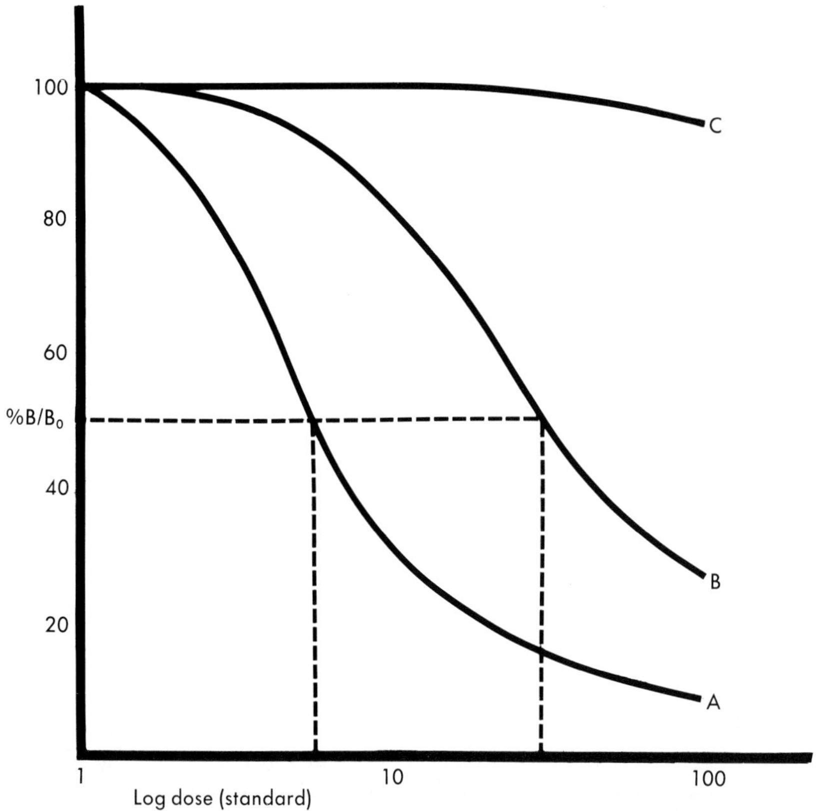

Percent cross reactivity = Ag dose at 50% displacement/ cross reacting substance dose at 50% displacement X100

Dose B/dose A × 100 = $\frac{6}{24}$ × 25% cross reactivity

Fig. 33-15. Demonstration of a cross-reactivity curve for the determination of specificity. Curve A is the standard curve for the ligand of interest. B is the curve generated by a cross-reacting substance showing a 25% cross reactivity. C is the curve for a substance with insignificant cross reactivity.

than 10^6 molecules. Although this theoretically is correct, there are several limitations. The amount of radioactivity detected is limited by the efficiency of the detection system; the specific activity is limited by the destruction of the ligand; and the ability of the binder to react with the labeled ligand is itself limited (there appears to be a saturation point for each binder at which no further increase in specific activity will affect the sensitivity). Another effect of the labeled ligand is the half-life of the radionuclide. The shorter the half-life, the greater the sensitivity. Again this is limited by the effective shelf life of the assay.

The antibody or binder affects sensitivity by the antibody dilution and affinity constant. Although an antibody dilution giving a maximum binding of 30% to 50% is used, Ekins has shown that as maximum binding approaches 0%, sensitivity becomes greater. However, the effective useful range of the assay also becomes shorter, limiting the usefulness of the curve. An antibody dilution giving 30% to 50% maximum binding appears to give greatest sensitivity with the most useful range for most assays. In CPB assays or RIAs, the limiting factor to sensitivity is the affinity or equilibrium constant of the antibody or binder. It has been shown that the minimum detectable dose approaches the reciprocal of the affinity constant:

$$\text{Minimum ligand concentration} \cong 1/K_a$$

This value can be determined by the use of a dose-response curve and the Scatchard plot. By performing the assay and plotting the response as T/B (on the X-axis) versus the dose (on the Y-axis) where T is total activity counts and B is the count in the bound fraction, the Y-intercept value and the concentration of the labeled ligand can be calculated, using the following formula:

$$p = -p^* + Cb\ T/B$$

which transforms to $Cb = (Cp + p^*)\ B/T$ where p and p* are unlabeled and labeled ligand, respectively, and the concentration of bound antigen (Cb) can be determined for each standard.

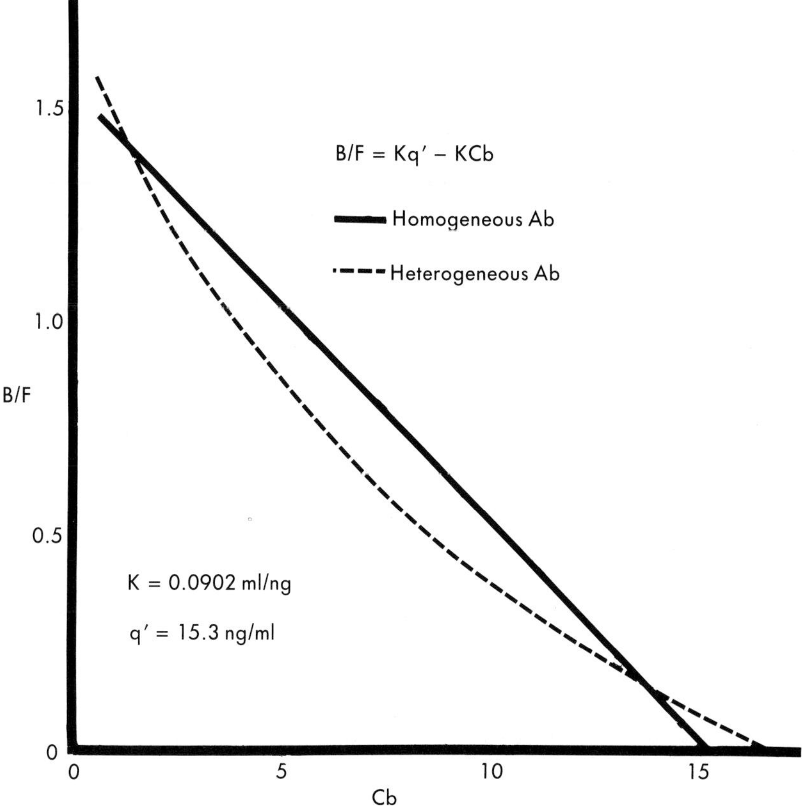

Fig. 33-16. Scatchard plot of a homogeneous and heterogeneous antibody demonstrating the calculation of the affinity constant *(K)* and concentration of binding sites *(q′)*. If a divalent antibody is assumed, then the concentration of Ab is $q'/2$.

The Scatchard plot can now be graphed by plotting the B/F ratio on the Y-axis versus Cb on the X-axis. The formula for the Scatchard plot is as follows:

$$B/F = K_{q'} - KCb$$

where B/F is the bound to free ratio, K is the equilibrium or affinity constant, q′ is the concentration of bound binding sites, and Cb is the concentration of bound antigen. By calculating the slope and determining the X-intercept, K and q can be calculated. From this the concentration of antibody can be determined by $q'/2$, since there are two binding sites for each antibody (Fig. 33-16). As can be seen from the Scatchard plot, several important factors about the assay can be determined:

1. $K = K_a$ = affinity constant. The greater the K_a, the better the antibody, the shorter the incubation time (time for equilibrium), and the more sensitive the assay, since sensitivity $\cong 1/K_a$. Thus this is another way of determining maximum sensitivity of the assay.
2. The concentration of binding sites and antibody can be determined.
3. The concentration of labeled ligand can be determined.
4. The heterogeneity of the antibody can be seen by the curvature of the graph. Fig. 33-16 indicates a straight line for homogeneous Ab and a curved line for heterogeneous Ab.

The Scatchard plot and the calculations shown here are more complicated and involved to be discussed further here; it is suggested that further reading in this area be pursued, since this type of data reduction has certain advantages:

1. Gross measuring errors can be readily identified and discarded.
2. Labeled antigen stability can be checked.
3. Deterioration of antibody can be detected.
4. Reagents and commercial kits can be simply and routinely evaluated.
5. A nearly constant slope indicates a nearly constant sensitivity throughout the curve.

Another type of sensitivity is the minimum difference between two values that can be shown to be significantly different from each other. This is not generally determined, since it is included in the precision of the assay and is dependent on the ability of the technologist and the errors in the instruments.

The overall limiting factor for sensitivity of an RIA and CPB is the antibody, but for IRMA assays the limiting factor is the specific activity of the labeled ligand, since antibody is used in excess.

Precision. Precision or reproducibility is the error associated with a result. This indicates how reliable your result is and also gives you some idea of the sensitivity or degree of differentiation between two results. Two types of precision parameters are usually calculated: intraassay and interassay precision.

The intraassay precision is a measure of the error expected for a sample value within an assay run. This value is determined by assaying sample pools, called *controls,* at three analyte values: low, normal, and high. Twenty individual samples of each level are assayed in the same run as unknowns. The results of the controls for each level are then subjected to statistical calculation to give the SD, CV (usually expressed as a percent), and mean.

$$SD = \pm\sqrt{\frac{\Sigma\,(x_i - \bar{x})^2}{n - 1}}$$

where:

xi = Individual values
$\bar{x}$ = Mean of all individual values
n = Number of individual determinations

$$CV\ (\%) = \frac{SD}{\bar{x}} \times 100$$

The intraassay precision, or CV, is a measure of the error caused by technique and reproducibility of the instruments used. Intraassay CVs should be less than 10% for good within-run reproducibility and reliability of results. This procedure is usually only performed when starting a new assay or lot or when evaluating a new kit.

The interassay precision is a measure of the variability or error associated with test results from day to day. This parameter is calculated as described earlier for the intraassay precision, or CV, except that the pooled samples or controls are only performed in duplicate each day or with each standard curve and usually calculated on a monthly basis. The interassay CV is not only affected by those variables described previously but also by the stability of the standards, antibodies, tracers, and buffers along with lot-to-lot variability caused by manufacturing. The values of the interassay CVs should also be less than 10%. This parameter will be discussed further in the next section.

Ekins has suggested the use of the *precision profile,* which is simply a plot of the CV values for each standard on the Y-axis against the standard values on the X-axis. By drawing this curve and plotting a straight line through the maximum CV value acceptable, several parameters can be determined:

1. The change in CV values throughout the curve
2. The acceptable range of the standard curve
3. The least detectable dose with an acceptable CV

Accuracy. Accuracy is the ability of an assay to detect all of the substance being assayed that is present in the sample. Accuracy can be divided into two sections: recovery and parallelism.

Recovery simply is the ability to detect, as closely as possible, 100% of a known quantity of analyte added to a serum sample. This is easily performed by preparing a pooled sample and assaying for the analyte to determine the baseline value. Then known amounts of pure analyte are added to the pooled samples at three levels: low, normal, and high. The samples are then assayed again for the analyte. The baseline value is subtracted from the result, and this value is divided by the known value for that sample times 100 to give a percent recovery. A good assay should result in 100 ± 3% recovery.

Parallelism can be considered as specificity, since it is usually used to determine if there are any substances in the serum causing immunochemical interference, affecting the unknown result. This is performed by making serial dilutions of the suspect sample and comparing the standard curve with the sample dilution curve. If there is no interference, the two curves will be parallel. Failure for the two curves to be parallel could mean that cross-reacting substances are present in the sample. This may indicate that this type of sample cannot be assayed without some type of extraction first.

Parallelism can also be used to determine the linearity or dilution effects of the assay. If an extremely high sample level has to be diluted, can this be done without disturbing the reaction or equilibrium? Parallelism can be used to determine this.

The effects of various substances can also be determined by the use of this technique. By performing parallelism on various samples containing different suspect interfering substances, the change in the slope of the curve can indicate whether the substance is inhibiting or enhancing binding.

Clinical correlation. Even if all other quality control parameters are acceptable, the ultimate test for the acceptance of an assay is its ability to diagnose the patient's disease correctly or give clinical correlation. This is performed by assaying a large number of patient samples that have been confirmed as positive or negative for the disease or diseases for which the assay is intended. Two correlation parameters must be determined: the ability to detect all positive patient samples (no false negatives—clinical sensitivity) and the ability to detect all negative patient samples (no false positives—clinical specificity). The combination of these two parameters will result in the determination of clinical accuracy.

Normal range. The usual method for determining a normal range in most laboratories is to select a group of healthy individuals, usually from the laboratory, on whom to perform the test. The results are analyzed by determining a mean ±2 SD for the normal range. This assumes a gaussian distribution for this analyte and automatically classifies 5% of the healthy individuals as abnormal.

Another method to establish a normal range is not to presuppose any shape curve (nongaussian) but rather gather data from a large group of normal individuals and determine a median and range of normals. This is also subject to error, since extremely high or low values will distort the curve, unless very large numbers of patient samples are tested. Some laboratories use patient samples sent for tests other than the test of interest as normals to establish a normal range. The problem is that these are not normal individuals, and although they do not have the disease for which the sample is being assayed, the disease they do have may have an effect on the analyte for which the normal range is being sought.

Every laboratory should establish its own normal range, often called the *reference range,* based on the patient population, environmental and physiologic conditions, techniques, and other miscellaneous parameters. This may not always be possible, at least in a short time; therefore most laboratories use the normal range established by the manufacturer until enough data are acquired to establish their own normal range.

■ DAILY ASSAY QUALITY CONTROL

Quality control used on a daily basis (day to day) is necessary to keep track of all aspects of assay performance. Daily quality assurance is generally monitored by the use of control samples and data reduction calculations from the curve itself.

■ Serum/plasma controls

There are many methods that can be used to evaluate the reliability of an assay. By far the most important controls are the serum or plasma controls that are assayed along with the patient's samples. There are three types of serum or plasma controls that can be used:

1. *Pooled controls.* These controls are made in the laboratory by pooling the serum or plasma samples that would ordinarily be discarded, aliquoting desired volumes, and freezing for daily use in the assays.
2. *Commercial controls.* These are either lyophilized sera or synthetic controls containing different levels of various substances. These controls are produced by pharmaceutical companies or companies engaged in the manufacture of radioassay kits. Values for the various substances in these controls and for different companies' kits are determined and published by the manufacturer.
3. *Recovery controls.* Recovery controls are made by adding known quantities of a substance to serum or saline solution containing enough protein to make it equivalent to patient serum samples.

It is absolutely necessary that a pooled and/or commercial control be included every time an assay is performed. Recovery controls are not generally used in the same way as pooled or commercial controls but are used primarily to determine the efficiency of a kit for the determination of a specific substance.

A normal control should always be included with every assay, usually around midrange. In addition, a high and/or low control should also be included, depending on whether the abnormal values for that assay are in the high or low range. Many laboratories advocate the use of a high, medium, and low control for all assays so that if one control is out of line, part of the curve may still be salvaged and the whole assay need not be repeated. If commercial controls are used, it is recommended that a pool control also be included.

A daily record of all control results should be kept and monthly (in the case of assays performed daily) or quarterly (in the case of weekly assays) statistics calculated (Fig. 33-17). The mean, SD, and CV can be determined from these data. The lower the CV, the better the assay. Any assay in which the controls are more than ±2 SDs from the mean should be evaluated further and repeated if necessary. The mean and ±2 SD lines can be drawn on a graph for each control (Fig. 33-18). The daily control values can then be plotted, and the daily and long-range performance of each assay can be seen at a glance, known as the Levy-Jennings chart. By using the right controls, the intraassay and interassay performance of the kit can be determined at all times.

The following are some general rules for using assay controls:

1. A standard curve must be run with each assay, except when otherwise indicated.
2. Reference controls must be included with each assay, preferably three different concentrations to cover the range of clinically important values (low, normal, and high).
3. Standards, reference controls, and patient samples should be run in duplicate, except when otherwise indicated.
4. When a new reference control serum is run, the data given by the manufacturer will be used during the initial period, until enough data accumulate from the values determined in the laboratory to calculate your own mean and SD. A new control chart will then be used for the reference control with the new mean and 2 SDs indicated.
5. Every time an assay is run, the reference control results must be plotted on Levy-Jennings charts, using the mean as the center line and ±2SD as 95% confidence limits.
6. Patient results are released if controls are inside the 2 SD range.
7. If one reference control value is outside the ±2SD

Daily quality control record

Month July Year 1984 Assay Digoxin

Day	Control value 01641	$\bar{x}-x$ 0.65 ±	$(\bar{x}-x)^2$ 0.06 ng/ml	Comment
7/1	0.67			
7/2	0.60			
7/3	0.64			
7/4	0.70			
7/5	0.72			acc. <3SD
7/6	0.61			
7/7	<0.5			Broken tube
7/8	0.63			
$\Sigma x =$		$\Sigma(\bar{x}-x)^2 =$		

$n =$

$\bar{x} =$

$SD = \sqrt{\Sigma(\bar{x} - x)^2 / n - 1} =$

$2\ SD =$

$\%\ CV = (SD/\bar{x})\ 100 = (\quad)\ 100 =$

Mean =

Range =

Fig. 33-17. Quality control record for the calculation of monthly CVs for each assay and control sample.

limits, a careful evaluation of the run should be made before releasing any patient results. If the run is approved for release, the reason must be stated and the work sheet signed by the person authorizing it. Any action taken is recorded on the quality-control sheet. Generally 5% of the time a control value will be outside 2 SDs.

8. If two reference control values are outside the ±2 SD limits, the patient results should not be released until carefully analyzed. Again, the reason for run acceptance should be recorded and signed.
9. Any run in which all reference control values fall outside the ±2 SD limits is clearly out of control and results should not be released. Appropriate action should be taken.
10. If a trend (seven successive points with increasing or decreasing values) or a shift (seven successive points on the same side of the mean) is noticed by the technologist performing the quality-control plotting, the patient results should not be released, since this could indicate a reagent or control problem. The problem must be reported immediately and troubleshooting started.

There are other quality-control parameters that can be used to determine the performance of an assay. By keeping a record of the counts, calculations, and results for all standards, patients, and controls, the following control monitors can be used.

■ Initial binding ($\%B_0$) or maximum binding

$\%B_0$ is the percent binding with zero or no standard and should be between 30% and 70% of the total activity. A change of greater than 5% throughout the life of the kit indicates a problem with antibody affinity, incubation time, or separation method.

■ Minimum binding or nonspecific binding (NSB)

NSB is the percent binding with an infinite standard dose or with what should be no binding at all. This should not be more than 5% binding. If it is greater than 5%, it may be caused by some reaction other than the immunologic one involved in your assay, such as sticking to the tube or trapping of labeled analyte.

■ Midrange dose (MRD)

One of the controls should be run at 50% intercept or halfway on the curve, or a midrange dose can be calculated from the curve. This point should not vary by more than ±2 SDs (preferably ±1 SD). This is a good interassay check on the kit and/or technique. A CV can also be calculated as described previously and should be maintained to check quality control.

■ Midrange CV

The midrange CV monitors the variation between duplicate samples within an assay and should be less than 5% (preferably 3%). It is a good check technique. The

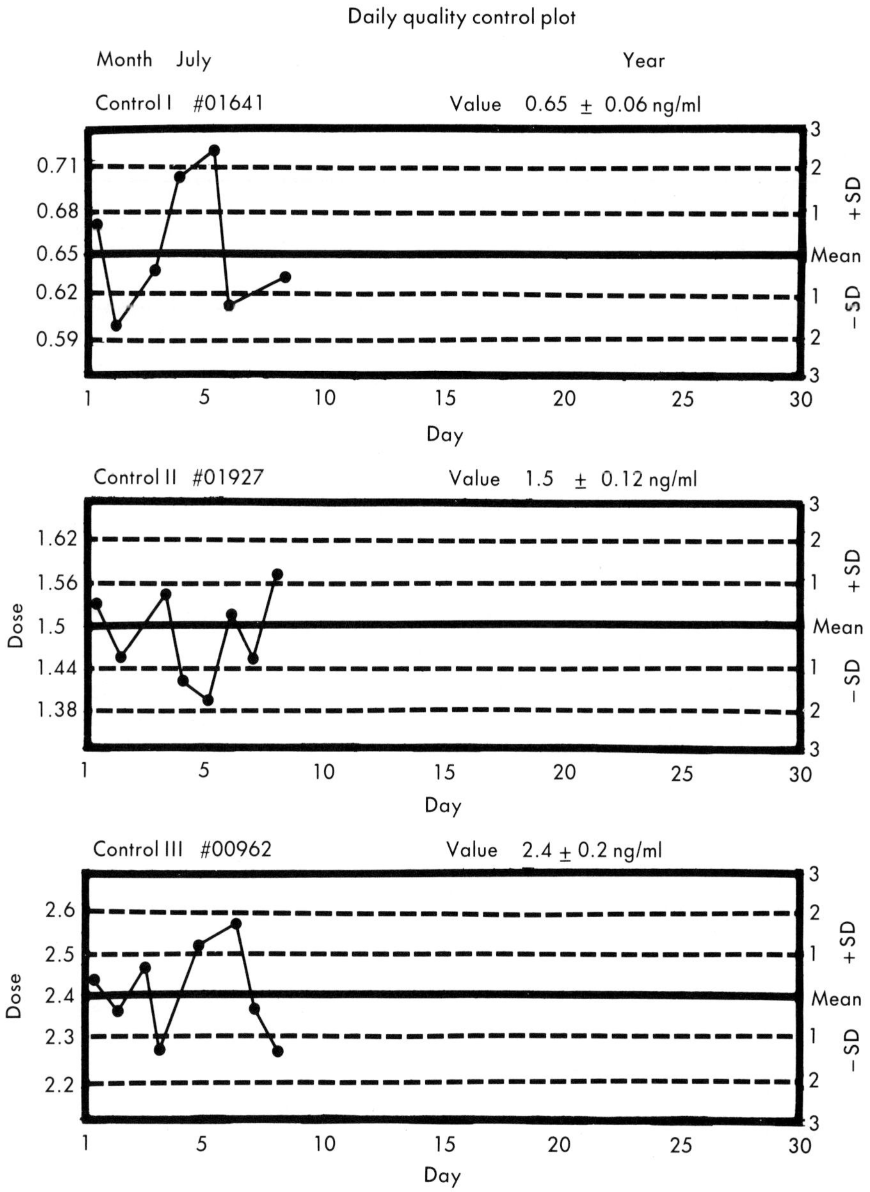

Fig. 33-18. Monthly Levy-Jennings plots for three levels of controls for each assay.

midrange dose, SD, CV, and CV of duplicates can also be calculated for the low and/or high control and thus used as a quality control monitor for any part of the curve.

■ Midrange slope

The midrange slope of the curve monitors interassay precision. The slope of the curve is an indication of the sensitivity of the assay. The steeper the slope, the more sensitive the assay. If the slope flattens out, this could indicate breakdown of the antibody or expiration of the kit.

■ Least detectable value

The value at 2 SDs from the zero standard value that can be significantly differentiated from zero. Most results should never be reported as zero but as less than the least detectable value.

■ Slope, y-intercept, and correlation coefficient of curve

The slope, Y-intercept, and correlation coefficient are usually not possible to determine, if performing the tests manually, but with the use of computers and programmable calculators, these values can be calculated. Most data-reduction systems give these values depending on the type of assay and the method of data reduction. The slope and Y-intercept should remain constant throughout the life of the kit, and a significant change could indicate a lack of stability or breakdown of reagents, or an error in the procedure. The correlation coefficient (R^2) is simply a statistical calculation to show how well the standards fit the standard curve. Standard curves should have an R^2 of greater than 95% for good precision and accuracy.

• • •

All of these quality control monitors are necessary for an efficient, well-run laboratory. They may someday be required of every laboratory. At times you may be tempted to skip some of these calculations, since they are time-consuming and add to the already high volume of paperwork in the laboratory. These problems can be solved very easily by the use of a computer system. All of these quality-control monitors can be used to evaluate new kits, which is a very important part of every laboratory.

So far, only internal quality control has been discussed. It is also necessary to perform external quality control. This is done simply by subscribing to a quality-control program from a reference laboratory such as the College of American Pathologists (CAP). They will send samples to evaluate on a quarterly basis and will compare your results to those of other laboratories around the country. Subscribing to a reference laboratory is a requirement of most regulatory agencies.

A good laboratory is one that follows a complete quality-control program, making it an efficient and accurate operation. This procedure will make the laboratory respected in your community, it will give the personnel pride in their laboratory and their work, and the laboratory will run more efficiently and economically. The following is a list of general rules, many of which are often ignored, which are necessary for a properly run and controlled laboratory:

1. A standard curve should be constructed for each set of unknowns to be tested.
2. Controls must be included with every run.
3. Reference controls or pooled serum or plasma control values differing by more than ±2 SD of the mean must be called to the supervisor's attention before reporting any values from that assay.
4. Samples with duplicate counts that do not have good agreement (within 10%) should be repeated.
5. Sterile distilled and/or deionized (depending on the assay) water should be used for reconstitution of reagents, standards, and controls.
6. Class A volumetric pipettes are used to reconstitute standards and controls.
7. Before reconstituting lyophilized material, vials should be tapped a few times to bring the contents to the bottom of the vial. The closure and stopper are removed carefully, taking care not to lose any small particles of freeze-dried material adhering to the stopper. The stopper should be inverted on a clean surface.
8. Lyophilized reagents are mixed gently by intermittent swirling and inversion until the contents have dissolved completely.
9. Standard curve, control, and patient samples should be run in duplicate.
10. Various lots of any kit component should not be mixed within an individual assay.
11. Components should not be used beyond the expiration date shown on the kit label.
12. When preparing reagents, standards, or controls, the reconstitution date should be written on the label.
13. Refrigerated reagents should be brought to room temperature and mixed gently before use in assays (unless otherwise specifically indicated, since certain tests may require that they be used cold).
14. Frozen samples should be thawed at room temperature and mixed gently before pipetting.
15. Samples should *never* be thawed in a heated water bath.
16. Freeze-thaw cycles and vigorous mixing should be avoided, since these procedures may result in denaturation of protein.
17. Frozen plasma samples should be allowed to thaw at room temperature, mixed well, and centrifuged to remove any particles before assaying.
18. The presence of contaminating radioactivity in the sample(s) of patients undergoing in vivo radionuclide diagnosis (or treatment) may give rise to false assay results. Before running an assay, a check is made (if tube has red tape) by counting the same amount of specimen that is going to be used in the assay. If contamination is found (and significant), a blank is run, or, if the technologist is in doubt, the procedure should be checked with your supervisor. Some tests (HCG, B_{12}, folate) should not be run. New specimen should be requested or the radioactivity allowed to decay.
19. The pipette tips should be moistened with the reagents or unknown before pipetting a series of aliquots.
20. Clean tips should be used for each new sample or reagent.
21. All samples and reagents are pipetted into the bottom of the assay tubes or as far down in the tube as possible, being careful not to touch any material already dispensed.
22. The sequence of reagent addition and the exposure time of the unlabeled and labeled substrate with the binding protein may affect the results. Instructions must be followed step by step.
23. Incubation temperature and time are critical in RIA testing.
24. When incubating an assay in a water bath, the temperature should be checked and the water level should be above the level of the reagents in the tube.

25. Standards, controls and unknowns—must be incubated under the same conditions.
26. Every time an assay is run, the control values should be recorded and plotted and the initials of the technologist who ran the test added to the quality control sheet.
27. After the technologist uses a repeating syringe for delivering a radioactive material, the syringe should be rinsed thoroughly with decontaminant and filled and rinsed at least five or six times with distilled water before being used again for another type of material.

■ MISCELLANEOUS

In recent years other nonradionuclide immunoassays (enzyme and florometric assays) have been developed as replacements for radioassays. They have been promoted by such statements as the following:

1. Less dangerous—no radioactivity
2. Longer shelf life—no waste
3. Easier to perform
4. No new equipment needed
5. Faster to perform—stat testing
6. Cheaper
7. Just as sensitive and specific
8. New equipment less expensive

However, all but one of these statements is false because of the tremendous developments in the radioassay field in recent years; for instance:

1. The amount of radioactivity used in the assay is insignificant. In 1985, it was deregulated by the Nuclear Regulatory Commission, which stated that up to 1 Ci of ^{125}I or ^{57}Co can be disposed of in the ordinary trash or down the sink in each facility under proper conditions. This amounts to over 100,000 radioassay kits per year.
2. Nonradionuclidic assays do have a longer shelf life; however, if a kit can not be used in 2 months, the shelf life of most radioassay kits, then it is not cost-effective to perform the test in-house.
3. Radioassay procedures are now, in most cases, easier, faster, and cheaper to perform than nonisotopic assays.
4. If radioassays are already being performed, no new equipment is needed to perform more assays, and any equipment that may be needed is in most cases less expensive than enzyme or fluorometric equipment.
5. In most cases enzyme and fluorometric tests are less sensitive and specific than radioassay methods because of the interfering substances in serum.

■ CLINICAL TESTS

The following is a list of the most familiar radioassay tests routinely performed today. The reference values presented are taken from the literature and specific manufacturers' kit data. Each laboratory should establish its own normal values since they are dependent on the reagents, geographic location, patient type, etc

• Adrenocorticotropic hormone (ACTH)

ACTH levels are clinically useful in the assessment of several disease states, including adrenal insufficiency; Cushing's syndrome secondary to pituitary tumors; Nelson's syndrome (pituitary enlargement following bilateral adrenalectomy); and ectopic production of ACTH, which occurs primarily in small cell carcinoma of the lung.

Reference values (pg/ml)		
Adults:	8 AM to 10 AM	20 to 140
	Midnight	10 to 70
Pediatric:	1 day old	47 to 71
	3 day old	43 to 75
	4 day old	37 to 71
	5 day old	37 to 65
	6 day old	28 to 46
	7 day old	29 to 41
	1 week	same as adults

Disease states*	
Cushing's syndrome (pituitary tumor)	98 to 480
Nelson's syndrome (pituitary insufficiency)	408 to 2000
Addison's disease	208 to 718
Ectopic ACTH (lung cancer)	120 to 14,000

*To further evaluate these disease states, various provocative tests are also used, such as: low and high dose dexamethasone suppression; vasopression stimulation; insulin stimulation; and metaprione stimulation.

Continued.

- **Aldosterone**

Aldosterone levels are useful for the differential diagnosis of hypertensive states (with plasma renin activity) and/or hyperaldosteronism both primary (Conn's syndrome) and secondary, and deficient secretion in Addison's disease. Plasma levels are dependent on sodium intake and whether the patient is supine or standing.

Reference values

Plasma or serum [normal sodium intake (ng/dl)]

Adult: Standing		4-31	
Supine		1-16	
		Mean	*2 SD*
Pediatric (years):	0 to 1	4.3	5 to 132
	1 to 4	26	5 to 60
	4 to 8	19	4 to 76
	8 to 12	10	3 to 28
	12 to 16	9	1 to 18

Urine (μg/day)

Adult: Normal diet	6 to 25
Low salt	17 to 44
High salt	0 to 6

- **Alpha fetoprotein (AFP)**

AFP levels in amniotic fluid and maternal serum above normal variation may be indicative of fetal maldevelopment resulting from open neural tube defects (such as spina bifida and anencephaly), amphalocele, and congenital nephrosis. Abnormal levels in nonmaternal serum may be indicative of hepatoma.

Reference values

Adults (nonmaternal serum): <10 IU/ml

Normal maternal serum

Gestational age (weeks)	*Range (IU/ml)*
14	7 to 43
15	9 to 58
16	11 to 68
17	12 to 78
18	15 to 93
19	18 to 110
20	20 to 128
21	24 to 148

Normal amniotic fluid

Gestational age (weeks)	*Range mean (kIU/ml) mean + 3 SD*
16	12.0 to 21.9
17	11.2 to 22.5
18	9.2 to 18.8
19	6.2 to 12.2

- **Amikacin**

Amikacin is an aminoglycoside antibiotic that is effective against most disease-causing members of the Enterobacteriacae. High levels of amikacin run a high risk of ototoxicity and nephrotoxicity.

Therapeutic levels: 4 to 16 μg/ml
Toxic level (at peak concentration) >35 μg/ml

- **Androstenedione**

Androstenedione is clinically useful in the diagnosis of premature adrenarche (premature sexual development), congenital adrenal hyperplasia (CAH), and hirsutism.

Reference values

Women:	85-275 ng/dl
Men:	75-205 ng/dl
Prepubertal children:	8-50 ng/dl
Postmenopausal women:	30-140 ng/dl

- **Angiotensin-converting enzyme**

Angiotensin-converting enzyme is responsible for the conversion of angiotensin I to angiotensin II. It is clinically useful in the diagnosis of Gaucher's disease and active sarcoidosis, and can be used to follow the progress of sarcoid disease in remission or therapy. Angiotensin-converting enzyme levels have been shown to be useful in the evaluation of lung cancer, emphysema, tuberculosis, and pulmonary embolism.

Reference values

Adults: 46 to 150 nmole/min/ml

- **Antidiuretic hormone (ADH)**

	Reference values
ADH (vasopressin) is a difficult test to perform and is not generally performed in the routine laboratory. However, ADH levels are useful in the diagnosis of hypothalamic and nephrogenic diabetes insipidus, psychogenic compulsive water ingestion, and syndrome of inappropriate ADH secretion (SIADH), which is the classic and common form of hyponatremia caused by pituitary or nonpituitary origin, such as an ectopic tumor.	Children and adults: Ad lib. fluids 0.4 to 5.3 μU/ml

- **Anti-DNA**

	Reference values
The anti-DNA assay is specifically directed against double-stranded DNA and is primarily useful for the diagnosis of systemic lupus erythematosus (SLE) and discoid lupus erythematosus. It has also been shown to be elevated in some patients with connective tissue disorders, Sjögren's syndrome, and chronic active hepatitis.	Adults: <25 U/ml or <1.4 μg/ml

- **B_{12}**

	Expected values
Low B_{12} levels are associated with lack of intrinsic factor, which is responsible for B_{12} absorption in the ileum (pernicious anemia) and other malabsorption syndromes in the ileum such as a blind loop syndrome. High levels are associated with hepatic and neoplastic diseases.	B_{12} deficiency: 0 to 130 pg/ml Indeterminate: 130 to 180 pg/ml Normal: 180 to 900 pg/ml

- **$Beta_2$ microglobulin**

	Reference values
$Beta_2$ microglobulin is useful for the assessment of renal function such as alterations in renal glomerular permeability, rejection of kidney transplants, nephrotoxicity, immune and malignant disorders, rheumatoid arthritis, and viral meningitis.	Serum: 0.54-2.75 ml/L Urine: 4 to 370 μg/L

- **Calcitonin**

Determination of calcitonin levels has been most useful for the differential diagnosis of medullary thyroid carcinoma and to monitor therapy and detect recurrences. Calcitonin levels may also provide an early indication of the presence of an ectopic tumor of neural crest or lung origin.

Reference values (pg/ml)

Adults: <100		
Children:	<1 yr	112 to 322
	1 to 2 yr	60 to 330
	3 to 4 yr	40 to 376
	5 to 6 yr	0 to 348
	7 to 8 yr	14 to 312
	9 to 10 yr	0 to 286
	11 to 13 yr	4 to 244
	14 to 18 yr	25 to 159

- **Carcinoembryonic antigen (CEA)**

CEA is best used for the follow-up management of patients with colorectal carcinoma and adenocarcinomas, and cancers in other digestive organs, lung, breast, and prostate.	Reference value: <3 ng/ml

- **Catecholamines**

Plasma catecholamines are abnormally high in essential hypertension and some phases of diabetes mellitus, but these measurements are more useful in diagnosis of pheochromocytoma, ganglioneuroma, neuroblastoma, and other neural crest tumors.

Reference values (supine)

Norepinephrine	104-548 pg/ml
Epinephrine	0-88 pg/ml
Dopamine	0-136 pg/ml
Total catecholamines	104-772 pg/ml

- **CK-MB**

The MB isoenzyme of creatine kinase is the most specific and sensitive indicator of an acute myocardial infarction (AMI)	Reference value: <5.0 EU/ml

Continued.

• Compound S (11-deoxycortisol)

Compound S is useful in the diagnosis of adrenal hyperplasia, Addison's disease, pituitary insufficiency, virilization, and hypertension.

Reference value
Specific 0-8 ng/ml
Direct (post metopirone) 80-250 ng/dl

• Cortisol

Cortisol levels are useful in the diagnosis of Cushing's syndrome (hyperadrenocorticalism) and Addison's disease (primary adrenal insufficiency). It is often used in conjunction with dexamethasone suppression or ACTH stimulation.

Reference values (serum)
Mornings: 7 to 25 μg/dl
Evenings: 2 to 9 μg/dl

• C peptide

C peptide is useful in the evaluation of beta cell function in diabetes with antibodies to exogenous insulin. It is also useful in detecting remission in transient diabetes mellitus and in separating people with insulin-dependent diabetes into those with and without some residual islet function. C peptide can also be useful in the diagnosis of insulin-secreting islet tumors or cancer, provocative testing of islet function, detection of residual tissue after pancreatectomy, testing for pancreatic transplant function, and diagnosis of hypoglycemia.

Reference value: 1.5 to 10 ng/ml

• Dehydroepiandrosterone sulfate (DHEA-S)

Serum DHEA-S levels are useful in evaluating conditions of adrenal androgen excess, as in hirsutism, the differential diagnosis of Cushing's syndrome, carcinomas and adenomas of the adrenal gland, and evaluation of bilateral adrenal cortical hyperplasia.

Reference values

Male: prepubertal	100 to 600 ng/ml
adult	2000 to 3350 ng/ml
Female: prepubertal	100 to 600 ng/ml
premenopausal	820 to 3380 ng/ml
term pregnancy	230 to 1170 ng/ml
postmenopausal	110 to 610 ng/ml
Newborns: both sexes	1670 to 3640 ng/ml

• Digoxin

Digoxin is a cardiac glycoside used in the treatment of congestive heart failure, atrial fibrillation, atrial flutter, and supraventricular tachycardias. It is necessary for serum levels to be monitored to maintain proper therapeutic levels without toxicity.

Therapeutic levels: 0.8 to 2.1 ng/ml
Toxic level: >2.1 ng/ml

• Estradiol

Estradiol levels are useful in the diagnosis of menstrual and/or ovarian dysfunction, ovarian tumors, ovulation induction, and infertility.

Reference values (pg/ml)

Females: Early follicular	10 to 150
late follicular	5 to 300
midcycle	250 to 600
luteal	50 to 300
Male: adult	10 to 50
prepubertal	<20

• **Estradiol (free and total)**

Estriol levels increase rapidly the third trimester of pregnancy and have been shown to be useful in monitoring fetal condition. Consistently low levels indicate fetal distress and the necessity for treatment.

Free estriol range by week of gestation (ng/ml)

Week	*Range*
25	3.5 to 10.0
28	4.0 to 12.5
30	4.5 to 14.0
32	5.0 to 16.0
34	5.5 to 18.5
35	6.0 to 21.0
36	7.0 to 25.0
37	8.0 to 28.0
38	9.0 to 32.0
39	10.0 to 34.0
40	10.5 to 25.0
41	10.5 to 25.0

• **Estrogens (total)**

This assay is used to evaluate estrogen status in children and adults, menstrual and/or ovarian dysfunction, ovarian tumors, and ovulation induction and infertility after human menstrual gonadotropin (HMG) therapy.

Reference values (pg/ml)

Prepubertal (male and female): <40		
Males:		40 to 205
Female cycle:	1 to 10 days	61-394
	11 to 20 days	122-437
	21 to 28 days	156-350
	Postmenopausal	<40
HMG treatment (therapeutic range): 400 to 800		

• **Ferritin**

Serum ferritin levels are useful in monitoring changes in iron stores in children during development and in iron deficiency in children and adults. Ferritin concentrations are increased with iron overload caused either by transfusional siderosis or primary idiopathic hemochromatosis.

Reference values

Male:	10 to 300 ng/ml
Female:	10 to 175 ng/ml

• **Folate**

Folic acid deficiency is present in patients suffering from megaloblastic anemia, anemia, hypersegmentation of the granulocytic nuclei, liver damage, and iron deficiency. RBC folate levels are used to verify folate deficiency and may also indicate B_{12} deficiency, which blocks the cells ability to retain folic acid.

Reference values

Folate deficiency	0 to 2 ng/ml
Indeterminate	2 to 3 ng/ml
Normal	3-17 ng/ml
RBC folate deficiency	0 to 200 ng/ml
RBC indeterminate	200 to 300 ng/ml
RBC normal folate	>300 ng/ml

• **Follicle-stimulating hormone (FSH)**

The measurement of FSH is important for the evaluation of disorders of the hypothalamic-pituitary-gonadal axis. When used in conjunction with luteinizing hormone (LH), it can be useful in differentiating between hypothalamic and pituitary disorders. FSH and LH levels are important for the differential diagnosis of hypogonadism, gonadal dysfunction and infertility, ovulation timing, and induction.

Reference values (mIU/ml)

Females: excluding midcycle peak	2.8 to 17.2
midcycle peak	15 to 35
postmenopausal females	24 to 170
Males	2.5 to 18.6
Prepubertal	<10

Continued.

• Gastrin

Serum gastrin levels are useful in the diagnosis of peptic ulcers, pernicious anemia, and Zollinger-Ellison (ZE) syndrome. It is particularly useful in ZE syndrome when used with a stimulation test to distinguish from peptic ulcers.

Reference range: <115 pg/ml

• Gentamicin

Gentamicin is a broad-spectrum aminoglycoside antibiotic with a narrow therapeutic range. Serious ototoxicity, nephrotoxicity, or both may occur if the therapeutic range is exceeded. Therefore careful serum levels must be monitored in patients undergoing gentamicin therapy.

Therapeutic range: Trough levels <3 μg/ml
Therapeutic or peak levels 3-10 μg/ml
Toxic levels (at peak): >12 μg/ml

• Glucagon

Glucagon has been shown to be useful in the diagnosis of diabetic hyperglycemia, which is mediated by elevated levels. There is also some evidence that glucagon levels may be useful in the evaluation of glucagon-secreting tumors of the pancreas.

Reference fasting levels: 50-150 pg/ml

• Hepatitis

These assays are useful for the evaluation of viral hepatitis, type A and B at different stages of the disease, or non-A, and non-B.

Hepatitis A-AB

Positive in the acute and recovery (years after exposure) phases of hepatitis A; may indicate previous disease and present immunity.

Hepatitis A-Ab-M

Diagnostic of the acute phase of hepatitis A; positive from 28 to 45 days after exposure.

Hepatitis Bs-Ag

Positive 13 to 14 weeks after exposure to hepatitis B and may remain positive for 2 weeks to 3 months. This is the earliest indication of hepatitis B infection and is an infectious period.

Hepatitis Bc-Ab

First indication of recovery; shows a rise in concentration about 4 months after exposure, reaches maximum about 6 to 9 months after, and remains high for years.

Hepatitis Bs-Ab

Last recovery response; rises approximately 6 months to 1 year after exposure, reaches maximum after several years, and shows gradual decline thereafter; indicates complete recovery and immunity.

Hepatitis Be-Ag

This is the second indication of hepatitis B infection (early acute phase) and remains positive for only a short period of time. This is also an infectious period. Persistently high levels indicate carrier state.

Hepatitis Be-Ab

Second recovery response; rises 5 months after exposure, with maximum 8 to 10 months after, and shows gradual decline after many years. No response or late response indicates a carrier state.

Hepatitis Bc-Ab-IGM

Also an early indication of recovery; rises 4 months after exposure, reaches maximum 6 to 9 months after, and is undetectable after 1 to 2 years.

Normal

All hepatitis assays should be negative; however, a positive on some tests does not necessarily indicate a current infection.

• Human chorionic gonadotropin-beta (HCG-beta)

The primary uses for HCG-beta is in the detection and follow-up of choriocarcinoma and hydatidiform moles, ectopic pregnancy, and threatened abortion. It is valuable in the detection of early pregnancy (10 days), especially in those patients for whom other diagnostic tests might be detrimental to the embryo. HCG-beta is also useful for the detection of HCG-secreting tumors such as ovarian cancer, testicular tumors, and cancers of the breast, prostate, lung, kidney, and gastrointestinal tract.

Reference values (mIU/ml)

Males: <5
Females: nonpregnant <5

Pregnant:	
first week	10 to 30
second week	30 to 100
third week	100 to 1,000
fourth week	1,000 to 10,000
second to third month	10,000 to 100,000
second trimester	2,000 to 45,000
third trimester	1,000 to 45,000

- **Human growth hormone (HGH)**

Serum human growth hormone (HGH) levels are important in the diagnosis of growth retardation (low levels), either idiopathic or acquired; pituitary insufficiency (low levels) caused by pituitary dysfunction or lack of hypothalamic stimulation: acromegaly, which is hypersecretion in adults; and giantism, which is hypersecretion in children.

Reference range: 0-5.6 ng/ml

- **Human placental lactogen (HPL)**

HPL, also known as human chorionic somatomammotropin (HCS), is growth hormone of placental origin. HPL levels are used to assess placental function, fetal well-being, and threatened abortion.

Reference values: levels increase throughout gestation to a maximum at 30 weeks. Levels < 4 μg/ml indicate risk of fetal distress or neonatal asphyxia.

- **IgE**

The immunoglobulin class IgE is responsible for allergic reactions and is elevated in most patients with asthma, hay fever, eczema, and other allergies.

Reference values	**(U/ml)**
6 weeks	0 to 2
6 months	0 to 7
1 yr	0 to 7
2 yr	0 to 9
3 yr	0 to 6
4 yr	0 to 24
7 yr	0 to 46
10 yr	0 to 116
14 yr	0 to 63
Adult	0 to 41

- **Insulin**

Measurement of insulin is useful in diagnosing hypoglycemia (including insulin-secreting pancreatic tumors or insulinomas), alimentary hypoglycemia, reactive hypoglycemia, and diabetes mellitus, usually used in conjunction with a glucose tolerance test.

Normal overnight fasting level: <20 μU/ml

- **Iron, serum, total iron binding capacity (TIBC) and unsaturated iron binding capacity (UIBC)**

Serum iron, TIBC, and UIBC are useful in the diagnosis of iron-deficiency anemias such as malabsorption, pregnancy, hemolysis, and blood loss. It may also be useful in the evaluation of chronic infections, cancer, rheumatic fever, Hodgkin's disease, and collagen vascular disease. High levels may be indicative of hemachromatosis, hemosiderosis, hepatic disease, bone-marrow hypoplasia, and megaloblastic anemias.

Reference values (μg/dl)
Serum iron: 35 to 178
TIBC: 254 to 466
UIBC: 141 to 366

- **Luteinizing hormone**

The measurement of LH is important for the evaluation of disorders of the hypothalamic-pituitary-gonadal axis. When used in conjunction with FSH, it can be useful in differentiating between hypothalamic and pituitary disorders. LH and FSH levels are important for the differential diagnosis of hypogonadism, gonadal dysfunction, and infertility.

Reference ranges (mIU/ml)	
Females: (excluding midcycle peak)	3.6 to 29.4
midcycle peak	58 to 204
postmenopausal	35 to 129
Males	3.9 to 22.6
Prepubertal	<10

- **Methotrexate**

Methotrexate is an effective antileukemic agent and is effective against other neoplastic diseases. To prevent toxicity, serum levels must be monitored during therapy.

Toxic levels: 24 hr: >10 μM/L or 4.5 μg/ml
48 hr: >1 μM/L or 0.45 μg/ml
72 hr: >0.1 μM/L or 0.045 μg/ml
Peak levels: 1 to 2 hr after infusion: 1000 μM/L or 450 μg/ml

Continued.

- **Myoglobin**

Myoglobin levels are elevated following myocardial infarction (MI) and usually peak 5 to 18 hours after onset of chest pain. Increased myoglobin levels are one of the earliest indications of MI.

Reference range: 6 to 85 ng/ml

- **Parathyroid hormone (PTH)**

PTH measurements are useful in the differential diagnosis and management of hypercalcemia and hypocalcemia; more specifically, in the diagnosis of tumors and hyperplasia of the parathyroid gland, hypoparathyroidism, renal osteodystrophy, and renal failure with hyperparathyroidism

Reference range (C terminal): 100 to 550 pg/ml with calcium at 8.8 to 10.4 μg/ml; depends on calcium levels

- **Phenytoin**

Phenytoin (DPH, Dilantin) is an anticonvulsant drug used in the treatment of epilepsy. Serum levels should be monitored to maintain therapeutic levels without toxicity.

Therapeutic levels: 10-20 μg/ml
Toxic level: >20 μg/ml

- **Progesterone**

Progesterone is important in the preparation for and maintenance of pregnancy. Serum levels are useful in detecting ovulation, luteal phase defects, and ovulation induction; monitoring replacement therapy; and detecting and evaluating high-risk pregnancies during the early weeks.

Reference values (ng/dl)

Males: <40 ng/dl	
Females: follicular	10 to 150
midluteal	570 to 2810
luteal	250 to 2810
over 60 yr	0 to 20
oral contraceptives	10 to 30
pregnancy	
first trimester	900 to 4700
second trimester	1680 to 14,600
third trimester	5500 to 25,500

- **Prolactin**

Serum prolactin measurement is necessary for evaluation of patients with infertility or suspected hypothalamic-pituitary dysfunction. Low prolactin levels are associated with microadenomas, hypothalamic-pituitary dysfunction, and a variety of drugs. High levels are associated with galactorrhea, amenorrhea, and infertility.

Reference values: females and males: 0 to 18.5 ng/ml

- **Prostatic acid phosphatase (PAP)**

Serum levels of PAP are useful in the diagnosis and management of prostatic cancer.

Reference values: <4.0 ng/ml
Borderline values: 4.0 to 5.0 ng/ml
Elevated values: >5.0 ng/ml

- **Renin activity, plasma (PRA)**

PRA levels are important in the diagnosis of primary and secondary aldosteronism in hypertensives and in the prognosis and therapy of patients with essential hypertension. They are also valuable in the evaluation of the renin-angiotensin system in disease states.

Reference values*
Range ± 1 SD (ng/ml/hr)
Supine 1.24 ± 1.09
Erect 2.63 ± 1.32

*Ad libitum salt intake

- **Testosterone (total)**

Testosterone measurement is helpful in evaluating hypogonadal states such as hypogonadism, orchidectomy, estrogen therapy, Klinefelter's syndrome, hypopituitarism, testicular feminization, and hepatic cirrhosis. Increased levels in females are caused by polycystic ovaries, ovarian tumors, adrenal tumors, adrenal hyperplasia, and virilization.

Reference values (ng/dl)	
Male: Prepubertal (late)	10 to 20
Adult	300 to 1000
Female: Prepubertal (late)	10 to 20
Follicular	20 to 80
Luteal	20 to 80
Postmenopausal	8 to 35

- **Theophylline**

Theophylline is a bronchodilator useful in the treatment of asthma. Serum levels are monitored to maintain a therapeutic level in the patient.

Subtherapeutic levels:	<10 μg/ml
Therapeutic levels:	10 to 20 μg/ml
Toxic levels:	<20 μg/ml

- **Thyroid function tests**

There are many thyroid function tests available today for the assessment of thyroid disease. They all have their own sensitivities, specificities, advantages, and disadvantages, so the choice of which test or tests to use is usually up to the requesting physician or laboratory. Their use is basically the same: to detect primary and secondary hypothyroidism, hypothalamic hypothyroidism, hyperthyroidism, T_3 thyrotoxicosis, and in the monitoring of thyroid replacement therapy.

Reference values	
T_3 uptake	25-37% T_3 U
T_3 RIA	90-120 ng/dl
Free T_3	3.0-8.6 p mol/L
T_4 RIA	4.5-12.5 μg/dl
Free T_4	0.7-1.8 ng/dl
Reverse T_3	20-53 ng/dl
TGB	12-30 μg/ml
TSH	0-7.6 μIU/ml

- **Tobramycin**

Tobramycin is an aminoglycoside antibiotic used in the treatment of gram-negative infections. Because of its potentially nephrotoxic and ototoxic effect, it is necessary to monitor serum levels.

Trough levels:	<3 ng/ml
Therapeutic levels:	3 to 10 ng/ml
Peak levels:	8 to 10 ng/ml
Toxic levels:	>10 ng/ml

BIBLIOGRAPHY

Al-Dujaili, E., and others: Evaluation and application of magnetizable charcoal for separation in radioimmunoassays, Clin. Chem. 25:1042-1405, 1979.

Allegra, J.C., and others: Estrogen receptor status: an important variable in predicting response to endocrine therapy in metastatic breast cancer, Eur. J. Cancer 16:323-331, 1980.

Al-Shawi, A., and others: Principles of labeled antibody immunoassays, Ligand Q. 4(4):43-51, 1981.

Baxter, J.D., and Funder, J.W.: Hormone receptors, N. Engl. J. Med. 301:1149-1161, 1979.

Berson, S.A., and Yalow, R.S.: Recent studies on binding antibodies, Ann. N.Y. Acad. Sci. 82:318-344, 1959.

Berson, S.A., and others: Insulin-^{131}I metabolism in human subjects: demonstration of insulin binding globulin in the circulation of insulin treated subjects, J. Clin. Invest. 35:170-190, 1956.

Berson, S.A., and others: Persistence of ^{131}I-labeled insulin in the blood of insulin-treated subjects, Northwest Med. 55:541-542, 1956.

Binoux, M.A., and Odell, W.D.: Use of dextran-coated charcoal to separate antibody-bound from free hormone: a critique, J. Clin. Endocrinol. Metab. 36:303-310, 1973.

Bio-Educational Publications Slide/Seminar Education Programs: Radioimmunoassay, Vols. 1-3, Rochester, N.Y., 1982, Bio Educational Publications.

Bolton, A.E.: Radioimmunoassay. In Voller, A., Bartlett, A., and Bidwell, D., editors: Baltimore, 1981, University Park Press, pp. 69-83.

Bowry, T.R.: Immunology simplified, New York, 1978, Oxford Book Co., Inc.

Brenner, W.S., and Chase, G.D.: Some concepts of RIA theory, data reduction, and quality control, IV. Binding mechanisms and nonlinear scotchard plots, Ligand Q. 3(1):21-27, 1980.

Brown, J.P., Hellstrom, K.E., and Hellstrom, I.: Use of monoclonal antibodies for quantitative analysis of antigens in normal and neoplastic tissues, Clin. Chem. 27:1592-1596, 1981.

Brown, T.R., and others: Pre-precipitated and solid-phase second antibody compared in radioimmunoassays, Clin. Chem. 26:503-507, 1980.

Brooker, G., Terasaki, W.L., and Price, M.G.: Gammaflow: a completely automated radioimmunoassay system, Science 194:270-276, 1976.

Cambiaso, C.L., and others: Glutaraldehyde-activated aminohexyl-derivative of sepharose 4B as a new versatile immunoabsorbent, Immunochemistry 12:273-278, 1975.

Catt, K., Niall, H.D., and Tregear, G.W.: Solid phase radioimmunoassay, Nature 213:825-827, 1967.

Catt, K., and Tregear, G.W.: Solid-phase radioimmunoassay in antibody-coated tubes, Science 158:1570-1572, 1967.

Cernosek, S.F.: Data reduction in radioimmunoassays. Part 1, Introduction, Ligand Rev. 1(1):34-37, 1979.

Cernosek, S.F.: Data reduction in radioimmunoassays. Part 2. Linearization of dose-response data, Ligand Rev. 1(2):22-24, 1979.

Cernosek, S.F.: Data-reduction in radioimmunoassays. Part 3. Weighted regression analysis, Ligand Rev. 2(1):56-60, 1980.

Cernosek, S.F.: Data reduction in radioimmunoassays. Part 4. Empirical curve fitting methods, Ligand Rev. 2(4):7-11, 1980.

Chard, T.: An introduction to radioimmunoassay and related techniques, New York, 1981, North-Holland Publishing Co.

Chase, G.: Some concepts of RIA theory, data reduction and quality control, I. Basic approaches to data reduction. II. The ideal RIA. Ligand Q. 2(3):25-33, 1979.

Chase, G.: Some concepts of RIA theory, data reduction, and quality control—the Scatchard plot and the equilibrium model, Ligand Q. 2(4):30-33, 1979.

Chen, I.-W.: Commercially available fully automated systems for radioligand assay. Part 1. Overview, Ligand Rev. 2(2):46-50, 1980.

Chen, I.-W.: Commercially available fully automated systems for radioligand assay. Part 2. Performance characteristics, Ligand Rev. 2(3):46-48, 1980.

Chiang, C.S.: A linear method for determining specific activity of tracers in radioimmunoassays, Clin. Chem. 33(7):1245-1247, 1987.

Clark, J.H., and Peck, E.J., Jr.: The analysis of hormone receptor systems: a primer, Ligand Rev. 2(2):23-28, 1980.

Daughday, W.H., and Jacobs, L.S.: Methods of separating antibody-bound from free antigen. In Odell, W.D., and Daughaday, W.H., editors: Principles of competitive protein binding assays, Philadelphia, 1971, J.B. Lippincott Co., pp. 303-316.

Demers, L.M., and Derck, D.D.: Centria system 2, Ligand Rev. 2(3):50-57, 1980.

Desbuquois, B., and Aurbach, G.D.: Use of polyethylene glycol to separate free and antibody-bound peptide hormones in radioimmunoassays, J. Clin. Endocrinol. 33:732-738, 1971.

De St. Groth, S.F., and Scheidegger, D.: Production of monoclonal antibodies: strategy and tactics, J. Immunol. Methods 35:1-21, 1980.

Diamond, B.A., Yelton, D.E., and Scharff, M.D.: Monoclonal antibodies: a new technology for producing serologic reagents, N. Engl. J. Med. 304:1344-1349, 1981.

Ekins, R.P.: The "precision profile": its use in RIA assessment and design, The Ligand Quarterly 4(2):33-44, 1981.

Ekins, R.P.: Radioimmunoassay and saturation analysis: basic principles and theory, Br. Med. Bull. 30:3-11, 1974.

Haynes, B.F., and Eisenbarth, G.S.: Monoclonal antibodies, probes for the study of autoimmunity and immunodeficiency, Orlando 1983, Academic Press, Inc.

Heal, A.: Safety and disposal changes that affect regulations in radioassay labs, Lab. World 32(12):50-53, 1981.

Hilliard, J.: Monoclonal antibody production with hybridoma lines: evaluation of technology and potential, Ligand Rev. 1(2):13, 1979.

Hurrel, J.G.R.: Monoclonal hybridoma antibodies: techniques and applications, Boca Raton, Fla., 1987, CRC Press, Inc.

Jacobs, P.M.: Separation methods in immunoassays, Ligand Q. 4(4):23-33, 1981.

Kahn, C.R.: Membrane receptors for hormones and neurotransmitters, J. Cell Biol. 70:261-286, 1976.

Kahn, C.R., and others: Receptors for peptide hormones: new insights into the pathophysiology of disease states in man, Ann. Intern. Med. 86:205-219, 1977.

Kajubi, S.K., and others: Differential effects of non-specific factors in several radioimmunoassay systems, Ligand Q. 4(2):63-66, 1981.

Kennett, R.H., McKearn, T.J., and Bechtol, K.B., editors: Monoclonal antibiotic, hybridomas: a new dimension in biological analyses, New York, 1980, Plenum Press.

Kiang, D.T., et al.: Estrogen receptors and responses to chemotherapy and hormonal therapy in advanced breast cancer, N. Engl. J. Med. 299:1330-1334, 1978.

King, A.C., and Cuatrecasas, P.: Peptide hormone-induced receptor mobility, aggregation, and internalization, N. Engl. J. Med. 305:77-88, 1981.

Kohler, G., and Milstein, C.: Continuous cultures of fused cells secreting antibody of predefined specificity, Nature 256:495-497, 1975.

Kricka, L.J., Ligand-binder assays—labels and analytical strategies. Clinical and Biochemical Analysis, Morton K. Schwartz, Editor, Vol. 17, New York, 1985, Marcel Dekker, Inc.

Kronvall, G., and Frommel, D.: Definition of staphylococcal protein A reactivity for human immunoglobulin G fragments, Immunochemistry 7:124-127, 1970.

Kronvall, G., and Williams, R.C.: Differences in antiprotein A activity among IgG subgroups, J. Immunol. 103:828-833, 1969.

Kronvall, G., and others: Phylogenetic insight into evolution of mammalian F_c fragment of a G globulin using staphylococcal protein A, J. Immunol. 104:140-147, 1970.

Lau, K.S., and others: Measurement of serum vitamin B12 level using radioisotope dilution and coated charcoal, Blood 26:202-214, 1965.

Leake, R.E.: Steroid receptor assays in the management of endocrine disorders, Ligand Rev. 3(3):23-35, 1981.

Leiva, W., and others: Sasant principles of radioimmunoassay RIA 101 & 102, Sloane Audio Visuals for Analysis and Training, Fullerton, Co., 1978.

Lerner, E.A.: How to make a hybridoma, Yale J. Biol. Med. 54:387-402, 1981.

Lippman, M.E., and Allegra, J.C.: Current concepts in cancer. Receptors in breast cancer, N. Engl. J. Med. 299:930-933, 1978.

Lippman, M.E., and others: The relation between estrogen receptors and response rate to cytotoxic chemotherapy in metastatic breast cancer, N. Engl. J. Med. 298:1223-1228, 1978.

Lo, D.H.: A quality control system in RIA, Ligand Q. 4(2):45-60, 1981.

Marchalonis, J.J.: An enzymatic method for the trace iodination of immunoglobulin and other proteins, Biochem. J. 113:299-305, 1969.

Meriadec, B., Jolu, J.P., and Henry, R.: A new and universal free/bound separation technique for the "CENTRIA" automated radioimmunoassay system, Clin. Chem. 25:1596-1599, 1979.

Miles, L.E.M., and Hales, C.N.: Labelled antibodies and immunological assay systems, Nature 219:186-189, 1968.

Milstein, C.: Monoclonal antibodies, Sci. Am. 243:66-74, 1980.

Mockus, M.B., and others: Estrogen-insensitive progresterone receptors in a human breast cancer cell line: characterization of receptors of a ligand exchange assay, Endocrinology 110:1564-1571, 1982.

Mortensen, E.: Separation of free and protein-bound ligand molecules by means of protein-coated charcoal, Clin. Chem. 20:1146-1149, 1974.

Motulsky, H.J., and Insel, P.A.: Adrenergic receptors in man: direct identification, physiologic regulation, and clinical alterations, N. Engl. J. Med. 307:18-29, 1982.

Murphy, B.E.P.: Application of the property of protein binding to the assay of minute quantities of hormones and other substances, Nature 201:679-682, 1964.

Murphy, B.E.P., Hood, A.B., and Pattee, C.J.: Clinical studies utilizing a new method for the serial determination of plasma corticoids, Can. Med. Assoc. J. 90:775-780, 1964.

Murphy, B.P., Engelberg, W., and Pattee, C.J.: A simple method for the determination of plasma corticoids, J. Clin. Endocrinol. Metab. 23:293-300, 1963.

Narra, R., and Miller, W.: Radioimmunoassay. In Early, P.J., Razzak, M.A., and Sodee, D.B., editors: Textbook of nuclear medicine technology, ed. 3, St. Louis, 1979, The C.V. Mosby Co., Chapter 30.

Nayak, P.N.: The kinetics of solid phase immunoassays, Ligand Q. 4(4):34-42, 1981.

Nordblom, G., and others: Ligand specificity and bridging phenomena in hapten radioimmunoassay, Ligand Q. 2(4):34-36, 1979.

Nye, L., and others: Solid-phase magnetic particle radioimmunoassay, Clin. Chim. Acta 69:387-396, 1976.

Odell, W.D., Silver, C., and Grover, P.K.: Competitive protein binding assays: methods of separation of bound from free. In Cameron, E.H.D., Hillers, S.G., and Griffiths, K., editors: Steroid immunoassay, London, 1975, Alpha Omega Publishing, Ltd., pp. 207-222.

Perlstein, M., and others: Parallelism: a useful tool for troubleshooting, Ligand Q. 3(1):34-36, 1980.

Peterson, M.A., and Swerdloff, R.S.: Separation of bound from free hormone in radioimmunoassay of lutropin and follitropin, Clin. Chem. 25:1239-1241, 1979.

Pichin, M.F., and Milgrom, E.: Characterization and assay of progesterone receptor in human mammary carcinoma, Cancer Res. 37:464-471, 1977.

Pierce, J.T., and Cochran, E.M.: Immunoassay in biological monitoring of occupationally exposed workers, ACPR, Feb. 1988, pp. 10-13.

Pollet, R.J., and Levey, G.S.: Principles of membrane receptor physiology and their application to clinical medicine, Ann. Intern. Med. 92:663-680, 1980.

Praither, J.D.: Basic principles of radioimmunoassay testing: a simple approach, J. Nucl. Med. Technol. 13(1):34-43, March 1985.

Price, C.P., and Newman, D.J.: Principles and practices of immunoassay, New York, 1992, Stockton Press.

Reese, M.G., and Johnson, L.R.: Automated measurement of serum thyrosine with the "ARIA II," as compared with competitive protein binding and radioimmunoassay, Clin. Chem. 24:342-344, 1978.

Rodbard, D., and others: Kinetics of two-site immunoradiometric ("sandwich") assays. II. Studies on the nature of the "high-dose hook effect," Immunochemistry 15:77-82, 1978.

Rodbard, D., Munson, P.J., and Thakun, A.K.: Quantitative characterization of hormone receptors, Cancer 46(suppl.):2907-2918, 1980.

Rodbard, D., Munson, P.J., and Delean, A.: Improved curve-fitting, parallelism testing, characterization of sensitivity and specificity, validation, and optimization for radioligand assays. In Symposium on Radioimmunoassay and Related Procedures in Medicine, IAEA, Vienna, 1977, pp. 469-514.

Romic-Stojkovic, R., and Gamulin, S.: Relationship of cytoplasmic and nuclear estrogen receptors and progesterone receptors in human breast cancer, Cancer Res. 40:4821-4825, 1980.

Rosenbaum, C., and others: Estrogen receptor status and response to chemotherapy in advanced breast cancer: the Tufts-Shattuck-Pondville experience, Cancer 46(suppl.):2919-2921, 1980.

Rubens, R.D., and Hayward, J.L.: Estrogen receptors and response to endocrine therapy and cytotoxic chemotherapy in advanced breast cancer, Cancer 46(suppl.):2922-2924, 1980.

Scatchard, G.: The attractions of proteins for small molecules and ions, Ann. N.Y. Acad. Sci. 51:660-672, 1949.

Smith, S.W., and Feldkamp, C.S.: Qualitative features of Scatchard plots: positive curvature, Ligand Q. 2(4):37-40, 1979.

Snyder, L., and others: Automated chemical analysis: update on continuous-flow approach, Anal. Chem. 48:942A-956A, 1976.

Special report: Antibody structure and function, Ligand Rev. 1(2):9, 1979.

Spelsberg, T.C., and Boyd-Leinen, P.A.: Identification of biologically active and inactive steroid receptors, Clin. Biochem. 5:198-203, 1980.

Thorell, J.I.: Internal sample attenuator counting (ISAC): a new technique for separating and measuring bound and free activity in radioimmunoassays, Clin. Chem. 27:1969-1973, 1981.

Travis, J.C.: Fundamentals of RIA and other ligand assays, Sci. Newsletter, Inc., Anaheim, Calif., 1979.

Updike, S.J., and others: Gel entrapment of antibody: a new strategy for facilitating both manual and automated radioimmunoassay, Clin. Chem. 19:1339-1344, 1973.

Wide, L., Bennich, H., and Johansson, S.G.: Diagnosis of allergy by in-vitro test for allergen antibodies, Lancet 2:1105-1107, 1967.

Witherspoon, L.: Immunoassay: is there a future role for nuclear medicine? J. Nucl. Med. 24:952-965, 1983.

Wittliff, J.L.: Steroid receptor interactions in human breast carcinoma, Cancer 46(suppl.):2953-2960, 1980.

Wittliff, J.L., and others: Specific estrogen-binding capacity of the cytoplasmic receptor in normal and neoplastic breast tissues of humans, Cancer Res. 32:1983-1992, 1972.

Yalow, R.S., and Berson, S.A.: Assay of plasma insulin in human subjects by immunological methods, Nature 184:1648-1649, 1959.

Yalow, R.S., and Berson, S.A.: Immunoassay of endogenous plasma insulin in man. J. Clin. Invest. 39:1157-1175, 1960.

Yalow, R.D., and Berson, S.A.: Introduction and general considerations. In Odell, W.D., and Danghaday, W.H., editors: Principles of competitive protein-binding assays, Philadelphia, 1971, J.B. Lippincott Co., pp. 1-21.

Young, P.C.M., Ehrlich, C.E., and Einhorn, L.H.: Relationship between steroid receptors and response to endocrine therapy and cytotoxic chemotherapy in metastatic breast cancer, Cancer 46(suppl.)2961-2963, 1980.

Zola, Heddy: Monoclonal antibodies: a manual of techniques, Boca Raton, Fla., 1987, CRC Press.

Chapter 34

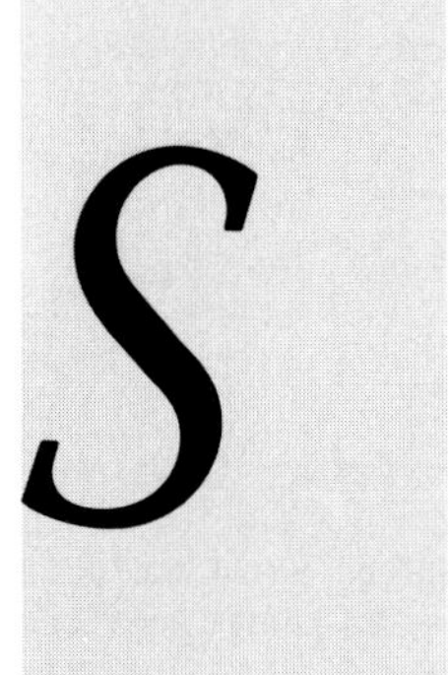

PECIAL IMAGING PROCEDURES

D. BRUCE SODEE

■ TESTICULAR IMAGING

LABORATORY APPLICATION

85

DETECTION OF TESTICULAR DISORDER/DISEASE

Purpose

Testicular imaging reveals the patency of the blood supply to the testes and any increased perfusion caused by inflammatory disease processes.

Torsion of the testes is a surgical emergency, as the testis becomes nonviable within 2 hours after disruption of its blood supply. Acute epididymoorchitis is difficult clinically to distinguish from torsion. Testicular imaging clearly separates these two entities.

Procedure

Materials

1. Scintillation camera with low-energy, medium-resolution collimator
2. ^{99m}Tc pertechnetate, 15 mCi (555 MBq)
3. Tape, towel, and pillow (used for positioning patient)

Patient preparation

1. No special preparation of the patient is required.
2. Explain the entire procedure to the patient. A professional and to-the-point manner should be used, since the patient's sense of modesty will be compromised.

Technique

1. Place the patient in a supine position with legs abducted. The penis should be taped up over the pubis to remove it from the field of view.
2. The testes should be supported by a towel placed over the thighs and underneath the testes. A pillow may also be used for support.
3. The testes may be separated by wedging a towel between them.
4. Place collimator parallel to and as close to the scrotum as possible.
5. Set camera and recording devices for a dynamic study with 5-second exposures.
6. Administer 15 mCi (555 MBq) of ^{99m}Tc pertechnetate to patient and begin imaging at 8 to 10 seconds.
7. Record six to eight 5-second images.
8. Follow flow immediately with two 500,000-count static images.

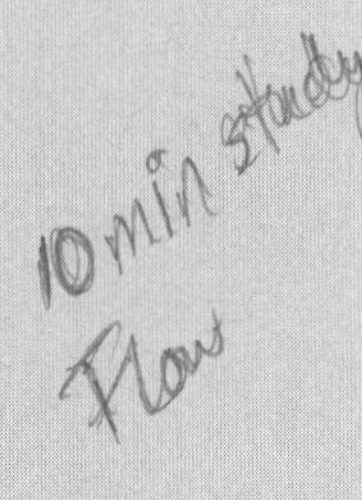

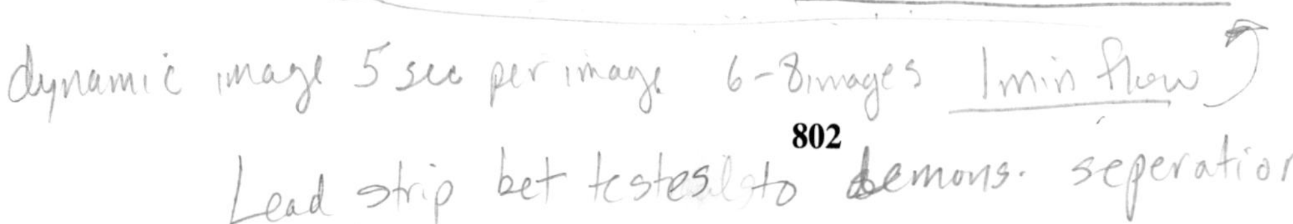

Diagnosis (Figs. 34-1 and 34-2)

	Perfusion	Static images
Torsion	None	Decreased activity in region of testes
Acute inflammation	Increased	Increased activity in inflamed region

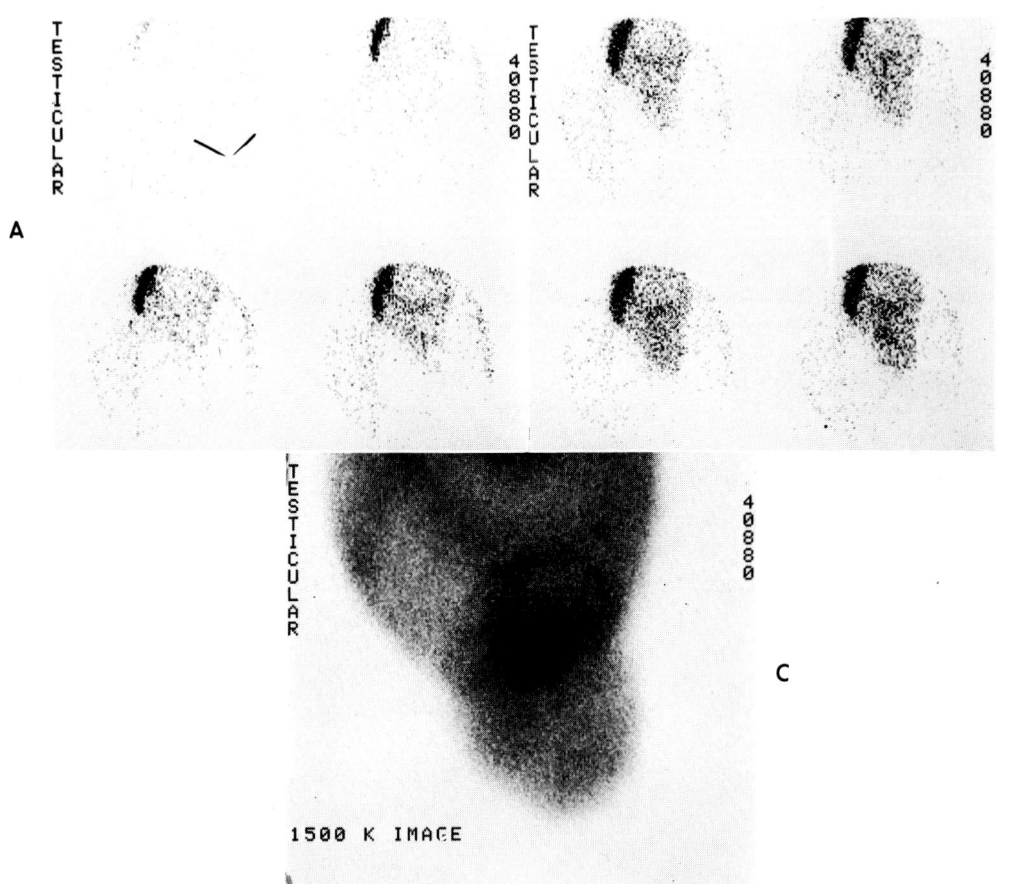

Fig. 34-1. Normal testicular image. Testicular imaging performed following intravenous administration of 15 mCi of ^{99m}Tc pertechnetate. **A,** and **B,** Dynamic phase reveals symmetric perfusion of both testes. **C,** Sequential 1-minute images for a period of 5 minutes revealed rather symmetric distribution of radionuclide in the scrota. No areas of increased or decreased concentration identified.

delays then 10 min
5 min

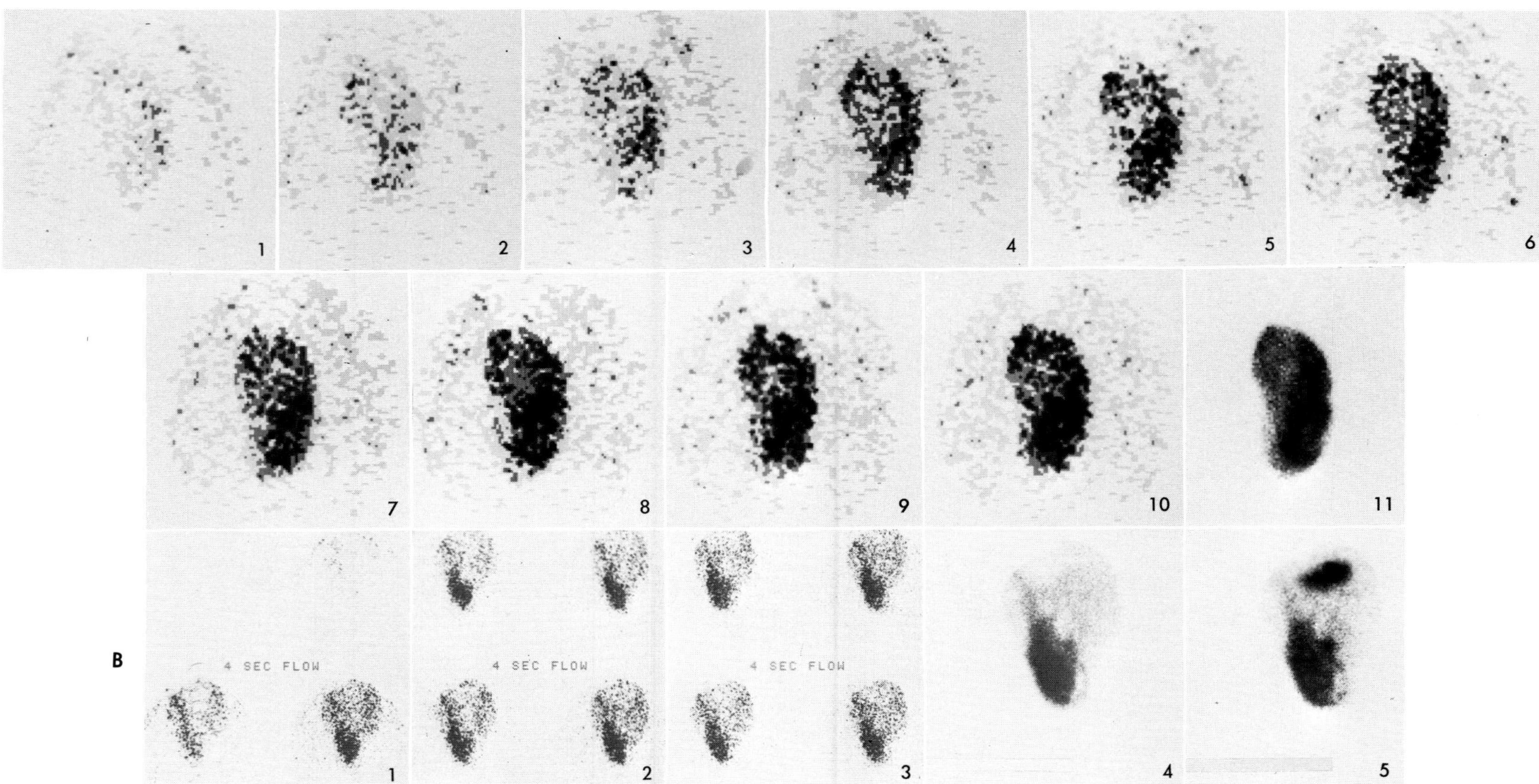

Fig. 34-2. Testicular image performed with 15 mCi of ^{99m}Tc pertechnetate administered intravenously. **A,** *1* to *10,* 4-second sequential perfusion study, 9-point computer smoothed. Perfusion study reveals increased perfusion of left epididymis. Note increased perfusion surrounding left testicle. *11,* Static image reveals diffusely increased concentration through epididymis and throughout left testicle, compatible with epididymitis and orchitis. Testicular tumor with associated epididymitis could not be ruled out from this study. **B,** *1* to *3,* Sequential 4-second perfusion study. Significantly increased perfusion of right epididymis. *4* and *5,* immediate static views reveal increased concentration of nuclide in region of swollen right epididymis. Note ring of activity surrounding right testicle, which by ultrasonography was shown to be a reactive hydrocele, secondary to orchitis.

■ SALIVARY GLAND IMAGING

LABORATORY APPLICATION

86

DETECTION OF SALIVARY GLAND DISORDER/DISEASE

Purpose

Salivary gland imaging is used to establish the functional capacity of salivary gland tissue and to demonstrate whether space-occupying lesions of the salivary gland are metastatic or primary.

^{99m}Tc pertechnetate is taken up by the functioning cells of the parotid and salivary glands. Therefore during the first 1 to 2 hours after dose administration, gross anatomic changes of this tissue may be visualized.

Indications

1. For study of salivary tissue function
2. For study of the function of palpable masses in parotid or salivary tissue

Procedure

Materials

1. Scintillation camera with low-energy, high-resolution collimator or 280-keV, medium-resolution collimator
2. ^{99m}Tc pertechnetate, 10 mCi (370 MBq)
3. Gum to stimulate the gland
4. Tape (½- or 1-inch) to secure patient's head
5. Pillow to place under patient's shoulders
6. Angle sponge (or pillows) to place under patient for lateral positioning

Patient preparation

1. Explain the entire procedure to the patient.
2. Have the patient chew gum.

Technique

1. Position the patient on a cart with a pillow under the shoulders to hyperextend the neck.
2. Place patient under the detector with suprasternal notch at the lower edge of the field of view. Mark the patient's left side with radioactive marker.
3. Set ^{99m}Tc pertechnetate peak.
4. Intravenously inject ^{99m}Tc pertechnetate.
5. Record 300,000-count images at the following intervals: 2, 5, 10, 15, 20, and 30 minutes after dosage administration. At 30 minutes obtain right and left lateral views with the head extended back slightly.
6. Any enlargement of the glands should be palpated at this time and marked on the image with a radioactive marker.
7. Check the images with the department physician, then continue with stimulation of the gland with gum. The patient should chew the gum for approximately 10 to 15 minutes.
8. Take an anterior image (post-stimulation) for 10 minutes and follow with lateral views.

Interpretation

Anterior and lateral images

Position	Normal, upward, or downward displacement
Shape	Normal parotid and salivary glands with smooth margins, apparent or not
Size	Normal, enlarged, or small
Space-occupying lesions, filling defects	1.5 to 2 cm in diameter; patchy decreases in activity in Sjögren's syndrome and in mixed tumor of the parotid No activity in metastatic tumors, abscesses and cysts

Continued.

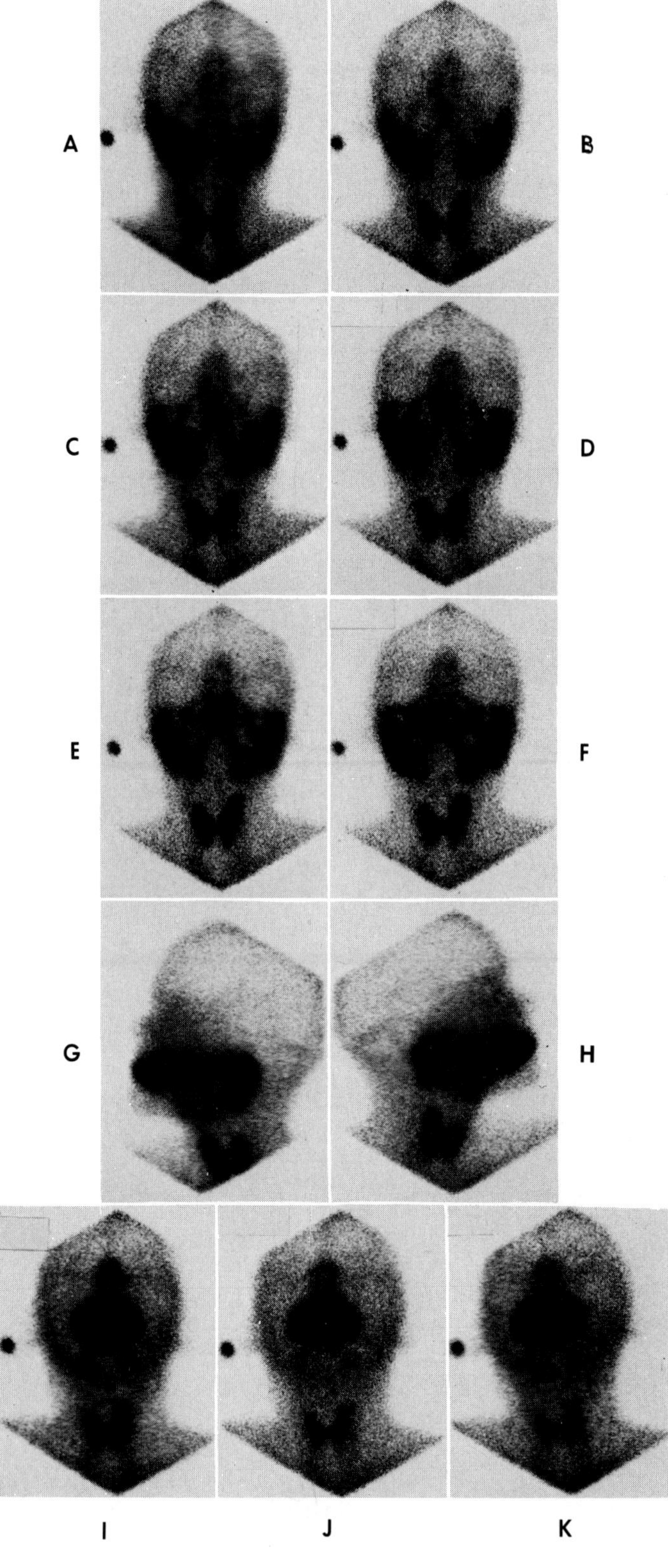

Fig. 34-3. Study performed with 10 mCi of ^{99m}Tc pertechnetate administered intravenously. **A** to **F,** Sequential images reveal rapid, even concentration of radioactivity in salivary and parotid glands. **G** and **H,** Thirty-minute static lateral images reveal even distribution in normal parotid glands. **I** to **K,** Postperchlorate discharge images reveal complete discharge of salivary and parotid glands.

Diagnosis

Interpretation of images (Figs. 34-3 and 34-4)

This procedure is not a commonly used study so there are only scattered case reports. With refinement, the procedure may be a definite aid in differential diagnosis related to parotid-salivary tissue.

Sjögren's syndrome

This syndrome is characterized by decreased activity in salivary tissue with patchy decreases in concentration.

In Sjögren's syndrome there are four levels of involvement.

Class I—Patients are normal.

Continued.

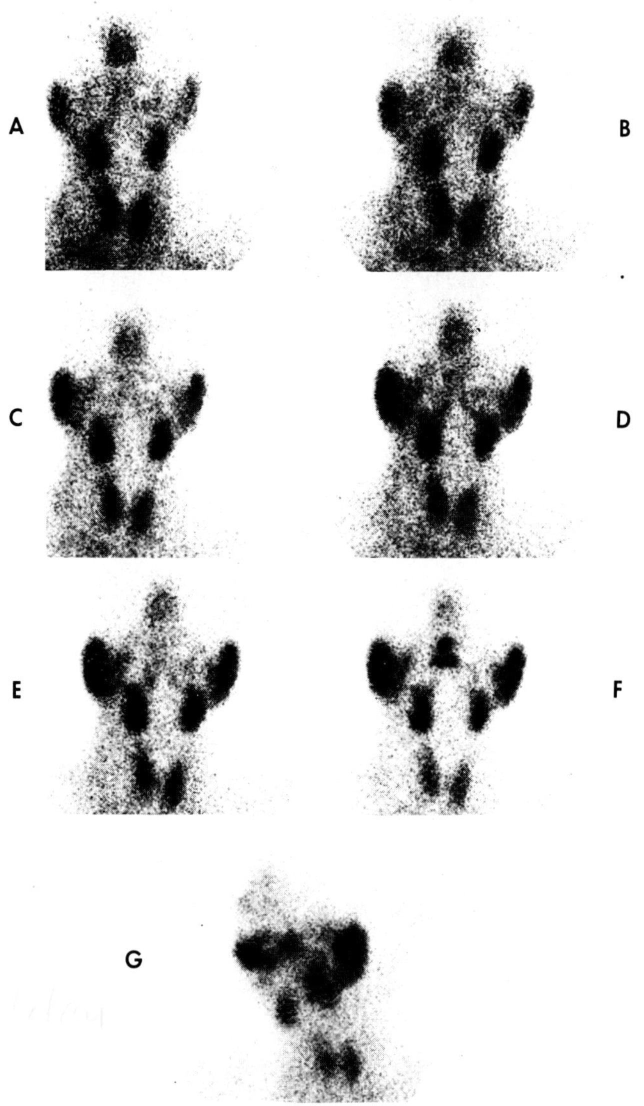

Fig. 34-4. Study performed with 10 mCi ^{99m}Tc pertechnetate administered intravenously. **A** to **F,** Sequential images (anterior view). Images reveal rapid uptake and discharge of pertechnetate from parotid-salivary tissue. There is a palpable 2-cm nodule in tail of right parotid, which is illustrated by a marker in **H** and **I.** The lesion has no function. **J** to **M,** Postperchlorate discharge images reveal slight retention of ^{99m}Tc in remaining portion of right parotid. This patient had carcinoma in tail of right parotid. *Continued.*

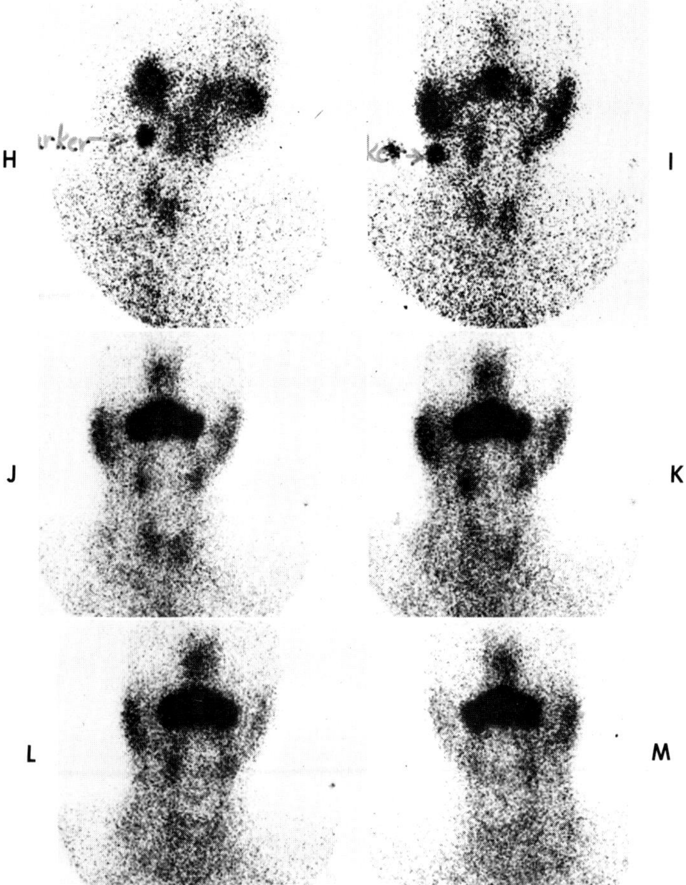

Fig. 34-4, cont'd. For legend see p. 807.

Class II—Patients' uptake dynamics may be normal with decreased concentration, uptake may be delayed with normal concentration, uptake may be delayed with normal concentration, or uptake may be diminished and delayed.

Class III—Patients reveal markedly delayed and diminished concentration with little oral activity.

Class IV—Patients reveal no parotid or salivary concentration.

Lymphomatous infiltration

Glands may have normal count rates with patchy areas of decreased concentration; with increasing infiltration, count rate decreases.

Mixed parotid tumors

There is a patchy decrease in activity in area of lesion; however, lesion may have normal or even increased count rate.

Warthin's tumor

There is increased concentration of nuclide with this tumor.

Metastatic lesions

Metastatic lesions are slightly ragged and space-occupying with absent activity.

Abscess

Abscesses are smooth and round, have an absence of activity, and are usually tender to palpation.

Cyst

Cysts are smooth and round, have an absence of activity, and are not tender.

Active concentration of ^{99m}Tc occurs in the parotid-salivary system within the first 19 minutes and becomes progressively concentrated over time. There is prompt excretion with visualization of the oral cavity between 20 and 40 minutes. At 1 hour the oral cavity is the "hottest" area.

The administration of potassium perchlorate 1 hour after administration of pertechnetate has added useful information to the salivary study. If there is no discharge of ^{99m}Tc from the salivary gland following administration of perchlorate, there has to be an element of ductal obstruction. This information is physiologic and may be masked by the catheterization technique of radiographic sialography.

■ LACRIMAL DUCT IMAGING

LABORATORY APPLICATION

87

PERFORMING A DACRYOCYSTOGRAM

Purpose

A simple noninvasive test for defining the patency of the lacrimal duct is accomplished with ^{99m}Tc pertechnetate dacryocystography. Functional obstruction can be visualized unlike the radiographic contrast study, in which the duct is catheterized.

Procedure

Materials

1. Scintillation camera with pinhole collimator and a 2-mm insert
2. ^{99m}Tc pertechnetate 200 μCi (6.4 MBq) per eye; this amount can be prepared by diluting 10 mCi (370 MBq) of ^{99m}Tc to 0.5 ml with normal saline solution; 10 drops in each eye delivers approximately 200 μCi (7.4 MBq)
3. Eye dropper

Patient preparation

1. No special preparation is required.
2. Explain the entire procedure to the patient.

Technique

1. Place the radioactive material in the form of drops, on the lower eyelid.
2. Quickly position the patient upright at a distance of 1.5 to 6.0 cm from camera. Distance depends on whether one or both eyes are to be imaged.
3. Perform 25,000-count images at the following times: immediately and 5, 10, and 15 minutes after administration of dose. Delayed images may be obtained, but lack of drainage 15 minutes after dose administration indicates blockage of the drainage system.

Interpretation (Fig. 34-5)

Normal images should show activity in the area of the nose in 10 to 15 minutes. The level of obstruction can be well demonstrated on images.

Continued.

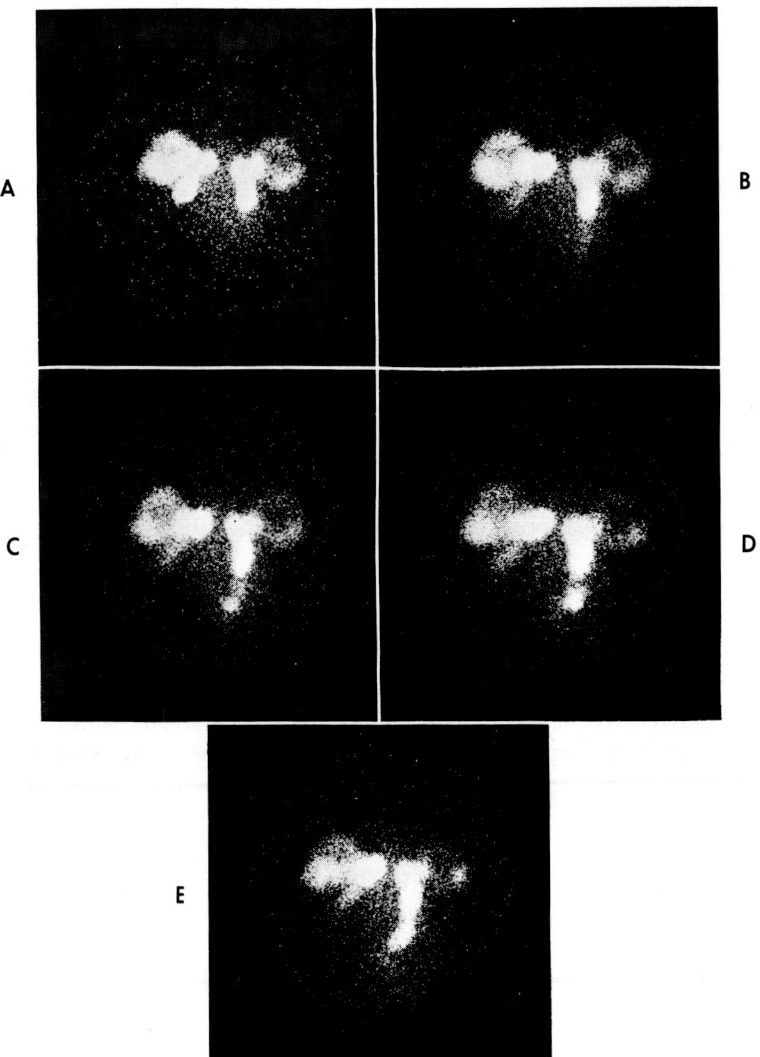

Fig. 34-5. Dacrocystography performed with 200 μCi of $^{99m}TcO^{-}_{4}$ per eye. **A** to **E,** Immediate views through view 15 minutes after installation of drops. Left eye drains normally with rapid visualization of nasal lacrimal duct. There is complete clearance at 15 minutes after dosage is administered. Examination of right eye reveals complete block of nasal lacrimal duct.

■ LYMPHATIC IMAGING

LABORATORY APPLICATION

88

DETECTION OF LYMPH NODE DISORDER/DISEASE

Purpose

The study is used to demonstrate the historeticular tissue of the retroperitoneal, axillary, parasternal, and cervical lymph nodes by interstitially administered radiocolloids. Because of their particle size, subcutaneously injected radiocolloids are transported by lymphatics. The most important factor for lymphatic transport is compression of lymphatic vessels by muscular contraction. Lymph node pathology causes diminished or absent flow or diminished and absent uptake of radiocolloids in nodal tissue.

Indications

1. For staging of known Hodgkin's disease
2. For study of diseases that involve nodal tissue (for example, lymphatic leukemia, and reticulum cell carcinoma)
3. For evaluation of lymphatic transport
4. To search for metastatic disease
5. For selection of endolymphatic radiotherapy

Procedure

Materials

1. Scintillation camera with high-resolution, 140-keV parallel-hole collimator
2. Imaging device and computer for data acquisition
3. ^{99m}Tc sulfur colloid (particle size between 0.2 and 0.5 micron), 0.5 to 1.0 mCi (18.5 to 37 MBq), in a volume not to exceed 0.25 ml per injection site
4. Tuberculin 1-ml syringe with 22-gauge needle

Patient preparation

1. Explain the entire procedure to the patient.
2. Place the patient in a supine position for the injections.
3. Areas to be visualized and injection sites are as follows:
   a. *Retroperitoneal lymph nodes.* Injection into medial two interdigital webs of the feet.
   b. *Axillary and apical lymph nodes.* Injection into medial two interdigital web of the hands.
   c. *Cervical lymph nodes.* Injection into dorsum of the processus mastoideus.
   d. *Internal mammary chain.* Injection into posterior rectus sheath below rib cage, angling toward the diaphragm (injection should be intramuscular (and not intraperitoneal) to obtain adequate visualization of the nodes).*
   e. *Iliopelvic lymph nodes.* Injection into perianal region just lateral to the anal margin at 3 o'clock and 9 o'clock. Patient should be in knee-to-chest position. Syringe should be parallel to the tabletop when injection is performed.†

Technique

1. Set camera for proper window (140 keV).
2. Prepare computer and photographic device for data acquisition.
3. Set proper orientation.
4. Press reset count and time.
5. Begin imaging as follows:
   a. *Retroperitoneal nodes* (including part of the liver). Imaging is begun 4 hours post injection. Position patient in supine position. Using the paralumbar lymph nodes as the focal area, take a 100,000-count view.
   b. *Axillary and apical nodes.* Imaging may be done 2 to 4 hours after injection. Position patient in supine position for upper chest and neck. Tilt chin back and secure patient's head. Take a 40,000-count view. For axillary image, flex arm at elbow and bring arm upward toward the head. Turn patient's face away from area being studied. Take a 40,000-count view.
   c. *Cervical nodes.* Imaging may be done 2 to 4 hours post injection. Position patient in supine position for anterior and anterior oblique views of the neck region. Take a 40,000-count view.
   d. *Internal mammary lymph nodes.* (Refer to article indicated under injection sites for complete procedure.)
   e. *Iliopelvic lymph nodes.* (Refer to article indicated under injection sites for complete procedures.)

*For detailed protocol, see Ege, G.N.: Lymphoscintigraphy—techniques and applications in the management of breast carcinoma, Semin. Nucl. Med. 13(1):26, 1983. Dufresne, E.N., and others: The application of internal mammary lymphoscintigraphy to planning of radiation therapy, J. Nucl. Med. 21(7):697, June 1980.
†For detailed protocol, see Kaplan, W.D.: Iliopelvic lymphoscintigraphy, Semin. Nucl. Med. 13(1):42, 1983.

Continued.

6. The count rate over the site of injection is very high in comparison with that of the lymph nodes. Do not set the image to this count rate, set the image away from the injection site.

Interpretation

Approximately 70% of the injected colloid is transported by the lymphatics. After 4 hours a chain of radioactivity can be seen on the image in the inguinal. iliac, and periaortic regions. Radioactivity is also accumulated in the liver in correspondance to the radiocolloid transported through the thoracic duct to the blood. Singular lymph nodes cannot be differentiated.

In the axillary and infraclavicular region the radioactivity is distributed in a circumscribed area.

Two to four lymph nodes are seen on each side of the internal mammary chain.

In the cervical area radioactivity is distributed as far as the supraclavicular region.

The image interpreter should take into consideration the normal variation of lymph nodes. Anatomic disturbances of flow can be detected by the radiocolloid technique more readily than the space-occupying lesions in nodes that may cause the shunting of flow. The images reveal physiologic or pathophysiologic lymphatic transport in contrast to x-ray lymphography. The direct infusion of a large amount of contrast media in x-ray lymphography opens up areas that may be occluded from normal lymphatic circulation.

For diagnosis one must pay attention to the following signs:

1. The continuity of the typical chain of activity (interruption through metastases, in postoperative states, or in physiologic variations).
2. The width of the iliac and paraaortic radioactive chain (enlargement through lymphoma or congestion by partial or total blockade of the lymphatics).
3. The intensity of the uptake (reduced in systemic diseases such as malignant lymphoma and increased through congestion and, in some cases, lymphadenitis).
4. The topographic distribution of the radioactivity (displacement of normal lymph nodes through metastases or collateral circulation of the lymphatics).
5. The radioactivity within the liver (missing in insufficient movement of the extremities or in lymphatic blockade).

This study is valuable in the preoperative evaluation of the expected lymph node drainage of tumors such as melanomas, where it is important to document expected or possible metastatic lymph node regions for radical surgery or external radiation therapy.

■ TUMOR IMAGING

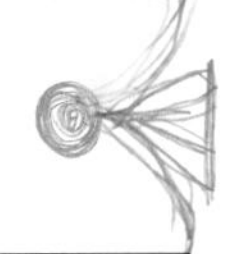

LABORATORY APPLICATION

89

TUMOR IMAGING WITH GALLIUM-67

Purpose

^{67}Ga citrate imaging is a widely used procedure to aid the physician in demonstrating specific primary carcinomas and their metastatic sites, as well as to localize, stage, and follow-up inflammatory disease states. In the majority of instances the gallium image is used as a correlative procedure with CT, ultrasonography, standard x-ray study, and magnetic resonance imaging.

^{67}Ga imaging has been found to be efficacious in a few histologic types of cancer. These include bronchogenic carcinoma, Hodgkin's and non-Hodgkin's lymphoma, and in primary hepatomas. The concentration of gallium may be found in other tumor types but with low specificity and sensitivity.

Indications

Staging and post therapy imaging in:

1. Lung carcinoma
2. Hodgkin's disease
3. Non-Hodgkin's lymphoma
4. Hepatocellular carcinoma

5. Melanoma
6. Leukemia

Procedure

Materials

1. Large field-of-view camera with medium energy collimator for the 184 and 296 keV energy emissions of gallium-67, and SPECT capability.
2. 5 to 10 mCi (185 to 370 MBq) ^{67}Ga citrate.

Patient preparation

1. Intravenously inject 5 to 10 mCi (185-370 MBq) ^{67}Ga. Imaging is begun 72 hours post-injection.
2. If the area of interest is in the abdomen, the patient should have cleansing enemas the day before and the morning of the examination.
3. Explain the entire procedure to the patient.

Technique

1. Whole body planar imaging is routine unless a limited exam is requested.
2. SPECT capability is desirable and frequently performed for better localization or identification of a region of abnormal uptake. (If SPECT is anticipated, a higher dose of gallium is desirable.)
3. Imaging is performed using medium energy collimation for the 184 and 296 keV energy emissions of gallium-67.
4. Windows of 25% around those peaks are set.
5. Images are acquired for 1000k counts, anteriorly and posteriorly to include the head, chest, abdomen, pelvis and extremities, as warranted.
6. If multihead detector equipment or scanning whole body table detector arrangements are available, the study time can be reduced.

Image diagnosis

Malignant tissue has an affinity for ^{67}Ga, therefore small lymph nodes involved with malignancy can be visualized well on whole body images but particularly well on high contrast SPECT images. On CT scans lymph nodes larger than 1 cm will be called abnormal; however, the ^{67}Ga images will visualize less than 1 cm nodes that are involved with malignancy. The ^{67}Ga study is well suited for the evaluation of patients before and after radiation or chemotherapy to determine therapy effect on the malignant tissue.

LABORATORY APPLICATION

90

TUMOR IMAGING WITH THALLIUM-201 AND TECHNETIUM-99m SESTAMIBI

Purpose

Thallium-201 localizes in malignant breast tissue and in metastatic breast carcinomatous sites. In many instances^{99m}Tc sestimibi has shown predeliction to concentrate in the same abnormal sites as ^{201}Tl with obvious improvement in count rate.

Procedure

Materials

1. 3 mCi(111 MBq) ^{201}Tl or 25 mCi (925 MBq) ^{99m}Tc sestimibi, administered intravenously.
2. Cobalt markers.
3. Scintillation camera with low energy high resolution collimator.
4. Low energy GAP collimator.

Patient preparation

1. None.
2. Explain entire procedure to the patient.

Continued.

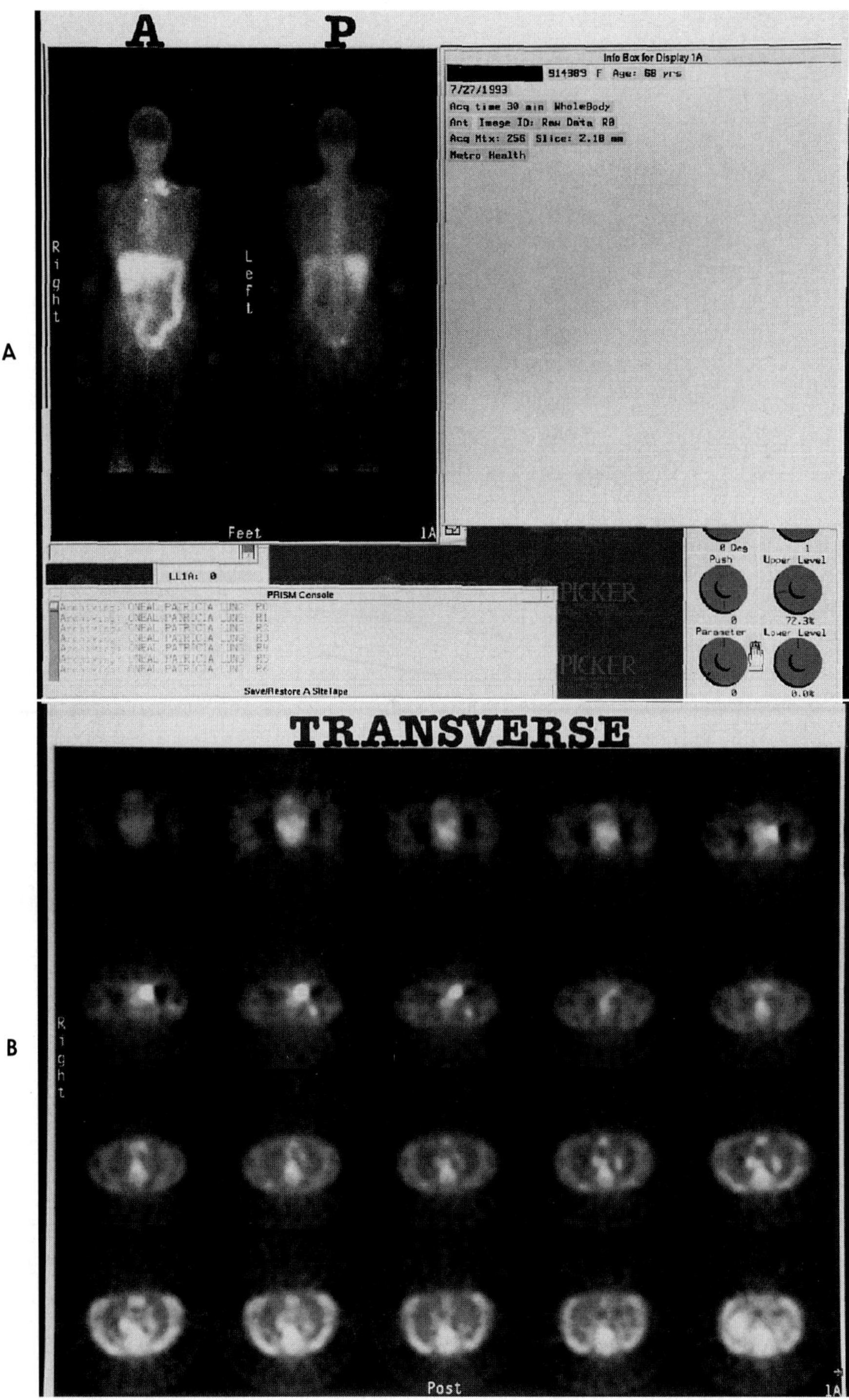

Fig. 34-6. This 68-year-old male presented with weight loss and palpable lymph nodes in the left supra-clavicular lymph node region. Biopsy revealed non-Hodgkin's lymphoma. CT scan identified the supraclavicular nodes, but the chest was normal. **A,** Whole-body images 48 hours post-administration intravenously of 5 mCi gallium-67 reveal the irregular increase in concentration in the left supraclavicular region, but also reveal an increase in both hilar regions. **B,** Transverse, **C,** sagittal, and **D,** coronal SPECT images reveal the marked involvement of the left supraclavicular region and further involvement beneath the left scapula and in the perihilar region bilaterally.

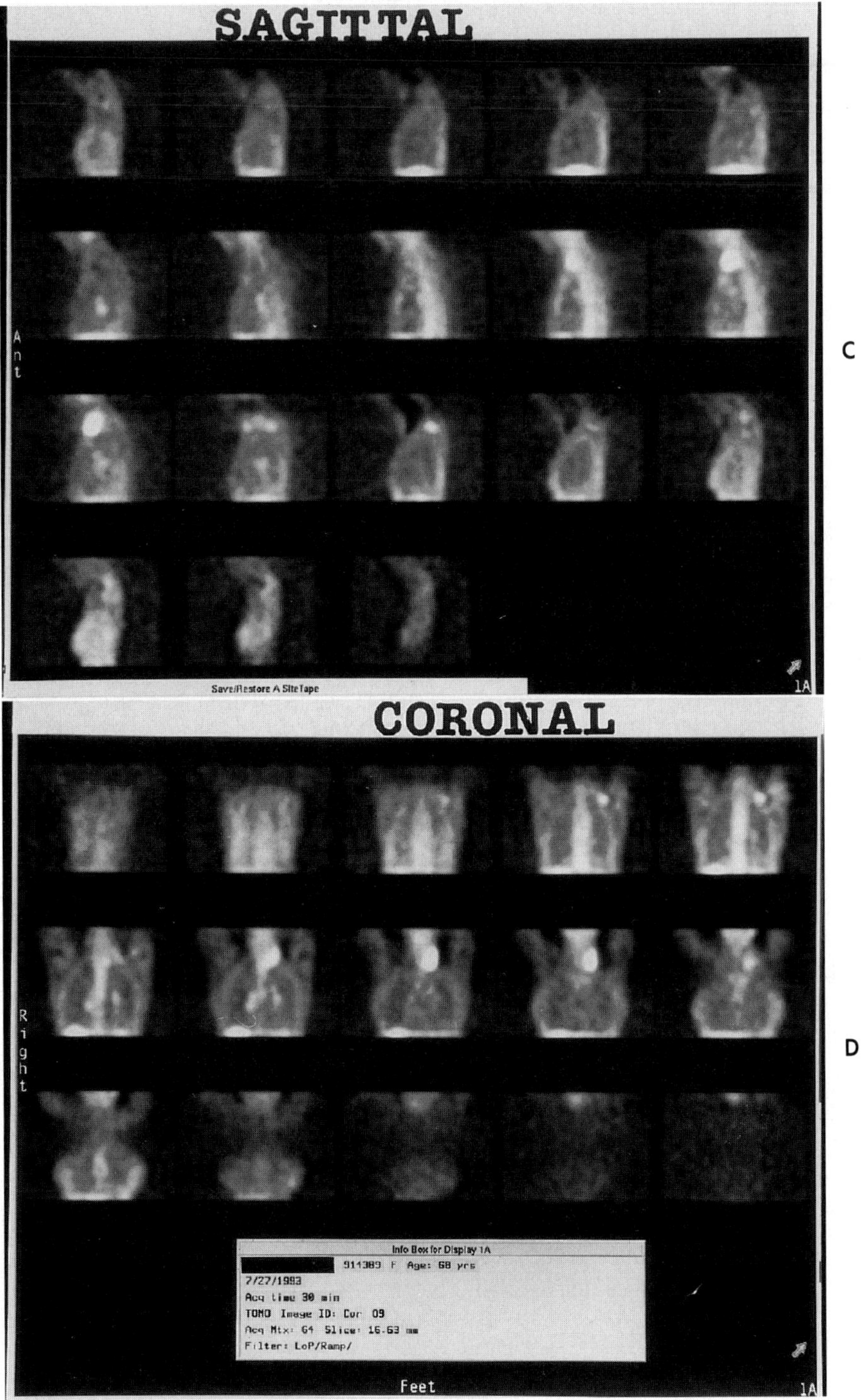

Fig. 34-6, cont'd. For legend see p. 814.

Continued.

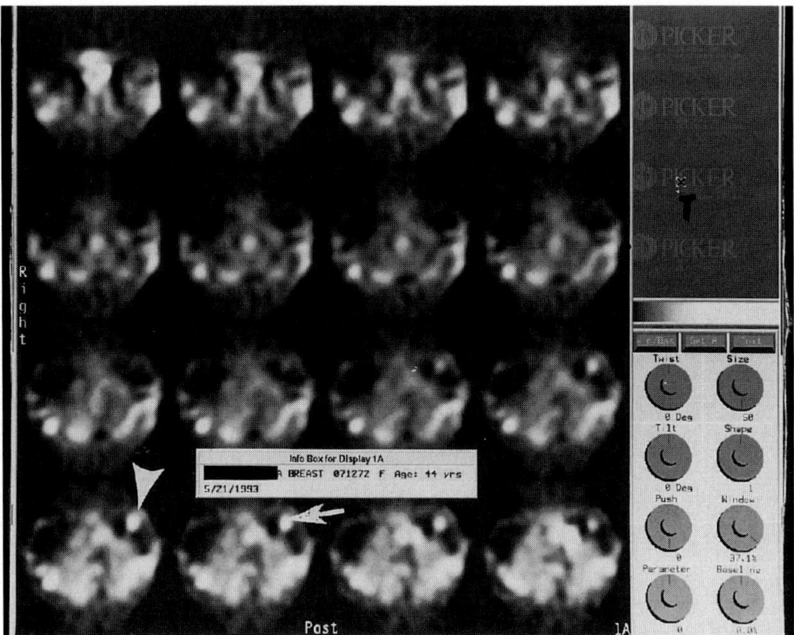

Fig. 34-7. A 44-year-old female with a newly palpable mass in the left breast. Mammography revealed a 1.8 cm slightly irregular mass in the left breast without microcalcification. Transverse SPECT sestimibi (25 mCi) images reveals marked concentration of nuclide in an ovoid lesion that appears to infiltrate the subcutaneous tissue overlying the lesions.

Technique: static imaging

1. Begin imaging 20 minutes post-injection.
2. Set camera for ^{201}Tl peak (80 keV) or ^{99m}Tc (140 keV).
3. Perform 1000k images over affected area with several views.

Technique: whole-body imaging

1. Begin imaging 20 minutes post-injection.
2. Set camera for ^{201}Tl peak (80 keV) or ^{99m}Tc (140 keV).
3. Perform 20 to 25 minute anterior and posterior whole-body images.

Technique: SPECT imaging

1. Preferably perform a continuous rotation (16 minutes via 4 rotations).
2. Perform a test orbit to ensure that no part of the patient touches the collimator.
3. If the area of interest is the brain, adjust the table height to ensure that all of the patient's head is included. Fan beam collimators are recommended.

Processing SPECT images

1. *Transverse reconstruction*—adjust reconstruction diameter as needed.
2. 3D post-filter—Try several different filters for best image.
3. Change slice thickness to 2 before you reconstruct the sagittal and coronal slices.

Technique: static breast imaging

1. Place patient in supine position and inject in the opposite arm of the affected breast.
2. With triple-head camera place one camera head in the anterior position and the other two heads in the oblique positions.
3. Inject patient intravenously with either 3 mCi ^{201}Tl or 25 mCi ^{99m}Tc sestimibi.
4. The arms should be over the patient's head. Include in the field of view the axillae and the breast. Compress with the anterior camera head.

5. Begin imaging 2 minutes post-dose and take 2 to 10 minute acquisitions.
6. Perform RAO and LAO views of the affected breast and axilla. Repeat these views for 2 minutes each with marker on suspected mass and nipple.
7. If needed, tape the breasts to avoid superimposition on liver or heart.

Image diagnosis

Preliminary work utilizing thallium-201 in breast carcinoma has a 96% sensitivity and no false positive results were obtained. There may be a place in the future for the radionuclide breast image, because mammography is not reliable in the dense or dysplastic breast and the negative mammogram may cause a delay in biopsy of the patient who is later shown to have carcinoma of the breast.

Thallium-201 and technetium-99m sestimibi have been shown to be efficatious in localizing many malignancies. These radionuclides have been extremely useful in finding malignant brain tumors with metabolically active remnants following radiation therapy. CT and MRI have been unable to differentiate remaining viable tumor from radiation effects in brain tissue.

BIBLIOGRAPHY

Testicular imaging

Chen, D.C.P., and others: Radionuclide scrotal imaging: further experience with 210 patients. I. Anatomy, pathophysiology, and methods, J. Nucl. Med. 24:735, 1983.

Clinical Nuclear Medicine Updates for Referring Physicians: Radionuclide scrotal imaging, Central Chapter of the Society of Nuclear Medicine, Aug. 1987.

Donoghue, G.D., and others: Early diagnosis of testicular tumor using Tc-99m pertechnetate scrotal imaging, Clin. Nucl. Med. 8(12):630, 1983.

Dunn, E.K., and others: Testicular scintigraphic findings two to three months after torsion: correlation with sonography and histopathology, Clin. Nucl. Med. 16(1):37-39, 1991.

Fenner, M.N., Roszhart, D.A., and Texter, J.H. Jr.: Testicular scanning: evaluating the acute scrotum in the clinical setting, Urology 38(3):237-241, 1991.

Haynes, B.E., and others: The diagnosis of testicular torson, JAMA 249:2522, 1983.

Heck, L.: Scrotal imaging. In Beckerman, C., and others, editors: Manual of pediatric and unusual nuclear medicine procedures, Crystal Lake, Ill., Central Chapter, of the Society of Nuclear Medicine.

Lutzker, L.G., and Zuckier, L.S.: Testicular scanning and other applications of radionuclide imaging of the genital tract, Semin. Nucl. Med. 20(2):159-188, 1990.

McCormack, J.L.: Radionuclide testicular scanning, J. Med. Soc. NJ 81(3):190, 1984.

Melton, J.W., Chung, C.J., and Gordon, L.: Pseudobullseye sign of the testicle: a window to the peritoneum, Clin. Nucl. Med. 16(8):604-605, 1991.

Middleton, W.D., and others: Acute scrotal disorders: prospective comparison of color Dopper US and testicular scintigraphy, Radiology 177(1):177-181, 1990.

Nakielny, R.A., and others: Radionuclide evaluation of acute scrotal disease, Clin. Radiol. 35(2):125, 1984.

Patel, B.R.: Radiological Seminar CCXLII: Role of scintigraphy and ultrasound in evaluation of scrotal mass, J. Miss. State Med. Assoc. 26(3):61, 1985.

Sty, J.R., and Starshak, R.J.: Tc-99m MDP scrotal image: testicular amyloidosis, Clin. Nucl. Med. 8(3):142, 1983.

Wasnick, R.J., and others: Testicular torsion and usefulness of radionuclide scanning, Urology 15:318, 1980.

Wise, P.A., and others: Scrotal scintigraphy: a review of 42 cases, Del. Med. J. 55(7):421, 1983.

Salivary gland imaging

Abd El Salam, Z.: Scanning of the major salivary glands by using scintigraphy after radiotherapy, Egyptian Dental Journal 35(4):347-358, 1989.

Becker, W., and others: Stimulated salivary clearance of technetium-99m pertechnetate (letter), J. Nucl. Med. 27(2):306, 1986.

Blue, P.W.: Failure of washout following gustatory stimulation in Warthin's tumour, Nucl. Med. Commun. 9(6):431, 1988.

Chaudhuri, T.K., and Stadalnik, R.C.: Salivary gland imaging, Semin. Nucl. Med. 10(4):400, 1980.

Chisin, R., and others: The clinical value of quantitative dynamic scintigraphy in salivary gland disorders, Int. J. Radiol. Appl. Instrum. (B) 15(3):313, 1988.

Clinical Nuclear Medicine Updates for Referring Physicians: Radionuclide salivary gland imaging, Central Chapter of the Society of Nuclear Medicine, Aug. 1987.

Copley, D.J., and Smith, R.: Salivary scintigraphy: decreased activity, Semin. Nucl. Med. 16(3):220, 1986.

Copley, D.J., and Smith, R.: Salivary scintigraphy: unilateral increased activity, Semin. Nucl. Med. 16(3):222, 1986.

Fossaluzza, V., DeVita, S., and Geatti, D.: Sequential salivary scintigraphy in Sjogren's syndrome: proposal for a new method of evaluation, Clin. Exp. Rheumatol. 8(5):469-474, 1990.

Hardoff, R., and Nachtigal, D.: Unilateral gallium-67 uptake in submandibular salivary gland following sialography, Clin. Nucl. Med. 14(1):65, 1989.

Kohn, W.G. and others: Salivary gland ^{99m}Tc-scintigraphy: a grading scale and correlation with major salivary gland flow rates, J. Oral Pathol. Med. 21(2):70-74, 1992.

Kosuda, S., and others: Radionuclide imaging for parotid oncocytoma, Clin. Nucl. Med. 12(2):150, 1987.

Luyk, N.H., Doyle, T., and Ferguson, M.M.: Recent trends in imaging the salivary glands, Dentomaxillofac. Radiol. 20(1):3-10, 1991.

Nakamura, T., and others: Salivary SPECT and factor analysis in Sjogren's syndrome, Acta Radiologica 32(5):406-410, 1991.Schroeder, B.A., and others: Salivary gland scintigraphy: cystic hydroma of the parotid, Clin. Nucl. Med. 12(6):485, 1987.

Siddiqui, A.R., and Weisberger, E.C.: Possible explanation of appearance of Warthin's tumor on I-123 and Tc-99m-pertechnetate scans, Clin. Nucl. Med. 6(6):258, 1981.

Singh, A.: Impaired trapping of Tc-99m pertechnetate in the salivary glands of patients with congenital hypothyroidism, Clin. Nucl. Med. 15(4):257-259, 1990.

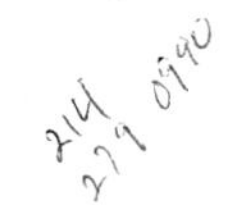

Sostre, S., and others: The various scintigraphic patterns of Warthin's tumor, Clin. Nucl. Med. 12(Aug.):620, 1987.

Sugihara, T., and Yoshimura, Y.: Scintigraphic evaluation of the salivary glands in patients with Sjorgren's syndrome, Int. J. Oral Maxillofac. Surg. 17(2):71, 1988.

Sulavik, S.B., spencer, R.P., and Castriotta, R.J.: Panda sign-avid and symmetrical radiogallium accumulation in the lacrimal and parotid glands, Semin. Nucl. Med. 21(4):339-340, 1991.

Wells, R.G., and others: Radionuclide angiography, Parotid hemangioma, Clin. Nucl. Med. 10(8):599, 1985.

Yamauchi, K., and others: Gallium-67 uptake in the salivary glands in chronic graft-versus-host disease after bone marrow transplantation, Clin. Nucl. Med. 14(5):330-332, 1989.

Yang, D.C., and others: Demonstration of parotid maxillary sinus nasal fistula by radionuclide salivary imaging, Clin. Nucl. Med. 12(5):411, 1987.

Dacryocystogram

Carlton, W.H., Trueblood, J.H., and Rossomondo, R.M.: Clinical evaluation of microscintigraphy of the lacrimal drainage apparatus. J. Nucl. Med. 14:89, 1973.

Chaudhuri, T.K.: Clinical evaluation of nuclear dacryocystography, Clin. Nucl. Med. 1:83, 1976.

Chaudhuri, T.K.: Nuclear dacryocystography, Appl. Radiol. 4:127, 1975.

Chaudhuri, T.K.: Technical aspects of nuclear dacryocystography, Appl. Radiol. 4:184, 1975.

Daubert, J., and others: Tear flow analysis through the upper and lower systems, Ophthal. Plast. Reconst. Surg. 6(3):193-196, 1990.

Denffer, H.V., and others: Lacrimal dacryoscintigraphy, Semin. Nucl. Med. 14(1):8, 1984.

Kadambi, V., and Williams, B.V.: Functional integrity of lacrimal drainage apparatus by radionuclide dacryocystography, Indian J. Ophthalmology 38(1):24-26, 1990.

Kim, C.K., and others: Serial dacryoscintigraphy before and after treatment with pseudoephedrine, Clin. Nucl. Med. 14(10):734-735, 1989.

Nixon, J., Birchall, I.W., and Virjee, J.: The role of dacryosystography in the management of patients with epiphora, British J. Radiol. 63(749):337-339, 1990.

Villaneuva-Meyer, J., and others: Lacrimal gland dosimetry for the brain imaging agent technetium-99m-HMPAO, J. Nucl. Med. 31(7):1237-1239, 1990.

Weir, J.: Radionuclide dacryocystography. In Beckerman, C., and others, editors: Manual of pediatric and unusual nuclear medicine procedures, Crystal lake, Ill., Central Chapter of the Society of Nuclear Medicine.

Lymphatic imaging

Aikou, T., and others: Lymph drainage originating from the lower esophagus and gastric cardia as measured by radioisotope uptake in the regional lymph nodes following lymphoscintigraphy, Lymphology 20(3):145, 1987.

Baulieu, F., and others: Visualization of the thoracic duct by lymphoscintigraphy, Eur. J. Nucl. Med. 13(5):264, 1987.

Dufresne, E.N., and others: The application of internal mammary lymphoscintigraphy to planning of radiation therapy, J. Nucl. Med. 21(7):697, June 1980.

Eberbach, M.A., and others: Utility of lymphoscintigraphy in directing surgical therapy for melanomas of the head, neck, and upper thorax, Surgery 102(3):433, 1987.

Ege, G.N.: Lymphoscintigraphy—techniques and applications in the management of breast carcinoma, Semin. Nucl. Med. 13(1):26, 1983.

Ege, G.N.: Radionuclide lymphoscintigraphy in neoplastic disease, Cancer Res. 40:3065, 1980.

Ege, G.N., and Clark, R.M.: Internal mammary lymphoscintigraphy in the conservative management of breast carcinoma, Clin. Radiol. 31:559, 1980.

Freeman, L.M., and Blaufox, M.D., editors: Interstitial lymphoscintigraphy, Semin. Nucl. Med. 13(1):(entire issue), 1983.

Gasparini, M., and others: Lack of efficacy of lymphoscintigraphy in detecting axillary lymph node metastases from breast cancer, Eur. J. Cancer Clin. Oncol., 23(5):475, 1987.

Gregg, D.C., and others: Lymphoscintigraphy: chylous ascites and lymphocele demonstration, Clin. Nucl. Med. 13(4):300, 1988.

Henze, E., and others: Lymphoscintigraphy with Tc-99m labeled dextran, J. Nucl. Med. 23:923, 1982.

Kaplan, W.D., and others: Iliopelvic radionuclide lymphoscintigraphy in patients with testicular cancer, Radiology 147(1):231, 1983.

Kaplan, W.D., and others: Mediastinal lymphoscintigraphy in ovarian cancer using intraperitoneal autologous Tc-99m labeled erythrocytes, Br. J. Radiol. 54:126, 1981.

Kaplan, W.D.: Iliopelvic lymphoscintigraphy, Semin. Nucl. Med. 13(1):42, 1983.

Karayalcin, B., and others: Parasternal lymphoscintigraphy using ^{99m}Tcm-dextran, Nucl. Med. Commun. 9(9):657, 1988.

Keenan, A.M., and others: Immunolymphoscintigraphy in patients with lymphoma after subcutaneous injection of indium-111-labeled T101 monoclonal antibody, J. Nucl. Med., 18(1):42, 1987.

Kontturi, M., and others: Radioimaging of lymph node involvement in prostatic carcinoma, Scand. J. Urol. Nephrol. Suppl. 110:1137, 1988.

Kramer, E.L., and others: The impact of intradermal lymphoscintigraphy on surgical management of clinical state I truncal malignant melanoma, J. Dermatol. Surg. Oncol. 13(5):508, 1987.

Mulshine, J.L., and others: Immunolymphoscintigraphy of pulmonary and mediastinal lymph nodes in dogs: a new approach to lung cancer imaging, Cancer Res. 47(13):3571, 1987.

Pettit, J., and Sawczuk, I.S.: Use of lymphoscintigraphy in chyluria, Urology 32(4):367, 1988.

Reicht, A., and others: Three-dimensional internal mammary lymphoscintigraphy: implications for radiation therapy treatment planning for breast carcinoma, Int. J. Radiat. Oncol. Biol. Phys. 14(3):477, 1988.

Sullivan, D.C., and others: Lymphoscintigraphy in malignant melanoma: Tc-99m antimony sulfur colloid, Am. J. Roentgenol. 137:847, 1981.

Wahl, R.L., and others: Radiolabeled antibodies, albumin and antimony sulfide colloid: a comparison as lymphoscintigraphic agents, Int. J. Rad. Appl. Instrum.(B), 15(3):243, 1988.

Weissleder, H., and Weissleder, R.: Lymphedema: evaluation of qualitative and quantitative lymphoscintigraphy in 238 patients, Radiology 167(3):729, 1988.

Tumor imaging

Sehweil, A.M., and others: Mechanism of ^{201}Tl uptake in tumors, Eur. J. Nucl. Med. 15(7):376, 1989.

Waxman, A.D.: Use of thallium-201 in tumor evaluation, West. J. of Med. 157(1):60, 1992.

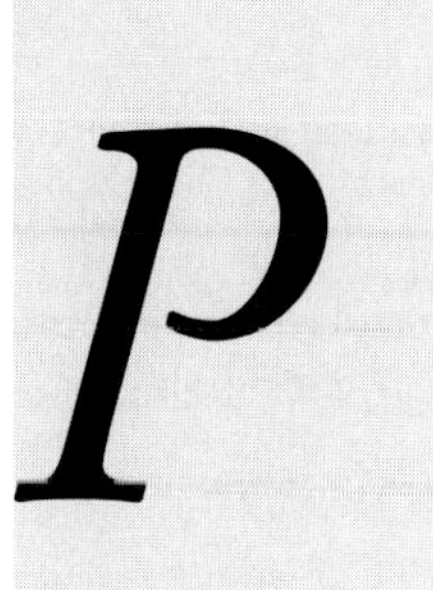

Chapter 35

RINCIPLES OF MANAGEMENT

JOHN H. BAUGHMAN

This chapter is designed to help chief technologists or managers in nuclear medicine departments better understand their roles as health-care leaders. For student technologists, this discussion should provide a better insight of what good managers must consider when developing and implementing plans and overseeing operations. Attention will be focused on planning, decision-making, organization, personnel management, leadership, and quality control of a nuclear medicine department. It is important for the reader to understand that this chapter is not designed to replace management texts, but rather to introduce important techniques in practical terms.

The need for improved management in health care was intensified through the government implementation of Diagnostic Related Groups (DRGs). When third-party insurers adopted similar reimbursement policies, hospitals rapidly recognized the need to improve efficiency and productivity in order to survive. These external pressures have challenged health-care providers to look for ways to cut costs without sacrificing quality patient care.

In an effort to increase efficiency and productivity in ancillary departments such as nuclear medicine, administrators now expect managers to be involved in the development and implementation of strategic plans. This in turn places greater responsibility and accountability directly on the manager and influences how he or she will staff the department, care for supplies, provide patient services, and plan for both operational and capital budgets. For managers to adapt to these new challenges, they must gain confidence through understanding basic management techniques, which in turn will enable greater productivity from both equipment and employees.

In the past, a chief technologist's primary duties were to oversee employee schedules and work loads, maintain orderly NRC records and keep radiopharmaceuticals in stock. These important duties now comprise only part of the chief technologist's responsibilities, which have been expanded to include development and implementation of productivity programs, understanding operating and capital budgets and, in all cases, being held accountable for expenditures and revenues generated by the nuclear medicine department.

While chief technologists/managers work in this type of environment, they should consider their role as a manager and what is expected to get this job done on a daily basis. The following sections will provide some of the answers to these basic questions.

■ PRINCIPLES OF EFFECTIVE MANAGEMENT

We live in a dynamic and demanding society, and we in the health-care field often find ourselves hurriedly performing routine duties and functions without stopping to find out why. A manager must question the operational steps of the management process and break it down into its basic parts. The process of management is, very simply, "getting things done through the use of people and other resources." To succeed, a manager must first separate activities into two main categories: doing and thinking. In some cases, the chief technologist who has had several years of technical experience can fall into the trap of spending too much time "doing" (in a technical sense) and not enough time "thinking" (in the management process). For effective management, the following six basic principles should be reviewed on a daily basis:

1. *Planning*—The process of setting goals and objectives for future operations, and developing a means to accomplish these goals and objectives.
2. *Decision making*—A critical function every health-care manager performs according to the level of authority in a given organization.
3. *Organization*—The process of coordinating employee activities so that goals and objectives are reached in an efficient and timely manner.
4. *Personnel management*—The process of assessing manpower needs, recruiting personnel, screening po-

tential employees, and educating those chosen for given positions.

5. *Leadership*—A people-oriented function that focuses on getting the job done in the organization. Activities include leading, motivating, communicating, and delegating. This is where a manager becomes a leader.
6. *Quality control*—A monitoring process that includes establishing measurable performance standards, scheduled evaluations, and systems for taking corrective action. One of the most important aspects of this system is *feedback and the timeliness of responding to this feedback*.

■ PLANNING

Careful planning is essential for the smooth operation of a department. Developing a defined, systematic approach to a given idea or project will greatly reduce your risks while increasing your chances for success. Because your plan is the road map that will take you to your goal, planning should precede all other management functions. A manager's success depends on the ability to think ahead.

A manager who plans for the future makes things happen efficiently and effectively. This individual is usually innovative. Rather than waiting for problems to dictate actions, a good planner anticipates problems and views them as opportunities to identify new and better ways to reach the organization's short-term and long-term goals. Goals and objectives are the steps by which an organization accomplishes its overall purpose or mission. In addition, a good planner gives consideration to forecasting the future and has the flexibility to quickly develop an alternative plan of action, reacting positively if circumstances change or the organization's objectives are suddenly altered because of internal or external influences. As an organization's goals and objectives are developed and announced, the nuclear medicine manager must plan the steps necessary to reach them. By successfully executing his stated plan, the manager demonstrates the ability to analyze current conditions, anticipate needs for the future, and make concrete decisions based on the information provided by senior management. In the planning process, a manager should consider these basic principles:

1. Obtain proper information from both superiors and subordinates.
2. Plan flexibly to allow for changes in working environment.
3. Include subordinates in planning. This keeps them informed and makes changes less traumatic.
4. Review plans in conjunction with goals and objectives.
5. Put plans in writing and in terms that others can understand.
6. Have specific target dates and meet the deadlines.
7. Establish a means of monitoring and controlling the newly implemented plan. Be ready to adjust as necessary.

■ DECISION MAKING

By developing good planning techniques, a manager is better able to make decisions in a proactive manner. As a manager investigates a situation needing a resolution, it is important that every alternative be considered during the decision-making process. For example, if considering purchase of new equipment, the following questions should be answered: Does the equipment need to be replaced? Can the equipment be replaced at a later time? Can another piece of equipment do the job? What kind of equipment should replace the old unit? Only after careful analysis of all information can the manager decide on the best alternative. In order to make the decision, the manager follows five steps in the problem/situation solving process:

1. Identify and define the problem.
2. Determine all possible solutions/alternatives.
3. Select the best possible solution.
4. Implement new solution.
5. Monitor results.

■ Identifying and defining the problem

Managers must collect data to correctly identify the problem. Many times it is easy to confuse the primary problem with secondary symptoms surrounding it. It is important for the manager to separate these two areas as rapidly as possible to target and treat both areas effectively.

■ Determining all possible solutions/alternatives

Once the two areas are identified, various possible solutions can be generated. Careful consideration by the manager will prepare them to make a final decision, which should be sensitive both to their own staff and to others working in the same system who might be influenced by it.

■ Selecting the best possible solution

After the manager reviews all possible alternatives, a decision must be made. This may be an independent decision or may involve several people, depending on the manager's style and the issue under consideration. Once the preferred solution is selected, it should be implemented promptly and confidently.

■ Implementation of new solution

Once the manager makes a decision, total commitment must be conveyed to the individuals involved. This same commitment should be conveyed when the decision is announced and implemented. A good manager will have already involved others in the decision-making process, when appropriate, and can anticipate support. Therefore, there are no surprises to those involved when the solution is implemented.

■ Monitoring results

The last step involves monitoring the effectiveness of the solution. This monitoring process gives the manager feedback on the effects of his decision, which indicate whether the decision was good or bad. In the event a wrong decision was made, it is important to admit to an error, reevaluate the situation, then move on to an alternative plan. Employees have a higher regard for managers who admit to their errors—normally the admitted mistakes will pass with time.

■ THE DECISION-MAKING PROCESS

An example of the decision-making process might go as follows:

- The chief technologist identifies the need to purchase an additional gamma camera because of increased patient volume.
- The data supporting the need for the additional gamma camera is passed to the chief technologist's supervisor, with the recommendation to purchase this new equipment.
- Additional information such as price, financial arrangements, adequate space, power requirements, and the need for air conditioning are then assessed.
- Data are collected from representative companies to be shared with the physicians and technical staff, and specific feedback is sought to help determine the appropriate equipment for purchase.
- Assuming space needs are adequate and the equipment falls within the capital budget, arrangements are then made to purchase the equipment.
- Before delivery, appropriate training is arranged for both technical and medical staff.
- As training is completed and the new equipment has become a functional unit within the standards set by the department, scheduling of patients can begin.
- Monitoring of this process should be ongoing. The chief technologist should be prepared to identify problem areas as they arise and make the appropriate adjustments as needed to keep the project on schedule.

The planning process can be approached in various ways, depending on the project and the manager's style. As indicated earlier, the key is for the manager to plan creatively, implement confidently, and monitor constantly. It becomes obvious with experience that these three management functions interact freely as the manager performs his or her duties.

■ ORGANIZATION

Organizing is the process of coordinating employee and department activities to ensure that an organization's goals and objectives are reached in a timely and effective manner. This extension of the planning function can also be defined as organizing the systematic use of available resources; namely, employees, equipment, and supplies. This is normally started when the organization states its mission, organizational philosophy, and purpose.

Generally, guidelines will be provided to department managers for use in writing their own goals and objectives so they support the overall goals of the mission statement. As managers define goals, they must take into consideration both long-term and short-term pursuits ("long-term" extending beyond the current fiscal year, and "short-term" to be accomplished before year's end). As the goals and objectives are better defined, the department will develop a strategy to achieve them. It is important for the manager to understand the overall organization mission to ensure that plans are carried out appropriately. Thus, the manager becomes a catalyst interacting with the staff, enabling them to work efficiently with patients and accomplish department goals/objectives at the same time.

To succeed in this process, a manager must establish clear lines of authority, responsibility, division of work flow, and a strong feedback system. This can be done through some degree of departmentalization, which will vary depending on the size of the nuclear medicine department. Larger departments may ask senior staff members to oversee the operation and function of other employees. In smaller departments, all supervision may be delegated to the chief technologist or manager. In either case, there is a need for assigning duties and coordinating efforts to ensure that the department runs smoothly. Means of accomplishing these activities will be discussed in further detail in the Personnel Management Leadership, and Quality Control sections of this chapter.

■ PERSONNEL MANAGEMENT

Manpower utilization is a key factor in running a cost-efficient nuclear medicine department. Labor expense (salaries and benefits) is usually one of the larger expenditures a department will face each year. It is also an area in which a good manager can constantly fine-tune the efficiency of the department. Carefully reassessing staffing needs is critical when going through the annual budgeting process. If the manager oversees a large department, areas such as employee mix (full-time employees [FTE] versus part-time employees [PTE]) can be adjusted to reduce expenses.

Once needs are determined, the manager can begin recruiting, keeping in mind current and future budget restraints as well as the department's goals and objectives. During the interviewing process, a job description should be provided to the technologist or support personnel. The manager should explain job duties and expectations in detail to the candidate. It is important to ask candidates to describe themselves and their abilities as a future employee. This gives the manager insight into how much a candidate can contribute to the job. In addition, it helps the manager determine how well this individual works with others. Anticipating personality conflicts is important since personnel problems are always very time-consuming and nonproductive. Communication and interaction should be given a high priority by managers. These factors alone can make the difference between an efficient operation and an inefficient one.

When an employee is hired, it is important to acquaint the individual with the departmental routine as quickly as possible. This helps the employee feel more at ease in becoming a part of the nuclear medicine team. This training can be accomplished in several different manners:

1. One-on-One. The new employee can be assigned to a responsible individual to start the in-service program. Best results will be obtained if the instructor is a supervisor or has equivalent abilities.
2. Lectures. This method can be used to give the new employee needed background information concerning department operations.
3. Informal Program Instruction. This can be done by viewing videotapes or by reading policy and procedure manuals, allowing the employee to work at his own pace.
4. On-the-Job Training. This is probably the best method available, considering the nuclear medicine technologist already has a formal education. This can be accomplished in a one-on-one atmosphere or in a group setting.

The manager should adapt his or her approach, depending on the size of the department, to the personality and training requirements of the new employee. The objective is to train the employee to the point at which he or she feels challenged by his new position without being intimidated, thereby creating a productive member of the nuclear medicine team.

During the training period, every new employee should be given an opportunity to read and discuss departmental and organizational policies and procedures, specifically emphasizing the section on "Disciplinary Action." Every organization has performance guidelines developed by the human resources or personnel department. Discipline, defined as the process of modifying behavior, is usually accomplished by some type of reprimand. Most guidelines recommend that discipline be given immediately and directed toward the *actions* of the employee. Equally important, discipline should be consistent for all employees. A manager who disciplines fairly and discreetly will be respected by the staff. Often, discipline becomes an effective means of reinforcing policy and demonstrating that appropriate and fair action does occur within the system. Having accomplished the above, a manager will know that the employees clearly understand what is expected of them on their jobs. Equally important is the need to compliment the new employee when he or she performs well.

■ LEADERSHIP

Types of managers vary as widely as the types of employees they manage. As discussed earlier, management is the process of getting things done through the use of human resources. The methods a manager uses to accomplish these goals are his "style." Douglas McGregor compares two styles of management, "theories X and Y." Theory X is autocratic and rational, while Theory Y is more humane and personal. McGregor formulates theory X as follows:

1. The average human being has an inherent dislike of work and will avoid it if possible.
2. Because of this human characteristic of dislike for work, most people must be forced, controlled, directed, and threatened with punishment to get them to put forth adequate effort toward the achievement of organizational objectives.
3. The average human prefers to be closely directed, wishes to avoid responsibility, has relatively little ambition and wants security above all.

In Theory Y, McGregor states:

1. The expenditure of physical and mental effort in work is as natural as play and rest. The average human being does not inherently dislike work. Depending on controllable conditions, work may be a source of satisfaction (and voluntarily performed), or a source of punishment (and avoided if possible).
2. External control and threat of punishment are not the only means for bringing about effort toward organizational objectives. People exercise self-direction and self-control and the service of objectives to which they are committed.
3. Commitment to objectives is a function of the rewards associated with their achievement. The most significant of such awards (e.g., satisfaction of ego and self-actualization needs) can be direct products of efforts directed towards organizational objectives.
4. The average human being, under proper conditions, learns not only to accept but to seek responsibility. Avoidance of responsibility, lack of ambition, and emphasis on security are generally consequences of experience, not inherent human characteristics.
5. The capacity to exercise a relatively high degree of imagination, ingenuity, and creativity in the solution of organizational problems is widely, not narrowly, distributed in the population.
6. Under conditions of moderate industrial life, the intellectual potentialities of the average human being are only partially utilized.

As one might expect in the health-care environment, most managers choose the approach presented in theory Y. It is designed to bring out the best performance in an employee, thus demonstrating the ability of both the organization and the manager to maximize employee potentials.

In recent years, W.G. Ouchi developed theory Z and contrasted it with McGregor's theories X and Y. The thrust of theory Z is that the involved worker is the key to obtaining quality and productivity gains. Ouchi describes five categories of the theory Z organization:

1. Lifetime employment relationships
2. Investment in organization-specific skills
3. Balance between explicit and implicit decision criteria
4. Participative decision making
5. A holistic view of people

This equates to a form of participative management, as opposed to the style in which the manager takes the command position. The manager becomes more involved with the employees; this in turn creates higher quality and productivity. Participative management does not reduce the authority of the manager but provides a method to develop a sense of trust in an organization. Unfortunately, this style of management can become time-consuming. As more people are drawn into the process of planning and decision making, more labor hours are used. Some managers feel the payoff from the enhanced performance will more than justify the cost incurred because of time.

The last style of leadership being discussed is the "laissez-faire" approach. This manager is usually not involved in the department's daily activities, and communication between the manager and employees is minimal. This style is not normally recommended, but it can be very effective if the manager is fortunate enough to be working with a highly motivated employee group.

As a manager, it is important to evaluate one's confidence in making decisions without the input and support of others. Occasions will arise when decisions must be made with authority and decisiveness.

It is difficult to state one style of leadership will work better than another. A good leader should possess most of the characteristics described in each of these categories, applying techniques appropriately to the circumstances at hand. Some employees need continual exchanges of information (participative leadership), while others would rather be given direction for a project and left alone (laissez-faire); each style can successfully reach organizational or departmental goals and objectives.

Regardless of style of leadership, a manager must be able to motivate employees. A direct indicator of a leader's effectiveness is his or her talent for motivating others. This may need to be learned. Moving from the technical ranks into a management position can be a difficult transition. Not all highly skilled and confident technologists have innate management ability. On the other hand, many have made the transition successfully. Those successful managers realize they must place a lower priority on technical aspects of their duties and begin dedicating more of their time to the leadership role.

Just as managers have expectations of their employees, so do employees have expectations of their managers. Employees need and expect their supervisors to be levelheaded, handling all matters in a fair and consistent manner. When a manager demonstrates consistency, they gain respect and loyalty from staff members.

Another important factor to be considered is recognition of the employee's job well done. Positive recognition will increase professional growth, wages, job security, fulfillment, and self-esteem. By meeting these needs, the manager in turn gives the employee a feeling of job satisfaction and a sense of being a part of a team. This helps to develop morale, motivation, and continued loyalty.

In contrast, a discontented employee can be a destructive force leading to increased absenteeism, increased turnover, and low productivity. One manifestation of a discontented or an undermotivated employee is negative outward reactions, demonstrating their needs are not being met.

In some cases, the manager may lack the ability to motivate the staff to strive toward planned goals. Listed below are several key demotivators managers should try to avoid when dealing with their employees:

1. *A feeling that no one cares about them.* With the vast number of changes the health-care field is now experiencing, employees may feel they have been left out, that no one cares. It is important to keep staff abreast of changes as decisions are made, preferably before their effective dates.
2. *Criticism without constructive suggestion.* One of the fastest ways to demotivate employees is to issue criticism without direction for corrective action.
3. *Poor communication of what is expected of them.* Again, with the tremendous changes health care is facing, communication is essential. Tell employees directly what is needed of them to succeed and meet the goals and objectives of the department. Do not avoid giving the employee the facts. This is also an opportune time for the manager to give and collect feedback to and from the employee.
4. *Inconsistent disciplinary action.* As indicated earlier, consistency in discipline is essential for gaining trust and loyalty of staff members.
5. *Setting goals too high or too low.* When working with staff members, it is important to recognize their unique needs and potentials. Once goals are set, it is important to review the employee's current status in relationship to the organizational and departmental goals.
6. *Insufficient tools for a given job.* Most nuclear medicine departments have the appropriate equipment to accomplish a given job. It is important for the manager to occasionally inspect and check for items that may have been broken and not reported. Sometimes minor problems can create or significantly increase employee frustration and, in turn, decrease productivity.
7. *Lack of recognition.* This area can be very difficult to address because different employees have different needs. Sending a simple letter to the individual's

home, which states specifically how this employee has contributed to the department, is an effective means of recognition. Giving a personal recognition for their efforts will reap positive dividends many times over. However, it is important for the manager to be sincere, whether it be a letter or a pat on the back for a job well done.

■ COMMUNICATION

Without good communication, a manager cannot be effective in planning, decision making, organization, personnel management, leadership or quality control. Each of these functions requires interaction with people. Planning cannot be carried out if the plan is not expressed to the employees by some means of communication (verbal or written), nor can a manager motivate employees without communication. When communicating to another individual, it is important for the sender to make his message clear enough so that the receiver can understand the message being conveyed. Also, if a spoken message is misinterpreted by the listener, the concept or view will be received improperly; therefore listening becomes equally important in the process of oral communication. There are many barriers and disturbances individuals must overcome when listening (noise, short attention span, clarity of the speaker, and individual thought processes). We live in a noisy society with constant commotion in our environment (radio, TV, equipment, etc.), and it is difficult to stay attentive when listening. In addition, a listener may either interrupt a conversation or allow his or her mind to drift off to another subject, missing what is being communicated. The speaker can be the cause of any one of these, depending on the ability to hold the listener's attention. In either case, the manager needs to develop good speaking and listening abilities when communicating with superiors, peers or subordinates.

Managers must also develop good writing skills. Communicating clearly in written form can be difficult, especially when dealing with a technical profession such as nuclear medicine. Every manager will need to assess his communication skills and discover ways to improve any weak areas. As deficiencies are confronted, improvement can begin. Further education may be a good start. Remember, neither the department nor the organization can meet its goals without good communication. Information must flow freely, and the person most responsible for successful departmental communication is the manager.

■ DELEGATION

As a manager's responsibilities increase, the need to delegate duties to others becomes necessary. This can be a difficult change to make if the manager is the type who wants to control all aspects of the daily operations of the department. As the manager continues to succeed and assumes greater responsibilities, total control will become more difficult. A good manager will thus view delegation as a means of staff development and will communicate this to the staff. Delegation allows the subordinate opportunities to gain better insight into department activities and increases their understanding of assignments. Areas for delegation might include routine tasks requiring little or no supervision, or tasks of low priority. Others may involve basic problem-solving skills in which the employee, with the proper information, can take on a challenging task and resolve it successfully. Delegation also provides managers an opportunity to realign departmental duties when their job duties change because of a promotion or because broader responsibilities have been delegated to them. Either of these situations might occur without notice; therefore it is important to learn delegation skills early. To assist the employee who has been assigned new duties, a manager should provide guidelines and expectations concerning the tasks delegated. As the employee begins the new duties, a manager should convey support by:

1. Informing co-workers of the employee's new responsibilities and why they were delegated. All staff involved must understand that the manager supports the individual completely.
2. Clarifying the individual's new level and scope of authority.
3. Encouraging the employee to try alternative routes if problems occur in relation to the new duties.
4. Remind the employee that you support his or her efforts completely.
5. Create a check system for feedback to determine progress, especially if the task is complicated or lengthy.
6. On completion of the task, give the individual credit for his or her performance.

The following are several occasions when a manager should *not* delegate responsibility:

1. Never delegate moral issues to others. This should be handled with full involvement of the director or manager.
2. Discipline should not be delegated; however, defined lines of authority should be followed.
3. Never delegate to employees who are incapable of performing the task (e.g., preparing a financial plan when the individual has only technical expertise).
4. If a task is highly confidential, it is better that the manager complete the task.
5. A controversial issue or a known problem area should be handled by the manager. "Passing the buck" to another creates resentment and guarantees negative results.

As a manager, through delegation, develops a relationship with subordinates, it is important for all parties to understand that the duties being delegated are above and be-

Table 35-1. City hospital income expense report

Current activity					Year-to-date			
Actual	**Budget**	**Variance**	**% Var.**	**Revenue**	**Actual**	**Budget**	**Variance**	**% Var.**
54,184−	55,859−	1,675−	3.0−	Inpatient	419,688−	446,881−	27,192−	6.1−
369−	344	24	7.2	Emergency	3,721−	2,757−	964	35.0
28,415−	20,515−	7,899−	38.5	Outpatient	182,838−	164,121−	18,717−	11.4
82,968−	76,719−	6,249	8.1	Total	606,249−	613,760−	7,511−	1.2−
				Statistics				
443−	476−	33−	6.9−	Inpatient	3,643−	3,816−	173−	4.5−
9−	7−	2	28.6	Emergency	56−	54−	2	3.7
51−	112−	61−	54.5−	Outpatient	883−	902−	19−	2.1
503−	595−	92−	15.5−	Total	4,582−	4,772−	190−	4.0−
				Productive Hours				
2,765	2,809	44−	1.6−	Regular	22,093	22,455	362−	1.6−
83	67	16	23.9	Overtime	964	526	438	83.3
2,848	2,876	28	1.0−	Total	23,057	22,981	76	0.3
				Nonproductive Hours				
0	19	19−	100.0−	Education	126	152	26−	17.1−
62	311	249−	80.1−	Benefit	1,897	2,471	574−	23.2−
62	330	268−	81.2−	Total	2,023	2,623	600−	22.9−
2,910	3,206	296−	9.2−	Total	25,080	25,604	524−	2.0
				Productive Salary & Wages				
22,571	23,740	1,169−	4.9−	Regular	178,395	189,900	11,505−	6.1−
1,097	1,078	19	1.8	Overtime	13,120	8,620	4,500	52.2
23,668	24,818	1,150	4.6	Total	191,516	198,520	7,004−	3.5−
				Nonproductive Salary & Wages				
0	236	236−	100.0	Education	1,115	1,884	769−	40.8−
341	3,217	2,876−	89.4	Benefits	18,071	25,714	7,643−	29.7−
341	3,453	3,112−	90.1−	Total	19,186	27,598	8,412−	30.5−
24,009	28,271	4,262−	15.1	**Total Salary/Wages Benefits**	210,702	226,118	15,416−	6.8−
21,483	16,857	4,626	27.4	**Total Supply**	103,780	134,834	31,054−	23.0−
2,209	5,284	3,075	58.2−	**Total Service**	49,997	42,264	7,733	18.3
172	476	304−	63.9−	**Total Other**	1,206	3,796	2,590−	68.2−
23,865	22,617	1,248	5.5	**Total Other Expense**	154,983	180,894	25,911−	14.3−
47,874	50,888	3,014	5.9	**Total Expenditure**	365,685	407,012	41,327	10.2

yond the call of duty. This can be demonstrated by praise, rewards, and most important, backing and respect from the manager.

If done properly, the employee will look forward to new assignments in the future, thereby improving morale and productivity within the department. In selecting candidates for delegation of duties, the manager may choose several employees, especially in larger departments. This can help develop a team spirit. By involving several individuals in the delegation process, they are more likely to respond positively to future changes.

■ QUALITY CONTROL

The final management function to be discussed is quality control. This is the process by which one monitors the use of departmental resources to achieve a given result. The manager may accomplish this by comparing known standards to current department activities. As examples, we will consider management information systems and quality assurance.

Management information systems deals with financial indicators such as budgets, accounting, and financial ratio analysis. Of these three, nuclear medicine managers will normally have greatest exposure to the budget process, which will include developing and monitoring an operating budget. Health-care managers use budget reports to numerically express how plans or programs are progressing in relation to goals of the department. These reports provide a concrete tool for monitoring and controlling costs, as well as awareness of the level of resource consumption in a given department or cost center. Some organizations subscribe to the method of "incremental budgeting," in which they review existing programs and build a new budget based on the previous year's activities. Others use an approach known as "zero base budgeting," which requires a thorough cost/benefit analysis as if all projects and activities were being newly activated. In other words, the manager must base the budget as if no money had even been allocated for the project.

Regardless of the approach, budgeting is a method of

Table 35-2. Sample cost analysis sheet

Department ________________ Number ________ Rating Date ________________

Procedure ________________ Number ________ Last Rating Date ________________

DIRECT COSTS

PERSONNEL

JOB CLASS No.	Description	Rate/Hr.	Hours	Personnel
123	Technologist	$10.00	1.0	10.00
321	Receptionist	7.00	0.1	.70
456	Secretary	9.00	0.2	1.80
654	Transporters	6.00	0.3	1.80
	Total Salaries			14.30

SUPPLIES AND OTHER

ITEM No.	Description	Units	Unit Price	Cost
	Film	6	1.00	6.00
	Radiopharmaceutical	1	8.00	8.00
	Syringe	1	.50	.50
	Needle	2	.20	.40
	Misc. Supplies	1	1.00	1.00
	Total Supplies and Other			$15.90

DEPRECIATION

EQUIPMENT No.	Description	Cost	Life	Volume	Cost/Unit
1	Gamma Camera	$300,000.00	5	13,000	23.07
	Total Direct Cost				53.27

Prepared By ________________________

		Proposed		Approved
Direct Cost		________		________
Indirect Cost (60%) of Direct Cost		________		________
Total Cost		________		________
Professional Fee		________		________
Margin		________		________
Prepared Proposed Rate		________		________
Hospital	________	________	________	________
Rate	________	________	________	________

Approved

________________________ Division Director ________________ Date

________________________ Medical Director ________________ Date

________________________ Director, Finance ________________ Date

________________________ Administration ________________ Date

Effective Date ________________________________

forecasting volume of service, cost of providing the service, and demonstrating revenues generated from the service. Monitoring is accomplished by comparing the actual cost to a predetermined standard. This variant indicates the positive or negative result on the invested funds. Through management information systems, a monthly income and expense report is generated so that the manager can compare current expenditure and revenue levels for that month and year-to-date against the budgeted amount. As the operating budget is reviewed, it is important to verify that actual dollars spent for materials and labor (line items) are accurate. Well-written management information systems reports will itemize revenues produced by in-patients, out-patients, and emergency-room procedures. The reports will also demonstrate expenses incurred to perform these services, such as salaries, wages and benefits, supplies, and maintenance agreements. The monthly report will be formatted to period (current activity) and will also provide the year-to-date activity (YTD). The income and expense report will follow a format similar to that shown in Table 35-1.

In addition to the income and expense report, nuclear medicine managers will need to periodically review the cost of performing specific procedures; this is known as cost analysis. The information generated from this process gives the accounting department a basis for developing the patient's charge per procedure, thereby covering the actual cost and also generating revenue. Each health-care organization has its own format for doing cost analysis. It is critical that managers know how their department resources are used. This knowledge will help the manager to predict the financial success of a program or project (see Cost Analysis Sheet, Table 35-2).

As managers become more familiar with their organizations, they will find other management information system reports that will assist in management (e.g., accounts payable, time and attendance, other departmental statements, patient admissions and discharges, etc.). These reports will assist the manager in running a more efficient and productive department.

The second management information system being discussed in relation to controlling is quality management (QM), which has become a function of paramount importance in all nuclear medicine departments. The Joint Commission for the Accreditation of Health Care Organizations (JCAHCO) has placed a great deal of emphasis on this management function. Because of the breadth of the subject of nuclear medicine, we will only be able to discuss it briefly here.

In general, quality management guidelines give the manager and the health-care organization means of developing criteria, or standards, for health-care practices. Through familiarity with predetermined standards, a health-care manager can monitor activities within his or her department (i.e., determining if an examination or procedure is ordered and performed appropriately). To establish parameters for the manager and the staff, guidelines that detail procedures, preventative and corrective measures, and appropriate tolerance levels must be provided. Getting a good QM program in place takes dedication and many months of concerted effort, but once put in place and properly applied, it becomes a very effective monitoring tool for both patients and employees.

The role of the nuclear medicine manager has undergone many changes in recent years, in both technical and administrative aspects. As the field of nuclear medicine becomes more complex, greater amounts of time must be dedicated to the activities of planning, decision making, organization, personnel management, leadership, and quality control, each of which influence patient care and the efficiency of the department. The manager of the future must possess the ability to evenly balance financial systems and patient care systems in both the in-patient and out-patient areas.

Good leaders will continue to explore new management techniques and to broaden their educational backgrounds, in turn enabling not only themselves but the managers of the future to change with the ever-changing and challenging health-care environment.

BIBLIOGRAPHY

Cleverly, W.O.: Essentials of hospital finance, ed. 1, Germantown, Md., 1978, Aspen Systems Corp.

McGregor, D.: The human side of enterprise, New York, 1960, McGraw-Hill Book Co.

Ouchi, W.G.: Theory Z: how American business can meet the Japanese challenge, Reading, Mass., 1981, Addison-Wesley.

Rakich, J.S., Longest, Jr., B.B., and Darr, K.: Managing health services organizations, ed. 3, Baltimore, Md., 1992, Health Professions Press.

Schermerhorn, J.R.: Management for productivity, ed. 2, New York, 1986, John Wiley & Sons, Inc.

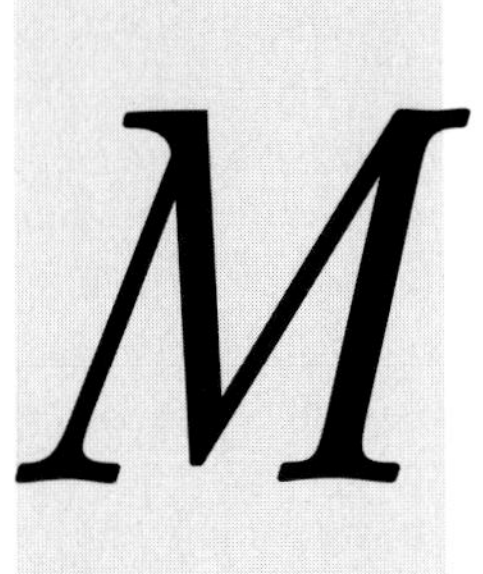

Chapter 36

MARKETING NUCLEAR MEDICINE SERVICES

RALPH G. ROBINSON
MYRON L. LECKLITNER

■ BASIC MARKETING CONCEPTS

Marketing a physician's services has often been looked on with scorn. However, most physicians have confused "marketing" with paid advertising. Paid advertising is *not* marketing. It may be one part of an overall marketing strategy, but it is often inappropriate for medical marketing in general and physician services in particular. In the opening section of this chapter we will describe a simple nine-point marketing program that outlines the elements of a successful nuclear medicine practice. In the later sections we will focus on public relations as a marketing approach, with a specific focus on the media to further increase nuclear medicine referrals.

Physicians have always marketed their services. For decades, the only marketing that was necessary was word of mouth. Today, the practice of medicine is no longer a win-win situation. The increasing number of physicians, the competition for quality practice, and increasing influence by third-party payers and government on the ability of the physician to make decisions concerning an individual patient's best interests make it necessary for the individual nuclear physician to present his or her services in the best possible way in the marketplace. Nuclear medicine, as a dynamic and growing specialty, has much to offer patients and referring physicians. The skills of nuclear medicine professionals will be wasted if no one knows who they are and what they can do.

Marketing is defined as all activities directed toward satisfying wants and needs of a buyer/consumer. Physician/patient can be substituted for buyer/consumer. If nuclear medicine professionals are to be successful in any marketing effort, they must understand the services and technologies they offer, and they must understand the potential buyers and consumers of that service. They must also understand the applications and limitations of the new diagnostic or therapeutic technique. They need to know the strengths and weaknesses of their own institution. With this knowledge, they need to define their market and develop a marketing plan. That plan needs to be tied to the promotional strategy of the hospital or health-care institution.

A nuclear medicine professional's market is the referring physician. Thus in almost all cases, the primary objective should be to increase communication with referring physicians. Nuclear medicine professionals need to tell physicians that they can help them do a better job of taking care of their patients and can reduce time-to-diagnosis. A nuclear medicine professional's service is the diagnostic procedure performed or the therapeutic treatment given the patient. Nuclear medicine professionals would like to think that the patient is the product. Certainly a satisfied patient is the medical and professional goal. The real product, however, is the information, the result, returned to the referring physician. Nuclear medicine professionals depend on that referral for survival.

The American College of Nuclear Physicians, through its Professional and Public Information Program, has developed a succinct nine-point marketing program. It is called "The Elements of a Successful Nuclear Medicine Practice." The main points are shown in Fig. 36-1. The elements of a successful nuclear medicine practice include:

1. *Imaging excellence*—Imaging technology should be updated, and knowledge and use of clinical applications and the right quality-control procedures should be current. Outdated imaging equipment needs to be replaced. The nuclear medicine professional should know competing modalities.
2. *Availability*—The presence of the nuclear medicine professional when studies are done makes a difference—they can get the images they need and can

MARKET YOUR NUCLEAR MEDICINE SERVICES THROUGH . . .

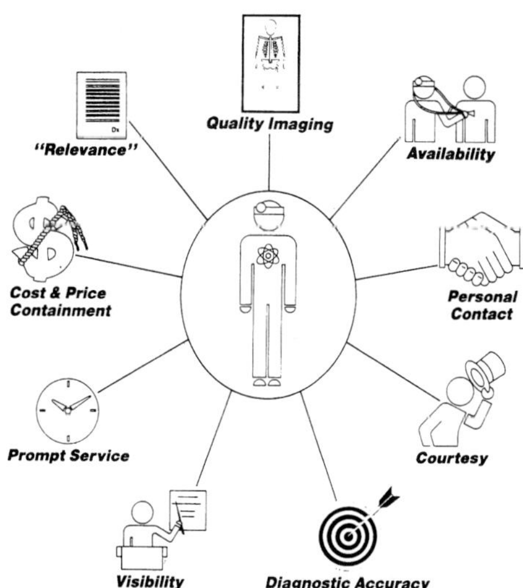

Fig. 36-1. Elements of a successful nuclear medicine practice. (From The elements of a successful nuclear medicine practice, American College of Nuclear Physicians, Suite 700, 1101 Connecticut Ave., N.W., Washington, D.C. 20036.)

correlate them with physical findings. Night and weekend on-call service should be provided.

3. *Courtesy*—The nuclear medicine professional is represented by every staff member. Patients should be treated with dignity and respect, and referring physicians should receive prompt and courteous attention.
4. *Visibility*—The nuclear medicine professional should attend and participate in medical conferences and staff meetings in his or her hospital. Conferences should be presented that show what nuclear medicine can do.
5. *Prompt service*—Same-day imaging service should be provided whenever possible; studies that are put off do not get performed. Reports should get out the same day the study is done.
6. *Relevancy*—A diagnosis should be put on every report. It should be short and concise, and the question that was asked should be answered. The patient's medical history should be known. If correlation with the history, physical findings, and/or imaging results is needed, the nuclear medicine professional should do this himself. Reports should be tailored to the clinician's language. A reference file should be maintained.
7. *Personal contact*—The nuclear medicine professional should call referring physicians with reports and should speak personally with patients. The hospital administrator should be dealt with personally and should be extended invitations to visit the nuclear medicine department and staff meetings.
8. *Cost and price containment*—Overpriced studies will not be ordered. Containing costs help keep prices down. New equipment should be justified before ordering.
9. *Diagnostic accuracy*—Previous hints will help increase referrals, but *diagnostic accuracy is the bottom line.*

Each of these nine elements of a successful nuclear medicine practice appears so rationally obvious; taken collectively, however, they describe an active, up-to-date, and, more important, accurate diagnostic imaging practice. They describe a practice that will be well respected in the hospital or clinic where it is used.

■ DEVELOPING A SUCCESSFUL MARKETING PROGRAM

The nine elements of a successful nuclear medicine practice combine elements of an overall marketing program (personal contact and increased visibility) with the provision of completely up-to-date and professional patient services. Once these concepts have been established in practice, a specific set of objectives, a 1- to 2-year short-range plan can be developed. A marketing plan establishes goals with an established time period, it establishes priorities, and it alerts other departments in a hospital or clinic that support in specific areas may be needed. A marketing objective might be to increase users' satisfaction by meeting their needs more efficiently than can competing institutions or modalities. The next step is to communicate this information. This involves marketing communications, defined as any method of spreading information about a product or service. Communicating this information persuades the referring physician and the patient to respond in a positive way.

■ COMMUNICATION

The nuclear medicine practitioner can increase communication with referring physicians in several ways. Paid advertising could be bought or sales incentives offered. Though these are classic marketing techniques, they may be inappropriate here. Instead, a message has to be developed to alter and improve the referring physician's perception of the services nuclear medicine can offer. It must be remembered that perception is reality.

Advertising is a nonpersonal, commercial message—a communication in which the sponsor is paying for an advertisement. *Advertising is not in itself marketing.* Advertising may be one part of an overall marketing strategy, but it is generally inappropriate for nuclear medicine practitioners.

Next, let us consider marketing through public relations, remembering that "advertising" is intrusive. Public relations, rather than being intrusive, involves stories about good things going on at your hospital and in the nuclear medicine department. This approach appeals to most people. Advertising is a direct influence, and as such is generally short-term in its effect. Readers may glance at the ads in the papers, but they will read stories generated by public relations. Public relations is an indirect influence. It has no time-specific message and is therefore a long-term investment. Good news travels far and "stays with you" a bit longer. Advertising is purchased, but public relations must be constantly sold. If someone has a message but is unable to get it out effectively, no one is going to hear it. Advertising does change consumer *behavior* on a more immediate level, but public relations modifies consumer *attitudes* on a long-term basis. This is the ongoing good feeling that nuclear medicine professionals are trying to create for their institutions or hospitals as well as for their specific services.

Specific promotions focusing on the referring physicians can be done with letters, personal contact, and presentations at grand rounds, all aimed at expressing the specific utility of nuclear medicine services to that physician or group. In essence, what can a new nuclear medicine procedure or technique offer that medical specialist? Once the elements of a successful nuclear medicine practice have been adopted, the nuclear medicine professional is ready to market his or her services by increasing competitive visibility.

■ CREATING COMPETITIVE VISIBILITY

In medicine, as in other facets of life, there is a difference between truth and the perception of truth. It follows that there is a difference between reality and the perception of reality. The challenge in medical diagnosis is to see through the veil (the perception) to obtain the truth. In marketing, the thinking is exactly the opposite: marketing executives are exquisitely sensitive to both the reality and the perception of reality, but they downplay the reality to the perception of reality. In marketing, the perception becomes the reality. According to a survey by a New York executive placement firm, 85% of fired executives shared one common trait: *not* calling attention to their abilities and achievements. Hence, they were perceived as not having any abilities or achievements. A second study by a Boston research firm found that successful managers know how to intensify their images through self-promotion. Do these same observations not apply equally to physicians and hospitals? They do, of course.

The current explosion of medical knowledge has fostered medical specialization. Unfortunately, specialization has been attended by a kind of physician "remoteness," which potentiates *perceived* haughtiness, if not *perceived* abject arrogance. Moreover, locational remoteness within the hospital or large multispecialty free-standing clinic aggravates medicosocial remoteness. Nuclear physicians typically practice far from the day-to-day clinical venue of referring physicians. Thus arises the double-whammy effect, so potentially deleterious to the practice of nuclear medicine: specialist remoteness and locational remoteness, leading to a lack of visibility. Nuclear medicine professionals must decide individually and collectively whether they will elect to become competitively visible.

In addition to organizing an occasional seminar or presenting a staff talk, a nuclear medicine professional should contact his or her hospital's public relations department and should generate newsworthy articles appropriate for his or her hospital, university (if applicable), and *local* newspapers. Subjects appropriate for printed media include new equipment and new services; grant awards and grant results; elected and appointed office; awards from county, state, regional, and national medical organizations; and prestigious talks before regional, national, and international learned societies, governmental agencies, and industrial groups.

A public relations department does not create news; it shapes, reports, and releases news. Nuclear medicine professionals must provide the substance of the story if they want their story to be seen or heard. Their accomplishments and successes go far to let referring physicians, health-care consumers, local public officials, and industrial leaders know that nuclear medicine is a hive of positive activity and progress. To allow these marketing opportunities to pass unnoticed is akin to winking in the dark; yes, something was accomplished, but nobody saw it, let alone appreciated it.

Physicians suffering from a lack of self-promotion may not approve of the behavior of the "high-profile physician," but those same physicians can easily recognize the benefits to be derived from successful self-promotion and image intensification. If nuclear medicine professionals elect to continue winking in the dark, they must unfortunately but necessarily be willing to be ignominously referred to as "those guys in the basement."

■ VALUE OF THE MEDIA IN MARKETING

About the only contact most nuclear medicine professionals have with the media is a request for an anecdotal response to events of the day, such as the accident at Chernobyl or the buildup of radon in personal dwellings. Nuclear medicine professionals have assumed a reactionist role limited to interviews or letters to the editor. In this section we will see the importance of looking at the media from a different if not totally new perspective: defining the role and power of the media, emphasizing the interface between nuclear physicians and the media, and providing a 12-point program for successfully using the media to tell the nuclear medicine story. Although most of the points are likewise applicable to electronic media (television and radio), the focus here is on telling one's nuclear medicine story in print.

How does communication media fit in the marketing plan? Under the new economic order sweeping both medicine and health-care delivery, diagnosis-related groups (DRGs), preferred-provider organizations (PPOs), health-maintenance organizations (HMOs), individual practice associations (IPAs), as well as protean physician-reimbursement policies of third-party carriers, physicians, and technologists are faced with a new challenge: survivability. Yet mere survivability in itself appears an abject reason for getting out of bed in the morning, for "surviving" means "to continue to exist."

For the purpose of this discussion, the use of the media will be viewed within the context of medical marketing. First, some definitions appear in order. Marketing is the goal of creating additional demand for a product (goods and/or service) where a previous demand did not exist. Although strategies of marketing include advertising, public relations, market share, market positioning, merchandising, and other activities, appreciating the different roles of advertising and public relations is of utmost importance. Although both are cost centers, advertising must be *purchased,* public relations must be *sold.* Advertising changes consumer buying *behavior* toward products; public relations modifies consumer *attitudes* toward the producer or provider of the product. Advertising is short-term; public relations is long-term. Advertising anticipates a *direct* positive influence on sales and services; public relations anticipates an *indirect* positive influence on sales and services.

Because both advertising and public relations are cost centers, would it not seem faster and less expensive to generate in-house advertising campaigns or retain an advertising agency to manage those facets of marketing? Perhaps. Some physicians go that route. But there are other considerations. In the mind of the public, advertising is *intrusive;* public relations channeled through the media is eye-catching and appealing. For example, to a person reading the newspaper, one often hears a second person inquire, "What's in the news?" But no one ever asks, "What's in the advertising?" A second consideration, equally important, is that news articles are seven to 10 times more credible than are advertisements. Finally, there is the element of control. Advertising, at least for hospitals, is well beyond the purview of most. On the other hand, newsworthy articles can be initiated by nuclear medicine practitioners and can relate specifically to our services.

Is the nuclear medicine story bona fide news? To answer this, nuclear medicine professionals should take stock of those assets that create medicine's magnetism in the eyes of the press. Medical imaging is high-tech, always holding appeal for the press and public. Though high-tech, is nuclear medicine practice high-touch?

Virtually any not-for-profit organization's *service* activities are readily regarded by the press as "legitimate news," in contrast to the hard-core selling activities (auto part sales, for example) of one who must *buy* advertising. It is safe to say that medical and paramedical individuals are viewed by the press as being experts and enjoy a high degree of *credibility.* In addition, the quality of *reliability* of the source (as is generally enjoyed by the medical professions) is of paramount importance to reporters. Because of these assets, the press assigns a high priority to medical and health-care articles in the form of "quick bits"—the maximum accuracy and length of printed story per unit of time and effort invested by the press. Most local reporters cover more than one story a day; medical stories can be completed without protracted expenditure of time and effort, hence the term, "quick bit."

And what exactly, for the purpose of this discussion, is the "power of the press?" As quoted by Thomas Carlyle in his work, *Heroes and Hero-Worship,* Burke said, "There are three Estates [nobility, clergy and commoners] in Parliament, but in the reporter's gallery yonder, there sat a Fourth Estate more important by far than they all." Indeed, as emphasized by Tony Schwartz, ". . . the media can change the course of a war, bring down a president or king, elevate the lowly, and humiliate the proud . . .".

Although most of this discussion focuses on the power of the print media to support the nuclear medicine profession, other media as well play an important role. How do the major television networks present the news? With very few exceptions, all address prioritized concerns: Is my world safe? Is my country safe? Is my family safe? Am I safe? When one considers news from the standpoint of "safety," then medicine and health-care delivery receive a whopping 20% of network air time. When the costs of air time and competition between major networks are considered, there can be little doubt that medicine and health care are deemed very newsworthy topics with a great deal of appeal to the public.

From the standpoint of the nuclear imaging facility, what activities would be considered newsworthy? Repeatedly, the old chestnut that "nothing ever happens at our hospital or clinic" is heard but should not be believed. There are several news stories each year at a nuclear imaging facility that go untold. Was someone appointed to chair a committee or elected to office in an important society or other association? Are there new facilities? Equipment? Services? Research grants? Research results? If none of these newsworthy activities has occurred in the past year or two, there may be more fundamental operational problems than those amenable to the challenges of medical marketing.

■ NUCLEAR MEDICINE AND THE MEDIA: A 12-POINT PROGRAM*

As a prelude to 12 practical points that will enhance the ability to tell the nuclear medicine story in the media, a caveat is in order: Don't shoot yourself in the foot. In the corporate world, this caveat reads "Don't shoot yourself in the purse." Can this actually happen? The answer is: effortlessly. The motto of medicine, *primum non noncere* ("first do not harm"), is as relevant to nuclear medicine's relations with the media as it is to health-care delivery. A

*Adapted with permission from Prospective nuclear medicine—nuclear medicine and the media: a 12-point program, *Current concepts in diagnostic nuclear medicine,* Summer 1987, MacMillan Healthcare Information.

good finished product in the media takes the same planning and attention to detail as does a good manuscript or good oral presentation. Furthermore, a nuclear medicine professional should not be caught up in undue expectation and excitement that could result in the premature release of the article—before the new service is really operational, for example, or before the new equipment has been acceptance-tested or even received. An untimely news release or article can only affect credibility and antagonize disappointed referring physicians if what was promised cannot be delivered.

■ 1. Work through your public relations department

Every hospital has a public relations department. Every large clinic should have an appointed spokesperson who has at least a nodding acquaintance with public relations personnel who are particularly capable in interfacing with the press. A sharp director of hospital public relations attends committee meetings at all organizational levels, particularly executive, policy-making sessions. Public relations directors and their associates know those hospital areas to be marketed, the priorities of marketable areas, the resources to be committed to each area, and the proper time to initiate interviews and to release stories. For example, featuring a hospital's helicopter capability is best deferred on a day when the wire services are buzzing with stories of the high number of hospital-owned helicopter crashes. This, in fact, recently happened. A good public relations department knows *when* to release the story.

As a nuclear medicine specialist, you may decide to go it alone and contact the press directly. It is important to think twice before doing so. The justification may be that this item has nothing to do with the hospital; it has to do only with your private office. More often than not, however, the reporter will tag the name of the hospital onto your name. This approach can definitely create conflict and ill will between you and the hospital; though the intent was simply to feature your private facility and your personal views, the hospital's position is that it has a virtually identical facility or a different opinion. The hospital will be perceived by the readers as endorsing your services and opinions, and the hospital will see its name appearing in the article as an unsolicited passive endorsement of a specific medical practice.

■ 2. The process begins with you

What exactly are the roles of public relations and the nuclear medicine specialist? You bring insight: what is the instrument's purpose and how does it work? is it cost effective? how does it lower morbidity? mortality? patient discomfort? Public relations brings marketing expertise to the joint venture. In most cases, PR personnel can say it better and add that certain journalistic style to your background material and key points. Your first hurdle is to convince your own public relations department that your bit is, in fact, newsworthy.

■ 3. Your bit must be newsworthy

The press is exquisitely sensitive to individuals, groups, and associations attempting to disguise advertising as bona fide news. In such cases, the press will refer these individuals to the newspaper's advertising department, and reasonably so. You are promoting, yes, but your bit must have general news appeal and interest to the public.

■ 4. Define the thrust of your article

Most topics that you want to release to the public will not be fast-breaking news. Take your time to organize your efforts. What is the focus of your story? Do you wish to be perceived as offering a very accurate diagnostic test? a safe test? a faster diagnostic test? or the best diagnostic test among various alternatives? Create appeal, but know in advance which appeal you desire to create.

■ 5. Control what you can: options

There are only two ways to have your story printed: interviews and press releases. Although an interview has more slice-of-life reader appeal than does a straight news story, the interview process is fraught with pitfalls and limitations. From the standpoint of an accurate recount by the reporter, what you *said* is irrelevant; it's what the reporter *heard* that will be printed. Interviews that generate hospital news should always be discussed with the hospital's public relations department for two reasons. First, this allows a jointly determined judgment on the propriety of the proposed article; second, it allows public relations to contact the press to schedule the interview, either one-on-one or in press-conference format. Also, public-relations—generated press releases allow in-house time to put the fine brush strokes on the piece; the copy can be reviewed and revised at leisure. There is not much a newspaper can do to misquote you or generate other substantive errors if the newspaper is furnished with the story as a well-written news release.

Working with the PR office, you have the right to review in-house press releases for inaccuracies in the final product before the release. On the other hand, do not be tempted to ask for the right of review of out-of-house preprint interviews; you would be infringing on the freedom of the press, a constitutional right closely guarded by the press.

■ 6. Doing your homework

Whether you are being interviewed or are releasing the story, you should emphasize only a few key points that you want to appear in print. Determine in advance what your major points will be. Interviews can waffle or degenerate into large delusional pools of prattle that truly distract from the thrust and appearance of your article. If necessary, have three to five main points written down and available to you during the interview. Present your key points early in the interview. Otherwise, the reporter can be out the door before you've told your story. There is a marketing expression that goes, "more is less, and less is more." Simply put, the expression means that attempting to stuff *more* facts into an article than is necessary will hold *less* appeal to the reader; a few well-chosen facts are actually more appealing.

■ 7. Bridge: they expect it

"Bridging" is an interview technique for focusing on those points that you want reflected in the printed piece. "Bridging" is an *interviewee's* technique. For instance, you have granted an interview concerning low-level radioactive waste, and the reporter requests your thoughts on Love Canal. You should respond, "Love Canal had to do with *chemical* waste, which I don't know much about. Now, concerning low-level *radioactive* waste, did you know that . . . ." Call it a parry, or side-stepping an irrelevant question; nonetheless, it is important to control the interview and make your major points known to the reporter.

■ 8. Don't throw rocks at others

In the eyes of readers, you will not win friends by putting down others, in effect attempting to denigrate the competition. Your argument must stand on its own merit. In a recent article highlighting several physicians, two of the medical luminaries volunteered such juicy recommendations as cleaning the crooks out of city hall and cleaning up that slum called downtown. The article then culminated with a comment concerning their hospital's full service with in-house physicians available 24 hours a day, unlike Brand X Hospital: "I'll bet you can't find a physician in Brand X after 10 p.m." Interestingly, the next issue of that periodical had a retraction of these statements, not by the physicians but by the editor. The point is: Had the original article done more harm than good in terms of public relations? The answer is clear.

■ 9. All comments are on the record

It seems a bit redundant to use the term *investigative reporter;* all reporters are investigative. They will always be looking for the story, the provocative, the news; that's their job. Never say anything to a reporter that you would not want to see in print in close proximity to your name. There simply is no such thing as an off-the-record comment to the press.

■ 10. Include a photograph

Discuss the suitability of a photograph with your public relations department, and let them arrange for a professional to acquire the pictures.

What kind of photograph? If the story is to feature an individual's accomplishments or achievements, then a head-and-shoulders photograph is appropriate. If the story is to feature new equipment or new services, then you should include an "action shot," a picture of the "big machine" with one employee acting in a supervisory role and another employee acting as the patient. A photograph augments the story and adds realistic and perceptional appeal. If the photographer will be taking the photographs, have a few good recommendations for "action shots" that will catch the essence of your key points and complement the article.

■ 11. Pray for a good headline

Good headlines can dramatically dress up an article, but good and bad headlines come with the luck of the draw. Because most people don't read the whole story unless they're especially interested in the subject, for the majority of readers the headline *is* the story. Nothing is more vexing than to be interviewed for the better part of a morning, only to open the newspaper several days later and find your article and your picture under some inane and ho-hum headline. Your sole means of controlling the headline is to give a good interview, bridging if necessary. The same statement holds true for a press release.

One must rise above the impulse to call the reporter and remonstrate against an inaccurate or pedestrian headline; the reporter doesn't select the headline. That selection is accomplished at the next higher organizational level of the press: the layout editor. There's not much you can do about that.

■ 12. Maximize your return on investment

You want your story to run where it will do your facility, your hospital or clinic, and you the most good. If you grant an interview, then you are locked in to that periodical. This does not mean that you cannot agree to multiple interviews. But why would you consider multiple outlets? Virtually all news stories that you initiate will ingratiate you with your referring physicians and other colleagues: run your bit in the hospital newspaper as well as county and state medical newsletters. If you provide services for a university-based PPO or an HMO and/or hold an appointment on the faculty of a university, there is a better than even chance that the university's employees constitute one of your large health contracts; run your story in the university's paper. If you are in private practice or belong to an IPA, your referring physicians and their spouses read the city newspaper; run your story in the city newspaper. If all three conditions apply, run it in all three newspapers as a news release. Again, maximize your return on investment.

Marketing has much to offer the nuclear medicine specialist who is willing to learn a few simple techniques. We are all familiar with the adage, "Out of sight, out of mind."

Yet that saying assumes more significance when put in the terms of marketing: "Out of mind, out of business." In the current economically challenging times of medicine and health-care delivery, proper use of the media can go far in maintaining or expanding your market share of nuclear medicine.

Bibliography

Robinson, R.G.: Nuclear medicine in the prospective payment environment: the need for individual and group initiatives, J. Nucl. Med, 17: 433-434, 1986.

Schwartz, T.: Media: the second god, Garden City, N.Y., 1983, Anchor Press/Doubleday, p. 2.

Appendix A

PHYSICAL DATA FOR RADIONUCLIDES USED IN NUCLEAR MEDICINE*

Element	Chemical symbol (X)	Atomic number (Z)	Mass number (A)	Half-life	Radiation	Principal gamma energy (MeV)
Arsenic	As	33	74	17.9d	EC, β^+, β^-, γ	0.596
Calcium	Ca	20	47	4.5d	β^-, γ	1.308
Carbon	C	6	11	20.3m	β^+	None
			14	5730y	β^-	None
Cesium (^{137m}Ba)	Cs	55	137	30y	β^-, γ	0.662
Chromium	Cr	24	51	27.8d	EC, γ	0.320
Cobalt	Co	27	57	270d	EC	0.122
			58	71.3d	EC, β^+, γ	0.810
			60	5.26y	β^-, γ	1.17, 1.33
Gallium	Ga	31	67	78h	EC, γ	0.091, 0.093 (38%) 0.184 (24%) 0.300 (16%) 0.394 (4%)
Gold	Au	79	195m	30.6s	IT, γ	0.200 (1.6%) 0.262 (68.2%)
			195	183d	EC, γ	0.099 (10.9%) 0.130 (0.8%)
			198	2.7d	β^-, γ	0.412
Iodine	I	53	123	13h	EC, γ	0.159
			125	60d	EC, γ	0.035 γ (7%) 0.027 x (1.15%) 0.031 x (25%)
			131	8.06d	β^-, γ	0.364
Iron	Fe	26	59	45d	β^-, γ	1.17, 1.33
Indium	In	49	111	2.8d	EC, γ	0.173 (89%) 0.247 (94%)
Krypton	Kr	36	79	1.45d	EC, γ	0.398, 0.606

*From Early, P.J., Razzak, M.A., and Sodee, D.B.: *Textbook of nuclear medicine technology,* ed 3, St. Louis, 1979, The CV Mosby Co.

Element	Chemical symbol (X)	Atomic number (Z)	Mass number (A)	Half-life	Radiation	Principal gamma energy (MeV)
Mercury	Hg	80	195m	41.6h	IT, EC, γ	0.262 (32.3%)
						0.388 (2.3%)
						0.560 (7.5%)
			195	9.9h	EC, γ	0.062 (6.4%)
						0.180 (2.0%)
						0.207 (1.6%)
						0.262 (1.6%)
						0.585 (2.0%)
						0.600 (1.8%)
						0.788 (7.0%)
						1.111 (1.5%)
						1.172 (1.3%)
			197	2.7d	EC, γ	0.077
			203	46.9d	β^-, γ	0.279
Molybdenum	Mo	42	99	2.78d	β^-, γ	0.740
Oxygen	O	8	15	2.1m	β^+	None
Phosphorus	P	15	32	14.3d	β^-	None
Rubidium	Rb	37	86	18.7d	β^-, γ	1.078
Selenium	Se	34	75	120d	EC, γ	0.265
Strontium	Sr	38	85	64d	EC, γ	0.514
			87m	2.83h	IT, γ	0.388
			90	27.7y	β^-	None
Technetium	Tc	43	99m	6h	IT, γ	0.140
			99	2.12 x10^5y	β	None
Thallium	Tl	81	201	73h	EC, γ, x	0.135 γ (3%)
						0.167 γ (10%)
						0.068 − 0.080 x (94.5%)
Tin	Sn	50	113	115d	EC, γ	0.255
Tritium	H	1	3	12.26y	β^-	None
Xenon	Xe	54	127	36.4d	EC, γ	0.172 (22%)
						0.203 (65%)
						0.375 (20%)
			133	5.31d	B^-, γ	0.08
Ytterbium	Yb	70	169	32d	EC, γ	0.177 (22%)
						0.198 (35%)

Appendix B

TABLE OF ATOMIC MASS UNITS

Symbol	Element	Atomic mass units (amu)
e	Electron	0.000549
n	Neutron	1.008665
p	Proton	1.007277
${}^{1}_{1}H$	Hydrogen	1.007825
${}^{2}_{1}H$	Deuterium	2.014102
${}^{3}_{1}H$	Tritium	3.016050
${}^{3}_{2}He$		3.016030
${}^{2}_{5}He$	Isotopes of helium	4.002603
${}^{5}_{2}He$		5.012297
${}^{6}_{2}He$		6.018893
${}^{10}_{6}C$		10.016810
${}^{11}_{6}C$		11.011432
${}^{12}_{6}C$	Isotopes of carbon	12.000000
${}^{13}_{6}C$		13.003354
${}^{14}_{6}C$		14.003242
${}^{15}_{6}C$		15.010600
${}^{12}_{5}B$	Isobars of mass 12	12.014354
${}^{12}_{6}C$		12.000000
${}^{12}_{7}N$		12.018641
${}^{16}_{8}O$	Oxygen	15.994915
${}^{32}_{15}P$	Isobars of mass 32	31.973910
${}^{32}_{16}S$		31.972074

Appendix C

PERSONNEL MONITORING TERMS

Assume a serious radiation accident with $Na^{131}I$ in which a film badge value of 1 rem of deep dose exposure (DDE) was received by a member of the nuclear medicine staff. Further, it was estimated that there was an uptake of 10 μCi from the volatilized ^{131}I breathed in by this nuclear medicine staff member. The purpose of the new philosophy embodied by new Part 20 is to determine not only the nonstochastic dose to the thyroid, but the risk of stochastic effects to the whole body as well. The procedure would be as follows:

■ Procedure

1. Perform a thyroid bioassay within 24 hours (assume bioassay = 10 μCi*).
2. Evaluate film badge (assume deep dose exposure (DDE) film badge result = 1 rem).
3. Dose ($D_{thyroid \leftarrow thyroid}$) = 5×10^2 mGy/MBq* × 0.0037 = 1.85 rad/μCi × 10 μCi = 18.5 rad

*This is an extremely large amount of ^{131}I to be taken up by the thyroid gland. The limits as dictated by the Nuclear Regulatory Commission (NRC) are much smaller. In accordance with Regulatory Guide 8.9 (NRC), two levels of concern must be established in regard to thyroid bioassays. The *evaluation level* will be any time the organ or tissue receives 2% of the ALI value. The ALI is the Annual Limit on Intake, which indicates the derived limit for the amount of radioactive material taken into the body of an adult worker by inhalation or ingestion in a year. ALI values for both inhalation and ingestion can be found in Table I, Columns 1 and 2 of Appendix B, 10CFR20. The nonstochastic value for inhaled ^{131}I is 50 μCi, with a stochastic value of 200 μCi. However, the thyroid intake retention factor (IRF) for ^{131}I at 24 hours is 0.133 (from NUREG 4884). Therefore, the evaluation level would be 0.133 μCi (50 μCi × 0.133 × 0.02). The *investigational level* is any time the person receives 10% of the ALI value, or 0.665 μCi. Based on the above IRF for a thyroid gland, to receive an uptake of 10 μCi, the person would have had to inhale 75 μCi of ^{131}I, a highly unlikely occurrence, especially in a routine nuclear medicine department.

■ Calculations

External: DDE = D × Q × N = 10 × 1 × 1 = 1.0 rem
Internal: CDE = D × Q × N = 18.5 × 1 × 1 = 18.5 rem
CEDE = CDE × w_T = 18.5 × 0.03† = 0.555 rem
TEDE (stochastic) = DDE + CEDE = 1.0 + 0.555 = 1.555 rem vs.
TODE (nonstochastic) = 18.5 rem + 1 rem = 19.5 rem

It is clear from the above calculation that while the internal radiation dose to the thyroid (from the thyroid) is alarming (18.5 rem) and since contributions from other organs are inconsequential, the equivalent stochastic risk to the whole body (TEDE) is only 1.555 rem. For every rem of exposure, one stochastic event (a fatal malignancy) occurs in every 20,000 people.‡ This radiation accident has increased that risk to 1.555 stochastic events/20,000 people.

See Fig. C-1 for a flow chart of personnel monitoring terms.

*Appendix F.
†Table 6-2.
‡BEIR V.

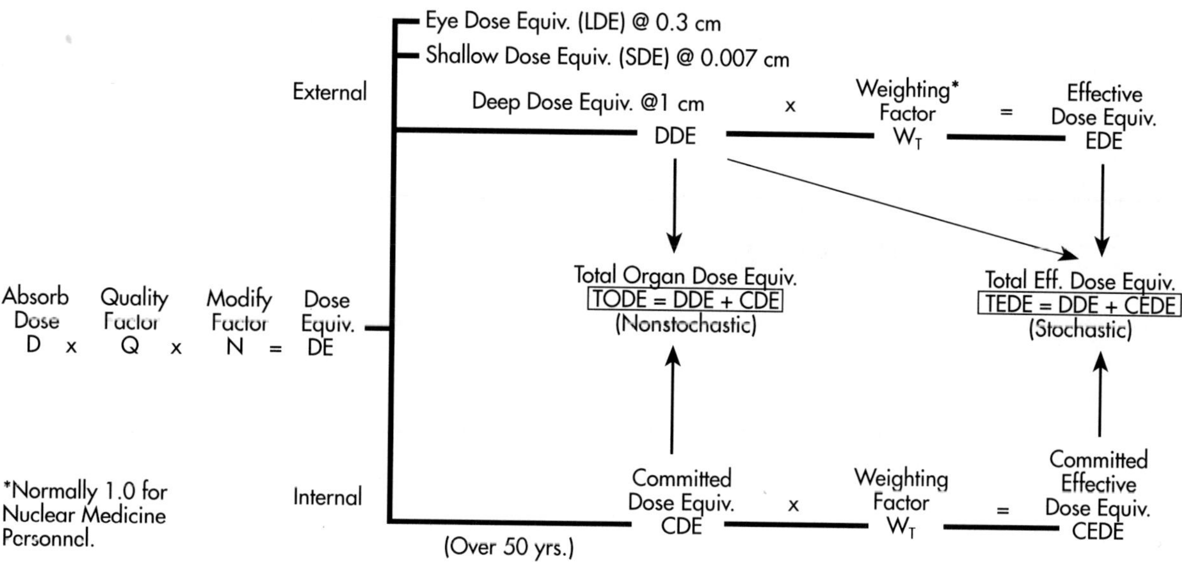

Fig. C-1. Flow chart of personnel monitoring terms.

Appendix D

DATA FOR DECAY OF RADIONUCLIDES USED IN NUCLEAR MEDICINE*

Radionuclide	$T_{1/2}$	$\overline{E}_\beta$(MeV)	Principal photon energies (MeV)	Fractional emission (n_i)	$\Delta_i\left(\frac{g \times rad}{\mu Ci \times hr}\right)$
^{18}F	110m	0.250	—	—	0.5157
			0.511	1.94	2.1115
^{24}Na	15h	0.555	—	—	1.180
			1.37	0.999	2.915
			2.75	0.999	5.861
^{32}P	14.3d	0.695	—	—	1.4799
^{51}Cr	27.8d	0.005	—	—	0.011
			0.320	0.102	0.0694
^{59}Fe	45d	0.117	—	—	0.255
			0.142	0.0096	0.003
			0.19	0.029	0.012
			0.033	0.002	0.002
			1.10	0.56	1.299
			1.29	0.44	1.214
^{60}Co	5.26y	0.093	—	—	0.202
			1.17	0.99	2.494
			1.33	0.99	2.838
^{67}Ga	78h	—	—	—	0.0685
			0.0933	0.3797	0.0754
			0.1845	0.2388	0.0939
			0.2090	0.0247	0.0110
			0.3002	0.1613	0.1031
			0.3936	0.0429	0.0359
			0.0086 (x-ray)	0.3075	0.0056
^{99m}Tc	6h	0.014	—	—	0.0371
			0.018 (x-ray)	0.044	0.0017
			0.021 (x-ray)	0.011	0.0004
			0.140	0.879	0.2630

*Data derived primarily from MIRD Supplement No. 2, Pamphlet 4, March 1969, and MIRD Supplement No. 4, Pamphlet 6, March, 1970, New York, Society of Nuclear Medicine.

Radionuclide	$T_{1/2}$	$\bar{E}_\beta$(MeV)	Principal photon energies (MeV)	Fractional emission (n_i)	$\Delta_i\left(\frac{g \times rad}{\mu Ci \times hr}\right)$
^{113}In	1.7h	0.133	—	—	0.277
			0.392	0.621	0.518
			0.024 (x-ray)	0.124	0.0064
^{123}I	13h	0.026	—	—	0.0602
			0.027 (x-ray)	0.71	0.0415
			0.159	0.84	0.2831
			0.53	0.01	0.0118
^{125}I	60d	0.014	—	—	0.0463
			0.027 (x-ray)	1.152	0.0671
			0.031 (x-ray)	0.248	0.0163
			0.035	0.07	0.0050
^{131}I	8.06d	0.188	—	—	0.4135
			0.080	0.026	0.004
			0.284	0.058	0.035
			0.364	0.820	0.637
			0.6367	0.065	0.0886
			0.723	0.017	0.027
^{133}Xe	5.31d	0.110	—	—	0.299
			0.031 (x-ray)	0.387	0.025
			0.081	0.36	0.062
$^{137}Cs(^{137m}Ba)$	30y	0.226	—	—	0.5367
			0.032 (x-ray)	0.059	0.0039
			0.66	0.898	1.266

Appendix E

DOSIMETRY FOR COMMON PROCEDURES

Radiopharmaceutical	Administered activity	WB (rads)	Gonads (rad)	Other (rad)
$^{99m}TcO_4^-$ (resting population)[1]	10 mCi	0.14	0.09 (testes) 0.22 (ovaries)	2.5 (stomach) 0.65 (large intestine) 1.3 (thyroid) 0.53 (bladder) 0.19 (red marrow)
^{99m}Tc Sn DTPA[2]	20 mCi	0.12	0.15 (testes) 0.22 (ovaries)	1.8 (kidneys)
^{99m}Tc sulfur colloid[3]	4 mCi	0.075	0.0044 (testes) 0.023 (ovaries)	1.35 (liver) 0.85 (spleen) 0.11 (bone marrow)
^{99m}Tc MAA[4] or ^{99m}Tc HAM	3 mCi	0.05	0.05 (testes) 0.06 (ovaries)	0.78 (lung) 0.08 (spleen) 0.09 (liver)
^{99m}Tc PYP[5]	15 mCi	0.13	0.15 (testes) 0.14 (ovaries)	0.59 (skeleton) 0.42 (bone marrow) 2.1 (kidneys)
^{99m}Tc gluco	15 mCi	0.11	0.15 (testes) 0.24 (ovaries)	2.55 (kidneys) 4.20 (bladder) 0.15 (liver)
^{99m}Tc HSA	5 mCi	0.073	0.079 (testes) 0.082 (ovaries)	0.166 (bladder) 0.063 (kidneys) 0.076 (red marrow)
^{99m}Tc Sestamibi[6]	30 mCi	(2 hr void) 0.5	0.3 (testes) 1.5 (ovaries)	5.4 (ULI wall) 3.9 (LLI wall) 3.0 (small intestine)
		(4-8 hr void) 0.5	0.4 (testes) 1.6 (ovaries)	5.4 (ULI wall) 4.2 (LLI wall) 4.2 (urin./bl. wall)
^{99m}Tc Choletec[7]	10 mCi	0.2	0.05 (testes) 1.01 (ovaries)	4.74 (ULI wall) 3.64 (LLI wall) 2.99 (small intestine)

Radiopharmaceutical	Administered activity	WB (rads)	Gonads (rad)	Other (rad)
Na ^{131}I[8]	10 μCi	0.005	0.001 (testes) 0.001 (ovaries)	8.0 (thyroid) 0.004 (liver) 0.002 (red marrow) 0.016 (stomach)
^{133}Xe (equilibrium study)[10]	10 mCi	0.001	—	0.30 (lung)
^{67}Ga citrate[11]	4 mCi	1.04	0.96 (testes) 1.12 (ovaries)	3.60 (lower colon) 2.24 (upper colon) 2.32 (bone marrow) 2.12 (spleen) 1.84 (liver) 1.64 (kidneys)
^{111}In DTPA (intrathecal injection)[12]	1 mCi	0.10	0.06 (testes) 0.07 (ovaries)	2.3 (brain) 1.3 (spinal cord) 0.12 (kidneys) 0.10 (red marrow)
^{111}In OncoScint[13]	5 mCi	2.7	1.4 (testes) 2.9 (ovaries)	16 (spleen) 15 (liver) 12 (red marrow) 9.7 (kidney)
^{201}Tl chloride[14]	1.5 mCi	0.36	0.81 (testes) 0.85 (ovaries)	0.51 (heart) 2.2 (kidneys) 1.12 (thyroid) 0.97 (small intestine) 0.93 (liver) 0.51 (red marrow)
Na ^{123}I (radioisotopically pure)[8]	200 μCi	0.005	0.002 (testes) 0.007 (ovaries)	1.5 (thyroid) 0.006 (liver) 0.006 (red marrow) 0.046 (stomach)
^{125}IHSA[9]	10 μCi	0.02	—	0.14 (blood)
^{51}Cr RBCs[15]	100 μCi	0.028	0.033 (testes) 0.033 (ovaries)	0.10 (blood) 1.32 (spleen)
^{131}I triolein[16]	25 μCi	0.004	0.005 (testes) 0.005 (ovaries)	
^{125}I oleic acid[17]	25 μCi	0.001	—	
^{57}Co cyanocobalamin[18]	0.5 μCi	0.005	0.0026 (testes) 0.0033 (ovaries)	0.065 (liver) 0.0003 (lower large intestine)
^{58}Co cyanocobalamin[18]	0.8 μCi	0.012	0.0074 (testes) 0.010 (ovaries)	0.14 (liver) 0.0018 (lower large intestine)

References

1. MIRD/dose estimate report No. 8; Summary of current radiation dose estimates to normal humans from ^{99m}Tc as sodium pertechnetate, Jan. 1976.
2. Package insert for DTPA (Sn) kit (chelate), Diagnostic Isotopes, Inc., Jan. 1977.
3. Package insert for Tesuloid technetium =99m sulfur colloid kit, ER Squibb & Sons, Inc., May 1978.
4. Package insert for Pulmolite technetium =99m aggregated albumin kit, New England Nuclear, Aug. 1976.
5. Package insert for TechneScan PYP kit, Mallinckrodt, Inc., March 1978.
6. Package insert for Cardiolite, DuPont Merck Pharmaceutical Co.
7. Package insert for Choletec, Squibb Diagnostics.
8. MIRD/dose estimate report No. 5: summary of current radiation dose estimates to humans from ^{123}I, ^{124}I, ^{125}I, ^{126}I, ^{130}I, ^{131}I, and ^{132}I as sodium iodide, Sept. 1975.
9. *Physician's desk reference for radiology and nuclear medicine,* Oradell, NJ, 1976, Medical Economics Co., pp 86-87.
10. Package insert for ^{133}Xe-V.S.S. (Ventilation Study System), Medi-Physics, Inc., Aug. 1978.
11. Gallium imaging, part 1, *Medi-Physics/Forum* 1(2), June 1975.
12. Proposed package insert for indium $^{-}$111 DTPA, Medi-Physics, Inc., Nov. 1975.
13. Package insert for OncoScint, Cytogen and Knoll.
14. Package insert for thallous chloride ^{201}Tl, New England Nuclear, Nov. 1977.

15. Package insert for sodium chromate ^{51}Cr injection, Mallinckrodt, Inc., July 1977.
16. Package insert for triolein ^{131}I capsules, Mallinckrodt, Inc., March 1978.
17. Package insert for oleic acid ^{125}I capsules, Mallinckrodt, Inc., March 1978.
18. Package insert for Dicopac kit, Amersham Corp., May 1978.

Appendix F

ABSORBED DOSE EQUIVALENT PER UNIT ADMINISTERED ACTIVITY IN NORMAL ADULTS

Function or organ examined	Radionuclide	Pharmaceutical	Most highly exposed organs: Organ I (mGy/MBq)*	Organ 2 (mGy/MBq)	Organ* (mGy/MBq)	Conceptus (mGy/MBq)	Effective dose equiv. (mSv/MBq)
Bone	^{99m}Tc	phosphate/phosphonate	6.3E-02 (bone surface)	5.0E-02 (bladder)	9.6E-03 (bone marrow)	6.1E-03	8.0E-03
Renal	^{51}Cr	EDTA	2.3E-02 (bladder)	2.8E-03 (uterus)	1.8E-03 (kidney)	2.8E-03	2.3E-03
	^{123}I	Hippuran	2.0E-01 (bladder)	1.7E-02 (uterus)	7.3E-03 (lower large intestine)	1.7E-02	1.5E-02
	^{131}I	Hippuran	9.6E-01 (bladder)	3.5E-02 (uterus)	3.0E-02 (kidney)	3.5E-02	6.6E-02
	^{99m}Tc	DTPA	6.5E-02 (bladder)	7.9E-03 (uterus)	4.4E-03 (kidney)	7.9E-03	6.3E-03
	^{99m}Tc	DMSA	1.7E-01 (kidney)	1.9E-02 (bladder)	1.3E-02 (adrenal, spleen)	4.6E-03	1.6E-02
Thyroid	^{99m}Tc	pertechnetate (no blocking)	6.2E-02 (upper large intestine)	2.9E-02 (stomach)	2.3E-02 (thyroid)	8.1E-03	1.3E-02
	^{131}I	iodide (35% uptake)	5.0E+02 (thyroid)	4.6E-01 (stomach)	4.0E-01 (bladder)	5.0E-02	1.5E+01
	^{123}I	iodide (35% uptake)	4.5E+00 (thyroid)	6.8E-02 (stomach)	6.0E-02 (bladder)	1.4E-02	1.5E-01
Liver (+ gall bladder)	^{99m}Tc	colloid (large)	7.7E-02 (spleen)	7.4E-02 (liver)	1.2E-02 (pancreas)	1.9E-03	1.4E-02
	^{99m}Tc	millimicrospheres	7.7E-02 (spleen)	7.4E-02 (liver)	1.5E-02 (bone marrow)	1.8E-03	1.4E-02
	^{99m}Tc	HIDA	1.1E-01 (gall bladder)	9.2E-02 (upper large intestine)	6.2E-02 (lower large intestine)	1.3E-02	2.4E-02
	^{57}Co	B_{12} (no carrier)	5.1E+01 (liver)	5.4E+00 (adrenals, pancreas)	5.0E+00 (kidney)	1.8E+00	5.8E+00
Brain	^{99m}Tc	pertechnetate (blocked thyroid)	3.2E-02 (bladder)	6.6E-03 (uterus)	4.7E-03 (kidney, ovary)	6.6E-03	5.3E-03
	^{99m}Tc	DTPA (lumbar)	4.6E-02 (spinal cord)	2.9E-02 (bone marrow)	1.7E-02 (kidney, bladder)	4.5E-03	1.1E-02
	^{99m}Tc	gluconate/glucoheptonate	5.6E-02 (bladder)	4.9E-02 (kidney)	7.7E-03 (uterus)	7.7E-03	9.0E-03
	^{18}F	FDG	1.7E-01 (bladder)	6.5E-02 (heart)	2.6E-02 (brain)	2.0E-02	2.7E-02

Function or organ examined	Radionuclide	Pharmaceutical	Most highly exposed organs: Organ I (mGy/MBq)*	Organ 2 (mGy/MBq)	Organ* (mGy/MBq)	Conceptus (mGy/MBq)	Effective dose equiv. (mSv/MBq)
Lung	^{99m}Tc	MAA	6.7E-02 (lung)	1.6E-02 (liver)	1.0E-02 (bladder)	2.4E-03	1.2E-02
	^{99m}Tc	aerosol (fast clearance)	4.7E-02 (bladder)	1.7E-02 (lung)	5.9E-03 (uterus)	5.9E-03	7.0E-03
		(slow clearance)	9.3E-02 (lung)	1.3E-02 (bladder)	6.4E-03 (breast)	1.7E-03	1.5E-02
	^{133}Xe	gas, 5 min (re-breathing)	1.1E-03 (lung)	8.4E-04 (bone marrow)	8.3E-04 (breast)	7.4E-04	8.0E-04
	^{133}Xe	gas, 30 s 1 breath	7.7E-04 (lung)	1.2E-04 (bone surfaces, bone marrow, breast)	1.1E-04 (small & large intestines, liver, pancreas, spleen, uterus)	1.1E-04	1.9E-04
	^{81m}Kr	gas	2.1E-04 (lung)	4.6E-06 (breast)	3.5E-06 (pancreas)	1.3E-07	2.7E-05
Heart	^{201}Tl	thallous ion	5.6E-01 (testes)	5.4E-01 (kidney)	3.6E-01 (lower large intestine)	5.0E-02	2.3E-01
	^{99m}Tc	RBC	2.3E-02 (heart)	1.5E-02 (spleen)	1.4E-02 (lung)	4.7E-03	8.5E-03
Abscess	^{111}In	white cells	5.5E+00 (spleen)	7.1E-01 (liver)	6.9E-01 (bone marrow)	1.2E-01	5.9E-01
	^{67}Ga	citrate	5.9E-01 (bone surface)	2.0E-01 (lower large intestine)	1.9E-01 (bone marrow)	7.9E-02	1.2E-01
Thrombi	^{125}I	fibrinogen (thyroid totally blocked)	3.2E-01 (heart)	2.4E-01 (spleen)	2.3E-01 (lung)	5.5E-02	1.2E-01
	^{111}In	platelets	7.5E+00 (spleen)	7.3E-01 (liver)	6.6E-01 (pancreas)	9.5E-02	7.0E-01
	^{51}Cr	platelets	2.6E+00 (spleen)	3.0E-01 (liver)	1.9E-01 (bone marrow)	2.8E-02	2.4E-01
Pancreas	^{75}Se	methionine	6.2E+00 (liver)	5.3E+00 (kidney)	3.9E+00 (spleen)	2.6E+00	3.0E+00
Adrenals	^{75}Se	methyl cholesterol	5.1E+00 (adrenals)	2.0E+00 (liver)	1.8E+00 (small intestine, pancreas, uterus, bone marrow)	1.8E+00	1.7E+00
	^{131}I	MIBG	8.4E-01 (liver)	5.9E-01 (bladder)	4.9E-01 (spleen)	7.7E-02	2.1E-01
Spleen	^{51}Cr	RBC denatured	5.6E+00 (spleen)	3.0E-01 (pancreas)	1.7E-01 (liver)	1.3E-02	4.0E-01
GIT	^{99m}Tc	pertechnetate (oral, no blocking agent)	7.4E-02 (upper large intestine)	5.0E-02 (stomach)	3.0E-02 (small intestine)	8.7E-03	1.5E-02

*mGy/MBq × 3.7 = rad/mCi

Appendix G

MISCELLANEOUS

■ RELATIONSHIPS BETWEEN "SPECIAL" UNITS AND THE SI UNITS

Quantity	Dimensions	Previous SI unit	New SI unit; name (abbreviation)	Relationships with special unit
Activity	s^{-1}	s^{-1}	becquerel (Bq)	1 Ci = 3.7×10^{10} Bq 1 Bq ≃ 2.703×10^{-11} Ci
Exposures	$s \cdot A \cdot kg^{-1}$	$C \cdot kg^{-1}$	—*	1 R = 2.58×10^{-4} C/kg 1 C/kg = 3.876×10^{3} R
Absorbed dose	$N \cdot m \cdot kg^{-1}$	$J \cdot kg^{-1}$	gray (Gy)	1 rad = 10^{-2} Gy 1 Gy = 100 rad
Dose equivalent	$N \cdot m \cdot kg^{-1}$	$J \cdot kg^{-1}$	sievert (Sv)	1 rem = 10^{-2} Sv 1 Sv = 100 rem

*No name proposed; it is anticipated that this unit will eventually disappear.

■ CONVERSION FACTORS FOR UNITS OF ACTIVITY (A) AND ABSORBED DOSE (D)

Activity (A)				
1 picocurie	(1 pCi)	= 10^{-12} Ci	= 37 millibecquerels	(37 mBq)
1 nanocurie	(1 nCi)	= 10^{-9} Ci	= 37 becquerels	(37 Bq)
1 microcurie	(1 μCi)	= 10^{-6} Ci	= 37 kilobecquerels	(37 kBq)
1 millicurie	(1 mCi)	= 10^{-3} Ci	= 37 megabecquerels	(37 MBq)
1 curie	(1 Ci)	= 1 Ci	= 37 gigabecquerels	(37 GBq)
1 kilocurie	(1 kCi)	= 10^{3} Ci	= 37 terabecquerels	(37 TBq)
1 megacurie	(1 MCi)	= 10^{6} Ci	= 37 petabecquerels	(37 PBq)
1 gigacurie	(1 GCi)	= 10^{9} Ci	= 37 exabecquerels	(37 EBq)
1 becquerel	(1 Bq)	= 1 Bq	= 27.03 picocuries	(27.03 pCi)
1 kilobecquerel	(1 kBq)	= 10^{3} Bq	= 27.03 nanocuries	(27.03 nCi)
1 megabecquerel	(1 MBq)	= 10^{6} Bq	= 27.03 microcuries	(27.03 μCi)
1 gigabecquerel	(1 GBq)	= 10^{9} Bq	= 27.03 millicuries	(27.03 mCi)
1 terabecquerel	(1 TBq)	= 10^{12} Bq	= 27.03 curies	(27.03 Ci)
1 petabecquerel	(1 PBq)	= 10^{15} Bq	= 27.03 kilocuries	(27.03 kCi)
1 exabecquerel	(1 EBq)	= 10^{18} Bq	= 27.03 megacuries	(27.03 MCi)

Absorbed dose (D)			Absorbed dose (D)		
1 millirad	(1 mrad) = 10^{-3} rad = 10 micrograys	(10 μGy)	1 microgray	(1 μGy) = 10^{-6} Gy = 100 microrad	(100 μrad)
1 rad	(1 rad) = 1 rad = 10 milligrays	(10 mGy)	1 milligray	(1 mGy) = 10^{-3} Gy = 100 millirad	(100 mrad)
1 kilorad	(1 krad) = 10^{3} rad = 10 grays	(10 Gy)	1 gray	(1 Gy) = 1 Gy = 100 rad	(100 rad)
1 megarad	(1 Mrad) = 10^{6} rad = 10 kilograys	(10 kGy)	1 kilogray	(1 kGy) = 10^{3} Gy = 100 kilorad	(100 krad)

GLOSSARY

aberrant deviated from normal structure.

ablation removal.

absorption the process by which radiation imparts some or all of its energy to any material through which it passes. (See *Compton effect, photoelectric effect,* and *pair production.*)

absorption coefficient fractional decrease in the intensity of a beam of radiation per unit thickness (linear absorption coefficient), per unit mass (mass absorption coefficient), or per atom (atomic absorption coefficient) of absorber.

accuracy the degree to which the experimentally obtained value agrees with the true value. See also *precision.*

acinus saccular terminal division of a compound gland having a narrow lumen, in contrast to an alveolus. Several acini combine to form a lobule.

acquisition in data processing, the tabulation of raw data, especially from a device such as a counter, teletype, or punched or magnetic tape.

activation analysis A method of chemical analysis especially for small traces of material, based on the detection of characteristic radionuclides following nuclear bombardment.

activity see *radioactivity.*

acute exposure term used to denote radiation exposure of short duration.

adenopathy any disease of the glands, especially lymph glands.

adjuvant a substance that increases the formation and persistence of antibodies when injected together with antigens.

  Freund's adjuvant in the incomplete form a mixture of neutral detergent and mineral oil; the complete form also contains killed mycobacteria.

adrenergic activated or transmitted by epinephrine. A term applied to those nerve fibers that liberate sympathin at a synapse when a nerve impulse passes (that is, the sympathetic fibers).

affinity related to the energy of reaction; most often used synonymously with avidity. The simple difference between these two terms is that avidity specifically refers to the quality of the antibody, whereas affinity reflects the quality of the antigen. Both avidity and affinity affect the overall binding in antigen/antibody complex formation.

affinity constant (K) for the reaction $A + BR \overset{K_a}{\rightleftarrows} A - BR$ between the total analyte (A) and binding regent (BR), then $K_a = \frac{(A - BR)}{(A)\,(BR)}$ at equilibrium under defined conditions, where [ ] indicates molar concentrations.

agglutination mass formed by the joining together or aggregation of suspended particles.

akinesis absence of motor function or activity.

allergy altered reaction capacity to a specified substance; acquired sensitivities to drugs and biologic substances.

alpha particle a helium nucleus, consisting of 2 protons and 2 neutrons; it has a double positive charge and possesses a mass of 4.00278 atomic mass units (amu).

alveolus designates a small saclike dilation; an air cell of the lung.

amplification as related to radiation detection instruments, the process (either gas or electronic or both) by which ionization effects are magnified to a degree suitable for measurement.

analyte the substance in the specimen to be analyzed in an assay.

ancillary departments a diagnostic or service area providing patient care (e.g., Nuclear Medicine, Laboratory, Radiology, Physical Therapy).

anemia deficiency of blood as a whole, or deficiency of hemoglobin or in the number of red blood cells.

angstrom unit (Å) 10^{-8} cm. Used to measure the wavelength of electromagnetic radiations.

anion negatively charged ion.

ankylosis abnormal immobility and consolidation of a joint.

annihilation radiation the photons produced when an electron and a positron unite and then cease to exist. The annihilation of a positron-electron pair results in the production of 2 photons; each has an energy of 0.51 MeV.

anode a positive electrode; the electrode to which negative ions (anions) are attracted.

anoxia oxygen deficiency; a condition that results from a diminished supply of oxygen to the tissues.

antecubital vein vein located in front of the elbow in each arm.

antibiotic a substance of biologic origin that inhibits the growth of or kills microorganisms. Common examples are penicillin, streptomycin, and aureomycin.

antibody protein of the immunoglobulin class produced in lymphoid cells in response to stimulation by immunogen and capable of combining in vivo with said antigenic substance as a defense mechanism, or of reacting in vitro for specific analysis of the antigen; or, a substance produced in response to an antigen that reacts specifically with that antigen.

anticoincidence circuit a circuit with two input terminals that delivers an output pulse if one input terminal receives a pulse but not if both input terminals receive a pulse either simultaneously or within a predetermined time interval. A principle used in pulse-height analysis.

antigen (Ag) any substance that can induce the formation of antibodies and that reacts specifically with the antibodies formed.

antigen/antibody complex the product of the joining of an antigen to an antibody. The complex has both chemical and physical properties different from either the antigen or the antibody.

antigenicity the ability of a substance to induce the immune response. Antigenicity of a substance depends on both its molecular size and its chemical composition. Certain substances, because of their small molecular size (for example, digoxin, angiotensin I, angiotensin II, triiodothyronine), will be able to induce the immune response only when they are coupled to larger molecules.

antiserum blood serum from an animal immunized against a specific antigen and therefore containing antibody to that antigen.

aplasia developmental defect or congenital absence of a part.

arrhythmia absence of rhythm.

arteriogram radiographic study of an artery following injection of contrast media.

arteriosclerosis hardening of the arteries.

assay a procedure to measure the presence or amount of test substance (for example, hormone in blood), usually by comparing the reactive behavior of sample to that of a standard or series of standards in which the amount of substance is known.

atheroma arteriosclerosis with significant degenerative changes.

atom the smallest particle of an element that is capable of entering into a chemical reaction.

atomic mass unit (amu) unit of mass equal to $\frac{1}{12}$ the arbitrary mass assigned to carbon 12. One amu is equivalent to 931.2 MeV of energy.

atomic number symbol: Z. The number of protons in the nucleus and therefore the number of positive charges in the nucleus. The atomic number also reflects the number of electrons outside the nucleus of a neutral atom.

atomic weight the relative weight of the atom of an element compared with the weight of one atom of oxygen taken as 16.

atrophy size reduction of an organ, cell, or tissue.

attenuation the process by which radiation is reduced in intensity when passing through some material. This is a combination of absorption and scattering processes.

autoimmune immunity directed against the body's own tissue.

autologous an immunologic term for "derived from self" (for example, skin graft, blood cells). Related terms are isologous (*synonym,* syngeneic), derived from identical twin (same genetic makeup); homologous, derived from the same species; and heterologous, derived from a different species. All may be related to immunochemical specificity.

autonomous self-governing, independent function.

autoradiograph the record of radiation from radioactive material in an object that is made by placing its surface in close proximity to a photographic emulsion.

avalanche the multiplicative process in which a single charged particle accelerated by a strong electric field produces additional charged particles through collision with neutral gas molecules.

average life (mean life) the average of the individual lives of all the atoms of a particular radioactive substance. This average is 1.443 times the radioactive half-life of the substance.

avidity represents the energy of binding between an antibody and its specific antigen.

Avogadro's number the number of molecules in a gram molecular weight of any substance (6.03×10^{23} molecules); also, the number of atoms in a gram atomic weight of any element.

B_0 in competitive binding analysis or other such assays using a standard curve, an index of the amount of tracer (for example, labeled antigen) reacting with binding reagent (for example, antibody) in the absence of any added test substance (unlabeled standard antigen).

background count that portion of the count displayed by the counter that is intrinsic to the measurement system but independent of the assay reaction.

background radiation radiation caused by cosmic rays, radioactive materials in the vicinity, and a slight radioactive contamination of the materials of which the instrument is made.

backscattering the process of scattering or deflecting into the sensitive volume of a measuring instrument radiations that originally had no motion in that direction. The process is dependent on the nature of the mounting material, the nature of the sample, the type and energy of the radiations, and the particular geometric arrangement.

barrier shields of radiation-absorbing material, such as lead and concrete.

batch a group unit in assay processing comprising controls, standards, and a set of test samples.

batch table in data processing by computer, a table defined by the user that lists parameters such as type, position, and number of replicates—in effect describing the makeup of an assay batch.

benign not malignant.

beta emission release of high-energy beta particles by disintegration of certain radioactive nuclides.

beta particle an elementary radioactive particle like an electron emitted from the atomic nucleus and most commonly measured in radioassay by liquid scintillation counting. High-energy positively or negatively charged electron.

betatron a device for accelerating electrons by means of magnetic induction.

binary scaler a scaler in which the scaling factor is 2 per stage. See *scaler*.

binding in competitive radioassay, the reactive forces between ligand and binding agent describable by the mass action law and measurable by the fraction of reagent tracer bound in the ligand-binding agent complex.

binding agent in competitive radioassay, the test reagent chosen, most commonly antibody, to react specifically with the substance under test via mass action, reversible reaction.

binding assay an in vitro test employing the principles of reversible reactions.

binding capacity the amount of specific binding sites available per quantity of binding reagent. The extrapolated point of the x-axis of a Scatchard plot performed under defined conditions.

binding energy the energy represented by the difference in mass between the actual mass of the nucleus and the sum of the component parts.

binding site site of specific attachment of macromolecules to one another. In immunoassay, antibody tends to be bivalent and antigen multivalent.

biologic half-life time required for an organism to eliminate one half of an administered dose of any substance by normal processes.

bivalent see *binding site*.

bleb a bubble (culla) or vesicle filled with fluid or air.

blood pigments pigments normally found in blood, such as hemoglobin and bilirubin.

bone marrow the soft material that fills the cavity in most bones and manufactures most of the formed elements of the blood.

bound in competitive binding assay, the fraction of tracer test substance recovered in or calculated to be in the ligand-binding agent complex (for example, antigen/antibody) at reactive completion. See also *free*.

Bremsstrahlung the secondary photon radiation produced by the deceleration of charged particles as they pass through matter.

budget a means of numerically expressing levels of resources expended and revenues generated over time, usually by month for a duration of 1 year, compared with a predetermined standard.

buffer(s) or buffer solution the ability of a system to resist changes in pH on the addition of acid or base or on diluting it with the solvent. pH may be defined as the negative logarithm of the hydrogen ion concentration. Mathematically it is written as [pH = −log(H+)]. A weak acid or weak base in the presence of one of its salts forms a buffer solution. Examples of typical buffer systems include the following: acetic acid (CH_3COONa), sodium dihydrogen phosphate (NaH_2Po_4), disodium hydrogen phosphate (Na_2HPo_4), ammonium hydroxide (NH_4OH), and ammonium chloride (NH_4Cl).

cancer popular terminology for any malignant neoplasm.

capillary small, hairlike vessel connecting arterioles and venules.

carcinogenic cancer-producing.

carcinoma malignant epithelial tumor.

carrier (1) a quantity of an element that may be mixed with its radioisotopes to give enough of a quantity to facilitate chemical operations. (2) A substance that, when associated with a trace of another substance, will carry the trace with it through a chemical or physical process.

carrier (cold compound) the unlabeled (nonradioactive) form of an element or compound.

carrier free a preparation of radioisotope of "high isotopic abundance," that is, one containing no carrier.

catabolism destructive phase of metabolism in which complex compounds are broken down by the cells of the body often with the liberation of energy; the opposite of anabolism.

cataract a clouding of the lens of the eye that obstructs the passage of light.

cathode a negative electrode; the electrode that attracts positive ions.

cation a positively charged ion.

CBA an abbreviation for competitive binding assay.

cell fundamental unit of structure and function in living organisms.

chain reaction any chemical or nuclear process in which some of the products of the process, including energy, are instrumental in the continuation or magnification of the process.

characteristic radiation radiation originating from an atom after the removal of an electron or excitation of the nucleus.

chromatoelectrophoresis method of separating bound from free based on differential migration in an electrical field (electrophoresis) in which the support medium exhibits a higher affinity for free ligand relative to bound complex.

channel in radioassay, the discriminator settings for the energy range selected for an isotope counted in a gamma or liquid scintillation counter.

channels ratio a method of quench correction in liquid scintillation counting.

chronic exposure the term used to denote radiation exposure of long duration.

cirrhosis chronic, progressive disease of the liver, essentially inflammatory, characterized by proliferation of connective tissue, degeneration of parenchymal cells, and distortion of architectural pattern. The liver may be either enlarged or reduced in size.

cleanup in radioassay, any preliminary treatment of test sample to remove interfering or competing substances.

clot retraction contraction or shrinkage of a blood clot resulting in the extrusion of serum.

cloud chamber a device for observing the paths of ionizing particles that is based on the principle that supersaturated vapor condenses readily on ions.

coagulation formation of a coagulum or clot, as in blood or milk.

coated tube a form of solid phase radioimmunoassay involving the attachment of antibody to a solid structure such as a test tube wall or plastic bead to facilitate separation.

cocktail in liquid scintillation counting, a system of organic solvents and fluors into which sample is dispensed for counting.

coincidence the occurrence of one or more ionizing events in one or more detectors simultaneously or within an assignable time interval.

coincidence circuit a circuit with two input terminals that delivers an output pulse only when both input terminals receive pulses simultaneously or within a predetermined time interval. A principle used in the detection of positron emitters.

collimator a device for confining the elements of a beam within an assigned solid angle.

competitive binding the underlying principle of RIA, namely, the competition between labeled (tracer) and unlabeled test substance molecules for binding sites on test reagent molecules during a reversible reaction.

competitive binding assay an in vitro test procedure using the principles of competitive binding, commonly employing but not limited to the use of radioactive isotope as a tracer, antigen as ligand, and antibody as binding agent.

competitive protein binding assay a competitive binding assay that uses for binding agent some protein other than antibody, commonly a serum or plasma protein.

Compton effect absorption effect observed for x- and gamma radiation in which the incident photon interacts with an orbital electron on the absorber atom to produce a recoil electron and a photon of energy less than the incident photon.

concentration the amount of a substance in weight or moles present in unit volume of a solution.

- ***molar concentration*** concentration expressed as moles per liter or millimoles per milliliter (1 mM = 0.001 mol). A mole is Avogadro's number (6.023×10^{23}) of molecules of a substance or mass numerically equal to the molecular weight. It is usually expressed as the gram molecular weight.

congenital existing at birth.

conservation of mass-energy energy and mass are interchangeable, as evidenced by the equation $E = mc^2$, where E is energy, m is mass, and c is velocity of light.

contamination, radioactive deposition of radioactive material in any place where its presence may be harmful. The harm may be in invalidating the experiment or procedure or in actually being a source of danger to personnel.

corpuscle (1) encapsulated sensory nerve end-organ, (2) old term for cell, especially a blood cell.

cosmic rays radiation, both particulate and electromagnetic, that originates outside the earth's atmosphere.

cost analysis an accounting process that identifies both direct and indirect costs incurred for providing a service. It is used to determine patient charges for services.

count (radiation measurements) external indication of a device designed to enumerate ionizing events. It may refer to a single detected event or to the total number that is registered in a given period of time.

count rate meter a device that gives a continuous indication of the average rate of ionizing events.

counting efficiency counts per minute/disintegrations per minute $\times$ 100 = Efficiency.

control samples samples of known composition run to check accuracy or correct for reaction vectors.

control tubes sets of tubes in an assay batch that permit taking critical parameters into account, namely TC, NSB, B_0, and standards.

conversation in data processing, the interaction between user and computer processor to list a set of instructions to be carried out by the computer system.

counter a general designation applied to radiation detection instruments.

cpm an abbreviation for counts per minute, the average rate of radioactive events in a test sample perceived and displayed by a gamma or liquid scintillation counting system.

CPB an abbreviation for competitive protein binding.

cross-reacting antibody antibody capable of combining with an antigen that did not specifically stimulate its production.

cross-reacting antigen antigen capable of combining with antibody produced in response to a different antigen.

cross reactivity closely resembles specificity. Reactions where antibodies react with two or more antigens of similar structure are known as cross reactions. Cross reactivity can occur between different hormones from the same species. For example, there is partial or complete cross reactivity between FSH, LH, and TSH and HGH and HPL.

cumulative dose (radiation) total dose resulting from repeated exposures. This may be radiation to the same region or to the whole body.

curie basic unit of radioactivity. One curie (Ci) = 2.22×10^{12} dpm.

current activity normally demonstrates a given activity's effect on a budget, over a specific time frame (e.g., current activity for the month of July) for the purpose of comparison.

curve fitting in competitive radioassay, the plotting in various ways of the fraction of tracer bound as a function of test substance concentration in the assay standards. Commonly, mathematical transformations are used to linearize these curves, which tend to be exponential, the most popular methods being Scatchard plots, logit, and hyperbolic transforms.

cyclotron a device for accelerating charged particles in a spiral fashion to high energies by means of an alternating electric field between electrodes placed in a constant magnetic field.

cytoplasm protoplasm of a cell other than that of the nucleus, as opposed to nucleoplasm.

daughter a synonym for a product of decay.

DCC an abbreviation for dextran-coated charcoal.

decade scaler a scaler that has a power of 10 for a scaling factor.

decay, radioactive the disintegration of the nucleus of an unstable atom by the spontaneous emission of charged particles and/or photons.

decay in radioassay, the spontaneous transformation of a radionuclide, resulting in a decrease with time of the number of radioactive events in a sample.

decay constant the fraction of the number of atoms of a radionuclide that decay in unit time.

decay curve a curve showing the relative amount of radioactive substance remaining after any given time.

default in data processing by computer, a value automatically assigned by the processor when the user does not assign a value in response to a conversation question.

densitometer an instrument using the photoelectric principle to determine the degree of darkening of developed photographic film.

density a term used to denote the degree of darkening of photographic film.

desquamation a shedding of the superficial epithelium, renal tubules, mucous membranes, and skin.

detoxify process, usually consisting of a series of reactions, by which a substance foreign to the body is changed to a compound or compounds more readily excreted.

deuterium ($^2_1$H) a heavy isotope of hydrogen having 1 protron and 1 neutron in the nucleus. It is sometimes called "heavy hydrogen."

deuteron the nucleus of a deuterium atom, containing 1 proton, 1 neutron, and no orbital electrons.

dextran-coated charcoal solution of cross-linked dextrans and activated charcoal used to separate bound from free in RBA absorbing free ligand.

diastole a period of relaxation and dilation of a heart chamber during which it fills with blood.

dilution (1) the difference in concentration of test substance between steps in a standard curve. (2) The addition of diluent to test sample to (a) match the concentration of standard(s) more closely or (b) minimize the effect of interfering substances.

direct costs costs that can be directly identified with a specific activity or cost center (e.g., supplies, services).

disintegration, nuclear spontaneous nuclear transformation (radioactivity) characterized by the emission of energy and/or mass from the nucleus.

disintegration constant the fraction of the number of atoms of a radionuclide that decay per unit time.

dispenser or dispenser/diluter a mechanical device to dispense reagents and/or dilute samples or standards as an aid in laboratory benchwork.

displacement analysis one of several general terms for competitive binding assay, most often used to refer to a variant technique wherein the addition of tracer is delayed to enhance assay sensitivity.

dose in competitive binding assay, the amount of test substance added to any given reference standard.

dose (dosage) according to current usage, the radiation delivered to the whole body or to a specified area or volume.

dose rate radiation dose delivered in unit of time.

dose rate meter any instrument that measures dose rate.

dose/response curve the plot of tracer bound in a competitive binding assay system as a function of test substance concentration.

dosimeter an instrument used to detect and measure an accumulated dose of radiation. In common usage, it is a pencil-size ionization chamber, with or without a built-in, self-reading electrometer used for personnel monitoring.

double antibody technique a technique of recovering bound tracer for measurement of CBA system wherein the separation agent is antibody, heterologous to the primary binding agent antibody.

double label the use of two tracer species (usually different radioisotopes in an assay system).

dpm an abbreviation for disintegrations per minute, the average rate of radioactive events occurring in a test sample.

dyskinesis impairment of motor function or activity.

dyspnea labored or difficult breathing.

ectopic away from normal position.

effective half-life the time required for a radionuclide introduced into a biologic system to be reduced to one half as a result of the combined action of radioactive decay and biologic elimination.

efficiency (of counters) a measure of the probability that a count will be recorded when radiation is "seen" by a detector.

efficiency in radioassay, the counts perceived by a gamma or beta counter relative to the known disintegration rate of a comparable standard radioactive source.

ejection fraction percent of difference between ventricular systolic and diastolic volume.

electrode either terminal or an electric source.

electrolyte substance that in solution is capable of conducting an electric current and is decomposed by it.

electron a negatively charged particle that is a constituent of every neutral atom. A unit of negative electricity equal to 4.80×10^{-10} electrostatic units. It has a mass of 0.000549 atomic mass units (amu).

electron capture a method of radioactive decay involving the capture of an orbital electron by its nucleus.

electron volt (eV) the amount of energy gained by an electron as it passes through a potential difference of 1 volt.

electrophoresis migration of charged colloidal particles through the medium in which they are dispersed when placed under the influence of an applied electric potential.

electroscope an instrument for detecting electric charges by deflection of charged bodies.

element a pure substance consisting of atoms of the same atomic number.

elution process of extraction of the absorbed substance from the solid adsorbing medium in chromatography.

embolus any foreign matter, as a blood clot or air bubble, brought by the blood through a larger vessel and forced into a smaller one obstructing circulation.

emphysema overdistension of the air spaces (alveoli) in the lungs.

endocrine internal secretion; pertaining to ductless glands that secrete substances directly into the bloodstream.

endogenous produced within or as a result of internal causes; applied to the formation of cells or of spores within the parent cell.

endothelium mesodermally derived, simple, squamous epithelium lining any closed cavity in the body.

energy the capacity to do work. Potential energy is the energy inherent in mass because of its position with reference to other masses. Kinetic energy is the energy possessed by mass because of its motion.

enriched material material in which the relative amount of one or more forms of an element has been increased.

enzyme substance formed by living cells, having the capacity to facilitate a chemical reaction.

epidermis the outer layer of the skin.

epilation the temporary or permanent loss of hair.

epithelium the cells lining all canals and surfaces having communication with external air; cells specialized for secretion in certain glands.

equilibrium the stage in a reaction where the concentration of the reactive species is no longer changing.

erg the unit of work done by a force of 1 dyne acting through a distance of 1 cm. The unit of energy that can exert a force of 1 dyne through a distance of 1 cm.

erythema redness of the skin produced by congestion of the capillaries, which may result from a variety of causes, the etiology or a special type of lesion often being indicated by a modifying term.

erythematous of the nature of erythema (red).

erythrocyte red blood corpuscle. A small, circular disc, with both faces concave, containing hemoglobin that carries oxygen to the body tissues.

erythrocytosis increased erythrocyte count of more than two standard deviations above mean normal as determined by use of the same method on blood of healthy persons of the patient's age and sex and associated with increased total blood volume.

erythroid of a red color; reddish; pertaining to a red cell series.

erythropoietin factor elaborated by the kidney (juxtaglomerular cells) that stimulates red cell production.

etiology the study of the causes of disease and mode of operation.

exocrine pertaining to glands that deliver their secretion or excretion to an epithelial surface, either directly or by means of ducts.

exophthalmos protrusion of eyeball from the orbit.

extracellular occurring outside the cell.

exudation passage of various constituents of blood through the walls of vessels into adjacent tissues or spaces in inflammation.

fibroblast stellate or spindle-shaped cell with a large, oval, flattened nucleus and a thin layer of cytoplasm found in fibrous tissue.

film badge photographic film used for the approximate measurement of radiation exposure for personnel monitoring purposes.

fission the splitting of a nucleus into two or more parts with the subsequent release of enormous amounts of energy.

fission products the elements resulting from fission.

flat-field collimator a collimator constructed so as to permit a broad area to be visualized by a radiation detector. It is usually made of lead with a single aperture that is either cylindrical or slightly conical in shape.

fluor in liquid scintillation counting, an organic compound that reacts indirectly to the energy of beta (or equivalent) radiation from sample material and in turn emanates light photons. In gamma counters the luminescent material is usually inorganic and referred to as scintillator or crystal.

fluorescence in radioassay, a term often used to denote intrinsic luminenscence noted in liquid scintillation counting independent of sample radioactivity. Phosphorescence is also used similarly.

focused collimator a collimator constructed so as to permit only a restricted area to be visualized at one time. It is usually made of lead with holes arranged in a honeycomb fashion and converging at some point distant to the face of the collimator.

follicle a small secretory or excretory sac or gland.

free in competitive binding assay, the fraction of tracer test substance not bound at reaction completion. See also *bound*.

FTE full-time employees, or full-time equivalent. (Two employees, each working a 24-hour part-time week, equals one FTE.)

fusion the act of combining two or more nuclei into one nucleus.

gamma counter solid scintillation counter (solid NaI crystal) used for counting radiation from gamma emitters.

gamma emitters radioactive substances that release photons (electromagnetic waves) on disintegration.

gamma globulin globulins of plasma that in neutral or alkaline solutions have the slowest electrophoretic mobility. Most antibodies are gamma globulins.

gamma rays high-energy, short-wavelength electromagnetic radiation emanating from the nucleus of some nuclides; similar in properties to x rays.

gas amplification the release of additional ions from neutral atoms caused by collisions of electrons that are set free in response to the paths of ionizing radiation and that have acquired high energies as a result of an increased electrical field. A phenomenon seen in proportional counters.

gas-flow counter a radiation detector in which an appropriate atmosphere is maintained in the counter tube by allowing a suitable gas to flow slowly through the sensitive volume.

Geiger counter one of the earliest forms of radiation detection instrument, employing a gas-filled tube.

Geiger region an ionization radiation detector whose operating voltage interval in which the charge collected per ionizing event is essentially independent of the number of primary ions produced in the initial ionizing event.

Geiger threshold the minimum voltage at which a Geiger-Mueller tube operates in the Geiger region.

Geiger-Mueller (G-M) counter tube a highly sensitive gas-filled, radiation-measuring device that operates at voltages in the region of avalanche ionization.

genetic effect of radiation inheritable changes (mutations) produced by the absorption of ionizing radiations.

geometry (1) The spatial configuration, pattern, or relationship of radioactive sample to detector. (2) Sometimes used with a percentage value to denote the portion of sample radiation that reaches the sensitive zone of a detector.

germ cells (genetic cells) the cells of an organism whose function is to reproduce its kind. These cells are characteristically haploid.

globulin class of proteins characterized by being insoluble in water but soluble in saline solutions.

glycogen a carbohydrate formed by and largely stored in the liver.

half-life the time required for disintegration of one half of the radioactive nuclei initially present.

half-value layer (half-thickness) the thickness of any material required to reduce the intensity of an x-ray or gamma-ray beam to half its original value.

hapten any substance unable to induce antibody formation by itself but able to incite antibody formation with antigenic specificity when joined to a large protein molecule.

Hashimoto's struma diffuse enlargement of the thyroid characterized by atrophy of the thyroid parenchyma, fibrosis, and excessive formation of lymphoid tissue.

hematopoiesis formation of blood cells.

hematuria urine containing blood.

hemolysis destruction of red cells and the resultant escape of hemoglobin.

heterologous see *autologous*.

homologous see *autologous*.

hyperbolic curve fit see *curve fitting*.

hormones substances secreted by the endocrine, or ductless, glands that influence the activity of the various organs of the body and thus regulate the metabolic processes. Chemically these represent a diverse group of compounds and can be divided into three classes: (1) Polypeptide or protein hormones, those secreted by pituitary, parathyroid, and pancreas (for example, thyrotropin, TSH, growth hormone, HGH, follicle-stimulating hormone, FSH, parathormone, calcitonin, and insulin). The molecular weights of these hormones range from approximately 1000 to 30,000 or more. (2) Steroid hormones, those produced by the adrenal cortex and gonads (for example, aldosterone, corticosterone, testosterone, progesterone, and estrogens). (3) Simple hormones, those produced by adrenal medulla and thyroid. These are neither protein nor steroid but simple amino acid derivatives (for example, epinephrine, triiodothyronine [T_3], and thyroxine [T_4]).

hydrocephalus increased volume of cerebrospinal fluid within the skull.

hypertonic above normal tension or strength.

hypertrophy increase in size.

hypochondrium upper lateral area of abdomen below the rib cage.

hypokinesis decreased motor function or activity.

hypotonic below normal tension or strength.

hypoxia oxygen want or deficiency, any state wherein a physiologically inadequate amount of oxygen is available to or used by tissue irrespective of cause or degree.

immunochemistry with special reference to competitive binding assay, biochemical techniques and concepts applied to the production, purification, and characterization of antigens and antibodies and to the manipulation of antigen/antibody reactions for analytic purposes.

immunogen a substance that elicits a general immune response, one that triggers the response mechanism without necessarily resulting in the production of specific antibody. Often synonymous with antigen but sometimes referring only to functional immunity against a pathogen.

immunogenicity see *antigenicity*.

immunoreactivity reaction that takes place between an antigen and its antibody.

immunology the biology and chemistry of the immune response (including the phenomena of antibody production), of the development of immunity, and of the mechanisms of immunologic tolerance.

immunosorbent an artificial solid-phase form of immunochemical reagent made by coupling antigen or antibody to a polymer or other insoluble matrix; used for either preparative or analytic purposes.

income/expense report a managing tool demonstrating monthly and year-to-date activities for statistics, revenue, and expenditures.

incremental addition a technique for preparing standards for a standard curve so that the last in a row of tubes contains the highest concentration of known test substances. See also *serial dilution*.

incubation refers to the antigen-antibody (ligand-binding agent) reaction and the conditions under which it is carried out.

indirect costs costs that usually cannot be directly identified with a specific activity, and are usually allocated among areas or departments, depending on such factors as space and utilization (e.g., electricity, heating).

induced radioactivity that activity produced in a substance after bombardment with neutrons or other particles.

inert lacking activity.

infarct an area of dead tissue produced by interference with bloodflow.

input device a data processing term for a device, such as a counter, used to feed data to another device, such as a cassette or computer processor.

insolubilized antibody antibody converted to insoluble form, such as a polymer before the RIA reaction (incubation) as a convenience in separating bound and free tracer.

integrating circuit an electronic circuit that records, at any time, an average value for the number of ionization events occurring per unit time, or an electrical circuit that records the total number of ions collected in a given time.

internal conversion a method of radioactive decay in which the gamma rays from excited nuclei cause the ejection of orbital electrons from the atom.

international reference materials (1) International biologic standard, a reference material of an international source serving as the prime reference or standard against which other reference preparations may be standardized. (2) International reference preparation; a reference preparation standardized against the international biologic standard may be used directly in an assay system.

interstitial (1) Situated between important parts; occupying the interspaces or interstices of a part. (2) Pertaining to the finest connective tissue of organs.

intrathecal within a sheath, particularly within the meninges into the subarachnoid space.

intrinsic factor substance produced by the stomach that combines with extrinsic factor (vitamin B_{12}) to yield an antianemic factor.

ion an atomic particle; an atom or chemical radical bearing an electric charge that is either positive or negative.

ion pair two particles of opposite charge; usually refers to the electron and positive atomic or molecular residue resulting after the interaction of radiation with the orbital electrons of atoms.

ionization the process or the result of any process by which a neutral atom or molecule acquires a charge, either positive or negative.

ionization chamber an instrument designed to measure the quantity of ionizing radiation in terms of the charge of electricity associated with ions that are produced within a defined volume.

ionization potential the potential necessary to separate one electron from an atom, resulting in the formation of an ion pair.

ionizing energy the average energy lost by ionizing radiation for the production of an ion pair in air—about 34 electron volts (eV).

ionizing event any process whereby an ion or group of ions is produced.

ionizing radiation any electromagnetic or particulate radiation capable of direct or indirect ion production in its passage through matter.

irradiation any exposure of matter to radiation.

ischemia local deficiency of blood supply associated with obstruction or functional constriction.

isobar one of two or more different nuclides having the same mass number.

isocount curves curves showing the distribution of radiation in a medium by means of lines or surfaces drawn through points receiving equal doses.

isomer one of several nuclides having the same number of neutrons and protons, but capable of existing for a measurable time in different energy states. Usually, the isomer of higher energy decays to one with lower energy by the process of isomeric transition.

isomeric transition (IT) the process by which a nuclide decays to an isomeric nuclide of lower energy state. Isomeric transitions proceed by gamma ray and/or internal conversion electron emission.

isoresponse curves see *isocount curves*.

isotone one of several nuclides having the same number of neutrons in their nuclei.

isotopes nuclides of the same element having different mass numbers (A) but the same atomic numbers (Z) (that is, same number of protons but different numbers of neutrons).

isotopic abundance in a mixture of isotopes of an element, the fraction or percentage of all atoms of the element that consists of one type of nuclide.

K capture a colloquialism for K electron capture; also loosely used to designate any orbital electron capture process.

keV one thousand electron volts (10^3 eV).

kinetic pertaining to motion; producing motion.

kit a complete system of calibrated reagents and aids prepackaged for convenient performance of an assay.

labeled compound a compound consisting, in part, of labeled molecules. By observations of radioactivity or isotopic composition, this compound or its fragments can be followed through various physical, chemical, or biologic processes.

labeled molecule a molecule containing one or more atoms distinguished by unnatural isotopic composition (with radioactive or stable isotopes).

lamella thin leaf or plate, as of bone.

LD_{50} (lethal dose) the dose of radiation that causes mortality in 50% of a species.

lead equivalent the thickness of lead that results in the same reduction in radiation dose rate under specified conditions as the material in question.

ligand from the Latin, "that which is bound"; in radioassay or competitive binding this term refers to the substance tested for, usually the smaller molecule.

ligation tying off, especially arteries, veins, or ducts.

linear absorption coefficient an expression of the fraction of a beam of radiation absorbed in unit thickness of material.

linear accelerator a device for accelerating charged particles, using alternate electrodes and gaps arranged in a straight line. These electrodes and gaps are so proportioned that when their potentials are varied in the proper amplitude and frequency, particles passing through them receive successive increments of energy.

linear amplifier a pulse amplifier in which the output pulse height has been amplified to a height that is proportional to the input pulse height.

liquid scintillation counter a counter used to measure the amount of radioactivity, usually beta, emitted from a sample dispersed in a liquid scintillation cocktail.

lobule small lobe or a subdivision of a lobe.

logit see *curve fitting*.

lyophilization freeze drying.

lysis dissolution, setting free, releasing, or destruction-decomposition.

macrophage phagocytic cell (not a leukocyte) belonging to the reticuloendothelial system. It has the capacity for storing in its cytoplasm certain aniline dyes in the form of granules.

marker, label, tracer the substance used to monitor the count of a binding assay.

mass absorption coefficient the linear absorption coefficient per centimeter divided by the density of the absorber in grams per cubic centimeter.

mass action, law of the mathematical description of reversible reactions that attain equilibrium, generally regarded as applicable to CBA.

mass defect the difference between the mass of the nucleus as a whole and the sum of the nuclear components weighed separately.

mass number symbol: A. The number of nucleons in the nucleus of an atom.

matrix basic material from which a thing develops.

maturation process of coming to full development.

maximum permissible dose (MPD) the maximum dose of radiation permitted for persons working with ionizing radiation. MPD for whole body = 5(N − 18) rems; N = age.

median lethal dose (MLD/30) the dose of radiation required to kill 50% of the individuals in a large group of animals or organisms within 30 days.

medulla the middle; the marrow.

megakaryocyte giant cell of the bone marrow containing a large, irregularly lobulated nucleus; the progenitor of blood platelets.

megaly denoting great size.

metabolism the sum of all the physical and chemical processes by which a living substance is produced and maintained and by which energy is made available for the uses of the organism.

metaplasia change in the type of adult cells in a tissue to a form that is not normal for that tissue.

metastable state an excited state of a nucleus that returns to its ground state by the emission of a gamma ray. Ground state is not achieved immediately, but over a measurable half-life.

metastatic pertaining to the spread of malignant cells.

MeV one million electron volts (10^6 eV).

microcurie (μCi) a unit of radioactivity defined as 37,000 disintegrations per second; one-millionth of a curie.

micromicrocurie (picocurie) (μμ Ci) 3.7×10^{-2} disintegrations per second (one millionth of a microcurie).

millicurie (mCi) 3.7×10^7 disintegrations per second (one thousandth of a curie).

millimicrocurie (Nanocurie) (mμCi) 37 disintegrations per second (one thousandth of a microcurie).

milliroentgen (mr) one thousandth of a roentgen.

MIS Management Information Systems.

mitral stenosis diseased valve causing obstruction of the blood flow through left atrioventricular opening.

molecule the ultimate unit of a compound that can exist by itself and retain all the properties of the original substance.

monitoring the periodic or continuous determination of the amount of ionizing radiation or radioactive contamination present in an occupied region.

area monitoring routine monitoring of the level of radiation or of radioactive contamination of any particular area, building, or room.

personnel monitoring monitoring of any part of an individual such as breath, excretions, or clothing.

monoenergetic radiation radiation of a given type in which all photons or particles have the same energy.

morphogenesis structural changes during development of an organism.

multivalent see *binding site*.

mutation a change in the characteristics of any organism as a result of an alteration of the usual hereditary pattern.

myelofibrosis replacement of the bone marrow by fibrous tissue occurring in association with a myeloproliferative disorder or another unrelated condition.

myeloid pertaining to, derived from, or resembling bone marrow.

myxedema swelling associated with hypothyroidism. A sallow, puffy appearance, particularly in hands and face, is characteristic.

necrosis decay or death of tissue as a result of loss of blood supply.

negatron (β^-) a particle having a mass and charge equal to that of an electron but originating from the nucleus. Its mass is 0.000548 amu. This term is not used in the United States.

neoplasia new growth, usually applied to a tumor.

nephritis inflammation of the kidneys.

neutrino a neutral particle of very small mass (approaches zero rest mass) emitted during various processes of decay.

neutron an elementary, electrically neutral nuclear particle with a mass approximately the same as that of a proton. Its mass is 1.00898 atomic mass units (amu).

nonproductive hours benefit hours (vacation, bereavement, sick time).

nonproductive salary and wages dollars expended for benefit hours (vacation, bereavement, sick time).

NSB (1) an abbreviation for nonspecific binding, meaning that portion of the tracer used in a CBA that is found in the bound fraction, independent of the binding reaction. (2) An assay batch control tube made up without binding agent (antibody) and treated in the same way as other assay tubes.

nonspecific binding see *NSB*.

nuclear reactor an apparatus in which the nuclear fission reaction may be self-sustaining.

nucleon a common term for a constituent particle of the nucleus; usually applies to protons and neutrons.

nucleus (of an atom) that part of an atom in which most of the mass and the total positive electric charge are concentrated.

nuclide a general term applicable to all atomic forms of the elements. See also *isotope*.

occult hidden; concealed; not evident as occult blood—the blood in excrement or secretion not clearly evident to the naked eye.

off-line a data processing term meaning data input to the computer processor directly from the counter.

on-line a data processing term for data input to the computer processor directly from the counter.

operating voltage the voltage across the electrodes in the detecting chamber required for proper detection of an ionizing event.

osmotic pressure pressure developed when a solution and its solvent component are separated by a membrane permeable to the solvent only or when two solutions of different concentration of the same solute are similarly separated.

ossification method by which fibrous tissue or cartilage is converted into bone or a bony substance.

osteoblast cell arising from a fibroblast that, as it matures, plays a role in the production of bone.

osteoid resembling bone. Also the organic matrix of bone; young uncalcified bone.

osteon basic unit of structure of compact bone; haversian canal and its concentrically arranged lamellae (four to 20, each 3 to 7 μ thick) in a single (haversian) system. Such units are directed mainly in the long axis of the bone.

osteoprogenitor cells forefather or ancestor of cells of the bone marrow.

pair production an absorption process for x- and gamma radiation in which the incident photon is annihilated in the vicinity of the nucleus of the absorbing atom, with subsequent release of a positron and a beta particle. This reaction cannot occur for incident radiation energies of less than 1.02 MeV.

panmyelosis multiplication of all the elements of the bone marrow.

parent a radionuclide that yields another nuclide on disintegration. The latter (the daughter) may be radioactive or stable.

patency open.

percent bound

$$\text{Of } B_O\text{: } \frac{\text{Bound CPM (sample)} \times 100}{\text{Bound CPM (0 standard)}}$$

$$\text{Of total: } \frac{\text{Bound CPM (sample)} \times 100}{\text{Total counts}}$$

pernicious anemia anemia that results from defects of the bone marrow, such as hypoplasia, euplasia, and degenerative changes. It is caused by a deficiency of red cells, hemoglobin, and granular cells, with a predominance of lymphocytes.

phagocytosis ingestion of foreign or other particles, principally bacteria, by certain cells.

photoelectric effect a process by which a photon ejects an electron from an atom and thereby is totally absorbed.

photographic dosimetry the determination of the accumulative radiation dosage by use of photographic film.

photomultiplier tube a tube in which small electron currents are amplified by a cascade process employing secondary emission.

photon a quantity of electromagnetic energy.

physical half-life (T_p or $T_{1/2}$) the time required for a source of radioactivity to lose 50% of its activity by decay.

piezeoelectric effect charges of electricity developed when pressure is applied to certain crystals.

pile see *nuclear reactor*.

pinocytosis absorption of liquids by cells.

Planck's constant a natural constant of proportionality *(h)* relating the frequency of a quantum of energy to the total energy of the quantum; equivalent to 6.61×10^{-7} erg-sec.

planimetry the measurement of level surfaces; plane geometry.

plateau as applied to radiation detector chambers, the level portion of the voltage curve at which changes in operating voltage introduce minimum changes in the counting rate.

pleomorphic widely different forms of the same species.

plication designating a fold or ridge.

positron a particle having a mass equal to the electron and having an equal but opposite charge. Its mass is 0.000548 atomic mass units (amu).

precision extent to which the obtained measurements of a defined substance agree with one another, usually stated as coefficient of variation, or confidence limits.

interassay precision determined by assaying the same sample *n* times in multiple assays.

intraassay precision determined by assaying the same sample *n* times in a single assay.

precordium area of the chest overlying the heart.

progenitor to bring forth.

processor a data processing term for the hardware computer unit used in the execution of instructions, reduction, and storage of data.

productive hours actual hours that employees work.

productive salary and wages dollars expended for actual hours worked.

prone lying with face downward.

proportional counter a gas-filled radiation detector in which the pulse produced is proportional to the number of ions formed in the gas by the primary ionizing particle.

proportional region the voltage range in which the gas amplification is greater than 1 and in which the charge collected is proportional to the initial ionizing event.

proteolysis enzymatic or hydrolytic conversion of proteins into simple substances.

protocol a detailed description of the exact manner in which an assay is to be performed.

proton an elementary nuclear particle with a positive electric charge equal numerically to the charge of the electron and having a mass of 1.00759 atomic mass units (amu).

PTE part-time employee (or part-time equivalent).

pterygium anything like a wing; disease of the eye in which a membrane grows over it from the inner corner.

ptosis (ptotic) falling down of an organ; prolapse; abnormal position.

pulse height analyzer any circuit designed to select and pass voltage pulses in a certain range of amplitudes.

pyknosis thickening; especially degeneration of a cell in which the nucleus decreases in size and the chromatin condenses.

quality control (1) See *control samples*. (2) repeated assay of known standard material and monitoring of reaction parameters to assure precision and accuracy.

QC an abbreviation for quality control.

quantum see *photon*.

quench in liquid scintillation counting, a decrease in counting efficiency resulting from physicochemical interferences in the scintillation process of attenuation of the photons produced.

quenching the processing of inhibiting discharge in a counter tube that uses gas amplification.

quenching gas a polyatomic gas used in Geiger-Mueller counters to quench or extinguish avalanche ionization.

radiation absorbed dose (rad) a measure of the amount of energy imparted to matter by ionizing radiation per unit mass of irradiated material at the place of interest; equivalent to 100 ergs of absorbed energy per gram of irradiated material.

radioactive half-life see *physical half-life*.

radioactivity the spontaneous disintegration of an unstable atomic nucleus resulting in the emission of ionizing radiation.

radioassay test for the presence or amount of substance, usually biologically active, by radioisotope techniques.

radiobinding assays a general method of analysis in which the concentration of a ligand (L) is measured by allowing L and a fixed amount of a similar radiolabeled ligand (L*) to react with a given amount of receptor reagent (R), resulting in a distribution of L* into two separable compartments (bound and unbound). The distribution of L*, which varies as a function of the total concentration of a ligand (L + L*) present, is estimated by the magnitude that the dilution L exerts on the label in the bound or free compartment or on some function of bound and free.

radiochemical purity the production of total activity of a radiochemical that is present as the stated radionuclide.

radioimmunoassay an RBA in which the receptor is an antibody or group of antibodies (or a CPB in which the protein is an antibody or group of antibodies) and the label is radioisotope.

radioisotope a specific form of an element of the periodic table whose nucleus disintegrates spontaneously.

radioligand a radiolabeled (tagged) ligand.

radionuclide a species of atom whose nucleus disintegrates spontaneously, emitting radiation in the form of alpha or beta rays.

radionuclide purity the proportion of total activity of a given radioactive material that is present as the stated nuclide.

radioreceptor assay a type of RBA in which the receptor is a structural component of a tissue.

radioresistance the relative resistance of cells, tissues, organs, or entire organisms to the injurious action of radiation.

radiosensitivity the relative susceptibility of cells, tissues, organs, entire organisms, or any substances to the injurious action of radiation. Radioresistance and radiosusceptibility are currently employed in a qualitative or comparative sense, rather than in a quantitative or absolute one.

RBA an abbreviation for radiobinding assays.

read-out a method of presenting a total count or rate of detected radiation events.

receptor binding reagent, found on or in cells, used in ligand assays.

relative biologic effectiveness (RBE) the ratio of x- or gamma ray dose to the dose that is required to produce the same biologic effect by the radiation in question.

relativistic mass the increased mass associated with a particle when its velocity is increased. The increase in mass becomes appreciable only at velocities approaching the velocity of light (3×10^{10} cm/sec).

replicate identical sample.

resolving time, counter the minimum time interval between two distinct ionization events that permits both to be counted.

revenue monies received for goods or services.

RIA an abbreviation for radioimmunoassay.

roentgen the quantity of x- or gamma radiation such that the associated corpuscular emission per 0.001293 gram of air produces, in air, ions carrying 1 electrostatic unit of electrical charge, either positive or negative.

roentgen equivalent, man (rem) a unit of human biologic dose as a result of exposure to one or many types of ionizing radiation. It is equal to the absorbed dose in rad times the RBE of the particular type of radiation being absorbed.

sample preparation a catchall phrase to denote any of the steps required to convert specimen material to samples appropriate for a given analytic protocol.

saturation analysis one of the general terms favored by some to connote competitive binding assay.

scaler an electronic device that produces an output voltage pulse whenever a prescribed number of input pulses has been received.

scanner a device used to display a two-dimensional portrayal of the variations of concentration of radioactivity in any volume of material.

scan speed the rate of travel of the scanner detector as it traverses the area being visualized.

Scatchard plot see *curve fitting*.

scattering the change of direction of particles or photons as a result of a collision or interaction.

scintillation emission of light flashes from certain materials as a result of interaction with ionizing radiation.

scintillation counter an instrument that measures radioactivity by way of a scintillation detector.

second antibody antibody heterologous to the antibody used as primary binding agent.

secondary radiation radiation originating as the result of interactions of other radiation in matter. It may be either electromagnetic or particulate in nature.

self-absorption the absorption of radiation by the matter in which the radioactive atoms are located; in particular, the absorption of radiation within the sample being assayed.

sensitivity (1) The lowest concentration of test substance measurable in an assay. (2) The minimal difference in test substance concentrations distinguishable by a given assay, usually a function of the steepness of the assay curve.

separation the technique used in removing ligand-binding agent complex to measure the extent of tracer bound during CBA (RIA).

separation agent reagent used to affect or aid in the separation of bound and free tracer in radioassay (for example, heterologous antibody, solid-phase antibody, protein-precipitating agent, or adsorbent).

sequential saturation modification of saturation assays in which the forward reaction is significantly favored so that, theoretically, the binding of ligand to binding reagent is irreversible.

sequestration separation.

serial dilution the progressive dilution of standard or sample in a row of tubes so that the first tube contains the highest concentration of test substance. See also *incremental addition*.

shunting alternate way, bypass.

software in computer data processing, instructions in the processor memory, or in a form to be put there, that direct the operations to be performed.

solid phase separation method in which the binding reagent is immobilized by coupling to an insoluble material (coated tubes, polymers, etc.).

somatic (1) Pertaining to the body. (2) Pertaining to the framework of the body and not to the viscera, such as the somatic musculature (the muscles of the body wall or somatopleure) as distinguished from the splanchnic musculature (the splanchnopleure).

somatic cells body cells, usually having two sets of chromosomes. Germ cells have only one set.

species specificity situation in which the same antigen from two different animal species exhibits different reactivity toward an antibody. Hormones exhibit species specificity to a high degree. When assaying these hormones, it is often necessary to use the same antigen for the preparation of tracer and standards and the production of antibodies. In these cases, of course, all the antiserum must be obtained from the same species.

specific activity (1) Of a compound: total radioactivity per gram of compound; (2) of an element: total radioactivity per gram of element; (3) of an isotope: total radioactivity per gram of radioisotope.

specific gravity measured mass of a substance with that of an equal volume of another taken as a standard. For gases, hydrogen of air may be the standard; for liquids and solids, distilled water at a specified temperature is the standard.

specificity the selective reactivity between binding agent and ligand and, by implication, the absence of reaction with other substances present.

spectrometer a device used to count an emission of radiation of a specific energy or range of energies to the exclusion of all other energies.

spondylitis inflammation of the spine with pathologic changes in the vertebrae and intravertebral joints.

spurious count the count caused by any agency other than the radiation desired to be detected.

stable isotope an isotope that is not radioactive.

standards a set of samples containing known amounts of test substance, used as a basis for measuring unknown amounts in assay samples.

standard curve a plot of tracer binding versus the known concentrations of test substance in a set of standards, usually prepared by serial dilution of incremental addition.

steatorrhea (1) Increased flow of the secretion of the sebaceous follicles. (2) Fatty stools.

steroids a type of hormone usually secreted by glands of mesodermal origin that possess in common a cyclopentenoperhydrophenanthrene ring.

stray radiation radiation serving no useful purpose.

supine lying on back with face upward.

synchrotron a device for accelerating particles, ordinarily electrons, in a circular orbit with frequency-modulated electric fields combined with an increasing magnetic field applied to synchronism with the orbital motion.

systole contraction of the heart chambers.

tachycardia excessive rapidity of the heart's action.

tagged compound see *labeled compound*.

TC an acronym for total count, which in radioassay represents that set of control tubes permitting estimation of the amount of radioactivity used in each sample.

threshold (1) Lower limit of stimulus capable of producing an impression on consciousness or of evoking a response in an irritable tissue. (2) Entrance of a canal.

thrombocytosis condition marked by the presence of a large number of blood platelets in the blood.

thrombosis formation of a clot of blood.

thyrotoxicosis hyperthyroidism of any type.

titer (1) A measure of antibody concentration in an antiserum. (2) In RIA, that dilution of an antiserum that binds a predetermined percentage (usually 50%) of tracer antigen in the absence of unlabeled antigen.

tracer test substance labeled with a marker such as radioactive isotope or a fluorescent compound, ideally in such manner as to have no discernible effect on the assay reaction.

transferrin siderophilin; a pseudoglobulin of blood, having molecular weight of about 90,000. It is capable of combining with 2 atoms of ferric iron to form a compound that serves as a transport form of iron in blood.

tritium (^3H or ^3T) an isotope of hydrogen having a mass number of 3 (1 proton, 2 neutrons).

vagus nerve parasympathetic pneumogastric nerve; the tenth cranial nerve, composed of both motor and sensory fibers. It has a wide distribution in the neck, thorax, and abdomen, and sends important branches to the heart, lungs, stomach, and other organs.

vascular pertaining to, consisting of, or provided with vessels.

viscus any one of the organs enclosed within one of the four great cavities; the cranium, thorax, abdomen, or pelvis, especially an organ within the abdominal cavity.

vitamin B_{12} essential vitamin needed for the normal maturation of cells of the erythrocytic series and for normal neurologic function. When given parenterally, it corrects both the hematologic and neurologic symptoms of pernicious anemia.

wavelength the distance between the same point on two subsequent electromagnetic waves.

window a term that describes the upper and lower limits of energy of radiation accepted for counting by a spectrometer; also termed *window width*.

x rays penetrating electromagnetic radiations having wavelengths much shorter than those of visible light.

zero dose the absence of added ligand, synonymous with B_0.

zero standard see *zero dose*.

zymogen inactive precursor of an enzyme that, on reaction with an appropriate kinase or other chemical agent, liberates the enzyme in active form.

■ PREFIXES

A prefix consists of one or two syllables placed before a word to modify the meaning. These syllables are often prepositions or adverbs.

a, an	Without, negative
ab	From, away from
ad	Adherence, increase, near, toward
ante, antero	Before, forward, front
anti	Against
auto, aut	Self
bi, bis	Twice, double
cata	Lower, down, negative
co, com, con	Together, with
contra	Against, counter, opposite
de	Down from
di	Double, twice
dia	Through, apart
dis	Apart, away from

dys	Painful, difficult
ec	Out of
ecto	Outside
em, en	In, into
end, endo	Within
entero	Intestine
epi	Upon, at, in addition to
ex, exo	Out, away from, over, outside
gastro	Stomach
hemi	Half
hemo	Blood
hyper	Above, excessive, beyond
hypo	Decreased, under
infra	Beneath, below
inter	Among, between
intra, intro	Into, within
macro	Large
micro	Small
multi	Many
myo	Muscle
neuro	Nerve
ortho	Straight, normal
pan	All, every
para	Around, beside, by, beyond, abnormal, near
patho	Disease
per	Through
peri	Around
poly	Many
post	After, behind
pre	Before, in front of
pro	In front of, forward
pseudo	False
py	Pus
re	Again, back
retro	Back, backward
semi	Half
steno	Narrow, contracted
sub	Under, below, beneath
super, supra	Above, beyond, superior
sym, syn	With, along, together, beside
tendo	Tendon
trans	Across, over, through
tri	Three
ultra	Excess, beyond

■ SUFFIXES

A suffix is a syllable or syllables added to the end of a word or root to modify its meaning.

algia	Pain
dynia	Pain
ectomy	Surgical removal of
genic	Origin, producing
genous	Kind
gram	Picture, tracing
lysis	Dissolution, breaking down
oid	Resembling, like
ology	Science of, study of
oscopy	Diagnostic examination
ostomy	Opening
otomy	Incision
penia	Lack, decrease
plegia	Paralysis
trophy	Nutrition
uria	Urine

■ DIAGNOSTIC SUFFIXES OR COMBINING FORMS

cele	Hernia, tumor
ectasis	Expansion, dilation
emia	Blood
iasis	Condition, presence of
itis	Inflammation
malacia	Softening
megaly	Enlargement
oma	Tumor
osis	Condition, disease
pathy	Disease
ptosis	Falling
rrhexis	Rupture

■ POSITION OR DIRECTION

anterior or ventral	Front of
posterior or dorsal	Back of
superior or upper	Situated above
inferior or lower	Situated beneath
cranial, craniad, cephalic	Nearest or toward the head
caudal, caudad	Away from the head, inferior in position
medial	Middle, internal
lateral	Side, to the side
proximal	Near the source or attachment
distal	Away from the source

INDEX

I

Q

R